This book is to be returned on or before
the last date stamped below.

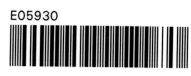

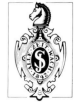

Paediatric Pathology

Edited by
Colin L. Berry

With Contributions by
Robert H. Anderson, Anton E. Becker, Mies J. Becker,
Christopher L. Brown, Jerry N. Cox, Jean W. Keeling, Brian D. Lake,
Peter A. Revell, R. Anthony Risdon, Joseph F. Smith, Michael Swash

With 673 Figures

Springer-Verlag
Berlin Heidelberg New York 1981

Colin L. Berry, MD, PhD, FRCPath,
Professor of Morbid Anatomy, Institute of
Pathology, The London Hospital Medical
College, Whitechapel, London, E1 1BB,
United Kingdom.

ISBN 3-540-10507-7 Springer-Verlag Berlin Heidelberg New York
ISBN 0-387-10507-7 Springer-Verlag New York Heidelberg Berlin

Library of Congress Cataloging in Publication Data
Main entry under title: Paediatric Pathology.
Bibliography: p. Includes index. 1. Pediatric pathology. I. Berry, Colin Leonard, 1937–. [DNLM: 1. Pathology – In
infancy and childhood. WS 200 P1255] RJ49.P3 618.92′007 81-2196
ISBN 0-387-10507-7 (U.S.) AACR2

Filmset and printed by BAS Printers Limited, Over Wallop, Hampshire, UK

2128/3916–543210

Preface

The increased provision of facilities for neonatal and paediatric care in the last 25 years has been accompanied only in part by appropriate developments in pathology. Specialist pathologists are many fewer than paediatric departments, and details of the advances in knowledge of the pathogenesis of diseases in childhood and of ways of investigating them are not uniformly available. In many institutions an individual with a special interest rather than a special training will be responsible for paediatric pathology and it is to this group of histopathologists that this text is addressed. For this reason it is not written as a comprehensive text and is not intended for use as a reference volume. Areas which may produce particular difficulties for the individual with little specialist knowledge of the very young (e.g., the lung) are dealt with in more detail and, in general, entities in which the histopathology does not differ greatly from that of the adult disease are considered briefly. A brief account of developmental processes is included where prenatal considerations are helpful in understanding a particular entity. A number of specialist topics which are known to trouble those who work in nonspecialist departments are described fully (diseases of muscle) or with guides to investigation (metabolic disease). The value of investigation and careful description of abnormalities of development is also emphasized.

The authors are from different backgrounds, paediatric pathologists (J. W. Keeling, J. Cox), pathologists in general departments with extensive experience in paediatric pathology (C. L. Berry, R. A. Risdon, M. Becker, J. Smith) or specialists with an interest in the manifestation of diseases of which they have expert knowledge in the young (P. A. Revell, R. H. Anderson, C. L. Brown, M. Swash, A. E. Becker, B. D. Lake). All are valued and respected friends, who have been asked to contribute in a particular way; any errors of 'design' are my own.

Acknowledgements

It is a pleasure to thank Professor A. E. Claireaux, a mentor of five of the authors, for his generosity in allowing us to use illustrations of many cases seen at The Hospital for Sick Children, Gt. Ormond Street. Our collective thanks are owed to Miss L. Singer who has made sense of many difficult manuscripts.

Mr Michael Jackson and Mrs J. Dodsworth of Springer-Verlag have been unfailingly generous with help and advice in the preparation of the text.

London, 1981   Colin L. Berry

List of Contributors

Robert H. Anderson, BSc, MD,
MRCPath, Professor in Paediatric Cardiac
Morphology, Cardiothoracic Institute,
Brompton Hospital, London; Honorary
Consultant, Brompton Hospital, London

Anton E. Becker, MD, Professor of
Pathology, University of Amsterdam;
Professor of Cardiovascular Pathology,
Interuniversity Cardiology Institute,
Amsterdam, The Netherlands

Mies J. Becker, MD, Pathologist, Stichting
de Heel Zaandam, St. Jams Gasthuis en
Streekziekenhuis West Friesland, Hoorn;
Consultant Pathologist, University of
Amsterdam, Wilhelmina Gasthuis,
Amsterdam, The Netherlands

Christopher L. Brown, MB, BS, FRCPath,
Senior Lecturer in Pathology, The
London Hospital Medical College;
Honorary Consultant Pathologist, The
London Hospital, London

Jerry N. Cox, MD, Consultant Paediatric
Pathologist, Hopital Cantonal, Geneva,
Switzerland

Jean W. Keeling, MB, BS, MRCPath,
Consultant Paediatric Pathologist, John
Radcliffe Hospital, Oxford

Brian D. Lake, BSC, PhD, MRCPath,
Reader in Histochemistry, Department
of Histopathology, Hospital for Sick
Children and Institute of Child Health,
Great Ormond Street, London

Peter A. Revell, BSc, MB, BS, PhD,
MRCPath, Senior Lecturer in Morbid
Anatomy, The London Hospital Medical
College, London

R. Anthony Risdon, MD, FRCPath,
Reader in Morbid Anatomy, The
London Hospital Medical College,
London

Joseph F. Smith, FRCPath, Professor of
Morbid Anatomy, University College
Hospital Medical School, London

Michael Swash, MD, FRCP, Consultant
Neurologist, The London Hospital,
London; Honorary Consultant
Neurologist, St. Mark's Hospital,
London; Honorary Senior Lecturer in
Neuropathology, The London Hospital
Medical College, London

Contents

Chapter 1

Examination of the Fetus

Colin L. Berry

In many pathology departments products of conception are not examined in detail and sections are taken only to confirm pregnancy. Much information can be obtained from these specimens, which may be of value in genetic counselling or in the management of future pregnancies. The occurrence of congenital heart disease, facial clefts, or neurospinal defects in embryos and early fetuses all have considerable predictive value in terms of the likely outcome of future pregnancies, and may help to ensure that screening techniques (e.g., α-fetoprotein determinations) are used in individuals at risk. Although many relatively complex procedures may be used on material from abortions, including cell culture with subsequent enzymatic or metabolic studies, these are not practicable in most instances or in any but a few laboratories. Nor is it desirable that they should be carried out in many centres; as Benson et al. (1979) have pointed out, there are considerable advantages in terms of experience and the control of assay techniques in carrying out tests for metabolic disease in only a few centres. It has also been estimated that less than 120 pregnancies will be known to be at risk of metabolic disease in the United Kingdom in a year, suggesting that a few centres could cope with the likely workload.

This figure contrasts sharply with the 15 000 or so infants delivered with major congenital defects each year. If the increased incidence of defects found in early pregnancies is considered (p. 68) it is evident that most histopathological laboratories receive abnormal fetuses every year, although few are documented in detail. An example of a defect that can be diagnosed by inspection in early pregnancy is shown in Fig. 1.1.

Simple morbid anatomy and histopathology will provide useful data on embryonic and fetal material, and require only a dissecting microscope and X-ray facilities. Specimens are often received incomplete,

fragmented, with or without the placenta, and usually fixed. The techniques recommended take note of these constraints. Detailed accounts of abnormalities are not given here, but can be found in the relevant chapters. Further technical details can be found in Berry (1980).

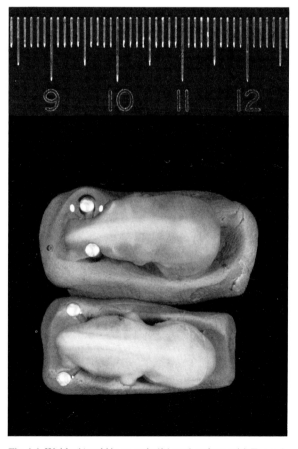

Fig. 1.1. Webbed 'neck' in an early (34-mm) embryo with Turner's syndrome. (45 ×) A control embryo is also shown.

1. History

As with all surgical specimens, a good history is important but not always provided. The date of the last menstrual period is an essential piece of information if findings are to be properly interpreted. Knowledge of previous reproductive performance is valuable, and the mode of induction of abortion should be stated, if it is not spontaneous.

2. Dimensions

Many measurements can be made on fetal and embryonic specimens, but there are considerable difficulties with a number of them. Crown–heel lengths measured by different observers under normal laboratory conditions vary considerably, as do crown–rump (CR) measurements. Table 1.1 provides average values for the latter variable, based

Table 1.1. Change in crown-rump length (CR) with age

Day	CR (mm)	Day	CR (mm)
35	8	127	134.5
42	15	134	146.0
49	22	141	156.5
56	29.5	148	167.0
63	40.0	155	177.5
70	50.5	162	188.0
77	61.0	169	198.5
84	71.5	176	209.0
91	81.5	183	219.5
98	92.0	190	230.0
105	103.0	197	240.5
113	113.5	204	251.0
120	124.0		

Table 1.2. Later gestational age–foot length correlations (Usher and McLean 1969)

Gestational age (weeks)	Foot length (mm)[a]
27–28	55.4 (3.08)
29–30	57.7 (2.12)
31–32	62.6 (3.32)
33	67.4 (4.78)
34	69.6 (3.76)
35	71.4 (3.76)
36	72.8 (4.12)
37	78.0 (3.91)
38	78.2 (4.11)
39	77.3 (3.56)
40	78.4 (3.45)

[a]Figures in parentheses give SD.

on a number of series. There is wide variation, however, which depends largely on the reproducibility of the position of the fetus and its degree of maceration. Careful studies such of those of Bagnall et al. (1975) and Birkbeck et al. (1975a) show the value of CR and crown–heel measurements, but for a pathological laboratory the measurement of foot length is simpler and provides comparable data. Foot length is not affected significantly by fixation or maceration, and an intact foot is often found where the fetus is received in fragments. Data relating foot length to CR length and gestational age, based on the work of Streeter (1920) and Trolle (1948), are shown in Fig. 1.2; figures for later pregnancy from Usher and McLean (1969) are shown in Table 1.2. Foot length has the additional advantage that it is seldom directly affected by malformation—for example anencephalic fetuses have normal foot lengths (Nañagus 1925) though they are otherwise difficult to measure.

3. Weights

The weights of the placenta and fetus should be determined. Determination of fetal age by weight alone is always imprecise (see Birkbeck et al. (1975b)), but marked disproportion between placental and fetal weight may be informative.

There is no doubt but that accurate measurement of placental weight is very difficult; different authors have trimmed different parts of the membranes, cut off the cord, drained blood from the organ before weighing, etc. The most accurate measurement of the weight of placental tissue is obtained after homogenization of the organ and estimation of the haemoglobin in the homogenate; if the value of haemoglobin in cord blood is assumed to be the same as that in the placenta a correction for the weight of the contained blood can be made.

This is clearly impracticable as a routine technique. In general the determination of placental weight in early pregnancy is unhelpful. Fetal weight is exceeded by placental weight until week 14–15 (100 mm CR length, 17 mm foot length), when the placental growth rate falls and that of the fetus increases rapidly. The data of Boyd and Hamilton (1970) are often cited for relative weight, and tables have been constructed from arithmetic regression based on their data. The scatter in the original observations is enormous and, in the author's view, permits only limited statements. At 200 g fetal weight the placenta usually weighs 120 ± 20 g, and at a fetal weight of 1000 g the placenta weighs 250 ± 50 g. For figures for later pregnancy (32 weeks onward) the data of Thomson et al. (1969) for gross placental weight, in which the placenta has not been manipulated or trimmed in any way, are preferred. Fetal and placental weights in early pregnancy are shown in Table 1.3.

Table 1.3. Fetal and placental weight (date from Boyd and Hamilton 1970)

Weeks	CR length (mm)	Fetal wt. (g)	Placental wt. (g)
4–8	5– 30	0.5– 2.9	5.0– 27.0
8–12	31– 60	2.7– 25.0	10.0– 80.0
12–16	61–100	11.0–135.0	28.0–134.0
16–20	101–155	57.0–350.0	55.0–198.0

4. Dating

External examination, careful measurement, infinite technical resources (serial sectioning), and precise historical details will allow most embryos and fetuses to be dated with accuracy. This is neither possible nor necessary in routine practice, and the 'markers' given here are those that any laboratory can determine readily. Dating should be carried out on the basis of several sources of data (history, external form, size, weight, morbid anatomy, and histological development).

5. Chronology of Early Pregnancy in Man

If day 1 is considered to be the day on which a fertilized egg is present in the Fallopian tube, on day 2 there will be a 2- or 4-celled mass present. On day 3, an 8- to 12-celled mass is found, on day 4 the blastocoele begins to develop, and on day 5 a free blastocyst is found in the uterus. The blastocyst begins to implant on day 6 and implantation is not complete until day 13–14.

Morphological developmental indicators found by certain times are shown in Tables 1.4 and 1.5. These are readily identifiable in selected blocks and demonstration of them does not require serial sectioning. Between 12 and 20 weeks axial skeletal development provides a useful guide (see Fig. 1.3).

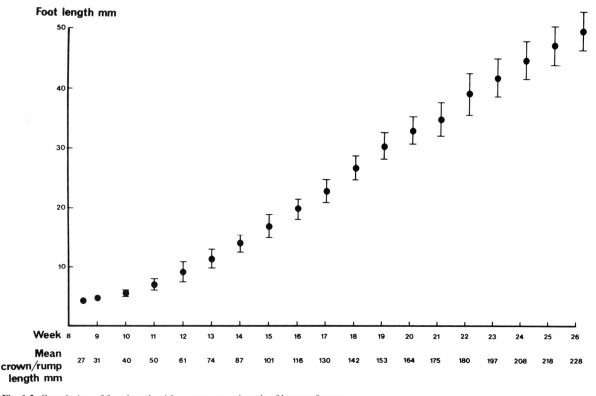

Fig. 1.2. Correlation of foot length with crown–rump length of human fetuses.

Table 1.4. Morphological markers of development

Time (days)	System					
	Central nervous	Cardiovascular	Urogenital	Gastrointestinal	Respiratory	Other markers
28	Anterior neuropore closed Cerebral vesicles present Lens placode reaches optic cup	Septum primum present	Metanephros forming	Oesophagus separated from trachea Liver bud present Dorsal pancreatic component present	Lung primordium established Trachea and primitive bronchi present	Thyroid in mid-line
35	Lens pocket closes	Ventricular septum and semilunar valves forming	Ureteric buds develop Germ cells in genital ridges			Spleen in dorsal mesogastrium
42	Semicircular canals Neurohypophysis develops	Truncus divides, septum secundum appears	Major calyces appear	Hepatic haematopoiesis begins Hernia of umbilical loop	Capillaries in lung parenchyma	Thymus and para-thyroids arise from branchial pouches Paddle-shaped hand
50	Lens vesicle a 'full' sphere Eyelids developing	Ventricular septum complete	Paramesonephric duct Seminiferous tubules as solid strands	Palatal shelves and salivary glands develop		Thymus invaded by lymphocytes Separate digits

Embryos can seldom be examined in sufficient detail in routine laboratories, although our knowledge of the morphology of early human malformations is scanty and such studies would be valuable. Serial sectioning is clearly impracticable, and if abnormal embryos are found they are often best examined in a laboratory with a special interest. What follows is a description of how best to deal with fetuses with CR lengths between approximately 30 and 200 mm.

6. External Examination

Abnormal facies may yield useful information, which can either be specific, as in Potter's syndrome (p. 397), or indicative of the presence of possible visceral abnormality (Fig. 1.4). Early in the external examination it is helpful to pass a probe into the nose to check the patency of the posterior nares, and to examine the palate.

It is then customary for us to X-ray the fetus, using a Faxitron cabinet. This simple device permits rapid X-ray pictures to be provided promptly within the department (a Polaroid attachment is available), and will identify bony anomalies, which are usually better examined by further X-ray after removal of the viscera (Figs. 1.5 and 1.6).

Table 1.5. Later morphological markers

Age in weeks	Finding
10	Fingerprints present
11	Gut loops return to abdomen
20	Bronchi cease budding
22–25	Three layers of primitive glomeruli present. Alveoli appear
25–28	Two layers of primitive glomeruli present. Eyelids open
28–30	One layer of primitive glomeruli present
31	Occasional primitive glomeruli seen
36	No further glomerulogenesis. Ears flat. Breast $\simeq 3$ mm diameter
40	Ears show cartilage ridges. Breast $\simeq 7$ mm diameter. Testes in scrotum. Full foot creases present. Ossification centres in lower femoral epiphysis, calcaneus and talus

7. Internal Examination

For all fetuses with CR length over 100 mm a mini-autopsy is probably the best procedure. However, the use of a modified Rokitansky technique is desirable, the kidneys, ureters, and bladder being left in situ while all other viscera are removed en bloc after examination of the reflections of the mesentery. This block can then be examined with the aid of the dissecting microscope when necessary.

For smaller fetuses a modification of the Wilson free-hand sectioning method (Wilson 1965) used extensively on rodents in teratological studies should

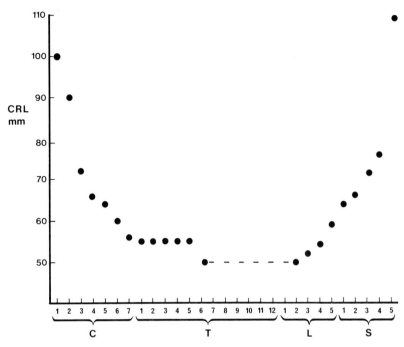

Fig. 1.3. Scheme of appearance of vertebral body ossification centres. These are first evident in the lower thoracic region, and spread up and down the spinal column as shown.

be employed. This involves cutting the trunk of the embryo into slices approximately 2–3 mm thick, which are examined from above and below by dissecting microscopy. This technique is simple and thorough (Figs. 1.7 and 1.8).

Following removal of the viscera the skeleton is again X-rayed. This gives a good picture of the axial skeleton, which apart from specific abnormalities provides useful information on dating.

Where any tissue appears abnormal, or any organ seems to be too large or too small, a block should be taken.

8. Abnormalities of Specific Systems

When macroscopic anomalies are found the standard technique is often abandoned.

8.1. Central Nervous System

In general, anomalous portions of the central nervous system should not be dissected as wet specimens. The cerebrospinal axis may be preserved as a unit, and cut in large sections or transversely in a number of blocks (see Fig. 1.9). Recent reports (Granchrow and Ornoy 1979) have emphasized the value of

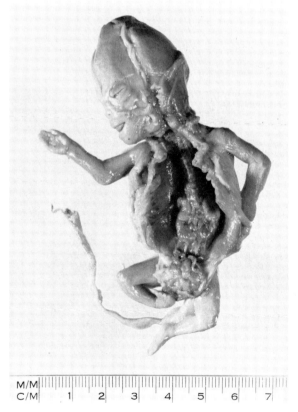

Fig. 1.4. Fetus affected by Meckel's syndrome. Encephalocoele is present and horseshoe kidneys, shown to be dysplastic, are also seen. The liver showed cystic bile ducts in histological sections.

histopathological examination of this type of speci-men, which has rarely been performed. Insights into or alternative suggestions for pathogenesis may follow accurate documentation of the changes found (Bell 1979). It must be remembered that examination of neurospinal malformations at term will illustrate the effects of injury or abnormality followed by up to 8 months of attempted repair and further growth. This type of examination, where only the 'late' stage of a lesion is studied, would yield little information about the pathogenesis of a contracted kidney, for example.

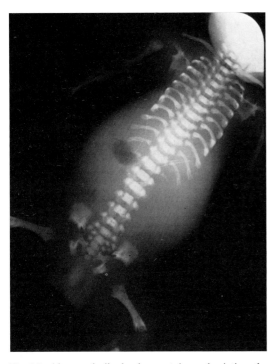

Fig. 1.5. Abnormal rib development in asphyxiating thoracic dystrophy. (Courtesy of Dr. A. B. Bain).

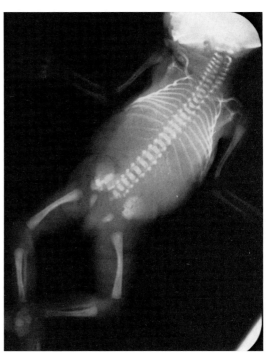

Fig. 1.6. Bell-shaped thorax in pulmonary hypoplasia, a change seen in several conditions, including Potter's syndrome.

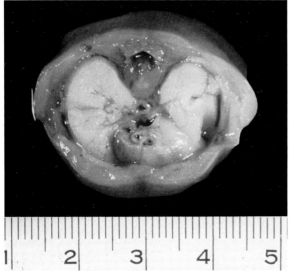

Fig. 1.7. Slice of fetus at the level of the great vessels.

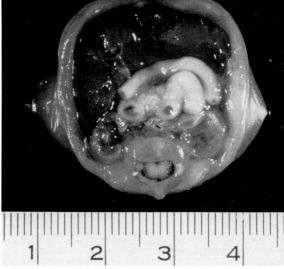

Fig. 1.8. Upper abdominal slice showing kidneys and liver, viewed from below.

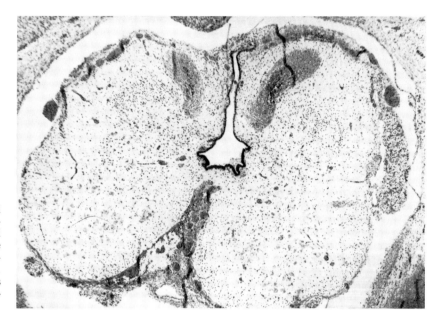

Fig. 1.9. Section of spinal cord above lumbo-sacral meningomyelocoele. The abnormal central canal and partial division of the cord extend dorsally for several vertebral bodies above the defect. From a fetus terminated at 20 weeks for dysraphism. (Methacrylate section; trichrome stain; × 40)

8.2. Cardiovascular System

Even without an extensive knowledge of the vastly complex field of congenital heart disease a useful assessment of anomalies can be made if the system of Tynan and his colleagues is used (see Tynan et al. 1979 and Chap. 4, where the method is described in detail). If the heart is classified in this way a description may be of considerable value to those expert in the field or for later checking, in an area where photography is difficult and where the heart may not always be kept.

8.3. Musculoskeletal System

Musculoskeletal abnormalities are well illustrated by X-ray, but valuable data can be obtained by section. For example, extra digits can be defined by checking muscle insertions to see whether a 'thumb' is really a finger. Abnormalities of the digits have not often been described so carefully, but the information obtained from this type of examination would permit more critical analysis of limb defects. Animal studies suggest that this would be valuable in man. [See, for example, the work of Theisen et al. (1979) with thalidomide.]

8.4. Urogenital System

After removal of the other viscera, the kidneys and ureters should be freed from the posterior abdominal wall. The pubes are then split and the pelvic viscera removed. Dissection, or fine probing, will then reveal where aberrant ureters drain, or whether fistulae exist. Fine polythene catheters, heat-sealed at their ends, make good probes.

8.5. Metabolic Abnormalities

Prenatal diagnoses are usually made in selected groups. These include women over 35 years of age being screened for chromosomal abnormalities and women who have previously given birth to an infant affected by a malformation, c.g., neurospinal dysraphism. Metabolic disorders are usually sought only after an affected child has been diagnosed, which emphasizes the value of examining abortion material. It is clearly absurd to suggest, however, that all abortuses are examined for possible metabolic disease, so the role of the pathologist is to look out for abnormalities that might be associated with metabolic disease. Foam cells in the placenta or central nervous system suggest lipidosis, while some of the skeletal anomalies of the mucopolysaccaridoses are recognizable in fetal material, as are some features of the glycogenoses. Seventeen types of lipidosis, 11 of mucopolysaccharidosis, 22 of amino-aciduria or related disorders, 11 defects of carbohydrate metabolism, and 26 miscellaneous disorders have been diagnosed antenatally; a further 7, 7, 17, 8, and 15 disorders are potentially diagnosable in each category, respectively (see Milunsky 1976).

Alerting a clinical colleague to the possibility of the presence of such a disorder is of major importance in preventive terms.

9. Blighted Ova

Examination of spontaneous abortuses reveals an intact or ruptured gestation sac without an embryo or fetus or with a stunted embryo or fusiform fetal mass in approximately 50% of cases. These 'blighted ova' indicate massive failure of early development. Microscopic examination of the placenta may show predominantly hydatidiform change or stromal fibrosis and vascular obliteration, two ends of a spectrum suggesting failure of establishment of an adequate maternal or villous circulation, respectively, with intermediate mixed findings being common (Rushton 1978). Chromosomal abnormalities are common in this group (Mikamo 1970), but history of recurrent abortion is not found at an enhanced frequency within it. Other placental features that accompany intrauterine death include collapse of the vasculature of the villi, obliterative endarteritis of the arteries of the stem villi, sclerosis of the villous stroma, increased perivillous and intervillous fibrin deposition, increased syncytial knotting, and calcification (see also Chap. 3).

10. Some Normal Histological Appearances During Development

Changes in histological appearance in various tissues or organs with time are illustrated in this section. This is not an attempt to provide an atlas of normal development, but rather a guide that any pathologist can use, taking only a few sections. The appearances are those found by a certain time in pregnancy, though in some instances the changes illustrated may be apparent earlier.

I *External Form of the Brain*

The progressive expansion of the cerebral hemispheres and their subsequent convolution occurs over a long period. The hemisphere expands caudally and ventrolaterally to form the temporal lobe (beginning at *10–11 weeks*). By *20 weeks* frontal and parietal lobes, separated by the central sulcus, are seen and the occipital lobe is demarcated medially. Further sulci appear (*24 weeks*) and at *36 weeks* the process of cerebral convolution is well advanced (see also p. 147).

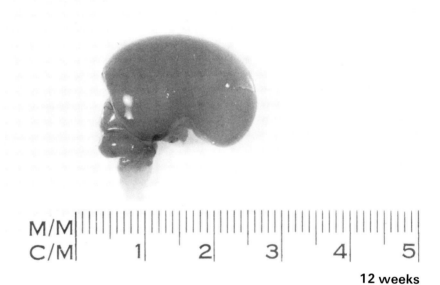

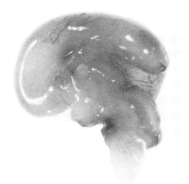

12 weeks

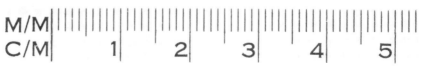

12 weeks

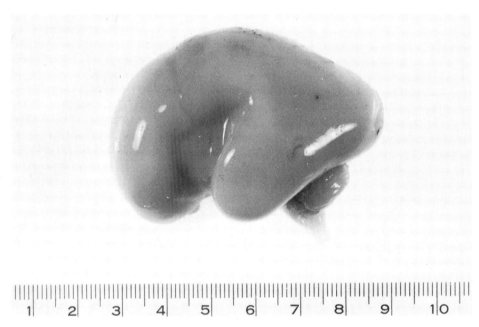

20 weeks

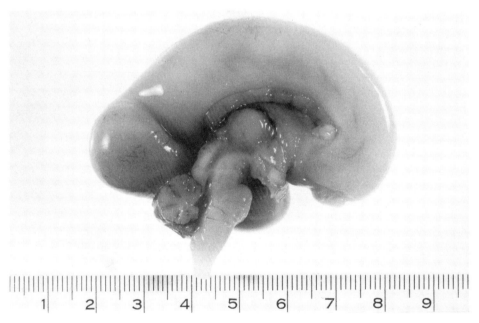

20 weeks

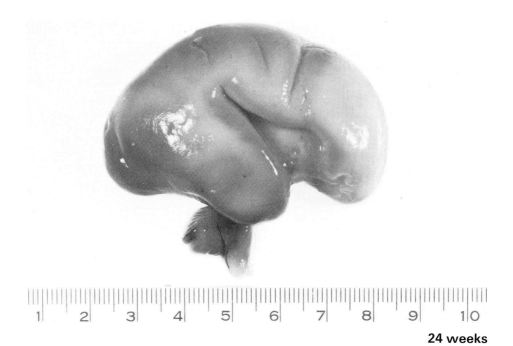

24 weeks

24 weeks

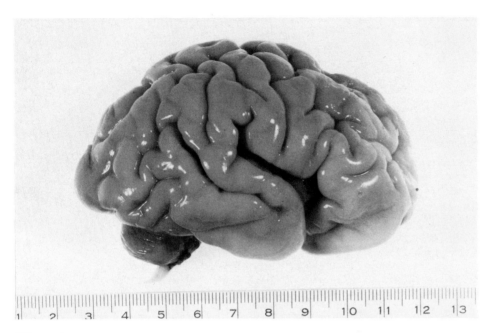

36 weeks

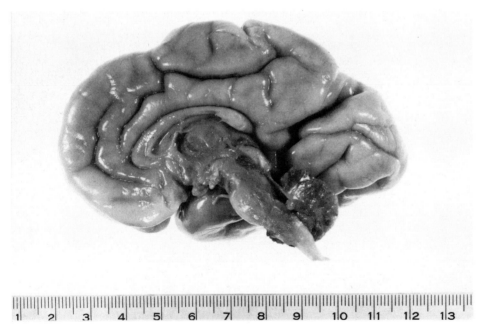

36 weeks

II *Lung* (see also p. 300)

10 weeks

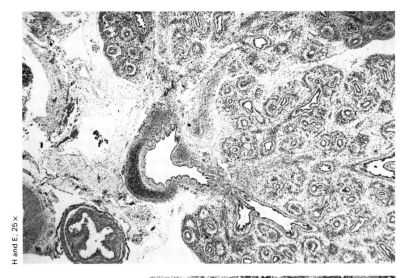

H and E: 25×

10 weeks

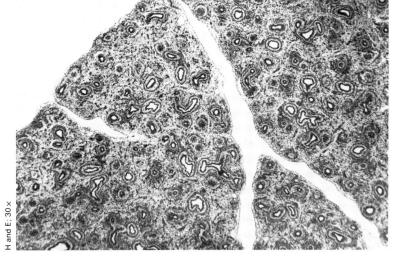

H and E: 30×

10 weeks

At *10 weeks* development is entirely bronchial, with large amounts of interbronchial mesenchyme. Cartilages have begun to form from precartilage. The bronchi are lined by nonciliated columnar epithelium, which may be pseudostratified.

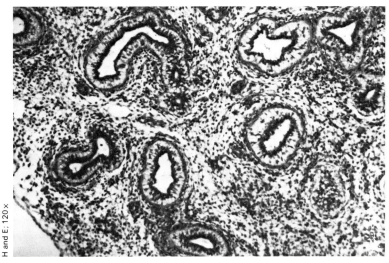

H and E: 120×

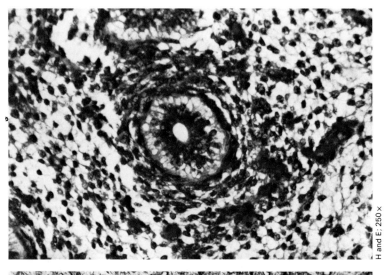

H and E; 250 ×

10 weeks

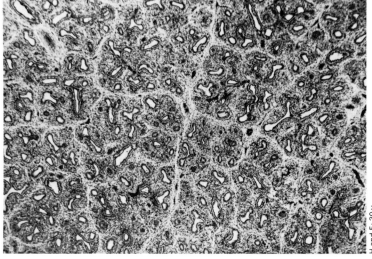

H and E; 30 ×

14 weeks

By *14 weeks* the interbronchial mesenchyme is diminishing in extent.

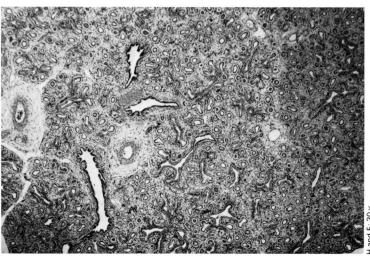

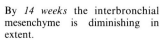

16 weeks

By *16 weeks* bronchial development is advanced; the epithelium has lost its pseudostratification and is ciliated.

16 weeks

16 weeks

22 weeks

At *22–26 weeks* development of the terminal airways begins, with terminal bronchioles giving rise to nonalveolated bronchioles, which will form terminal respiratory bronchioles. Rudimentary alveolar development occurs but the lining epithelium is prominent.

H and E; 120 ×

H and E; 120 ×

H and E; 30 ×

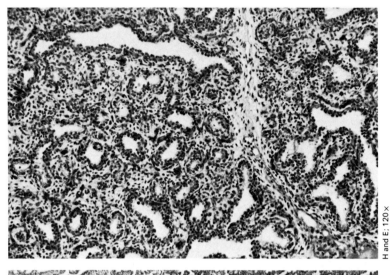

H and E; 120 ×

22 weeks

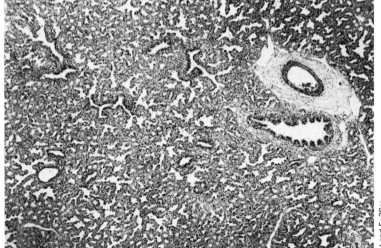

H and E; 30 ×

26 weeks

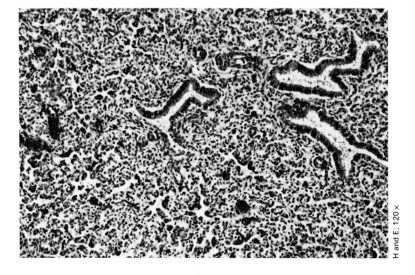

H and E; 120 ×

26 weeks

III *Kidney*

12 weeks

12 weeks

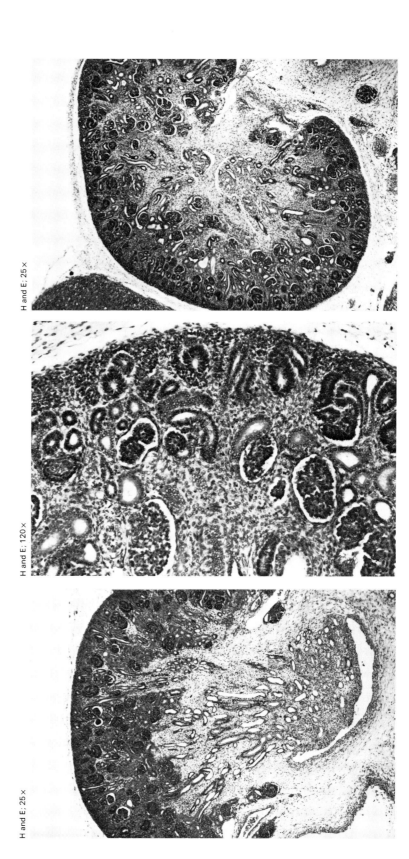

H and E; 25 ×

H and E; 120 ×

H and E; 25 ×

16 weeks

The kidney has some corticomedullary demarcation by *12 weeks*, with fetal glomeruli and S-form tubules present. By *16–20* weeks the development of the pyramids is advanced, and cortical and papillary development encroach on the loose mesenchyme in the central part of the kidney.

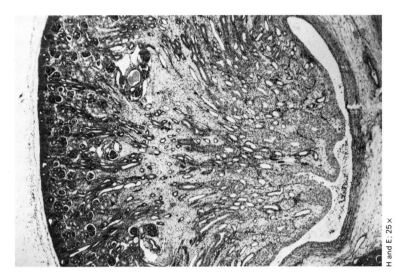

20 weeks

H and E; 25 ×

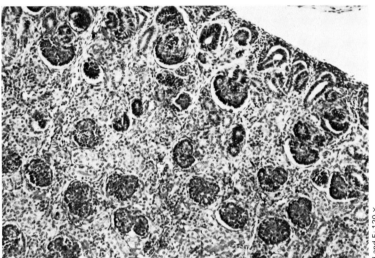

22 weeks

H and E; 120 ×

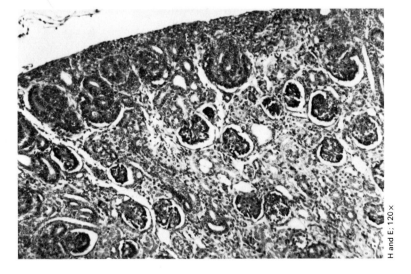

26 weeks

Between *22 and 36* weeks the number of layers of primitive glomeruli diminishes from three to two (*26 weeks*) and subsequently to one (*34 weeks*) and finally to zero. Glomerulogenesis ceases at *36 weeks*. It must be emphasized that a wide expanse of cortex should be scanned to allow an impression of how many layers are present.

H and E; 120 ×

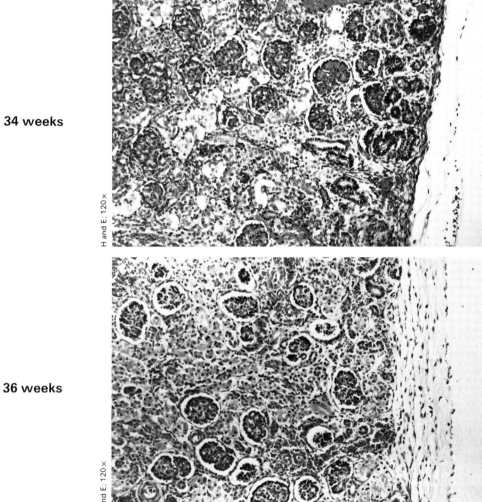

34 weeks

H and E; 120×

36 weeks

H and E; 120×

IV *Gonads (Testis)*

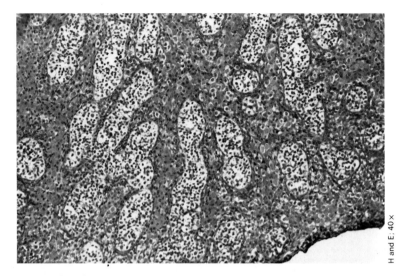

H and E; 40 ×

10 weeks

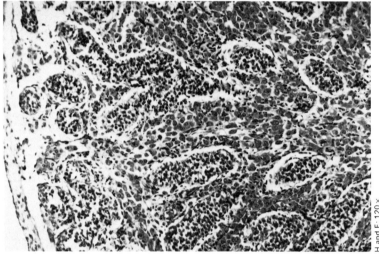

H and E; 120 ×

16 weeks

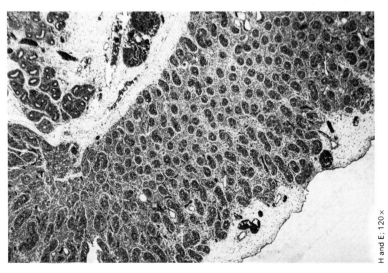

H and E; 120 ×

20 weeks

It is often not possible to distinguish between the two gonads before *10 weeks* of age. The cords of germ cells are then said to be continuous in males and interrupted in females, but this may be difficult to assess. By *16 weeks* this change is obvious and Leydig cells are present in large numbers in the developing testis, where the tubules are canalized. Stromal development in both gonads occurs later.

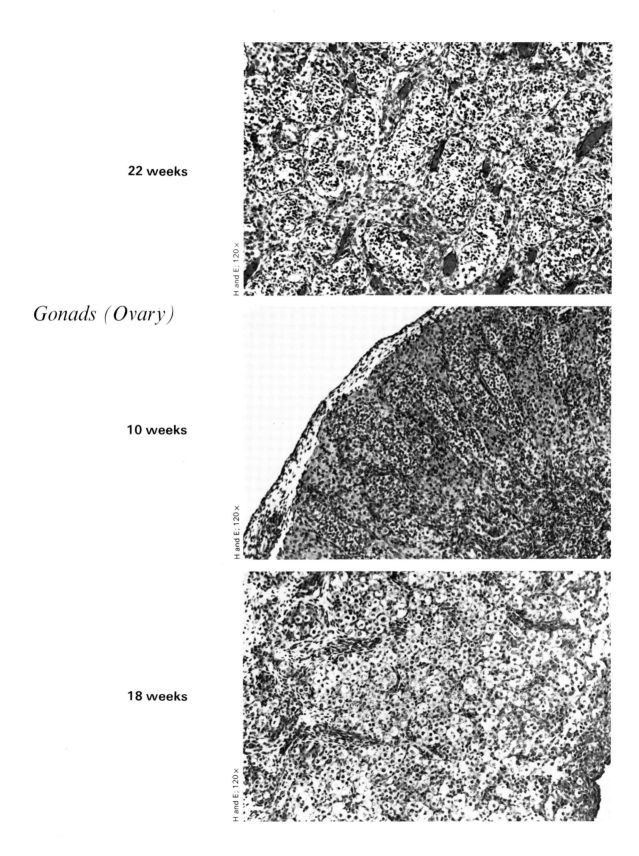

22 weeks

Gonads (Ovary)

10 weeks

18 weeks

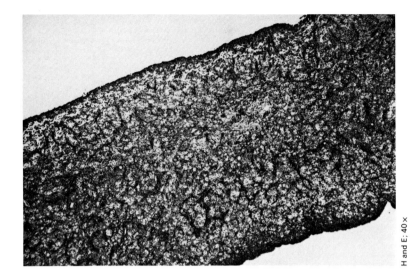

20 weeks

H and E; 40 ×

V *Stomach*

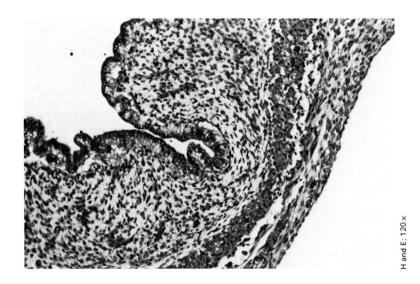

10 weeks

At *10 weeks* the stomach has well-defined muscle coats and a broad loose submucosa. Mucosal folding and early gland formation are seen by *14–16* weeks and a more organized mucosal pattern by *20 weeks*.

H and E; 120 ×

14 weeks

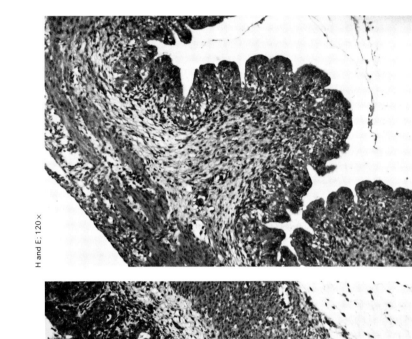

H and E; 120×

16 weeks

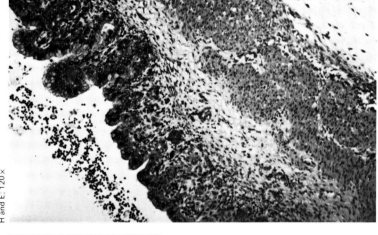

H and E; 120×

20 weeks

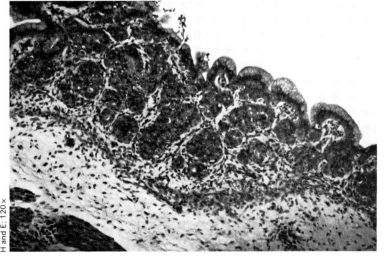

H and E; 120×

VI *Colon*

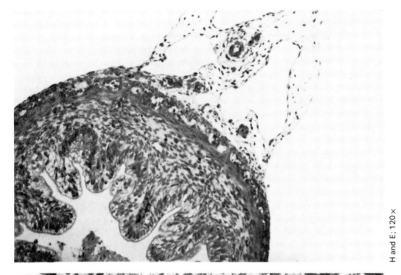

10 weeks

H and E; 120×

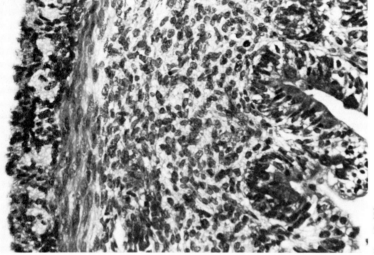

14 weeks

H and E; 250×

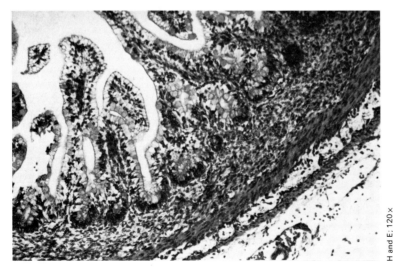

18 weeks

H and E; 120×

At *10 weeks* ganglia are readily seen in the myenteric plexus, being apparently more numerous on the mesenteric border. At *14 weeks* the submucosa is still cellular and broad, but by *18 weeks* this appearance is changing fast. Muscle coats thicken by *20–22* weeks.

22 weeks

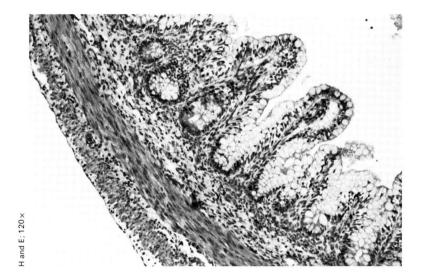

H and E; 120×

VII *Pancreas*

10 weeks

Initially composed of ducts (*10 weeks*), acinar structures begin to form relatively early (*12–14 weeks*). The gland has an abundant stroma at this stage. In the author's experience later development is very variable, and islet tissue, although visible from *16 weeks* on, may vary considerably in amount.

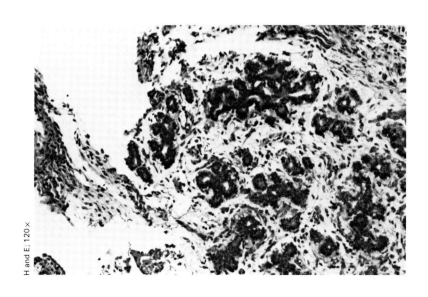

H and E; 120×

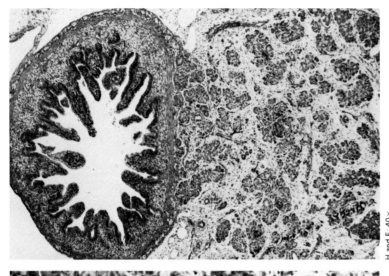

H and E; 40 ×

12 weeks

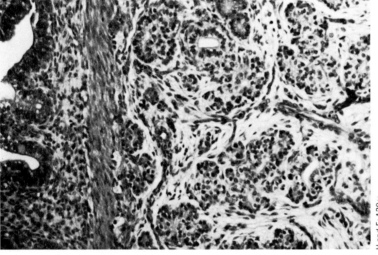

H and E; 120 ×

12 weeks

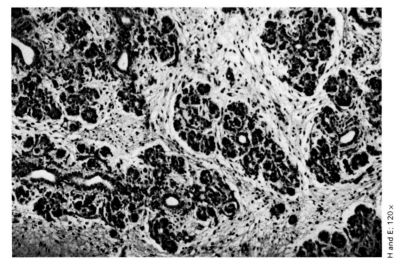

H and E; 120 ×

14 weeks

16 weeks

18 weeks

20 weeks

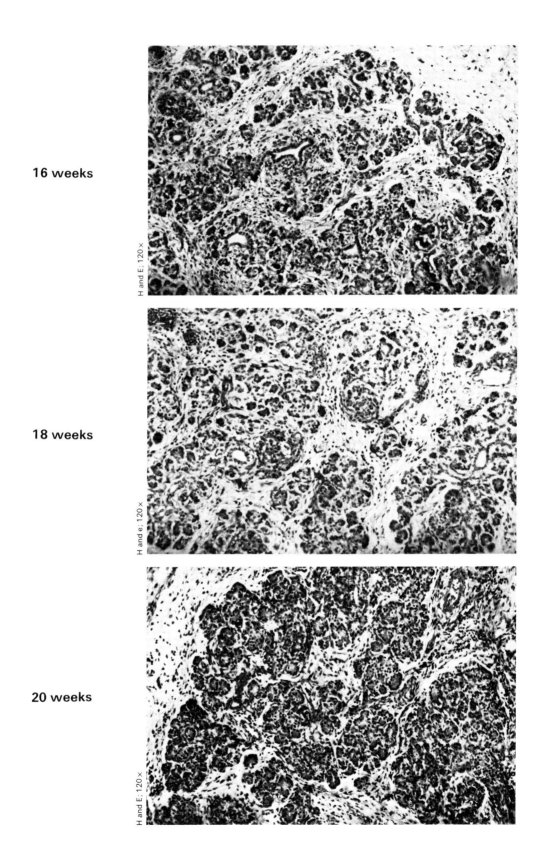

H and E; 120 ×

H and e; 120 ×

H and E; 120 ×

VIII *Liver*

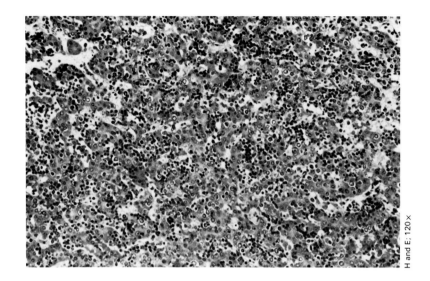

H and E; 120×

Haematopoiesis is established in the liver from *8 weeks*. By *10 weeks* the appearance (shown here) resembles that found at term.

IX *Trachea and Oesophagus*

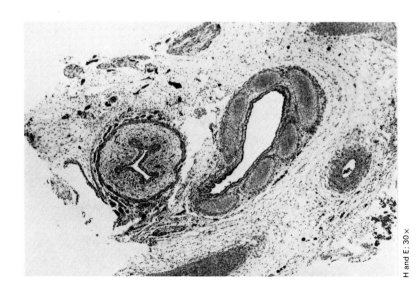

H and E; 30×

10 weeks

By *10 weeks* the trachea and oesophagus are distinct but the muscle coats of the latter are thin. Complete tracheal rings are found.

Colin L. Berry

29

10 weeks

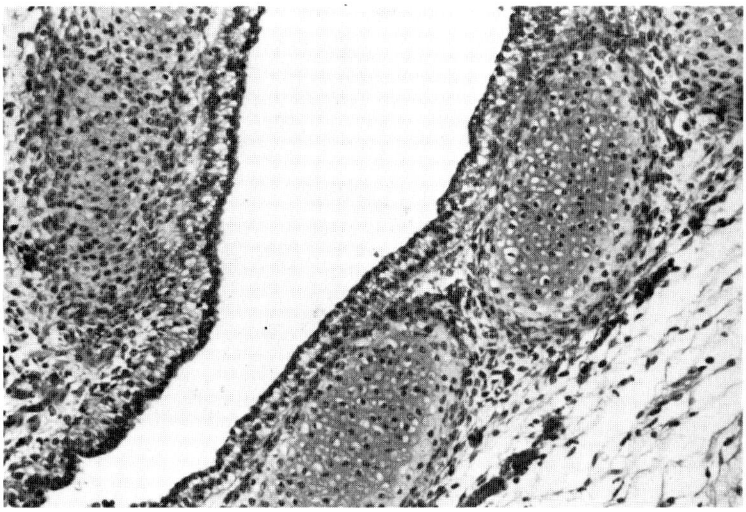

H and E; 120×

10 weeks

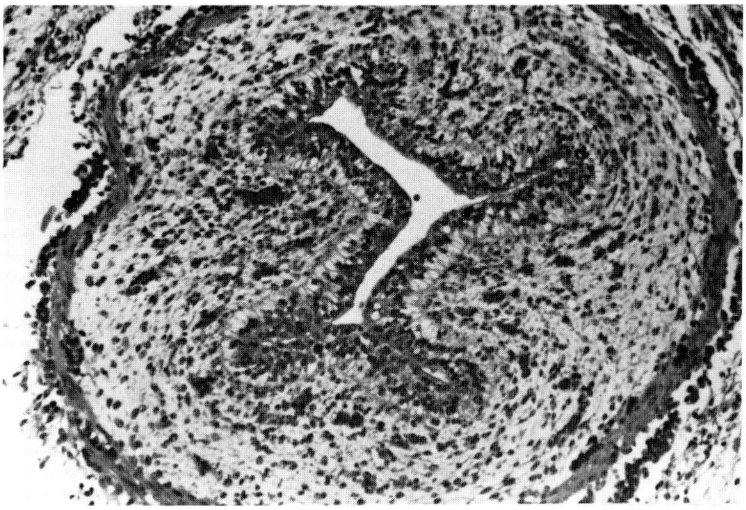

H and E; 120×

12 weeks

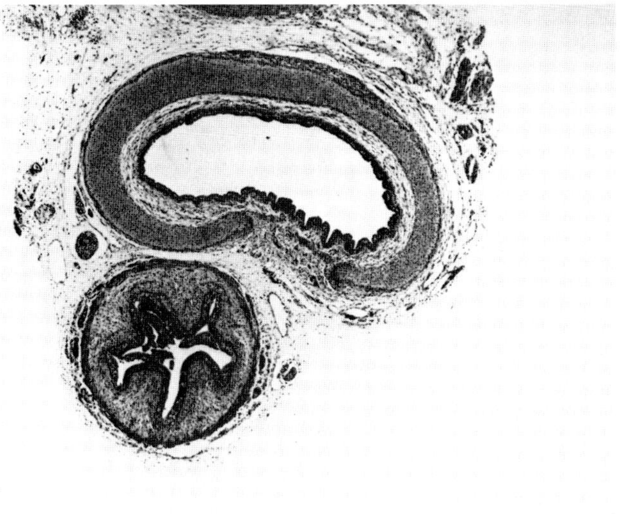

At *12 weeks*, both structures have well-defined wall components and epithelia are maturing.

H and E; 30×

X *Skin*

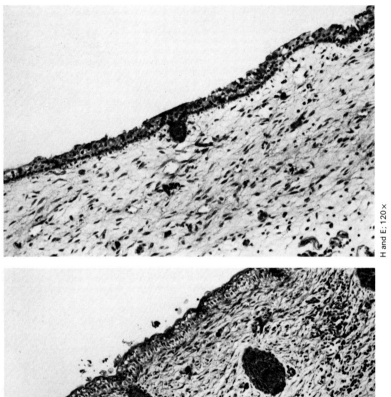

H and E; 120 ×

12 weeks

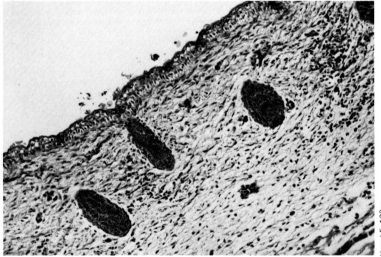

H and E; 120 ×

18 weeks

Hair follicles are seen in the skin by
12 weeks, and are more abundant at
18 weeks.

References

Bagnall KM, Jones PRM, Harris PF (1975) Estimating the age of the human foetus from crown–rump measurements. Ann Hum Biol 2: 387

Bell JE (1979) Fused suprarenal glands in association with central nervous system defects in the first half of fetal life. J Pathol 127: 191

Benson PF, Fensom AH, Polani PE (1979) Prenatal diagnosis of metabolic errors. Lancet 1: 161

Berry CL (1980) The examination of embryonic and fetal material in diagnostic histopathology laboratories. J Clin Pathol 33: 317

Birkbeck JA, Billewicz WZ, Thomson AM (1975a) Human foetal measurements between 50 and 150 days of gestation, in relation to crown–heel length. Ann Hum Biol 2: 173

Birkbeck JA, Billewicz WZ, Thomson AM (1975b) Foetal growth from 50 to 150 days of gestation. Ann Hum Biol 2: 319

Boyd JD, Hamilton WJ (1970) The human placenta. Heffer, Cambridge.

Granchrow D, Ornoy A (1979) Possible evidence for secondary degeneration of central nervous system in the etiology of anencephaly and brain dysraphia. A study in young human fetuses. Virchows Arch [Pathol Anat] 384: 285

Mikamo K (1970) Anatomical and chromosomal anomalies in spontaneous abortion. Possible correlation with overripeness of oocytes. Am J Obstet Gynecol 106: 243

Milunsky A (1976) Prenatal diagnosis of genetic disorders. N Engl J Med 295: 377

Nañagus JC (1925) A comparison of the growth of the body dimensions of anencephalic human fetuses with normal fetal growth as determined by graphic analysis and empirical formulae. Am J Anat 35: 455

Rushton DI (1978) Simplified classification of spontaneous abortions. J Med Genet 15: 1

Streeter GL (1920) Weight, sitting height, head size, foot length and menstrual age of the human embryo. Carnegie Institute Contributions to Embryology 11: 143

Theisen CT, Bodin JD, Svododa JA, Pettinelli MW (1979) Unusual muscle abnormalities associated with thalidomide treatment in a Rhesus monkey: a case report. Teratology 19: 313

Thomson AM, Billewicz WZ, Hytten FE (1969) The weight of the placenta in relation to birthweight. J Obstet Gynecol Br Cwlth 76: 865

Tynan MJ, Becker AE, Macartney FJ, Jimenez MQ, Shinebourne EA, Anderson RH (1979) Nomenclature and classification of congenital heart disease. Br Heart J 41: 544

Trolle D (1948) Age of foetus determined from its measures. Acta Obstet Gynecol Scand 27: 327

Usher R, McLean F (1969) Intrauterine growth of liveborn caucasion infants at sea level: Standards obtained from measurements in 7 dimensions of infants born between 25 and 44 weeks of gestation. J Pediatr 74: 901

Wilson JG (1965) Methods for administering agents and detecting malformations in experimental animals. In: Wilson JG, Warkany J (ed) Teratology—Principles and techniques. University of Chicago Press, Chicago

Chapter 2

Placental and Abortion Pathology

Mies J. Becker

1. General Comments

The placenta is of major importance in the in-trauterine development of the fetus. For this reason a thorough knowledge of its structure is necessary in the study of the pathology of stillbirth and of many of the neonatal problems that arise in the early postnatal period.

From a practical point of view a distinction is made between 'early' and 'late' gestation, with the turning point around the 12th week. It should be realized, of course, that such a sharp distinction cannot really be made. We have nevertheless chosen such a distinct categorization for two reasons. Firstly, early and late gestational periods differ in the incidence of the various pathological abnormalities of the placenta (Fig. 2.1). Secondly, the material usually available for study from the two periods is quite different, the placenta itself not having

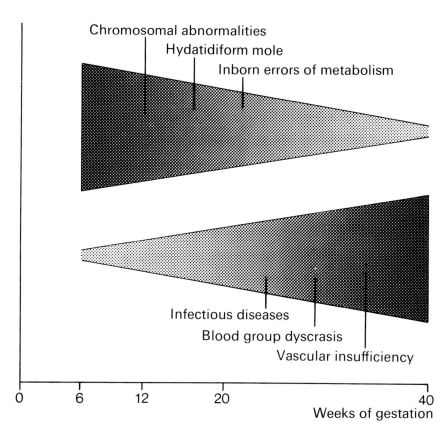

Fig. 2.1. Schema showing various pathogenic mechanisms affecting the placenta, with reference to gestational age.

obtained its definitive form before the 12th week. In the early period, therefore, the material is mostly obtained from abortions and consists of either a placental sac or fragmented placental and embryonal tissues, while in later stages of development a well-defined placenta is usually available. Thorough knowledge of the developmental aspects of the placenta is thus mandatory. Moreover, after the intrauterine death of a fetus the placenta will remain viable for a prolonged period, so that the pathologist should be trained to distinguish true pathological changes from those that occur after fetal death. Study of the placenta may thus yield important information, but the investigator should be aware of the difficulties. It is beyond the scope of this book to give a detailed account of placental pathology. In this particular chapter a survey is given of those abnormalities of the placenta that are of prime interest for routine investigations in paediatric cases. For further studies the reader is referred to the comprehensive studies by Strauss et al. (1967) and Fox (1978).

2. Handling of Tissues

The way in which placental tissues are handled depends on the state in which the material is obtained. The material should preferably be inspected unfixed; for further processing routine fixatives can be used.

Abortion material will usually consist of a placental sac, which may be intact but which in the majority of cases will consist of fragments of placental tissue. A fetus may be present within this material, and careful examination of specimens is therefore indicated. The material is best displayed by spreading it on a flat surface, to facilitate the distinction between blood clots and fragments of placenta. Some pathologists prefer to examine fragments in water. Decidual tissue and villous structures are recognized from their red-brown colour, having a firmer consistency than blood clots (Fig. 2.2a). Nevertheless, microscopical examination of selected fragments may only reveal decidual tissue, without villi. It is thus advisable to

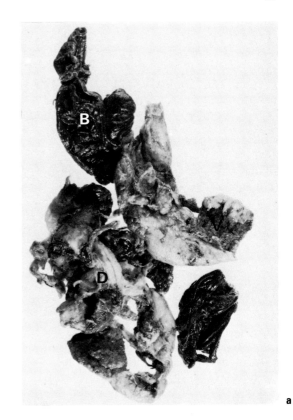

a

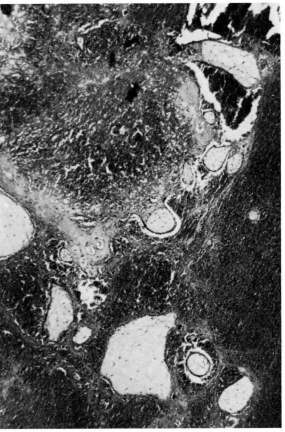

b

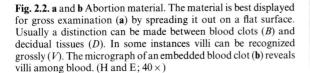

Fig. 2.2. a and **b** Abortion material. The material is best displayed for gross examination (**a**) by spreading it out on a flat surface. Usually a distinction can be made between blood clots (*B*) and decidual tissues (*D*). In some instances villi can be recognized grossly (*V*). The micrograph of an embedded blood clot (**b**) reveals villi among blood. (H and E; 40 ×)

include pieces of blood clot for histological processing, since these may contain villi (Fig. 2.2b). Inspection of the fragmented material may also reveal membrane-like structures, some of which should always be examined histologically. Fetal structures are only rarely recognized with certainty among the fragmented material. It is important to embed a large quantity of material, to increase the chance of identifying fetal parts.

In 'spontaneous' abortions the placental sac is usually intact when expelled. It can be recognized among the remaining blood clots because of its dark brown colour and its peculiar shape. It is usually pear-shaped, representing a cast of the uterine cavity (Fig. 2.3). The outer aspect of the sac displays a fibrillar structure caused by the adherent decidua (Fig. 2.3a). The dimensions of the placental sac should be determined as a reference point for the developmental state of the fetus. Opening of the sac is best performed from the 'cervical' side, i.e., the elongated part of the sac. Great care should be taken not to damage the fetus or separate it from the placenta. Its position can then be determined (Fig. 2.3b). The umbilical cord and fetus should be inspected in situ. In some instances the fetus is identified only as a tiny knob-like thickening at the end of a small cord-like structure (Fig. 2.3b). If there is a marked discrepancy between the size of the placental sac and that of the fetus a diagnosis of missed abortion can be made (Fig. 2b). Congenital

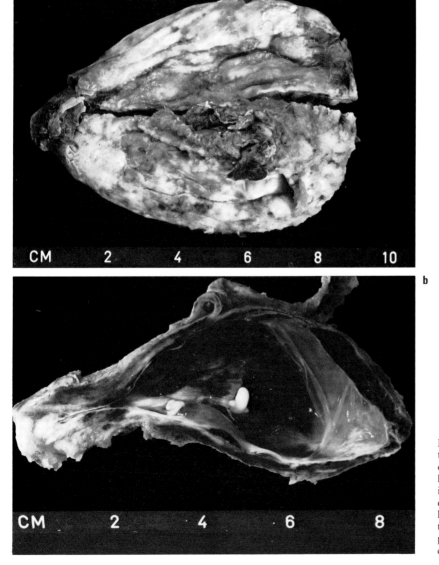

Fig. 2.3. a and b A placental sac: a the intact specimen with its rough outer surface caused by the adherent decidua. Note the characteristic pear shape; b the inner aspect of the sac, revealing the fetus as a knob-like thickening at the end of the small cord-like structure. This particular appearance is indicative of missed abortion.

malformation in a fetus can only be detected by extensive serial histological sectioning, which is beyond the resources of most departments.

The handling of a well-formed placenta obtained from later gestational periods is relatively simple, in that inspection is the most important aspect (see p. 50). If the placenta is obtained in toto, with membranes and umbilical cord, the site of the tear in the membranes should be determined and the site of insertion of the membranes relative to the placenta should be inspected. Only after complete examination should the membranes be removed along their line of insertion. They are then coiled and fixed in a routine fixative. After fixation transverse sections can be taken, which will facilitate the study of a relatively large surface area of membranes in only a few slides (Fig. 2.4).

The umbilical cord is examined and measured, and particular attention is given to the number of vessels within it. The degree of twist in the cord is observed, with particular reference to the presence of torsion and umbilical knots (see p. 50).

Haemorrhages and oedema should be looked for. The placental insertion of the umbilical cord needs careful inspection. Sections are taken routinely from the site of the placental insertion; additional sections may be taken from sites suspected of showing abnormalities.

The placenta itself is first examined from its fetal side. A normal membrane surface should give a glistening reflection, being transparent and slightly greyish in colour (Fig. 2.5a). Cloudiness or any other change in colour should alert the pathologist to an abnormality. Normally the vessels will radiate from the umbilical cord insertion towards the periphery, and they are usually of similar size and filled with blood. Dilated and tortuous or extremely attenuated vessels suggest a pathological condition. Abnormalities in vascular configuration should always be looked for. The maternal side of the placenta is then examined (Fig. 2.5b). The presence of cotyledons

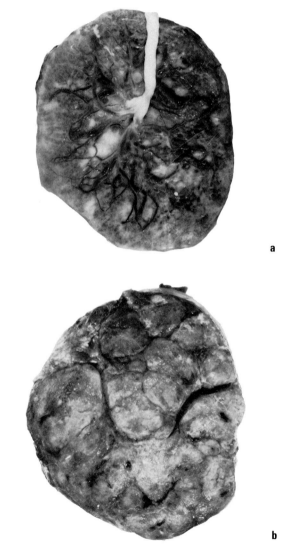

a

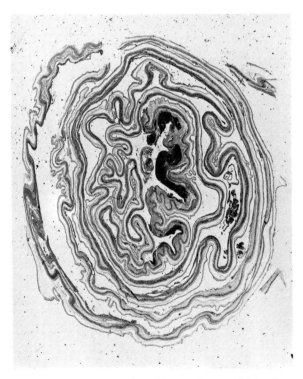

Fig. 2.4. Microscopical section of the membrane, which has been fixed in a coiled position to allow the study of a large surface area in only a small number of slides. (H and E; 7 ×)

b

Fig. 2.5. a and **b** Specimen of placenta: **a** the fetal aspect, covered by membranes that give the surface its glistening aspect. Note the central insertion of the umbilical cord and the radiating vessels from the site of insertion; **b** the maternal aspect, revealing the presence of cotyledons, which gives the maternal surface its lobulated aspect.

normally gives this surface a lobulated aspect. Particular care should be given to the inspection of the completeness of the cotyledons, which is not easy because of blood clots and tears that may have occurred during delivery. Concavities on the maternal surface may reveal the presence of a retroplacental haemorrhage. Calcification can normally be identified on the maternal side of the placenta, but unusually large amounts of calcific material should always suggest the presence of disease.

The placenta is then weighed, without its membranes and cord. The significance of the weight recorded, however, is debatable.

For further examination the placenta is cut into parallel slices approximately 1 cm thick. The incisions are best made from the maternal side, with the organ resting on its fetal membrane surface (Fig. 2.6). Each slice should be carefully inspected for abnormalities. When abnormalities are present, an attempt should be made to evaluate whether they are localized or diffuse. Moreover, an attempt should be made to express their extent as a percentage of the total placental tissue. Routine histological investigations should be carried out on sections from the membranous and decidual sites of the placenta and the peripheral and central areas. Further sectioning is only indicated when abnormalities have been noted during examination.

Bacteriological and virological studies can only be carried out on fresh tissues, and strict precautions should be taken not to contaminate the material. Chromosomal studies of the placenta also need optimal circumstances for reliable results to be obtained.

3. Developmental Morphology

Before the abnormal placenta can be evaluated it is necessary to be acquainted with the developmental changes that affect the placental villi. In the early period, i.e., in the first 12 weeks of gestation, the placenta grows mainly because of an increase in the numbers of villi. Thereafter, growth is accompanied by a process of differentiation within the villi themselves. Thus, various morphological stages of maturity can be recognized, which correlate with clinical subdivisions such as immaturity and prematurity. A sharp distinction on morphological criteria alone is not always feasible, however.

In early gestation the placental tissues consist mainly of stem villi. These are relatively simple structures, each composed of a broad core of loosely textured mesenchyme, covered with trophoblast. Blood vessels are present centrally. Tissue macrophages with foamy cytoplasm, the so-called Hofbauer cells, are scattered within the mesenchyme. The trophoblast is composed of a layer of two or more cells, the inner layer of which is made up of cuboid or polyhedral cells with well-defined cell boundaries and relatively large, pale-staining nuclei with a finely dispersed chromatin network. The layer composed of these cells is the *cytotrophoblast*, and the cells composing the layer are known as Langhans' cells (Fig. 2.7). The outer layer of cells is the *syncytiotrophoblast* (Fig. 2.7). It is composed of flattened cells with ill-defined cell boundaries, whose nuclei are smaller and stain more darkly than those of Langhans' cells. The cell cytoplasm is sometimes slightly vacuolated and, particularly in the very

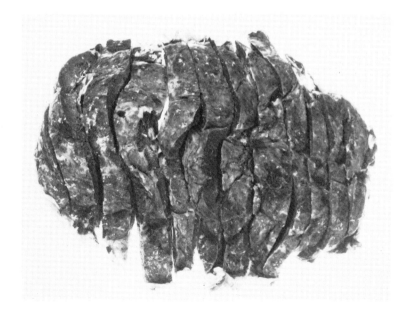

Fig. 2.6. Photograph to illustrate how the placenta is incised for further examinations. Two slices are made at approximately 1 cm. This allows close inspection of the cut surface at different levels.

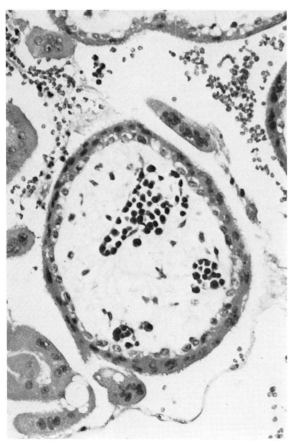

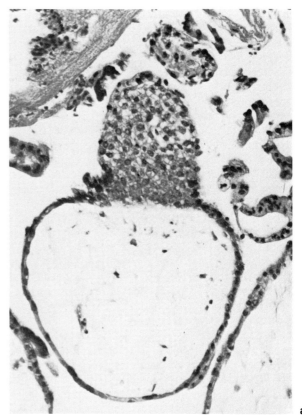

Fig. 2.7. A placental villus of approximately 12 weeks of gestation. The surface layer is composed of a double layer of cells. The inner layer shows a vacuolated cytoplasm and is composed to so-called Langhans cells. The layer itself is termed the cytotrophoblast. The outer layer is termed the syncytial trophoblast, being composed of a more flattened layer of cells. The nuclei of this layer are more darkly stained than those of the cytotrophoblast. (H and E; 80 ×)

young villi, the cells of the syncytiotrophoblast may show a brush border at their surface. Placental tissues obtained from abortions usually contain villi with these structural characteristics.

The growth of the placenta is established mainly by a process of 'budding' of the cells of the trophoblast, with the original stem villi as the point of departure (Fig. 2.8a). A core of mesenchyme will gradually 'invade' this cell mass, to be followed in later stages by capillaries (Fig. 2.8b). In the mature placenta the number of cotyledons reflects the number of stem villi from which further develop-

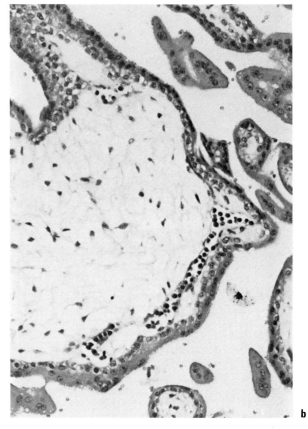

Fig. 2.8. a and b A growing placenta, showing the process of budding of cells of the trophoblast (a) and a later stage in which a core of mesenchyme has invaded this cell bud (b). (H and E; a 200 ×, b 50 ×)

ment has sprung. The newly formed sprouts initially show a similar architecture to that described for the stem villi. Through a continuous process of budding further villi are formed, until the stage of maturity is reached. With each generation of newly formed villi their diameter gets smaller, while that of the ingrowing capillaries remains the same, so that the volume occupied by these capillaries increases markedly. As a consequence of continuous budding, an increasing number of villi will exhibit vascular spaces in direct contact with the overlying trophoblast (Fig. 2.9). The placenta is full-grown at aproximately 32 weeks' gestation.

Simultaneously with growth, a process of differentiation occurs within the villi. This is first recognized by an increase in cellularity in the core of stem villi, a phenomenon that is most probably due to differentiation of fibroblasts, expressed as a gradual increase in connective tissue fibres. Initially, these changes occur centrally in the core, particularly in perivascular locations. The central vessels themselves develop a distinct wall of smooth-muscle cells. Nucleated red cells are present.

In these early stages of development the cells of both cytotrophoblast and syncytiotrophoblast, together composing the trophoblast, are still easily identified. This feature can be considered 'typical' for a placenta of up to approximately 28 weeks of gestation. With increasing gestational age, the placenta will increase the number of mature villi, which are characterized by their minute size and relatively wide vascular spaces in contact with the surface layer (Fig. 2.10). Moreover, owing to a continuous process of fibrosis the stem villi are gradually transformed into fibrous stalks (Fig. 2.10a). Fibrous tissue will gradually spread out within the newly formed villi, so that the mature placenta will show collagen fibres extending into the terminal villi. Concomitant with this mesenchymal differentiation, changes occur within the trophoblast. The layer of Langhans' cells gradually becomes inconspicuous (Fig. 2.10b), a feature that correlates with decreased activity of budding villi. The cells flatten and become dispersed between those of the syncytiotrophoblast. The remaining cells are considered to represent inactive reserve cells that may

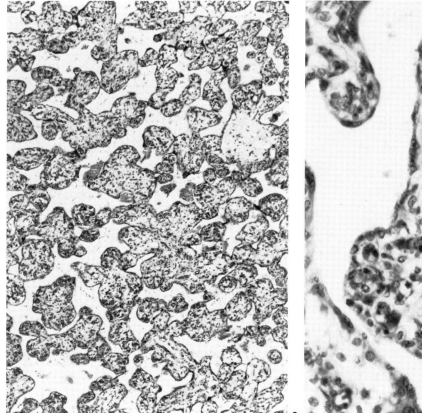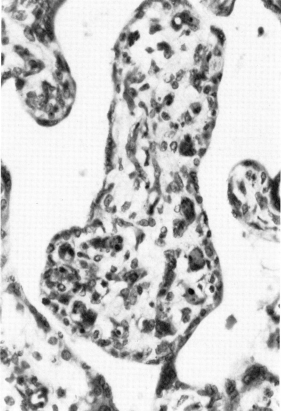

Fig. 2.9. a and **b** A placenta of approximately 26 weeks of gestation, showing a low-power view that still reveals the sprouting of newly formed villi from more centrally located, 'older' villi (**a**) and a detail of one of these newly formed villi (**b**). The trophoblast has thinned considerably but the Langhans cells are still recognizable. Moreover, the capillaries are in a more peripheral position, though the total surface area taken by capillaries is still minimal. (H and E; **a** 56 ×, **b** 350 ×)

replace the cells of the syncytiotrophoblast when necessary. The latter layer is flat, and the cells show irregularly dispersed nuclei. In the fully matured placenta the cells composing the syncytiotrophoblast may become so attenuated that in places a cellular coating is no longer recognizable. Nuclear material, moreover, may aggregate to form clumps, the so-called syncytial knots. These knots appear gradually in the premature placenta but they increase in number, so that in the mature placenta they are a striking histological feature (Fig. 2.10a).

A fully matured placenta is thus characterized by fibrous stalks, which represent the original stem villi and are located centrally in each cotyledon, and a compact arrangement of villi of various generations, ranging from large-sized structures with relatively few vessels and a high collagen content to minute villi with wide vascular spaces in contiguity with the surface coating and hardly any collagen. The surface coating of these villi shows a single layer of syncytiotrophoblast, in which syncytial knots are an outstanding feature.

In the mature placenta, moreover, parts of the surface of the villi are coated by clumps of fibrin, particularly at sites where the syncytiotrophoblast is absent (Fig. 2.11). Occasionally, such depositions can be observed in a premature placenta, but they are invariably present in full-term placentas and are more conspicuous in those defined as postmature. Indeed, the deposition of fibrin may become so extensive, particularly at the periphery, that whole clusters of villi appear glued together. This pheno-

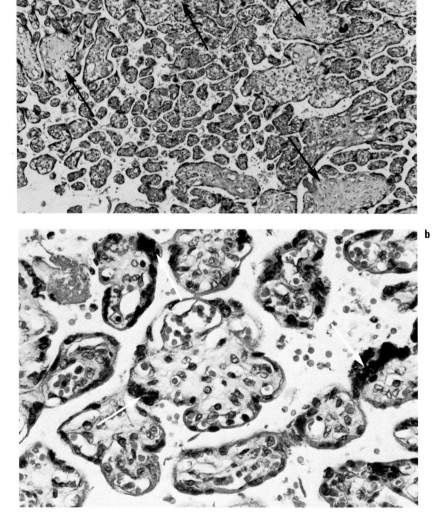

Fig. 2.10. a and b A mature placenta. H & E a A low-power view in which the fibrous stalks in the larger villi are clearly identified (*arrows*). 35 × b The villi in more detail. The surface area taken up by capillaries has definitely increased at the expense of the stromal component. Moreover, the trophoblast layer is composed mainly of the syncytiotrophoblast. There are many nuclear aggregates, forming the so-called syncytial knots (*arrows*). (88 ×)

menon needs to be differentiated from placental infarction (p. 57). The pathogenesis of fibrin deposition remains unclear.

The process of placental maturation is often accompanied by a deposition of calcium. It usually appears first in the late gestational period and then affects primarily the stem villi. In the mature and postmature placenta it is common to find prominent calcium deposits at these sites. They take the form of coarse granules and are usually intimately related to areas of fibrosis (Fig. 2.12). Occasionally, one may find such deposits in terminal villi, but under these circumstances these alterations are almost always associated with degenerative changes (see p. 43).

4. Post-mortem Placental Changes

Following intrauterine death of the fetus the placenta does not die but remains vital until it is expelled. During this period, however, its morphology alters considerably. The alterations observed are collectively referred to as post-mortem changes and their proper identification is important, since they may obscure pathological changes present at the time of fetal death. Unfortunately, postmortem changes resemble those that occur normally in a growing and maturing placenta. They also resemble those that occur secondary to vascular insufficiency, which is in itself a common cause of intrauterine death. It is of practical significance, therefore to remember that primary vascular placen-

tal insufficiency tends to result in *focal* abnormalities of the placenta, affecting both the maternal and the fetal compartments, whereas post-mortem changes tend to be diffuse, affecting primarily fetal structures. This phenomenon is related to the fact that the fetal circulation will come to a complete standstill after intrauterine death. This affects all villi, and the changes that occur are diffuse. Their nature, however, is such that with an increasing time lapse between the death of the fetus and the expulsion of the placenta it becomes increasingly difficult to obtain an adequate impression of pre-existent placental pathology. Even with vast experience it may sometimes no longer be feasible to ascertain the true nature of the placental abnormalities found. The distribution of changes may then be the only indicator of their pathogenesis: focal lesions suggest a pre-existent abnormality.

Since it is mainly the fetal compartment of the placenta that is affected the description will focus on the alterations that occur in the villi.

4.1 Vascular Changes

As stated above, fetal death results in a complete interruption of the fetal circulation. The vascular spaces within the villi are therefore empty and collapsed. After some weeks they are no longer recognizable within the altered villi (see below). Larger vessels, which have already developed a distinct muscular wall, will remain open for a long time and some of these vessels may still contain blood. In the majority, however, a fine meshwork of fibrin and platelets occludes the lumen (Fig. 2.13). Within weeks these intravascular clots will become

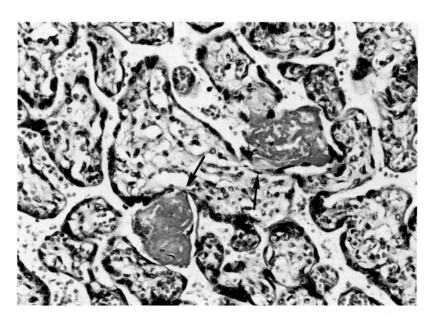

Fig. 2.11. A mature placenta, showing villi with fibrin depositions adherent to the surface. At these sites the syncytiotrophoblast appears to be absent (*arrows*). (H and E; 200 ×)

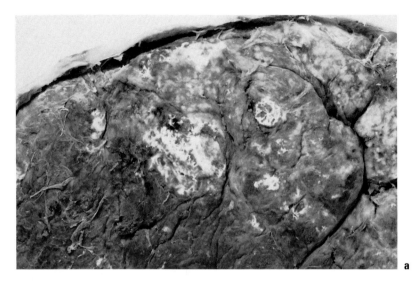

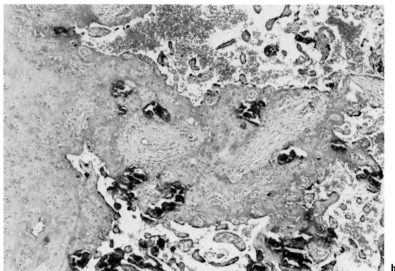

Fig. 2.12. a and b A mature placenta, showing deposition of calcific material. **a** Maternal aspect of the placenta with grossly recognizable calcifications; **b** Coarse calcific deposits are present in stem villi. (H and E; 56 ×)

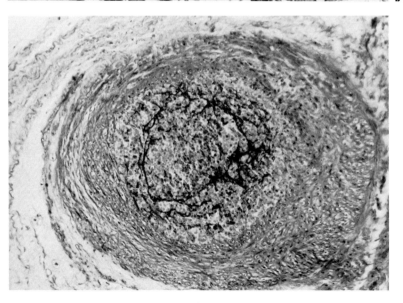

Fig. 2.13. A chorionic vessel, showing an occluded lumen with a fine meshwork of fibrin and platelets. (PTAH; 140 ×)

organized by ingrowth of fibroblasts, so that the vessels ultimately become completely obliterated by fibrous tissue. In our experience, classic thrombosis does not occur. In time, the muscular wall of the larger blood vessels also become fibrotic. Thus, several weeks after intrauterine fetal death the larger blood vessels are totally transformed into fibrous strands, which appear as fibrous nodules on histological cross sections.

4.2 Stromal Changes

Concomitant with the vascular changes, the stroma of the villi changes. In the very young placenta, i.e., before the 20th week of gestation, some of the peripheral villi may exhibit liquefaction of the stroma (Fig. 2.14). This alteration is often referred to as a cyst-like change (see p. 47). In the older placenta the changes affecting the villi are mainly characterized by fibrosis, which first appears in the larger villi and concentrates around collapsed vessels, often showing concentric layering (Fig. 2.15). In time, fibrosis occurs in the more peripheral villi, so that

ultimately almost all terminal villi are affected. At this stage it is extremely difficult to recognize the pre-existent villous capillaries. In some instances they can be traced as slit-like spaces with an endothelial lining, embedded in otherwise totally fibrosed villi. In its initial stages the fibrotic change is cellular, with only sparse connective tissue fibres. However, with time the pattern reverses, so that eventually dense fibrosis dominates the microscopical appearance (Fig. 2.16). At this stage it is practically impossible to distinguish such a post-mortem stromal change from alterations that occur in patients with primary circulatory insufficiency of the placenta. Again, in these circumstances the most reliable means of distinguishing between the two conditions is that post-mortem changes are generally diffusely present throughout the placenta, affecting all villi, whereas a primary circulatory insufficiency tends to be focal.

Calcification may be observed in addition to fibrosis as a post-mortem change within villi. This calcification presents as fine granules (Fig. 2.17), and therefore contrasts with the coarse deposits that sometimes occur in villi during physiological maturation (cf. Figs. 2.12 and 2.17). The identification

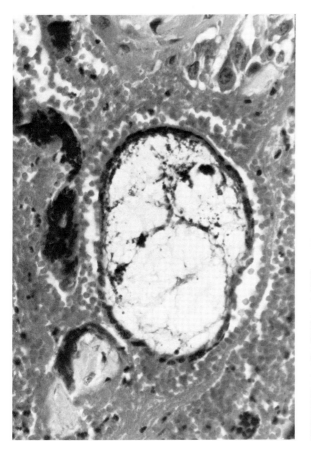

Fig. 2.14. A villus, showing liquefaction of the stroma. (H and E; 350 ×)

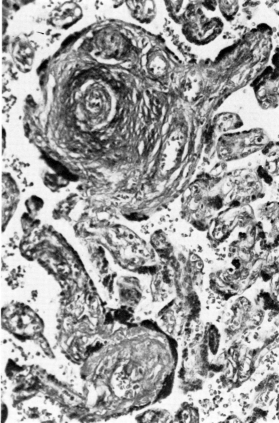

Fig. 2.15. Villi, showing concentric layering of collagen fibres around the vessels within them. (H and E; 200 ×)

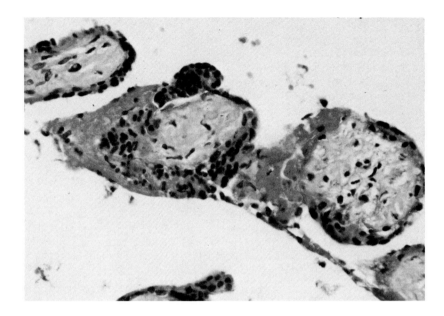

Fig. 2.16. A terminal villus, showing completely fibrosed stroma without recognizable capillaries. In addition there is a pronounced proliferation of trophoblastic cells and deposition of fibrin at the surface. (H and E; 350×)

of this particular type of calcification is thus a reliable indicator that one is dealing with a post-mortem change and not a pre-existent deposition. These fine granules of calcium are deposited along the basal membrane of the trophoblast (Fig. 2.17) and occasionally may outline remnants of stromal cells and endothelial cells. In most instances, moreover, the calcium depositions are mixed with precipitates of iron. It is of practical significance to study these finely granular depositions and to distinguish them from the larger, coarse deposits, which occur either as part of a normal maturation process or at sites of necrosis.

4.3. Trophoblastic Changes

The changes that occur in the trophoblast are late and depend on circulatory changes within the maternal compartment. The fetal circulation may come to an abrupt stop but the circulation in the intervillous spaces will only gradually diminish. This phenomenon also explains why post-mortem trophoblastic changes are very similar to those that occur in the placenta with primary circulatory insufficiency. In both conditions the trophoblast exhibits enhancement of what appears to be a normal maturation process. In other words, an excessive formation of trophoblastic knots appears (Fig. 2.18). Again, the major recognizable difference between the two conditions is that post-mortem changes are usually diffuse, whereas primary vascular insufficiency is focal.

The fact that the intervillous blood spaces contain less blood than might be expected is difficult to evaluate and is thus of no practical significance. It is

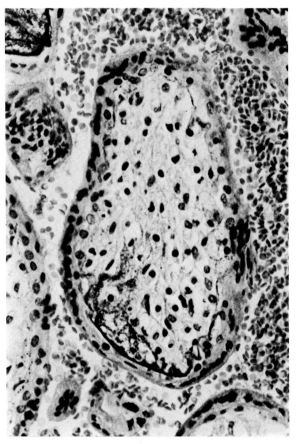

Fig. 2.17. A villus, showing fine calcific granules, which in part outline the stromal cells and in part have impregnated the basal membrane of the trophoblast. (H and E; 350×)

important to note that classic intervillous thrombosis (see below) does *not* occur as a post-mortem change; when observed it is *always* an indication of a pre-existing abnormality. Fibrin deposition, on the other hand, does occur and indeed can become so extensive that vast areas of fibrous villi may become completely encased within fibrin (Fig. 2.19). On gross examination such placentas are firm and greyish-white on their cut surface. It is in this final stage, which occurs after some months, that a precise interpretation of the abnormalities is no longer feasible. It should be re-emphasized, however, that close examination of the placenta, with particular attention to the pattern of distribution of the lesions, may still give some clue as to the true nature of the abnormalities observed.

5. Placental Pathology in Early Gestation

At present there is much uncertainty in the interpretation of the findings in placental tissues from early gestation, i.e., before the 12th week. Our knowledge is based mainly on abortions performed because of prenatal detection of a congenital disorder; the categories of chromosomal abnormalities or inborn errors of metabolism are most frequently concerned. Correlations have been made with morphological abnormalities, but our knowledge is still not adequate.

In this section we will describe some of the more common changes known to be related to certain pathological conditions.

5.1 Gross Features

As stated before, careful examination of the material obtained at abortion is of major importance. If an

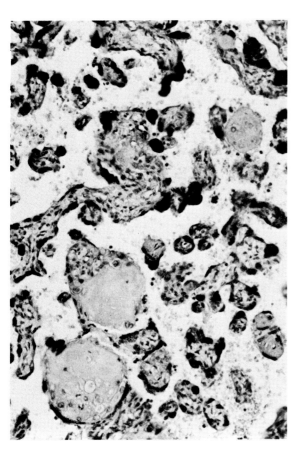

Fig. 2.18. A placenta, showing excessive formation of trophoblastic knots. (H and E; 200 ×)

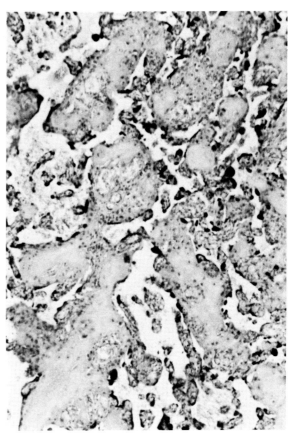

Fig. 2.19. A placenta, showing fibrous villi encased within fibrin. (H and E; 80 ×)

amniotic sac can be identified, it is necessary to evaluate whether or not there is a discrepancy between the size of the amniotic sac and that of the fetus. Marked discrepancies are indicative of missed abortion (see Fig. 2.3) (Boué et al. 1976). It should be emphasized that this discrepancy is so far the most reliable diagnostic sign for missed abortion. If fetal structures cannot be identified one has to rely on a discrepancy between the microscopical aspect of the placenta and the anticipated gestational age. This requires full and detailed knowledge of the maturation morphology of the placenta.

Another important observation is obtained from inspection of the cut surface of the placental tissues. In normal development the placenta should have a diffuse homogeneous and finely granular appearance. However, cyst-like structures (see below) are sometimes observed scattered among otherwise normal placental tissues (Fig. 2.20). Such an observation is highly suggestive of chromosomal triploidy. As yet, no other chromosomal abnormalities have been described with this particular appearance.

Finally, close inspection of the abortion material may reveal the presence of a hydatidiform mole.

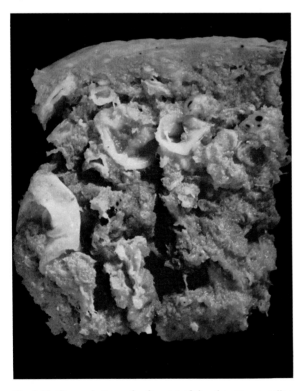

Fig. 2.20. Gross photograph of a part of the placenta, revealing cyst-like structures in a placenta of otherwise normal appearance. This observation is highly suggestive for a chromosomal triploidy.

5.2. Microscopical Features

Most microscopical changes affect the villi. One of the most striking alterations is the occurrence of cyst-like villi. They represent areas of stromal liquefaction without an epithelial lining, and are therefore not true cysts. They are filled with a clear watery fluid and in most microscopical sections they appear empty. The observation of cyst-like changes in villi is of importance, since there are three major circumstances in which these changes can be observed. These are (1) after death, e.g., in cases of missed abortion; (2) among patients with triploidy; and (3) in hydatidiform mole. In evaluating these possibilities it is important to realize that further classification depends both on the distribution of the abnormality within the placenta itself and on detailed microscopical features. In the case of postmortem change the cyst-like villi are randomly distributed throughout the placenta, although not all villi are affected to the same degree. However, villi exhibiting cysts will also show stigmata that are clearly definable as post-mortem alterations. In other words, such villi also show collapsed vascular spaces, at least the larger ones, while the trophoblast may exhibit accelerated maturation with excessive syncytial knots. In addition, the occurence of a fine granular calcium deposition in these villi is a most reliable indicator for a post-mortem change (see Fig. 3.14).

In triploidy, one of the most striking features is that the cystic alterations appear to be focal instead of diffuse (Fig. 2.20). Moreover, the detailed histology of the villi will reveal a viable stroma with vascular spaces containing blood (Fig. 2.21a) (Leschot et al. 1978). Centrally within the villi a variable degree of liquefaction of the stroma may be found. The trophoblast shows focal hyperplasia of trophoblastic cells, almost all of which appear viable. In between these compact and solid areas of cells one may find strands of fibrin (Fig. 2.21b), but these do not dominate the picture and there is no indication of an increased number of syncytial knots, such as may be observed in cases with postmortem change. In fact, it is a distinctive feature that the trophoblast of the cystic villi is not much different from that observed in the nonaffected villi. These accumulated data make it possible to distinguish the cyst-like villi in triploidy from those in other conditions.

In hydatidiform mole it is usual for all placental tissues to be similarly affected and a fetus is usually absent. Recognition of a molar pregnancy is of particular significance, since it can be followed by an overt malignancy. In the western world a mole occurs in approximately one in 2000 pregnancies, but in other parts of the world (e.g., Taiwan) the incidence can be as high as approximately one in 125 (Wei and Ouyang 1963; Hertig and Sheldon 1947; Smalbraak 1957). Hydatidiform mole is an early developmental aberration of the placenta that is characterized by an excessive development of stroma and trophoblast in the absence of an embryo. In the typical case a molar pregnancy terminates spontaneously before the 20th week of gestation. The material available for the pathologist is highly characteristic and the diagnosis can be made on gross examination (Fig. 2.22a). The material consists only of cysts, which may vary in size from approximately 1 or 2 mm in diameter to approximately 10 mm (Fig. 2.22b). The cysts are shiny and contain clear fluid. It is important to note that normal placental tissues are virtually absent and fetal parts are never recognized. Microscopical examination of the tissues reveals a decidual layer but no stem villi anchored into it. There is an abrupt transition from the decidua to abnormal villi. The larger ones show liquefaction of the inner stromal compartment, which results in cyst-like spaces, bordered by a rim of

mucoid stroma without vessels (Fig. 2.23). In small villi sometimes only an absence of capillaries is noted, but cystic changes may be absent or only present in some parts (Fig. 2.24). The trophoblast of these abnormal villi may show a variable picture. In some instances there is a single- or double-layered trophoblast, without other apparent abnormalities (Fig. 2.25a). Other villi, however, may show an excessive proliferation of trophoblastic cells (Fig. 2.25b), sometimes to such an extensive degree that the stromal component may be barely recognizable in the histological sections. One may also observe villi that are partly covered by a flat and rather inconspicuous layer of trophoblast while elsewhere there is an abrupt transition to excessive trophoblastic proliferation. The diagnosis of a hydatiform mole can thus always be made with certainty, since all tissue samples examined show these abnormalities.

When confronted with a mole the pathologist will have to face the question as to whether or not the particular example is potentially malignant. It is generally accepted that as yet there are no definite

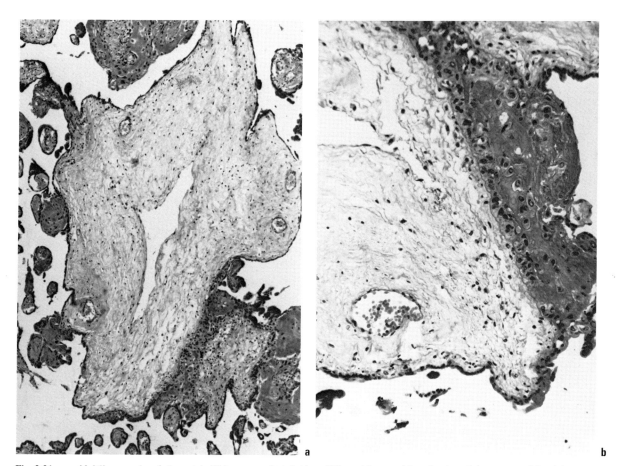

Fig. 2.21. a and **b** Micrographs of placental villi in a case of triploidy. **a** Villus with central liquefaction of the stroma, giving it its cyst-like appearance. (55 ×) **b** Detail of such a villus with focal hypoplasia of trophoblastic cells, which appear viable. Note how these cells are embedded within fibrin at the surface. The stroma, although fibrous in appearance, contains blood vessels. (140 ×)

histological criteria for this change (Elston and Bagshawe 1972). Nevertheless, experience has shown that certain histological and cytological features may be of relevance. The degree of trophoblastic proliferation, the degree of atypia of cells and nuclei, and the number of mitoses all play a role in this respect. In general, an increase in each of these variables correlates positively with an increased malignant potential. However, it is not yet possible to give quantitative data on which a prognosis can be based with certainty. One therefore has to rely on experience, and it seems wise to request a follow-up in every case of hydatidiform mole.

It is not appropriate to discuss the relationship between mole and chorion epithelioma here; texts of gynaecological pathology will supply additional information.

Finally, we have observed that in patients in whom early fetal death is associated with an XO chromosomal abnormality the placenta sometimes exhibits excessive post-mortem changes, far more severe than would be expected from the presumed time of intrauterine death of the fetus. There is as yet no satisfactory explanation for this observation.

In cases of trisomy one may encounter some large villi amidst the normal ones. The abnormal villi exhibit a loosely textured mesenchyme with marked hypovascularity and a thin trophoblastic layer (Honore et al. 1976). Such abnormal villi are randomly distributed throughout the placenta. Difficulties may arise in distinguishing these changes from those that occur as post-mortem alterations.

Inborn errors of metabolism, such as gangliosidosis and mucolipidoses, may give rise to typical cellular abnormalities within villi. These are characterized by vacuolization of Hofbauer cells and the cells of the cytotrophoblast (Fig. 2.26a and b) (Powell and Bernirschke 1976). This change should thus alert the pathologist to the possibility of an inborn error necessitating further investigation.

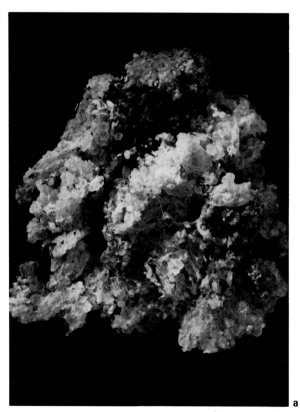

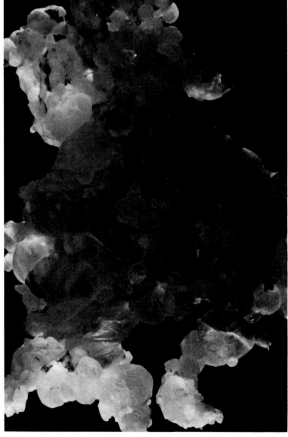

Fig. 2.22. a and **b** Specimen of hydatidiform mole. **a** The gross specimen characterized by a multitude of cysts, which may vary considerably in size. **b** Detail of part of these cyst-like villi.

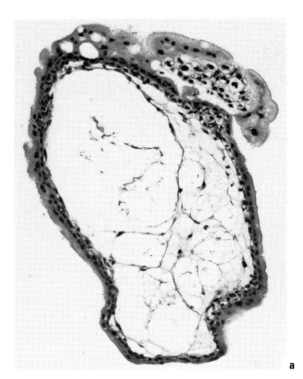

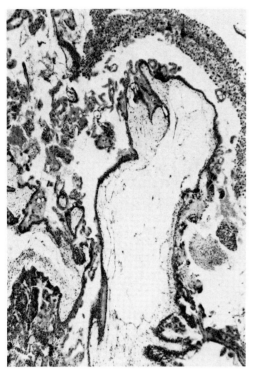

Fig. 2.23. Cystic villus in a case of hydatidiform mole. The stroma shows extensive liquefaction, which gives the villus its cyst-like appearance. (H and E; 35 ×)

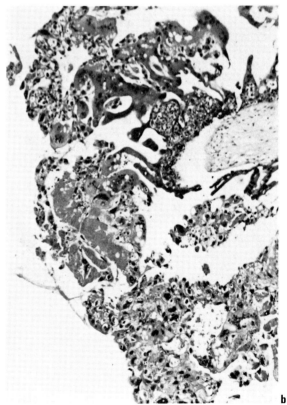

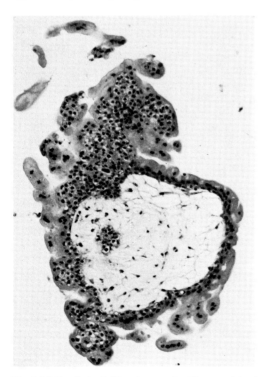

Fig. 2.24. Small-sized villus characterized by complete absence of capillaries. Note that in this small villus no cystic changes have occurred. There is a localized extensive proliferation of trophoblast cells. (H and E; 140 ×)

Fig. 2.25. a and **b** Villi in a case of Hydatidiform mole. H and E **a** A small villus with liquefaction of the stroma. There is localized proliferation of trophoblast cells, but otherwise the trophoblast is normal. (200 ×) **b** A villus with extensive trophoblast cell proliferation dominating the picture. (64 ×)

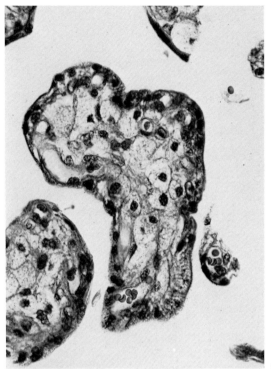

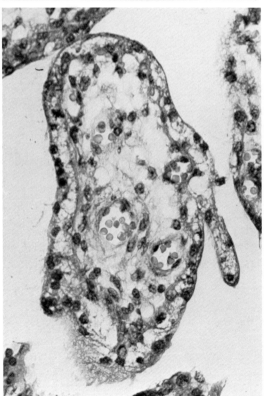

Fig. 2.26. a and **b** Placental villi in a case of gangliosidosis. H & E; 350 × **a** A villus with extensive vacuolization of Hofbauer cells within the stroma. **b** A villus with distinct vacuolization of the trophoblast cells. Courtesy of Dr J. L. J. Gaillard, Erasmus University, Rotterdam.

6. Placental Pathology in Late Gestation

Where fetal casualties occur late in gestation the placenta with membranes and umbilical cord should be available for study. It has been shown that when a fetus is stillborn, study of the complete placenta together with the fetus provides important information regarding the pathogenesis of intrauterine death. In fact, in such circumstances the pathologist should emphasize the necessity for a complete investigation (Becker 1976; Becker and Becker 1976).

This section describes the pathology of the umbilical cord, the membranes, and the placenta proper as separate units, but all of these should be regarded as integral parts of a functional whole.

6.1 Umbilical Cord

Abnormalities of the umbilical cord are difficult to interpret with regard to their functional significance, although recent work suggests their importance may have been underestimated. The length of the cord is important, since cases have been reported in which an umbilical cord of considerable length has caused strangulation of the fetus, leading to stillbirth (Strauss et al. 1967). This is extremely rare, but one should always be aware of the possibility. In contrast, an extremely short umbilical cord can also cause problems, which usually do not become apparent until the time of delivery.

The significance of umbilical knots is a controversial topic, and a clear distinction should be made between false and true knots. The former are varicose dilatations of umbilical vessels, mimicking knots, and they have no functional significance. True knots, on the other hand, can cause impaired flow in the umbilical cord and may thus affect the fetus. However, one should be cautious in attributing functional significance to a true knot, since in many instances it appears as an incidental finding at delivery. The pathologist should therefore look for manifestations of a circulatory disturbance. True knots that have caused a circulatory disorder are always accompanied by oedema within the cord on one side of the knot (Fig. 2.27). Histological examination may also reveal small haemorrhages and/or iron depositions as a result of previous bleeding. These features, in our opinion, are the most reliable indicators that the knot has been of functional significance. Awareness of this possibility may occasionally give a clue to the cause of stillbirth, even in the presence of a severely macerated fetus.

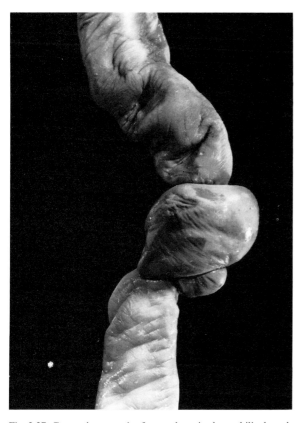

Fig. 2.27. Gross photograph of a true knot in the umbilical cord. The discoloration at one side of the knot is indicative of a circulatory disturbance.

Torsion of the umbilical cord can also affect the fetus. To determine whether torsion has occurred, the pathologist has to rely upon secondary phenomena, such as oedema and haemorrhages, as described for true knots. In this respect, it may be helpful to recall that torsion of the umbilical cord almost always occurs close to its site of origin or insertion, i.e., close to either fetus or placenta.

Haemorrhages may occur within the umbilical cord and it is generally accepted that haematomas larger than 1 cm in diameter can cause impaired umbilical cord flow (Fig. 2.28). The pathogenesis of this type of bleeding is uncertain, but a traumatic origin is considered to be most likely.

The pathologist should also note the site and mode of placental insertion of the cord. Marginal or velamentous insertions may underlie excessive and sometimes lethal haemorrhages during delivery, since large-calibre fetal vessels may traverse the site of membrane rupture (Fig. 2.29). Furthermore, marginal insertion has been considered to be a potential cause of neonatal dysmaturity, because both the fetal and the maternal compartments in the marginal zone show regressive alterations during maturation (see p. 40). Even in cases where the placenta exhibits a 'normal' site of insertion of the umbilical cord, one should always try to evaluate the actual site of insertion critically, since extensive haemorrhages or infarctions at this particular point may have a different connotation from those found elsewhere in the placenta (see below).

Finally, the umbilical cord may contain tumours, or tumour-like lesions. The most common types are of vascular origin (angiomas, angiomyxomas, and aneurysms) (Barry et al. 1951). Circulatory disturbances, such as hydramnios or fetal hydrops, appear to be the main clinical manifestations.

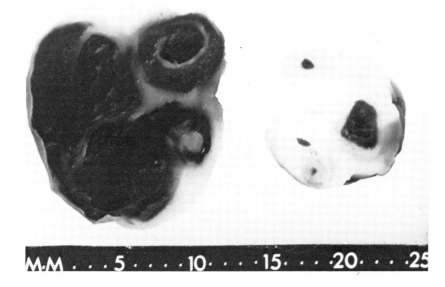

Fig. 2.28. Gross photographs of the cut surface of the umbilical cord, showing an extensive haemorrhage causing functional impairment.

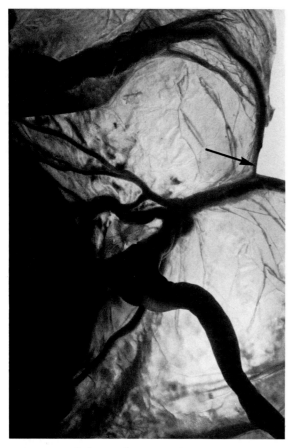

Fig. 2.29. Detail of gross photograph of a velamentous insertion of umbilical vessels. The rupture in the membrane has torn one of these vessels (*arrow*).

6.2 Membranes

The membranes are usually inserted at the very margin of the placenta. In some instances, however, membrane insertion is displaced centrally, leaving part of the periphery of the placenta devoid of membranous coverage (Fig. 2.30). Lamellated thrombosis is often present in this area, frequently accompanied by fibrosis of the underlying placenta. These changes may occur gradually; indeed, placenta circumvalata is often considered to be the end-result of early rupture of membranes.

Membranes are normally transparent, with a greyish colour. Small yellow plaques a few millimetres in diameter can sometimes be identified close to the periphery of the placenta, and these appear to be remnants of the original yolk sac. These vestiges have no functional consequences. Amnion nodosum, on the other hand, is significant, and its recognition provides useful information. In this condition the fetal surface of the membranes exhibits a fine granular appearance with slightly elevated grey nodules (Fig. 2.31) a maximum of a few millimetres in diameter. Microscopical examination reveals that the nodules consist of fibrin and embedded squamous epithelial cells. Moreover, one occasionally observes proliferation of the epithelial cells of the amnion, which in some instances may exhibit squamous metaplasia. Amnion nodosum most frequently occurs in association with oligohydramnios, and the possibility of serious congenital malformations affecting the renal system or the digestive tract should be considered.

An opalescent appearance of the membranes is almost always due to cellular infiltration. The membranes are oedematous and on microscopical examination reveal a cellular infiltrate of polymorphonuclear leucocytes (Fig. 2.32). Most of these are located directly underneath the layer of amniotic epithelial cells and they sometimes extend into the base of the chorionic plate. Chorionic vessels may be affected by a cellular infiltrate, particularly at the site of the amniotic cavity. Such a cellular infiltration does not necessarily imply an infectious disease. Any type of irritation can provoke a cellular reaction, and only microbiological studies can distinguish between a noninfectious and an infectious origin. The major problem in this respect will be to obtain noncontaminated cultures, and the results of routine microbiological studies should be carefully evaluated.

Green discoloration of the membranes is most probably due to staining by meconium. Microscopical studies in these cases reveal macrophages loaded with eosinophilic granular material These observations indicate periods of fetal stress.

Brown discoloration of membranes is indicative of impregnation by iron pigments, usually the end result of previous haemorrhages. Microscopy reveals iron-loaded macrophages and, occasionally, minute recent haemorrhages. It is generally accepted that such minor haemorrhages are of no functional significance, in contrast to haemorrhages caused by rupture of larger chorionic vessels. Indeed, the pathologist should always give particular attention to the pattern of the larger chorionic vessels. In rare cases accessory placental lobes connected to the main placental mass by membranes harbouring large vessels are encountered. Disruption during delivery can cause fetal haemorrhages, which may be fatal, like those that occur with velamentous insertion (see Fig.). One should also be aware of anomalous and potentially hazardous vascular patterns in cases of multiple pregnancy. Occasionally chorionic vessels running from one umbilical cord directly towards the other, by-passing the corresponding placental tissues, are observed (Fig. 2.33). Most often, however, such anomalous vascular connections are embedded deep within the

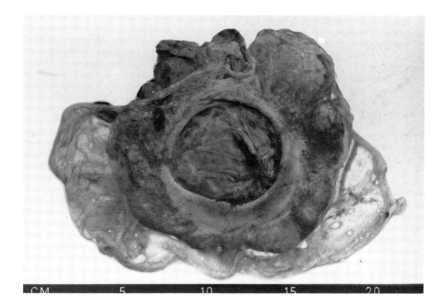

Fig. 2.30. Specimen of placenta circumvallata, viewed from the fetal side.

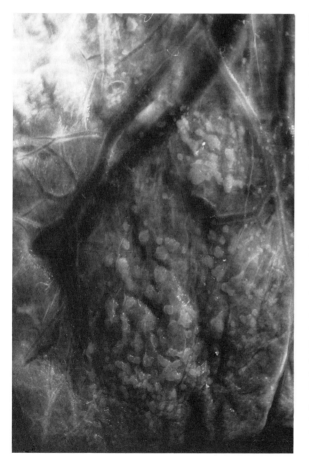

Fig. 2.31. Gross detailed view of the fetal surface of the placenta, showing the fine granular appearance of slightly elevated nodules. This appearance is characteristic for amnion nodosum.

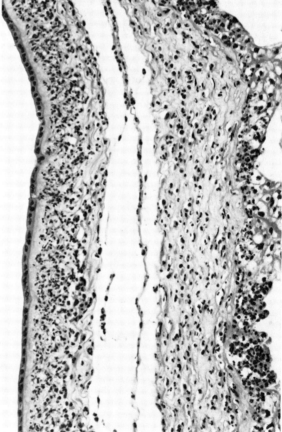

Fig. 2.32. Photomicrograph of the membrane, showing a dense cellular infiltration of polymorphonuclear leucocytes. The cellular infiltrate extends from just underneath the amniotic epithelial cells into a base of the chorionic plate. (H and E; 230 ×)

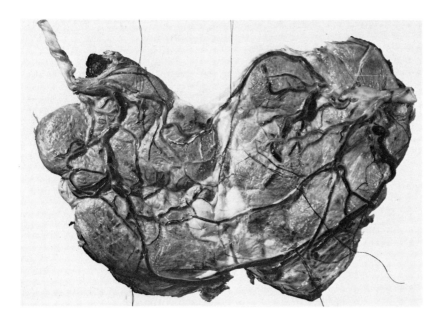

Fig. 2.33. Placenta of a twin pregnancy, showing chorionic vessels that traverse the 'barrier' between the two structures.

placenta and are only revealed by post-delivery injection or corrosion techniques. Inspection of the chorionic vascular pattern may also reveal tortuous or dilated vessels (Fig. 2.34a), which can sometimes be occluded by a thrombus. It is generally accepted that such localized vascular deformities may underlie intramembranous haemorrhages, which when extensive can cause fetal damage or death. Such vascular abnormalities seen on the surface may be part of a concealed vascular hamartoma embedded within the placenta itself (Fig. 2.34b). However, rupture and thrombosis of chorionic vessels can occur without previous deformity. Indeed, there are occasional cases where dysmaturity, or even stillbirth, is associated with extensive spontaneous haemorrhages or thrombosis of chorionic vessels (Fig. 2.35).

In rare circumstances cysts of the membranes are found (Fig. 2.36). Such cysts are of variable diameter, but seldom exceed 5 cm. They are filled with a clear fluid and are usually located between the amniotic and chorionic layers (Fig. 2.36). Their functional significance remains uncertain.

a

b

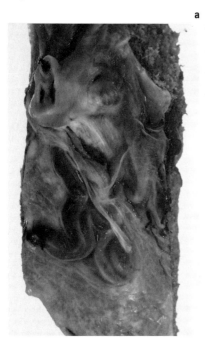
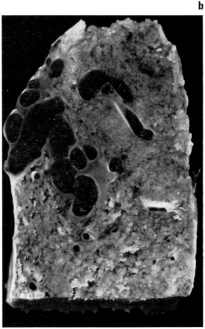

Fig. 2.34. a and b Placenta with tortuous chorionic vessels: a fetal aspect, revealing these dilated vessels; b cut surface; it appears that the vessels extend into the placenta. This anomaly is sometimes considered to represent a hamartoma.

Fig. 2.35. a and **b** The placenta in a case of stillbirth, showing 'spontaneous' thrombosis of chorionic vessels: **a** gross appearance on cut surface; **b** photomicrograph of one of the chorionic vessels, totally occluded by a lamellated thrombus. (H and E; **b** 9 ×)

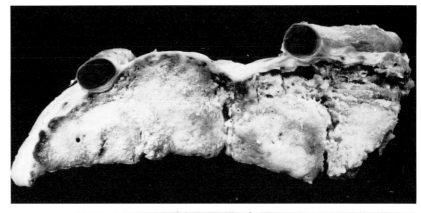

a

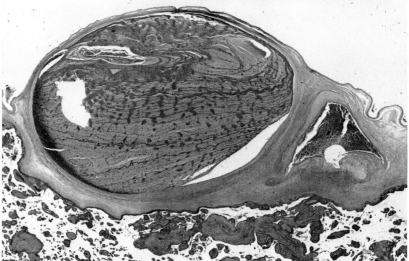

b

Fig. 2.36. (*below*) Example of a cyst of the membranes, located between the amniotic and chorionic layers, at the site of insertion of the umbilical cord.
▽

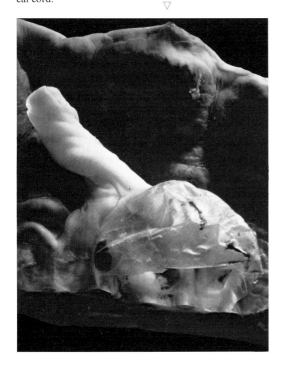

6.3. Placenta

The placenta can show a variety of changes in the late gestational period, some of which are well recognized as having a profound functional effect while the significance of others remains obscure. A major problem in evaluating the functional significance of placental pathology is the general uncertainty as to what percentage of noninvolved tissue is necessary to guarantee adequate function. It is generally accepted that fetal development becomes impaired when approximately 10 % of the placenta is affected by major alterations, such as infarctions and/or fibrosis.

Most of the pathology of the placenta in developed countries is a consequence of circulatory disturbances. The majority of abnormalities described are thus related to such disorders. It is important to determine whether changes are focal or diffuse, although affected areas may be randomly distributed throughout the placenta.

We have chosen to describe placental pathology by taking grossly recognizable and microscopically detected abnormalities as points of departure. We felt this to be a pragmatic approach, in accordance with the task faced by the pathologist when confronted with the examination of this organ. For each category we will try to indicate the most likely causative factors.

6.3.1. Gross Abnormalities

There are three grossly indentifiable major changes that affect the placenta, each of which relates to a circulatory disturbance.

6.3.1.1. Haemorrhage. Placental haemorrhages occur in the intervillous spaces, which normally contain circulating maternal blood. The precise definition of bleeding within this compartment is therefore difficult, and its pathogenesis is mysterious. Nevertheless, placental haemorrhages are most marked on gross examination, when a mass of blood compressing surrounding placental tissues is seen. Microscopical examination simply endorses this impression. The extent of the bleeding is of functional significance, as is its location. Classically, a distinction can be made between retroplacental haemorrhages and intraplacental bleeding.

In its typical form, the retroplacental haemorrhage presents as a centrally located haemorrhage separating the placenta from its maternal bed. This change underlies the classic abruptio placentae. Examination of such a placenta will reveal abnormalities at the maternal side. In cases with extensive bleeding all the cotyledons will be flattened, whereas in localized haemorrhage retroplacental indentation is present (Fig. 2.37). In other instances of retroplacental haemorrhage the bleeding may be localized at the periphery of the placenta. This will lead to a continuous loss of blood, but the extent of undermining of the placenta may vary from one individual to another. It is this change that may underlie the clinical condition of so-called atypical abruptio. Again, careful examination of the placenta may reveal a localized flattening of the contour of the cotyledons.

An intraplacental haemorrhage usually takes the form of a rounded mass compressing the surrounding tissues. These haemorrhages are, in most instances, restricted in size and may thus be an incidental finding during examination. Older haemorrhages of this type are sometimes recognized by the finding of a cyst-like cavity (Fig. 2.38), the microscopy of which reveals its origin as a haemorrhage. In rare circumstances intraplacental haemorrhages may be so extensive that one has to attribute a functional significance to them (Fig. 2.39).

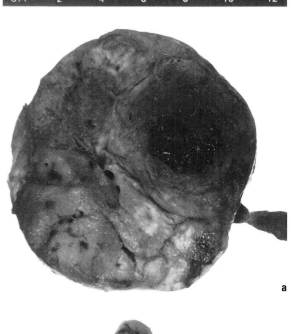

a

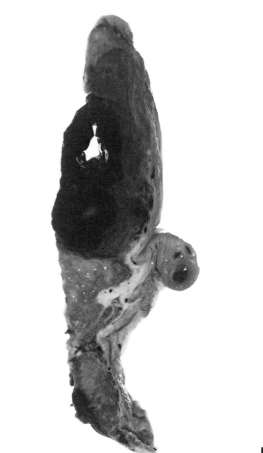

b

Fig. 2.37. a and **b** An example of a retroplacental haemorrhage underlying classic abruptio placentae: **a** maternal aspect of the placenta with the localized haemorrhage; **b** cut surface of the placenta at the site of the haemorrhage.

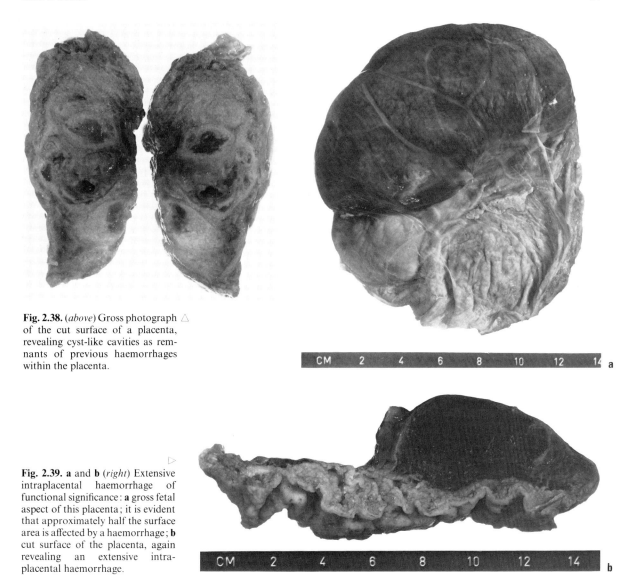

Fig. 2.38. (*above*) Gross photograph △ of the cut surface of a placenta, revealing cyst-like cavities as remnants of previous haemorrhages within the placenta.

▷

Fig. 2.39. a and **b** (*right*) Extensive intraplacental haemorrhage of functional significance: **a** gross fetal aspect of this placenta; it is evident that approximately half the surface area is affected by a haemorrhage; **b** cut surface of the placenta, again revealing an extensive intraplacental haemorrhage.

6.3.1.2. Infarcts. A placental infarct constitutes an area of necrosis of villi. The pathogenesis of these infarcts is a circulatory disturbance, although it is uncertain why and how placental infarcts develop. The general consensus is that the circulatory abnormality affects the maternal compartment first, rather than the fetal circulation. Grossly, the identification of an infarct depends largely upon its age. A recent infarct is characterized by a dark red colour, due to extensive localized congestion, and thus a recent infarct may not be easily recognized against the haemorrhagic aspect of a normal placenta. Microscopic examination will reveal that the vascular spaces within the villi are dilated and congested wtih blood. In some villi extravasation of blood may have already occurred. The intervillous spaces show

hardly any abnormality at this stage. In later stages the reparative response will affect the villi and will alter the gross aspect. In the end stage the affected area has a greyish-white colour and a more or less triangular shape with its base at the site of the decidual plate (Fig. 2.40a). Microscopical examination will reveal fibrosed villi (Fig. 2.40b). By this stage, these have clumped together encased in fibrin, and may actually appear as 'ghosts' amidst the homogeneous eosinophilic material (Fig. 2.41). Moreover, coarse calcification may be present (Fig. 2.41). It is this particular microscopic picture that needs differentiation from that seen in the postmature placenta (see p. 41). When sufficient attention is given to the detailed features, however, differentiation will not be too difficult.

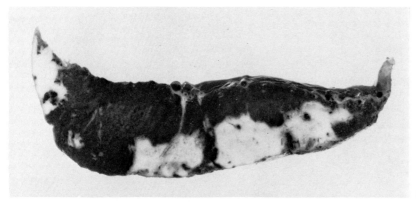

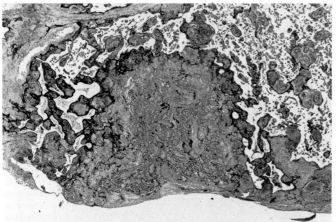

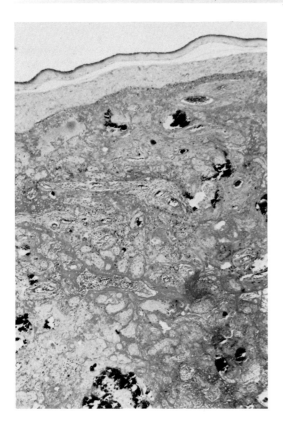

◁ **Fig. 2.40. a** and **b** Example of an old placental infarct: **a** gross aspect of the cut surface of the placenta, in which the infarct is recognized as a greyish-white zone, more or less triangular in shape, with its base at the maternal side; **b** micrograph of such an area, in which completely fibrosed villi are glued together by fibrin. (PTAH; 12 ×)

6.3.1.3. Intervillous Thrombosis. Like placental haemorrhages, intervillous thrombosis affects primarily the maternal compartment. It is easily recognized from the gross aspect, since the thrombosis exhibits all the classic features to be expected (Fig. 2.42). It is clear that such a lesion reflects a circulatory disturbance, but again it is not clear what mechanisms may have triggered its development. Intervillous thrombosis can be an accidental finding restricted to a minute area somewhere within the placenta, or it can present as a multitude of thrombosed regions, sometimes affecting a high percentage of the total placental tissue; the latter finding is extremely rare.

Intervillous thrombosis has a predilection for occurring within the placental mass, but occasionally occurs in a subchorial location, where it is often associated with placenta circumvallata (see p. 53) and is probably related to a process of continuous laceration occurring in the marginal area affected. In any case of intervillous thrombosis, the pathologist faces the difficulty of evaluating its

◁ **Fig. 2.41.** Photomicrograph of an old placental infarct, which shows the ghost of placental villi amidst homogeneous eosinophilic material and coarse calcifications. (H and E; 35 ×)

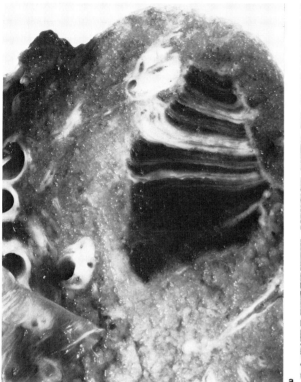
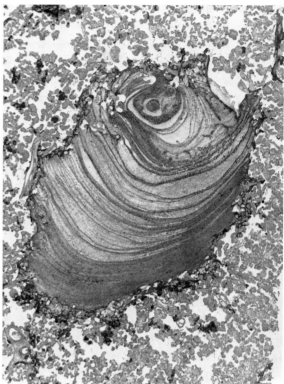

Fig. 2.42. a and **b** Example of intervillous thrombosis: **a** gross aspect, in which the characteristics of a thrombus are already identifiable; **b** histological picture, again revealing the characteristic layered appearance of a thrombus. (PTAH; 12×)

pathogenesis and significance. It is only from careful observation that we can hope to gain a better insight into this phenomenon. It is of interest that intervillous thrombosis is the only placental pathology present in a personal series of cases of the fetomaternal transfusion syndrome.

6.3.2. Microscopical Abnormalities

Microscopical examination of placental tissue taken from sites other than those already grossly identified as being abnormal (see above) may also reveal abnormalities. The significance of these changes must be evaluated in the light of other abnormalities and in relation to their extent.

6.3.2.1. Fibrin Exudation. Exudation of fibrin is characterized by an extensive deposition of fibrin in the intervillous spaces, encasing the villi. The origin and pathogenesis of this change is unknown, but it is generally accepted that it is one of the features of a circulatory disturbance. On the other hand, these changes are occasionally observed as a feature of postmaturity. Close correlation with clinical and other morphological data is mandatory.

Excessive fibrin exudation is also seen in the rare condition of early maturation of the placenta, so-called maturitas praecox. This peculiar developmental abnormality of the placenta is characterized by a discrepancy between the gestational period and the histological maturation of the placenta. Usually the placenta exhibits signs of full-term development, while the fetus is still premature. The pathogenesis of this disorder is uncertain, but the condition is often associated with toxaemia of pregnancy and dysmaturity of the neonate, suggesting that vascular insufficiency may play a paramount role. It is obvious that this diagnosis can only be made when accurate clinical data are available and the gestational age does not exceed 36 weeks.

6.3.2.2. Avascular Villi. When avascular villi are present the placenta is characterized by groups of villi that exhibit all the stigmata of post-mortem change, such as fibrosis, excessive formation of syncytial knots, etc., whereas the remainder of the surrounding placental tissues are within normal limits (Fig. 2.43). Fibrin deposition in these areas is not conspicuous. The change in the villi needs to be distinguished from true necrosis (see Section 6.3.2.3). The cause of this peculiar abnormality is considered to be occlusion of fetal vessels, although this concept is still controversial (Fox 1978).

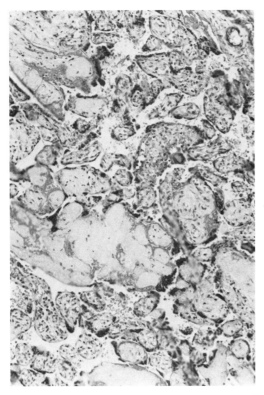

Fig. 2.43. Photomicrograph showing avascular villi, amidst villi with a normal appearance. (H and E; 140 ×)

6.3.2.3. Necrosis of Villi. Necrosis of villi is a most interesting abnormality, which may be considered as a sort of microinfarction. Usually, the condition is characterized by small groups of villi exhibiting all the features of necrosis. They are invaded by polymorphonuclear leucocytes, which seem to be derived from the maternal compartment (Fig. 2.44). In almost all instances micro-infarcts appear to accompany larger infarct zones and it is therefore accepted that these micro changes have a similar aetiology. When such a micro-infarct is encountered during routine histological examination of a placenta it is advisable to re-examine the gross aspect of the placenta and take additional sections. This is particularly true for recent infarcts, which can easily be missed during gross examination because of their less clearly defined margins.

6.3.2.4. Oedema of Villi. Oedema must be regarded as a circulatory disturbance. It can manifest itself in the placental villi in one of two forms. Firstly, placental oedema can occur as a localized accumulation of fluid in the subtrophoblastic area, creating large bullae filled with clear watery fluid (Fig. 2.45). The villi are otherwise normal, apart from a slight stromal compression due to the bullae themselves. It is our opinion that this type of villous oedema is seen particularly in *acute* processes, such as haemor-

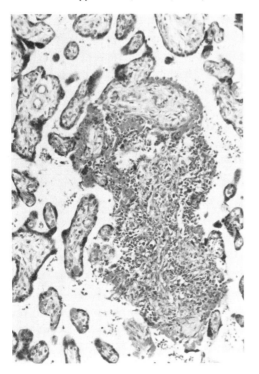

Fig. 2.44. Photomicrograph of villous necrosis, characterized by a massive infiltration of polymorphonuclear leucocytes, which appear to be derived from the maternal compartment. (H and E; 140 ×)

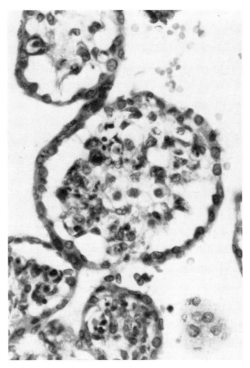

Fig. 2.45. Placental villus with distinct oedema. This shows as a localized accumulation of fluid in the subtrophoblastic area creating large bullae, which appear as empty spaces. (H and E; 400 ×)

rhage. The second form of oedema is characterized by a diffuse oedematous change in all villi. In these circumstances the villous stroma shows separation of the otherwise normal stromal components. Moreover, macrophages may be present and accumulate fluid, judging from their vacuolated cytoplasm (Fig. 2.46b). It is this particular form of oedema that occurs in conditions of chronic circulatory disturbance of a more generalized nature. Moreover, similar oedematous villous changes can be observed in cases of infectious diseases affecting the placenta, blood group incompatibilities, renal disease of the fetus, and diabetes mellitus in the mother. Recognition of this placental change is thus of major significance for further investigations.

6.3.2.5. Blood Disorders. In the early stages of placental development it is usual to find immature erythrocytes and leucocytes within the fetal capillaries. With advancing maturation of the fetus and the placenta, their number decreases in proportion to the number of mature cells. Around the 20th week of gestation nucleated red cells become inconspicuous. Thus an abundance of immature blood cells after the 20th week of gestation is almost always an expression of underlying disease (Fig. 2.47), and in general it can be said to indicate excessive haematopoiesis in the fetus. One of the most common underlying conditions is blood group incompatibility; however, any other disease that provokes a similar fetal reaction can result in a similar microscopical picture in the placental villi. Among these conditions, infectious diseases rank high.

Congenital leukaemia in the fetus is extremely rare, but when present may give a similar microscopical picture.

Other abnormalities, such as sickle cell disease of the mother, can be recognized within the placenta.

6.3.2.6. Inflammatory Infiltrates. In the presence of an inflammatory cell infiltrate a clear distinction should be made between infiltrates that are limited to the intervillous spaces and those that affect the villi. In the former situation one is dealing with a so-called intervillositis, which in itself is a nonspecific finding (Fig. 2.48) and may be an expression of leucocytosis in the mother. It does not necessarily mean that the fetal part of the placenta is affected, or that the development of the fetus is impaired. Recognition of intervillositis is nevertheless important, since the infiltrates are an expression of maternal disease, which may trigger the early onset of labour.

Cellular inflammatory infiltrates that affect villi are almost always an indication of the existence of an infectious disease. Its type and the mode of infiltration are nonspecific as far as the pathogenetic

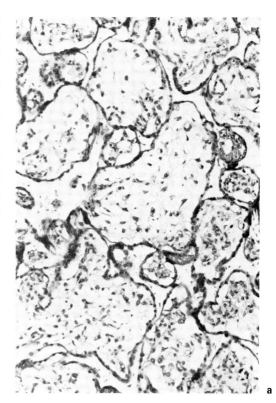

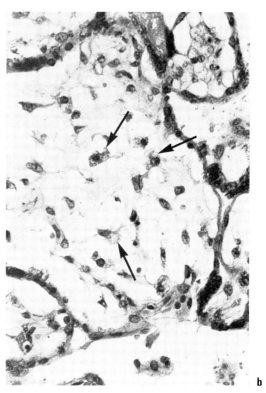

Fig. 2.46. a and **b** Diffuse oedema of villi: **a** low-power view in which the swollen and oedematous villi are apparent; **b** detail of a villus, showing macrophages with a vacuolated cytoplasm (*arrows*). (H and E; **a** 140×, **b** 350×)

organism is concerned in the vast majority of cases. In a few instances the histology may give a clue to the nature of the underlying infection. A cellular infiltrate composed mainly of plasma cells should always arouse suspicion of a syphilitic infection. Vasculitis with fibrinoid necrosis and cellular infiltration composed mainly of lymphocytes and plasma cells should suggest a viral infection. Cytomegalic inclusion body disease has a typical cytopathogenic effect on stromal cells, with the formation of giant cells with both nuclear and cytoplasmic inclusion bodies (Fig. 2.49). Toxoplasma gondii may occasionally affect the placenta and can be recognized by the formation of cyst-like structures that contain the micro-organisms. The disease has a distinct tendency to affect the membranes (Fig. 2.50a), and if toxoplasma infection is suspected one should always be prepared to study the membranes extensively. In rare circumstances toxoplasmic lesions are also found within the villi of the placenta (Fig. 2.50b).

Listeria monocytogenes may also affect the placenta, where it can give rise to minute areas of necrosis (Fig. 2.51). Within these necrotic foci it may sometimes be possible to identify the rod-shaped bacilli responsible for the infection.

Infectious diseases that affect the developing fetus do not necessarily provoke a marked cellular infiltrate. This reaction depends upon the maturation of the immune mechanisms and may not be fully developed when infection occurs. The extent of the cellular reaction is a poor variable by which to judge the severity of the infectious process.

6.2.3.7. Placental Tumours.

Primary placental tumours are exceedingly rare. The most common primary tumour is chorangioma (Fig. 2.52) (Fox 1978; Strauss et al. 1967). This is a tumour, or tumour-like lesion, characterized by large villi composed mainly of a proliferation of vascular spaces (Fig. 2.52b). The endothelial cells are inconspicuous. The lesion is very much like that seen in ordinary

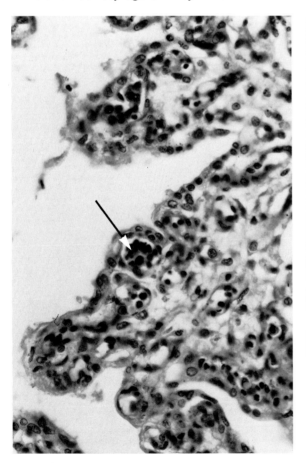

Fig. 2.47. Photomicrograph of an almost mature placental villus. The subtrophoblastic capillaries contain dense accumulations of nucleated red cells (*arrow*), which are indicative of an excessive haematopoiesis in the fetus. (H and E; 350 ×)

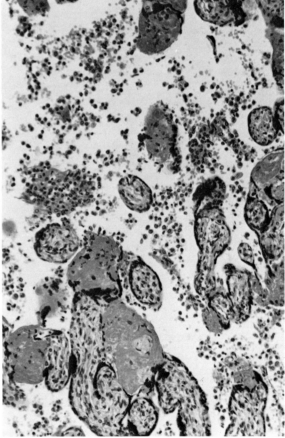

Fig. 2.48. Intervillositis, characterized by a large number of polymorphonuclear leucocytes in the maternal compartment. (H and E; 140 ×)

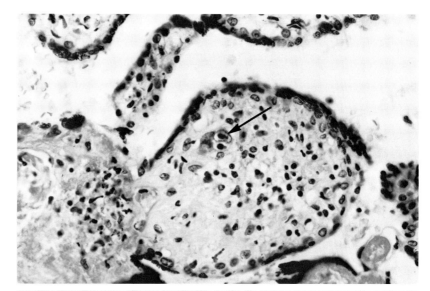

Fig. 2.49. A placenta with a cytomegalic inclusion body disease infection. Note the transformed stromal cells with nuclear inclusion bodies (*arrow*). (H and E; 350 ×)

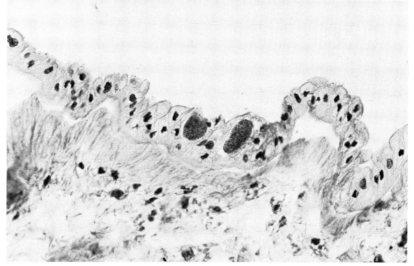

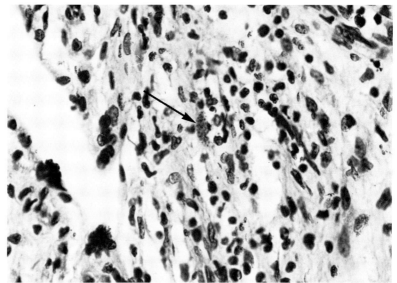

Fig. 2.50. a and **b** A placenta affected by *Toxoplasma gondii*: **a** with cyst-like structures containing the micro-organisms within the amniotic cells; **b** detailed view of a placental villus with the micro-organisms in an endothelial cell (*arrow*) (H and E; **a** 350 ×, **b** 500 ×)

a

b

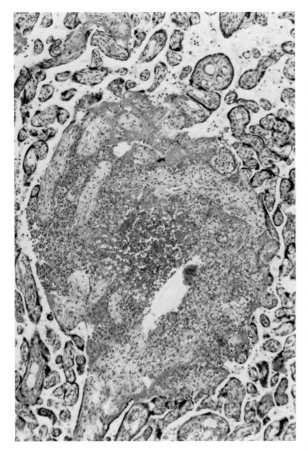

Fig. 2.51. The placenta in a listeria monocytogenes infection. There is a small area of necrosis affecting a number of villi, which are embedded within fibrin and invaded by polymorphonuclear leucocytes. (H and E; 64 ×)

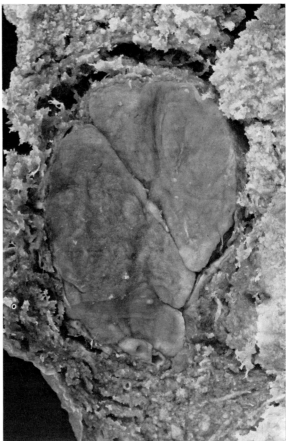

a

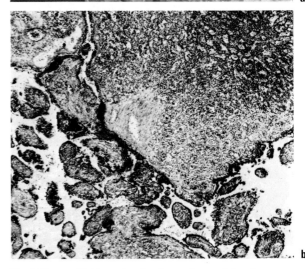

b

Fig. 2.52. a and **b** Example of a chorangioma of the placenta. **a** Gross aspect of the lesion, embedded within placental tissue of normal appearance; **b** micrograph of the lesion, characterized by a proliferation of vascular spaces within large villi. (H and E; **b** 55 ×)

haemangiomas elsewhere in the body. Chorangiomas vary considerably in size and their functional significance can also vary. Small lesions may sometimes escape notice during gross examination of the placenta and subsequently be an accidental finding on microscopy. Larger masses are usually identified during gross examination, and these lesions can actually cause functional disturbances leading to hydramnios and oedema of the fetus. The term diffuse chorangiomatosis is used for an ill-defined situation where most villi appear to contain more vascular spaces than usual, and should be applied very critically.

Secondary tumours are even less common. Metastatic tumours described in the placenta include melanoma and mammary carcinoma, but other tumours can also give rise to placental deposits. Malignant lymphoma and leukaemia can also affect the placenta. Occasionally a primary tumour of the fetus (e.g., neuroblastoma) may metastasize into the placenta (Fox 1978; Strauss et al. 1967).

References

Barry FE, McCoy CP, Callahan WP (1951) Haemangioma of the umbilical cord. Am J Obstet Gynecol 62: 675

Becker MJ (1976) Intra-uteriene vruchtdood. Thesis, Amsterdam

Becker MJ, Becker AE (1976) Fat distribution in the adrenal cortex as an indication of the mode of intrauterine death. Hum Pathol 7: 495

Boué J, Philippe E, Giroud A, Boué A (1976) Phenotypic expression of lethal chromosomal anomalies in human abortuses. Teratology 14: 3

Elston CW, Bagshawe KD (1972) The value of histological grading in the management of hydatidiform mole. J Obstet Gynaecol Br Cwlth 79: 717

Fox H (1978) Pathology of the placenta. Saunders, Philadelphia London Toronto (Major Problems in Pathology, Vol VII)

Hertig AT, Sheldon WH (1947) Hydatidiform mole: a pathologico-clinical correlation of 200 cases. Am J Obstet Gynecol 53:

Honore LH, Dill FJ, Poland BJ (1976) Placental morphology in spontaneous human abortuses with normal and abnormal karyotypes. Teratology 14: 151

Leschot NJ, Treffers PE, Becker-Bloemkolk MJ, de Leeuw R, Otten JA (1978) Human triploidy. Case history and relevance in obstetrics. Eur J Obstet Gyneco Reprod Biol 8: 295

Powell HC, Bernirschke K (1976) Foamy changes of placental cells in fetal storage disorders. Virchows Arch [Pathol Anat] 369: 191

Smalbraak J (1957) Trophoblastic growths. Elsevier, Amsterdam

Strauss F, Bernirschke K, Driscoll SG (1967) Handbuch der speziellen Pathologischen Anatomie und Histologie. Placenta. Springer, Berlin Heidelberg New York

Wei PY, Ouyang PC (1963) Trophoblastic diseases in Taiwan. A review of 157 cases in a 10 year period. Am J Obstet Gynecol 85: 844

Chapter 3

Congenital Malformations

Colin L. Berry

This chapter is primarily concerned with congenital abnormalities as defined by McKeown and Record (1960): 'macroscopic abnormalities of structures attributable to faulty development and present at birth'. This definition excludes metabolic defects such as glycogen storage disease and the haemoglobinopathies; these abnormalities, which are caused by single genes of large effect, inherited according to Mendelian patterns, collectively account for less than 1% of human malformations and are not described in this account, although many are described elsewhere in the book. We shall consider here the larger groups of malformations and, in particular, the ways in which various epidemiological and other studies have contributed to knowledge of their pathogenesis. It should be emphasized that accurate pathological identification of malformation and malformation syndromes is an essential step in identifying aetiological factors, and one where the pathologist has a large part to play.

The incidence of congenital malformations has been studied for many years, usually in ways that prevent direct comparisons between the work of different groups. Some data are collected retrospectively, others prospectively; some studies have 1 year and some 5 years of follow-up; often the definition of what constitutes a malformation is not clear; and the source of records (death certificates, nursing reports, hospital notes, questionnaires) varies widely. Kennedy (1967), in reviewing 238 reports between 1901 and 1966 on a total of more than 20 million births, emphasized many of these difficulties.

A fundamental point that is sometimes ignored in discussions of the incidence of congenital malformations is the way in which figures vary at different stages of pregnancy. There is ample evidence to illustrate this. Nishimura, in a series of studies of abortions, has shown that in Japan, where the incidence of neural tube defects is low (around 1 per 1000 births) such abnormalities occur in over 13 per 1000 aborted embryos (see Nishimura 1970). Many of these abnormal embryos (20%–30%) have an abnormal karyotype, a finding confirmed in other studies, including that of Carr (1972), which suggests that most chromosomally abnormal fetuses abort. Machin (1974) has shown that chromosomal abnormalities are common in all perinatal deaths, notably in the malformed. Roberts and Lowe (1975) have estimated that 78% of all human conceptions abort, a figure in general agreement with the earlier studies of Witschi (1969). It seems likely that the normal outcome of human pregnancy is abortion, and that this represents an effective mechanism for the prevention of defects. Figure 3.1, taken from Witschi, shows the probable cause of these losses at the various stages of pregnancy.

The frequency of specific defects varies considerably from country to country. Within countries it varies from region to region and among different social classes. Thus, central nervous system defects are much commoner in England and Wales than in the West Indies or Japan; they are three times commoner in infants of social class V than in infants of social classes I and II; and they are three times commoner in the valleys of South Wales than along its coastal plain (Lowe 1972; Richards et al. 1972). These are important variations and may give valuable clues to aetiology, but as previously emphasized, the figures must be regarded with some caution in terms of the *incidence* of defects.

In contrast to the variability in the incidence of specific defects, total malformation rates for differing groups *at birth* appear to be roughly comparable (Table 3.1). This finding even applies to primitive South American Indian groups (Neel 1974). Neel has suggested that this general consistency supports the concept that the malformed

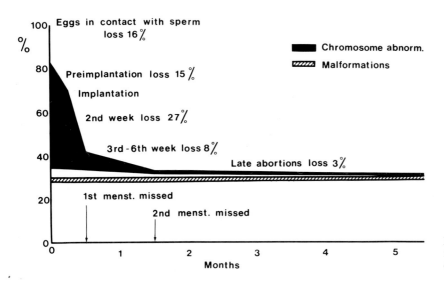

Fig. 3.1. Chronology and possible reasons for the loss of 70% of human conceptions. After Witschi 1969.

represent that percentage of individuals in every generation that falls below the threshold of the obligate proportion of loci needed, in a heterozygous state, to ensure normal development.

Deaths due to congenital malformations in England and Wales in 1975 are shown in Table 3.2. In consideration of these figures some caution should be exercised. A case of a patient with anencephalus dying between 25 and 29 years is recorded and an atrial septal defect was the apparent cause of death in an individual in the 90–94 year age group. In general, of 918 deaths attributable to congenital malformations outside the paediatric age group, the majority resulted from defects of the cardiovascular and urinary systems. The approximate frequency of the various types of defect and their sex ratio are given by Carter (1976), and Table 3.3 is based on this information.

Table 3.1. Prevalence of some external malformations in 3000 embryos and fetuses compared with prevalence at birth[a]

Malformation	Prevalence per 1000		% Loss
	Abortions	Birth	
Neural tube	13.1	1.0	92
Cleft lip and palate	24.4	2.7	87
Polydactyly	9.0	0.9	90
Cyclopia and cebocephaly	6.2	0.1	98

[a] Data from several sources, including Nishimura 1970.

Table 3.2. Deaths resulting from congenital malformations (England and Wales) 1975[a]

Deaths due to	All ages	Under 1 year	1–4 years	5–9 years	10–14 years
All causes	582 841	9488	1699	1140	1046
All malformations	3804	2303	319	163	102
All CNS malformations (excluding neurofibromatosis)	1025	826	66	53	27
All malformations of the heart and great vessels	1693	885	200	192	56
All malformations of the urinary system	331	108	9	3	6
All gastrointestinal malformations	195	109	22	7	1

[a] Data from Mortality Statistics (cause), Series DH2 no.2. Office of Population Censuses and Surveys.

Table 3.3. Approximate frequency and sex ratio of the more common major congenital malformations in Great Britain

Malformation	Frequency/1000 live and stillbirths	Approximate sex ratio (M:F)
Spina bifida cystica	2.5	0.6
Anencephaly	2.0	0.3
Congenital heart defects	6.0	1.0
Pyloric stenosis	3.0	4.0
Cleft lip ($\pm$ cleft palate)	1.0	1.8
Congenital dislocation of the hip	1.0	0.14

1. Genetics of Common Malformations

The largest groups of defects in man (those of the central nervous system, musculoskeletal system, and cardiovascular system) are found to have a number of characteristics in common when studied epidemiologically. The defects are common; familial aggregates are found; there is variation in prevalence with birth rank and parental age; variation also occurs with season of birth and with geographical localization. The recurrence rate in siblings is of the order of 1 %–5 %, much higher than the prevalence in the general population but too low for any simple 'Mendelian' explanation. Finally, the recurrence rate in dizygotic twins is the same as that in siblings, whilst that in monozygotic twins is 20 %–50 %. These findings suggest that both genetic and environmental factors affect the prevalence of the anomalies.

The data have been used to construct a model of polygenic or multifactorial inheritance of congenital abnormality, described by Carter (1965, 1969) and subsequently modified by Falconer (1965) and Edwards (1969). The hypothesis can best be explained as follows:

Where two or more alleles are present at a gene locus with a frequency of more than 1 %, genetic polymorphism is said to exist. If the character to be studied is several steps away from the primary product of gene activity it is likely that the different products of many genes are involved in the observed variation of the character. If there is polymorphism at several of these gene loci the character is likely to be continuously and normally distributed (see Fig. 3.2). If the expression of the gene is further modified by local factors acting via the environment these will provide a further source of variation of the character concerned. Height, intelligence, blood pressure, and fingerprint ridge count (Fig. 3.3) all show continuous variation with normal distribution. Although the degree of polymorphism necessary under the hypothesis is high, biochemical studies have shown that it exists in man. This polymorphism is central to the hypothesis presented and enables it to be tested in a number of ways.

In characters on which environmental factors have little influence it is possible to predict the degree to which the relatives of index cases will resemble them. A monozygotic twin with all genes in common with the index patient will have a regression coefficient of 1.0 (complete resemblance). A parent passes on half his or her genes to a child, with a resultant regression coefficient of 0.5 (child on parent). Siblings will inherit the same member of a gene pair from one parent in half the possible instances on average, so that their regression on the index patient will also be 0.5. Uncles, nephews, and grandparents (second-degree relatives) have an average of a quarter of their genes in common with the index patient, so that their regression coefficients are 0.25. Third-degree relatives (cousins) have an average of 1 in 8 of their genes in common, with a resultant regression coefficient of 0.125.

The original model of polygenic inheritance proposed by Carter separated genetic and environmental factors, using the distribution of genetic predisposition to a defect to indicate a population at risk for the triggering effect of environmental factors (Fig. 3.4). He assumed that the distribution of predisposition in relatives would be 'normal' with a scale that gave a normal curve in the general population, and also that the variance in relatives was the same as that in the general population. Neither of these assumptions is true, but they do not introduce large errors.

Malformations are unlike the continuously variable characteristics we have discussed above, in that they are threshold in type, i.e., present or absent. Thus since first-degree relatives have a genetic correlation of 0.5 with the index patients they will have a curve of distribution about a mean approximately half-way between that of the general population and the index patients beyond the threshold. The position of the mean for second-degree relatives would be shifted one-quarter of the distance between the general population mean and the index patients; that for third-degree relatives would be shifted one-eighth of the distance from the population mean towards the index patients.

As an example, in a defect occurring at a population frequency of 1 in 100 for which we assume a 100 % heritability, the proportion of first-degree relatives beyond the threshold—and thus, in this example, affected—will be 8 %. For second-

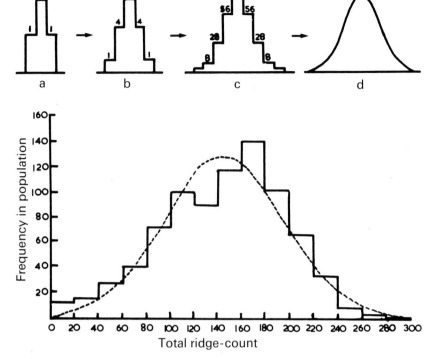

Fig. 3.2. a–d The effect of increasing the number of additive alleles at two loci on the phenotype. Where more than four genes are involved the character is likely to be normally distributed. **a** two alleles at one locus; **b** two alleles at each of two loci; **c** three alleles at each of two loci; **d** normal curve from alleles at many gene loci.

Fig. 3.3. Fingerprint ridge count in a population of 825 British males with the calculated 'normal' curve with the same mean and standard deviation. After Holt 1961.

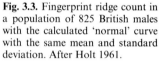

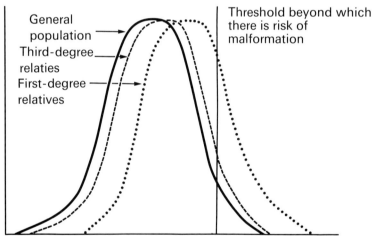

Fig. 3.4. Carter's model. The curve for second-degree relatives is omitted for the sake of clarity.

degree relatives the figure is 1.2%, and for third-degree relatives, 0.4%. Taking the example of cleft lip with or without cleft palate, we would have calculated correlations of 0.5, 0.25 and 0.125 for first-, second-, and third-degree relatives, respectively. The observed figures indicate correlations of about 0.35, 0.19, and 0.085, suggesting a heritability (see below) of about 70%, which is supported by twin studies.

In the improved polygenic model of Falconer (Fig. 3.5) the liability to produce a defect, composed of both genetic and environmental factors, is shown along the x-axis. Since environmental factors are included it is appropriate to consider all those

beyond the threshold as affected and to estimate an upper limit of the heritability of the malformation from the birth frequency in the general population and the proportion of the relatives affected. With this type of model it has been calculated that heritability for pyloric stenosis is about 60%, estimated from the first-degree relatives of male patients, and 90% for female relatives of female patients. For neural tube malformations heritability is about 60%, with similar values for talipes equinovarus.

Extensive studies of polygenically determined defects have shown up certain other characteristics, which are important to the pathologist in his role in providing documentation for those involved in genetic counselling. These are:

1) The more severe the malformation in the index patient, the greater the risk to relatives

2) If there is a preponderance of one sex in affected individuals the risk will be higher for the relatives of the less frequently affected sex

3) The risks to relatives are likely to be higher where the index patient already has one near relative affected, since the presence of two patients is an indication of a high-risk family.

1.1. Variance and Heritability

The two concepts of variance and heritability are important in consideration of the causation of many human malformations. The familiar concepts of normal distribution and standard deviation will not be considered further here, but the square of the standard deviation, the variance (σ^2), is used in population genetics because it can be partitioned or fractionated into additive components by analysis of variance. The phenotypic variance (σp^2) of a particular trait in a population is the result of different genotypic effects and their interaction with environmental influences. From an analysis of variance the genetic (σ_G^2) and environmental (σ_E^2) components can be calculated. From this it is evident that

$$\sigma p^2 = \sigma_G^2 + \sigma_E^2.$$

Both genetic and environmental components can be further fractionated into other specific contributions

(e.g., climatic, age-dependent, or birth rank effects and additive, epistatic (interaction), or dominance-genetic effects).

In attempts to attribute the various causative factors in any malformation to genetic or environmental factors, estimates of heritability are of great importance. Heritability is the ratio of the genetic variance to the phenotypic variance

$$h^2 = \frac{\sigma_G^2}{\sigma p^2}.$$

σ_G^2 includes all types of genetic factors. However, only additive variance has predictive value, and heritability is thus often defined as

$$h^2 = \frac{\sigma_A^2}{\sigma p^2}.$$

The reasons for adopting this narrowed concept are as follows:

Additive effects are seen when a gene contributes a constant increment to the phenotype whenever it is present in the genotype and where heterozygotes have a phenotype exactly intermediate between the two homozygotes. If an allele exhibits partial dominance when present in the heterozygote the extent of this effect can be determined by analysis of variance, which will also identify additive effects in genes showing various degrees of interaction. If, as frequently occurs, there is a multiple allelic series, with varying degrees of dominance,

$$A^1 > A^2 > A^3 > A^4$$

the gene A^3, which will be dominant in one parent ($A^3 A^4$), may be combined with a gene (A^2) that was

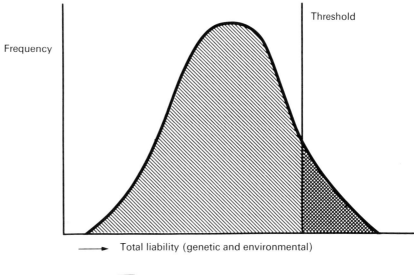

Fig. 3.5. Falconer's model.

Frequency

Threshold

Total liability (genetic and environmental)

Frequency distribution in the population

Distribution in those affected

recessive in the other parent ($A^1 A^2$). In the offspring ($A^2 A^3$), A^2 now appears as a dominant allele. In other words, when dominance or complex interactions are involved, one cannot predict the contribution a parent will make to the phenotype of its offspring.

Heritability is valuable in the study of large populations. If all the phenotypic variability for a given trait is attributable to environmental factors the heritability will be zero. If all the variability is of genetic origin (e.g., blood groups) it is 100%. Most traits in outbred populations have intermediate values.

Heritability in metric traits can be calculated from correlations between offspring and the mid-parent value (the mean of the two parents) since the progeny receive half their genes from each parent: alternatively, it can be calculated from twice the correlation between offspring and one parent ($h^2 = 2r$). The same relationship is valid for siblings (sharing half their genes). Half-sibs have only a 25% genetic relationship; therefore $h^2 = 4r$ (see Fig. 3.6).

Accurate determination of regression coefficients in mono- and dizygotic twins can be used to estimate the heritability of a defect. The use of twin studies to calculate heritabilities depends on the fact that the variance within dizygotic twin pairs is caused by half the additive genetic variation in the population, plus the variation attributable to environmental differences between the two members of the twin pair, whereas the variance within monozygotic twins is caused entirely by environmental differences.

As an example of such a study, Table 3.4 shows the results of examination of fingerprint ridge count, which of the characters showing a normal distribution shows the highest value for calculated heritability in man, 92%.

Table 3.4. Observed correlations of relatives for total fingerprint ridge count compared with the theoretical correlations expected with simple additive inheritance. After Holt 1961

Type of relationship	Observed correlation	Theoretical correlation
Husband–wife	0.05 ± 0.007	0.00
Monozygotic twins	0.95 ± 0.07	1.00
Dizygotic twins	0.49 ± 0.08	0.50
Sib–sib	0.50 ± 0.04	0.50
Parent–child	0.48 ± 0.03	0.50

1.2. Abnormalities of Neural Tube Closure

A vast descriptive literature exists on defects of the development of the neural tube (their terminology is discussed in detail in Chap. 5. In most epide-

miological studies two large groups are considered, 'anencephaly', including craniorachischisis (combined anencephaly and spina bifida), and 'spina bifida', which includes meningocele, myelocele, and encephalocele.

Variations in reported incidence in various countries are extreme (see Table 3.5). In Great Britain the prevalence varies from around 1.4–1.5 per 1000 total births for the two groups of defects in London, to rates approximately three times as high in Belfast. Few rates higher than about 1 per 1000 have been reported except from the British Isles, Northeastern North America, and the Middle East. Some Sikh

Table 3.5. Range of highest to lowest frequencies in congenital defects of the central nervous system in single births in various countries. Data from Lilienfeld 1969

| Malformation | Frequency/1000 total births | | Centre with | |
	Lowest	Highest	Lowest	Highest
Anencephalus	0.11	0.49	Bogota	Belfast
Anencephalus and spina bifida	0.03	0.61	Santiago	Alexandria
Hydrocephalus	0.05	1.99	Calcutta	Alexandria
Hydrocephalus and spina bifida	0.03	1.64	Bogota Manila	Belfast
Spina bifida	0.03	2.59	Manila	Belfast
All neural tube defects	0.61	10.21	Medellin	Belfast

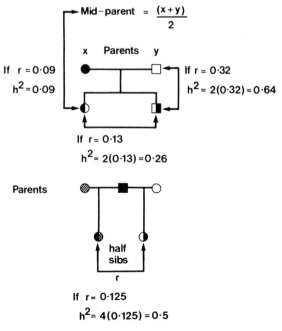

Fig. 3.6. Heritability in various relationships.

communities have frequencies of about 3 per 1000 (see Leck 1974).

From studies of the epidemiology of these two groups of defects it is evident that they must have related causes, since they show such similar variations in incidence. Furthermore, these causes must be partly environmental, since in children of the same genetic background there is marked variation with place, time, maternal age and parity, and socioeconomic status. The relatively low incidence in the offspring of Jewish women born in Israel after their parents had migrated there from other Middle Eastern countries, whilst high rates were seen in the children of mothers who were themselves born elsewhere in the Middle East (Naggan 1971), supports the suggestion that both environmental and genetic influences may be important in pathogenesis. Leck suggests that the stability of the rates for Sikhs and Ashkenazim could also be of environmental origin. The low rates for Negroes may also be related to maternal factors rather than fetal genes, since the rates for children of Negro fathers and European mothers may be as high as those for Europeans (Leck 1972). Where detailed studies of the incidence of anencephalus have been made some interesting trends have developed with time. In two investigations, Edwards (1958) and Fedrick (1976) examined the incidence of anencephalus in Scotland. A considerable variation in differing geographical locations had persisted, although relative frequencies had changed and there was an overall decline in the incidence of the lesion, most marked in those under 20 years of age and in the lower social classes. There was little seasonal variation in the time of delivery, but years with excessive numbers of cases have occurred (1961, 1971). Similar episodes have occurred in New England, Berlin, and Birmingham (see Leck 1974). In Great Britain a prolonged 'epidemic' may have lasted from 1920 to the late 1940s.

Seasonal variation in prevalence presents a very confused picture. For spina bifida there is a peak in children conceived in mid-spring and a trough in early autumn conceptions, but anencephalus may show this or other patterns. The picture is more clear-cut when variation in maternal age and parity is considered. Associations between these variables are found whenever large series are studied (see Leck 1974 for bibliography). In all instances there is agreement that the defects are least common in second births. Among births after the second the tendency for most countries is for the prevalence to increase with parity, and there is a tendency for increasing prevalence with increasing maternal age. Variations with social class are less clear-cut and the higher prevalence in lower social classes has been found to be less marked in recent studies and to be very variable in extent.

The sex ratio (male to female) for the defects is around $0.7:1$ and $0.8:1$ for spina bifida and $0.45:1$ for anencephaly in Great Britain, rising to unity in oriental populations. The female anencephalic rate appears to be both higher and more variable than the male rate (Rogers and Morris 1973).

Family studies show that concordance is less common in twins than is recurrence in sibships. Apart from this hazard the sibs of index cases are particularly liable to be aborted, and may have spina bifida occulta more often than other children (Carter et al. 1968; Carter and Evans 1973). It seems that both parental and maternal effects can affect prevalence, and in areas of high prevalence consanguinity can more than double the risk.

Various estimates suggest that about half of all embryos for fetuses with CNS defects are aborted. This may account for the paradox that neural tube defects are less common in the twins of children with those defects than in other sibs.

A number of possible environmental causative factors will be considered briefly later. However, a recent survey of the incidence of central nervous system anomalies in British Columbia (Trimble and Baird 1978) shows that total rates for these anomalies have remained constant at around 3 per 1000 births (anencephalus 0.6 per 1000; spina bifida 0.8 per 1000). Microcephalus had apparently decreased remarkably in frequency, but the authors point out that the introduction of measurement and well-defined criteria for this defect were probably of primary importance in this apparent change.

1.3. Cleft Lip and Palate

Cleft lip and palate combined (CL + P) and cleft lip alone (CL) are closer to each other, in aetiological terms, than to cleft palate alone (CP) (see review by Leck 1976). Approximately 20% of children with facial clefts have associated major malformations, the proportion of individuals with CP and associated defects being the highest in the group.

The lips develop during the 4th to 7th weeks of intrauterine life, the palate from the 4th to 8th weeks—these dates depending a little on the starting point assumed. Genetic data suggest that a mechanism altering lip development may have a secondary effect on palatal development, but that the latter may be affected independently of the former (Woolf 1971) and that both these processes increase in frequency with parental age.

All studies in which data are adequate show between 0.6 and 1.35 per 1000 total births for Caucasians, but Mongoloids have higher rates and Negroids considerably lower. Hawaiian studies show that children of mixed genetic background have an intermediate liability to CL + P (Ching and Chung 1974). Fraser and Pashayan (1970) suggested that differences in facial shape were important in determining this malformation, as has been shown for the mouse, a suggestion supported by more recent work in man (see Kurisu et al. 1974).

The frequency of CL alone varies considerably in different regions of England and Wales (25 %–33 % in most studies but up to 47 % in Northeast England: Knox and Braithwaite 1962), a variability also seen in Mongoloid races. In both groups unilateral clefts of the lip are commoner than bilateral ones, and about two-thirds are left-sided. In addition, CL shows some evidence of clustering (see Leck 1976 for bibliography), although investigation of seasonal variations does not suggest a specific pattern or provide evidence for specific aetiological factors, e.g., influenza.

There is a marked trend for the prevalence of (CL + P) to rise with maternal age; in CL alone this effect is much less marked (Hay and Barbano 1972). Parity appears to have little effect regardless of age.

1.3.1. Cleft Palate Alone

Rates for cleft palate range from 0.4 to 0.8 per 1000 in Caucasians (see Leck 1976 for bibliography). Face shape is also probably important in this defect; in Finland Saxen (1975) has shown that the prevalence is highest in the east of the country, where faces are wider. The prevalence of CL increases with maternal age, as does that of CL + P, but there is some evidence to suggest that an independent paternal effect may also be important.

1.3.2. Family Patterns of Occurrence

For CL + P, if we assume a general population incidence of 1 per 1000, the concurrence rate for monozygotic twins is 400 times the population figure and the rates for first-, second-, and third-degree relatives are 40, 7, and 3 times this figure, respectively.

1.4. Congenital Heart Defects

The problem of the prevalence of defects is nowhere more difficult to resolve than in the large group of abnormalities that affect the heart and great vessels. Prolonged follow-up and sophisticated study is necessary for proper ascertainment, and investigations that satisfy these major criteria are few. Rates of 6–8 per 1000 births are generally found (e.g., Frederick et al. 1971; Yerushalmy 1970). The

prevalence at birth of all defects increases with maternal age and is high in monozygotic twin pairs (Mitchell et al. 1971; Kenna et al. 1975). The increased incidence with high maternal age persists even when allowance is made for the well-documented association of Down's syndrome with congenital heart disease. The eight commonest lesions (ventricular septal defect, patent ductus arteriosus, aortic stenosis, atrial septal defect, coarctation of the aorta, Fallot's tetralogy, pulmonary stenosis, and the transposition complexes) account for about 80 % of all defects. Defects of the ventricular septum are the commonest single group (approximately 30 % of the total in most series). From a number of studies patent ductus arteriosus appears to be more common in females, whilst transposition, coarctation of the aorta, and aortic stenosis are commoner in males.

A possible aetiological factor, hypoxia, has been identified from surveys of patent ductus arteriosus. This defect has been shown to increase with altitude, and at places over 4500 m high it occurs at 30 times the frequency observed at sea level (Peñaloza et al. 1964). It seems likely, however, that other factors, perhaps involving hypoxia are involved. Short gestation, low birth weight, and fetal or neonatal asphyxia are also associated with increased frequency of the diagnosis.

Other cardiac defects show no convincing seasonal or geographical associations.

1.5. Infantile Hypertrophic Pyloric Stenosis

Rates of between 2 and 4 per 1000 births have been recorded for infantile hypertrophic pyloric stenosis in Great Britain, significantly higher than the 1–3 or less per 1000 recorded for other countries (see Leck 1976 for bibliography). Again, there are diagnostic difficulties, particularly in establishing the relationship of true hypertrophic pyloric stenosis, treated surgically, to 'pylorospasm', which can be conservatively managed. The male:female ratio is 4:1 or 5:1 in all studies, and there is a significant excess of first-born children. In a recent report, Bear (1978) has shown that an excess of male births over females is also found among unaffected members of sibships in which more than one case of pyloric stenosis has occurred.

Tumour size in pyloric stenosis tends to increase with age, suggesting postnatal development of the muscular hypertrophy. Dodge (1971, 1973) considers that feeding frequency and habits may affect the development of the anomaly, and that gastrin, which can produce pyloric hypertrophy in puppies, may play an important role. Some cases of pyloric stenosis have apparently had their origin at birth and have required operative intervention in the first weeks of life (Laurence 1963; Powell 1962; Lloyd Davies 1963), but this is uncommon, the mean age at operation being 7 weeks.

The disease shows the characteristics of polygenic inheritance (Carter 1969), with heritability of 68% (sons–fathers), 54% (brothers–brothers), or 90% (daughters–mothers). This illustrates the general point that when one sex is seldom affected, individuals of that sex who do express the defect have a higher genetic 'load' tending to produce the abnormality.

1.6. Musculoskeletal System Defects

1.6.1. Club Foot

In abnormalities of the club foot type it is extremely difficult to obtain accurate data, since many apparent defects disappear in the first weeks of life. If these infants are disregarded, and cases of talipes equinovarus (TEV) with other defects are excluded, then in Caucasoid races the prevalence is between 2–4 per 1000 with TEV and 1 per 1000 each for talipes calcaneovalgus (TCV) and metatarsus virus (MV) (Wynne-Davies 1964; Chung and Myrianthopolus 1968). Within-series comparisons suggest that TEV is half as common in children of Oriental origin and six times as common in Polynesian children as in Caucasoids (Ching et al. 1969).

Significant trends have been reported with season of birth, multiple births, and maternal age and parity (Hay and Wehrung 1970; Dunn 1976). Dunn has suggested that this defect may be a manifestation of postural moulding in utero, and that multiple births will enhance this tendency.

1.6.2. Congenital Dislocation of the Hip

In recent years there have been wide swings in the supposed frequency of occurrence of congenital dislocation of the hip, owing in part to difficulties in diagnosis and variation in the diagnostic criteria used. However, both unstable hip and congenital dislocation show similar epidemiological trends; namely a four- to six-fold excess of females over males, a preponderance of bilateral cases, relatively high rates in first-born children and among those born in winter, a frequent history of breech delivery and an association between the defect and high social class (see Leck 1976 for bibliography). Dunn (1976) also considers moulding important in this defect, suggesting that breech delivery following

oligohydramnios may be an important aetiological factor. The female excess is thought to be the result of hormone-induced joint laxity.

Carter and Wilkinson (1964) first emphasized the role of both acetabular dysplasia (inherited polygenically) and dominantly inherited persistent joint laxity in the genesis of the defect. The importance of these factors was confirmed by the later studies of Wynne-Davies (1970a, b). In her work she found a higher proportion of affected individuals in first-degree than in second- and third-degree relatives, and also showed that patients with the highest degree of acetabular dyplasia had the highest proportion of affected children. These individuals tended to be in the last diagnostic group; patients diagnosed early were more likely to show persistent joint laxity. However, in most cases both causative factors were thought to be important.

2. Chromosomal Abnormality and Malformations

It has already been emphasized that the bulk of embryos with chromosomal abnormalities are aborted. Between 3 and 5 liveborn infants per 100 are chromosomally abnormal, with Down's syndrome (47, +22), Klinefelter's syndrome (47XXY), and 47XYY and 47XXX all having frequencies greater than 1 per 1000. The predominance of sex chromosome anomalies in these syndromes is probably related to the relative paucity of genetic information in them—loss or duplication of an autosome having much more serious effects on development.

The general effects of chromosome anomalies are growth retardation, mental retardation, and impaired fertility. Phenotypically, generalizations of this kind are impossible.

The classic study on the incidence of chromosomal defects in recent years is that of Bové et al. (1975), who carried out retrospective and prospective studies on 1500 karyotyped spontaneous human abortions. Concentrating on abortuses of less than 12 weeks' gestational age, they found 577 normal and 921 abnormal karyotypes. In the normal group they found morphological abnormalities, which suggested undetected zygotic causes. Structural chromosomal anomalies were rare (3.8% of defects), the bulk of the abnormalities being numerical and the result of errors at the time of gametogenesis (nondisjunction at meiosis), at the time of fertilization (triploidy caused by digyny or dispermy), or during the early division of the fertilized ovum (tetraploidy or mosiacism). The incidence of chromosome anomalies remained stable over the 6 years studied. There was no evidence of a collective or singular tendency for anomalies to show evidence of seasonal variation.

From this work it appears that 61.5% of spontaneous abortions have chromosomal defects, a figure in good general agreement with those given in the other recent studies of Therkelsen et al. (1974) (54.7%) and Kajii et al. (1973) (59%). As reported by other groups, almost all monosomies were monosomy X (about 15% of the anomalies studied). Trisomy 16 was the most frequent autosomal trisomy. It must be emphasized that even studies of this type are selected and demonstrate only some of the total errors that may occur in early development. The blighted ovum familiar to pathologists examining abortuses is a manifestation of massive developmental failure. The accompanying placental changes can give useful indicators of possible anomalies (see p. 46); Bové et al. 1976).

The numbers of chromosomal abnormalities at term have been demonstrated by Machin (1974). He found that 9% of macerated stillbirths, 4% of fresh stillbirths, and 6% of early neonatal deaths had an abnormal karyotpye—this despite the fact that adequate cultures were obtained from only 18% of macerated stillbirths, 76% of fresh stillbirths (intrapartum death), and 90% of early neonatal deaths. Again a striking maternal age effect was found, with mothers over 40 having a much greater risk of bearing a chromosomally abnormal child.

2.1. Some Common Syndromes

2.1.1. Trisomy 18 (Edwards' Syndrome)

Trisomy 18 is commoner in females (4:1) with a greatly increased frequency with advancing maternal age. Affected infants are small with a narrow pinched face and marked micrognathia. The hands are often clenched, with digits II and V overriding III and IV. Rocker-bottom feet are seen. Dermatoglyphic changes include the presence of arches on all fingertips. Most affected infants die within 6 months of birth (Fig. 3.7; see also p. 279).

2.1.2. 5p- (Cri-du-chat Syndrome)

In the cri-du-chat syndrome a variable amount of material is lost from the short arm of chromosome 5. There is microcephaly and gross hypertelorism. The name is derived from a peculiar mewing cry, which is gradually lost if the child survives (Fig. 3.8).

2.1.3. Trisomy 13 (Patau's Syndrome)

Midline facial defects, micropthalmia, and anophthalmia or cyclops are found in trisomy 13; the nose is often large and bulbous. Holoprosencephaly may occur. Polydactyly is common and the individuals are usually profoundly mentally retarded (Fig. 3.9; see also p. 157).

2.1.4. Trisomy 21 (Down's Sydrome)

Classically trisomy 21 is characterized by a small head with flattened occiput, low-set ears with rolled-over helix, flattened nasal bridge, slanting eyes, and prominent epicanthic folds. The mouth is open, with the tongue protruding. Hands are short and spatulate, a transverse palmar crease is present with an incurved fourth finger, and dermatoglyphic abnormalities are seen. Wide separation of the great and second toes is found in some cases (Fig. 3.10).

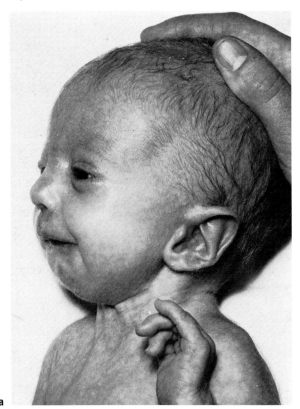

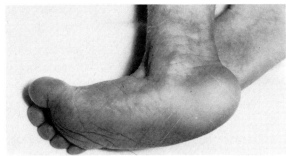

Fig. 3.7. a and **b** Trisomy 18. **a** Micrognathia and the pinched face are evident; **b** rocker-bottom foot. Courtesy of Prof. P. Polani.

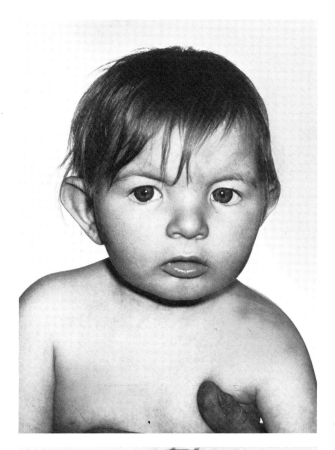

Fig. 3.8. (*left*) Cri-du-chat syndrome with marked hypertelorism. Courtesy of Prof. P. Polani.

Fig. 3.9. a Facial defects in Patau's syndrome. **b** Polydactyly. Courtesy of Prof. P. Polani.

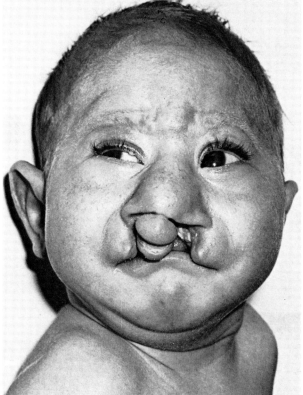

a

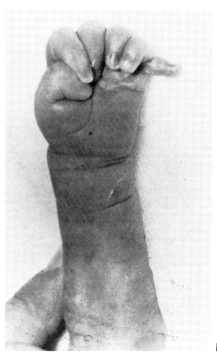

b

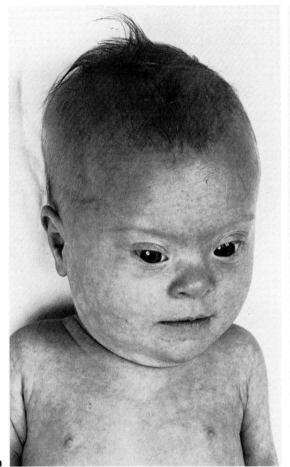

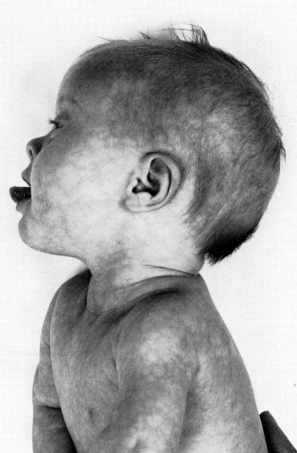

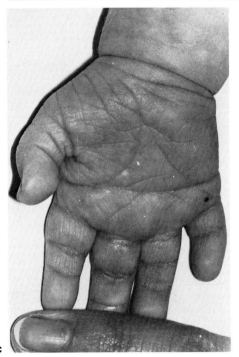

Fig. 3.10. a–c Down's syndrome. **a** Typical facies; **b** prominent tongue; **c** spatulate hand with transverse palmar crease and incurved fourth finger. Courtesy of Prof. P. Polani.

3. Specific Human Teratogens

In view of the complex genetic and environmental factors involved in the causation of malformations it is evident that establishing the role of potential teratogens is difficult. Heritability for the large groups of human defects is in excess of 60%, and maternal age, birth rank, season, altitude, etc. all add some loading, providing a background against which teratogens must be assessed. Undoubted teratogens exist for man; these will be considered briefly below. Despite extensive testing of compounds it is likely that unknown teratogens of small and possibly cumulative effect are introduced into the environment from time to time. We may console ourselves with the fact that the prevalence of malformation has changed very little with time, so that such effects are probably not large. Nevertheless, the approach of Smithells and Sheppard (1978) is eminently sensible. They point out that avoidance of unnecessary medication in pregnancy, particularly in the first trimester, is prudent but that there will always be occasions where the health of the mother (and hence the fetus) requires drug administration. Most drugs in day-to-day use have not been examined for possible teratogenic effects in man, and in view of the difficulties of extrapolating animal data it is doubtful whether they should be. Testing can be carried out by examining centralized prescription records and following up births to mothers taking a particular medicine in a particular period. Smithells and Sheppard have described this technique and discussed its merits clearly, in demonstrating the absence of a teratogenic effect from Bendectin.

3.1 Human Teratogens

The reports that first drew attention to a number of noninfectious human teratogens are shown in Table 3.6.

In general the pattern of their recognition has been that one case is reported, followed by a study of a larger group. Since the thalidomide disaster many compounds have been suspected of being teratogens, but relatively few appear to have such effects after adequate investigation.

3.2 Radiation

Murphy (1929) reported on the outcome of 625 pregnancies in which women were exposed to 'pelvic radium therapy' or roentgen irradiation either before or after conception, collecting his data from a review and a questionnaire sent to 1700 gynaecologists and radiologists. Radiation was therapeutic rather than diagnostic, and in some cases it had been used in a direct attempt to induce sterility. Approximately a quarter of the 625 pregnancies ended in abortion; in this respect preconception irradiation was less likely to induce abortion than postconception treatment. Neither the stillbirth rate nor the infant mortality was increased by preconception irradiation. Malformations in 402 term infants in this group included one case each of microcephaly, anencephaly, phocomelia, tracheal stenosis, and congenital heart disease. A parietal bony defect was noted and one child was recorded as 'deformed', with no further description provided. These figures suggest little real effect on the incidence of major malformation.

There were no stillbirths after postconception irradiation. Of the 74 full-term infants born after this treatment 17 had microcephaly, two had hydrocephalus, one was blind and growth-retarded, one had spina bifida and club feet, one had a 'malformation of the head', and one had deformed upper extremities. A divergent squint was seen in one further child and a case of Down's syndrome was recorded in a child whose mother had had only a diagnostic X-ray.

Although there are faults in this early study, it clearly established the importance of high-dose irradiation in the production of microcephaly and mental retardation, an association unhappily confirmed at Hiroshima and Nagasaki, where Blot and Miller (1973) found that children irradiated in utero had an increased chance of being microcephalic or retarded, or both. Many isolated reports have been well reviewed by Brent (1977).

It will be evident that therapeutic radiation has usually been given in ignorance of pregancy (e.g., in ankylosing spondylitis) and reports of this are now, happily, rare. There appears to be no evidence to suggest that present levels of diagnostic irradiation are associated with an increased frequency of congenital defects. The role of radiation in childhood oncogenesis is less certain (see pp. 602, 666).

3.3 Cytotoxic Drugs

Following the early reports of abnormalities induced by a folic acid antogonist (see Table 3.6), a number of experimental studies have confirmed the expected teratogenicity of cytotoxic compounds—these studies have been ably reviewed by Connors (1975). Methotrexate, azathioprine, and cyclophosphamide are all teratogenic in animals and might be administered to pregnant women. In general, however, such compounds are not given in pregnancy unless for compelling clinical reasons such as malignant disease in the mother. The few data available suggest that early treatment at high doses usually results in abortion rather than the production of a live child with malformations. A report of myeloschisis in a leukaemic woman treated with busulphan has recently been published by Abramovici et al. (1978).

3.4 Thalidomide

The details of the thalidomine incident are now well documented. The general morphological features are shown in Table 3.7 and the compound will not be considered in detail here. Later reports of the affected children (Stephenson 1976) suggest that a

greater degree of central nervous system damage may have occurred than was first thought.

3.5 Warfarin

In 1966 De Saia described a female infant with bilateral optic atrophy, mental retardation, and nasal malformation, born to a mother with a history of ingestion of several drugs during pregnancy, including warfarin. Further reports (Kerber et al. 1968), including a follow-up of the original case (Becker et al. 1975), resulted in the identification of further characteristics of the syndrome and retrospective reviews of many cases (see Warkany 1976 for bibliography).

In general, the anticoagulant has been given to

Table 3.6 Some definite human teratogens

Agent	Authors and date	Cases	Comment
Radiation	Aschenheim (1920)	1	Child with microcephaly and mental retardation
	Murphy (1929)	625 pregnancies	Microcephaly noted in offspring irradiated in utero
Folic acid antagonist (4-amino-PGA)	Thiersch (1952)	3	Growth retardation, anencephaly, hydrocephaly, cleft lip and palate, skull defects were produced. Later reports included similar malformation syndromes in individuals using these drugs as abortifacients
Testosterone and synthetic progestogens	Grunwaldt and Bates (1957)	1	Virilization of female fetus with production of atypical genitalia
	Wilkins (1960)	70 cases (review)	Similar changes to those noted with testosterone, ethisterone being the drug most often used
Thalidomide	McBride (1961)		Noted 'increased incidence of multiple malformations in babies of women given Distaval'
	Lenz (1962)	52	Response to McBride's letter
	Lenz and Knapp (1962)	Approx. 300	Detailed description of syndrome, with timing of critical events
Warfarin	Di Saia (1966)	1	Nasal and facial abnormalities, stippled epiphyses
	Becker (1975)	5	
Alcohol	Lemoine et al. (1967)	127	Abnormal facies, microcephaly, oblique palpebral fissures, pre- and postnatal growth retardation
Anticonvulsants	Meadow (1968)	6	Cleft lip and palate and congenital heart disease, minor skeletal abnormalities
Methylmercury	Amin-Zaki et al. (1974)	6	Blindness, deafness, hyperactive reflexes. Impairment of motor and intellectual development in some offspring affected by foodstuffs treated with mercury-based antifungal agents

Table 3.7. Abnormalities in thalidomide-affected children

Defects of the upper limbs	1.	Amelia—arm absent
	2.	Short phocomelia—flipper only present
	3.	Long phocomelia—humerus and ulna both present but short
	4.	Short forearm—upper arm normal
	5.	Radial aplasia—normal ulna or hypoplasia
	6.	Absence of radial digits
	7.	Hypoplasia of thumb or thenar muscles or both
	8.	Triphalangeal thumb
Defects of the lower limbs	1.	Phocomelia—rudimentary bone present between pelvis and foot
	2.	Femoral hypoplasia—lower limb normal
	3.	Deformities of tibia and/or fibula
	4.	Deformities of feet only
	5.	Congenital dislocation of the hip
Defects of internal organs	1.	Congenital heart disease
	2.	Anomalies of the kidneys
	3.	Anomalies of the alimentary tract
	4.	Choanal atresia
Defects of the eyes and ears	1.	Anotia—absence of the pinna
	2.	Microtia—small deformed pinna
	3.	Facial palsy—may be associated with 1 and 2
	4.	External ophthalmoplegia—may be associated with 3
	5.	Anophthalmos
	6.	Microphthalmos
	7.	Coloboma

women with prosthetic heart valves during pregnancy or to those suffering from deep vein thrombosis. The majority of infants born to women treated in this way are normal, but abnormalities found include nasal malformations (hypoplasia of nasal bridge, choanal stenosis), optic atrophy, microcephaly and mental retardation, hypotonia, and, in one instance, agenesis of the corpus callosum (Holzgreve et al. 1976). A distinctive finding is the so-called stippled epiphysis, a change resembling Conradi–Hünermann disease or chondrodystrophia congenita calcificans. Discrete punctate areas of calcification are seen in the epiphyses of long bones, and are thought to be the result of local haemorrhage.

3.6 Alcohol and Fetus

Warnings about the effects of alcohol on development have been given since biblical times (Judges 13, 7) but despite an interesting description of the offspring of alcoholic mothers in a report of a select committee of the House of Commons (1834) the syndrome now associated with excessive alcohol intake in pregnancy was not recognized until the observations of Lemoine et al. (1968) and Jones et al. (1973). The specific syndrome is well documented, and various studies have shown that the frequent abuse of other drugs by alcoholics are not central to its production. Approximately 250 cases have been reported in the literature to date, but the various estimates of incidence seem to be based on inadequate data.

The features of the syndrome are as shown in Table 3.8. In addition to these features, the babies are light and their linear growth rate and average weight gain are both greatly reduced despite adequate caloric intakes. Catch-up growth does not occur. Histopathological study of the brain shows altered neuronal and glial migration with cerebellar dysplasia and heterotopic cell clusters on the surface of the brain (Clarren et al. 1978).

The effects of 'nonalcoholic' patterns of alcohol ingestion on the outcome of pregnancy have not yet been adequately studied.

3.7 Anticonvulsants

Meadow's report (1968) was the first to associate congenital abnormalities and anticonvulsants when he described six infants with cleft lip and palate and certain other anomalies born to mothers taking these compounds during pregnancy. Janz and Fuchs (1964) had previously reported five malformations (including three cases of cleft lip and palate) in 225 epileptic mothers taking anticonvulsants, but concluded that the difference between their study group and controls was not significant. Smithells (1976), in reviewing the many studies that have followed these observations, considers that there is a real association between the drugs and malformation, that it is drug ingestion rather than the epileptic condition that is critical, that phenytoin is more teratogenic than phenobarbitone, and that the two combined are more teratogenic than either alone. Primidone is

Table 3.8 Fetal alcohol syndrome

Growth	Below 2 SD from mean, adipose tissue disproportionally affected
Central nervous system	Microcephaly, hypotonia, mental retardation. May be irritable or hyperactive infants
Heart	Atrial septal defects common
Facies	Short palpebral fissures—may be ptosis, epicanthic folds prominent
Nose	Short and up-turned
Mouth	Thinned vermillion border of upper lip, diminished philtrum

largely metabolized to phenobarbitone in the body, and probably has similar effects. In treated epileptics the incidence of cleft lip and palate is about 12 times and that of congenital heart disease about 3 times that in the general population. Phalangeal hypoplasia (mainly the terminal phalanx) and hypoplasia of the finger- and toenails may also occur. Facial abnormalities, including a short nose with a broad depressed bridge and prominent epicanthic folds, have also been described (Hanson 1976).

Speidel and Meadow (1974) pointed out that defects have been reported in association with other anticonvulsants, but a recent specific trimethadione syndrome has been identified by Goldman and Yaffe (1978), which differs from that described above in the presence of V-shaped eyebrows and low-set ears with an anteriorly folded helix. Phalangeal hypoplasia does not occur.

3.8. Methylmercury Compounds

The effects of the release of organic mercury compounds into Minamata Bay in the 1960s were manifest in the subsequent birth of children with cerebral palsy and mental retardation to mothers who had ingested heavily contaminated shellfish from the bay. Following a disastrous outbreak of methylmercury poisoning in rural Iraq in 1972 due to the ingestion of home-made bread made from wheat treated with a methylmercury fungicide, it has been found that methylmercury passes readily from mother to fetus and may also be transmitted via breast milk. Gross impairment of motor and mental development has occurred in some individuals (Amin-Zaki et al. 1974).

Although methylmercury is not teratogenic in the sense of producing congenital anomalies of the type formally defined at the beginning of this chapter, neuropathological changes have been found to occur in affected individuals (Matsumoto et al. 1965).

3.9. Hyperthermia

From the experimental work of a number of authors, notably Edwards (see review by Edwards and Wanner 1977), it is evident that short periods of hyperthermia are teratogenic in animals. Studies in man have suggested that this may also be true in our species (Miller et al. 1978), although serious reservations have been expressed about most of the reported observations (Leck 1978). The present position is uncertain; a number of prospective studies are in progress, but it is possible that change in body temperature may help to explain the

inconsistent associations of malformations reported for some infections.

3.10. The Operating Room Environment

There is evidence to support the contention that spontaneous abortion rates are higher than normal in women working in surgical theatres (see Smithells 1976 for bibliography). Data for malformation rates are not convincing, however; skin naevi, malabsorption syndrome, and hernias have been included as malformations in some series (Corbett et al. 1974). No prospective study has been reported to date.

3.11. Cumulative Teratogens of Small Effect

There is increasing concern over the possible effects of teratogens introduced into the environment as food additives, preservatives, cosmetics, etc. Whilst such concern is probably ill-founded—overall malformation rates appear to change little with time—it is true to say that there is no effective system for the examination of teratogens of small effect. It has already been emphasized that the causation of most human malformations involves a large genetic component, and that the predisposition to malformation is distributed polygenically. From the model shown in Fig. 3.6 it will be evident that a small change in the position of the threshold may produce a large change in the frequency of expression of a defect. Substances of minor effect may act in this way, and if cumulative in their action, may have significant effects. Test systems to identify this type of agent are necessary and are discussed elsewhere (Berry and Nickols 1979).

3.12. Smoking and the Fetus

Simpson (1957) first drew attention to the problems of smoking in pregnancy in a preliminary report. The general conclusions that can be drawn from the many publications on the subject since are that smokers' babies weigh between 150 and 250 g less than those of nonsmokers and that twice as many infants under 2500 g are born to smokers. There is a direct relationship between the number of cigarettes smoked and the reduction in weight, and this reduction is independent of other infant and maternal factors known to influence birth weight (Meyer et al. 1976).

These effects have been accompanied by an increasing awareness of the effects of smoking in early pregnancy, where in the study of Boué et al.

(1975) (see Chap. 2) it was found that 50% of the fetuses aborted by mothers who smoked and inhaled had normal karyotypes, suggesting an enhanced loss of normal conceptuses in these individuals. From the large Ontario Perinatal Mortality Study it is evident that after controlling for a number of variables (maternal height, weight, birthplace, age, parity, etc.) smoking less than one packet of cigarettes a day increased perinatal mortality by 20%; this increase rose to 35% for those smoking more than one packet. Increased risk of in utero death in the 20–28 week period and deaths in premature infants born in this period were associated with increases in the rate of placenta praevia and abruptio placentae. (See Fielding 1978 for bibliography.)

4. Infectious Causes of Abnormal Development

4.1. Rubella

Maternal rubella infection has been associated with fetal infection rates of approximately 90% in the first 8–10 weeks in some series (Rawles et al. 1968), and on the basis of this fact and other data the number of abnormal fetuses produced suggests that some are infected without damage. By the 3rd and 4th months the rate of infection may be below 10%.

Fetal rubella may be associated both with congenital malformations and with chronic infection that persists for months or years after birth. Rubella virus may be isolated from an abortus, from the placenta or amniotic fluid, and from most viscera. In the liveborn child the virus can be recovered from the throat, urine, meconium, and conjunctival and cerebrospinal fluids. Reports of positive culture from cataract material, liver biopsies, and ductal tissue have also been made.

The features of congenital rubella include a general failure of growth, manifest both pre- and postnatally, eye changes (cataracts, usually bilateral, microphthalmia, pigmentary retinopathy), CNS changes (microcephaly, retardation, progressive panencephalitis), congenital heart disease (patent ductus arteriosus, pulmonary artery lesions including localized stenosis and hypoplasia, aortic stenosis, ventricular septal defects, Fallot's tetralogy, myocarditis), defects of hearing, hepatitis, interstitial pneumonitis, a chronic rash, and persistent lymphadenopathy. Bone changes may also occur.

The pathological findings have been described in detail by Singer et al. (1967).

4.2. Congenital Syphilis

Although adequate antenatal care should prevent congenital syphilis, recent increases in its frequency in several countries should alert pathologists to the possibility of the diagnosis. The manifestations are protean, and range from hydrops with hepatosplenomegaly and haemolytic anaemia, periostitis, and meningitis to those defects identified in childhood, namely interstitial keratitis, eighth-nerve deafness, bony defects (abnormal teeth, saddle nose, frontal bossing), cutaneous lesions, and hepatic fibrosis.

4.3 Toxoplasmosis

Infection with *Toxoplasma gondii* is said to occur in half the population of the United States of America (Krick and Remington 1978), and may be responsible for up to 3000 abnormal births per year there. The infection is a zoonosis, members of the cat family being the definitive hosts.

Congenital toxoplasmosis occurs when a previously uninfected woman is infected during pregnancy. The protozoans are then transmitted across the placenta to the fetus, where they cause multiple lesions in many organs. Early reports emphasized the importance of central nervous system involvement with the production of microcephalus, hydrocephalus, microphthalmus, and chorioretinitis. Periventricular calcification was considered to be a specific feature (see p. 183). More recently it has been realized that newborn infants with active disease may have fever, convulsions, maculopapular skin rash, lymphadenopathy, hepatosplenomegaly, icterus, and thrombocytopenia. Such symptoms are associated with a 40% mortality. As with other infections, early (first-trimester) infections are associated with the most tissue damage.

4.4. Cytomegalovirus (CMV) Infection

Infection by CMV is probably the commonest viral infection of the human fetus, occurring in 4–10 infants per 1000 births (Dudgeon 1976). Congenital abnormalities occur less frequently in this disease than in rubella, with CNS involvement a major feature. A classic presentation in the newborn is with hepatosplenomegaly, jaundice and petechial haemorrhages (often with thrombocytopenia). This picture is not incompatible with recovery, but if respiratory or CNS involvement is evident the prognosis is worsened. A destructive encephalitis with calcification may occur; microcephaly is sometimes evident and fits and spasticity may develop.

It is generally assumed that infection occurs following maternal infection in early pregnancy, but this is uncertain and many woman carry the virus in the cervix. It has been shown that placental infection without involvement of the fetus may occur.

4.5. Other Virus Infections

Isolated cases of malformation associated with Herpes simplex virus (HSV) have been reported, usually involving the central nervous system. In one instance HSV has been isolated from the cerebrospinal fluid. Microcephaly, cerebral calcification, microphthalmia, and skin rashes have all been reported (South et al. 1969).

Evidence for the association of mumps or enterovirus infections is not good. Similarly, despite extensive studies no convincing association of influenza and subsequent malformation has been demonstrated (see Leck [1963] and Dudgeon [1976] for more detailed discussions).

5. Antenatal Diagnosis of Congenital Abnormalities

Techniques for the detection of abnormalities include various physical methods (radiology, ultrasound, fetoscopy), the use of amniotic fluid cultures permitting the diagnosis of chromosomal anomalies, sex-linked disorders, inherited biochemical defects (some 80 can be diagnosed in this way), and chemical methods, including determination of α-fetoprotein levels in amniotic fluid and maternal blood.

The problems of diagnosis and of amniocentesis are specialized topics, and recent reviews of the major topics have been published by Laurence and Gregory (1976), MacVicar (1976), and Brock (1976). Screening for neural tube defects was discussed in a recent leader in *The Lancet* (1977).

References

Abramovici A, Shaklai M, Pinkhas J (1978) Myeloschisis in a six weeks embryo of a leukaemic woman treated by busulphan. Teratology 18: 241

Amin-Zaki L, Elhassani S, Majeed MA, Clarkson TW, Doherty RA, Greenwood M (1974) Intrauterine methylmercury poisoning in Iraq. Pediatrics 54: 587

Aschenheim E (1920) Schädigung einer menschlichen Frucht durch Röntgenstrahlen. Arch Kinderheilkd 68: 131

Bear JC (1978) The association of sex ratio anomalies with pyeloric stenosis. Teratology 17: 19

Becker MH, Genieser NB, Finegold M, Miranda D, Spackman T (1975) Chondrodysplasia punctata: is maternal warfarin therapy a factor? Am J Dis Child 129: 356

Berry CL, Nickols CD (1979) The effects of aspirin on the development of the mouse third molar. A potential screening system for weak teratogens. Arch Toxicol 42: 185

Blot WJ, Miller RW (1973) Mental retardation following in utero exposure to the atomic bombs of Hiroshima and Nagasaki. Radiology 106: 617

Boué J, Boué A, Lazar P (1975) Retrospective epidemiological studies of 1500 karyotyped spontaneous human abortions. Teratology 12: 11

Bové J, Phillipe E, Giroud A, Bové A (1976) Phenotypic expression of lethal chromosome anomalies in human abortuses. Teratology 14: 3

Brent RL (1977) Radiation and other physical agents. In: Wilson JG, Clarke Fraser F (eds) General principles and etiology. Plenum Press, New York London (Handbook of teratology, vol I, p 153).

Brock DJH (1976) Pre-natal diagnosis, chemical methods. Br Med Bull 32: 16

Carr DH (1972) Cytogenic aspects of induced and spontaneous abortions. Clin Obstet Gynaecol 15: 203

Carter CO (1965) The inheritance of common congenital malformations. Prog Med Genet 4: 59

Carter CO (1969) Genetics of common disorders. Br Med Bull 25: 52

Carter CO (1976) Genetics of common single malformations. Br Med Bull 32: 21

Carter CO, Evans K (1973) Spina bifida and anencephalus in Greater London. J Med Genet 10: 209

Carter CO, Wilkinson JA (1964) Genetic and environmental factors in the aetiology of congenital dislocation of the hip. Clin Orthop 33: 119

Carter CO, David PA, Laurence KM (1968) A family study of major central nervous system malformations in South Wales. J Med Genet 5: 81

Ching GHS, Chung CS (1974) A genetic study of cleft lip and palate in Hawaii. I. Interracial crosses. Am J Hum Genet 26: 162

Ching GHS, Chung CS, Nemechek RW (1969) Genetic and epidemiological studies of clubfoot in Hawaii: ascertainment and incidence. Am J Hum Genet 21: 566

Chung CS, Myrianthopolus NC (1968) Racial and prenatal factors in major congenital malformations. Am J Hum Genet 20: 44

Clarren SK, Alvord EC, Sumi SM (1978) Brain malformations related to prenatal exposure to ethanol. J Pediatr 92: 64

Connors TA (1975) Cytotoxic agents in teratogenic research. In: Berry CL, Poswillo DE (eds) Teratology: trends and applications. Springer, Berlin Heidelberg New York, p 49

Corbett TH, Cornell RG, Endres JL, Weding K (1974) Birth defects among children of nurse-anesthetists. Anesthesiology 41: 341

Di Saia J (1966) Pregnancy and delivery of a patient with a Starr–Edwards mitral valve prosthesis. Report of a case. Obstet Gynecol 28: 469

Dodge JA (1971) Abnormal distribution of ABO blood groups in infantile pyloric stenosis. J Med Genet 8: 468

Dodge JA (1973) Infantile pyloric stenosis. Inheritance, psyche and soma. Ir J Med Sci 142: 6

Dudgeon JA (1976) Infective causes of human malformations. Br Med Bull 32: 77

Dunn PM (1976) Congenital postural deformities. Br Med Bull 32: 71

Edwards JH (1958) Congenital malformations of the central nervous system in Scotland. Br J Prev Soc Med 12: 115

Edwards JH (1969) Familial predisposition in man. Br Med Bull 25: 58

Edwards MJ, Wanner RA (1977) Extremes of temperature. In: Wilson JG, Clarke Fraser F (eds) General principles and etiology, Plenum, New York London (Handbook of teratology, vol. I, p 421)

Falconer DS (1965) The inheritance of liability to certain diseases, estimated from the incidence among relatives. Ann Hum Genet 29: 51

Fielding JE (1978) Smoking and pregnancy. New Engl J Med 298: 337

Fraser FC, Pashayan H (1970) Relation of face shape to susceptibility to congenital cleft lip. A preliminary case report. J Med Genet 7: 112

Fedrick J (1976) Anencephalus in Scotland 1961–1972. Br J Prev Soc Med 30: 132

Frederick J, Alberman ED, Goldstein H (1971) Possible teratogenic effect of cigarette smoking. Nature 231: 529

Goldman AS, Yaffe SJ (1978) Fetal trimethadione syndrome. Teratology 17: 103

Grunwaldt E, Bates T (1957) Nonadrenal female pseudohermaphrodism after administration of testosterone to mother during pregnancy. Pediatrics 20: 503

Hanson JWM (1976) Fetal hydantoin syndrome. Teratology 13: 185

Hay S, Barbano SH (1972) Independent effects of maternal age and birth order on the incidence of selected congenital malformations. Teratology 6: 271

Hay S, Wehring DA (1970) Congenital malformations in twins. Am J Hum Genet 22: 622

Holt SB (1961) Quantitative genetics of finger-print patterns. Br Med Bull 17(3): 247

Holzgreve W. Garey JC, Hall BD (1976) Warfarin-induced fetal abnormalities (Letter). Lancet 2: 914

Janz D, Fuchs U (1964) Sind antiepileptische Medikamente während der Schwangerschaft schädlich? Dtsch Med Wochenschr 89: 241

Jones KL, Smith DW, Ulleland CB, Streissguth AP (1973) Pattern of malformation in offspring of chronic alcoholic mothers. Lancet 1: 1267

Kajii T, Chama K, Nukawa N, Ferrier A, Avirachan S (1973) Banding analysis of chromosomal karyotypes in spontaneous abortion. Am J Hum Genet 25: 539

Kenna AP, Smithells RW, Fielding DW (1975) Congenital heart disease in Liverpool 1960–1969. Q J Med 44 (173): 17

Kennedy WP (1967) Epidemiologic aspects of the problems of congenital malformations. Birth Defects 3: 1

Kerber IJ, Warr OS, Richardson CJ (1968) Pregnancy in a patient with a prosthetic mitral valve. Association with a fetal anomaly attributed to warfarin sodium. JAMA 203: 223

Knox G, Braithwaite F (1962) Cleft lip and palates in Northumberland and Durham. Arch Dis Child 38: 66

Krick JA, Remington JS (1978) Toxoplasmosis in the adult, an overview. JAMA 298: 550

Kurisu K, Niswander JD, Johnston MC, Maxaheri M (1974) Facial morphology as an indicator of genetic predisposition to cleft lip and palate. Am J Hum Genet 26: 703

Lancet Leader (1977) Screening for neural-tube defects. Lancet 1: 1345

Laurence KM (1963) Hypertrophic pyloric stenosis. Lancet 1: 224

Laurence KM, Gregory P (1976) Prenatal diagnosis of chromosome disorders. Br Med Bull 32: 9

Leck I (1963) Incidence of malformations following influenza epidemics. Br J Prev Soc Med 17: 70

Leck I (1972) The etiology of human malformations. Insights from epidemiology. Teratology 5: 303

Leck I (1974) Causation of neural tube defects: clues from epidemiology. Br Med Bull 30: 158

Leck I (1976) Descriptive epidemiology of common malformations (excluding central nervous system defects). Br Med Bull 32: 45

Leck I (1978) Maternal hyperthermia and anencephaly. Lancet 1: 671

Lemoine P, Harousseau H, Borteyni JP (1968) Les enfants de parents alcooliques: anomalies observées. Quest Med 25: 476

Lenz W (1962) Thalidomide and congenital abnormalities. Lancet 1: 45

Lenz W, Knapp K (1962) Foetal malformations due to thalidomide. German Medical Monthly 7: 253

Lilienfeld AM (1969) Population differences in frequency of malformation at birth. In: Fraser FC, McKusick VA (eds) Congenital malformations. Proceedings of the Third International Congress. Exerpta Medica, Amsterdam New York, p 251

Lloyd-Davies RW (1963) Hypertrophic pyloric stenosis. Lancet 1: 110

Lowe CR (1972) Congenital malformations and the problems of their control. Br Med J 3: 515

Machin GA (1974) Chromosome abnormality and perinatal death. Lancet 1: 594

MacVicar J (1976) Ante-natal detection of fetal abnormality—physical methods. Br Med Bull 32: 4

Matsumoto H, Koya G, Takeuchi T (1965) Fetal minamata disease. A neuropathological study of two cases of intrauterine intoxication by a methylmercury compound. J Neuropathol Exp Neurol 24: 563

McBride WG (1961) Thalidomide and congenital abnormalities. Lancet 2: 1358

McKeown T, Record RC (1960) Malformations in a population observed for five years after birth. In: Wolstenholme GEW, O'Connor CM (eds) Ciba Foundation Symposium on Congenital Malformations. Churchill, London, p 2

Meadow SR (1968) Anticonvulsant drugs and congenital abnormalities. Lancet 2: 1296

Meyer MB, Jonas BS, Tonascia JA (1976) Perinatal events associated with maternal smoking during pregnancy. Am J Epidemiol 103: 464

Miller P, Smith DW, Shepard TH (1978) Maternal hyperthermia as a possible cause of anencephaly. Lancet 1: 519

Mitchell SC, Sellman AH, Westphal MC, Park J (1971) Etiologic correlates in a study of congenital heart disease in 56,109 births. Am J Cardiol 28: 653

Murphy DP (1929) The outcome of 625 pregnancies in women subjected to pelvic radium or roentgen irradiation. Am J Obstet Gynecol 18: 179

Naggan L (1971) Anencephaly and spina bifida in Israel. Pediatrics 47: 577

Neel JV (1974) A note on congenital defects in two unacculturated Indian tribes. In: Janerich DT, Skalko RG, Porter IH (ed) Congenital defects, new directions in research. Academic, New York London, p 3

Nishimura H (1970) Incidence of malformations in abortions. In: Fraser FC, McKusick A (ed) Congenital malformations. Proceedings of the Third International Congress. Exerpta Medica, Amsterdam New York, p 275

Ontario Perinatal Study Committee (1967) Second report of the perinatal mortality study in ten university teaching hospitals, vol I. Ontario Department of Health, Toronto

Peñaloza D, Arias-Stella J, Sime F, Recavarren S, Marticorena E (1964) The heart and pulmonary circulation in children at high altitudes: physiological, anatomical and clinical observations. Pediatrics 34: 568

Powell BW (1962) Hypertrophic pyloric stenosis. Lancet 2: 1326

Rawles WE, Desmyter J, Melnick JL (1968) Serological diagnosis and fetal involvement in maternal rubella. Criteria for abortions. JAMA 203: 627

Richards IDG, Roberts CJ, Lloyd S (1972) Dolichol phosphates as acceptors of manrose from guanosine diphosphate manrose in liver systems. Br J Prev Soc Med 26: 89

Roberts CJ, Lowe CR (1975) Where have all the conceptions gone? Lancet 1: 498

Rogers SC, Morris M (1973) Anencephalus: a changing sex ratio. Br J Prev Soc Med 27: 81

Saxén I (1975) Epidemiology of cleft lip and palate. An attempt to rule out chance correlations. Br J Prev Soc Med 29: 103

Screening for neural tube defects (1977) Annotation. Lancet 1: 1345

Select Committee on Drunkenness (1834) Report on drunkenness presented to the House of Commons

Simpson WJA (1957) A preliminary report on cigarette smoking and the incidence of prematurity. Am J Obstet Gynecol 73: 808

Singer DB, Rudolph AJ, Rosenberg HS, Rawles WE, Noniuk M (1967) Pathology of the congenital rubella syndrome. J Pediatr 71: 665

Smithells RW (1973) Defects and disabilities of thalidomide children. Br Med J 1: 269

Smithells RW (1976) Environmental teratogens of man. Br Med Bull 32: 27

Smithells RW, Sheppard S (1978) Teratogenicity testing in humans. A method demonstrating safety of Bendectin. Teratology 17: 31

South MA, Tompkins WAF, Morris CR, Rawles WE (1969) Congenital malformation of the central nervous system associated with genital type (type 2) herpesvirus. J Pediatr 75: 13

Speidel BD, Meadow SR (1974) Epilepsy, anticonvulsants and congenital malformations. Drugs 8: 354

Stephenson JBP (1976) Epilepsy: a neurological complication of thalidomide embryopathy. Dev Med Child Neurol 18: 189

Therkelson AJ, Grunnet N, Hjort T, Myhre O, Jensen J, Jonasson J, Lauritson JG, Lindsten B, Petersen B (1974) Studies on spontaneous abortions. In: Bové A, Thibault C (eds) Chromosomal errors in relation to reproductive failure. Institut National de la Santé et de la Recherche Médicale, Paris

Thiersch JB (1952) Therapeutic abortions with a folic acid antagonist, 4-aminopterolyglutamic acid (4-amino-PGA). Am J Obstet Gynecol 63: 1298

Trimble BK, Baird PA (1978) Congenital anomalies of the central nervous system. Incidence in British Columbia 1952–1972. Teratology 17: 43

Warkany J (1976) Warfarin embryopathology. Teratology 14: 205

Wilkins L (1960) Masculinisation of female fetus due to use of orally given progestins. JAMA 172: 1028

Witschi E (1969) Teratogenic effects from overripeness of the egg. In: Fraser FC, McKusick A (eds) Congenital malformations. Proceedings of the Third International Conference. Exerpta Medica, Amsterdam New York, p 157

Woolf CM (1971) Congenital cleft lip. A genetic study of 496 propositi. J Med Genet 8: 65

Wynne-Davies R (1964) Family studies and the cause of congenital club foot. Talipes equinovarus, talipes calcaneovalgus and metatarsus varus. J Bone Joint Surg [Br] 46: 445

Wynne-Davies R (1970a) A family study of neonatal and late-diagnosis congenital dislocation of the hip. J Med Genet 7: 315

Wynne-Davies R (1970b) Acetabular dysplasia and familial joint laxity: two etiological factors in congenital dislocation of the hip. A review of 589 patients and their families. J Bone Joint Surg [Br] 52: 704

Yerushalmy J (1970) The California Child Health and Development Studies. Study design and some illustrative findings on congenital heart disease. In: Fraser FC, McKusick A (eds) Congenital malformations. Proceedings of the Third International Conference. Exerpta Medica, Amsterdam New York, p 199

Chapter 4

Cardiac Pathology

Anton E. Becker and Robert H. Anderson

The pathology of the heart in the paediatric age group can be divided into congenital lesions and postnatally acquired heart disease.

The first category is by far the larger, but experience has shown that many pathologists consider a congenitally malformed heart a mystery, a notion based on the misconception that profound knowledge of embryology is a prerequisite for its understanding. However, it is still possible, without any knowledge of cardiac embryogenesis, to classify a congenitally malformed heart and to understand the pathophysiology from the anatomy observed.

In recent years, interest in congenital disease has revived, owing mainly to the surgeon's urge for a detailed and unambiguous description of congenital cardiac malformations. This 'renaissance' has led to the development of segmental analysis of the congenitally malformed heart. In this section we will employ a purely descriptive system of segmental analysis, in this way avoiding matters of controversial interpretation.

Postnatally acquired heart disease in the paediatric age group is of minor importance in the West. However, acquired disease in the setting of congenital heart disease is achieving increasing significance.

1. Autopsy Technique

It is not our purpose to describe a full autopsy technique in detail, but simply to point out some steps that are of particular significance in patients with congenital heart disease.

1.1. Examination of the Visceral Situs

Particular attention should be given to the abdominal and thoracic visceral situs, since important information can immediately be obtained. Thus, abdominal heterotaxia is almost always associated with an abnormal thoracic situs and abnormalities of the heart. The finding of *absence of the spleen* should therefore immediately alert the pathologist to the likelihood of an abnormal thoracic situs. Nearly always 'asplenia' is accompanied by bilateral symmetry of the tracheobronchial tree resulting in the presence of paired eparterial (morphologically right) bronchi and usually of paired trilobed lungs (Fig. 4.1; see also p. 95. In turn, the presence of bilateral eparterial bronchi (dextroisomerism of the bronchi) is nearly always associated with an abnormal atrial situs in which both atria show anatomical features of a morphologically right atrium, evidenced externally by the presence of a morphologically right atrial appendage on both the right and the left side. One can then anticipate severe abnormalities in the cardiovascular system.

Identification of *polysplenia* is also of significance. In this condition multiple spleens are present, located on both sides of the mesogastrium (Fig. 4.2a). This finding must, of course, be distinguished from accessory spleens, which are always present on the left side of the mesogastrium, as is the normal spleen. Polysplenia has a tendency to be associated with symmetrical development of left-sided structures, so that the lungs show two lobes on either side, with bilateral hyparterial bronchi (Fig. 4.2b). As with dextroisomerism, this levoisomerism is usually accompanied by symmetrical development of the atria, both of which show left-sided characteristics; this is particularly obvious in the atrial appendages. Recognition of this condition will again serve as an indicator of the presence of cardiovascular abnormalities (p. 92).

The pathophysiological consequences of symmetrical development of the viscera reach far beyond the splenic abnormalities themselves. For this reason, the term 'visceral symmetry syndrome' has been introduced (p. 139), which is preferred to 'asplenia syndrome' and 'polysplenia syndrome'. The syndrome in fact describes an additional situs, namely situs ambiguus (Van Mierop et al. 1970), and this can be dextroisomeric or levoisomeric. Recognition of situs ambiguus at autopsy makes in situ preparation of the systemic and pulmonic venous systems mandatory.

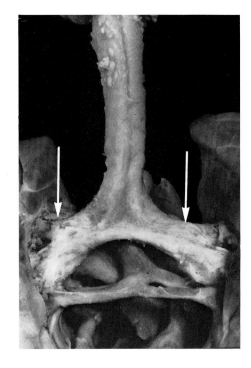

Fig. 4.1. Photograph illustrating the presence of paired eparterial ▷ bronchi (*arrows*) in a patient with absence of the spleen. Heart–lung preparation viewed from behind, showing in detail the artery to the lower lobes on both sides passing beneath the upper lobe bronchus. Cf. Fig. 4.2b.

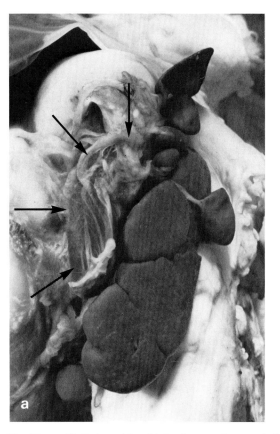

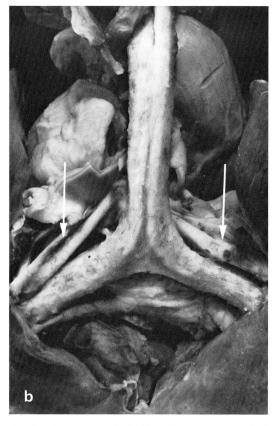

Fig. 4.2. a and **b.** Patient with multiple spleens: **a** photograph showing the splenic mass on both sides of the mesogastrium in detail. It is made up of multiple spleens, the ones on the right (*arrows*) being covered by the mesentery; **b** lungs of the same patient. The lower lobe pulmonary arteries on both sides cross over the upper lobe bronchi (*arrows*). Cf. Fig. 4.1.

1.2. Examination of the Heart

The position of the cardiac apex can give clues to the likelihood of intracardiac malformations, but in itself does not constitute a cardiac anomaly. Meso-cardia, a situation in which the apex points downwards in the mid-line, should suggest the possibility of some sort of rotational disturbance, particularly when associated with abdominal het-erotaxia. Dextrocardia, i.e., the heart in the right side of the chest with the apex pointing to the right, can exist with any atrial situs. In the presence of situs solitus of the thoracic organs and atria it is often associated with 'inversion' of the ventricles and abnormal connections of the great arteries. The finding of levocardia in situs inversus should alert the pathologist to similar possibilties (p. 95).

Proceeding to the systemic and pulmonary venous systems, two points can be made. Firstly, the finding of a suprahepatic segment of the inferior caval vein does not always indicate the presence of normal drainage of the abdominal inferior vena cava. Indeed, drainage of the infrahepatic inferior caval vein via the azygos venous system into the superior caval vein frequently occurs in the presence of a normal suprahepatic cava. This arrangement, if found, should raise suspicion of the visceral sym-metry syndrome. The second point relates to the type of pulmonary venous connection. When normally connected the heart is restricted in its mobility after the pericardium has been opened. However, in most instances of abnormal pulmonary venous con-nections the heart can easily be lifted out of its posterior pericardial bed, immediately alerting the surgeon to the presence of this condition (Fig. 4.3).

The morphology of the atrial appendages is of particular significance, raising the suspicion of the presence of abnormal visceral situs, as outlined above (p. 87). Juxtaposition of atrial appendages, defined as the situation in which both appendages are positioned at the same side of the arterial pedicle, whether right or left (Fig. 4.4), is an important feature indicating serious additional cardiac malfor-mations in most instances (Menhuish and Van Praagh 1968).

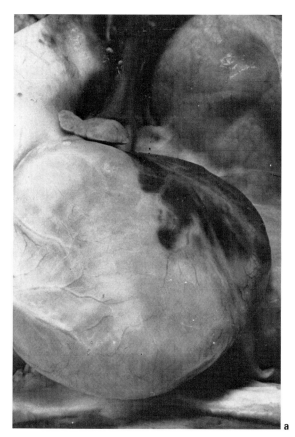
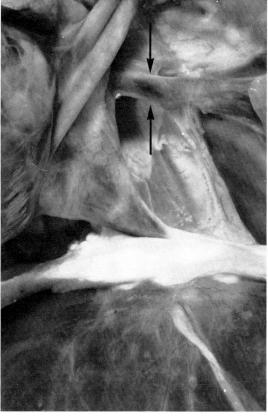

Fig. 4.3 a and **b** Patient with multiple spleens: **a** photograph showing the splenic mass on both sides of the mesogastrium in detail. It is its pericardial bed, since the left atrium is no longer anchored by normally connected pulmonary veins: **a** the heart in situ; **b** the heart tilted ventrally and to the right. Note the anomalous common channel (*arrows*) draining the left lung.

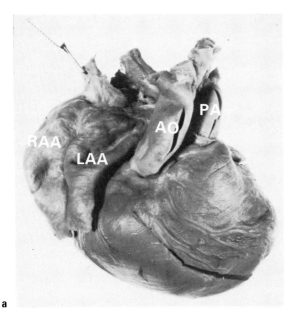

a

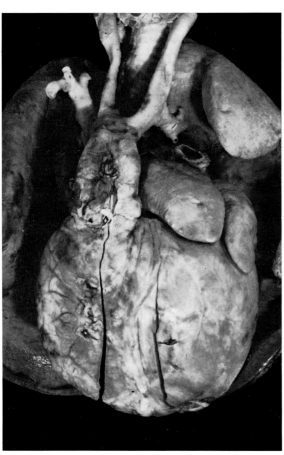

b

Fig. 4.4. a and **b** Photographs illustrating juxtaposition of the atrial appendages: **a** both appendages (*RAA, LAA*) are located to the right of the arterial pedicle (*Ao, PA*); so-called right juxtaposition; **b** left juxtaposition.

The epicardial course of the coronary arteries is particularly useful in determining the position and size of the ventricles. In hearts with a marked ventricular underdevelopment the anterior and posterior descending coronary arteries clearly indicate the plane of the interventricular septum and the position of the diminutive ventricle. Similarly, in other complicated cardiac malformations, such as hearts with straddling atrioventricular valves or univentricular hearts with rudimentary chambers, the surface anatomy of the coronary arteries is an excellent guide to the position of the septum.

Finally, examination of the heart should focus on the great arteries. An abnormal relationship between the aorta and pulmonary trunk tends to indicate an abnormal connection between arteries and ventricles, although it is necessary to emphasize that an abnormal relationship in itself is not indicative of any particular ventriculo–arterial connection or of a specific underlying ventricular anatomy.

1.3. Dissection of Veins and Arteries

As stated above, when situs ambiguus of the thoracic viscera is present, an in situ dissection of veins in both thorax and abdomen is desirable. In situ dissection of the aortic arch and its main branches is also advisable. In this fashion an aberrant subclavian artery will be identified *before* it is severed. Moreover, careful dissection will reveal the presence or absence of systemic collateral vessels to the lungs; this observation is significant in the pathophysiology of any case, but particularly in the presence of pulmonary atresia. The state of the ductus arteriosus needs careful evaluation. A reliable impression of its functional status can be obtained from inspection of its exterior, particularly its size relative to the pulmonary trunk and aortic arch. In our experience, probing of the ductus arteriosus is not strictly necessary and may indeed give a false impression of its functional significance. Too often a ductus is found to be 'probe patent', with the connotation of being functionally open, while the pathologist has in fact pushed a probe through a constricted lumen. Moreover, probing the ductus will damage its interior and may thus hamper histological investigations regarding its state of closure.

1.4. Dissection of the Heart

The heart and lungs, together with the great arteries and the trachea, should preferably be removed en bloc. This technique has the advantage that the various interrelationships are preserved, while a careful dissection in more pleasant surroundings

than are usually provided by an autopsy room is
then possible.

The heart should be opened in such a way as to
minimize the risk of damaging the internal architecture or the conduction system. To this end, the
following guidelines are suggested, although one
should always be prepared to adjust the method
according to the findings observed on examination
and during opening.

The right atrium can be opened through an
incision starting in the right atrial appendage and
curving down towards the right atrioventricular
junctional area, thereby skirting the sulcus terminalis (Fig. 4.5a). Septal structures and sinus
venosus valves are thus left intact. Moreover,
abnormal structures within the right atrial cavity are
not directly compromised, while a good display of
the interior of the right atrium is obtained. The left
atrium is opened by incising the roof of the cavity
between the two lower lobe veins (Fig. 4.5b). The
incision can be extended into these veins, thereby
creating a good view of the rest of the atrium. Ostial
stenosis of pulmonary veins or an unexpected cor
triatriatum can thus be diagnosed before irreversible
damage has been inflicted, and such an incision will
not open a persistent left superior vena cava. The
right-sided ventricle is best opened by incising its
anterior wall guided by a probe through an arterial
outlet (Fig. 4.5c). Extension of the incision will
depend upon the architecture encountered. A similar
approach is appropriate for the left-sided ventricle
(Fig. 4.5d). If no arterial outlet is present the
ventricular cavity can be opened in its inlet part,
leaving the atrioventricular junctional area intact.
Similarly, the ventriculo–arterial junction should be
inspected prior to incision.

1.5. The Conduction System

In some instances full pathological examination of
the heart may require a study of the conduction
system. This is another topic that is shrouded in
mystery for many pathologists, but we feel this
attitude is unjustified, since the examination is not
difficult to perform. In the normal heart the sinus
node is located in the sulcus terminalis lateral to the
junction of the superior vena cava and the right
atrium. The atrioventricular conduction tissues are

Fig. 4.5. a–d Photographs to illustrate the initial incisions for
opening of the atria and ventricles in a normally connected heart:
a right atrial incision. b left atrial incision, connecting the ostia of
the right and left lower lobe pulmonary veins. Both incisions
enable a clear inspection of the interior of the atria and atrioventricular orifices with a minimal chance of damaging important
structures. c incision of the right ventricular anterior wall, guided
by a probe.

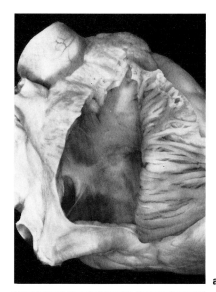
a

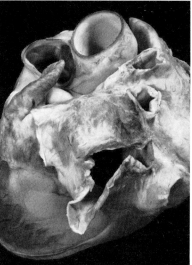
b

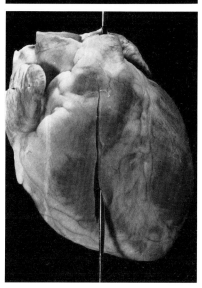
c

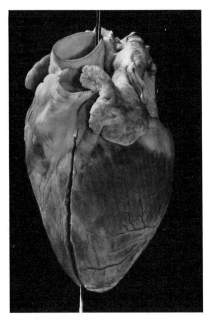

d

Fig. 4.5. (*continued*) **d** shows a similar left ventricular incision. The initial incision should be made approximately halfway along the right ventricular outflow and close to the apex in the left ventricle. Elongation of the incision should always be accompanied by close inspection.

located in the atrial septum adjacent to the central fibrous body, and the atrioventricular bundle (of His) is found between the membranous and muscular components of the ventricular septum. Removal of the entire right atrium in neonatal hearts will permit study of the conduction system by either serial or subserial sectioning (Fig. 4.6). In larger hearts separate blocks containing the sinus node and the atrioventricular conduction tissues can be removed and sectioned in a similar fashion. It is our opinion that insistence on the necessity of full serial sectioning in any study of the conduction system deters investigators from this task. While such a technique is clearly ideal, a considerable amount of information can be obtained by using subserial methods (Davies 1971: Smith et al. 1977; Becker et al. 1978c). Conduction tissue in malformed hearts will be discussed briefly in the appropriate sections. For study in these hearts, it is necessary to examine any union of a ventricular septal structure, if present, with the atrioventricular junctions.

2. Segmental Analysis of the Heart

Segmental analysis of the heart (Van Praagh 1972; Shinebourne et al. 1976; Brandt and Calder 1977) is based on the identification of the various 'building blocks' that constitute the heart and the way in which these segments are connected. In other words, a basic flow pattern through the heart is established through a number of sequential steps. We will discuss these steps in order, beginning with chamber identification, followed by the connections and relations at different junctional levels (Tynan et al. 1979).

2.1. Chamber Identification

The identification of cardiac chambers is based on morphological criteria (Figs. 4.7 and 4.8).

The fundamental criterion distinguishing between right and left atria is the morphological aspect of the atrial appendages (Fig. 4.9). The right atrial appendage has a broad pedicle and is blunt, while the left atrial appendage has a narrow pedicle and is more narrow and hooked (Fig. 4.9). Other features, such as venous connections and septal characteristics, are highly variable and may not be much help when the anomaly is complex. In complex cases the clinician generally relies on tracheobronchial anatomy, as visualized by a penetrating chest roentgenogram, to establish atrial situs. This approach is based on the premise that tracheobronchial and atrial anatomy are concordant (Macartney et al. 1978). Few exceptions to this rule have been described (Caruso and Becker 1979).

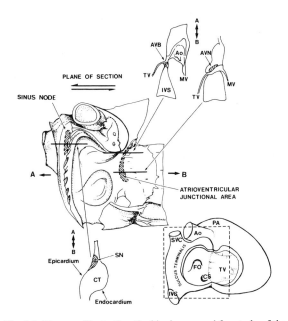

Fig. 4.6. Diagram illustrating the block removed for study of the conduction tissues from the neonatal heart and representative sections through the sinus node and atrioventricular conduction axis.

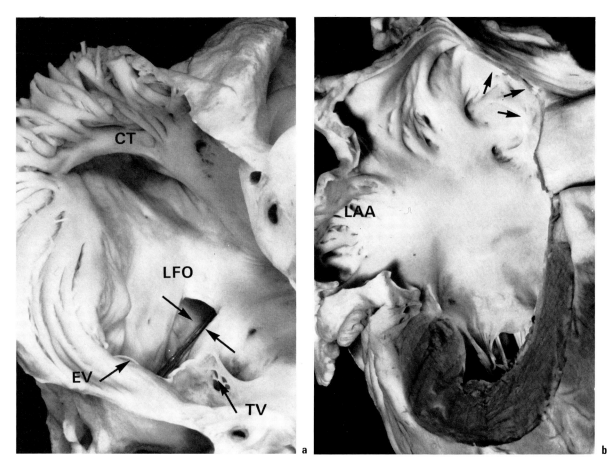

Fig. 4.7. a and **b** Anatomical characteristics of morphological right and left atria. **a** Opened right atrium with an extensive crista terminalis (*CT*) with radiating pectinate muscles. The limbus of the fossa ovalis (*LFO*) delineates the area of the foramen ovale through which a probe has been passed (*arrows*). Note also the remnants of the right sinus venosus valve, recognizable as the Eustachian (*EV*) and Thebesian (*TV*) valves. **b** Left atrium and left atrial appendage (*LAA*). There is no crista terminalis and the flap valve of the fossa ovalis is seen on the roughened septal surface (*arrows*).

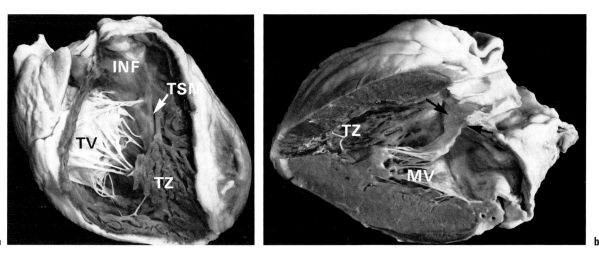

Fig. 4.8. a and **b** Photographs showing the anatomical characteristics of the right and left ventricles. **a** Opened right ventricle with the tricuspid valve (*TV*) in its inlet portion, the coarse trabecular zone (*TZ*), the complete muscular infundibulum (*INF*) and the trabecula septomarginalis (*TSM*) on the septal surface. **b** Opened left ventricle containing the mitral valve (*MV*) in its inlet portion, the fine trabecular zone (*TZ*), the smooth septal surface, and the arterial valve in fibrous continuity with the mitral valve (*arrows*).

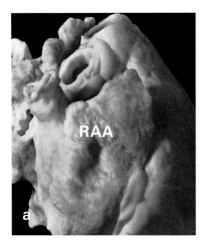
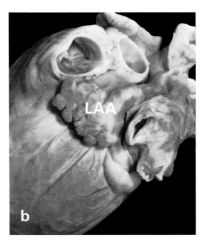

Fig. 4.9. a and b Photographs illustrating the difference in morphology between the right (*RAA*, a) and left (*LAA*, b) atrial appendages.

Identification of the morphologically right and left ventricles is based predominantly on the pattern of the ventricular trabeculae and on the architecture of the atrioventricular valve apparatus. It is important to appreciate that a normal ventricle has *three* anatomic components (Figs. 4.8 and 4.10). These are the inlet, that part related to and supporting the atrioventricular valve; the apical trabecular component; and the outlet, that part supporting the arterial valve. As will be seen, this tripartite ventricular division is of major significance in categorization of the univentricular heart and hearts with straddling valves.

2.2. Atrial Situs

Once the morphology of the atria has been identified the situs can be established. Situs solitus is present when the morphologically right atrium is on the right and the morphologically left atrium is on the left. Situs inversus of atria is the mirror-image situation (Fig. 4.11). Situs ambiguus characterizes the situation in which both atria exhibit morphological features of either a morphologically right or a morphologically left atrium. Situs ambiguus of the atria is therefore subclassified into 'bilateral right' (dextroisomeric) and 'bilateral left' (levoisomeric) types (Fig. 4.12).

When atrial situs has been established additional anomalies need a separate specification, e.g., 'persistent left superior caval vein connected to the coronary sinus' or 'unilateral total anomalous pulmonary venous connection to right atrium', etc.

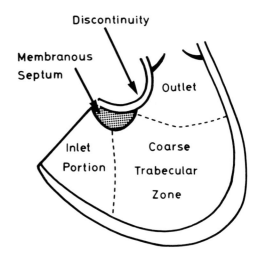

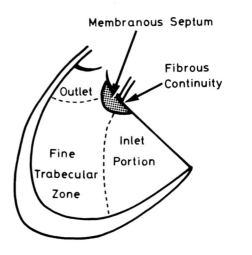

Fig. 4.10. Diagram illustrating the anatomical zones of the (a) right and left (b) ventricles. Cf. Fig. 4.8.

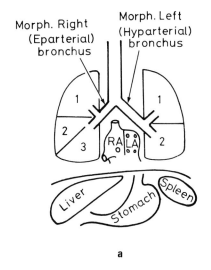

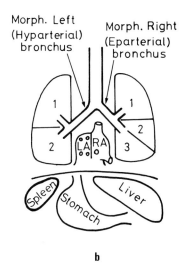

Fig. 4.11. **a** and **b** Diagrams illustrating the arrangement of thoracic and abdominal viscera in situs solitus (**a**) and situs inversus (**b**).

a   **b**

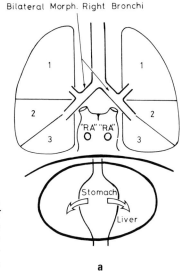

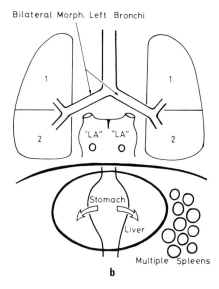

Fig. 4.12. **a** and **b** Diagrams illustrating the usual arrangement of thoraco-abdominal viscera in the two forms of situs ambiguus, dextroisomerism, usually with asplenia (**a**) and levoisomerism, usually with polysplenia (**b**).

a   **b**

2.3. Atrioventricular Junction

In the normal heart the atrioventricular connection is *concordant*; i.e., the morphologically right atrium connects to the morphologically right ventricle through the tricuspid valve and the left atrium connects to the left ventricle through the mitral valve (Fig. 4.13a). In congenital heart malformations, however, one should be prepared for the finding of an abnormal type of atrioventricular connection. If the right atrium connects to a morphologically left ventricle and the left atrium to a morphologically right ventricle the connection is termed *discordant* (Fig. 4.13b). Another possibility is that both atria connect to the same ventricle, a situation termed *double inlet atrioventricular connection* (Fig. 4.13d). One of the atrial chambers may have no connection,

either actual or potential, with the underlying chambers, a situation defined as *absence of one atrioventricular connection* (Fig. 4.13e). Very rarely one of the two atria may discharge its blood through two atrioventricular valves into the underlying ventricles, the contralateral atrium having no atrioventricular connection. This condition is defined as *double outlet atrium.*

From the above definitions it follows that a connection can only be classified as either concordant or discordant when positive identification of *both* atria and ventricles has been established. In the case of situs ambiguus of the atria (p. 94), any connection between the atria and the two underlying ventricles is classified by necessity as an *ambiguous connection* (Fig. 4.13c). The position of the ventricles is then added to give a full account of the situation,

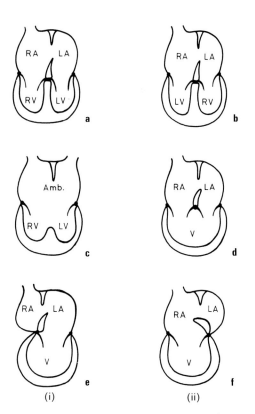

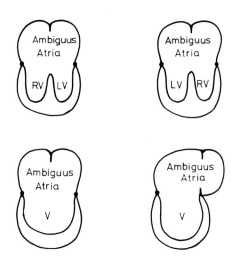

Fig. 4.14. Diagrams illustrating the ventricular relationships and atrioventricular connections possible with situs ambiguus. *Above,* ambiguous atrioventricular connections; *below left,* double-inlet ventricle; *below right,* absent left AV connection. It can also exist with absent right atrioventricular connection. Abbreviations as in Fig. 4.13.

Fig. 4.13. a–e Diagrams illustrating the five basic types of atrioventricular connection. RA, right atrium; LA, left atrium; AMB, ambiguus atria; RV, right ventricle; LV, left ventricle; V, ventricle of univentricular heart. **a** concordant; **b** discordant; **c** ambiguous; **d** double inlet; **e** absent right (i) or left (ii) connection.

for instance 'ambiguous atrioventricular connection with the right ventricle to the right' (Fig. 4.14). However, ambiguous atria may connect to only one underlying chamber, either via a double inlet connection or because of the absence of one connection (Fig. 4.14). In these circumstances, the appropriate connection can be defined accordingly. Indeed, hearts with situs solitus or inversus and either double inlet connection or absence of one connection have the additional feature that only one chamber in the ventricular mass receives the atrial inlets (with the exceedingly rare exception of double outlet atrium). We have used this fact to categorize all such hearts as *univentricular hearts.* This does not mean that all univentricular hearts contain only one chamber in their ventricular mass. What it does mean is that the chamber receiving the inlets is designated the *ventricle* while the chamber that does not receive an atrial inlet is categorized as a *rudimentary chamber.* As in biventricular hearts, both ventricles and rudimentary chambers in univentricular hearts possess trabecular components (Fig. 4.15). When the ventricle exhibits trabecular characteristics of the left ventricle the rudimentary

chamber is of right ventricular pattern and vice versa. The appropriate term for such hearts would then be 'univentricular heart of left ventricular or right ventricular type with rudimentary chamber'. The relationships of rudimentary chambers to ventricles should also be specified in simple descriptive terms.

It should be emphasized that thus far only the *type* of atrioventricular connection has been considered, together with the consequences it has for ventricular morphology and terminology. As a second step, the *mode* of the connection should be established (Fig. 4.16). In the normal heart the connection is established through two 'perforate' atrioventricular ostia. However, in the malformed heart one of the two connections may be composed of an imperforate membrane. In this situation the atrium will still be in potential connection with the underlying ventricle. This situation is therefore basically different, as far as the anatomy is concerned, from an absent connection, in which not even a potential connection is present (Fig. 4.17). An *imperforate valve* may thus coincide with concordant, discordant ambiguous, or double inlet atrioventricular connections. Another

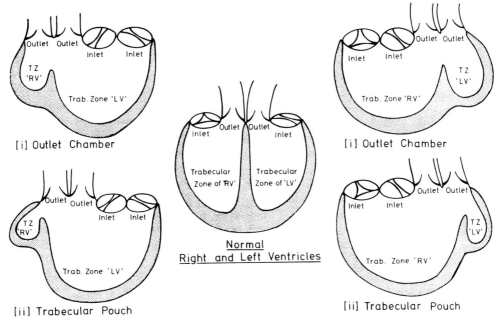

[i] Outlet Chamber

[ii] Trabecular Pouch

A. Rudimentary Chambers of RV Type
in Univentricular Heart LV Type

Normal
Right and Left Ventricles

[i] Outlet Chamber

[ii] Trabecular Pouch

B. Rudimentary Chambers of LV Type
in Univentricular Heart RV Type

Fig. 4.15. a and **b** Diagrams illustrating the components of ventricles and rudimentary chambers and the way they can be arranged to form univentricular hearts. Reproduced from Tynan et al. (1979), by permission of the editor of the *British Heart Journal.*

mode of connection is that characterized by presence of a *common atrioventricular valve*. If such a 'common valve' occurs with a concordant atrioventricular connection, the right atrium still connects to the right ventricle and the left atrium to the left ventricle. However, in more complicated conditions a discordant or double inlet connection can be present through a common atrioventricular valve. We would not use the term common valve in hearts with an absent atrioventricular connection, because in such hearts the valve present connects to only one atrium. We accept that in some circumstances the single valve may resemble a common valve in terms of morphology, but we prefer to utilize the connection as our criterion. A third, and more complicated, mode of connection is the one in which the tension apparatus of an atrioventricular valve is attached to both sides of an underlying ventricular septum; a condition defined as *straddling atrioventricular* valve. This condition will raise problems in classification of the heart, because the degree of overriding may vary considerably. It is for this reason that a 50% rule has been introduced (Tynan et al. 1979). If an atrioventricular valve overrides a ventricular septum by 50% or more the orifice is considered to belong to the ventricle receiving the greater part of its circumference, because the degree of overriding determines the type of connection. For instance, if the right atrioventricular valve connects through a straddling valve for the major part to a left

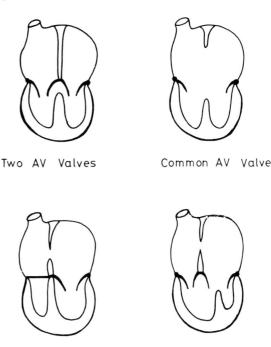

Two AV Valves   Common AV Valve

Imperforate AV Valve   Straddling AV Valve

Fig. 4.16. Diagram illustrating the four different modes of atrioventricular connection that can exist with the various types of connection. Note that the imperforate valve should be distinguished from an absent atrioventricular connection (cf. Fig. 4.17). Reproduced from Shinebourne and Anderson, *Concise Paediatric Cardiology* (1979), by permission of Oxford University Press.

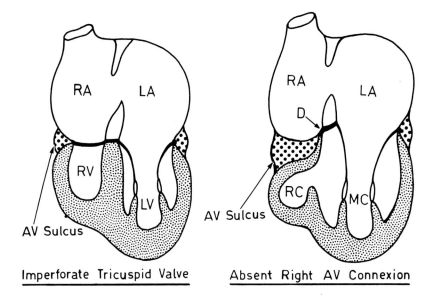

Fig. 4.17. Diagram illustrating the difference between an imperforate tricuspid valve (mode of connection) and an absent right atrioventricular connection (type of connection). In the latter the dimple (*D*) in the right atrial (*RA*) floor points to the main chamber (*MC*). The other chamber is rudimentary (*RC*) and the heart is univentricular. Reproduced from Anderson et al. (1979), by permission of the editors of *Paediatric Cardiology*.

ventricular chamber, which also receives the left atrioventricular valve, the connection is then 'double inlet with a straddling right atrioventricular valve' (Fig. 4.18a). If, however, a similar architecture is present, but with the straddling right atrioventricular valve committed mainly to the right ventricle, the situation would be 'concordant with a straddling right atrioventricular valve' (Fig. 4.18b). This approach may seem cumbersome at first glance, but it has the advantage that it accounts for a basic pattern of flow and circumvents many problems of semantics, e.g., the problem of how to define a ventricle. Instead of the size of the chamber, we advocate use of the inlet part of the chamber as the definitive variable. With the 50% rule a chamber is then considered to be a ventricle when it receives

50% or more of an atrioventricular inlet. Thus, in the example of the straddling right atrioventricular valve (Fig. 4.18), the degree of overriding not only changes the type of connection but also alters the terminology applicable to the underlying chambers. In case of a double inlet atrioventricular connection, by definition one of the underlying chambers receives more than half of both inlets and should therefore be designated as a *ventricle*. The other chamber, receiving less than 50% of the straddler, is then no longer a ventricle but is a *rudimentary chamber* (Fig. 4.18).

As indicated above, when the type and mode of atrioventricular connections have been established, attention should be given to the relationships of chambers in the ventricular mass. For instance,

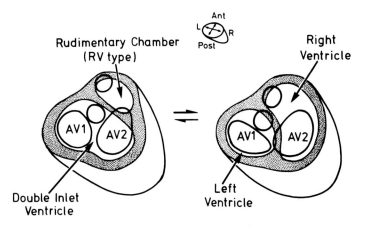

LESS THAN 50% STRADDLING   MORE THAN 50% STRADDLING
∴VENTRICLE & RUDIMENTARY CHAMBER   ∴LEFT VENTRICLE & RIGHT VENTRICLE

Fig. 4.18. Diagrams illustrating the effect that straddling of an atrioventricular valve has on the atrioventricular connection and hence on the terminology of ventricular chambers. Reproduced from Tynan et al. (1979), by permission of the editors of the *British Heart Journal*.

rotational disturbances during the development of the heart may result in a situation where the atrioventricular ostia and ventricles have acquired an abnormal spatial position. This may lead to peculiar relative positions, such as the 'criss-cross' atrioventricular relationship or the 'supero-inferior' or 'upstairs-downstairs' atrioventricular relationships. These conditions can occur with any atrioventricular connection and with all modes of atrioventricular connection.

2.4. Arterial Junction

In the normal heart, the morphologically right ventricle conveys blood into the pulmonary trunk and the left ventricle into the aorta. The arterial junctions are guarded by semilunar valves, each having three cusps. The pulmonary valve is usually widely separated from the tricuspid valve by a bar of muscle, the crista supraventricularis (Fig 5.8a), while the aortic valve shows fibrous continuity with the mitral valve (Fig. 5.8b). The pulmonary ostium is normally anterior and slightly to the left of the aortic ostium. In this situation the type of arterial connection is designated as *concordant* (Fig. 4.19a) with normal relationships. In some rare forms of congenital heart disease a concordant arterial connection may be present, but with an abnormal relationship, e.g., with the pulmonary trunk posterior and to the right and the aorta anterior and to the left. This condition has been termed 'anatomically corrected malposition'.

In the situation where the aorta arises from the right ventricle and the pulmonary trunk from the left, the connection is defined as *discordant* (Fig. 4.19b). Usually this particular condition is designated 'transposition of the great arteries'. However, the term 'transposition' is highly controversial and not unanimously interpreted (Becker 1978). For this reason we will only use the term transposition when further qualified by such terms as 'complete' or 'corrected' (see p. 119). The relationships of the great arteries in a discordant connection also need further specification, like 'aorta anterior and to the right', or 'to the left', etc. (Fig. 4.20).

Other types of arterial connections are *double outlet* (Fig. 4.21) and *single outlet of the heart* (Fig. 4.22). In double outlet, both great arteries arise from one chamber, which can be a ventricle or rudimentary chamber of right or left morphology. On examination of such an outlet it usually appears that the two ostia are separated from each other by a shelf of muscle, the infundibular septum.

In the condition termed single outlet heart there is only one great artery connected to the ventricles. The pathologist has an advantage over the clinician in that he will be able, at least in most instances, to specify this condition further. There are three possibilities: (a) true truncus arteriosus; (b) pulmonary atresia with the aorta as the single arterial trunk; and (c) aortic atresia, with a single pulmonary trunk (Fig. 4.22).

As with the atrioventricular connections, each type of arterial connection needs further specification, according to the mode of connection. Valvar atresia of, for example, a pulmonary valve, may coincide with any of the afore-mentioned types of connection except single outlet. The clinician may have classified a cardiac condition as 'single outlet,

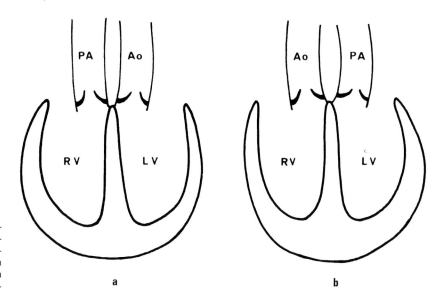

Fig. 4.19. a and **b.** Diagrams illustrating the difference between a concordant (**a**) and discordant (**b**) arterial connection. Reproduced from Tynan et al. (1978), by permission of Churchill Livingstone, Edinburgh.

large ventricular septal defect and pulmonary atresia', but the pathologist may be able to show a potential concordant, discordant or double outlet connection. In other instances of single outlet heart, however, even the pathologist will be unable to find any connection between the atretic trunk and the ventricular chambers on examination of the heart, and these are cases of true single outlet of the heart.

An *overriding arterial valve* creates a similar problem with respect to the classification of the type of connection, as described for the atrioventricular junction. Again, a 50% rule has been advocated (Kirklin et al. 1973). An artery is considered to arise from a ventricle or chamber when 50% or more of its circumference is committed to that chamber (Fig. 4.23). In other words, a double outlet arterial connection could occur with two overriding arterial valves, both committed mainly to the same chamber. Similarly, concordant (Fig 4.23) and discordant arterial connections may coincide with an overriding semilunar valve.

Any description of the arterial junction is incomplete without identification of any abnormal relationships, such as the relative position of the great arteries (Fig. 4.20) and the morphology of the

ventricular outflow tracts, i.e., presence or absence of a subaortic infundibulum or subpulmonary infundibulum.

2.5. Use of Segmental Analysis

With the use of the segmental cardiac analysis depicted above, any type of congenitally malformed heart can be described, irrespective of its complexity. Moreover it avoids controversial matters where different schools of opinion collide and where the same term may have different connotations.

It should be emphasized, however, that the segmental analysis presently advocated (Tynan et al. 1979) is not put forward as a system for classifying congenital heart diseases, or to replace current classifications. It merely facilitates a descriptive approach to the malformed heart, which will enable anyone to discuss a complex case in full knowledge of how the various building blocks have been put together, irrespective of pre-existing detailed knowledge regarding the 'official name' coined for the condition concerned.

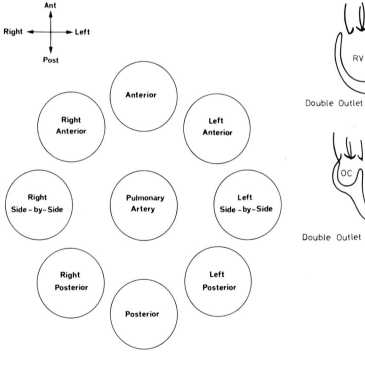

AORTIC POSITIONS

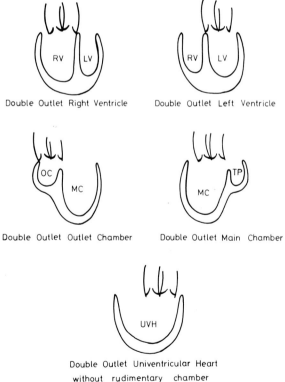

Double Outlet Univentricular Heart
without rudimentary chamber

Fig. 4.20. Diagram illustrating the variability in aortic position relative to the pulmonary artery with any arterial connection. Reproduced from Tynan et al. (1978), *Paediatric Cardiology 1977*, by permission of Churchill Livingstone, Edinburgh.

Fig. 4.21. Diagram illustrating the various types of double outlet chamber. Reproduced from Shinebourne and Anderson (1979), *Concise Paediatric Cardiology* by permission of Oxford University Press.

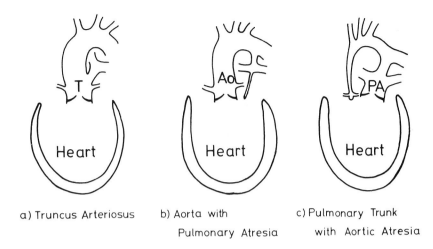

a) Truncus Arteriosus

b) Aorta with Pulmonary Atresia

c) Pulmonary Trunk with Aortic Atresia

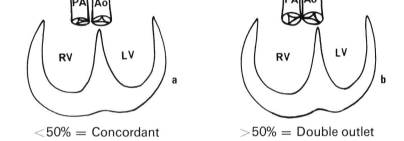

Fig. 4.23. Diagram illustrating the effect of an over riding arterial valve on the arterial connection. **a** <50%, i.e., concordant; **b** >50%, i.e., double outlet.

<50% = Concordant

>50% = Double outlet

3. Congenital Heart Disease

In the Western World, approximately eight newborns per thousand have congenital heart disease (Kerrebijn 1964; Campbell 1968). The most frequent conditions existing in the neonatal period are ventricular septal defect; patent ductus arteriosus; atrial septal defect; aortic coarctation; complete transposition of the great arteries; Fallot's tetralogy; pulmonary stenosis, and aortic stenosis in descending order of frequency (Campbell 1968). However, the significance of these malformations for mortality varies considerably. It can be said that approximately 30% of babies born with a congenital heart defect will die within the first year of life. The malformations that carry the highest early mortality risk are, in descending order of frequency aortic coarctation; left heart hypoplasia; complete transposition of the great arteries; extreme forms of Fallot's tetralogy; right heart hypoplasia and double-outlet right ventricle (Rowe and Mehrizi 1968).

The pathological aspects of these and other malformations will be discussed briefly in the sections below. A subdivision is made, into conditions with a basically normal segmental arrangement and those with an abnormal arrangement.

3.1. Congenital Heart Malformations with Normal Junctional Connections

All defects to be discussed in this section will show *concordant* atrioventricular and arterial connections, with a situs solitus anatomy of the atria assumed for the purpose of description. They can of course all exist with situs inversus and concordant connections, but this is exceedingly rare.

3.1.1. Anomalous Systemic Venous Connections

The most common anomalous systemic venous connection is a *persistent left superior caval vein* (Fig. 4.24), a condition that in itself has no functional significance. The vein runs to the heart anterior to the lung hilum as a continuation of the left innominate vein and usually connects to the coronary sinus. The ostium of the coronary sinus is

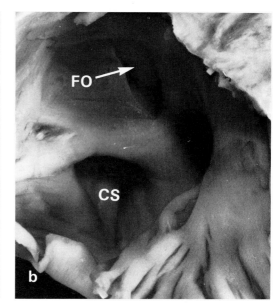

Fig. 4.24. a and **b** Photographs of persistent left superior caval vein. **a** Course of the vein (*LSVC*) as it descends ventral to the hilum of the left lung. The vein continues as the coronary sinus (*CS*). For a good display the heart has been lifted out of its pericardial bed, a procedure facililated by an anomalous pulmonary venous connection (same case as illustrated in Fig. 4.3). **b** Enlarged ostium of the coronary sinus (*CS*) in the opened right atrium. *FO*, foramen ovale.

larger than normal (Fig. 4.24b) and this observation may alert the pathologist to the presence of the anomaly if it has been missed during the initial inspection of the exterior of the heart.

More rarely, a persistent left superior caval vein connects directly to the left atrium. In these instances the coronary sinus is unroofed. As a consequence, an 'atrial septal defect' of the coronary sinus type (p. 105) is usually present. This particular condition, however, is often part of a more complex malformation. In rare cases the persistent left superior caval vein, draining into a coronary sinus, can be associated with absence or atresia of the usual right-sided superior caval vein. The persistent left superior caval vein is then the sole channel for the systemic venous return to the heart, the venous system of the neck and upper mediastinum being a mirror-image of the normal.

Abnormalities of the connections of the inferior caval vein are rare and almost always accompany a complex cardiac malformation.

At the site of the ostium of the inferior caval vein an extensive remnant of the right sinus venosus valve may be present, the so-called Chiari network (Fig. 4.25). In rare instances a sail-like membrane is observed, causing an inlet obstruction to the right ventricle, representing the entire embryonic valve of the sinus venosus. The anomaly may be termed cor triatriatum dexter (Doucette and Knoblich 1963).

The ostium of the coronary sinus in the right

atrium is occasionally occluded or congenitally narrowed. The functional significance of this condition remains speculative.

3.1.2. Anomalous Pulmonary Venous Connections

There is a vast variety of anatomical arrangements of anomalous pulmonary venous connections. Basically, the anomalies can be divided into *bilateral* and *unilateral* types, each of which may display *total* or *partial* involvement of the venous connections. If inspection of the heart has aroused suspicion of an abnormality in the pulmonary venous connections, in situ preparation is mandatory and the pathologist should be prepared to dissect a complex system of venous connections. *Bilateral total anomalous pulmonary venous connection* is characterized by total absence of a direct connection to the left atrium. In the usual instance the pulmonary veins join together behind the left atrium in a confluence. A distinct channel connects the confluence to the systemic venous side of the heart. The most common locations for such an abnormal connection are, in descending order, the left innominate (brachiocephalic) vein; the coronary sinus; the superior caval vein; and the right atrium itself (Fig. 4.26). In rare instances the anomalous connection is established below the diaphragm (Fig. 4.27a). In these cases

Fig. 4.25. Photograph of a chiari ▷ network guarding the ostium of the inferior caval vein.

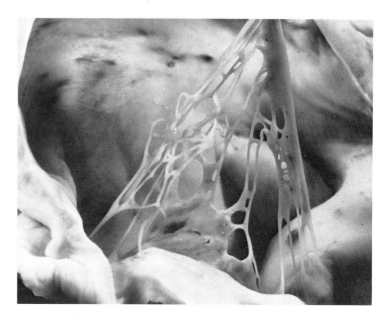

Fig. 4.26. Diagram illustrating the most common sites for an ▷ abnormal connection, in patients with bilateral total anomalous pulmonary venous connection. From Anderson and Ashley (1974) In: *Scientific Foundations of Paediatrics*, by permission of William Heinemann Medical Books Ltd.

Fig. 4.27. a and **b** (*bottom*) Photographs of two specimens with bilateral total anomalous pulmonary venous connection. **a** A case in which the right and left pulmonary veins (*arrows*) join into a common channel which passes through the diaphragm and is connected to the portal vein. The anomalous connection has been divided at the level of the diaphragm. Note the increased mobility of the heart, since the left atrium is no longer anchored posteriorly by pulmonary veins. Fig. 4.3. **b** Example of bilateral total anomalous pulmonary venous connection, in which the veins for the right lung and the vein draining the left lower lobe (*LL*) are connected to the coronary sinus (*CS*). The left upper lobe vein (*LU*) takes a separate route connecting to the left innominate vein. A tiny vein interconnects the two systems (between *arrows*). ▽

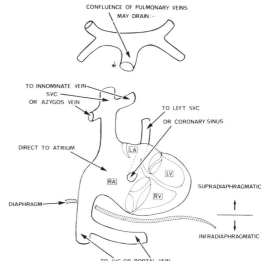

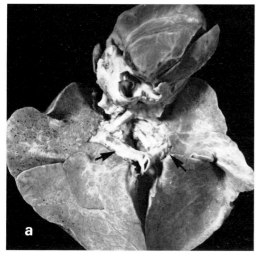

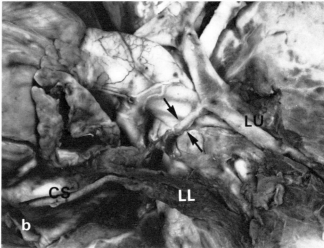

there is a long venous channel, generally accompanying the oesophagus on its way through the diaphragm, which then connects to the portal venous system or inferior vena cava. Generally, infradiaphragmatic connections have an extremely poor prognosis, because they result in a severe obstruction to pulmonary venous drainage. Early mortality, often without proper diagnosis, may occur. The pathologist should therefore be alerted to this arrangement, particularly when his examination of the viscera has suggested the presence of a visceral symmetry syndrome (p. 139). In the presence of a bilateral (or unilateral) total anomalous pulmonary venous connection, different sites of drainage of ' parts of the venous system may be found in the same patient. In particular, in patients with a bilateral total anomalous pulmonary venous connection to the coronary sinus, the left upper lobe of the lung can have a separate venous connection to the left innominate vein with or without additional interconnections with the main pulmonary venous route (Fig. 4.27b).

A particular form of *unilateral anomalous pulmonary venous connection* is the so-called Scimitar syndrome. In this malformation, frequently associated with other anomalies, the pulmonary veins of the right lung, or more frequently of the right lower lobe, connect through a single venous trunk to the inferior caval vein.

It is important for the pathologist also to realize that the clinical symptomatology and prognosis depend mostly on the presence or absence of obstructed drainage. Such obstructions usually result from intrinsic abnormalities, such as the presence of a long narrow channel conveying blood from the confluence to the systemic venous side or drainage into a relatively high-resistance area, e.g., the portal venous system. Rare instances of obstruction owing to external compression can occur when the connecting vein runs between a pulmonary artery and a main bronchus.

3.1.3. Cor Triatriatum Sinister

In cor triatriatum sinister the pulmonary veins connect to a distinct chamber, located posterior to the left atrium. The venous confluence communicates with the left atrium through an opening, which can vary considerably in size but is usually 'pin-hole' size (Fig. 4.28). Because of the restriction of pulmonary venous flow, pulmonary congestion occurs with right heart overload and a low cardiac output. The anatomical counterpart of these haemodynamic consequences is expressed in hypertrophy of right heart structures and the wall of the 'extra' atrium, while the pulmonary veins reveal 'arterialization' (p. 136).

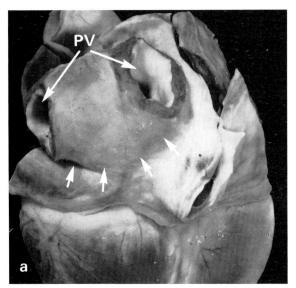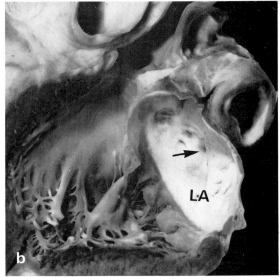

Fig. 4.28. a and **b** Heart specimen exhibiting cor triatriatum sinister. **a** Posterior aspect of the heart. The confluence of the pulmonary veins is vaguely outlined (*arrows*) from the inferior part of the left atrium. Note the marked myocardial hypertrophy at the site where the pulmoary venous connections (*PV*) have been cut. **b** Left side of this heart after removal of the anterolateral wall. A pinhole-size opening (*arrow*) is present between the inferior part of the left atrium (*LA*) and the 'extra' atrium. Note the difference in myocardial thickness between the two chambers.

3.1.4. Atrial Septal Defects

A defect can occur at different locations within the atrial septum. The most common type is an *atrial septal defect of the fossa ovalis type* (also called secundum type). This defect is present at the site of the fossa ovalis and can range in extent from localized small fenestrations in the floor of the fossa, just underneath the limbus, to a large defect extending almost down to the level of the atrio-ventricular valves (Fig. 4.29a). Such defects should not be confused with a probe-patent foramen ovale or a defect secondary to atrial stretch. The latter occurs when excessive dilatation of the left atrium stretches the floor of the fossa ovalis (i.e., the embryonic septum primum), creating a functional defect beneath the limbus. Conditions accompanied by an excessive left atrial overload can lead to herniation of the free edge of the septum primum into the right atrium. In hearts with aortic or mitral atresia this is a common finding, while right atrial

overload, e.g., in tricuspid atresia, may cause aneurysm of the floor of the fossa into the left atrium. A defect of the fossa ovalis type may be associated with anatomical abnormalities of the mitral valve apparatus with aortic coarctation.

Rarely, an atrial septal defect of the fossa ovalis type is located in a more posterior position extending towards the site of entrance of the inferior caval vein. This type of defect has been termed 'posterior defect', although we believe that the term 'fossa ovalis-type defect with posterior extension' would be preferable.

An even rarer type of defect can occur at the site of the anticipated ostium of the coronary sinus, the so-called atrial septal defect of the coronary sinus type. It is almost associated with a persistent left superior caval vein draining directly into the left atrium (p. 102). It is questionable whether such a communication should be classified as an atrial septal defect, but in extremely rare circumstances the coronary sinus may have developed in part, so that

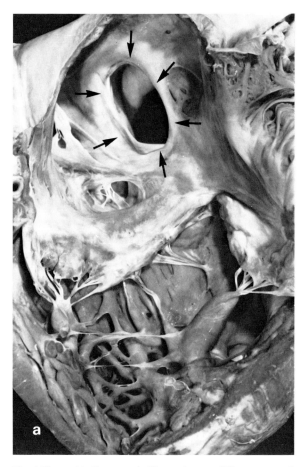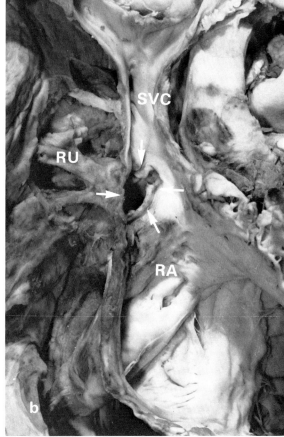

Fig. 4.29. a and **b.** Photographs illustrating two different types of atrial septal defect: **a** a large atrial septal defect of the fossa ovalis type (*arrows*); **b** a sinus venosus type defect (*arrows*), located at the base of the superior caval vein (*SVC*) where it enters the right atrium (*RA*). The ostium of the right upper lobe vein (*RU*) is intimately related to the defect.

bidirectional shunting between the atria can occur through its ostium in the right atrium. If the coronary sinus is better developed, windows may be present between coronary sinus and left atrium, permitting similar shunts (Fig. 4.30).

A special form of atrial septal defect is the so-called *sinus venosus type*. In this condition the defect is situated at the base of the superior caval vein, where it enters the right atrium. The ostium of the right upper lobe pulmonary vein is intimately related to the defect and usually overrides the atrial septum (Fig. 4.29b).

The *primum type of atrial septal defect* will be discussed under the heading of atrioventricular defects (p. 108).

An atrial septal defect will lead to an obligatory left-to-right shunt and an augmented pulmonary blood flow. The natural course of the disease will ultimately lead to irreversible pulmonary hypertension due to plexogenic pulmonary arteriopathy.

3.1.5. *Ventricular Septal Defects*

The terminology of different types of ventricular septal defects is complicated and not uniformly accepted (Becu et al. 1956; Warden et al. 1957; Lev 1959; Goor et al. 1970).

The classification of ventricular septal defects used in this section (Fig. 4.31) is new and has only

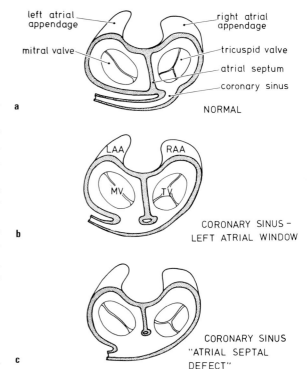

Fig. 4.30. a–c. Diagrams illustrating the close relationship between an atrial septal defect of the coronary sinus type (**c**) associated with a persistent left superior caval vein draining into the left atrium, and the situation in which the wall of the coronary sinus has only partially developed, so that bidirectional atrial shunting in a similar anatomical location is possible (**b**).

Fig. 4.31. Diagram illustrating the basic types of ventricular septal defects.

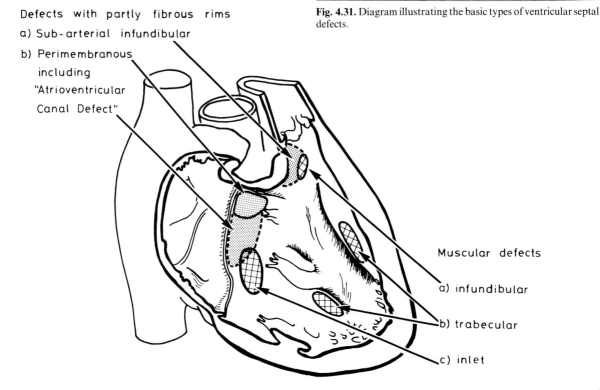

Defects with partly fibrous rims
a) Sub-arterial infundibular
b) Perimembranous
   including
   "Atrioventricular
   Canal Defect"

Muscular defects
a) infundibular
b) trabecular
c) inlet

recently been proposed (Soto et al. 1979). It is based upon the premise that the muscular ventricular septum, as with the ventricles, is composed of three parts, i.e., an inlet part, a trabecular part, and an outlet or infundibulum part (Fig. 4.10). The three parts join at the site of the right fibrous trigone, from which the interventricular part of the membranous septum is derived.

Three basic types of septal defect are then recognized (Fig. 4.31).

A *perimembranous defect* is defined as one in which the membranous septum, either its atrio-ventricular component or a remnant of its inter-ventricular component, forms part of the rim (Fig. 4.32). Perimembranous defects can extend into any of the three septal components, a feature permitting further subclassification if required. When the defect extends into the inlet septum, it is frequently termed an 'atrioventricular canal-type defect' (Neufeld et al. 1961). The significance of recognizing a defect as perimembranous in nature is that irrespective of its main direction of extension, the main axis of the atrioventricular conduction system will be present in its inferior rim, a feature of paramount interest to the surgeon. Perimembranous defects are frequently termed 'infracristal'.

Muscular ventricular septal defects are defined as those completely surrounded by musculature. Again, the subclassification of this type of defect is based on the localization of the defect according to the three parts of the ventricular septum. In other words, a muscular defect can occur in the inlet, trabecular or outlet septa and should be designated accordingly (Fig. 4.31). Muscular defects in the inlet septum may have the atrioventricular conduction axis close to their anterosuperior rim. Defects in the outlet part or trabecular part of the ventricular septum remain remote from the atrioventricular conduction bundle.

The third category is the *subarterial ventricular septal defect* (Fig. 4.33). This defect occurs in the infundibular septum but borders immediately on the arterial junction, so that the conjoined arterial valves constitute its upper rim. This particular type of defect is prone to develop early prolapse of the aortic

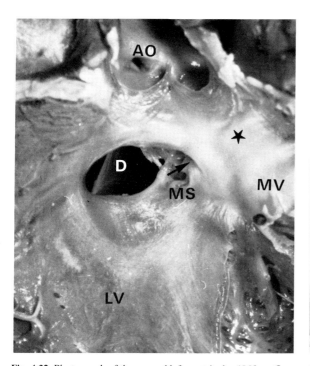

Fig. 4.32. Photograph of the opened left ventricular (*LV*) outflow revealing a perimembranous defect (*D*) with a remnant of the membranous septum (*MS*) in its posterior rim. Components of the tricuspid valve are visible through the defect. The area of fibrous continuity between the aorta (*AO*) and the mitral valve (*MO*) is indicated by an *asterisk*.

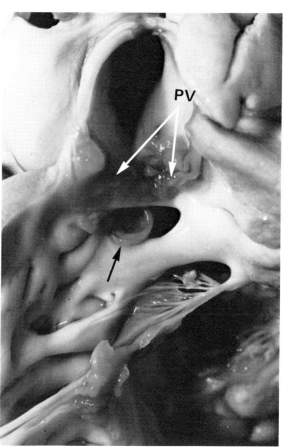

Fig. 4.33. Photograph of the opened right ventricular outflow, revealing a subarterial ventricular septal defect and a prolapsed aortic valve cusp (*arrow*). *PV*, pulmonary valve.

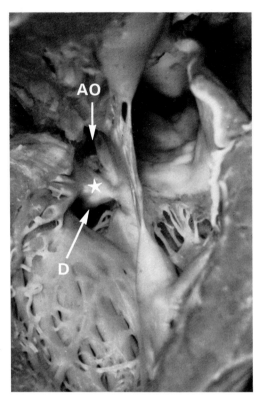

Fig. 4.34. Photograph illustrating the combined occurrence of a ventricular septal defect (*D*) and subvalvar aortic stenosis, due to leftward deviation of the infundibular septum (*asterisk*). *AO*, aorta.

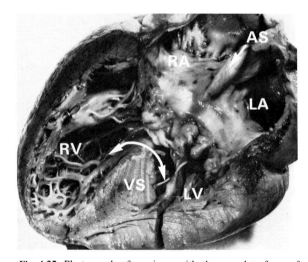

Fig. 4.35. Photograph of specimen with the complete form of atrioventricular defect. The anterior part of the heart is viewed from the posterior side. There is a common atrioventricular orifice through which the right atrium (*RA*) connects to the right ventricle (*RV*) and the left atrium (*LA*) to the left ventricle (*LV*). Underneath the bridging anterior leaflet a deficient ventricular septum (*VS*) is present, contributing to an interventricular communication (*double arrow*). The atrial septum (*AS*) is also highly deficient.

valve. Subarterial defect occurs much more frequently in Japan than in any other part of the world. It is frequently termed a 'supracristal' defect. The crest of the septum is formed by the trabecula septomarginalis, which buttresses the conduction system from the rim.

The frequency of *spontaneous closure* of a ventricular septal defect is high, as deduced from the marked discrepancy between postnatally, clinically identified ventricular septal defects and those that eventually need surgical repair or come to autopsy. The small muscular type may close spontaneously with growth of the heart and hypertrophy of muscle cells. In small perimembranous defects an aneurysm of the interventricular remnant of the membranous septum may form, which may become adherent to the edges of the defect. The adjacent part of the tricuspid valve may become involved in this process.

In some patients a ventricular septal defect is part of a more complicated cardiovascular abnormality. A particular association is seen in patients with a ventricular septal defect, subvalvar aortic stenosis owing to leftward deviation of the infundibular septum, and an interrupted aortic arch (Fig. 4.34). Moreover, aortic coarctation in a symptomatic neonate is often associated with a ventricular septal defect, the flow hypothesis to explain the occurrence of aortic coarctation being related in part to this common association (p. 131).

The presence of a ventricular septal defect will lead to an obligatory left-to-right shunt. The right ventricle will have to accommodate a high pressure, and this will be reflected in changes in the pulmonary circulation. The natural history of a patient with such a defect will thus become complicated by plexogenic pulmonary arteriopathy at a much earlier date than in patients with atrial septal defect. In the case of an otherwise uncomplicated ventricular septal defect it is generally accepted that it is unlikely for pulmonary hypertension to become irreversible before the age of 2 years.

3.1.6. Atrioventricular Defects

The anomalies grouped under this heading are also collectively referred to as 'atrioventricular canal malformations' or 'endocardial cushion defects', or by various other terms (Somerville 1978).

The hallmark of these conditions is variable 'persistence' of an early embryonic state of the atrioventricular junction. In its *complete form* the atrioventricular junction is characterized by the presence of a common atrioventricular orifice, through which each of the two atria communicates with its respective ventricle (Fig. 4.35). The orifice is guarded by a common valve in the sense that the components guarding the right and left sides of the common ostium are continuous along the anterior and posterior parts of its circumference. The abnormality is almost always further complicated by atrial and ventricular septal defects. Both defects are due to failure of septation processes, which in themselves may relate to the developmental abnormality of differentiation of the embryonic atrioventricular canal. The atrial septal defect is thus characterized by an incomplete downward extension of the atrial septum. In most cases a limbus of the fossa ovalis is present, as well as the cranial part of the septum primum, but the latter will form the upper rim of a semi-oval atrial septal defect. The lower part of the atrial defect, the so-called primum type, is formed by the plane of the common atrioventricular ostium. In some cases such a defect may be absent. Below the level of the atrioventricular valve the ventricular septum shows a deficiency, so that a perimembranous interventricular communication is found underneath the valve leaflets. In complete atrioventricular defect, the bridging anterior leaflet is variably attached to the right ventricular papillary muscles and crest of the ventricular septum, providing a system for subclassification (Rastelli et al. 1966). The posterior bridging leaflet, on the other hand, usually shows dispersed chordal attachments to the crest of the ventricular septum, although the interchordal spaces may still permit posterior interventricular communications.

The developmental abnormality at the level of the atrioventricular junction also affects the arterial pole of the heart. Thus, the aorta is unable to obtain its usual 'wedge' position between the two atrioventricular ostia. As a consequence, an elongated left ventricular outflow tract is found. This tract, together with the deficient outlet part of the ventricular septum and the attachments of the common atrioventricular valve, accounts for the peculiar left ventricular outflow tract anatomy seen on left ventricular angiograms and designated the 'goose-neck' deformity.

The *transitional form* of atrioventricular defect is characterized by the fact that, within a basic anatomical arrangement as outlined above, both the anterior and posterior bridging leaflets possess chordal attachments to the ventricular septum and that both can extend over the crest of the septum to meet in the middle (Fig. 4.36). One approach to the transitional forms, which undoubtedly exist, is to classify them as complete in the presence of a common annulus, but as partial (see below) if the anterior and posterior leaflets fuse to form separate orifices. The anatomy suggests an arrest at a later stage of development. The left ventricular outflow tract is still malformed, showing the basic characteristics outlined for the complete variety (Fig. 4.36b).

The *partial or incomplete form* of atrioventricular defect is usually characterized by a cleft left atrioventricular valve and an ostium primum defect (Fig. 4.37a). The right atrioventricular valve sometimes appears normal but may be cleft. In most cases, the primum defect is small and an interventricular septal defect is no longer present. The left ventricular outflow will nevertheless reveal the characteristics of the developmental anomaly (Fig. 4.37b). In rare cases; isolated primum defects without cleft valves, or isolated cleft left atrioventricular valve without ostium primum defect may also be found, with all the stigmata of atrioventricular defects.

It should be understood from the above developmental description that atrioventricular defects constitute an anatomical spectrum, so that categorization into types is somewhat artificial.

In the usual case the condition gives rise to an obligatory left-to-right shunt with development of early pulmonary hypertension. In fact, plexogenic pulmonary arteriopathy can occur before the second year of life in the complete variety of this syndrome. The possibility of left heart hypoplasia should also be borne in mind, since this is a serious complication with a major impact on attempts to correct the lesion surgically. In rare circumstances an atrioventricular defect can be associated with a Fallot-type outflow tract pathology (Lev et al. 1961a), in the sense that the aorta overrides the ventricular septum while the pulmonary outflow tract is considerably narrowed (p. 124). It may also occur with Ebstein's malformation (p. 110) of the right ventricular (tricuspid) component of the common valve (Caruso et al. 1978). Both associated conditions will dramatically alter the course of the disease.

The abnormality at the level of the atrioventricular junction also influences the topography of the atrioventricular conduction tissue axis (Lev 1958; Feldt et al. 1970). The atrioventricular node is displaced posteriorly by virtue of the large septal defect. The atrioventricular (His) bundle, however, is elongated, running along the crest of the ventricular septum. The left bundle branches show an early 'take-off', thereby creating a widened gap between them and the final evolution of the right bundle branch. This peculiar anatomy probably underlies the characteristic vectorcardiogram, which indicates early activation of the posterior left ventricular wall (Durrer et al. 1966). The course of the bundle, moreover, may explain why early degenerative changes can occur, providing an anatomical basis for the frequent occurrence of 'spontaneous' atrioventricular dissociation in the natural course of the disease.

Complete atrioventricular defects are the most common cardiac conditions occurring with the trisomy-21 syndrome (p. 76).

3.1.7. Tricuspid Valve Abnormalities

The right atrioventricular orifice can be diminished in size, a feature which in most cases indicates hypoplasia of the right ventricle, often associated with pulmonary atresia. Frequently the tricuspid valve guarding such a hypoplastic ostium shows features of Ebstein's malformation (see below).

Tricuspid atresia is the situation in which the right atrium has no outlet other than the foramen ovale or a true atrial septal defect. Two types can be recognized. In the classic form of tricuspid atresia there is no potential communication between the right atrium and the underlying ventricular mass. From an anatomical point of view, this type of malformation belongs to the category of univentricular hearts, and will be discussed under that heading (p. 126). The second form of tricuspid atresia is extremely rare. It consists of an imperforate

membrane separating the right atrium from an underlying right ventricle (Fig. 4.17). This imperforate membrane may show evidence of Ebstein's malformation. The fundamental difference between this condition and classic tricuspid atresia is the fact that a formed but usually hypoplastic right ventricle is present, in proper alignment with the right atrium.

Ebstein's anomaly of the tricuspid valve is characterized by the combined occurrence of distal displacement of some of the tricuspid valve attachments and dysplasia of the valve leaflets (Fig. 4.38). Both these features vary in extent (Becker et al. 1971). Distal displacement always affects the septal attachment of the valve but may include the posterolateral insertions. However, the anterior leaflet will always be attached to the annulus fibrosus. The distal displacement of part of the valve creates an 'atrialized part' of the right ventricle.

Dysplasia of valve leaflets is characterized by a

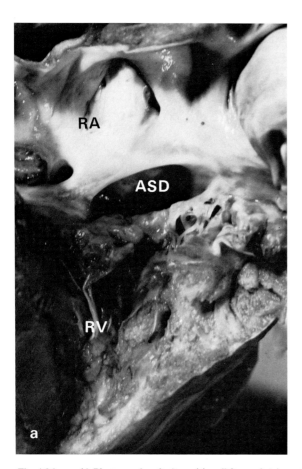 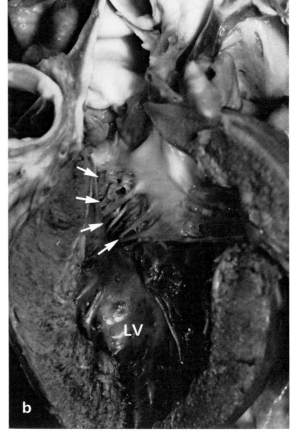

Fig. 4.36. a and **b** Photographs of a 'transitional' form of atrioventricular defect. **a** Opened right atrium (*RA*) and right ventricle (*RV*). Atrioventricular valve tissues insert over the crest of the ventricular septum and meet in the middle. An atrial septal defect (*ASD*) of the so-called primum type is present. **b** Opened left ventricle (*LV*) and outflow tract. Chordae for the anterior leaflet are anchored to the crest of the septum (*arrows*), but interventricular communications are still present. The anatomy is basically the same as that seen in the complete variety.

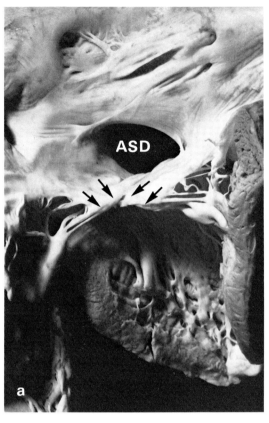

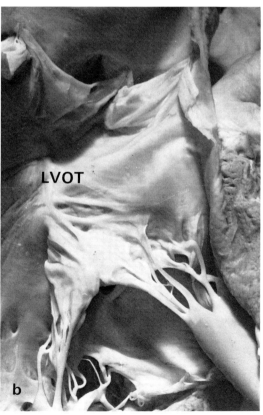

◁ **Fig. 4.37. a** and **b** Photographs of the partial form of atrioventricular defect. **a** left side of the heart with the cleft mitral valve (*arrows*), closely related to an atrial septal defect (*ASD*) of the primum type. **b** outflow of the left ventricle (*LVOT*), with basically the same malformation as seen in the complete variety, though interventricular communications are no longer present.

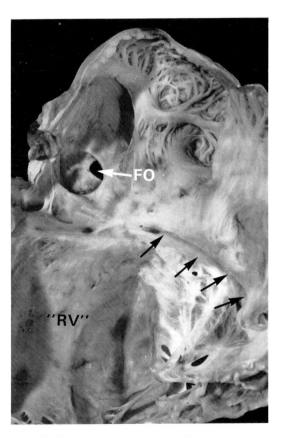

Fig. 4.38. Photograph of a heart with Ebstein's anomaly of the tricuspid valve. There is distal displacement of the basal attachments of the septal and posterior leaflets, creating a large 'atrial' part of the right ventricle (*RV*). The anterior leaflet takes origin from the annulus fibrosus (*arrows*), but is curtain-like and has many direct insertions into the ventricular wall. *FO*, foramen ovale.

curtain-like appearance, with valve leaflets having direct insertions into the ventricular wall. Fusion of leaflets may occur, so that a small orifice remains as the only inlet to the right ventricle. In fact, as indicated above, some forms of imperforate right valve are basically imperforate Ebstein's malformations. Moreover, the dysplastic valve leaflets can contain bands of myocardium.

Ebstein's anomaly of the tricuspid valve is often associated with an atrial septal defect of the fossa ovalis type, together with pulmonary valve abnormalities. In some instances a ventricular septal defect can co-exist.

In hearts with atrioventricular discordance, such as congenitally corrected transposition of the great arteries (p. 219), there is a relatively high incidence of Ebstein-like malformation of the 'inverted' tricuspid valve.

3.1.8. Mitral Valve Abnormalities

Isolated mitral valve abnormalities are rare. *Mitral atresia* is the most common form. In a majority of cases, however, the atrioventricular junction is characterized by an absent atrioventricular connection, so that the architecture is similar to that seen in hearts with classic tricuspid atresia (p. 110). Such hearts are again best considered univentricular. Congenital mitral stenosis can take various forms (Ruckman and Van Praagh 1978).

Parachute mitral valve is the condition where all chordae of the valve insert into one papillary muscle, thereby creating a funnel-type ventricular inlet. This condition can occur as an isolated lesion but is frequently part of a more complex malformation, which includes additional anomalies like aortic coarctation, muscular subaortic stenosis and supra-valvar stenosing ring of the left atrium (Shone et al. 1963).

Abnormal chordal attachments of the mitral valve apparatus may occur in isolation, although in most instances the abnormality is part of a complex form of atrioventricular defect.

3.1.9. Pulmonary Valve Abnormalities

Bicuspid and quadricuspid pulmonary valves can occur and are themselves of no or of only limited clinical significance.

Pulmonary valve stenosis in isolation is frequent. The valve in this condition nearly always shows a dome-shaped stenosis (Fig. 4.39). The pulmonary trunk reveals a post-stenotic dilatation. The ventricular septum is mostly intact. At the atrial level a patent foramen ovale or a 'true' atrial septal defect

may be present, facilitating decompression of right heart chambers. The term 'trilogy of Fallot' has been used, inappropriately, for the latter situation.

The condition leads to colossal right ventricular hypertrophy, particularly in cases without an atrial vent. Hypertrophy may ultimately also affect the left ventricular wall (Harinck et al. 1977). In long-standing cases fibrosis of right ventricular myocardium can occur, affecting right ventricular compliance.

In *pulmonary valve dysplasia* the valve consists of three cusps, which are thickened and have a gelatinous aspect. The condition can occur in isolation but is more frequently part of Noonan's syndrome (p. 140).

Pulmonary atresia with intact ventricular septum takes various forms, the most common being that in which a membrane-like structure is present at the level of the arterial junction (Fig. 4.40a); in other cases a muscular segment intervenes between ventricle and pulmonary trunk (Fig. 4.40b). The pulmonary trunk is nearly always small, in contrast to the dilated pulmonary trunk in patients with isolated pulmonary valve stenosis. The pulmonary blood supply is dependent upon the ductus arteriosus,

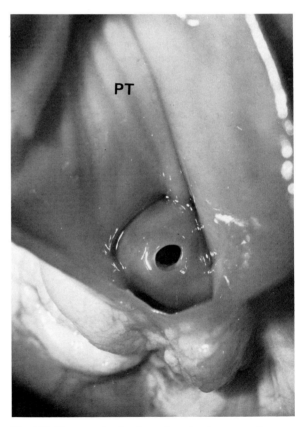

Fig. 4.39. Photograph of a dome-shaped pulmonary valve stenosis, viewed from above after opening of the pulmonary trunk (*PT*).

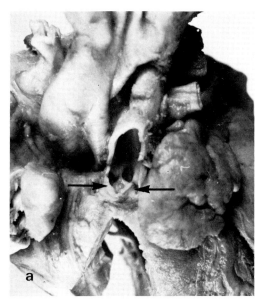 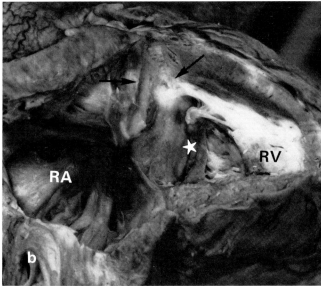

Fig. 4.40. a and **b** Photographs of heart specimens with pulmonary atresia and intact ventricular septum. **a** membrane-like structure at the level of the arterial junction (*arrows*); **b** an example of an intervening muscular segment (*arrows*). The anterior free wall has been removed, revealing a minute, thick-walled right ventricle (*RV*). Note the hypoplastic tricuspid ostium, guarded by a valve showing septal displacement (*asterisk*) characteristic for Ebstein's malformation, a frequently associated anomaly in this condition. *RA*, right atrium.

which in these instances is characteristically elongated, taking a curved course from its aortic site to the truncal bifurcation. The intrapulmonary arteries are thin-walled, as in all instances of diminished pulmonary flow. The number of peripheral arteries is probably lower than normal. The right ventricle can be small or of normal size, although occasionally a dilated right ventricular cavity is seen. Myocardial sinusoids may be present, connecting the right ventricular cavity to branches of the coronary arteries and serving as an outlet for the right ventricle. In such instances examination of the heart will reveal tortuous dilated epicardial coronary arteries.

Pulmonary atresia with ventricular septal defect. In the presence of a septal defect, pulmonary atresia is usually infundibular. The aorta, being the only outlet for the heart, usually overrides the septum to a varying degree, and the situation closely resembles an extreme degree of Fallot's tetralogy, except that the deviation of the infundibular septum is complete, producing atresia of the right ventricular outflow tract (Fig. 4.41). While the pulmonary blood supply may be duct-dependent, aortopulmonary collateral vessels are frequently found supplying all or part of the lungs, either with the pulmonary arteries or in isolation.

3.1.10. Aortic Valve Abnormalities

A bicuspid aortic valve has no functional significance in the paediatric age group; the pathological consequences of this valve anomaly may appear later in life. Quadricuspid aortic valve is extremely rare and most probably has no functional significance.

Aortic stenosis of valvar origin is nearly always caused by so-called unicommissural, unicuspid aortic valve (Fig. 4.42a). When viewed from its aortic aspect the valve has a modified dome-shaped appearance with a sort of key-hole orifice. From its commissural insertion the valve executes a U-turn without inserting into the aortic wall, and re-inserts at the site of the initial commissure (Fig. 4.42a). In the base of the valve an occasional shallow raphé can be present. This condition can be associated with either a small or a normal-sized left ventricle. In most instances the ventricular septum is intact, but a ventricular septal defect can be present. In all cases left ventricular hypertrophy is manifest. At an early age ischaemia will affect the myocardium, so that subendocardial infarction of the left ventricular wall will appear (Fig. 4.42b). Myocardial ischaemia underlies sudden death, which is a common finding in these patients. Moreover, left ventricular scarring will affect the pump function, so that left heart failure can appear early in the disease. Dilated left heart chambers and structural changes in the pul-

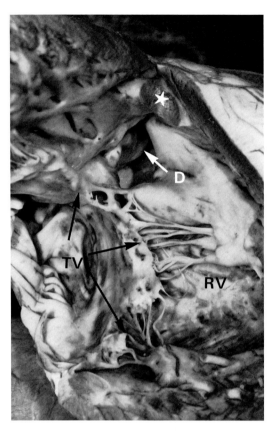

monary vasculature may underline this sequence of events.

Aortic valve dysplasia is a rare condition, which like pulmonary valve dysplasia (p. 140), is often part of Noonan's syndrome.

In *aortic atresia* the ascending aorta is a narrow channel, which conducts blood retrogradely to the coronary arteries. Coronary arterial flow and blood flow to the head and upper body depend on patency of the ductus, hence the early high mortality associated with this lesion. Usually aortic atresia is accompanied by hypoplasia of the left heart. This exists in two discrete forms. In the first the left

◁ **Fig. 4.41.** (*left*) Photograph of the opened right ventricle (*RV*) in a heart with pulmonary atresia and ventricular septal defect (*D*). The outflow part shows a striking similarity with that in classic Fallot's tetralogy (cf. Fig. 4.56b), hence the term 'extreme Fallot'. The infundibular septum (*asterisk*) shows an extreme anterior deviation producing atresia of the pulmonary outflow tract. The aorta is seen to override the defect. *TV*, tricuspid valve.

Fig. 4.42. a and **b** Heart specimen with a unicommissural, unicuspid aortic valve. **a** The stenotic unicommissural (*arrow*), viewed from its aortic aspect. **b** Marked left ventricular (*LV*) myocardial hypertrophy with extensive subendocardial fibrosis owing to impaired myocardial perfusion.
▽

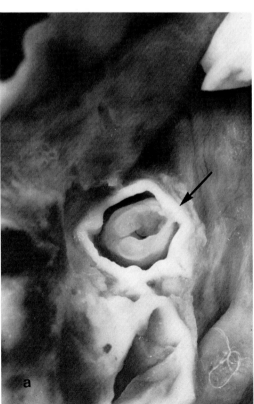

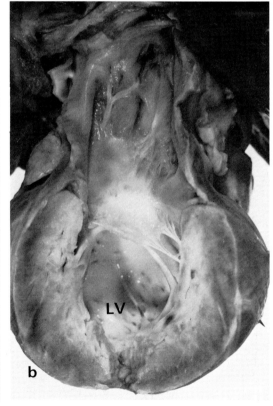

atrioventricular connection is absent and the left ventricular chamber is simply a trabecular pouch (p. 127). In the other form there is mitral stenosis because of a small valve apparatus and the ventricular chamber shows considerable endocardial fibroelastosis (Fig. 4.43). In rare instances aortic atresia is associated with a ventricular septal defect and a normally sized left ventricle and mitral valve.

3.1.11. Supravalvar Aortic Stenosis

Supravalvar aortic stenosis is characterized by an obstruction in the aorta beyond the level of the aortic valve. There are three types of supravalvar aortic stenosis. The most common form is the so-called hourglass type, in which a funnel-shaped stenosis is present (Fig. 4.44). The aortic media in the affected region shows a mosaic pattern, i.e., a disorderly arrangement of the lamellar aortic units. A second form of supravalvar aortic stenosis is the segmental type, which is characterized by a uniform thickening of the wall affecting the greater part of the ascending aorta. In some cases the diseased wall may extend into the innominate (brachiocephalic), carotid and subclavian arteries. The least common type of supravalvar aortic stenosis is that in which a perforate membrane obstructs the ascending aorta.

Location of the obstruction distal to the origin of the coronary arteries, so that the latter originate

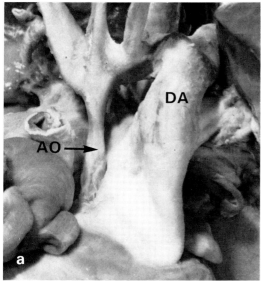

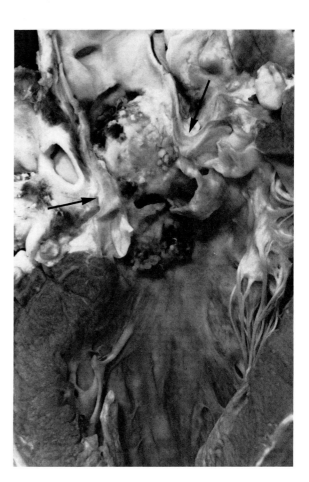

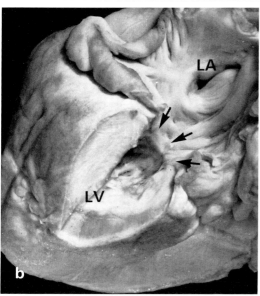

Fig. 4.44. (*above*) Specimen showing supravalvar aortic stenosis of the so-called hourglass type.

Fig. 4.43. a and **b** (*left*) Heart specimen with aortic atresia. **a** The hypoplastic ascending aorta (*Ao*). Systemic flow depends upon patency of the ductus arteriosus (*DA*); **b** extreme hypoplasia of the left ventricle (*LV*) connected to the left atrium (*LA*) through a minute mitral orifice (*arrows*) guarded by a basically normal mitral valve.

from a high pressure chamber, is common to all forms. In rare circumstances supravalvar aortic stenosis may be associated with similar structural changes in the pulmonary trunk and/or central pulmonary arteries. If the latter circumstance prevails the aortic abnormality is most often part of a nonfamilial, but otherwise complex syndrome, which consists of mental retardation and a particular facies, often in association with a syndrome of hypercalcaemia (p. 593). A familiar form can occur, which lacks these additional features but in which multiple aortic stenoses can be present.

3.1.12. Subvalvar Aortic Stenosis

Subaortic stenosis can have various substrates. At present the classification advocated is that based on the functional characteristics of the stenotic site. Three major types are distinguished: a dynamic type, a fixed type, and a mixed type. The first category shows, anatomically, a muscular thickening of the ventricular septum just below the level of the aortic valve. Not all conditions with a dynamic subaortic stenosis reveal a distinct abnormality at autopsy; most reveal a localized endocardial thickening of the ventricular septum as a sort of imprint of the anterior mitral valve leaflet. Histological examination of the affected region may reveal marked myocardial cell hypertrophy, often accompanied by an irregular arrangement of fibres and interstitial fibrosis. None of these changes, however, can be considered as pathognomonic for the dynamic type. The clinical terms ASH (asymmetric septal hypertrophy), IHSS (idiopathic hypertrophic subaortic stenosis), and HOCM (hypertrophic obstructive cardiomyopathy) are often used interchangeably for this still enigmatic disease. It occurs in familial and nonfamilial forms. Some infants may be 'primarily' affected by this condition, while other infants may gradually develop signs of a dynamic subaortic obstruction in the course of various types of congenital heart malformations.

Fixed types of subaortic stenosis can take several forms. The most common type is that in which a discrete subvalvar shelf-like fibrous ridge is present on the ventricular septal surface, continuing on to the ventricular aspect of the anterior mitral leaflet. In many instances this fibrous ridge is intimately related to one of the aortic semilunar valve cusps (Fig. 4.45). This *diaphragmatic* or 'membranous' type of subaortic stenosis is usually mild and carries a favourable prognosis. In contrast, the *tunnel type* of subaortic stenosis has a more serious outlook. In this condition a fibromuscular tunnel is present underneath the aortic valve. The abnormal segment has an intimate relation with the mitral valve and in

most instances intervenes between the mitral and aortic valves. Another form of fixed subvalvar aortic stenosis is that characterized by abnormal septal attachments of the mitral valve apparatus, a condition often associated with an atrioventricular defect.

The third type of subaortic stenosis is a combination of dynamic and fixed forms. Thus, in many instances of a dynamic outflow tract obstruction a marked fibrous thickening of the overlying endocardium occurs, contributing to the degree of stenosis.

3.1.13. Aortopulmonary Window

From a pathogenetic point of view, aortopulmonary window is closely related to truncus arteriosus (p. 126).

The condition is characterized by a 'window-like' communication between adjacent parts of the walls

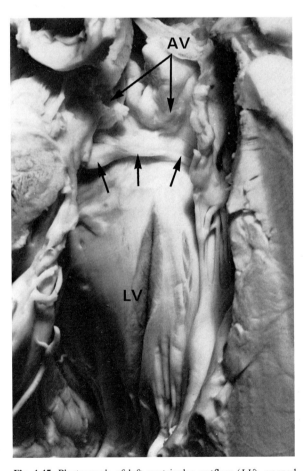

Fig. 4.45. Photograph of left ventricular outflow (*LV*), opened from the apex through the anterior mitral leaflet. The outflow tract is obstructed by a fibrous ridge (*arrows*), intimately related to the aortic valve (*AV*).

of the pulmonary trunk and ascending aorta (Fig. 4.46). The window is situated above the level of the semilunar valves in the region between the ostia of the right and left coronary arteries. Viewed from the pulmonary trunk the window is present in the posterolateral area, just underneath and anterior to the origin of the right pulmonary artery.

Both great arteries display separate semilunar valves, unlike the situation in classic truncus arteriosus. Moreover, the ventricular septum is usually intact.

An obligatory left-to-right shunt occurs, which usually leads to early plexogenic pulmonary arteriopathy and irreversible pulmonary hypertension.

3.1.14. Abnormalities of the Ductus Arteriosus

Premature closure of the ductus arteriosus has occasionally been reported as a cause of intrauterine death. Careful inspection of the ductus, particularly during an autopsy on a stillborn fetus, may further substantiate the potential significance of this observation.

More commonly, problems arise from *persistent patency of the ductus arteriosus*. In the mature neonate the ductus is usually permanently closed at approximately 3 weeks. In prematurely born neonates, however, the ductus may remain patent for some months after birth. It is generally accepted that a ductus that is still patent at 3 months of age will only rarely close spontaneously. The precise mechanisms of closure are not fully understood at present, and neither is the reason for persistent patency. Recent histological studies of patent ductus arteriosus have revealed an abnormal structural characteristic in the sense of an uninterrupted internal elastic lamina at the site of intimal cushions and in some instances 'aorticization' of the wall (Gittenberger–de Groot 1977).

In recent years the administration of prostaglandins has been advocated to prevent the ductus from closing where the life of the baby depends upon a functioning ductus (e.g., in patients with pulmonary atresia and intact ventricular septum). Prostaglandins decrease the vascular tone of the vessel. Histological studies have shown that the wall becomes oedematous and the danger of intimal tears, dissection, and rupture is real; the pathologist should be aware of this while examining the ductus (Gittenberger–de Groot et al. 1978).

Patent ductus arteriosus usually causes an aortico-to-pulmonary shunt with pulmonary hypertension as a result. In time irreversible pulmonary vascular changes can appear.

3.1.15. Abnormalities of the Coronary Arteries

Congenital abnormalities of the coronary arteries have been divided into two categories, constituting minor and major forms (Ogden 1970).

Minor congenital abnormalities consist of reduplication of coronary ostia, translocation of ostia, or abnormalities in the proximal course of the coronary arteries. It has been suggested that some of these so-called minor variations are less minor than initially thought. Translocation of the ostium of the left coronary artery to the right coronary sinus can lead to a situation in which the main stem of the left coronary artery runs between the pulmonary trunk and the aortic root. Cases of sudden death associated with this condition have been reported. Moreover, translocation of an ostium to the side of the commissural attachment may result in a slit-like ostium, which in time may become compromised by

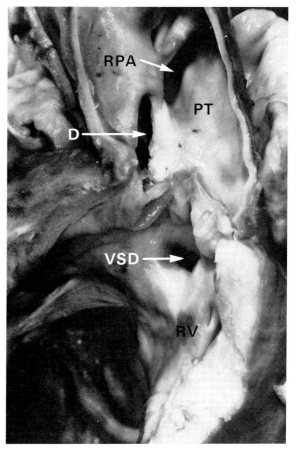

Fig. 4.46. Photograph of heart specimen with aorticopulmonary window, viewed through the opened right ventricular outflow (*RV*) and pulmonary trunk (*PT*). The defect (*D*) is located in the posterolateral area, just underneath and anterior to the origin of the right pulmonary artery (*RPA*). Note the presence of a ventricular septal defect (*VSD*).

degenerative aortic wall changes leading to ostial stenosis.

The most common abnormal course is that in which the left circumflex artery originates from the proximal segment of the right coronary artery and runs posterior to the aortic root before it takes its usual course in the left atrioventricular groove.

In hearts with abnormal relationships of the great arteries, abnormalities in the course of the coronary arteries are more common.

Major forms of congenital coronary artery abnormalities generally have direct functional consequences.

Aberrant origin of the left coronary artery from the pulmonary trunk (Bland et al. 1933) is of major clinical significance (Fig. 4.47a). Owing to the pressure drop in the pulmonary trunk after birth and the concomitant hypertrophy of the myocardial cells of the left ventricle, a decrease in flow in the left coronary artery is established and ischaemia or left ventricular myocardial infarction occur, often with mitral insufficiency as the leading symptom. If the neonate survives this initial period, recurrent ischaemic attacks may occur at later ages. In these instances abundant collateral arteries will have developed between the right coronary artery, normally originating from the aorta, and the aberrant left coronary artery. These collaterals can result in a preferential shunting of blood from the coronary arterial system to the pulmonary trunk. Large areas of left ventricular myocardium may thus be deprived of an adequate blood supply (Fig. 4.47b). In all instances of sudden death in an adolescent the pathologist should look for this particular congenital abnormality.

Aberrant right coronary artery from the pulmonary

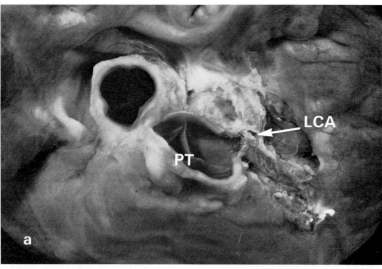

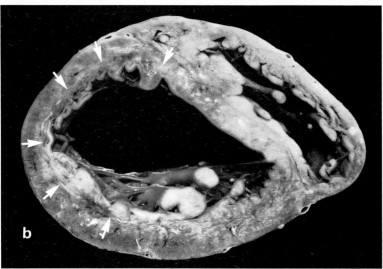

Fig. 4.47. a and **b** Heart specimen with aberrant origin of the left coronary artery from the pulmonary trunk: **a** site of origin of the left coronary artery (*LCA*) from the pulmonary trunk (*PT*); **b** transsection of the left ventricle, showing extensive, mainly subendocardial, myocardial necrosis (*arrows*) of the left ventricle.

trunk is extremely rare and usually has no consequences in the paediatric or adolescent age groups.

Coronary arterial fistulas can occur between the right and left ventricular chambers and the epicardial coronary arteries. Such fistulas often accompany conditions with increased intracavitary pressures, such as arterial valve atresia, but occasionally occur as isolated lesions. Usually such fistulas have limited functional significance. Examination of the heart may reveal the condition from the presence of dilated and tortuous epicardial coronary arteries.

3.2. Congenital Heart Malformations with Abnormal Junctional Connections

The malformations discussed in this section all involve at least one abnormal junctional connection. They can exist with situs inversus, but such cases are rare. They will therefore be described with situs solitus anatomy of the atria assumed.

3.2.1. Congenitally Corrected Transposition of the Great Arteries

Congenitally corrected transposition of the great arteries is characterized by a *dis*cordant atrioventricular connection, in association with a *dis*cordant arterial connection. In other words, the right atrium connects to the morphologically left ventricle, from which the pulmonary trunk arises, while the left atrium connects to the morphologically right ventricle, from which the aorta arises (Fig. 4.48). This situation usually occurs with the atria in situs solitus, but the same configuration may occur with a situs inversus anatomy of atria. Basically, the flow pattern is such that systemic venous blood is conveyed into the pulmonary trunk, albeit by way of the 'wrong' ventricle, while the pulmonary venous blood is directed into the systemic circulation, again along an abnormal route. The 'transposition' of the great arteries, in the sense of a discordant arterial connection, is thus 'corrected' because of inversion of ventricles, in the sense of a discordant atrioventricular connection; hence the name 'congenitally corrected transposition of the great arteries'.

The condition is usually complicated by additional anomalies (Lev and Rowlatt 1961b; Allwork et al. 1976). The most common associated abnormalities are ventricular septal defect, pulmonary outflow obstruction, and Ebstein-like malformation of the inverted (left-sided) tricuspid valve. The natural course of the disease is greatly influenced by these anomalies.

The condition is further complicated by an abnormal disposition of the atrioventricular conduction tissues (Anderson et al. 1974, 1975). Because of the malalignment between the interatrial septum and the inflow part of the interventricular septum, a regularly positioned posterior node is usually unable to contact the ventricular myocardium. It is known that during development a complete ring of conduction tissue surrounds the tricuspid orifice, with an expansion at the anterolateral margin. In corrected transposition this anterolateral node takes over as the connecting atrioventricular node, and from it a penetrating atrioventricular bundle descends on to the ventricular septum. This bundle is closely related to the fibrous annulus of the mitral valve and takes an elongated course, encircling the pulmonary outflow tract anteriorly to descend along the anterior rim of a ventricular septal defect if present. The abnormal disposition of the atrioventricular conduction axis is surgically very significant. Moreover, the attenuated course of the bundle, in close contact to the mitral valve attachment, may explain the high frequency of 'spontaneous' atrioventricular dissociation that occurs in the natural history of this condition.

3.2.2. Complete Transposition of the Great Arteries

Complete transposition of the great arteries is characterized by a *dis*cordant arterial connection, while the atrioventricular connection is *con*cordant (Fig. 4.49). Thus, the right atrium connects to a right ventricle, from which the aorta arises, while the left atrium connects to the left ventricle, which gives rise to the pulmonary trunk. This situation can occur with either a situs solitus or a situs inversus anatomy of atria.

In the usual case of complete transposition of the great arteries the aorta is positioned anterior to and to the right of the pulmonary trunk. However, it is not uncommon to find the aorta either in front or to the left of the pulmonary trunk, although the internal arrangement characterized by the discordant arterial connection is not altered. As a consequence of the abnormal aortic position, the left coronary artery will often run anterior to the pulmonary trunk, a situation that can be anticipated in all hearts with an anteriorly positioned aorta.

Basically, the anatomical arrangements in complete transposition of the great arteries result in two separate circulatory pathways. Therefore life can only be sustained if some sort of an exchange of blood between the two circulations can occur. Most cases of complete transposition of the great arteries will display a 'shunt possibility' at atrial level, either through a patent foramen ovale or through a 'true' atrial septal defect. Other sites of possible interchange between the two circulations are a ventricular septal defect or a persistent ductus arteriosus.

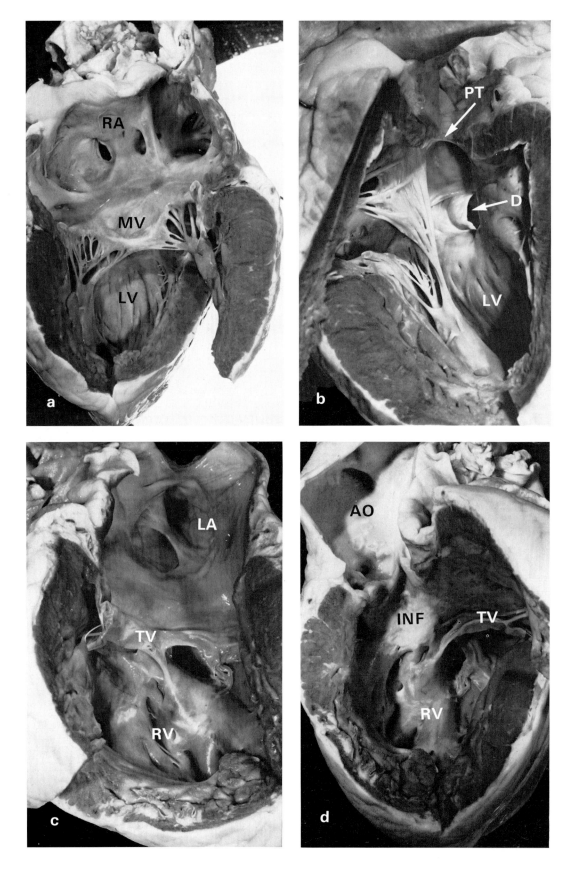

Complete transposition of the great arteries can be subdivided into three categories, those with an intact ventricular septum, those with a ventricular septal defect, and those with a ventricular septal defect and pulmonary stenosis.

The ventricular septal defects in these hearts can be located in similar sites to isolated defects although infundibular malalignment defects are more frequent (Fig. 4.50).

Pulmonary stenosis can be of valvar origin, but quite often a subvalvar outflow tract obstruction is also present (Fig. 4.51). Pulmonary stenosis can provide protection against the development of pulmonary vascular disease, which is a common and early complication in patients with complete transposition of the great arteries and a ventricular septal defect without pulmonary stenosis.

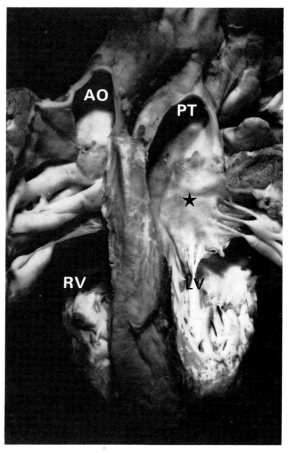

◁ **Fig. 4.48. a–d** Photographs of heart specimens with congenitally corrected transposition of the great arteries and a situs solitus anatomy of the atria: **a** opened right side of the heart. The right atrium (*RA*) connects to the morphologically left ventricle (*LV*). The atrioventricular junction is guarded by the mitral valve (*MV*); **b** outflow tract of the left ventricle (*LV*) into the pulmonary trunk (*PT*), which is in a posterior location. There is a large ventricular septal defect (*D*); **c** opened left side of the heart. The left atrium (*LA*) connects to the morphologically right ventricle (*RV*) via the tricuspid valve (*TV*); **d** outflow tract of the right ventricle (*RV*) leading into an anteriorly positioned aorta (*Ao*) separated from the tricuspid valve (*TV*) by the infundibulum (*INF*).

Fig. 4.49. Heart specimen showing the characteristics of complete transposition of the great arteries. A concordant atrioventricular connection is complicated by a discordant arterial connection. The aorta (*Ao*) arises from the right ventricle (*RV*), the two being separated by an infundibulum. The pulmonary trunk (*PT*) arises from the left ventricle (*LV*) and there is fibrous continuity (*asterisk*) between the pulmonary and mitral valves.

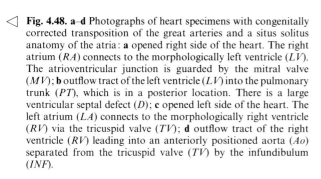

Fig. 4.50. Diagram showing the various sites of a ventricular septal defect in complete transposition of the great arteries. The condition shows a relatively high incidence of infundibular malalignment defects.

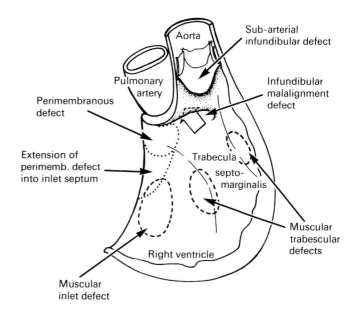

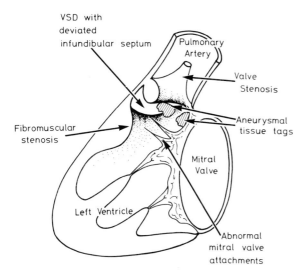

Fig. 4.51. Diagram illustrating the various types of left ventricular outflow obstruction as they may occur in complete transposition of the great arteries.

A brief note should be added on the surgical repair of complete transposition of the great arteries, because it is likely that the pathologist, at least in centres where cardiac surgery is performed, will be confronted with a corrected specimen.

The operative procedure most commonly followed is the Mustard operation. The essence of this repair is to convey the venous returns to their appropriate great arteries, by redirecting their atrial routes. The atrial septum is removed and a baffle is constructed inside the 'common' atrium in such a way that the pulmonary venous return is conveyed into the right ventricle (Fig. 4.52a), while the systemic venous blood is directed into the left ventricle (Fig. 4.52b). In most centres the baffle is constructed from either pericardium or a synthetic material.

A similar procedure is the Senning operation, in which flaps of atrial tissue are used for the re-routing of blood.

More recently an 'arterial switch' operation has been advocated, in which the great arteries are

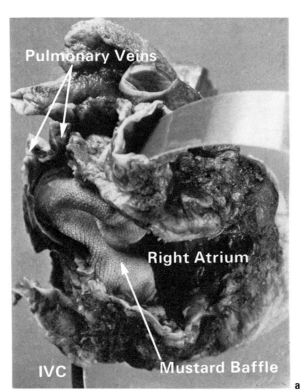

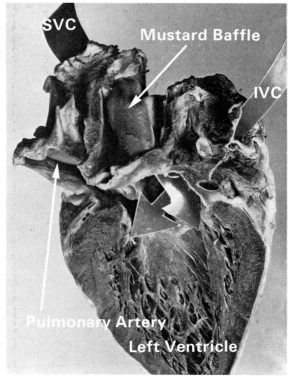

Fig. 4.52 a and b Heart specimen of complete transposition of the great arteries after a Mustard's procedure has been completed. a Posterior view of the heart. The posterolateral wall of the atria has been opened from the pulmonary venous ostia into the right atrial appendage. This reveals the baffle that has been constructed within a common atrium after removal of the atrial septum. The pulmonary venous return is thus conveyed into the right ventricle and hence into the aorta. b Left side of the heart. The systemic venous return from the superior (SVC) and inferior (IVC) caval veins, indicated by *arrows*, is re-routed via the baffle into the left ventricle and hence into the pulmonary artery.

divided and switched back to the appropriate ventricles, with relocation of the coronary arteries in the 'new' aortic root.

3.2.3. Double Outlet Right Ventricle

In double outlet right ventricle both great arteries arise mainly from the right ventricle. In most cases the aorta is to the right of the pulmonary trunk, in a side-by-side relationship (Fig. 4.53). When inspected from the interior the two arterial outlets are separated by a distinct rim of muscle, the infundibular septum (Fig. 4.53).

Subclassification is based on the position of the ventricular septal defect which may be subaortic (Fig. 5.53a), subpulmonary (Fig. 4.53b), doubly committed, or noncommitted.

In double outlet right ventricle with subpulmonary defect (Fig. 4.53b), the pulmonary trunk is closely related to the ventricular septum and in some instances may indeed straddle the septum. The so-called Taussig–Bing heart is the classic example in

this category (Taussig and Bing 1949). It is also from this particular specimen that the paradigm of a bilateral infundibulum ('double conus') has been set (Van Praagh 1968). It has been advocated for a long time that for a heart to be classified as double-outlet right ventricle the arterial valve should be separated from the mitral valve by a rim of muscle and the two arterial valves should be positioned at the same level. Meanwhile, however, many specimens have been observed that show fibrous continuity between the atrioventricular and arterial valves, but otherwise fulfil all criteria of a true double outlet (Lev et al. 1972). The classification of the heart as a double outlet, therefore, to our minds no longer depends upon the presence of such a 'bilateral infundibulum', but on the arterial connection of the great arteries.

The clinical significance of double outlet right ventricle with a subpulmonary defect is that preferential shunting of blood may occur from the left ventricle into the pulmonary trunk. From a functional point of view, this closely resembles the position in complete transposition of the great

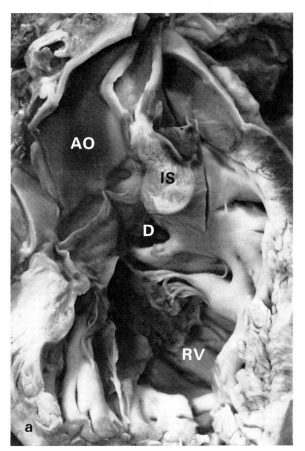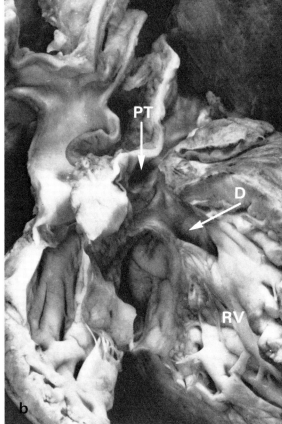

Fig. 4.53. a and **b** Heart specimens with double outlet right ventricle, in which the right ventricle (*RV*) and arterial outlets have been opened. The two great arteries show a side-by-side relationship, both outlets being separated by the infundibular septum (*IS*): **a** ventricular septal defect (*D*) in a subaortic (*Ao*) position; **b** defect (**D**) underneath the pulmonary trunk (*PT*).

arteries with ventricular septal defect. In contrast, double outlet right ventricle with subaortic defect can involve preferential shunting from the left ventricle into the aorta and clinically the case can thus resemble an ordinary ventricular septal defect or a tetralogy of Fallot.

A doubly committed defect is present underneath both arterial ostia, while a noncommitted defect is remote from the arterial outlets.

Double outlet right ventricle can be complicated by additional anomalies. Thus pulmonary stenosis frequently occurs with a subaortic defect, while narrowing of the subaortic outflow tract is frequent with subpulmonary defect, the latter often being associated with coarctation of the aorta. Straddling mitral valve is also frequent with subpulmonary defects (Kitamura et al. 1974).

3.2.4. Tetralogy of Fallot

Tetralogy of Fallot is characterized by the combined presence of a dextroposed aorta, a malalignment type of ventricular septal defect, pulmonary infundibular stenosis and right ventricular hypertrophy. The hallmark of the condition is the abnormal relationship of structures composing the outflow parts of the hearts (Becker et al. 1975; Becker and Anderson 1978b). The aorta is dextroposed and has a more anterior position than normal (Fig. 4.54). In addition, the infundibular septum is deviated anteriorly, thereby creating the infundibular outflow tract stenosis of the right ventricle (Fig. 4.55). At the same time, the abnormally positioned infundibular septum contributes to the presence of the 'malalignment' type of defect, which

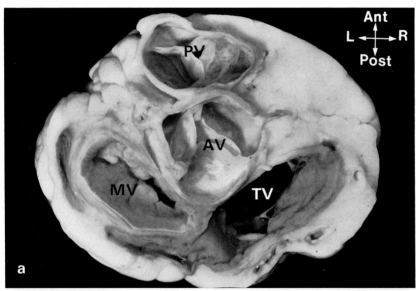

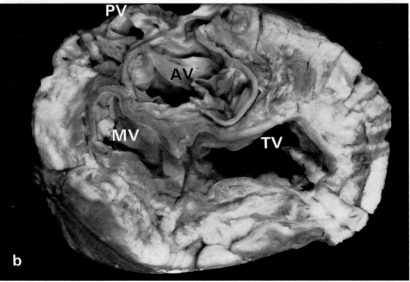

Fig. 4.54. a and **b** Photographs illustrating the abnormal position of the aortic root in Fallot's tetralogy. **a** Base of a *normally* constructed heart after removal of both atria and the great arteries. The aortic valve (*AV*) takes a wedge position between the tricuspid (*TV*) and mitral (*MV*) valves; **b** similar dissection in a heart with Fallot's tetralogy. The aortic valve (*AV*) is slightly dextroposed and displaced anteriorly. Note the position of the aortic valve relative to that of the pulmonary valve (*PV*), as compared with that in the normal heart (**a**). Reproduced from Becker and Anderson (1978), in: *Paediatric Cardiology* 1977, by permission of Churchill Livingstone, Edinburgh.

is usually but not always perimembranous. The tetralogy of Fallot is therefore characterized by the morphology of the outflow parts of both ventricles. From the point of view of the *arterial connections*, however, the condition can occur with either arterial concordance or double outlet ventricle, depending on the degree of aortic override (Shinebourne and Anderson 1978). In our opinion the term 'tetralogy of Fallot' should be restricted to hearts that fulfil the anatomic criteria outlined above. Most cases exhibit fibrous continuity between the mitral valve and the dextroposed aortic valve, but this feature is not crucial to the diagnosis.

From the brief description of the anatomy it follows that the malformation varies in its degree of severity. The degree of anterior deviation of the infundibular septum also differs from one case to the other, while induced hypertrophy may in time aggrevate the severity of the stenosis. Insight into these anatomical features may explain a clinical spectrum of Fallot's tetralogy, ranging from 'pink' Fallots to the classic deeply cyanotic infant.

An understanding of the basic structural abnormality of Fallot's tetralogy will also clarify the association of a 'Fallot-type' outflow tract pathology with other cardiac malformations, such as

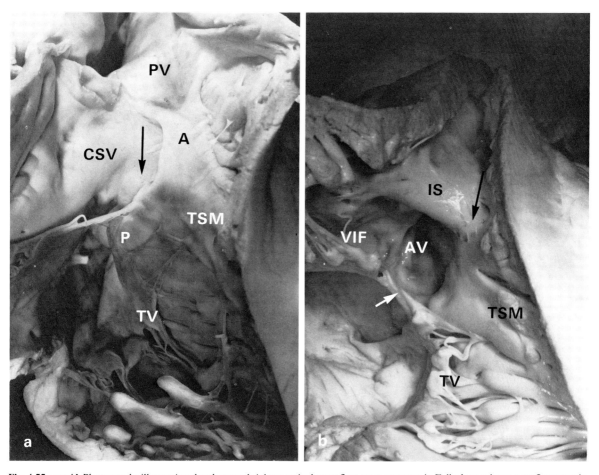

Fig. 4.55. a and b Photographs illustrating the abnormal right ventricular outflow tract anatomy in Fallot's tetralogy: a outflow tract in a *normally* constructed heart. The trabecula septomarginalis (*TSM*) shows anterior (*A*) and posterior (*P*) extensions, which embrace (*black arrow*) the crista supraventricularis (*CSV*); b anatomy in Fallot's tetralogy. The infundibular septum (*IS*) is deviated anteriorly and the relationship with the trabecula septomarginalis (*TSM*) has altered considerably (cf. *black arrows* in a and b). The infundibular septum (*IS*) has separated from the ventriculo-infundibular folds (*VIF*), both of which merge inconspicuously in the normally constructed heart, forming the crista supraventricularis (cf. a). A large ventricular septal defect is present, through which the aortic valve (*AV*) is readily identified as overriding the ventricular septum. The aortic valve and the tricuspid valve (*TV*) are brought into close proximity (*white arrow*). Reproduced from Becker and Anderson (1978), in: *Paediatric Cardiology* 1977, by permission of Churchill Livingstone, Edinburgh.

atrioventricular defects (p. 108). In a proportion of cases the ventricular septal defect has an entirely muscular rim owing to the fusion of the trabecula septomarginalis with the right-sided ventriculo-infundibular fold.

In approximately 25% of cases of tetralogy of Fallot a right-sided aortic arch is present.

3.2.5. Truncus Arteriosus

This condition is characterized by a single arterial trunk as the only outlet from the heart. It gives rise to the coronary arteries, at least one of the pulmonary arteries, and the ascending aorta (Crupi et al. 1977). There is one arterial orifice (Fig. 4.56) guarded by a semilunar valve, which in the majority of cases is composed of three cusps. A truncal valve with a different number of cusps is encountered in about 30% of cases. Immediately underneath the valve a septal defect is present (Fig. 4.56). The truncus

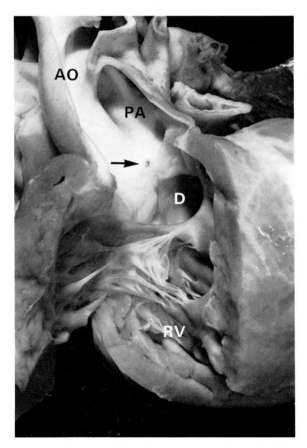

Fig. 4.56. Photograph illustrating truncus arteriosus. The right ventricle (*RV*) has been opened. The heart has one arterial orifice, which overrides a ventricular septal defect (*D*). A single arterial trunk gives rise to the coronary arteries (*arrow* points to an anomously located single ostium), the pulmonary trunk and arteries (*PA*), and the aorta (*Ao*).

overrides the ventricular septum, showing a slight preference for the right ventricle, although its position varies considerably. In the usual case the truncal valve is in direct fibrous continuity with the mitral valve, but is separated from the tricuspid valve by a rim of muscle (the right ventriculo-infundibular fold).

Two major anatomical types of truncus arteriosus can be recognized, depending on the origin of the pulmonary arteries. The first type is characterized by a common pulmonary trunk, from which the right and left pulmonary arteries arise (type I according to the classification of Collett and Edwards 1949). The second variety shows separate origins of the two pulmonary arteries from the truncus (types II and III in the classification of Collett and Edwards).

In rare instances, one of the pulmonary arteries originates from the aorta after its separation from the common truncus.

A particular type of truncus is that in which the pulmonary blood supply originates from the descending thoracic aorta. This particular anomaly is not uniformly accepted as a true truncus. At present the discussion around this anomaly is focussed on the question as to whether or not central pulmonary arteries (i.e., pulmonary arteries within the pericardial sac) are present in this particular condition (Thiene et al. 1976; Sotomora and Edwards 1978). The pathologist will play a major role in settling the question.

Truncus arteriosus shows a distinct tendency to be associated with a right-sided aortic arch, which occurs in approximately 40% of cases.

From a functional point of view, pulmonary hypertension is likely to occur with early development of plexogenic pulmonary arteriopathy.

3.2.6. Univentricular Hearts

Univentricular hearts are characterized by the fact that the atrial inlet portions are committed to a single chamber in the ventricular mass, so that an inlet septum is absent (Anderson et al. 1979). As outlined in Section 2, this condition can be present with two perforate atrioventricular valves, one perforate and one imperforate atrioventricular valve, a common atrioventricular valve, a straddling atrioventricular valve as long as the major circumference of the straddler connecting to the main chamber, or with absence of the right or left atrioventricular connection.

Further classification of univentricular hearts is based on the morphology of the chambers and the presence or absence of a rudimentary chamber within the ventricular mass and the arterial connections (Fig. 4.57).

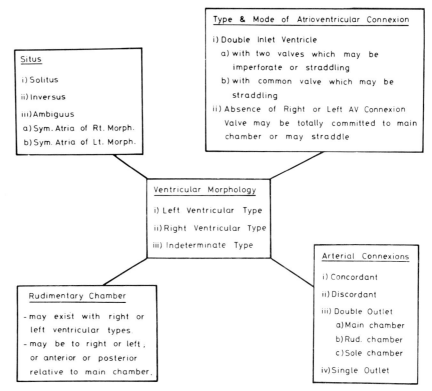

Fig. 4.57. Diagram illustrating the classification of univentricular hearts as based upon the morphology of the chambers, the presence or absence of a rudimentary chamber, and the arterial connections.

The most common form of univentricular heart is the one designated *double inlet univentricular heart of left ventricular type with a rudimentary chamber of right ventricular type* (synonym, single or common ventricle of left ventricular type). In this anomaly the two atria connect to the ventricle, which displays a trabecular pattern of left ventricular characteristics (Fig. 4.58b). A small rudimentary chamber not receiving an atrial inlet is positioned anteriorly in the ventricular mass (Fig. 4.58a). This chamber may be located on the right anterior shoulder of the heart, but it can also be positioned directly anterior or on the left shoulder. The rudimentary chamber connects to the main chamber via a defect, the outlet foramen, which may vary in size. In the usual condition the rudimentary chamber acts as an *outlet chamber* in the sense that the aorta arises from it. The aorta is thus positioned anterior to the pulmonary trunk, which originates from the main chamber (Fig. 4.58). The relationship between aorta and pulmonary trunk, however, can vary according to the position of the outlet chamber. Less commonly the pulmonary artery or both arteries arise from the outlet chamber, or both arteries arise from the ventricle, in which case the rudimentary chamber is simply a trabecular pouch.

The location of the outlet chamber is significant for surgical correction. The conduction tissue always arises from an anterior node, as in corrected transposition.

The second major type of univentricular heart is *double-inlet univentricular heart of right ventricular type, with rudimentary chamber of left ventricular type*, characterized by a ventricle with right ventricular trabecular characteristics (Fig. 4.59a). The rudimentary chamber is usually positioned posteriorly and displays the left ventricular travecular characteristics (Fig. 4.59b). In most cases the rudimentary chamber in this position does not act as an outlet chamber, but is a trabecular pouch with both great arteries originating from the main chamber. The conducting tissue is usually positioned posteriorly because the trabecular septum extends to the crux cordis.

The third major category is *univentricular heart of indeterminate type*. In this condition the trabecular characteristics of the sole chamber cannot be recognized as either right ventricular or left ventricular. In addition, the heart possesses only one chamber within the ventricular mass, which receives both atrial inputs and supports both great arteries. There is no rudimentary chamber.

The conduction tissue in these hearts can be anywhere, but usually arises from an anterior node.

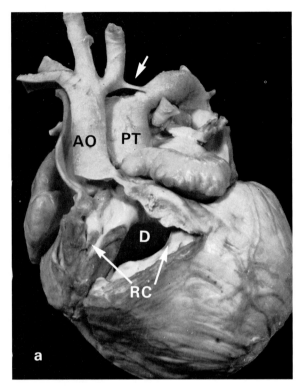 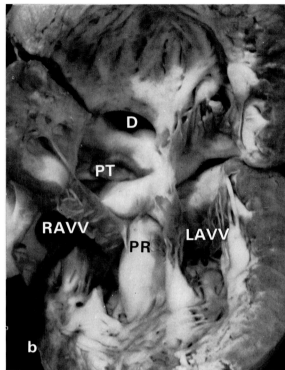

Fig. 4.58. a and **b** Photographs of a heart specimen classified as double-inlet univentricular heart of left ventricular type with a rudimentary chamber of right ventricular type. **a** Anterior view of the heart specimen. A rudimentary chamber (*RC*) is present in the right anterior shoulder of the heart and gives rise to the aorta (*Ao*), which is anterior and to the right of the pulmonary trunk (*PT*). The latter arises from the main chamber (see **b**). The outlet foramen through which the main chamber and rudimentary chamber are connected is clearly seen (*D*). There is atresia of the aortic arch (*arrow*) in this particular specimen. **b** Interior of the main chamber after the heart has been opened like a shell. The right (*RAVV*) and left (*LAVV*) atrioventricular valves enter the main chamber from which the pulmonary trunk (*PT*) arises. There is a posterior ridge (*PR*) between the two valves, but the absence of an inlet septum is conspicuous. The septum separating the rudimentary chamber from the main chamber is anterior and shows the fine trabeculations reminiscent of a morphological left ventricle. The rudimentary chamber receives no atrial inlets, as can be seen from the position of the outlet foramen (*D*) relative to both atrioventricular valves.

3.2.6.1. Tricuspid Atresia. 'Classic' tricuspid atresia is a form of univentricular heart, characterized by an absent right atrioventricular connection (Anderson et al. 1977b). Thus, a deep furrow is present between the right atrium and the underlying ventricular mass, so that there is not even a potential connection between the right atrium and the right ventricular chamber (Fig. 4.60). The only outlet of the right atrium is by way of a patent foramen ovale or an atrial septal defect. The left atrium connects to a main chamber. The ventricular morphology is that of univentricular heart of left ventricular type with a rudimentary chamber of right ventricular type, usually carried on the right anterior shoulder of the heart. This chamber communicates with the ventricle via an outlet foramen. An important difference with double inlet univentricular heart of left ventricular type concerns the arterial connection. In most cases of classic tricuspid atresia a rudimentary chamber supports the pulmonary trunk, the aorta arising from the main chamber (Fig. 4.60). The reverse usually occurs in univentricular heart of left ventricular type and double inlet (Fig. 4.58). However, in a minority of hearts with the arrangement of classic tricuspid atresia a discordant arterial connection can be present. Very rarely there is a double outlet or single outlet connection running either from the rudimentary chamber or from the main chamber.

The type of arterial connection seen in classic tricuspid atresia largely determines the clinical profile of the case. In patients with a concordant arterial connection (the common situation) a diminished pulmonary flow is usually present, while patients with a discordant arterial connection often develop hyperkinetic pulmonary hypertension.

3.2.6.2. Mitral Atresia. Most examples of atresia of the left atrioventricular orifice are due to absence of the left atrioventricular connection, and such hearts, like those with classic tricuspid atresia, are also

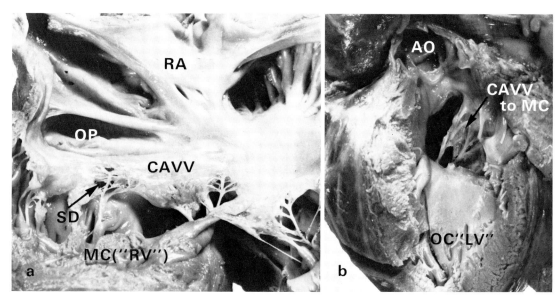

Fig. 4.59. a and **b** Photographs of univentricular heart of right ventricular type with rudimentary chamber of left ventricular type. **a** Opened main chamber of right ventricular type (*MC 'RV'*), receiving almost all of both atrial inlets through a common atrioventricular valve (*AVV*). Underneath the valve a defect is present (*SD*), through which a probe could be passed into a minute chamber with left ventricular characteristics (see **b**). There is an 'ostium primum' (*OP*) atrial septal defect. *RA*, right atrium. **b** The rudimentary chamber of left ventricular morphology (*OC 'LV'*) from which the aorta (*Ao*) arises is shown. The minute portion of the common atrioventricular valve related to this outlet chamber is indicated (*CAVV* to *MC*). From Keeton et al. (1979), by permission of the editors of *Circulation*.

univentricular. Usually absence of the left connection is associated with aortic atresia and an intact septum, and frequently the atretic aorta cannot be traced to the hypoplastic left ventricular chamber, which is a trabecular pouch. In the presence of a septal defect, the chamber is larger and may be in potential communication with the atretic aorta. This type of mitral atresia is therefore a univentricular heart of right ventricular type. Absence of the left connection also occurs in univentricular hearts of left ventricular type with left-sided rudimentary chambers. It is arguable whether this anomaly is mitral or tricuspid atresia. It is unequivocally absence of the left atrioventricular connection, and underlines the significance of the descriptive approach to segmental analysis.

Mitral atresia can also occur with an imperforate valve. This in itself is extremely rare, but when it occurs tends to be associated with double outlet right ventricle.

4. Congenital Malformations of the Aorta

The principal malformations affecting the aortic arch are aortic coarctation, interrupted aortic arch, and vascular rings.

4.1. Coarctation of the Thoracic Aorta

In classic coarctation a shelf-like obstruction is present in the aortic arch, which projects into the lumen from the posterosuperior wall and is situated immediately beyond the origin of the left subclavian artery (Fig. 4.61). Histological examination at the site of obstruction will reveal an infolding of the media (Fig. 4.61b), accentuated on the internal surface by an intimal thickening, which in the infant has a mucoid appearance similar to ductal tissue but in older children and adults is a thick layer of collagen and elastin fibres. In a vast majority of cases the site of obstruction is opposite the aortic orifice of the ductus arteriosus (or ligamentum) and adjacent to the proximal aortic segment. A coarctation in this position is therefore classified as 'juxtaductal'. It is extremely rare for a coarctation to occur distal to the orifice of the ductus arteriosus; in fact the occurrence of coarctation in this particular location is

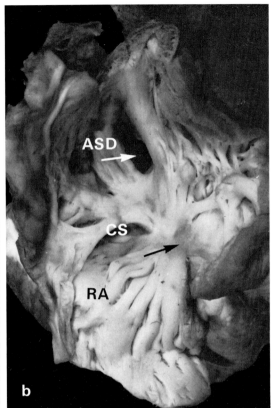

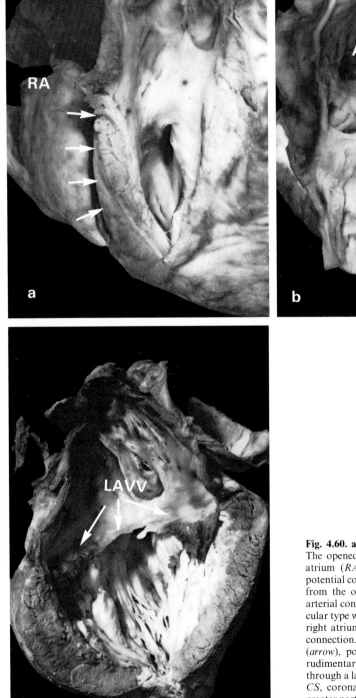

Fig. 4.60. a–c Heart specimen with 'classic' tricuspid atresia. **a** The opened outlet chamber, which is separated from the right atrium (*RA*) by a deep furrow (*arrows*), so that not even a potential connection is present. The pulmonary trunk (*PT*) arises from the outlet chamber, in contrast to the usual discordant arterial connection present in univentricular hearts of left ventricular type with a double atrial inlet (cf. Fig. 4.58a). **b** The opened right atrium (*RA*), revealing the absence of an atrioventricular connection. A dimple is present in the floor of the right atrium (*arrow*), pointing towards the main chamber rather than the rudimentary chamber. The only outlet of the right atrium is through a large atrial septal defect of the fossa ovalis type (*ASD*). *CS*, coronary sinus. **c** The opened left side of the heart. The greater part of the left atrioventricular valve (*LAVV*) has been cut away to reveal the trabecular pattern reminiscent of left ventricular morphology present in the main chamber. The site of the outlet foramen (*arrow*) is barely visible.

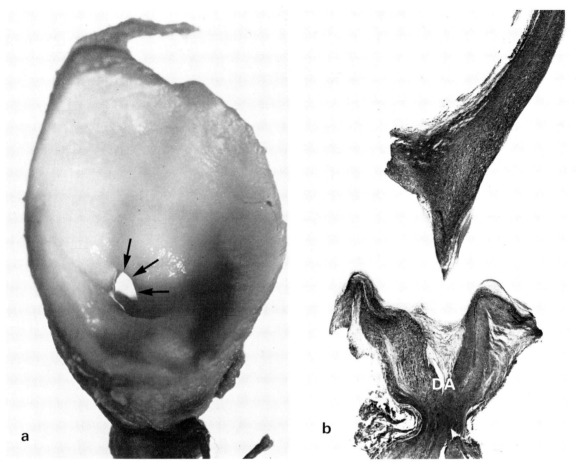

Fig. 4.61. a and **b** Surgically resected specimen of 'classic' aortic coarctation: **a** the gross specimen, viewed from the distal aortic end. A shelf-like infolding projects into the lumen from the postero-superior wall (*arrows*); **b** a histological section from this specimen. The infolding of the media is opposite the site of insertion of the ductus arteriosus (*DA*). (Elastin tissue stain; 8 ×)

questionable. The terms pre- and postductal coarctation have previously been used in relation to the site of obstruction relative to the ductus arteriosus. In such a terminology 'preductal coarctation' has often been considered synonymous with 'infantile coarctation'. However, in the symptomatic neonate the situation is usually much more complicated. In these instances it is common for a segment of the aortic arch to be underdeveloped; a condition termed 'tubular hypoplasia' or 'aortic arch hypoplasia' (Fig. 4.62). The hypoplastic segment is most commonly present between the origin of the left subclavian artery and the site of insertion of the ductus arteriosus, but other sites can be affected. Tubular hypoplasia frequently co-exists with a discrete shelf-like coarctation, and is also frequently associated with a ventricular septal defect and additional left ventricular inlet and/or outlet obstructions. It is this combination of anomalies that

underlies the serious prognosis of a symptomatic coarctation in infancy.

The pathogenesis of coarctation is still controversial. The original Skodaic concept that ductal tissue extends into the aortic wall, leading to constriction may indeed be operative in cases with classic coarctation in the sense of localized shelf-like obstruction. It has been suggested (Rudolph et al. 1972) that reduced flow through the aortic arch during development could lead to insufficient vascular development. This concept, which relates to the common occurrence of additional anomalies, could explain the presence of tubular hypoplasia.

In early infancy coarctation of the aorta results in biventricular hypertrophy. The secondary effects on the systemic vessels, both proximal and distal to the obstruction, will develop in time.

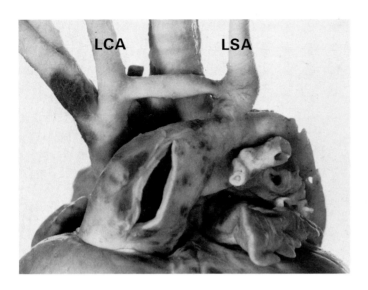

Fig. 4.62. Photograph illustrating tubular hypoplasia of the aortic arch between the left common carotid artery (*LCA*) and the left subclavian artery (*LSA*).

4.2. Interrupted Aortic Arch

This condition is characterized by complete interruption of the arch, most commonly localized immediately distal to the left subclavian artery. Other sites, however, may also be affected. The descending thoracic aorta is fed through a patent ductus arteriosus. The condition is nearly always associated with a ventricular septal defect (p. 106). In *atresia* of the aortic arch a fibrous strand connects the proximal and distal segments of the aorta, whereas in interrupted aortic arch no such remnant can be identified.

4.3. Vascular Rings

So-called vascular rings form a complex group of anomalies of the aortic arch system. The various anomalies can be understood from the developmental scheme of aortic arches (Stewart et al. 1964). The most common type of vascular ring develops when an aberrant subclavian artery originates from the descending aorta beyond the aortic arch. The initial part of this aberrant artery is formed by the dorsal segment of the contralateral arch system. In most cases the subclavian artery will run behind the oesophagus, leaving a slight impression, but the anomaly has no clinical significance. True 'dysphagia lusoria' develops when the aberrant artery connects to the contralateral pulmonary artery by way of a ductus or ligamentum arteriosum. In these instances the vascular anomaly constitutes a ring compressing the enclosed trachea and oesophagus.

Other types of vascular ring are extremely rare and will not be discussed further.

5. Congenital Malformations of the Central Pulmonary Arteries

Developmental anomalies of the central pulmonary arteries are rare. Unilateral absence of a pulmonary artery can occur. In most of these cases the contralateral lung is supplied through a separate 'pulmonary' artery which originates from the aorta.

The term *vascular sling* is reserved for the rare event in which the left pulmonary artery originates from the right pulmonary artery (Lubbers et al. 1975). From this aberrant origin the artery courses to the left lung hilum and passes between the trachea and oesophagus, producing an impression in the anterior wall of the oesophagus.

6. 'Isolated' Congenital Abnormalities of Endo-, Myo-, and Pericardium

Isolated congenital abnormalities of the endo-, myo-, and pericardium are rare lesions, which do not fit any of the previous headings. The lesions appear to be isolated, but further study may show that this is not so.

6.1. Endocardium

Fibroelastosis of the endocardium is a common finding in hearts exhibiting other congenital anomalies that lead to an increased volume or pressure within a cardiac chamber. However, primary endocardial fibroelastosis occurs without associated cardiac anomalies. Primary endocardial fibroelastosis most commonly affects the left ventricle. The endocardium is greatly thickened, giving the inner surface of the left ventricle a whitish appearance (Fig. 4.63a). Histological studies show that the thickening is composed of alternating layers of collagen and elastin (Fig. 4.63b). The underlying myocardium reveals no abnormalities. This histological appearance is not pathognomonic for primary endocardial fibroelastosis, however, since a similar architecture is found in hearts with secondary fibroelastosis, e.g., in hypoplastic left hearts associated with aortic valve anomalies (p. 113).

Primary endocardial fibroelastosis is subdivided into a dilated type, in which the left ventricular chamber is of normal size or enlarged, and a contracted type characterized by a small left ventricular cavity. Differentiation of the latter condition from isolated left ventricular hypoplasia becomes arbitrary. Because of the fibroelastic endocardial layer, the papillary muscle groups of the mitral valve apparatus appear to originate at a higher level than usual. This is most probably an illusion, but it is undoubtedly true that in a high percentage of cases the mitral valve apparatus has been involved by the endocardial process so that mitral valve insufficiency has occurred.

The nature of the disease remains obscure. Several aetiological factors have been suggested, such as a primary myocardial disorder with compensatory endocardial thickening, impaired lymphatic drainage of the heart, and a possible relationship with mumps (Edwards 1968).

6.2. Myocardium

Congenital aneurysms or diverticula of the heart occur. These abnormalities show a predilection for the region of the cardiac apex and the atrioventricular junctional area. Diverticular in the former site have a tendency to be associated with defects in the pericardium and diaphragm.

Uhl's disease (synonym, parchment heart: Uhl 1952) is characterized by focal absence of myocardium of the right ventricular wall, so that endocardium and epicardium become adherent. The condition was originally reported as an isolated lesion, but has since been described with various other anomalies, particularly those affecting the tricuspid valve.

6.3. Pericardium

Congenital defects of the pericardium can be partial or complete. In the case of total absence of the pericardium, the heart and lung lie together within one serous cavity. In a partial defect part of the heart may herniate into the defect, a condition that may become symptomatic.

Pericardial cysts and diverticula occur as a form of developmental anomaly showing preference for the cardiophenic angle. *Epicardial cysts* do occur but are extremely rare.

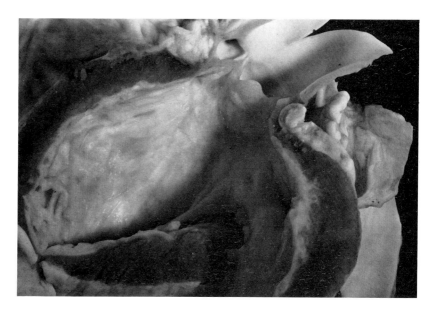

Fig. 4.63. Heart specimen with primary endocardial fibroelastosis. The opened left ventricle exhibits diffuse thickening of the endocardium.

7. Congenital Heart Block

Understanding of the developmental anomalies that can underlie congenital heart block develops from the knowledge that the normal atrioventricular conduction axis develops in situ from different embryological sources (Anderson et al. 1977a). The atrioventricular node and proximal part of the bundle develop on top of the developing inlet part of the ventricular septum, from an invaginated segment of the specialized tissues of the embryonic atrio-ventricular ring. The distal parts develop on the crest of the trabecular septum. These different anlagen are enveloped in embryonic mesenchymal tissue, the so-called sulcus tissues, which in part disappear and in part differentiate into the fibrous tissue of the annulus fibrosus.

Proper formation of the atrioventricular conduction axis thus depends upon normal cardiac septation with proper alignment of atrial and ventricular septa, and apposition of the different segments of the developing atrioventricular conduction axis with proper differentiation of the enveloping sulcus tissues.

It follows that congenital heart block can occur in hearts with a major developmental anomaly of septation, but also in hearts with a failure of proper apposition of the segments, or in which the sulcus tissue has not disappeared. In these the heart may be otherwise normal.

The first category includes conditions such as congenitally corrected transposition of the great arteries (p. 119) and univentricular hearts. The second category can be subdivided according to the level of the developmental anomaly. Two basic varieties are recognized, *atrionodal* discontinuity and *nodoventricular* discontinuity (Becker et al. 1978d) (Fig. 4.64). In the atrionodal form the proximal part of the conduction axis is poorly developed and devoid of atrial inputs whereas the distal parts of the atrioventricular conduction axis are well formed and normally located. In nodo-ventricular discontinuity the proximal and distal segments of the atrioventricular conduction are well formed, but the two are completely separated by dense fibrous tissue of the annulus fibrosus. His-tological studies are the only means of distinguishing between these varieties of congenital heart block.

8. Complications of Congenital Heart Disease

One of the major hazards of a congenitally mal-formed heart is that the anomaly may induce further pathological changes both in the heart itself and in other organ systems. These changes relate primarily to abnormal circulatory pathways, e.g., situations where systemic venous blood is conveyed directly into the aorta or conditions with left-to-right shunts with an increased pulmonary circulation; to a low cardiac output with insufficient perfusion of such organs as the brain, the kidneys and the heart itself; to compensatory myocardial hypertrophy, which may in some instances aggravate the functional consequences of the malformation; or to sites of laceration within the heart resulting from the underlying malformation, rendering certain struc-tures in the heart susceptible to infectious endo-carditis.

In view of all this it is advisable to perform a complete autopsy on any individual who has died of 'congenital heart disease' to obtain full insight into the pathophysiology of the disease.

8.1. Systemic Thromboemboli and Thrombosis

Paradoxical thromboemboli are a potential danger in all conditions in which right-to-left shunts exist. Emboli that originate in the systemic venous site of the circulation may cross into the systemic arterial circulation at all levels where mixing of the greater and lesser circulations occurs. Moreover, in the grossly desaturated (cyanotic) patient with a mar-kedly increased haematocrit, 'spontaneous' throm-bosis can occur, leading to irreversible changes in such vital organs as the brain.

8.2. Brain Abscess

The complication of a brain abscess is particularly likely in patients with a right-to-left shunt, whatever the anatomy of the underlying cardiac condition. In most cases the heart itself does not contain an infectious focus. The development of the brain abscess relates to the abnormal circulatory path-ways. Infected systemic venous blood is no longer 'filtered' in the lungs, but is in part conveyed directly into the systemic arterial circulation. This abnormal flow pattern will also lead to systemic arterial desaturation and hypoxia of the brain, a situation that renders the brain particularly vulnerable to an infection with anaerobic micro-organisms.

8.3. Renal Pathology

Renal insufficiency may appear clinically, particularly in patients suffering from low cardiac output (e.g., aortic stenosis) or in those with diminished perfusion of the kidneys (e.g., coarctation of the aorta). In some instances histological examination of the kidney reveals pathological changes consistent with renal ischaemia. Careful examination of the

glomeruli may reveal the existence of a process of intravascular clotting consequent on the cardiac disorder. Severe cyanosis is usually associated with glomerular hypertrophy.

8.4. Myocardial Pathology

It has long been known that in many patients with congenital heart malformations the myocardium contains areas of necrosis (Berry 1967; Franciosi and Blanc 1968). Both recent necrosis and various stages of repair can be encountered. In some instances it is evident that the changes must have

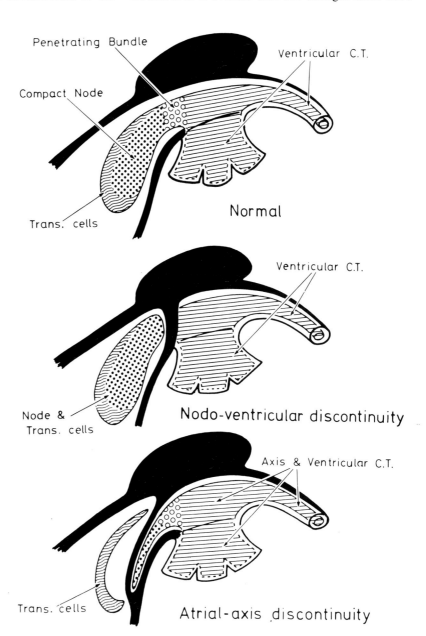

Fig. 4.64. Diagrams illustrating the two basic anatomical varieties of congenitally complete heart block in otherwise normal hearts. Reproduced from Becker et al. (1978), in: *Proceedings of the Symposium in Neonatal Cardiology*, by permission of Churchill Livingstone, Edinburgh.

occurred in utero, since extensive scarring, often accompanied by calcific deposits, can be present at birth. In such circumstances it is not immediately apparent whether myocardial cell death has been caused by a circulatory insufficiency or by other mechanisms, such as acquired intrauterine toxic or infectious diseases.

In other patients, who have lived with a congenital heart defect for a variable period, it is sometimes evident that actual *myocardial infarction* has occurred. This is a particularly frequent finding in hearts where coronary perfusion has been minimal, above all when combined with marked myocardial hypertrophy. Long-standing myocardial hypertrophy is nearly always accompanied by focal intramural fibrosis, which is most probably related to these mechanisms.

The significance of secondary degenerative changes in the natural history of patients who have undergone surgical 'correction' of their congenital heart defect remains speculative. However, there is accumulating clinical evidence that myocardial dysfunction in survivors becomes a major problem. In other conditions compensatory myocardial hypertrophy can have a deleterious effect in aggravating the clinical course of the disease. The outflow tract stenosis in tetralogy of Fallot can be cited as an example in this respect. The infundibulum is narrow at birth, due to an intrinsic abnormality of septal structures (p. 124), but it may become further narrowed because of myocardial hypertrophy and secondary endocardial fibroelastosis. The disease may thus gradually progress towards functional pulmonary atresia. In other conditions, e.g., classic tricuspid atresia or double inlet univentricular hearts with outlet chamber, the outlet foramen may diminish in size owing to myocardial hypertrophy and fibroelastosis, and diminished flow in the corresponding great artery will result. In some individuals suffering from various types of congenital heart disease, myocardial hypertrophy may develop to such an extent that hypertrophic (obstructive) cardiomyopathy appears. The precise pathogenetic mechanisms underlying this disorder are still not known.

Similarly, primarily induced right ventricular hypertrophy (e.g., in patients with 'isolated' pulmonary valve stenosis and intact ventricular septum) may in time lead to left ventricular myocardial hypertrophy and, rarely to left ventricular outflow tract obstruction. The pathogenetic mechanisms in these cases are probably related to alterations in the geometry of the left ventricular cavity.

8.5. Infectious Endocarditis

Infectious endocarditis in congenital heart disease usually affects sites of laceration, these being a direct consequence of the haemodynamic abnormalities resulting from the defect. In ventricular septal defects, the edges of affected sites reveal endocardial thickening. Similarly the tricuspid valve can become involved, as can parts of the right ventricular septum and free wall. Early structural changes are induced within the leaflets of anatomically abnormal valves, rendering them susceptible to infection. Bicuspid aortic valve is a classic example, although complications of this condition are rarely significant in the paediatric age group.

8.6. Pulmonary Vascular Pathology

It is important to realize that the pulmonary vascular bed should be considered to be intimately associated with any cardiac abnormality. Indeed, the 'success' of most surgical corrections in congenital heart disease depends upon the state of the pulmonary vascular bed prior to operation.

In childhood there are three major categories of induced pulmonary vascular changes to consider. These occur firstly in conditions with an increased pulmonary *arterial* flow, secondly in those with decreased flow, and finally in situations with primarily pulmonary *venous* hypertension.

Increased pulmonary flow. In these conditions a left-to-right shunt is nearly always present. The pulmonary vascular bed will initially adapt to the increased flow, enabling a large percentage of total cardiac output to pass through the lungs. However, in time structural changes will occur, the first expression of which is medial hypertrophy of muscular pulmonary arteries. These changes may gradually become complicated by a proliferation of intimal cells, leading to a concentric lamellar type of intimal fibrosis (Fig. 4.65a). The pulmonary arteries may ultimately develop fibrinoid necrosis and plexiform lesions (Fig. 4.66b). The term *plexogenic pulmonary arteriopathy* has been introduced to indicate this morphological pattern (World Health Organization 1975; Wagenvoort 1977). In the fully developed state, plexiform lesions will be present, but in less advanced instances the only change indicative of the onset of this train of events is medial hypertrophy, which is considered to be reversible in nature. In contrast, it is generally accepted that fibrinoid necrosis and plexiform lesions represent irreversible damage to pulmonary arteries. There is evidence that pulmonary hypertension with early plexogenic changes, such as cellular intimal pro-

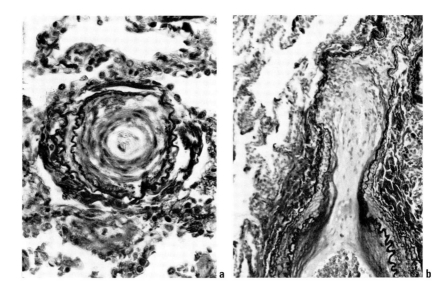

Fig. 4.65. a and b Micrographs showing two stages of plexogenic pulmonary arteriopathy: a pulmonary artery with a concentric lamellar type of intimal fibrosis (**a**, 350 ×) and a plexiform lesion (**b**, 140 ×) (Elastin tissue stain)

liferation, and with limited intimal fibrosis can still be reversible.

The structural characteristics of plexogenic pulmonary arteriopathy do not depend on the type of shunt. Thus, the structural changes are similar whether the patient has an atrial or a ventricular septal defect, a persistent ductus arteriosus, or a truncus arteriosus. The major difference is that irreversible arteriopathy will develop much later in patients with an atrial septal defect than in those with a 'post-tricuspid' shunt.

Decreased pulmonary flow. In patients with pulmonary stenosis, irrespective of the underlying cause, the pulmonary arteries are characteristically thin-walled and often dilated. Intravascular thrombosis and subsequent organization may result in cushion-like intimal fibrosis and the formation of intravascular fibrous septa.

Pulmonary venous hypertension. A variety of congenital cardiac malformations can lead to pulmonary venous congestion and hypertension. This in turn leads to medial hypertrophy of pulmonary veins, which in some instances (e.g., aortic atresia) can be present even before birth. The media of these veins may develop a structural rearrangement of elastin fibres, so that distinct internal and external laminae are formed. This process is called 'arterialization' and can be regarded as a reliable indicator of elevated pulmonary venous pressure (Fig. 4.66). The main feature of the pulmonary arteries in children with pulmonary venous hypertension is medial hypertrophy and muscularization of small arterioles; these arteries are devoid of easily recognizable media under normal circumstances. Plexiform lesions do not develop.

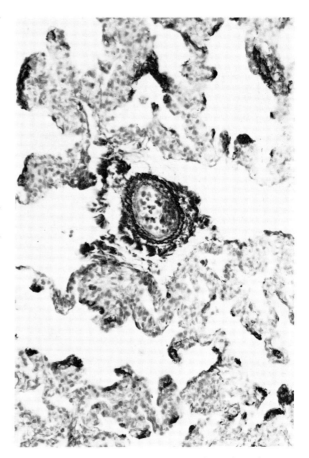

Fig. 4.66. Micrograph showing 'arterialization' of a pulmonary vein. (Elastin tissue stain; 65 ×)

8.7. Bronchial Compression

In a minority of patients with a left-to-right shunt, respiratory symptoms may not be caused primarily by the development of pulmonary vascular disease, but by compression of bronchi secondary to dilatation of pulmonary arteries. The anatomy of the pulmonary arterial tree in relation to that of the tracheobronchial tree shows certain sites of predilection for bronchial compression. These are the left main stem bronchus and the site of origin of the left upper lobe bronchus, and the right-sided intermediate bronchus and site of origin of the right middle lobe bronchus.

Dilatation of pulmonary arteries with increased intraluminal pressure may lead to external compression of the bronchi at these sites, which may result in either hyperinflation or atelectasis of the corresponding lobes.

8.8 Postnatally Acquired Heart Disease

The abnormalities described above are acquired, but still relate directly to the presence of an underlying congenital heart malformation. The heart may also be involved in many other disease processes, none of which is specific to the heart.

The most important group is that of the *infectious diseases*. Myocarditis and pericarditis can complicate almost any infectious disease, whether acquired in the prenatal or the postnatal period. The inflammatory process in the heart is usually nonspecific, and a definitive diagnosis depends on a full autopsy and bacteriological and virological studies. With the early recognition and treatment of most infectious diseases, at least in the West, their significance for cardial pathology has declined. The same applies to rheumatic fever, which in Europe no longer plays an important role in early morbidity and mortality.

Infantile periarteritis nodosa needs a brief discussion. This disease of unknown aetiology has a marked tendency to affect the coronary arteries. In such patients arteritis, with a predominantly mononuclear cellular infiltrate, and thrombosis can lead to myocardial infarction and death. Moreover, the disease may lead to the formation of coronary aneurysms, which may ultimately rupture, causing cardiac tamponade (Fig. 4.67). A positive diagnosis of infantile periarteritis nodosa always depends on histological verification, since the clinical spectrum

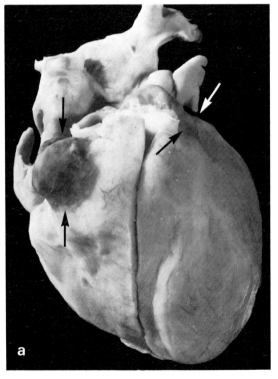
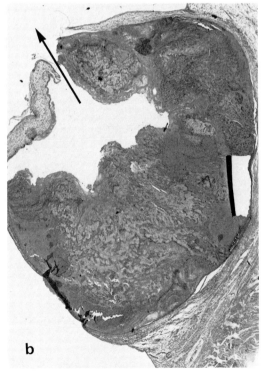

Fig. 4.67. a and **b.** Photographs illustrating a case of infantile periarteritis nodosa affecting the coronary arteries: **a** mycotic aneurysms in the proximal segments of both coronary arteries (*arrows*). The infant died of cardiac tamponade due to a rupture of the aneurysm in the right coronary artery; **b** histology of the aneurysm at the site of rupture (*arrow*). (Elastin tissue stain; 7×)

is rather complex and is considered nonspecific.

A 'new' disease entity has recently been reported, called *Kawasaki's disease* (synonym mucocutaneous lymph node syndrome) (Kawasaki 1974; Tanaka et al. 1976; Fujiwara and Hamashima 1978), which in Japan appears to be one of the most frequent causes of cardiovascular disease in infancy. The diagnosis of Kawasaki's disease is made primarily on clinical grounds. It is of interest, therefore, that patients who die of the disease (approximately 1%–2% of those affected) show pathological changes that cannot be distinguished from those of infantile periarteritis nodosa. Coronary arteritis with thrombosis and coronary aneurysms are present in nearly all instances. Furthermore, histologically nonspecific interstitial myocarditis is also identified in some cases. It is suggestive, therefore, that the medium-sized arteries constitute the target organ for an immune disorder, the nature of which remains unclear. Infantile periarteritis nodosa, being a descriptive term, could therefore be regarded as the pathological substrate of Kawasaki's disease (Becker 1976).

9. Syndromes Commonly Associated with Cardiovascular Malformations

Syndromes will only be discussed where a cardiovascular anomaly plays a major role in the disease. The type of anomaly will be mentioned: further details regarding the syndromes are given in the relevant chapters.

9.1. Visceral Symmetry Syndromes

Syndromes of visceral symmetry constitute a complex developmental disorder, and they have a profound tendency to be associated with anomalies of the cardiovascular system. Recognition of abdominal visceral heterotaxia and situs ambiguus of the thoracic organs should immediately alert the pathologist to these syndromes.

Visceral symmetry syndrome of bilateral right-sided type (dextroisomerism) is nearly always associated with an absent spleen, hence the term asplenia syndrome (synonym, Ivemark's syndrome) (Van Mierop et al. 1972).

The abdominal viscera in over 50% of cases show a bilaterally symmetrical liver with the gallbladder, stomach, duodenum, and pancreas on the right side, accompanied by varying degrees of malrotation of the intestines. The thoracic situs may reveal bilateral *tri*lobed lungs, and dissection of the tracheobronchial anatomy will show bilateral eparterial bronchi in nearly all cases. The cardiovascular system is highly abnormal in these instances. Bilateral superior caval veins, both draining to their respective atria, are present in the majority of cases. The abdominal part of the inferior caval vein ascends on either the right or left side of the spine, in close association with the abdominal aorta, and enters the atrium on its corresponding side. It is often accompanied by a common hepatic vein, which connects to the contralateral atrium. Bilateral total anomalous pulmonary venous connections are the rule. Even in the cases where the pulmonary veins enter an atrium they do so in the intercaval part derived from the sinus venosus, and therefore connect in an anomalous way. The heart in the vast majority of cases shows major abnormalities. The two atria, apart from the anomalous systemic and pulmonary venous connections, show isomeric atrial appendages of the right-sided type. The coronary sinus is usually absent, in keeping with the high incidence of a persistent left superior caval vein draining directly into the left-sided atrium. The atrial septum is abnormal and in most cases consists of a small triangular muscular band, which originates from the postero-inferior atrial wall and inserts with its apex into the anterior atrial wall. This band bridges a common atrioventricular orifice, which is almost invariably present. In the majority of patients a form of univentricular heart (Sect. 3.2.6.1) is present. Usually, the relative positions of the great arteries are abnormal, with the aorta anterior to the pulmonary trunk, while pulmonary stenosis and atresia are commonly associated anomalies.

A high degree of consistency in the pattern of the cardiovascular abnormalities is present in the dextroisomeric form of visceral symmetry syndrome.

Visceral symmetry syndrome of the bilateral left-sided type (levoisomerism) is nearly always associated with multiple spleens located to both sides of the dorsal mesogastrium (p. 224); hence the name 'polysplenia syndrome' (Van Mierop et al. 1972).

The abdominal viscera reveal isomerism of the liver in approximately 25% of cases. In the remainder the major lobe is more commonly found on the left than on the right side. The gall-bladder has a tendency to be associated with the major lobe, but it can be positioned in the mid-line or absent. In the majority of cases, the stomach, duodenum and pancreas are found on the right side. Malrotation of the intestines is a frequent condition. The thoracic situs may show bilateral *bi*lobed lungs, though bilateral hyparterial bronchi are a more consistent finding. In most instances the cardiovascular system will show abnormalities. Bilateral superior caval veins occur in less than 50% of cases. A single superior caval vein is more commonly found on the right than on the left side. In the majority of patients the inferior caval vein connects to the azygos venous system whether right- or left-sided, and drains by way of it into the superior caval vein. The separate common hepatic vein connects the liver to the right- or the left-sided atrium. Juxtaposition of the abdominal segment of the inferior caval vein and the aorta may occur, albeit less frequently than in cases with dextroisomerism. In some instances the right and left pulmonary veins connect to their respective sides of the atria, the sites of entrance being widely separated and often indicated by a groove in the postero-inferior atrial wall. In other cases the right and left pulmonary veins connect to one of the atria. In rare instances the pulmonary veins connect to a systemic vein. In some cases the atrial septum is intact, but the majority of patients have some sort of an atrial septal defect. At the level of the atrioventricular junction a common atrioventricular valve will be present in approximately 50% of cases. Two ventricles are almost always present, with a high frequency of double outlet right ventricle. Some type of a ventricular septal defect is almost always present. Pulmonary valve anomalies, on the other hand, are rare.

In the levoisomeric variety of visceral symmetry syndrome the spectrum of cardiovascular anomalies is much wider than in the dextroisomeric form, and includes a higher percentage of potentially correctable lesions.

9.2. Syndromes with Autosomal Chromosomal Anomalies (see also p. 76)

A variety of syndromes involve autosomal chromosomal anomalies, and the majority of them present a complex constellation of malformations. It is rare for cardiovascular anomalies to present as the leading clinical feature.

Trisomy 13–15 (D syndrome). The predominant cardiovascular anomaly is ventricular septal defect although other malformations, such as tetralogy of Fallot, can be present. The combination of polydactyy with cheilognathopalatoschisis should suggest the possibility of this particular trisomy.

Trisomy 16–18 (E syndrome). The major cardiovascular anomalies that accompany the other malformations present in this syndrome are ventricular septal defect and patent ductus arteriosus.

Trisomy 21 (Down's syndrome; mongolism). In about 40% of affected patients, trisomy 21 is associated with a congenital malformation of the heart. The most common conditions are atrioventricular defects and isolated ventricular septal defects.

9.3. Syndromes with Sex Chromosomal Anomalies

Among the various syndromes with sex chromosomal anomalies, *Turner's syndrome* may involve major cardiovascular anomalies with distinct clinical significance. The most commonly associated conditions are lymphoedema, caused by abnormalities in the development of the lymphatic system, and aortic coarctation and ventricular septal defect.

9.4. Noonan's Syndrome

A familial syndrome with an autosomal dominant trait, Noonan's syndrome is phenotypically closely related to Turner's syndrome, but with a normal karyotype. Cardiac abnormalities are apparent in approximately 50%–60% of patients. The most frequent abnormality is pulmonary stenosis, resulting from valve dysplasia. However, other abnormalities may be present, such as dysplasia of the aortic valve, patent ductus arteriosus, anomalous pulmonary venous connections and aortic coarctation. Recent reports emphasize a high frequency of hypertrophic cardiomyopathy underlying a dynamic type of left ventricular outflow tract obstruction (p. 116).

9.5. Glycogen Storage Diseases (see also p. 552)

The glycogen storage diseases are characterized by a genetically determined abnormality of the carbohydrate metabolism, which results in an intracellular accumulation of glycogen. Different forms exist, of which type II (Pompe's disease) is the one that primarily affects the heart. The condition is due to a deficiency of the enzyme acid maltase and is characterized grossly by cardiomegaly. Histological studies reveal massive accumulation of glycogen in all myocardial cells, which on routinely processed sections stained with haematoxylin and eosin exhibit extensive vacuolization of myocytes (Fig. 4.68).

9.6. Muscopolysaccharidosis (see pp. 464 and 621)

The various types of mucopolysaccharidosis are characterized by an abnormal accumulation of mucopolysaccharides present in large vacuolated

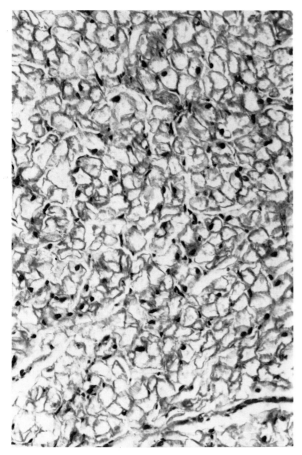

Fig. 4.68. Micrograph showing extensive vacuolization of the myocardial cells in a case of glycogen storage disease. (H and E; 230 ×)

cells. Different types exist, of which type I (Hurler's disease) and type II (Hunter's disease) affect the heart. Both conditions lead to dwarfism, with a characteristic facial appearance. Type I is transmitted as an autosomal recessive trait, in contrast to type II, which is an X-linked recessive. In both conditions the abnormal products accumulated are chondroitin suplhate B and heparin sulphate.

The cardiac valves are the structures mainly affected. On gross examination they show marked fibrosis, with thickened chordae; in this the condition is reminiscent of rheumatic valve disease, from which it should be differentiated. Histological studies reveal the large vacuolated clear cells. Fresh tissue is needed to demonstrate the accumulated mucopolysaccharides, since the abnormal products are water-soluble.

The abnormalities are not restricted to the valves, but can present focally in the myocardium and coronary arteries.

9.7. Marfan's Syndrome

Marfan's syndrome is characterized by defective connective tissues, the precise pathogenesis of which is still undetermined. The abnormalities that occur within the cardiovascular system all relate to the disorder of the supportive tissues. An early sign of the disease is dilatation of the aortic root. The most characteristic cardiac lesions are 'floppy' valves, in the sense of large redundant valve leaflets and attenuated chordae, leading to valve prolapse and insufficiency. The symptoms relate mainly to affected aortic and mitral valves. A common complication is dissecting aneurysm of the aorta. However, cardiovascular symptoms rarely occur in children.

9.8. Ehlers–Danlos Syndrome

An autosomal dominant disease, Ehlers–Danlos syndrome is characterized by a connective tissue abnormality that can affect the cardiovascular system. The changes, therefore, are like those which occur in Marfan's disease. A specific morphological change is as yet unknown. The coarse fragmented elastin fibres seen with the light microscope are probably an expression of an underlying primary collagen disorder. Clinical manifestations of this disease in childhood are rare.

9.9. Holt–Oram Syndrome

Holt–Oram syndrome is an inherited disease, showing an autosomal dominant trait. It is characterized by skeletal abnormalities, the most striking of which is an abnormal, often elongated thumb. The most frequently associated cardiac anomaly is atrial septal defect of the fossa ovalis type.

9.10. Osteogenesis Imperfecta (p. 461)

Similar abnormalities to those in Marfan's syndrome have been described in osteogenesis imperfecta, although the cardiovascular problems in osteogenesis imperfecta rarely dominate the clinical symptomatology.

9.11. Neuromuscular Disorders

In some instances a skeletal myopathy is associated with cardiac abnormalities. This is particularly true for *Friedreich's ataxia*, in which electrocardiographic abnormalities and heart failure can occur at a young age. Histological studies reveal nonspecific interstitial fibrosis with regressive changes of myocytes. Similar changes have been reported to occur in the myocardium of patients suffering from dystrophia myotonica and forms of progressive muscular dystrophy.

10. Cardiac Tumours

Primary cardiac tumours are extremely rare. Secondary or metastatic tumours of the heart are also rare in children, malignant lymphoma and neuroblastoma being the least uncommon. Leukaemic deposits are often found in the heart if carefully looked for.

The primary cardiac tumours that most frequently become symptomatic in the paediatric age group are rhabdomyomas, fibromas and vascular lesions.

10.1. Rhabdomyoma

Rhabdomyomas of the heart occur as circumscribed nodules, of a greyish tan colour within an otherwise normal-appearing myocardium (Fig. 4.69a). On microscopic examination the affected area shows markedly swollen myocytes with an irregular vacuolization. The vacuoles differ in size and are separated by thin strands of cytoplasm in which cross-striations may sometimes be identified. This architecture gives the characteristic appearance of the so-called spider cell (Fig. 4.69b). A diastase-resistant polysaccharide can sometimes be demonstrated within the cells. Microscopial studies of other areas of the myocardium, which grossly appear unaffected, will often reveal additional minute foci of a similar architecture. The nature of these lesions remains unclear. Because of the polysaccharide content of the cells it has been suggested that rhabdomyoma constitutes a particular type of glycogen storage disease. However, the markedly

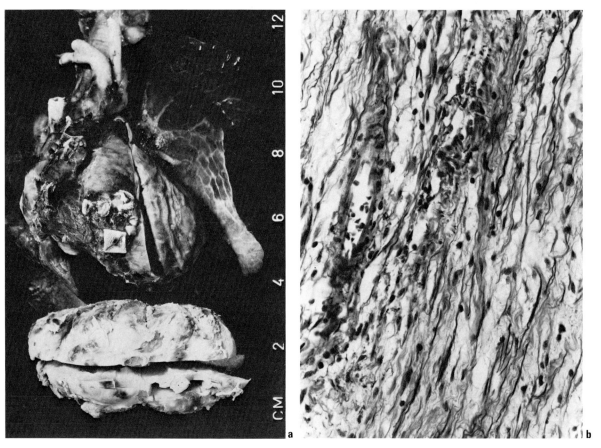

Fig. 4.69. a and **b** Illustrations of a cardiac fibroma. **a** the post-mortem specimen of the heart, in relation to the surgically removed fibroma. The latter was located in the right ventricular free wall and extended into the ventricular septum. At surgery the lesion appeared well delineated; **b** micrograph exhibiting the characteristic compact arrangement of wavy collagen fibres. (Elastin tissue stain, counterstained with Van Gieson stain; 350 ×)

dissimilar histological appearance makes this unlikely. It is of interest that cardiac rhabdomyoma has a strong tendency to be associated with tuberous sclerosis (p. 158).

As a rule rhabdomyoma of the heart leads to symptoms in early childhood.

10.2. Cardiac Fibroma

There is no consensus on the categorization of cardiac fibroma as a true neoplasm or hamartoma. Cardiac fibroma occurs predominantly in the left ventricular free wall or the ventricular septum (Figure 4.70). Gross examination reveals an apparently circumscribed lesion (Fig. 4.70a), which appears homogeneous and whitish on its cut surface. Microscopic studies reveal a compact arrangement of wavy collagen fibres with sparse vascularity (Fig. 4.70b). At the periphery the lesion may interdigitate with pre-existent myocardial fibres. Cardiac fibroma may occur in association with generalized fibromatosis. The symptomatology is largely related to the size and site of the lesion. Successful extirpation of cardiac fibromas has been reported (Geha et al. 1967).

10.3. Vascular Lesions

All histological types of haemangioma (cavernous, capillary, and mixed types) have been incidental findings at autopsy, but occasionally such a vascular anomaly can cause haemopericardium and tamponade.

The suspicion that a cardiac lesion may be an haemangioma is usually aroused by its gross aspect. Some haemangiomas appear to be circumscribed, but extensive spread is often present between pre-existent myocardial fibres.

10.4. Miscellaneous Lesions

Other primary cardiac tumours can occur in the paediatric age group, but they seldom become symptomatic. This applies in particular to the most common type of cardiac tumour, the *cardiac myxoma*. Only rarely will this tumour give rise to symptoms in children. Similarly, myxomatous papillary lesions can occur on the valves, but again are hardly ever of clinical significance in the young. *Mesothelioma of the atrioventricular node* deserves mention because this unique tumour can underlie conduction abnormalities (atrioventricular dissociation) and sudden death. The lesion replaces in part the atrioventricular node and is composed of

tubules lined by a single or multiple layer of predominantly flat cuboid cells. The tubules are embedded in a fibrous stroma. The histological appearance is somewhat reminiscent of that seen in mesothelioma. The nature of the lesion, however, remains speculative.

There have been isolated reports of primary *malignant* cardiac tumours, such as rhabdomyosarcoma and fibrosarcoma, occurring in the paediatric age group.

Blood cysts are small red nodules that appear predominantly on the mitral and tricuspid valves in

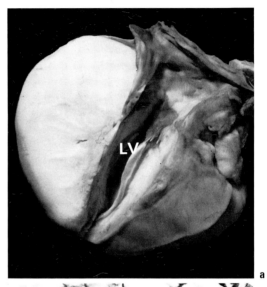

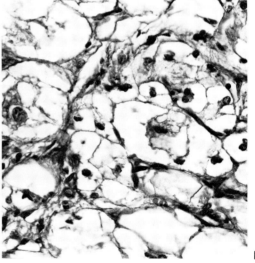

Fig. 4.70. a and **b** Illustrations of a cardiac rhabdomyoma: **a** incised left ventricle (*LV*) with the rhabdomyoma located in its anterior wall extending into the ventricular septum thereby reducing the left ventricular cavity to a slit-like space; **b** micrograph·revealing the spider cell architecture characteristic for rhabdomyoma. (H and E; 350 ×)

almost any neonatal heart. The 'cyst' is formed by crevices in the valve leaflets, filled with 'trapped' blood giving the characteristic appearance. The lesions tend to disappear with time and are completely benign.

References

Allwork SP, Bentall HH, Becker AE, Cameron H, Gerlis LM, Wilkinson JL, Anderson RH (1976) Congenitally corrected transposition of the great arteries: morphologic study of 32 cases. J Cardiol 38: 910

Anderson RH, Becker AE, Arnold R, Wilkinson JL (1974) The conducting tissues in congenitally corrected transposition. Circulation 50: 911

Anderson RH, Becker AE, Gerlis LM (1975) The pulmonary outflow tract in classically corrected transposition. J Thorac Cardiovasc Surg 69: 747

Anderson RH, Wenink ACG, Losekoot TG, Becker AE (1977a) Congenitally complete heart block. Developmental aspects. Circulation 56: 90

Anderson RH, Wilkinson JL, Gerlis LM, Smith A, Becker AE (1977b) Atresia of the right atrioventricular orifice. Br Heart J 39: 414

Anderson RH, Tynan MJ, Freedom RM, Quero-Jimenez M, Macartney FJ, Shinebourne EA, Van Mierop LHS, Wilkinson JL, Becker AE (1979) Ventricular morphology in the univentricular heart. Herz 4: 184

Becker AE, Becker MJ, Edwards JE (1971) Pathologic spectrum of dysplasia of the tricuspid valve. Features in common with Ebsteins' malformation. Arch Pathol 91: 167

Becker AE, Connon M, Anderson RH (1975) Tetralogy of Fallot. A morphometric and geometric study. Am J Cardiol 35: 402

Becker AE (1976) Kawasaki disease. Lancet 1: 864

Becker AE (1978) Transposition of the great arteries: introductory remarks. In: Van Mierop LHS, Oppenheimer-Dekker A, Bruins CLDC (eds) Embryology and teratology of the heart and the great arteries. Martinus Nijhoff, The Hague, p 91

Becker AE, Anderson RH (1978) Fallot's tetralogy—developmental aspects, anatomy and conducting tissues. In: Anderson RH, Shinebourne EA (eds) Paediatric cardiology 1977. Churchill-Livingstone, Edinburgh, p 245

Becker AE, Lie KI, Anderson RH (1978a) Bundle-branch block in the setting of acute anteroseptal myocardial infarction. Br Heart J 40: 773

Becker AE, Losekoot TG, Anderson RH (1978b) The conducting tissues in congenitally complete heart block. Clinico-pathologic correlation in three patients. In: Van Mierop LHS, Oppenheimer-Dekker A, Bruins CLDC (eds) Embryology and teratology of the heart and the great arteries. Martinus Nijhoff, The Hague, p 43

Becu LM, Fontana RS, DuShane JW, Kirklin JW, Burchell HB, Edwards JE (1956) Anatomic and pathologic studies in ventricular septal defects. Circulation 14: 349

Berry CL (1967) Myocardial ischemia in infancy and childhood. J Clin Pathol 20: 38

Bland EF, White PD, Garland J (1933) Congenital anomalies of the coronary arteries: report of an unusual case associated with cardiac hypertrophy. Am Heart J 8: 787

Brandt PWT, Calder AL (1977) Cardiac connections: the segmental approach to radiologic diagnosis in congenital heart disease. Current Problems in Diagnostic Radiology 7: 3

Campbell M (1968) The incidence and later distribution of malformations of the heart. In: Watson H (ed) Paediatric cardiology. London

Caruso G, Losekoot TG, Becker AE (1978) Ebstein's anomaly in persistent common atrioventricular canal. Br Heart J 40: 1275

Caruso G, Becker AE (1979) How to determine atrial situs? Considerations initiated by three cases of absent spleen with a discordant anatomy between bronchi and atria. Br Heart J 41: 559

Collett RW, Edwards JE (1949) Persistent truncus arteriosus: a classification according to anatomic types. Surg Clin North Am 29: 1245

Crupi G, Macartney FJ, Anderson RH (1977) Persistent truncus arteriosus. A study of 66 autopsy cases with sepecial reference to definition and morphogenesis. Am J Cardiol 40: 569

Davies MJ (1971) Pathology of conducting tissue of the heart. Butterworths, London

Doucette J, Knoblich R (1963) Persistent right valve of the sinus venosus. So-called cor triatriatum dextrum: review of the literature and report of a case. Arch Pathol 75: 105

Durrer D, Roos JR, van Dam RT (1966) The genesis of the electrocardiogram of patients with ostium primum defects (ventral atrial septal defects). Am Heart J 71: 642

Edwards JE (1968) Congenital malformations of the heart and great vessels. In: Gould SE (ed) Pathology of the heart and blood vessels, 3rd edn. Thomas, Springfield, p 373

Feldt RH, DuShane JW, Titus JL (1970) The atrioventricular conduction system in persistent common atrioventricular canal defect: correlations with electrocardiogram. Circulation 42: 437

Franciosi RA, Blanc WA (1968) Myocardial infarcts in infants and children. I. A necropsy study in congenital heart disease. J Pediatr 73: 309

Fujiwara H, Hamashima Y (1978) Pathology of the heart in Kawasaki disease. Pediatrics 61: 100

Geha AS, Weidman WH, Soule EH, McGoon DC (1967) Intramural ventricular cardiac fibroma. Successful removal in two cases and review of the literature. Circulation 36: 427

Gittenberger-de Groot AC (1977) Persistent ductus arteriosus: most probably a primary congenital malformation. Br Heart J 39: 610

Gittenberger-de Groot AC, Moulaert AJ, Harinck E, Becker AE (1978) Histopathology of the ductus arteriosus after prostaglandin E_1 administration in ductus dependent cardiac anomalies. Br Heart J 40: 215

Goor DA, Lillehei CW, Rees R, Edwards JE (1970) Isolated ventricular septal defect. Development basis for various types and presentation of classification. Chest 58: 468

Harinck E, Becker AE, Gittenberger-de Groot AC, Oppenheimer-Dekker A, Versprille A (1977) The left ventricle in congenital isolated pulmonary valve stenosis. A morphological study. Br Heart J 39: 429

Kawasaki T, Kosaki F, Okawa S, Shigematsu I, Yanagawa H (1974) A new infantile acute febrile mucocutaneous lymphnode syndrome (MCLS) prevailing in Japan. Pediatrics 54: 271

Keeton BR, Macartney FJ, Hunter S, Mortera C, Rees P, Shinebourne EA, Tynan M, Wilkinson JL, Anderson RH (1979) Univentricular heart of right ventricular type with double or common inlet. Circulation 59: 403

Kerrebijn KF (1964) Kindercardiologie in Nederland. Groen, Leiden

Kirklin JW, Pacifico AD, Bargeron LM, Soto B (1973) Cardiac repair in anatomically corrected malposition of the great arteries. Circulation 48: 153

Kitamura N, Takao A, Ando M (1974) Taussig–Bing heart with mitral valve straddling: case reports and postmortem study. Circulation 49: 761

Lev M (1958) The architecture of the conduction system in congenital heart disease. I. Common atrioventricular orifice. Arch Pathol 65: 174

Lev M (1959) The pathologic anatomy of ventricular septal defects. Dis Chest 35: 533

Lev M, Agustsson MH, Arcilla R (1961) The pathologic anatomy of common atrioventricular orifice associated with tetralogy of Fallot. J Clin Pathol 36: 408

Lev M, Rowlatt UF (1961) Pathological anatomy of mixed levocardia. A review of thirteen cases of atrial or ventricular inversion with or without corrected transposition. Am J Cardiol 8: 216

Lev M, Bharati S, Meng CCL, Liberthson RR, Paul MH, Idriss F (1972) A concept of double outlet right ventricle. J Thorac Cardiovasc Surg 64: 271

Lubbers WJ, Tegelaers WHH, Losekoot TG, Becker AE (1975) Aberrant origin of left pulmonary artery (vascular sling). Report of the clinical and anatomic features in three patients. Eur J Cardiol 2: 477

Macartney FJ, Partridge JB, Shinebourne EA, Tynan MJ, Anderson RH (1978) Identification of atrial situs. In: Anderson RH, Shinebourne EA (eds) Paediatric cardiology 1977. Churchill-Livingstone, Edinburgh, p 16

Melhuish BP, Van Praagh R (1968) Juxtaposition of the atrial appendages: a sign of severe cyanotic congenital heart disease. Br Heart J 30: 269

Neufeld HN, Titus JL, DuShane JW, Burchell HB, Edwards JE (1961) Isolated ventricular septal defect of the persistent common atrioventricular canal type. Circulation 23: 685

Ogden JA (1970) Congenital anomalies of the coronary arteries. Am J Cardiol 25: 474

Rastelli GC, Kirklin JW, Titus JL (1966) Anatomic observations on complete form of persistent common atrioventricular canal with special reference to atrioventricular valves. Mayo Clin Proc 41: 296

Rowe RD, Mehrizi A (1968) The neonate with congenital heart disease. Philadelphia

Ruckman RN, Van Praagh R (1978) Anatomic types of congenital mitral stenosis. Report of 49 autopsy cases with consideration of diagnosis and surgical implications. Am J Cardiol 42: 592

Rudolph AM, Heymann MA, Spitznas U (1972) Hemodynamic considerations in the development of narrowing of the aorta. Am J Cardiol 30: 514

Shinebourne AE, Anderson RH (1978) Fallot's tetralogy—angiographic-anatomic correlations. In: Anderson RH, Shinebourne EA (eds) Paediatric cardiology 1977. Churchill-Livingstone, Edinburgh, p 258

Shinebourne EA, Macartney FJ, Anderson RH (1976) Sequential chamber localization—logical approach to diagnosis in congenital heart disease. Br Heart J 38: 327

Shone JD, Sellers RD, Anderson RC, Adams P Jr, Lillehei CW, Edwards JE (1963) The developmental complex of 'parachute mitral valve', supravalvular ring of left atrium, subaortic stenosis, and coarctation of aorta. Am J Cardiol 11: 714

Smith A, Ho SY, Anderson RH (1977) Histological study of the cardiac conducting system as a routine procedure. Med Lab Sci 34: 223

Somerville J (1978) Introduction: atrioventricular canal malformations. In: Anderson RH, Shinebourne EA (eds) Paediatric cardiology 1977. Churchill-Livingstone, Edinburgh, p 417

Soto B, Becker AE, Moulaert AJ, Lie JT, Anderson RH (1980) Classification of isolated ventricular septal defects. Br Heart J 43: 332

Sotomora RF, Edwards JE (1978) Anatomic identification of so-called absent pulmonary artery. Circulation 57: 624

Stewart JR, Kincaid OW, Edwards JE (1964) An atlas of vascular rings and related malformation of the aortic arch system. Thomas, Springfield

Tanaka N, Sekimoto K, Naoe S (1976) Kawasaki disease. Relationship with infantile periarteritis nodosa. Arch Pathol Lab Med 100: 81

Taussig HB, Bing RJ (1949) Complete transposition of aorta and levoposition of the pulmonary artery: clinical, physiological and pathological findings. Am Heart J 37: 551

Thiene G, Bortolotti U, Gallucci V, Terribile V, Pellegrino PA (1976) Anatomical study of truncus arteriosus communis with embryological and surgical considerations. Br Heart J 38: 1109

Tynan MJ, Becker AE, Macartney FJ, Quero-Jimenez M, Shinebourne EA, Anderson RH (1979) The nomenclature and classification of congenital heart disease. Br Heart J 41: 544

Uhl HSM (1952) A previously congenital malformation of the right ventricle. Bull Johns Hopkins Hospital 91: 197

Van Mierop LHS, Eisen S, Schiebler GL (1970) The radiographic appearance of the tracheobronchial tree as an indicator of visceral situs. Am J Cardiol 26: 432

Van Mierop LHS, Gessner IH, Schiebler GL (1972) Asplenia and polysplenia syndromes. Birth Defects 8: 36

Van Praagh R (1968) What is the Taussig–Bing malformation? Circulation 38: 445

Van Praagh R (1972) The sequential approach to diagnosis in congenital heart disease. Birth Defects 8: 4

Wagenvoort CA, Wagenvoort N (1977) Pathology of pulmonary hypertension. Wiley, New York

Warden HE, DeWall RA, Cohen M, Varco RB, Lillehei CW (1957) A surgical pathologic classification for isolated ventricular septal defects and for those in Fallot's tetralogy based on observations made on 120 patients during repair under direct vision. J Thorac Cardiovasc Surg 33: 21

World Health Organization (1975) Primary pulmonary hypertension. Report on a WHO meeting. Hatano S, Strasser T (eds). WHO, Geneva

Chapter 5

Central Nervous System

Joseph F. Smith

1. Development

A knowledge of the development and maturation of the brain is essential for the understanding of anatomical malformations and the possible effects of environmental processes on the brain in late fetal and early neonatal life. Integration of the variables of organogenesis, histogenesis, myelination, and vascular formation is complex, as are the underlying chemical and enzymatic changes. In description it is necessary to deal with them consecutively, always bearing in mind that changes develop concurrently.

The essential features of the external structure of the brain develop in the first 3 months of life, starting with the formation of the neural plate in the late presomite stage. A groove follows with the appearance of somites, and becomes a tube at 7 somites (3 mm). The anterior end of this tube closes at 20 somites (3.5 mm, 24 days), the posterior end at 21–29 somites (3.5–5.5 mm, 26 days). By the time of anterior closure the three dilatations that will become the cavities of the fore-, mid- and hind-brain are present in the cephalic end of the tube. The optic vesicles, which are diverticula from the fore-brain, become optic cups by 7.5 mm (5 weeks). About this time the cerebral or telencephalic vesicles appear on either side of the fore-brain and the flexures between the main parts are accentuated. At 15 mm (6 weeks) the medulla oblongata with caudal cranial nerves and the primordium of cerebellum and cerebral hemispheres can be distinguished. The latter grow backwards over the diencephalon and mid-brain, so that their posterior ends are close to the future cerebellum, from which they are separated by a condensation of connective tissue which will become the tentorium. By 50 mm (12 weeks) the future lobes of the cerebral hemispheres can be roughly identified

and a depressed area on the lateral aspect of each indicates the future insula.

During the second trimester the cerebral hemispheres increase in size and become clearly demarcated by the primary sulci—the sylvian and the central on the lateral aspect, the calcarine and parieto-occipital on the medial aspect. Further growth of the cortex will lead to the development of more sulci with consequent gyri, which has the effect of accommodating more grey matter in a given surface area. The appearance of sulci in relation to gestational age is shown in Table 5.1, and is often valuable in assessing the latter.

During the process of early development the shape of the telencephalic vesicles becomes modified by the formation of such central nuclear masses as the basal ganglia, thalamus and mid-brain, all of which, together with the internal capsule, are recognizable in outline by the end of the first trimester. The posterior corpus callosum is present by 16 weeks and the ventricular system now has its future outline, although it will undergo considerable reduction in relative size by term. (An appreciation of its size is important before a diagnosis of hydrocephalus by ultrasound is attempted during life. The detailed illustrations of Larroche [1977] are most useful.) The choroid plexuses have formed early (14–18 mm), following the invagination of ependymal roof plates into the ventricular cavities by blood vessels of the pia mater. The abundant glycogen in their cytoplasm is a feature shared with some other fetal epithelia, e.g., the primitive pneumocytes, and may be correlated with an anaerobic metabolism at this stage; it disappears in later fetal life. The exits from the ventricular system in the fourth ventricle usually open between 3 and 5 months and some circulation of cerebrospinal fluid is then possible. Separation of the pia and arachnoid follows but is not completed until birth.

Table 5.1. Factors useful in assessment of maturity in the brain of premature babies[a]

Gestation (weeks)	Weight (g)	Frontal–occipital length (mm)	Sulci	Myelination
24	90	70	Sylvian, central, calcarine,	Spinal cord roots,
28	150	80	parieto-occipital, hippocampal Superior temporal	posterior columns Medial and lateral lemnisci, brain stem cranial nerves
32	220	90	Pre- and postcentral, middle temporal, superior and inferior frontal	Subthalamic nucleus and adjacent fibres, colliculi, superior cerebellar peduncles
36	300	110	Further ramification. About 8–10 gyri from frontal to occipital pole	Posterior limb of internal capsule. Optic chiasma and tracts
40	400	120	About 12–14 gyri from frontal to occipital pole	Thalamocortical radiation

[a]Pathology (e.g., intraventricular haemorrhage) has a very marked effect on brain weight; the other factors are more reliable. Further details have been recorded by Larroche (1977).

Myelination starts in the ventral roots of the spinal cord at the 4th month of fetal life and soon spreads to the dorsal roots, then to the fibre systems of the nuclear zone in the substance of cord and brain, proceeding in a cephalad direction but not reaching beyond the thalamus until after birth. Many of the cranial nerves are myelinated in the 6th and 7th fetal months, and by 7 months the process has started in the spinocerebellar and vestibular tracts. It can be detected on naked-eye examination in the medial lemniscus in the pons at 32 weeks and in the posterior limb of the internal capsule at 36 weeks. At term it is commencing in the thalamo-cortical radiation (Fig. 5.1) but is still very scanty in the hemispheres. This accounts for the gelatinous consistency of the cerebrum in the newborn (water content is 90%) and the poor demarcation of white and grey matter. For details of myelination, which is not complete until 2 years of life, the texts of Yakovlev and Lecours (1967) and Larroche (1977) should be consulted. A summary of some of the chief landmarks useful in assessing maturity is presented in Table 5.1.

It is generally agreed that the extents of gyral and myelin maturation are more accurate indices of fetal maturation than any others. The brain weight will be less in a small-for-dates infant than in the normal infant, but these indices will indicate the true maturity. The overall length from frontal to occipital pole is considered by Larroche (1977) to give consistent information about brain size—the figures she gives are in Table 5.1.

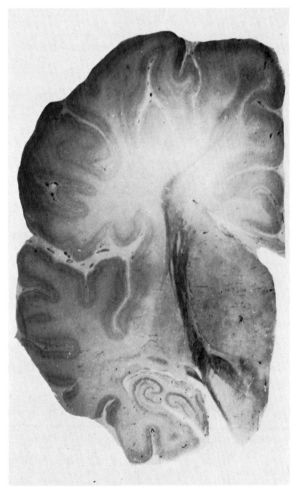

Fig. 5.1. Myelination in internal capsule and starting in thalamo-cortical radiation at 40 weeks. (LFB Neutral Red; 1.5×)

1.1 Cytological

The primitive epithelial lining of the neural tube is the source of all subsequent nerve cells except the microglia. It soon differentiates into an inner marginal or ependymal layer, an intermediate nuclear or mantle layer, and an outer marginal zone, which is at first devoid of nuclei. The neuroblasts of the inner layers will multiply and migrate to form the central nuclear masses and the future cortex, which is laid down from within outwards. Larroche (1977) has illustrated the further differentiation of these layers beautifully. By the end of the second trimester most of the neurones of the cortex are in place, closely packed and without significant cytoplasm apparent by light microscopy. Rakic and Sidman (1968) state that the majority of neurones have been formed by 18 weeks and reside as postmitotic neuroblasts in various stages of migration and differentiation in the mantle zone, presumptive white matter, cerebral cortical plate, and cerebellar cortex.

By 24 weeks (Fig. 5.2) the inner cellular marginal zone is confined to the lateral regions of the anterior and temporal horns and the vestibules of the lateral ventricles and is composed of small dark cells; mitoses are not seen here. At this time some of the neurones of the brain stem and central nuclear masses have differentiated to form cytoplasmic organelles, such as the Nissl substance, which are visible with the light microscope. However, the layering of the cerebral cortex cannot be recognized until 28 weeks, after which the cells become more

spaced out from one another as dendrites and axons develop. The development of dendrites probably starts much earlier (Fig. 5.3), but studies of cell connections with the electron microscope in embryonic and early fetal life are few. Nissl substance is recognizable in the Betz cells at 36 weeks.

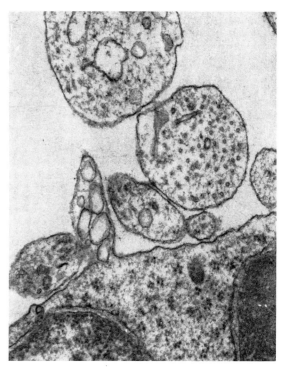

Fig. 5.3. Electron micrograph of developing dendrites at 16 weeks. (× 40000)

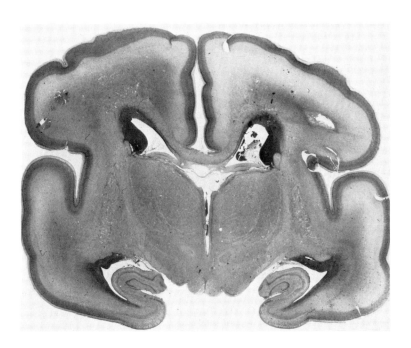

Fig. 5.2. Cross-section of hemispheres at 24 weeks. Note cellular subependymal region in lateral ventricles and temporal horns. The ventricles are relatively dilated at this age. (H and E; 1 ×)

In addition to neurones the primitive neuroblasts of the inner matrix give rise to glia cells. In embryonic life the long processes of some of these are said to act as guidelines for migration of neuroblasts to the presumptive cortex (Rakic 1972). The glia cells will also mature into astrocytes and oligodendroglia, but the existence of intermediate forms of these two cells is still debated.

In dealing with material likely to be examined by pathologists it is necessary to emphasize only a few points from this vast subject. The subependymal matrix of closely packed cells (Fig. 5.4) is a zone in which support for blood vessels is slight and haemorrhage into this area is especiallly likely to occur in the period between 24–36 weeks if pressure relationships oscillate critically. (See section on subependymal plate and intraventricular haemorrhage on p. 169.) After 28 weeks the cellularity gradually decreases in this matrix, some cells with light staining nuclei—probably future glia cells—become visible (Fig. 5.4), and the great majority of the cells have migrated elsewhere by full term. In this migration some cells may travel around vessels in the corona radiata and should never be confused with an inflammatory reaction (Fig. 5.5).

There is a considerable increase in cell numbers in the brain in late fetal life. This is the 'glia spurt' associated with and mainly preceding myelination. Most of the cells taking part are active oligodendrocytes, which line up in rows in the tissue before

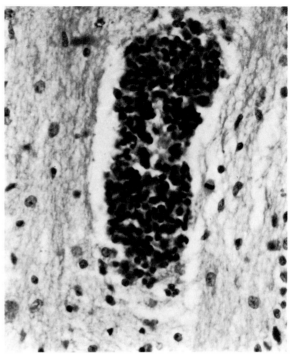

Fig. 5.5. Migrating neuroblasts around vessels in corona radiata at 36 weeks. Note an astrocyte in mitosis. (H and E; 400 ×)

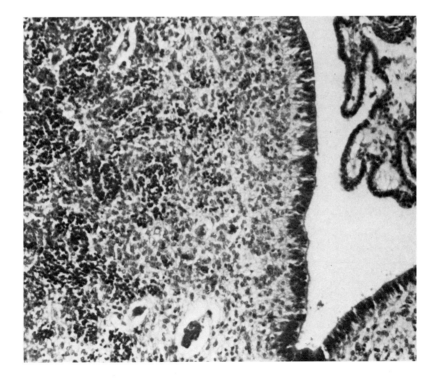

Fig. 5.4. Subependymal plate at 32 weeks. Most of the cells are small neuroblasts; some have differentiated to paler primitive glia cells. (H and E; 100 ×)

and during early myelination (Fig. 5.6). The cytoplasm of these cells is faintly pyronophilic and electron microscopy reveals moderate numbers of mitochondria, profiles of rough endoplasmic reticulum, and occasional lysosomes. Mitoses are not seen in human material but are occasionally caught in astrocytes (Fig. 5.5), which increase less markedly in numbers. With the light microscope the nuclear characteristics help to distinguish the two cell types (Fig. 5.7) if metallic impregnation methods are not available.

Del Rio-Hortega was the first to demonstrate clearly the identity of the microglia as a third glia cell type, with his silver impregnation method (Fig. 5.8). He considered them to be derived from the mesoderm and described their immigration into the brain from sites where mesoderm and developing brain are in close contact, e.g., the pia arachnoid forming the tela choroidea of the ventricles and the pia over the cerebral peduncles. In recent years there have been suggestions that many of the microglia are derived from the monocytes of the blood; on the other hand some workers have suggested an origin from the subependymal plate. A good discussion is that of Cavanagh (1970).

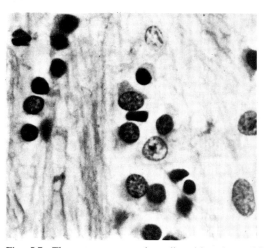

Fig. 5.7. The astroytes are the cells with pale nuclei; the oligodendrocytes have nuclei with a dense chromatin pattern. (H and E; 920 ×)

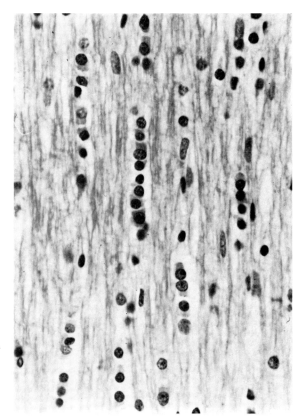

Fig. 5.6. The glia spurt in the internal capsule at 36 weeks. The oligodendrocytes are arranged in rows and some have active cytoplasm. (H and E; 400 ×)

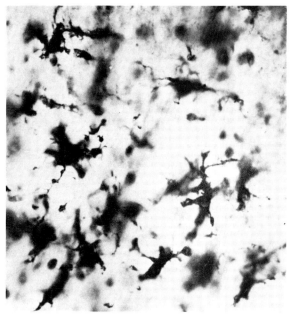

Fig. 5.8. Microglia cells in cerebellar white matter. (Weil–Davenport silver impregnation; 400 ×)

2. Reactions to Injury in the Nervous System

It is useful to summarize the changes that can be seen in the fully developed nervous system of the child following environmental injury. Differences in the reaction in the fetus and in the newborn will be considered before the pathological processes are described separately.

2.1. Nerve Cell

The detection of regressive changes in human pathology is beset by the problem that some similar alterations may result from autolysis or poor handling and fixation of tissues. Nevertheless, their observation is often useful, particularly if it is possible to compare damaged with unaltered areas.

Chromatolysis refers to the loss of cytoplasmic Nissl substance and may occur in a variety of conditions such as poliomyelitis and ischaemia; it is reversible. The ischaemic cell change may be regarded as a form of necrosis in which the cell body is shrunken, the nucleus is shrunken and pyknotic,

the cytoplasm stains darkly, but Nissl substance is not visible (Fig. 5.9). Ultrastructural details of this classic lesion (Fig. 5.10) are described by Brown (1977).

The homogenizing change is a form of necrosis in which the neurone may remain of normal size or shrink, the nucleus is usually pyknotic, but the cytoplasm is highly eosinophilic (Fig. 5.11). Ultrastructural observations show decreased electron density of nucleus and cytoplasm, with loss of distinctive organelles in the latter. In areas of necrosis some neurones may become shrunken with a very basophilic outline—this is mineralization resulting from incorporation of iron or calcium or both into the dead cell body. The accumulation of lipofuchsin pigment in cytoplasm as a nonspecific ageing change is rarely seen in children (Fig. 5.12), but the exaggeration of this phenomenon is the cardinal morphological change in neuronal ceroid lipofuchsinosis when a characteristic fingerprint inclusion is demonstrable with the electron microscope (see p. 632). Accumulation of other forms of lipid in cytoplasm is characteristic of the lipidoses. The study of ultrastructural and histochemical changes in recent years have aided in their clearer definition, together with an appreciation of the specific enzyme deficiencies responsible.

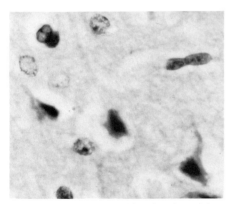

Fig. 5.9. Triangular cells with pyknotic nuclei are neurones showing ischaemic change. The pale nuclei are astrocytic. (H and E; 900 ×)

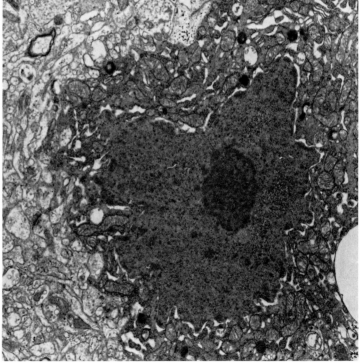

Fig. 5.10. Electron micrograph of ischaemic cell change showing pyknotic nucleus, dilated cisternae, but persisting preservation of some mitochondria. (11500 ×)

Joseph F. Smith

153

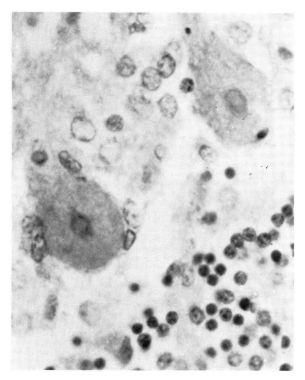

Fig. 5.11. Purkinje cells showing homogenizing change. (PAS; 400 ×)

In both the premature and the full-term newborn the most useful indication of neuronal necrosis is karyorrhexis of nuclei (Fig. 5.13), which appears to be a much more common reaction to ischaemia or hypoxia than at other times of life. In the premature baby the separation of severe hypoxic changes from autolytic ones can be especially difficult.

The diagnosis of injury is facilitated if there is a glial reaction as well as regressive changes in neurones. The cells taking part are the microglia and astrocytes. In paraffin sections distinction between the two is facilitated by the smaller size, darker nuclei, and sometimes kidney or oval shape of the microglia. When reacting, these cells become rounded, their cytoplasm is often distended by lipid or pigment, and the nucleus is pushed to one side and shrunken (Fig. 5.14). Their number is increased and in early stages they may be found around vessels. In early astrocytic reactions in the newborn the cells have large open nuclei with little visible cytoplasm, while in later reactions their cytoplasm is more evident and homogeneous. The detection of astrocytic processes with PTAH or Holzer stains in paraffin sections and with Cajal's gold chloride method in frozen sections (Fig. 5.15) may be necessary in cases of doubt. The use of immunological techniques to demonstrate glia fibrillary acidic

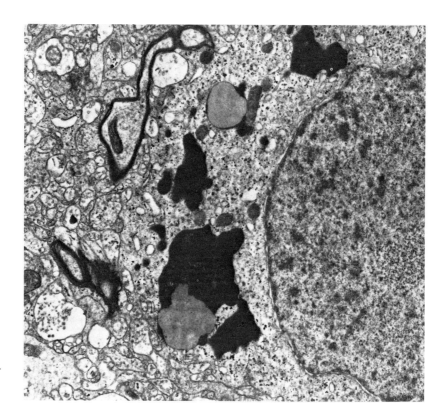

Fig. 5.12. Electron micrograph of neurone with excessive lipofuchsin. (14500 ×)

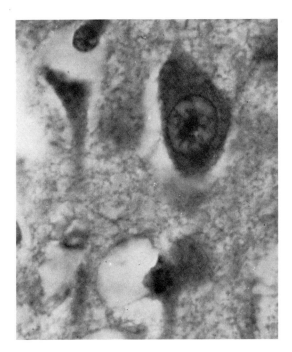

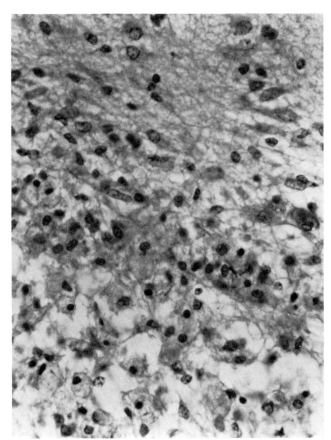

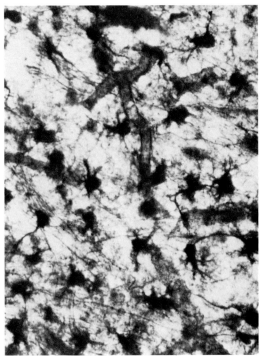

Fig. 5.13. Karyorrhexis of pontine neuronal nuclei in a full-term infant dying at 4 days with hypoxia from congenital heart disease (H and E; 1000 ×)

Fig. 5.14. Microglia and astrocytic reaction in periventricular leuco-malacia. Some of the microglia have become foam cells (lower third); others with dark nuclei are in the centre while astrocytes with open nuclei are above. (H and E; 400 ×)

Fig. 5.15. Astrocytes in subthalamic nucleus in kernic-terus at 9 days. (Cajal's gold chloride; 400 ×)

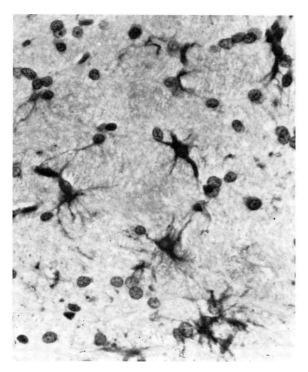

Fig. 5.16. Astrocytes in rat cerebellar white matter demonstrated by peroxidase method with antibody to glia fibrillary acidic protein. (H and E; 400 ×)

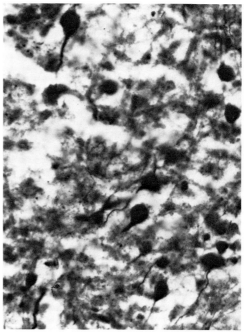

Fig. 5.17. Retraction balls on damaged axis cylinders in peri-ventricular leucomalacia. (Glees; 400 ×)

protein is now possible (Fig. 5.16). In confirming that microglia cells are laden with lipid the use of frozen sections stained with Oil Red O may be conclusive if lipid is abundant, but care must be taken not to confuse such phagocytic cells with the oligodendroglia containing scanty lipid that may be found in some stages of myelin formation.

Damage to myelinated fibres may be detected by focal swelling of the sheaths in LFB stains in early stages and by pallor or lack of staining in well-developed lesions. The demonstration of retraction balls on damaged axis cylinders that are not myelinated is useful in the diagnosis of peri-ventricular leukomalacia (Fig. 5.17).

In destruction of nervous tissue caused by in-fective agents all the changes so far described may be present, but there is usually, in addition, a reaction by lymphocytes and sometimes by plasma cells in the nervous tissue, Virchow Robin spaces, or the meninges, or in all three sites. In specific infections the causal agent may be demonstrable (see Sect. 9). The principles of reaction in meningitis are similar to those in other infections and will be considered in the appropriate section.

3. Malformations

The importance of anatomical malformations and the considerable incidence of those affecting the central nervous system have been discussed (p. 72). Defects in the formation of the neural tube include anencephaly, exencephaly (or encephalocoele), and spina bifida.

Anencephaly (Fig. 5.18) is lethal—most of the brain, including at least both cerebral hemispheres, is absent, the cerebellum is usually absent, and even the brain stem is malformed with reduction in its neurones. The spinal cord may be absent, ribbon-like, or split if the condition is associated with rachischisis. A mass of vascular tissue represents the defective hemispheres; in this glia and choroid plexus can be detected. The optic nerves are absent but the eyes are surprisingly well developed, as are the spinal ganglia and peripheral nerves. Most of the vault of the skull is absent, including the frontal bones above the supraorbital ridges and the parietal and squamous portions of the temporal bones. The occipital bones are underdeveloped and the obser-vations of Marin-Padilla (1965) indicate defects in the base of the skull in which it is difficult to identify individual components.

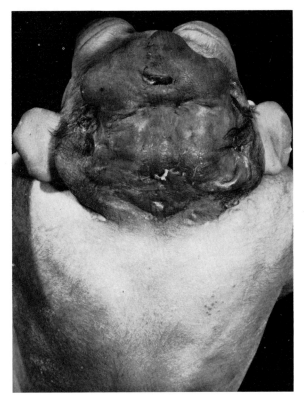

Fig. 5.18. Anencephalic fetus from above and behind. A mass of vascular tissue represents the brain.

It may be difficult to demarcate the shallow sella turcica, in which area some anterior but no posterior pituitary is present. The intermediate lobe is sometimes identifiable on histological examination. The adrenals are small because of the absence of the fetal cortex.

Exencephaly is a much rarer condition and involves a protrusion of part of the brain through a defect with smooth edges in the skull. This is most commonly seen in the occipitocervical region but parietal encephalocoele is also a well-recognized clinical problem. Anterior encephalocele is most frequent at the bridge of the nose; in occasional cases the protrusion is ventral, into the nasopharynx. Skin or a thin membrane may cover the variable amount of residual cerebral tissue in the protrusion, which may contain a cavity communicating with the ventricular system. However, the brain within the skull is usually well formed.

The degrees of spina bifida recognized are (a) spina bifida occulta, in which there is a deficiency only of the bony neural arches; (b) meningocele, in which the meninges are incorporated into the overlying skin and may show cystic distension; (c) myelomeningocele, in which both meninges and cord are incorporated into the overlying skin; and (d) myelocele, in which the cord lies exposed on the surface as a disorganized structure. The last three degrees can be grouped together as spina bifida cystica; this is useful for statistical purposes. Of this group meningoceles account for 5%–10%. However, it is often difficult to separate myelomeningocele from myelocele, because some cases of the latter become covered by epidermis and scar tissue, simulating myelomeningocele (Cameron 1956). Over 60% of patients with meningocele have no neurological abnormality, but in the larger group of spina bifida cystica with ectodermal defect there is almost universal morbidity and a high mortality from associated meningitis, hydrocephalus, and progressive renal failure following paraplegia and sphincter disturbances (Fig. 5.19). The neuromuscular effects are due to involvement of the cord, cauda equina, and nerves in the rachischistic lesion, which is most commonly sited in the lumbar and

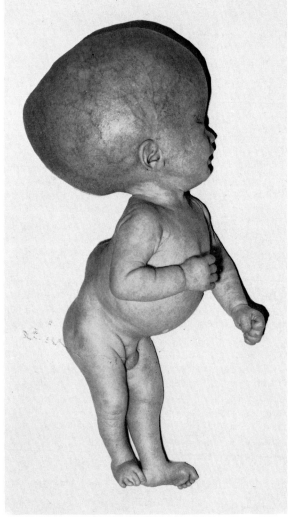

Fig. 5.19. Hydrocephalus associated with spina bifida cystica in a newborn.

lumbosacral region (70% of cases). Hydrocephalus is detected by the end of the first month in 50% of cases, and is nearly always due to the Arnold–Chiari malformation (p. 202 and Fig. 5.20).

For many years the orthodox view of the pathogenesis of anencephaly was a failure of closure of the anterior neuropore and that of spina bifida as a failure of closure of the posterior neuropore. However, Keiller had suggested a defect in the overlying mesoderm as an explanation for spina bifida in 1922, and this was also proposed for exencephaly by Emery and Kalhan (1970). Padget (1970) demonstrated the possibility of rupture of the neural tube from an examination of the embryos of Streeter's collection at the Carnegie Institute; an initial bleb raised the overlying ectoderm, which could necrose and rupture in severe lesions. Marin-Padilla (1978) has summarized his own extensive observations of the importance of the mesoderm in all defects of the neural tube. He considers that the primary defect is in the mesoderm, leading to malformations of the bones and dermis with secondary destruction of neural tissue as a result of its exposure to the amniotic fluid. It is difficult to reproduce the lesion of anencephaly in animals because of the short time of development of the brain in those investigated, which means that the consequences of exposure are not so severe as in humans.

Of other important but rare malformations, attention has been directed to failures of cleavage of the anterior fore-brain in recent years, because of the association with trisomy either 13–15 and 17–18 and its occurrence in the infants of diabetic mothers. The extent of the anatomical lesion varies widely, depending upon the degree of failure of separation of the prosencephalon. In the most severe type cyclops is present, with a single ventricle in the impaired brain. A less severe lesion is arrhinencephaly, in which absence of the olfactory tracts and bulbs may be the only lesion, or this defect may occur together with microphthalmic paired eyes, some separation of the hemispheres and a cerebral single ventricle (Fig. 5.21).

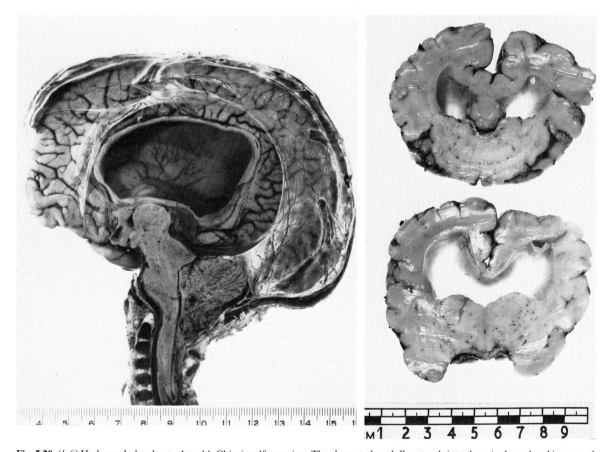

Fig. 5.20. (*left*) Hydrocephalus due to Arnold–Chiari malformation. The elongated medulla extends into the spinal canal and is covered posteriorly by cerebellar tonsils. The medulla and tonsils cause obstruction to circulation of the CSF at the foramen magnum (cf. Fig. 5.85).

Fig. 5.21. (*right*) Arrhinencephaly with a single ventricle in trisomy 13–15.

Many maintain that isolated agenesis of the corpus callosum is asymptomatic. The corpus callosum begins to develop in the 3rd month and is complete by the end of 4 months, although myelination does not occur until after birth. If agenesis is associated with other abnormalities of the medial aspect of the hemisphere, such as an absence or inward displacement of the cingulate gyrus and a separation of the parieto-occipital from the calcarine fissure, or defects elsewhere in the brain there may be clinical manifestation of these other defects.

Abnormalities of gyration include lissencephaly (pachygyria) and micropolygyria. In the former the number of cortical gyri is greatly reduced with the outer surface of the brain completely smooth in the extreme form (agyria). In a general way the microscopical appearance is similar to that of a 3–4 month fetus with four cell layers and a disturbance in neuronal migration indicated by the presence of heterotopias in the white matter. Richman et al. (1973) comment on the absence of the most superficial layer (II) of cells. They suggest that this is the result of a destructive injury restricted to the relatively acellular areas between the heterotopias of the inner zone interrupting cellular migration along the radial glia fibres and thereby producing the heterotopias. Clinical evidence of such injury is lacking for lissencephaly but is present in some examples of the very different macroscopic brain of micropolygyria in which, paradoxically, the microscopical features superficially resemble those of lissencephaly. However, although there are only four layers of the cortex in micropolygyria, the absent or cell-poor layer is the middle layer; the most superficial layer II is present, in contrast to the situation in lissencephaly. Richman et al. (1974) suggest that this is explained by an injury occurring when neuronal migration is complete, possibly intrauterine hypoxia or inadequate perfusion. The brain is not necessarily small, although it may be, as in some examples recorded in association with maternal cytomegalic inclusion disease or as a sequel to carbon monoxide poisoning of the mother in the 5th month of pregnancy. It is sometimes present in association with the Arnold-Chiari malformation which suggests an interference with development earlier in fetal life than the 5th month.

An abnormally small brain may result from a large number of destructive brain processes, which are described elsewhere. The term microcephaly can be used in description in these circumstances, but it is preferable to reserve it for conditions in which it is associated with stigmata of maldevelopment or evidence of inheritance. Familial microcephaly (Penrose 1963) is a Mendelian recessive condition in which the brain is small with reduced sulci and no indication of a destructive process. Survival into

adult life with mental retardation may occur. Other examples in which the mode of inheritance is less well defined are microcephaly with sudanophilic leucodystrophy and microcephaly with widespread calcification.

The term 'porencephaly' was originally used to mean a congenital abnormality in which a cavity extended from the cortical surface to the ventricle in any part of the brain. It is now restricted to such cavities that are the result of destructive disease, usually vascular or hypoxic in origin (p. 173) in fetal or neonatal life. Hydrancephaly is an extreme form of porencephaly (p. 175).

Schizencephaly is a true malformation in which bilateral cavities extending backwards and forwards from the region of the Sylvian fissures are surrounded by neural tissue in which there is no evidence of disease. Yakovlev and Wadsworth (1946) considered that the abnormality originated before the 2nd month of fetal life. If the infant survives mental retardation and quadriplegia are likely.

Various abnormalities of the cerebellum have been described under such terms as agenesis, hemiagenesis, and hypoplasia. They are all rare, as is the Dandy-Walker syndrome, which is a cause of obstructive hydrocephalus. The essential lesion in the Dandy–Walker syndrome is a posterior cystic dilatation of the fourth ventricle, lined by ependyma but with little normal tissue in the wall. The view that it results from failure of the foramina of the fourth ventricle to open has not been supported by experimental work, which indicates that the fundamental lesion is a persistence of the ovum membranacea superior—normally a transitory structure impermeable to cerebrospinal fluid and situated between the posterior fold of the cerebellum and the anterior fold of the choroid plexus of the fourth ventricle. The cerebellar hemispheres are small, the foramina of Majendie and Luschka may or may not be patent, and there is dilatation of all of the ventricular system proximally. In about 70% of cases there are associated abnormalities, such as micropolygyria, agenesis of the corpus callosum, and syringomyelia (Hart et al. 1972).

The term neurocutaneous syndrome is preferred to phakomatosis to describe conditions involving both the skin and the nervous system that originate as malformations, although their main manifestations occur in childhood or adult life. Tuberose sclerosis, encephalofacial angiomatosis, ataxic telangiectasia, and neurofibromatosis are considered here.

Tuberose sclerosis is transmitted as a Mendelian dominant (Gunther and Penrose 1935), although 80% of cases arise as mutants. It exhibits complex malformations in the brain, kidneys, breast, skin, lung, and sometimes bones. These may be affected in various combinations, the brain being the most frequently involved, the kidneys next (p. 410). Clinical manifestations are more frequent in childhood or adolescence, but retardation and epilepsy can present earlier.

In the brain, the swellings or tubers in the cortical gyri are firm, sometimes protuberant, smooth or partly granular, and up to 3 cm in diameter (Fig. 5.22); those in the ependyma of the ventricles may produce a 'candle guttering' appearance. Similar lesions can occur in the central grey matter, brain stem, or cerebellum. Histologically these lesions exhibit a mixed proliferation of glia cells and neurones, some of which may be abnormally large. In the tubers the abnormality is clear-cut, but the disturbance is often widespread and merges in places with normal brain. A well-recognized complication is the development of true tumours from an abnormal area. These may be gliomas or gangliogliomas.

Lesions in the retina are similar to those in the subependymal region and are known as phakomas (Fig. 5.23). In the kidney benign cortical tumours may be composed of a mixture of mesenchymal cells or may be epithelial, i.e., adenomas. Polycystic disease of the kidneys (Paulson and Lyle 1966) has been described, but it is not clear whether the condition differs from the normal adult form. The cardiac lesions described include rhabdomyomas, the constituent cells of which resemble the fetal heart muscle cells of Purkinje, and more diffuse lesions in which fibrous tissue and fat are more conspicuous. The most obvious of the somatic manifestations is adenoma sebaceum, the reddish-brown papular skin lesion on the face in which hyperplasia of sebaceous glands is the salient feature. Radiological changes in bones have been described by Dickerson (1955) and attributed to a fibrous dysplasia. The similarity of the radiological picture to that seen in occasional cases of neurofibromatosis has been used to suggest that the two conditions are allied, a concept for which there is no foundation. The pulmonary changes in tuberose sclerosis, which include cysts and hyperplasia of fibrous tissue and smooth muscle in the walls of air spaces, are infrequent in cases in which cerebral involvement is marked.

The nature of the disease has been the subject of considerable speculation. Bourneville's concept (1880) of an encephalitis occurring during fetal

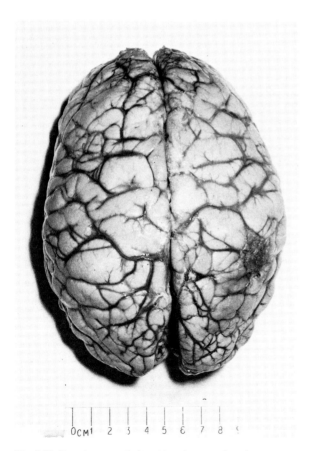

Fig. 5.22. Prominent cortical gyri in tuberose sclerosis.

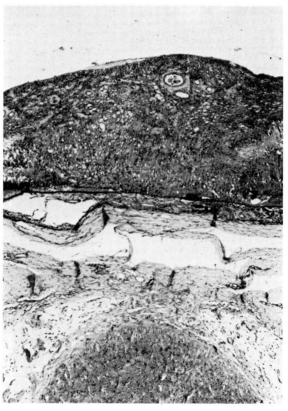

Fig. 5.23. Retinal phakoma in tuberose sclerosis. (H and E; 40 ×)

development cannot be sustained. A dysontogenesis of variable extent and genetic origin appears a more reasonable explanation at the present time. Borberg's (1951) study of the genetic aspects of tuberose sclerosis and neurofibromatosis concluded with the opinion that the two are genetically independent diseases and that any similarity is due to genes producing developmental anomalies of the same embryonic tissues.

In encephalofacial angeiomatosis (Sturge–Weber disease), Alexander and Norman (1960) stress the cutaneous angeiomatosis of the face, including the upper part in every case, epilepsy, gyriform calcification becoming radiologically visible after infancy (Fig. 5.24), and mental retardation. Hemiparesis of the side opposite to the cutaneous lesion is often present and homonomous hemianopia may sometimes be detected. This is due to involvement of the visual cortex but angeiomatosis may involve the choroid of the eye (Nellhaus et al. 1967).

Pathologically the distinctive features are the facial naevus, usually involving the ophthalmic and maxillary divisions of the trigeminal nerve, and a leptomeningeal angeiomatosis in which there is a dense network of small thin-walled vessels (Fig. 5.25). The dura and skull are very rarely involved. Beneath this excessively vascular area, which is normally in one occipital or occipitoparietal region, there is calcification in the underlying brain, which affects the white matter initially, later being severe in the grey matter and accompanied by neuronal loss. The abnormal vessels rarely penetrate into the brain and the mechanism by which they are related to the calcification is uncertain. Nevertheless it appears that there must be some relationship between the two. Most explanations have invoked an abnormal development of the embryo's blood vessels (Thieffry et al. 1961). Alexander and Norman were sceptical of the existence of formes frustes. There is no evidence of genetic inheritance.

Ataxia telangiectasia is inherited on an autosomal recessive basis, becoming manifest in early childhood with cerebellar ataxia and cutaneous and conjunctival telangiectasia. It was first clearly described by Louis-Bar in 1941 and numerous cases have been recognized in the last 20 years, when additional interest has been aroused by the findings of abnormal cellular and humoral immunity in some. An impaired development of the thymus is often present (p. 549) and levels of IgA and IgE in the blood may be low. There is an increased incidence of lymphomas and a cerebellar medulloblastoma complicated one of the cases reported by Shuster et al. (1966). Death is usual before adult life, often with a lung infection.

Strich (1966) gave a detailed account of the

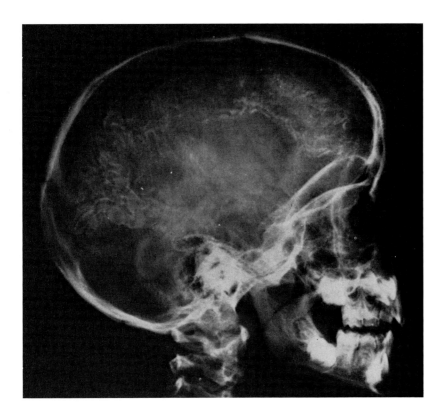

Fig. 5.24. Sturge–Weber disease. Radiograph showing calcification of cortex in skull in a 15-year-old boy.

pathological changes in three cases, emphasizing the degeneration of the cerebellar cortex, which is atrophic to the naked eve, loss of myelinated fibres in the posterior columns of the cord, diminution in the satellite cells in the posterior root ganglia, and enlargement of Schwann cell nuclei. The presence of an increased serum α-fetoprotein has been used in support of the theory that in this complex disease there is a primary defect of tissue differentiation.

Neurofibromatosis is the most common of the neurocutaneous syndromes and is inherited as a Mendelian dominant. In children the usual adult lesions of multiple peripheral neoplasms and skin pigmentation may be less obvious; it is possible for the presenting lesion to be an optic nerve or third ventricle glioma or a hamartomatous lesion in the nervous system. Schwann cell proliferation in the spinal cord and meningiomatosis of the cortex are examples of both. Very occasionally there is some degree of mental defect, which has been attributed to the abnormalities of cortical development following interference with neuronal migration in embryonic or fetal life.

The chromosomal abnormalities responsible for Down's disease have been discussed on p 76. Anatomical changes described in the brain include some abnormal roundness of the frontal and occipital poles, with a relative decrease in the size of the cerebellum and a narrow superior temporal gyrus. In recent years there have been several descriptions of ultrastructural changes in the cortical neurones, such as the presence of neurofibrillary tangles and senile plaques in the brains of young

adults. Marin-Padilla (1974) has described a decrease in the neuronal connections by dendrites following a Golgi study.

4. Deprivational and Toxic Lesions

Although some degree of apathy is common in nutritional deficiency in infancy and childhood there is little specific pathology of the nervous system. Worldwide the commonest nutritional deficiency is probably kwashiorkor, in which protein intake is low and fatty change in the liver is considerable and reversible with therapy (p. 287). Even in cases that develop acute encephalopathy with coma and death specific changes have not been described.

If hypoglycaemia is severe and prolonged following galactosaemia, glycogen storage disease, or hyperinsulinaemia caused by islet cell tumour, it is possible for neuronal changes similar to those produced by ischaemia or hypoxia to develop in the cortex. The question as to whether neonatal hypoglycaemia produces a specific pattern of neuronal damage, as described by Anderson et al. (1967) in acute cases and in cases surviving a few months by Banker (1967), has not yet been decided. It is possible that the areas affected are those selectively damaged by hypoxia in the neonate.

The occurrence of lesions as disparate as those of beri-beri and Wernicke's encephalopathy in adults

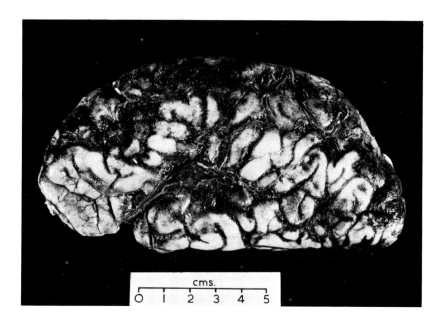

Fig. 5.25. Leptomeningeal angeiomatosis in same case as Fig. 5.24.

as a result of thiamine (vitamin B_1) deficiency is well known. The neuropathy of beri-beri is unusual in children and the classic causes of the encephalopathy of Wernicke (1881) are absent. However, the encephalopathy was described many years ago by Tanaka (1934) in an infant who was the child of a mother with latent beri-beri. This is the only record of the anatomical changes in the breastmilk intoxication described in many Far Eastern countries. The essential change in Wernicke's disease is a capillary proliferation and dilatation accompanied by astrocytic and microglial proliferation; damage to nerve cells is slight and haemorrhage is sometimes present in the walls of the third and fourth ventricles, including the corpora mammillaria.

The changes seen in infantile subacute necrotizing encephalopathy—Leigh's disease—are similar but the distribution of lesions is different. Furthermore, the condition is progressive, usually leading to death in a few months. A rare familial form has been described with inheritance as a Mendelian recessive.

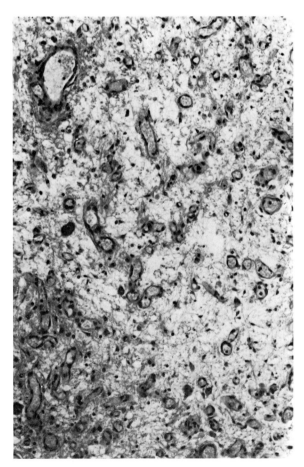

Fig. 5.26. Leigh's disease or infantile subacute necrotizing encephalopathy. Glia and vascular proliferation in the pons together with neuronal degeneration. (H and E; 200 ×)

Lesions are present in the grey matter of the brain stem, particularly the pons, and degeneration of neurones is present in affected areas (Fig. 5.26).

The most important metabolic poisonings to affect the nervous system in children are those of lead, mercury, and iron. Acute lead encephalopathy occurs predominantly in the age group 6 months to 3 years, rarely in older children. The mortality of the florid disease is high and neurological sequelae with retardation are common in survivors; the possibility of subclinical disease causing mental defect is constantly under consideration. The severe form of encephalopathy is rare in the British Isles but more frequent in large cities in the United States and Asia— the ingestion of paint from wooden houses or toys is a well-known source of lead poisoning. Toxic effects are likely if the blood level rises to 50 μg or more; this, together with punctate basophilia of red cells, aminoaciduria, increased urinary coproporphyrin, lead inclusions in epithelial cells in the urinary deposit, and a characteristic radiological change in long bones may be helpful in diagnosis. The presenting symptoms of irritability and gastrointestinal upset are often followed by convulsions and coma owing to the acute cerebral swelling with considerably raised intracranial pressure.

The brain is uniformly swollen (Fig. 5.27) and sometimes so soft that it disintegrates on handling. Both grey and white matter are involved and the ventricles are compressed. Although bilateral uncinate herniation is often present, mid-brain and pontine haemorrhage is not seen, probably because asymmetrical swelling is necessary for shearing stresses to develop in the brain stem arteries (p. 168).

Microscopically the appearances are variable

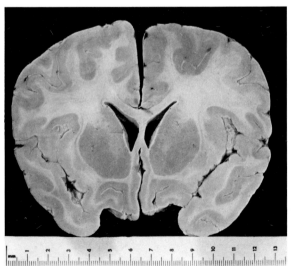

Fig. 5.27. Lead encephalopathy. Brain swelling with narrowed sulci and compressed ventricles.

(Smith et al. 1960). In severe cases the appearances are those of massive early necrosis, while in the less severe the changes are surprisingly slight—some perivascular exudation of plasma and a very few collections of lymphocytes or microglial cells may be associated with focal cerebellar atrophy and baso-philic impregnation of small vessels, indicative of damage preceding the final illness. Intranuclear inclusions that give reactions for cystine or cysteine (Fig. 5.28) may be present in the kidney tubular epithelium; these are useful in diagnosis.

The motor neuropathy that can develop in older children as a result of lead poisoning is described on p. 530. Pink's disease, in which a neuropathy associated with erythema resulted from mercury poisoning is no longer seen since the use of teething powders or worm cures containing calomel has been discontinued. Minamata disease is a form of mercury poisoning described in Japan as a result of eating fish contaminated by a methyl-mercury compound discharged into the water of the bay from a factory. Cases have been reported in newborns as a result of intrauterine intoxication. Changes were present in the cerebellum and cerebral cortex.

Although convulsions and coma can occur in children as a result of accidental ingestion of excessive amounts of iron or salicylates there are no well-documented accounts of changes in the nervous system.

In recent decades the subject of chronic de-generation of the nervous system has been elucidated considerably with the greater understanding of the genetically determined metabolic diseases of the nervous system, the diagnosis and biochemical lesions of which are considered in Chap. 14. A short description of important structural changes in some of the examples is included here. In both Tay–Sachs (GM$_2$ gangliosidosis) and Batten's (neuronal ceroid lipofuscinosis) diseases the brain is usually small, with the cerebellum more con-sistently shrunken in the latter (Fig. 5.29). In occasional cases of Tay–Sachs disease surviving for a long period—several years—the brain may be swollen, with cystic disintegration of some of the white matter of the hemispheres (Aronson et al. 1955). The accumulation of the same ganglioside as that present in neurones of the alimentary tract described on p. 629 is of course responsible for the distension of cytoplasm of neurones in the brain and spinal cord. The number affected at different sites is variable, and neuronal loss is more severe in cases of longer duration. Distension of neuronal processes with ganglioside is responsible for the characteristic 'torpedoes' (Fig. 5.30). Degeneration of the myelin-ated fibres of the brain and cord is mainly of the Wallerian type and there may be a reactive gliosis in relation to this.

In Batten's disease the distension of neurones is not so marked and their loss is most striking in the granular layer of the cerebellum. The specific biochemical abnormality has not yet been eluci-dated (p. 629).

In some of the mucopolysaccharidoses the neu-rones may be distended to some extent by lipid, and accumulation of stored material in macrophages in the leptomeninges may lead to fibrosis and obstruc-tive communicating hydrocephalus (Russell 1949).

Galactosaemia was not considered in Chap. 14 (because it cannot be diagnosed by histochemical methods). It is, however, one of the more common inherited errors of metabolism—1 in 20000 births (Hansen et al. 1964)—and is attributable to de-ficiency of the liver enzyme galactose-1-phosphate uridyl transferase. This results in accumulation of galactose-1-phosphate in the liver and galactose in the blood. The mechanism by which this is as-sociated with liver and brain damage, renal defects, and cataracts is uncertain. If galactose is not withheld from the diet death may follow quickly. Patchy astrocytic proliferation in grey and white matter is the only structural change in the brain in such cases but in those who survive for long periods there may be slight micrencephaly with gliosis in the white matter and cerebellar molecular layer together with loss of cells in the cerebellar cortex (Crome 1962).

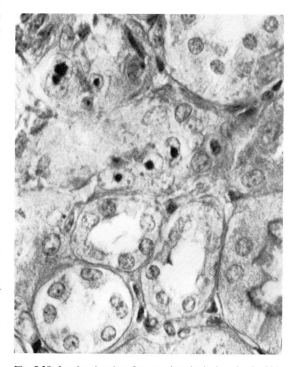

Fig. 5.28. Lead poisoning. Intranuclear inclusions in the kidney tubular epithelium. (Aldehyde Fuchsin after oxidation; 650 ×)

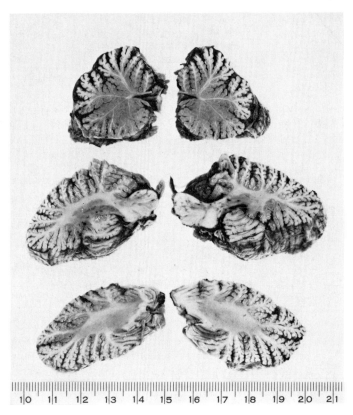

Fig. 5.29. Batten's disease. Atrophic folia of the cebellar cortex.

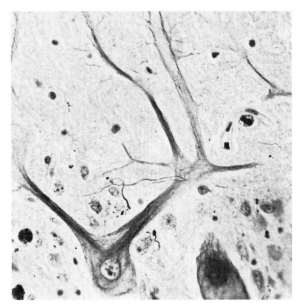

Fig. 5.30. Tay–Sachs disease (GM$_2$ gangliosidosis). Distension of cytoplasm and processes of Purkinje cells in the cerebellar cortex. (Glees; $200 \times$)

In long-standing phenylketonuria deficiency of myelination and some gliosis may be present in the white matter, together with focal cortical scars; these scars could be caused by convulsions. In several degenerative conditions the aetiology is still unknown, and it is convenient to consider these under lesions of the white matter and grey matter. Although Schilder's original description of his disease included three different types of case, the name is retained for the disease form in which there is a progressive demyelination and sclerosis of the white matter which is nonfamilial; it can be classified as a form of multiple sclerosis occurring in children or adolescents (in whom the classic disease is rarely seen) or as a sudanophilic leucodystrophy. It differs pathologically from multiple sclerosis only in the more extensive and diffuse involvement of the white matter of the cerebral hemispheres (which is not quite symmetrical), the lesser involvement of the brain stem and spinal cord, and the greater degree of axonal damage. The clinical picture is progressive rather than remitting, with intellectual impairment, pareses, cortical blindness, and possibly convulsions. The demyelination is accompanied by the appearance of sudanophilic lipids within and outside phagocytes, and astrocytic gliosis is conspicuous (Fig. 5.31).

There is a rare condition—familial sudanophilic leucodystrophy—in which the involvement of cerebral and cerebellar white matter is more uniform than in Schilder's disease; the cortical and subcortical U

fibres are spared and the descending tracts of the brain stem and cord may show evidence of secondary degeneration. Such leucodystrophy may be associated with microcephaly.

A form of leucodystrophy in which there is some evidence for sex-linked inheritance is Pelizaeus–Merzbacher disease. In this condition the demyelinating process is irregular with preservation

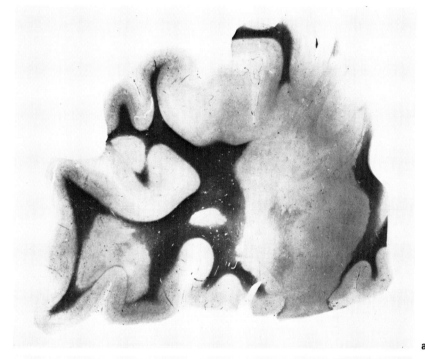

a

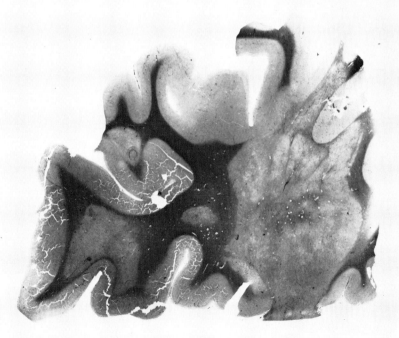

5.31. a and **b** Schilder's disease: **a** extensive demyelination in white matter of frontal lobe. (LFB; 2 ×) **b** gliosis in the demyelinated areas. (PTAH; 2 ×)

b

of islands of myelinated fibres. In contrast to sudanophilic demyelination the term dysmyelination is sometimes used for those conditions, such as sulphatide leucodystrophy (p. 626) and Krabbe's disease (p. 618), in which there is evidence of a defective synthesis of normal myelin—which may in turn break down more readily.

Other rare diseases of the white matter are spongy degeneration or Canavan's disease, maple syrup urine disease, and central pontine myelinolysis. In spongy degeneration there is evidence of autosomal homozygous inheritance with a prevalence in Jewish families. There is retardation of myelination, a spongy state at the junction of grey and white matter, and astrocytic proliferation in which Alzheimer type II cells may be prominent (Fig. 5.32). Involvement of the cores of cerebellar folia is sometimes conspicuous (Fig. 5.33). A similar spongy state is found in the white matter in newborns dying from maple syrup urine disease. Central pontine myelinolysis is unusual in that the extensive destruction of myelin is confined to the pons. Although this condition was first described in adults, cases have been recognized in children, who are usually debilitated or have had treatment with antileukaemic drugs.

Progressive degeneration of the cerebral cortex in infancy is also rare and is sometimes called Alpers' disease (Alpers 1931). The onset is some months or years after birth and there is extensive and continuing degeneration of neurones in all layers of the cerebral cortex with glial reaction. Familial cases have been recorded and in some there has been involvement of the brain stem and cerebellum as well as the cortex.

Fig. 5.33. Spongy degeneration in cerebellar folia. (H and E; 90 ×)

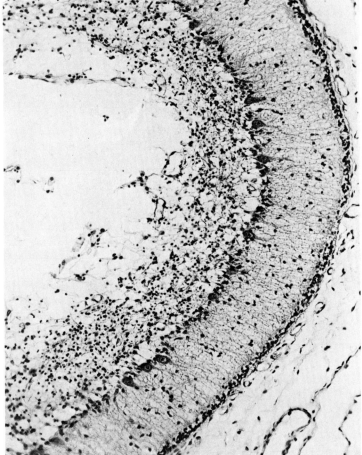

Fig. 5.32. Spongy degeneration of the nervous system. The astrocytes have the open nucleus characteristic of reacting cells in the newborn or of Alzheimer's type II cells. (LFB; 400 ×)

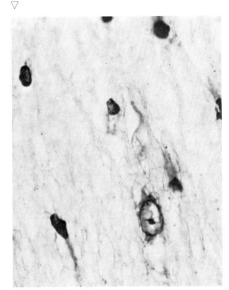

5. Kernicterus

Brain damage in neonatal jaundice was first described more than 100 years ago (Orth 1875). The name kernicterus was introduced by Schmorl (1904) in 1903 to describe the yellow staining of nuclear masses in the basal ganglia and brain stem. With the fact of its association with erythroblastosis fetalis came the recognition that damage by what we now know as unconjugated bilirubin was important. This was disputed for a time, as the change might occur with many causes of jaundice in the neonatal period, but the discovery of the same condition in the genetically determined hyperbilirubinemia named after Crigler and Najjar and a similar condition in the Gurr stain of rats with an inherited deficiency of glucoronyl transferase is convincing proof that excess unconjugated bilirubin in the tissues is the essential pathogenetic factor. Glucoronyl transferase was found by Billing and Lathe (1956) to be necessary for conversion of the type of bilirubin that is bound to plasma albumin and reacts indirectly in the van den Berg reaction to the type that reacts directly. Drugs that interfere with glucoronyl transferase (vitamin K analogues and streptomycin) may also exacerbate kernicterus. In the newborn infant, particularly the premature infant, the amount of this enzyme in the liver is small and excessive haemolysis, as in erythroblastosis fetalis, can lead to excessive accumulation of unconjugated bilirubin in the plasma and the tissues. Other factors that may be important for the production of cerebral damage are the facility with which the lipid-soluble unconjugated bilirubin passes through the blood–brain barrier into nervous tissue (direct conjugated bilirubin does not), the level of plasma albumin available to bind the unconjugated bilirubin in the blood, and the presence of drugs in the bloodstream such as sulphisoxazole (Silverman et al. 1956), salicylates, and caffeine, which interfere with the binding of bilirubin to albumin.

Whether unconjugated bilirubin is the essential cause of kernicterus or merely an indication or mark of neuronal damage from other causes is disputed by some. Experiments with kittens (Rozdilsky and Olszewski 1961) showed that IV injection of bilirubin alone would produce kernicterus, whereas in monkeys (Lucey et al. 1964) and baby rabbits (Chen et al. 1965) such injections only resulted in lesions when combined with asphyxia. The recent reports of Gartner et al. (1970) and Ackerman et al. (1970) of kernicterus in premature infants with a much lower serum bilirubin than 340 mmol/litre (the previous threshold value) has lent some support to the view that anoxia is a factor that may facilitate the lesions of bilirubin encephalopathy (a term sometimes used as a synonym for kernicterus). However, in Crigler–Najjar disease damage can occur without clinical evidence of anoxia.

In a typical acute case of kernicterus the sites most commonly jaundiced are the subthalamic nuclei, the globus pallidus, Ammon's horn, the dentate nuclei of the cerebellum, and the nuclei in the floor of the fourth ventricle, with the thalamus, putamen, and grey matter of the spinal cord affected less commonly and the cerebral cortex rarely. In full-term infants it is very unusual for the central white matter to be involved, but in prematures the sites of 'periventricular leucoencephalomalacia' can be stained. In involved areas the neurones may show nuclear pyknosis and vacuolation, cytoplasmic eosinophilia, or yellow staining—this last more clearly seen in frozen than paraffin sections (Fig. 5.34). Sometimes crystals can be identified in frozen sections. There are lesser changes in astrocytes and little reaction in acute fatal cases. Electron microscopic observations of the experimental lesions in newborn rabbits show nuclear and cytoplasmic changes in neurones and milder changes in astrocytes (Chen et al. 1966).

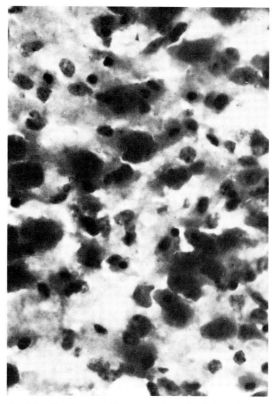

Fig. 5.34. Kernicterus. Frozen section of subthalamic nucleus. The paler cells with pyknotic nuclei are bile-stained neurones. (H and E; 400×)

In survivors with permanent brain damage the common clinical features are mental retardation with deafness and choreoathetoid movements. The pathological changes accompanying this condition are neuronal and fibre loss with gliosis, which is maximal in the globus pallidus and subthalamic nuclei and the hippocampus (Fitzgerald et al. 1939) but can affect a variety of areas including the cortex (Crome 1955). Gardner and Konigsmark (1969) have reported a case of the Crigler–Najjar syndrome in which death occurred at 15 years. Bile staining was present in the lungs, liver, kidneys, and heart. In the brain there was neuronal loss in thalamus, basal ganglia, and mid-brain, with minimal loss in the cerebral and cerebellar cortices and subependymal gliosis in the medulla. No pigment was demonstrable in the brain and those areas most severely affected in the infant appeared to be relatively spared.

6. Vascular and Hypoxic Damage

At present the most important causes of brain damage in the newborn are subependymal plate haemorrhage and hypoxic damage, which itself is often partly ischaemic—the phrase hypoxic ischaemic damage (abbreviated to HID) is useful when the separate contribution of the two factors is difficult to assess. There is evidence from animal experiments that hypoxia may lead to local cerebral ischaemia (Brierley 1971), but whether this is true in neonates is not yet known. The term 'birth trauma' is best avoided as it would include not only mechanical injury to the skull (now fortunately rare) but ischaemic, hypoxic, and haemorrhagic lesions occurring in the perinatal period, which are considered individually in this section.

In the consideration of ischaemic and haemorrhagic conditions in the neonate and the child it is useful to mention first a few concepts, the details of which must be found in textbooks of neuropathology or review articles. The boundary zones (or last fields) are areas of the parieto-occipital cortex lying between the territories of the anterior, middle, and posterior cerebral arteries, areas between anterior and middle cerebral territory (including parts of pre- and postcentral gyri), and between the middle and the posterior cerebral supply (passing from lateral occipital to temporal cortex). Whereas such zones are likely to be spared if one of the three main cerebral arteries is occluded because of meningeal anastomoses, they are more likely to show evidence of damage if there is general vascular

insufficiency as in cardiac arrest of neonatal shock.

Selective vulnerability is the term used to indicate that certain areas of the brain are more susceptible to damage than others in, for example, hypoxia, but also following other insults. Boundary zone lesions are one form of such selective vulnerability, where a vascular explanation of the localization of the hypoxic damage is possible. There are other lesions, e.g., the brain damage in kernicterus, where this type of explanation is less convincing.

In description the terms cerebral swelling, cerebral oedema, and the effects of internal herniation are often used. Cerebral swelling indicates an increase in the volume of the brain with flattening of convolutions, narrowed sulci, and compressed ventricles; cerebral oedema indicates a swelling in which there is excess fluid in the extracellular space or in unzipped myelin sheaths. The term cerebral swelling thus includes cerebral oedema, but also other conditions, in which both grey and white matter may be involved and in which intracellular and extracellular increase of fluid is possible. It would include, in a purely descriptive sense, the early stage of cerebral infarction, in which cellular membrane changes lead to retention of fluid within cells, and degenerative states short of infarction, in which a similar intracellular oedema develops. Such swelling of varied aetiology may sometimes lead to vascular compression in the manner postulated by Lindenberg (1955), with subsequent necrosis in such areas as the temporal lobe, thalamus and calcarine cortex.

Unilateral cerebral swelling is likely to cause internal herniations of the affected hemisphere and displacement of the mid-line structures. The cingulate gyrus may protrude beneath the falx across the mid-line; the hippocampal gyrus may be displaced through the tentorial opening to compress the mid-brain and third nerve. The grooving of the hippocampal gyrus by the free edge of the tentorium is an important, but not invariable, indication that such herniation has occurred—it may not be seen if the brain is soft.

When such hippocampal herniation occurs haemorrhage in the mid-brain and rostral pons is common in adults, and may be slight or extensive with a 'butterfly' configuration. It is less common in children and rare in infants, but hypoxic effects may occur in this area. This haemorrhage or necrosis may be caused by the caudal displacement of the mid-brain, which is elongated anteroposteriorly, and by displacement of the caudal part of the brain stem by the herniated hippocampus. These movements contribute to abnormal stresses on the mid-brain and pontine arteries, which cannot move caudally with the brain stem as they are anchored rostrally.

If the whole brain or the cerebral hemispheres alone are swollen there may be cerebellar tonsillar

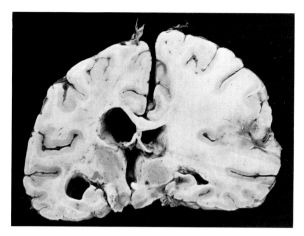

Fig. 5.35. Cerebral oedema around a small area of tumour.

herniation with the danger of medullary compression about the foramen magnum. In rare cases in the neonate or infant haemorrhagic necrosis of the tonsils and medulla may occur as a result of venous occlusion in the tissue impacted in the foramen.

The macroscopic and microscopic features of swelling caused by acute infarction are described on p. 172. When it is a prenecrotic state due to anoxia there is a uniform expansion of grey and white matter. When, however, the swelling is due to oedema of the white matter—and this is seen around tumours, abscesses, and local haematomas—the appearance is often distinctive. There is a marked expansion of the white matter relative to the grey (Fig. 5.35); in many cases it is firm and dry but in some it is moist and tends to disintegrate. In some cases there is a faint lemon yellow tint to the mainly white cut surface. Microscopically the most striking feature is the pallor of myelin staining, which spares the subcortical fibres. The myelin sheaths are separated and show focal swelling but there is no evidence of myelin catabolism. The cause is uncertain but is probably a metabolic change; the absence of grey matter involvement makes ischaemia or anoxia unlikely. A similar white-matter oedema is produced by alkyl tin poisoning in animals, and here the water accumulates between the layers of the myelin sheaths (Aleu et al. 1963).

Hippocampal herniation and mid-brain displacement can occur not only with cerebral swelling and oedema but as a consequence of extradural and subdural haemorrhage (see p. 170). Whatever the cause it is responsible for progressive unconsciousness, coma, and death through damage to the mid-brain and rostral pons. Its prevention is therefore of great importance.

The pressure of the cerebrospinal fluid is of less direct importance in the pathogenesis of the lesions described than in hydrocephalus (p. 201). However, it is significant when cerebral perfusion pressure and

tissue perfusion pressure are considered. Cerebral perfusion pressure is defined as the difference between mean arterial blood pressure and cerebral venous pressure and in practice is often simplified to the difference between mean arterial blood pressure and intracranial pressure—the latter being measured by the cerebrospinal fluid pressure. The tissue perfusion pressure is the difference between the tissue blood pressure (i.e., in the tissue arterioles) and the intracranial pressure, and is the effective pressure that determines whether blood flow in a particular region of the brain is adequate. Thus the blood flow in the boundary zones or in local areas of swollen brain may be inadequate when it is satisfactory elsewhere. The oxygenation of tissue depends upon both the blood flow and the oxygen saturation of the blood as well as the local metabolism. As mentioned earlier, it is possible that the blood flow may be affected by hypoxia.

6.1. Haemorrhagic Lesions

The most important cause of neonatal death in prematures is *intraventricular haemorrhage*. This is usually the result of haemorrhage in the subependymal plate of the lateral ventricle (Fig. 5.36) and occasionally follows haemorrhage into the choroid plexus.

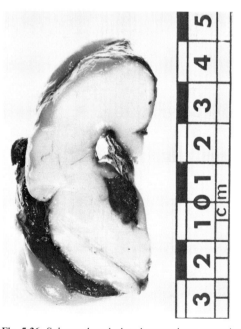

Fig. 5.36. Subependymal plate haemorrhage rupturing into lateral ventricle from which clot has been removed. The blood passed from the exits of the fourth ventricle into the subarachnoid space and in retrograde fashion frontally to the Sylvian fissures.

In the period between 24 and 32 weeks and to some extent up to 36 weeks of fetal life the subependymal plate is a very cellular tissue that gives poor support to veins and arteries within it; after this period it is much less cellular and fibrillary stabilization is present. The tissue texture is the dominant factor in rendering the area susceptible to haemorrhage (which can be bilateral) if there is damage to the walls of the vessels within it from hypoxia, stasis, or raised pressure. I favour the majority view that the haemorrhage comes from veins and capillaries, but Hambleton and Wigglesworth (1976) have produced evidence for capillary bleeding following a rise in arterial pressure. The infants in whom the catastrophe occurs often have hyaline membrane disease.

Once established, the haemorrhage may remain small, extend into the surrounding tissue with serious effects, or rupture into the ventricle. The last event is usually devastating, and it is more likely to occur after a few days of life (Harrison et al. 1968), possibly after prolonged hypoxia, intermittent changes in blood pressure, or neonatal heart failure. A small leak into the ventricular fluid may lead to hydrocephalus as a result of blockage of the aqueduct by a clot or by organization of an inflammatory reaction in the basal meninges to which blood is taken by the cerebrospinal fluid (Larroche 1972) (Fig. 5.89).

If the haemorrhage is confined to the subependymal plate it may become organized by a slow glial reaction (Sherwood et al. 1978) (Fig. 5.37); the effects of such a lesion on brain development are not yet known. An unusual feature seen in cases surviving 5–15 days is the occasional development of foci of extravascular haemopoiesis in adjacent tissue (Fig. 5.38).

When intraventricular haemorrhage is severe it extends to form a mass of clot throughout the ventricular system, and to fill the cisterna magna, cover the ventral surface of the hind-brain in the subarachnoid space, and even extend in a retrograde fashion towards the Sylvian fissures and lateral aspects of the hemispheres (Fig. 5.36).

However, *subarachnoid haemorrhage* as a distinct entity is also important in the neonate. It may occur in multiple areas, but distinct haematomas related to the temporal lobes (Fig. 5.39) or the posterior borders of the cerebellar hemispheres are sometimes seen. It is much commoner in premature babies but may be a manifestation of intrapartum or neonatal hypoxia in a full-term infant.

Subdural haemorrhage is occasionally seen in prematures. More typically it is found in a full-term baby as a complication of laceration of the falx or tentorium cerebelli with damage to bridging veins, the straight sinus, or the vein of Galen. It occurs when labour is prolonged, with ample opportunity for excessive moulding during passage of the head through the pelvic canal and the possibility of the development of asymmetrical forces if the infant is over-sized, if the presentation is abnormal, or if instruments are used incorrectly. Modern developments in obstetrics, in particular the more frequent use of caesarian section where prolonged labour is anticipated, have led to a diminution in its incidence. However, in the British perinatal mortality survey (Butler and Bonham 1963) cerebral birth trauma of this type had an appreciable incidence. When it

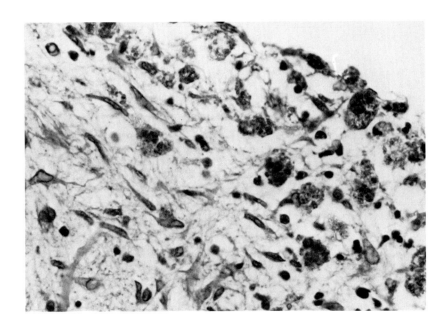

Fig. 5.37. Wall of subependymal plate haematoma at 35 days. Inner iron-pigmented macrophages are surrounded by proliferating astrocytes. (H and E; 400 ×)

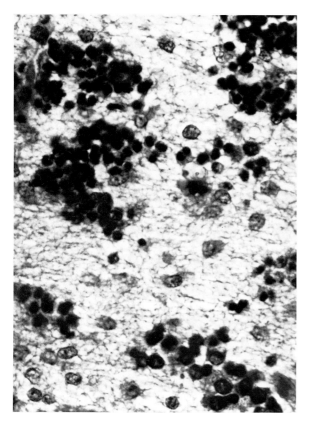

Fig. 5.38. Foci of extramedullary haematopoiesis in brain adjacent to a 14-day-old subependymal plate haematoma. (H and E; 400 ×)

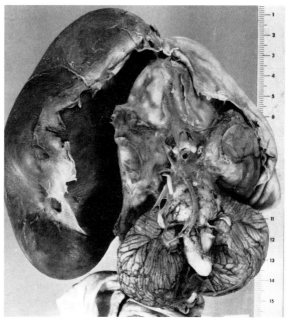

Fig. 5.40. Chronic subdural haematoma.

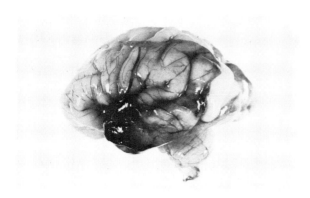

Fig. 5.39. Subarachnoid haematoma over temporal pole.

occurs in the posterior fossa it is often fatal; over the lateral side of a hemisphere it is less likely to be fatal but may be bilateral and lead to enlargement of the head in the neonatal period and in infancy. As in the comparable lesion in an adult the haemorrhage becomes enclosed by a proliferation over its surface of endothelial and fibrous tissue from the dura, the inner membrane being thinner than the outer. The content of the sac so formed may increase as a result of fresh bleeding from newly formed vessels or from

osmotic effects (Fig. 5.40). Ingraham and Matson (1944) postulated that such effusions could interfere with the normal growth of the frontal lobes, Rabe et al. (1962) discuss the mechanism by which such effusions and those of infective origin persist.

Intracerebral haemorrhage is not common in newborns, apart from the extension of a subependymal plate haemorrhage. A single large haemorrhage is likely to be due to rupture from a vascular malformation (p. 198), but this may be difficult to detect if there is extensive tissue destruction. Multiple small haemorrhages throughout the white matter are much rarer in my experience than in that of Schwarz (1961), who attributed them to variations in cerebral venous pressure during delivery. When they occur they are perhaps a variant of periventricular leucomalacia (see p. 172). The only blood dyscrasias that cause haemorrhage in fetal life or the neonatal period are neonatal thrombocytopenic purpura (Pearson et al. 1964) and haemorrhagic disease of the newborn.

6.2. Necrosis

Necrotic lesions in the neonate include extensive devastation, localized infarction, and scattered neuronal or white matter necroses. Extensive devastation may be seen in an acute or chronic form. The acute form is that described by Larroche (1968) as 'nécrose cérébrale massive'.

It is seen as a complication of severe HID from cardiac arrest, severe neonatal shock or possibly retroplacental haematoma. The changes are more easily detected if the infant survives a day or more— and this is common with modern therapy. The brain is swollen, the convolutions flat, and the sulci narrow; in addition there may be downward displacement of the tentorium with concavity of the superior surface of the cerebellar hemispheres and herniation of cerebellar tonsils into the foramen magnum. On section the brain is soft, even after fixation, the ventricles are compressed, and there may be patchy blotchy areas. Microscopically, neuronal necrosis is extensive and widespread, manifested by pyknosis and karyorrhexes of neuronal nuclei with amoeboid swelling of astrocytes and some microglial and astrocytic proliferation if survival continues for a few days or more. White-matter damage is present but in one personally observed severe case a remarkable feature was the preservation of active oligodendrocytes in the internal capsule. In mature babies in whom necrosis is less extensive, sites of election for neuronal damage include the cingulate gyrus, the dorsomedial thalamus, H_1 of the hippocampal cortex (Fig. 5.41), the internal granular layer of the cerebellar cortex, and above all the ventral pons (Fig. 5.13) (described as the griseum pontis by some authors).

Damage to the inferior colliculi of the mid-brain is less extensive and severe than might be expected from the experiments of Ranck and Windle (1959), who produced acute total anoxia in newborn monkeys and found that in survivors maximal lesions were present in the sensory nuclei and centres of the brain stem. This selective vulnerability was explained by Myers (1972) as an illustration of damage to the areas whose metabolic rate at the time of the injury was greatest. Myers emphasized that total asphyxia produced in this way did not resemble human perinatal damage, which he endeavoured to reproduce in full-term monkeys by partial asphyxia. A gradually progressive mixed respiratory and metabolic acidosis ensued with episodes of bradycardia. Cerebral swelling and necrosis in the hemispheres were the pathological sequelae, the extent of the latter depending on the duration of partial asphyxia.

In premature babies with such severe HID survival is less likely and the reaction patterns are less clear-cut. It is also more difficult to distinguish between autolytic and pathological effects. Thus a common finding is a soft brain with widespread shrinkage of neurones surrounded by halos. A similar appearance may result from imperfect fixation or autolysis. In such circumstances the presence of karyorrhexes in such sites as H_1 of the hippocampal cortex, the ventral pons and the

internal granular layer of the cerebellum is a good indication of HID.

6.3. Leucomalacia

In the premature baby it is common for grey matter lesions of the type just described to be associated with damage in the central future white matter of the hemispheres although this lesion, called periventricular leucomalacia by Banker and Larroche (1962), can occur on its own. They describe the naked eye appearance of characteristic 'white spots' often symmetrical in three zones, anterior to the anterior horn, in the corona radiata lateral to the superolateral angle of the lateral ventricle and lateral to the vestibules and occipital horns. With survival for a week or more these areas of coagulative necrosis may become cystic (Fig. 5.42). The most useful histological changes in diagnosis are the eosinophilia and positive periodic acid-Schiff reaction of the central necrotic zone (Fig. 5.43), the microglia and astrocytic reaction seen within hours, the vascular proliferation visible after 24 h and macrophage activity evident after 5 days (Fig. 5.14).

Banker and Larroche postulate that this lesion is the anatomical basis for Little's disease, in which

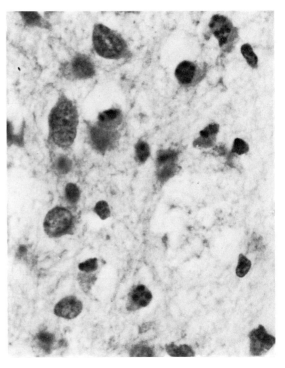

Fig.5.41. Karryorhexis of nuclei and shrinkage of cell bodies in hippocampal cortex in HID (H and E; 920 ×)

diplegia and mental retardation follow complications of delivery (Little 1861). They include in their series two cases in which survival for at least 1 month after the anoxic episode was followed by spasticity and retarded development. They suggest that this affection of these zones of the neonatal white matter (incidentally it is not yet white matter in many cases, as myelination is incomplete) is due to their location at the boundary zones between the areas supplied by the three main cerebral arteries. Abrahamowicz (1964) has provided some experimental support for this view by obliterating the basilar and carotid arteries in adult cats thereby producing periventricular necrosis without damage to the cortical grey matter. He suggests that in lower animals and in the immature human brain the main blood supply of the deep white matter comes from penetrating arteries which have few collaterals and no anastomoses; by contrast there are enough anastomoses in the fetal cortex to maintain oxygenation more easily.

Banker and Larroche (1962) give an interesting historical review of relevant observations including a discussion of the view of Schwarz (1961), who attributed such lesions to a differential pressure during delivery causing a similar effect on the superficial and deep venous system. This, he thought, resulted in both haemorrhagic and non-haemorrhagic lesions. Points against the view of Schwarz are the occurrence of such lesions in babies delivered by caesarean section without trial labour, the safe use of the vacuum extractor in obstetrics, and the fact that most of the lesions are non-haemorrhagic.

6.4. Late Effects of HID at Birth

Infarct-like lesions include sclerotic gyri—ulegyria, focal subcortical cystic lesions, paraventricular sclerosis, and multilocular cystic lesions or porencephaly. In all these there is necrosis of tissue with glia reaction, and circumstantial evidence indicates that the necrosis is due to anoxia or ischaemia or both. Ulegyria and focal subcortical lesions are probably more often due to arterial insufficiency and rarely to occlusion of the superior longitudinal sinus. Small cystic softenings in the deeper white matter, e.g., in the paraventricular white matter, can be a sequel to periventricular leukomalacia. The explanation of extensive multilocular cystic lesions is not clear. Wolf and Cowen (1956), after detailed consideration of this group, suggest a stasis in the Galenic system of veins, although this hypothesis is supported only by indirect evidence. In some brains there is a combination of lesions.

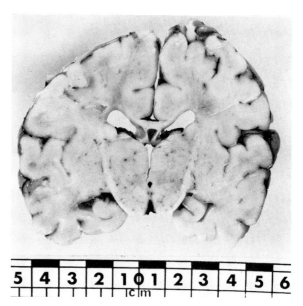

Fig. 5.42. Periventricular leucomalacia (PVL) at 11 days. Small cystic areas above and lateral to angles of ventricles.

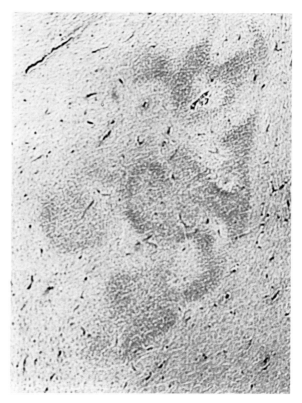

Fig. 5.43. A small acute area of PVL. (PAS; 400×)

Many of these lesions are found in the brains of older children (Fig. 5.44) and of adults who die after a lifetime of mental deficiency with perhaps paralysis and fits or other focal nervous system disturbances. The fact that the onset of the illness dates from a birth in which there was an indication of abnormal delivery or fetal or neonatal distress is taken to indicate that the lesion started at that time. They are sometimes found in infants dying within the first few weeks of life but rarely in infants dying in the first few days; this correlates with the fact that they all represent well-developed necrosis with reaction, a lesion that takes several days to evolve. Exceptional cases reported indicate that the onset can be in fetal life (Smith and Rodeck 1976).

'*Ulegyria*' (*atrophic sclerosis*) is the term used to describe areas of shrunken sclerotic gyri in which loss of tissue is maximal at the sides and minimal at the summit of a convolution, so that the term 'mushroom gyrus' is apt. Microscopically, loss of nerve cells is again maximal at the sides of the gyri or in the depths of a sulcus. Gliosis is present in the areas of neuronal loss as well as in the poorly myelinated areas of the gyri. Meyer (1949) has described intimal fibrosis in the leptomeningeal arteries over such areas; these may be the healing stage of the causal lesion. When areas of ulegyria occur in the boundary zones it is probable that they are due to arterial insufficiency; when they are bilateral and adjacent to the superior longitudinal sinus an old thrombosis of that channel should be

looked for and the possibility of venous stasis at delivery borne in mind if evidence of thrombosis is not found.

Focal subcortical cystic lesions often occur in the boundary zones between the middle, anterior, and posterior cerebral areas of supply. Of all the lesions in this group they are perhaps most like those cases of encephalomalacia seen in the adult, where an arterial block can be demonstrated. The cystic area involves the subcortical white matter predominantly; the deeper cortex is also affected. Astrocytic proliferation is often very marked, even in cases in which the infant is only a few weeks old at death. The possibility of paradoxical embolism following umbilical artery thrombosis should be considered in cases developing in early infancy after such parenteral therapy (Smith et al. 1974).

Paraventricular softening has been extensively reported by Norman (1963), who described it as 'the most characteristic cerebral lesion of birth trauma, almost its hall-mark'. His observations were mainly recorded in children and adults dying in a hospital for the mentally retarded. We have seen this change in infants in association with residua of sub-ependymal plate haemorrhage and periventricular leucomalacia (Sherwood et al. 1978) (Fig. 5.45).

Multilocular cystic encephalomalacia is characterized by extensive cystic cavities in the white matter, but there is always some destruction of the deeper grey matter, as in the focal subcortical lesions. Because of this, the conclusion of Wolf and Cowen

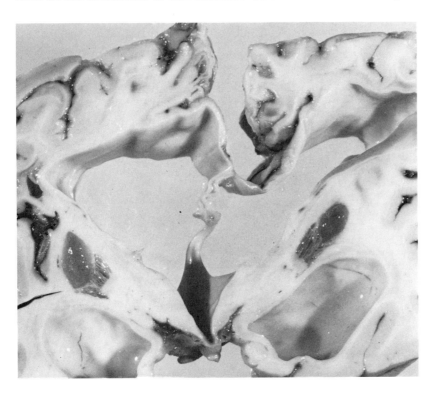

Fig. 5.44. Brain damage in a child dying at 4½ years after severe and prolonged birth hypoxia. There are shrunken and infarcted gyri on the medial aspect of the frontal lobes, cystic areas in the striatum, atrophy of the corpus callosum, and ventricular dilatation consequent to loss of tissue.

(1956) that the condition is anoxic in origin is preferred to the suggestion that it is a degeneration of white matter, comparable to diffuse sclerosis. The comparison with 'swayback' in animals is false, as in that condition the cortex is not involved. Astrocytic proliferation and foam cell reaction around the cavities are often conspicuous. The basic architecture of the cerebrum is still recognizable in most cases.

Hydranencephaly is included here because it is regarded as an extreme variety of multilocular cystic encephalomalacia with a similar aetiology. The cerebral hemispheres are reduced to membranous sacs, the outer wall of which is composed of leptomeninges and a thin remnant of cortex in which glia cells are more numerous than neurones. Internally the sacs are contiguous with the ventricular system, but there is no ependymal lining; this distinguishes the condition from congenital hydrocephalus. Lindenberg and Swanson (1967) describe cases in infants in which they postulate that the arterial supply is occluded by the pressure of swollen brain tissue, which can develop in a variety of ways. The basal parts of the brain and the hindbrain are preserved, indicating that the lesion is due to carotid insufficiency while the vertebral supply is preserved. An important clinical point, again distinguishing the condition from congenital hydrocephalus, is the fact that the head is not enlarged at birth but becomes big in the first few weeks of life.

Etat marbré is the hypermyelination of the basal ganglia and thalamus that is sometimes found in infants who have athetoid movements following birth injury. It may be associated with any of the lesions already described. A similar hypermyelination may be found in associated sclerotic gyri.

Other lesions. In mild degrees of cerebral birth injury with anoxia it is possible that gross damage will not occur but that there may be some patchy or diffuse loss of neurones or a varying degree of gliosis in the white matter. Courville (1953) has suggested that many examples of diffuse sclerosis in children are the result of anoxia at birth; this view is not generally accepted.

6.5. Cerebral Haemorrhage

Many examples of subdural, subarachnoid, and intracerebral haemorrhage and of the rare extradural bleed in childhood are traumatic. Small haemorrhages in the meninges and in the brain substance can occur in association with leukaemia and thrombocytopenic purpura—such cases are often terminal. Very rare causes are Schönlein-Henoch purpura, uraemia, and haemophilia. Manifestations of haemorrhage will be present in other tissues. Multiple small haemorrhages visible on naked eye examination of the white matter can occur in acute haemorrhagic leukoencephalitis (a type of allergic encephalitis: p. 188) and in fat embolism.

Subarachnoid haemorrhage in children due to a rupture of a congenital aneurysm of the circle of Willis is extremely rare, as is intracerebral haemorrhage due to hypertension. A more common cause of both types of haemorrhage in this age group is rupture of a congenital vascular malformation (p. 198).

Cerebral infarction in infancy and childhood. In addition to those examples described as consequences of HID infarction of a type more similar to that seen in adults can develop in childhood. Arteriosclerosis is practically never a cause, but embolism and rarely thrombosis of arteries can be, while thrombosis of veins and venous sinuses is also significant.

Congenital heart disease is the most common association. Thus in a series of 555 autopsies on children over 20 months of age at the Children's Medical Center, Boston, Banker (1961) found 48 with cerebral vascular disease. The autopsies included 133 with congenital heart disease, 11.3% of which had occlusive vascular disease. In a review of

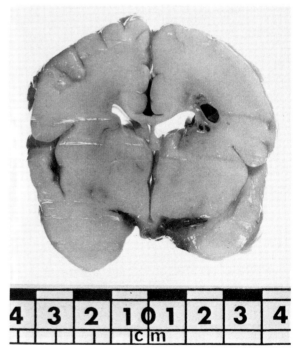

Fig. 5.45. A cystic paraventricular lesion due to fusion of paraventricular leucomalacia and subependymal plate haemorrhage in a 28-week baby who survived 27 days.

autopsies on 162 cases of congenital heart disease of all ages Berthrong and Sabiston (1951) found 25 of the 135 with cyanotic heart disease had cerebral infarcts and five had a brain abscess. The cerebral infarcts were more often due to venous thrombosis (Fig. 5.46) than arterial occlusion, which when it occurred could be thrombotic or embolic. All observers agree that the polycythaemia of congenital cyanotic heart disease is an important predisposing factor in cerebral thrombosis, and in the differential diagnosis of cerebral catastrophes in this group thrombosis is the important lesion before the age of 2 years, after which abscess must also be considered. Bacterial endocarditis complicating rheumatic or congenital heart disease in children is now rare, but embolism from such a source must still be considered as a cause of cerebral infarction or of mycotic aneurysm.

Other rare causes of cerebral arterial occlusion are polyarteritis nodosa and lupus erythematosus. Small vessels may become thrombosed in sickle-cell anaemia, and small arteries may be involved in pneumococcal and tuberculous meningitis, rarely in that due to *H. influenzae*. Medium-sized and small arteries are occasionally involved in fungal infections, particularly that due to Mucor.

In the acute stage of infarction resulting from arterial occlusion the affected zone is swollen with a patchy blush on the cut surface of the grey matter and a disintegrating white matter. At this time there is evidence of necrosis of neurones and some amoeboid swelling of astrocytes. A distinct glia reaction starts after about 2 days with mobilization of microglia cells and reinforcement of their number from blood monocytes to take part in phagocytosis of lipid from necrotic myelin. This results in the accumulation of lipid macrophages (foam cells) around vessels and between proliferating capillaries. An increase in astrocytes soon follows. Within a week the swollen area has decreased to normal size, thereafter it shrinks further and an old infarct may show a narrow rim of 'cortex' in which glia cells have

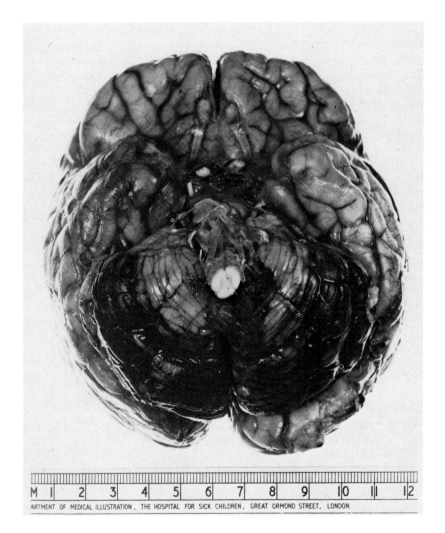

M 1 2 3 4 5 6 7 8 9 10 11 12

ARTMENT OF MEDICAL ILLUSTRATION, THE HOSPITAL FOR SICK CHILDREN, GREAT ORMOND STREET, LONDON.

Fig. 5.46. Haemorrhagic infarction of the cerebellum due to venous thrombosis in a child with congenital heart disease. (Female aged 20 months, transposition of the great arteries.)

replaced neurones and a partly cystic 'white matter' with similar cells and their fibres replacing nerve fibres.

This description applies to an infarct that is mainly anaemic. Some infarcts following arterial embolic occlusion are more frankly haemorrhagic, approaching the state described under that due to venous occlusion (see p. 175). If the infarct is caused by an infected embolus from a vegetation on a heart valve there may be more severe inflammatory reaction in the area of necrosis, or even abscess formation. Such an embolus may also cause pyogenic necrosis of the wall of the artery in which it lodges—a mycotic aneurysm whose rupture may cause subarachnoid and/or intracerebral haemorrhage.

If a child with a large infarct of one cerebral hemisphere survives for several years gross cystic change may develop in the white matter over a large area, so that a state resembling unilateral porencephaly develops. In other examples there is marked shrinkage of white and grey matter without much cystic change and with sparing of areas supplied by other arteries. Such specimens are sometimes removed at hemispherectomy years after the initial illness. It is then difficult to detect the causal vascular lesion. Bertrand and Bargeton (1955) have described conspicuous intimal fibrosis without changes in the media or adventitia in the middle cerebral artery in such specimens, and have discussed whether this 'endarteritis' is a sequal to old inflammation or thrombosis; they favoured the former.

The areas of cerebral necrosis due to occlusive arterial lesions in which an arteritis, sometimes with thrombosis, complicate meningitis, are smaller and may be multiple.

Haemorrhagic infarction due to venous sinus thrombosis is now rare in the United Kingdom. Superior sagittal sinus thrombosis used to be a rare complication of the dehydration produced by severe gastroenteritis, epidemics of which have almost disappeared. If the occlusion involved some of the draining veins as well as the sinus or a good length of the sinus, purplish red haemorrhagic infarction of the parietal lobes (and sometimes adjacent lobes) developed, with disintegration of the tissue.

Acute vascular encephalopathy is perhaps the most useful term to describe an acute illness with convulsions and impairment of consciousness, sometimes with paralysis and sensory loss in infancy or early childhood. It can be fatal within days, or a variable degree of recovery can occur; a more localized form can lead to a temporary or permanent hemiplegia. Some patients with such a hemiplegia may develop repeated and severe convulsions together with behavioural disturbances in later childhood and adolescence.

It is probable that the acute and chronic lesions found in such patients develop on the basis of vascular insufficiency, which can have more than one mechanism. The condition can arise de novo or be preceded by a short febrile illness or a recent inoculation, particularly with pertussis vaccine. The vascular pathogenesis is not universally accepted; thus the title 'acute encephalopathy of obscure origin in infants and children' was used by Lyon et al. (1961) for a wider spectrum of cases than those considered here. Acute toxic encephalopathy is another term employed, and 'encephalopathy and fatty degeneration of the viscera' (Reye et al. 1963) is an allied condition.

In the severe generalized form the brain is swollen; the weight can be considerably increased, the convolutions flattened, the ventricles compressed, and the tissue congested. Hippocampal and cerebellar tonsillar herniation may be present, and this may be sufficiently severe to produce haemorrhagic necrosis of the cerebellar tonsils, which have impacted in the foramen magnum. However, midbrain or rostral pontine haemorrhage is not seen in this condition or in other examples of bilateral and symmetrical cerebral swelling in children. Microscopically there is widespread neuronal necrosis (Fig. 5.47) and degeneration with variable astrocytic and microglia reaction. The cause of the swollen brain may be vascular insufficiency or stagnant anoxia

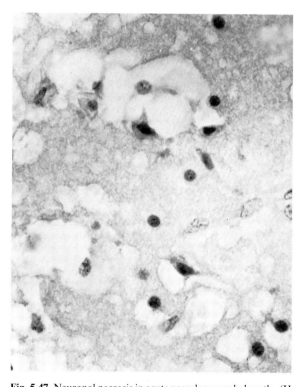

Fig. 5.47. Neuronal necrosis in acute vascular encephalopathy (H and E; 160 ×)

leading to intracellular oedema; Lindenberg (1963) stressed the importance of intracellular acidosis.

If hemiplegia is the dominant clinical feature death rarely occurs until years later, and even then the demonstration of an occlusion of a vessel is unusual. Norman and Urich (1957) demonstrated a dissecting aneurysm of the middle cerebral artery in a case in which death occurred 14 years after an acute episode at 6 months of age.

Some information about this general group of cases can be found from an examination of hemispherectomy specimens removed from patients with repeated convulsions and hemiplegia.

In a review of 50 cases subjected to hemispherectomy Wilson (1970) found the onset of the illness to be associated with perinatal trauma or hypoxia in 54%, and to have followed an acute febrile illness between 1 and 4 years in 30%; the remaining 16% were a miscellaneous group. Both Wilson (1970) and Carmichael (1966) drew upon the mainly upublished work of Mair (his findings in 17 cases were described in 1952), who found the perinatal group to have middle cerebral artery lesions—interruption of the internal elastic lamina, intimal proliferation or recanalized thrombus—with old infarction in the middle cerebral territory, often with a gross porencephalic cyst. In the late infantile group there were diffuse arterial lesions similar to the localized ones, with associated patchy infarction in the removed hemisphere. In the only case examined personally there was patchy old infarction of the lateral and anterior frontal cortex, the anterior superior temporal gyrus, and the lateral occipital and posterior temporal cortex, which was associated with extensive damage to the white matter but spared those fibres already myelinated at or soon after birth (Fig. 5.48). Vascular lesions were not detected. Venous occlusion was considered to be a possible cause in this case but it could not be proved; this possibility has also been put forward by Gastaut et al. (1960). The view of Aguilar and Rasmussen (1960) that the lesions in these cases are due to chronic encephalitis is not generally accepted. Some of the brain damage may be due to repeated convulsions and this is considered in the next section.

7. Epilepsy

An essential problem lies in distinguishing brain lesions that cause fits from those that are the result of fits. The historical aspects and a good discussion of the whole subject are found in work by Corsellis and Meldrum (1976).

Many of the organic lesions described in this chapter can cause convulsions, e.g., encephalitis, meningitis, lead encephalopathy, vascular lesions, the sequelae of head injury and tumours, and metabolic disturbances. It is estimated that approximately 5% of infants and young children affected by acute febrile illness develop fits during its course. There is no clear evidence of brain lesions causing the majority of such attacks, but if fits recur brain damage may result.

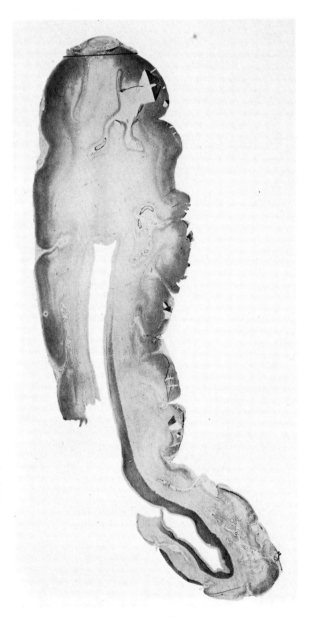

Fig. 5.48. Section at level of vestibule in a hemispherectomy specimen from a 21-year-old man in whom fits started at 1 year. There is extensive infarction of the lateral occipital and posterior temporal lobes but myelination in the optic radiation (developed before the fits) has remained. (LFB; 1 ×)

The lesion that has caused considerable controversy is the sclerosis of Ammon's horn in the anterior temporal lobe, which was thought by Earle et al. (1953) and Gastaut et al. (1959) to be the cause of fits in many subjects. It was postulated that the damage to this region developed at birth as a result of compression of the blood supply to it during hippocampal herniation produced in a difficult labour or of some other cause of acute unilateral brain swelling in infancy. This view has not gained general acceptance, and it is now thought that the hippocampal sclerosis is a manifestation of one of the many areas of brain damage that occur if convulsions are prolonged. The view that relative hypoxia or other metabolic abnormalities of the areas developing during the convulsive period are the cause of damage is widely supported. Undoubtedly, the fact that brain tissue in the temporal lobe damaged in this way may act as an epileptogenic focus with the possibility of further damage is generally accepted.

In temporal lobe epilepsy an association of a characteristic electroencephalogram present between psychomotor attacks has been associated with pathological lesions in the medial parts of the temporal lobes. These include tumours, areas of gliosis, and hamartomas, as well as the sclerosis described above. Excision of the affected area is often beneficial.

Norman (1964) has described the neuropathology of status epilepticus in young children, finding old and recent lesions affecting neurones. Neuronal loss or hypoxia was found in many areas in most cases, the cortex being affected in all, Ammon's horn in ten of the eleven, and the thalamus in nine of the eleven. Norman (1963) also reviewed a small group of cases in which cerebral hemiatrophy developed with convulsions and appeared to accept that such a state can result from the convulsions. He does fall back upon an initial vascular lesion, however, to describe the group called hemiatrophy with status spongiosus. This lesion appears to be similar to the changes found in some of the diffuse hemispherectomy specimens.

8. Trauma

Trauma is the most important cause of death in childhood after the first year of life. Falls and battering by adults are the more significant antecedents in infancy, while in children traffic accidents are the major problem. Subdural and subarachnoid haemorrhage, cerebral contusion and intracerebral haematoma are all fairly frequent; furthermore,

various combinations may occur in injury, usually, but not always, in association with fracture of the skull. Extradural haemorrhage is less common but may occur as a solitary lesion or with other forms of haemorrhage in severe trauma. Oedema is a well-recognized complication of intracerebral haematoma and may be relevant in the production of unilateral cerebral swelling. This in turn leads to hippocampal herniation with the danger of associated mid-brain haemorrhage. Generalized swelling without an appreciable local contusion or haematoma of the brain is exceptionally rare, but is sometimes found in children who die a few days after head injury: it is difficult to be certain in such circumstances whether the swelling is a direct reaction to trauma or to a complicating hypoxic episode.

9. Infections

9.1. Bacterial

Bacterial meningitis is the commonest infection of the nervous system in newborns, infants, and children, although epidemics of viral disease may occur. Fungal and protozoal infections are rare but some will be mentioned briefly.

The important causes of bacterial meningitis are gram-negative infections and *Str. pyogenes* in the newborn, *H. influenzae* between 4 months and 4 years, and *Str. pneumoniae* and *N. meningitidis* after that age. Worldwide *N. meningitidis* is the most important, epidemics still continuing in parts of Africa and elsewhere. *Myco. tuberculosis* is much less significant than a few decades ago.

The routes of infection include droplet spread from human carriers, when the organisms may pass from the nasopharynx, middle ears, or sinuses to the meninges, or via the bloodstream after entering the lungs. In recent years the possibility of infection via a myelomeningocele has continued, and the infection of Spitz–Holter valves used in hydrocephalic shunts is a fresh hazard. Terminal meningitis is occasionally seen in infants and children under treatment with immunosuppressive drugs and in those with immune deficiency syndromes.

All the bacteria mentioned (except *Myco. tuberculosis*, which will be considered separately) cause a rapidly spreading acute inflammation. In a florid case, dying after 2–4 days, the brain is swollen and congested. The subarachnoid space is distended by thick yellow pus in the basal cisterns, spreading to a variable extent over the convexities and the dorsum of the cerebellum but not extending onto the superficial aspect of the arachnoid. The spinal cord is coated with similar exudate, which may plug the exits from the fourth ventricle and the aqueduct of Sylvius, lie in flakes on the congested ependyma, or make the choroid plexus stiff. On microscopical examination the predominant cell initially is the polymorphonuclear leucocyte (except when the organism is *L. monocytogenes*); organisms are present inside and outside cells.

After 2 days the proportion of macrophages in the exudate increases, becoming greater than 50% by 7 days, when lymphocytes and plasma cells may also be present. The walls of veins are frequently involved in the reaction; arteritis is less common except in infections due to *Str. pneumoniae*, which may cause fibrinoid necrosis.

Fewer cells are seen in overwhelming infections and in cases where there has been some response to treatment. Thus in the severe septicaemic form of infection by *N. meningitidis* the cerebrospinal fluid may be only faintly opalescent; in such cases it will contain few cells but may teem with organisms. Exudate may then be limited to a few streaks alongside veins or in sulci. Death in these cases is

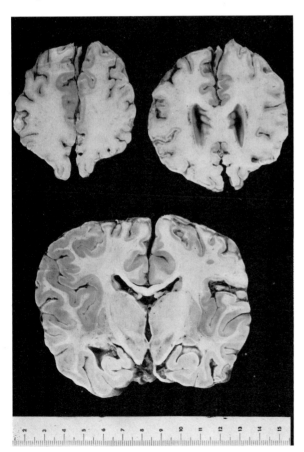

Fig. 5.49. Cortical atrophy and necrosis in frontal lobes following *H. influenzae* meningitis.

usually associated with haemorrhagic necrosis of the adrenal glands—the Waterhouse–Friderichsen syndrome.

In the first few days there is often some increase of cerebral volume resulting from cerebral swelling, which compresses the ventricles. As the swelling subsides inspissated exudate blocking the flow of cerebrospinal fluid at such critical places as the aqueduct of Sylvius, the exits from the fourth ventricle, or the cisterna ambiens may cause acute hydrocephalus.

Although death may occur from an overwhelming infection in the first 24 h, as already noted, or from toxaemia or the effects of the infection on other systems in the first week, most cases recover with modern therapy, except in the neonate, where the outcome is less certain.

In infants a subdural effusion may develop which contains few inflammatory cells and is thought to be the result of an extension of the infection along the sheaths of bridging veins. This effusion may become localized, usually in the frontal region, by the formation of a thin membrane from the undersurface of the dura. If fluid then persists or increases in volume the normal development of the frontal lobes may be arrested (Fig. 5.49).

All series emphasize the high mortality of neonatal meningitis (Fig. 5.50) (it is about 70%) and the high incidence of neurological defects in survivors. Whereas gram-negative rods such as *E. coli* and *Ps. pyocyaneus* were the most important organisms in this age group for many years, in the last decade there have been numerous cases of infection by *Str. pyogenes*.

Tuberculous meningitis has declined substantially in incidence in the last 50 years, mainly as a result of the better control of tuberculosis by the public health and therapeutic measures continued from earlier decades, but accentuated by the more effective specific therapy developed since 1947. The mortality is still 30%–40%.

Tuberculous meningitis in children is due to bloodstream dissemination from a primary complex in the lungs. In the florid case the basal cisterns contain a gelatinous yellowish-grey tissue, which extends into the stems of the Sylvian fissures. Pinhead or slightly smaller miliary tubercles are often scattered over the lateral surfaces of the cerebrum and the dorsum of the cerebellum; they may be seen along vessels (Fig. 5.51). Careful section of the fixed brain may reveal a small tuberculoma in the cerebral tissue with access to the cerebrospinal fluid. Rich and McCordock (1933) attributed the development of the meningitis to the discharge of bacilli from such small tuberculomas into hypersensitive meninges.

Microscopical examination shows eosinophilic

areas borded by or intermingled with epithelioid cells, lymphocytes and plasma cells; Langhans giant cells may be sparse. It is difficult to assess how much of the eosinophilic background is caseation and how much is fibrin without special stains for the latter. The epithelioid cells may form coronas about medium-sized or small arteries and in some examples the media of these vessels show fibrinoid necrosis (Fig. 5.52). Endarteritis fibrosa reducing the size of the lumen is a more common finding and may lead to vascular occlusion with or without thrombosis. This acute vascular and exudative component is much more frequent in the meningitis than in the primary tuberculous lesion or miliary lesions elsewhere, and may in fact reflect the reaction of bacilli with sensitized meninges.

Cases seen at necropsy now have often been treated. In these cases a few grey areas of thickening in the leptomeninges may be the only naked-eye abnormality, and extensive microscopical examination is sometimes required to detect more than a sprinkling of round cells in fibrous tissue (Fig. 5.53). In other cases, however, which may have survived for months or years, focal cerebral infarction will be found in association with thrombosis of inflamed arteries, together with hydrocephalus resulting from fibrosis in the meninges.

The number of cases with sequelae producing neurological deficit in most forms of meningitis has diminished with modern therapy, probably because the duration and amount of exudation is decreased, vascular involvement with thrombosis is less, and

complications such as subdural effusion and hydrocephalus are recognized and treated earlier. In addition to the problems following infection by *M. tuberculosis* sequelae can occur after influenzal and pneumococcal meningitis and neonatal infections. Vascular lesions, the mechanical effect of the exudate, subdural effusions, acute brain swelling at the height of infection, bacterial toxins, and metabolic changes have all been considered to be contributory factors.

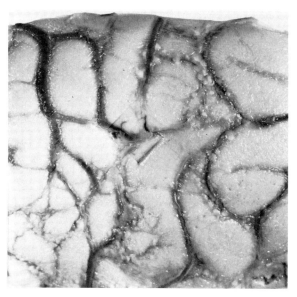

Fig. 5.51. Pinhead miliary tubercles on the surface of the brain in tuberculous meningitis.

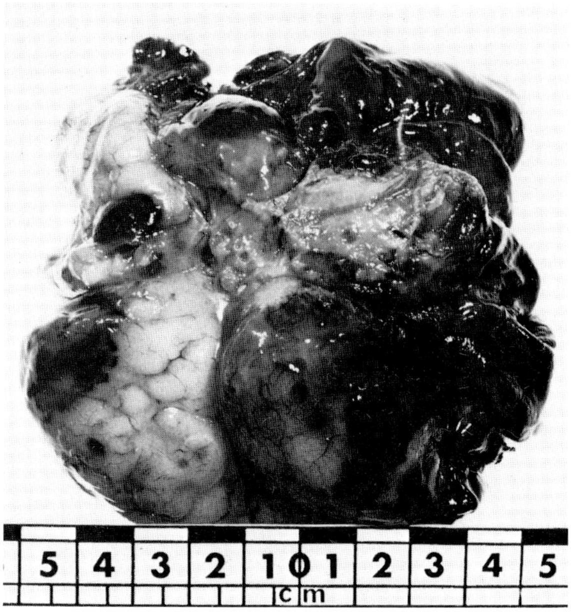

Fig. 5.50. Haemorrhagic infarction of the brain due to vasculitis in *E. coli* meningitis in a newborn.

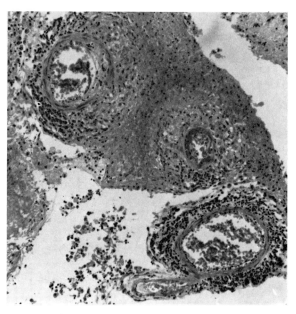

Fig. 5.52. Fibrinoid necrosis of artery in tuberculous meningitis with surrounding epithelioid cells. (H and E; 400 ×)

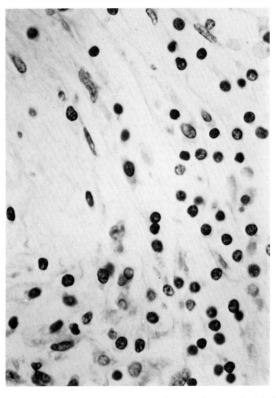

Fig. 5.53. Residual reaction in treated tuberculous meningitis. (H and E; 400 ×)

Local infarction has been attributed to arteritis in *Str. pneumoniae* meningitis (Smith et al. 1957) and in one of a series of 34 cases of *H. influenzae* meningitis (Smith and Landing 1960). The latter observers found venous occlusion to be a more significant factor: it caused infarction in five of the 34 cases. Berman and Barber (1966) described arteritis and phlebitis in 28 of 29 cases of neonatal meningitis and considered these lesions to be responsible for the four cases in which infarction developed. A diffuse necrosis of the white matter of the cerebral hemispheres in a case of *E. coli* meningitis was thought to be due to vasculitis by Buchan and Alvard (1969). Vascular occlusion resulting from compression by acute cerebral swelling developing in the course of meningitis was considered to be a possibility by Smith and Landing, who thought temporary venous compression occurred in some *H. influenzae* infections, and by Lindenberg and Swanson (1967), who attributed hydranencephaly in two infants to compression of the internal carotid arteries in the course of meningitis.

The question of diffuse neuronal damage occurring in the course of meningitis is discussed by Adams et al. (1948) as well as by Smith and Landing. It is not possible to be sure whether the shrinkage of cortical neurones, when occurring alone in fatal cases of meningitis, is a terminal event or due to hypoxia or metabolic change. When it is accompanied by neuronal loss and glia proliferation (Fig. 5.54) it obviously antedates the terminal hours of illness. Smith and Landing considered the possibilities of

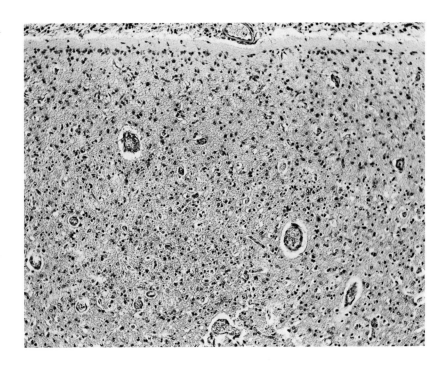

Fig. 5.54. Neuronal loss and glia proliferation in cortex beneath thick exudate in *H. influenzae* meningitis (H and E; 100 ×)

extension of infection into the cerebrum, diffusion of bacterial toxins into the brain, vascular factors, the effects of a thick exudate, acute cerebral swelling, and the age of the patients in explaining such diffuse damage. They were unable to come to a definite conclusion but favoured mechanical factors, such as the thick exudate and cerebral swelling acting in combination to produce temporary or intermittent venous occlusion; they also stressed the fact that such damage was restricted to infants under 1 year old in their series. Berman and Banker (1966) thought that a metabolic explanation was more likely in their neonatal group; in particular, anoxia following circulatory collapse. There appears little doubt that the hazard of diffuse damage is greater in meningitis occurring in the neonatal period. This may be due in part to the greater metabolic requirements and vulnerability of the maturing brain.

Intracerebral abscess is now rarely seen as a complication of inflammation in the ear, mastoid, accessory nasal sinuses, or chest. At present many of the cases seen in children and adolescents in developed countries arise as a complication of congenital heart disease (Fig. 5.55). An exception was the series of Wright and Ballantyne (1967), who found that in 30 cases seen between 1946 and 1965 the most common antecedent was chronic otitis, which was present in 11 of the 30.

Abscesses arising from bloodstream spread are more frequent in the cerebral hemispheres; they are rarely multiple. In congenital heart disease cerebral abscess is unusual before the age of 2 years, before which vascular thrombosis is more common. The fact that the abscess is a complication of heart disease with right-to-left intracardiac shunts leads to the hypothesis that the infection is caused by organisms which escape the lung filter. As a complication of local suppurative disease abscesses are likely to occur in the frontal lobe after sinusitis and in the temporal lobe or cerebellum with middle ear or mastoid disease. The organisms commonly spread along perforating vessels, and the initial lesion is a small area of necrosis surrounded by polymorphonuclear leucocytes at the junction of grey and white matter. In experimental material Falconer et al. (1943) demonstrated a more rapid spread from the initial lesion into the white matter than the grey, and correlated this with the poorer blood supply of the former. Hence in a well-developed abscess the central areas of pus is apt to be surrounded on the side of the grey matter by a well-developed inner reddish-yellow zone of granulation tissue interspersed with foam cells and an outer grey zone of proliferating glia as tissue reactions are better developed here. In the deeper white matter this barrier may be incomplete or loculation may be

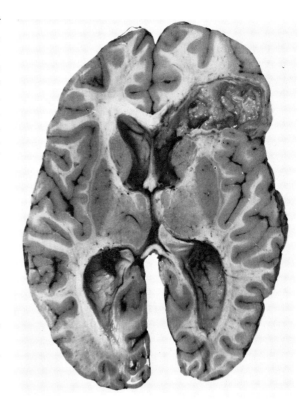

Fig. 5.55. Frontal lobe abscess extending to ventricle in a case of congenital heart disease.

seen, indicating that a fresh wave of suppuration and necrosis has extended through a partly developed barrier. In rare cases this form of spread may result in rupture into the ventricle. A zone of oedematous white matter with a lemon yellow tint is common around an abscess; it may, with the abscess, cause unilateral cerebral swelling and dangerous herniation.

The treatment of choice is excision of the abscess under antibiotic cover. The timing of such excision is disputed. Some argue that it should be done when localization is complete, while others (Wright and Ballantyne 1967) maintain that excision as soon as the diagnosis is definite is preferable.

9.2. Protozoal and Fungal

Protozoal and fungal infections are also found in infants. *Toxoplasmosis* entailing damage to the nervous system of a newborn infant was first described by Wolf and Cowen in 1937. There is evidence that organisms pass from mother to fetus, and in animals placental lesions have been demonstrated. The time at which infection of the fetus occurs is variable; there is some evidence that damage to the fetus is more likely if the transmission takes place between 2 and 6 months of fetal life (Desmonts and Couvreur 1974).

The baby may be stillborn, live for a few months, or survive until adult life with neurological damage; in some instances the nervous system may not be vulnerable to the organism, as cases are on record in which only one of twins has been affected. In those affected severely there is extensive meningoencephalitis and ependymitis with hydrocephalus and sometimes microcephaly. Damaged surface areas appear as shrunken gyri covered by thickened meninges. Yellow areas may be found in the depths of the cerebrum or the brain stem. On microscopic examination there is necrosis, often with patchy calcification, surrounded by diffuse inflammatory reaction and miliary granulomas. Microglia cells, histiocytes, plasma cells, lymphocytes, and astrocytes may all take part in the reaction. The organisms are found both intra- and extra-cellularly. In the latter (Fig. 5.56) position they are about 2.5 × µm, oval or round, and with a nuclear mass at one end of the cell. In haematoxylin and eosin preparations the cytoplasm stains a lighter blue than the nucleus, while in methylene blue eosin sections the cytoplasm is red. Collections of organisms are found in cysts, which can be up to 20–30 µm in diameter. Organisms in such cysts are compressed together; if identified in the cerebrospinal fluid or smears they are somewhat larger than in sections and

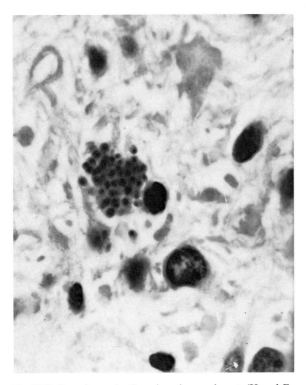

Fig. 5.56. Toxoplasmosis. Organisms in pseudocyst. (H and E; 1400 ×)

may appear crescentic or boat-shaped. Involvement of the ciliary body, choroid, and retina is often found in association with damage to the central nervous system, and there may be granulomas in other organs.

Infection acquired after birth rarely gives rise to clinical manifestations in the nervous system (see p. 83). An acute form of meningoencephalitis has been described, after which complete recovery is more common than residual brain damage (Degen and Elbel 1966).

Fungal infections of the nervous system are not very important numerically, but have become more significant with the advent of therapeutic immunosuppression. Disseminated candidiasis is occasionally seen in premature babies.

Infection by *Cryptococcus neoformans*, a yeast-like, non-spore-forming, budding fungus, which forms a distinctive capsule in tissues and in culture, is called torulosis. The central oval body is usually 2–4 µm in diameter, and the thicker capsule contains a complex mucopolysaccharide that stains both with alcian blue and the periodic acid Schiff method. The infection may be generalized and lung involvement is not uncommon. However, the central nervous system disease is likely to be dominant, and it frequently presents as a meningitis resembling tuberculous meningitis in many ways. The changes in the cerebrospinal fluid are similar to those in tuberculosis, but occasionally they are absent. The cryptococcus can usually be demonstrated in smears or cultures if it is looked for.

The organisms extend along perivascular spaces and may produce focal granulomas in grey and white matter. At post-mortem there is grey thickening of leptomeninges and focal white pinheads. If organisms are abundant the exudate in the subarachnoid space may have a slimy consistency. A characteristic finding on section of the brain are small cysts, up to 1 cm diameter, in the grey and white matter of the temporal lobes and in the basal ganglia. Microscopical examination shows a chronic inflammatory infiltrate with giant cells and organisms. These are more abundant in the cerebrum than in the meninges and may be found within giant cells. In some cases reaction is minimal or even absent.

Infection of the meninges by the common mucors (mucormycosis) has been more widely recognized in recent decades. Although most examples are seen in diabetics and patients on prolonged steroid therapy, there have been a few reports of infection in debilitated infants. The fungi are identified in tissues by their large, branching, nonseptate hyphae. These are seen in meninges, nervous tissue, and vessel walls. In the latter, as elsewhere, an inflammatory reaction may be present and vessels are sometimes occluded, with consequent infarction. Similar vascular invasion is seen in other organs of the body.

Where histoplasmosis is endemic it may produce a disseminated illness in infants in which meningitis or granulomas within the brain are present. Shapiro et al. (1955) reported lesions of the nervous system of six of eleven fatal cases in Tennessee and emphasized the similarity of the lesions to those in tuberculosis of the nervous system. Four of the six cases were infants. The organisms are basophilic, usually round or oval, 2–5 µm in diameter and surrounded by a halo. They are seen most convincingly in macrophages, which they often fill. The PAS method stains the inner capsule of the organisms but not the halo. Oppenheimer et al. (1973) have reported histoplasmosis as a complication of acute leukaemia in childhood and discuss the relationship of dissemination to the immunological status.

Newborn babies may develop cutaneous or alimentary tract candidiasis as a result of infection from the mother. Dissemination of monilia may occur in premature babies if the silastic catheters used for parenteral feeding become infected. The organisms are seen in the vicinity of small vessels in the brain and meninges. An unusual feature may be a macrophage response without other inflammatory cells (Fig. 5.57). The immunological significance of this is not clear. In older children dissemination may occur when there is immunological paralysis from disease or therapy, but involvement of the brain is rare.

9.3. Viral

Viral infections of the nervous system are more common in children than adults; the latter often have circulating antibody following previous subclinical infection by any given virus. While it is necessary to have a fairly comprehensive classification of infections such as that in Table 5.2, it is profitable to approach their pathological effects with three main categories in mind:

a) Those infections in which nervous system damage results mainly from the replication of virus within nerve cells, e.g., poliomyelitis
b) Those in which lesions result mainly from immunological reactions after the peak of the general infection—the postinfectious encephalitides
c) Slow virus infections, in which the manifestations occur months or years after the initial infection.

This classification, like many others, is not exclusive, as the categories overlap. Most of the encephalitides in Table 5.2 would fall into category

(a), and description will be limited to poliomyelitis, herpes simplex, rubella, measles, and (briefly) rabies. Even these few are now seen rarely by pathologists in the United Kingdom.

Table 5.2. Viruses causing disease of the nervous system

Symmetry		RNA	DNA
Cubic	Enteroviruses	Poliomyelitis	Herpes virus hominis
		Coxsackie	Herpes virus varicellae
		Echo	Cytomegalo-virus
Helical	Orthomyxovirus	Influenza	
	Rhabdoviridae	Rabies	
	Paramyxoviruses	Mumps	
	Morbilli	Measles	
Complex	Pox viruses		Variola
			Vaccinia
Uncertain	Arboviruses	Group A	
		Western equine	
		Eastern equine	
		Venezualan equine	
		Group B	
		Mosquito-borne	
		Japanese B	
		Murray Valley	
		St Louis	
		Tick-borne	
		Russian spring summer	
		Central European	
		Louping—ill	
	Arena viruses	Lymphocytic choriomeningitis	
		Lassa fever	

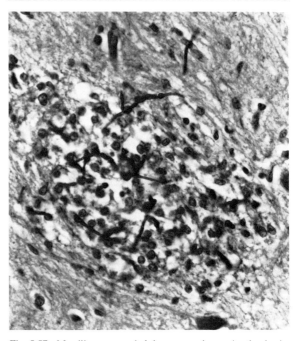

Fig. 5.57. Monilia surrounded by macrophages in the brain. Infection following parenteral feeding in a premature baby. (PAS; 400 ×)

The poliovirus, the most important of the enteroviruses, is one of the smallest. Three antigenic types are known, of which types I and III can cause paralytic disease. After proliferation in the lymphoid tissue of the alimentary tract following infection the virus reaches the bloodstream, crosses the blood–brain barrier, and replicates in motor neurones, particularly those of the cord and brain stem. In a fatal case the brain and cord will be congested but may show few macroscopical changes—possibly the odd petechial haemorrhage in the medulla or anterior horns of the spinal cord. Microscopically there will be neuronal necrosis and chromatolysis with neuronophagia (Fig. 5.58), in which dead and dying neurones are surrounded by macrophages. In the first few days polymorphonuclear leucocytes may be present between dilated vessels but these soon become sparse, to be replaced by lymphocytes, macrophages, and occasional plasma cells. The macrophages may form small collections or 'knots', and the lymphocytes are often aggregated around small vessels. Loss of neurones may be considerable and in severe cases micronecrosis is present (Fig. 5.59), although this is not sufficient to be detectable to the naked eye. In the brain stem the infiltration may extend among sensory neurones, but these do not show necrosis. If the hemispheres are involved lesions are likely to be confined to the thalamus and motor cortex. The areas damaged in the spinal cord correspond to those innervating paralysed muscles during life.

In chronic cases the cord is somewhat shrunken and there is loss of motor neurones, particularly the medial groups in the spinal cord, together with neurogenic atrophy in innervated muscles. In cases dying after a few months residual intranuclear inclusion bodies (Cowdry type B) in otherwise normal neurones are stated to be evidence of cell recovery.

In principle, all viral encephalitides in which lesions result from replication of the organisms within cells will lead to a similar type of reaction to that in poliomyelitis. Differences will depend on the affinity of different viruses for different groups of neurones, and the fact that in some infections there is considerable tissue necrosis. From these facts the pathologist may be able to make a fairly definite diagnosis in some cases, but in coming to this it is necessary to be aware of the clinical picture and the knowledge of sporadicity or epidemicity. Isolation of virus from cerebrospinal fluid may be achieved in some cases during life or from nervous tissue after death. Serological investigations during life and electron microscopy may be helpful in some examples.

Herpes simplex is described in outline because although rare in children it is one of the few forms of encephalitis in which there is often conspicuous local

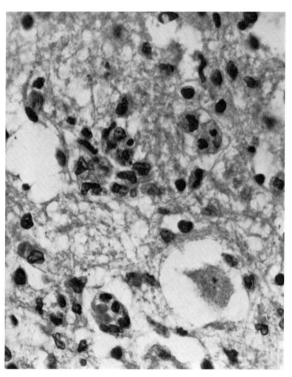

Fig. 5.58. Neuronophagia in anterior poliomyelitis. (H and E; 500 ×)

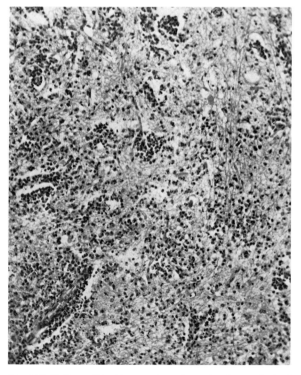

Fig. 5.59. Poliomyelitis. Devastation of anterior horn of spinal cord. (H and E; 125 ×)

macroscopic damage to the brain. This applies to the form in which the clinical presentation is that of a unilateral space-occupying lesion of rapid onset. If death occurs within a few weeks the affected hemisphere will be swollen and soft with a tendency to haemorrhage and disintegration in the frontotemporal region on handling (Fig. 5.60). Microscopically in these areas there may be a mixture of the changes of infarction and inflammatory reaction, with numerous lymphocytes mingling with masses of lipid-laden macrophages. Plasma cells may also be present. In the areas of astrocytic proliferation some cells, with swollen nuclei, may show eosinophilic intranuclear inclusions (Cowdry type A) (Fig. 5.61). Careful and prolonged search with the electron microscope is often necessary to demonstrate the characteristic double-contoured virus particles, about 100 nm in diameter (Fig. 5.62). They may also be demonstrated with fluorescent antibodies by means of appropriate techniques. The perivascular lymphocytic reaction may be found in many other parts of the nervous system.

Herpes simplex in this form is due to antigenic type I and is a characteristic example of a necrotizing encephalitis. Adams (1976) records that it was possible to demonstrate inclusion bodies in a minority of 25 personal cases. The rare disseminated infection in the newborn is due to Herpes simplex type II, and in this disease a meningoencephalitis may be associated with necrotic granulomas in liver, spleen, and adrenals. The brain may show widespread necrosis.

Rubella very rarely causes damage to the nervous system of child or adult except for the occasional case of postinfectious encephalitis (see p. 188). Its role in the aetiology of congenital malformations is referred to on page 83. With the severe rubella epidemics in the USA in 1963–1964 came the realization that this virus could not only be teratogenic but also persist after infection of the fetus in the first trimester, to cause a disease with widespread manifestations in the newborn. In this rubella syndrome meningoencephalitis sometimes occurred with thrombocytopenic purpura, hepatosplenomegaly , myocarditis, and bone lesions. Follow-up

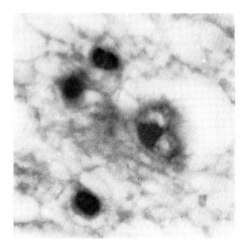

Fig. 5.61. Intranuclear inclusion in astrocyte in herpes simplex. (H and E; 1000 ×)

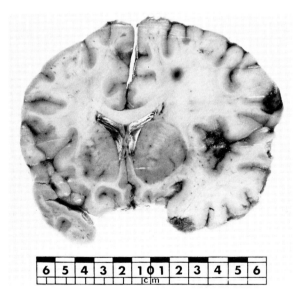

Fig. 5.60. Herpes simplex encephalitis showing swelling of right frontal and temporal lobes with areas of haemorrhage and necrosis.

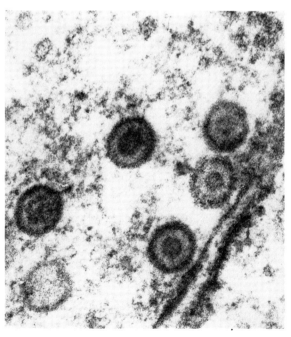

Fig. 5.62. Electronmicrograph of herpes simplex virus. (186 400 ×)

studies on cases of the rubella syndome indicate that mental retardation with microcephaly is a considerable hazard. Meningitis, vasculitis, and foci of necrosis have been described at post-mortem. Figures 5.63 and 5.64 show periventricular damage and reaction in an 11-day-old neonate with the syndrome.

Rabies was the first disease in which a viral cause was demonstrated. The intracytoplasmic inclusion in neurones—the Negri body (Fig. 5.65)—is diagnostic. The disease is still seen in many countries. The incubation period following a bite by a rabid animal is usually several weeks, which allows for protection by vaccination during the incubation period. The pathological reaction, apart from the specific inclusion bodies, does not differ from that in many other forms of encephalitis.

So far we have considered viral infections in which the encephalitis is dominant although a meningitis can be a part of the disease. There are some viral infections in which the converse is true. Mumps is the most common of these and fatal cases are rare. The association of a lymphocytosis in the cerebrospinal fluid with the clinical picture of meningitis complicating mumps is sufficient for a diagnosis;

recovery is usually complete. The virus can be demonstrated in the cerebrospinal fluid and rises in antibody titre may also be useful in cases where diagnosis is difficult. Histological changes are not specific, and lymphocytic infiltration of meninges and around vessels in the brain is not associated with neuronal necrosis.

The pathological changes in lymphocytic choriomeningitis, in which the lesions are confined to the meninges, are similar to those in mumps; the disease is more common in young adults than in children.

An encephalitis may develop at the height of the disease in measles and chicken pox. However, nervous system involvement in these exanthemas and in rubella is more likely to be a postinfectious encephalitis similar to the form that occasionally complicates vaccination against smallpox. Exanthema-associated encephalitis is probably the commonest form of childhood encephalitis when epidemics are absent. The pathology is that of a perivascular demyelination accompanied by lymphocytic, plasma cell, and macrophage infiltration around small veins in the white matter, brain stem, and spinal cord (Turnbull and McIntosh (1926). The

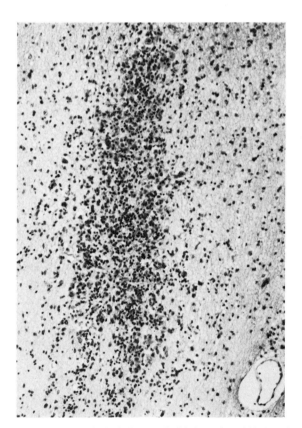

Fig. 5.63. Congenital rubella encephalitis in 11-day-old baby. The cellular infiltration is mainly of lymphocytes and plasma cells (H and E; 100 ×)

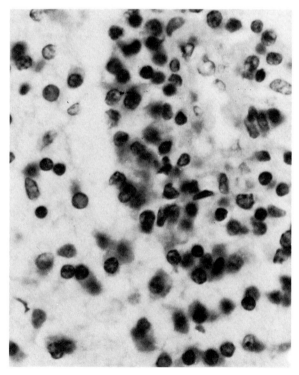

Fig. 5.64. Congenital rubella. Lymphocytic and plasma cell infiltrate. (H and E; 920 ×)

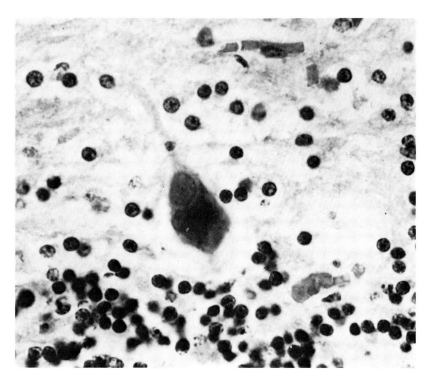

Fig. 5.65. Rabies. Cytoplasmic inclusion. Negi body in Purkinje cell. (H and E; 400 ×)

experimental model is experimental allergic encephalomyelitis (EAM), which is produced in animals by the repeated injection of brain tissue and Freund's adjuvant. In both the human and experimental disease the immunological basis is probably a delayed hypersensitivity reaction, as it is in the encephalomyelitis that complicates rabies vaccination in rare cases. The antigen is apparently nerve tissue that has been altered by the virus and thereby made antigenic to the host.

The example of category (c) is subacute sclerosing panencephalitis (SSPE), a very rare disease in children or young adults, with a duration of months to a few years. Damage to grey and white matter is associated with gliosis, lymphocytic and plasma cell infiltration about vessels, and microglia reaction. The lesions may be widely distributed in the brain and cord, usually with sparing of the cerebellum. Intranuclear inclusions (Cowdry type A), often surrounded by a halo, in glia cells and neurones are a diagnostic feature (Fig. 5.66). Ultrastructurally, collections of paramyxovirus particles are found (Fig. 5.67). Their description by Bouteille et al. (1965) disproved an earlier view that the disease was a manifestation of Herpes simplex infection. The subsequent finding of high levels of antibody to measles virus in the blood and CSF of patients with SSPE, the demonstration of measles antigen in neurones and glia cells in biopsy material by fluorescent methods, and finally the isolation of measles virus from a biopsy (Horta Barbosa et al. 1969) have led to acceptance of the view that this

virus is the causal agent. In many cases there is a history of measles in the first 2 years of life, but in 15% there is no history of a classic attack. Another interesting finding is a preponderance of cases in rural areas.

There is general agreement that the disease is caused by the entry of measles virus into nervous tissue and its slow replication there over a period of years. It is also thought that this occurs because of an abnormal immunological response in affected individuals. There has been much discussion about this, but the simple view of Burnet (1970) that the thymus-dependent system fails to function and prevent cell-to-cell infection within the CNS in the presence of high levels of antibody has not gained general acceptance.

Herpes zoster is rare in children but as in adults is due to the persistence of the varicella (chicken pox) virus in posterior root ganglia for months or years after the initial infection.

10. Tumours

Tumours of the nervous system are the most common form of solid neoplasm in children. Primary brain tumours and neuroblastomas of the autonomic system account for the great majority of cases; tumours of the spinal cord are rare and those of the meninges even more so.

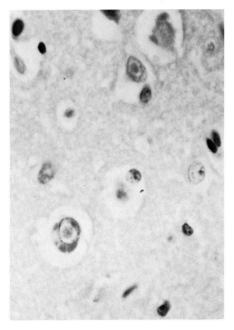

Fig. 5.66. Intranuclear inclusion with characteristic halo in subacute sclerosing porencephalitis (SSPE). (H and E; 400 ×)

The general aspects of the pathogenesis of neoplasms in childhood have been discussed (p. 641). In the nervous system genetic factors operate in a minority, those associated with the phakomatoses (p. 158) and retinoblastoma. There is good evidence that medulloblastoma may be congenital (p. 649) and that most cases arise from groups of migratory cells from the fetal granular layer. Other tumours which may develop from foci of misplaced cells in development are those associated with the phakomatoses and the craniopharyngeomas. The commonest tumours—those of the astrocytic series—probably arise from transformed cells in the same way as those of adult life. The most interesting experimental observations relevant to tumours in children are those concerning the production of a wide variety of central and peripheral tumours in the offspring of pregnant animals following the administration of nitrosamines (Druckrey et al. 1966).

10.1. Classification

The decision as to whether to use a grading system or one with individual types related to but not entirely dependent on a developmental basis has to be a personal one. My objections to grading are that it is unreliable on biopsy material, which is usually only a small sample of a tumour, it tends to suggest that the behaviour of a tumour remains fixed, and it gives more importance than is justified to limited histology in the assessment of treatment.

Table 5.3 is based on the classification of Russell and Rubinstein (1977). The figures are adapted from the personal series of Matson (1969) of 750 cases, in which he used astrocytoma grades III and IV for the more malignant forms and also mixed glioma; these

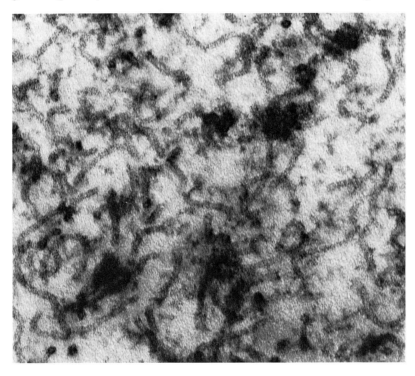

Fig. 5.67. Electron micrograph of Paramyxovirus particles. (SSPE; 115000 ×)

Table 5.3. Tumours of the central nervous system

A. Tumours of the glia series		
I. Astrocytic group		
1. Astrocytoma	202 + 79 + 27	41 %
2. Astroblastoma		
3. Polar spongioblastoma		
II. Oligodendroglia		
Oligodendroglioma		
III. Ependyma and its homologues		
1. Ependymoma.		
Subependymoma	66	9 %
2. Choroid plexus papilloma	23	3 %
3. 'Colloid cyst'		
IV. Glioblastoma multiforme	64	8.5 %
B. Pineal parenchyma		
1. Pineoblastoma	32	
2. Pineocytoma		
C. Retina (primitive epithelium)		
Retinoblastoma		
D. Tumours of neurone series		
1. Medulloblastoma	139	18.5 %
2. Medulloepithelioma		
3. Neuroblastoma	6	1 %
4. Ganglioneuroma and		
ganglioglioma		
Craniopharyngioma	79	10.5 %

have been equated with glioblastoma multiforme. Rubinstein (1972) gives a fuller discussion of the problems of classification and grading. Most series record 60%–70% of childhood gliomas as occurring below the tentorium, although a slightly increased incidence above was given in the series of Fossard (1968). Many of the subtentorial neoplasms are in the mid-line so that disturbances in cerebrospinal fluid circulation with alterations in pressure are often responsible for presenting symptoms and signs.

Astrocytomas, according to the published data, are the commonest cerebral tumours in children. Traditionally they have been classified, on a histogenetic basis, into protoplasmic and fibrillary forms, with the piloid tumour a subvariety of the latter. However, many tumours, particularly those of the cerebellum, show a mixture of forms so it is more profitable to group them on a regional basis.

Of Matson's 202 astrocytomas, 132 were in the cerebellum (66%). This slightly exceeded the number of medulloblastomas located in the posterior fossa, viz. 126. Of all glial tumours they are the most amenable to cure, partly because of their surgical accessibility and partly because in this site they are often well circumscribed. About half these neoplasms are solid and about half are cystic. In many instances the cyst wall is thin and devoid of tumour tissue, the cyst being essentially outside the tumour.

In younger children rather more of these tumours are in the mid-line than in one hemisphere; some extend from the mid-line to the hemisphere (Fig. 5.68). Microscopical examination frequently shows a meshwork of fibrillary astrocytes (Fig. 5.69); in some the cells are predominantly piloid, while in others microcysts are prominent and surrounded by protoplasmic astrocytes; calcification is rare but haemorrhage can occur into the tumour nodule or the cyst. Russell and Rubinstein (1977) do not regard the occasional presence of hyperchromatic nuclei and giant cells in these tumours as evidence of anaplasia in the absence of mitotic activity. Infiltration of the meninges and extension to the brain stem can occur but metastasis is rare.

In children, astrocytomas of the cerebrum may be cystic or solid and diffusely infiltrating. Cystic forms are less well circumscribed than the cerebellar examples and this, together with the tendency to involve deep structures, makes operative cure unlikely. In general, their microscopical features are similar to those of the cerebellar tumours.

In this age group the third ventricle is a well-recognized site for astrocytomas, which can often be demarcated laterally and superiorly but may blend with the chiasm and infundibular structures below. They may be associated with von Recklinghausen's disease (Fig. 5.70); the cut surface can be gelatinous, and the cell type is then a small astrocyte lying in a microcystic matrix. Gliomas of the optic chiasm and the optic nerve are normally pildod astrocytomas and may also be a manifestation of von Recklinghausen's disease.

The common concept of glioma of the brain stem is that of a uniform expansion of the pons by grey glia tissue; hence the old and misleading name: diffuse hypertrophy of the pons. Occasionally they are found higher or lower in the brain stem, and very rarely an example is limited to one half of the pons. On section they are mainly grey, but foci of haemorrhagic or darker grey tissue are seen in many. Corresponding to these naked eye features the predominant picture is a diffuse astrocytic proliferation, often of uniform piloid astrocytes. The darker areas show evidence of anaplasia with mitotic activity, increased cellularity and vascular proliferation (Fig. 5.71).

The concept of anaplasia is less pertinent to childhood astrocytomas than to those of adult life, with the exception of the brain stem group. When areas of a grey firm astrocytoma are found to be replaced by a more vascular or even haemorrhagic tissue it can be predicted that microscopical examination will show these areas to be more cellular, the cells to be larger with nuclear variation and mitotic activity, than in the remainder of the tumour, which

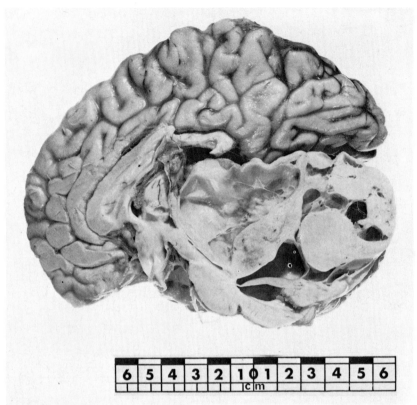

Fig. 5.68. Astrocytoma of cerebellum.

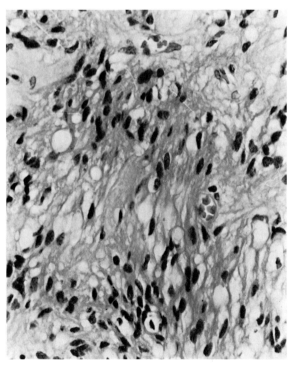

Fig. 5.69. Fibrillary astrocytes in well-differentiated tumour. (H and E; 400 ×)

shows the uniform picture of an astrocytoma. It is postulated that such areas have arisen as a result of de-differentiation or anaplasia in a slowly growing neoplasm and reflect a more rapid growth pattern. Matson classified 79 of the 750 intracranial tumours as brain stem gliomas but did not separate them further, as several in this particular group had not been confirmed histologically. The facts that clinical diagnosis of tumour in this situation in this age group can be made confidently and that surgical treatment is hopeless obviate the use of biopsy diagnosis.

Gliomas of the optic nerve are uncommon but they occur more frequently in childhood than at any other time. They are sometimes a manifestation of von Recklinghausen's neurofibromatosis, of which they may be the presenting feature. The tumours cause a uniform expansion of the optic nerve (Fig. 5.72), sometimes with a dumbbell extension through the foramen into the cranium or occasionally a diffuse infiltration back into the optic chiasm. Extension into the surrounding sheath can occur with reticulin production. The predominant cell type is the astrocyte and the variety of histological pattern possible is similar to that of astrocytomas elsewhere. Russell and Rubinstein consider that in many cases there is a mixed astrocytic and oligodendroglia proliferation.

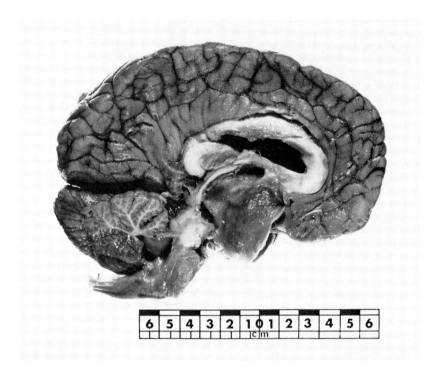

Fig. 5.70. Third ventricle astrocytoma in neurofibromatosis.

Oligodendrogliomas usually occur in the cerebral hemispheres, are often better defined than astrocytomas, and may show evidence of haemorrhage or calcification on a pinkish-grey cut surface. The microscopical appearance of box-like cells with clear cytoplasm is characteristic in paraffin sections; it is said to depend on acute swelling of the cells. The demonstration of the characteristic cell body and processes of oligodendroglia cells with silver impregnation methods is often difficult. In a review of 165 cases, Earnest et al. (1950) recorded seven in the first decade of life and 19 in the second.

Glioblastoma multiforme is the term reserved for a poorly defined tumour with a variegated cut surface with a characteristic histology illustrated in Fig. 5.73. The tumour illustrated is a parietal neoplasm in a child of 12, which metastasized via the cerebrospinal fluid to other parts of the brain, including the pons and medulla; death occurred within 4 months of diagnosis and 8 months from the onset of symptoms. The considerable cellularity, mitoses, giant cells, and vascular proliferation indicated the diagnosis, and these features were maintained in the distant deposits. Such a picture is rare in childhood neoplasms and when found it is usually in a supratentorial lesion. Those brain stem tumours with foci of such anaplastic growth against

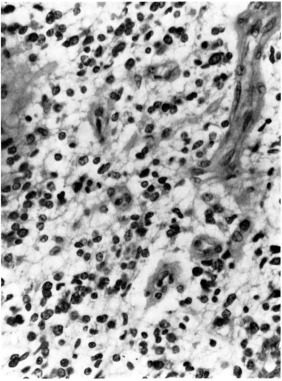

Fig. 5.71. Closely packed but uniform cells in pontine glioma. Some vascular proliferation and a mitosis are present. (H and E; 400 ×)

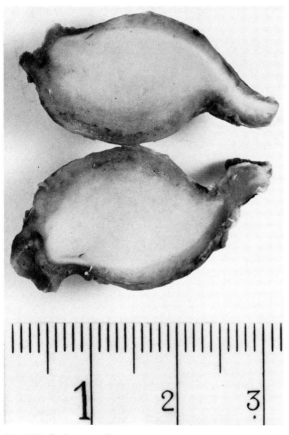

Fig. 5.72. Optic nerve glioma.

an astrocytic background have been classified as astrocytomas. The distinction of the glioblastoma multiforme, which has a rapidly growing pattern throughout and a rapid clinical course by its specific name, from the brain stem astrocytoma, with its longer history and a mixed histological pattern, is helpful in accurate description of the behaviour of these types. Metastasis outside the nervous system is extremely rare, but has been recorded occasionally in recent years in adult cases. The majority of extracranial deposits follow surgical treatment such as the insertion of ventriculopleural shunts (Brust et al. 1968), but rare examples without such treatment have been recorded (Rubinstein 1967).

Ependymomas were recorded in 66 of Matson's 750 intracranial tumours, 34 in the posterior fossa and 32 above the tentorium (Matson 1969). Wherever they arise there is usually some attachment to the ventricular lining (Fig. 5.74). In those tumours occurring in the posterior fossa the attachment is to the wall of the fourth ventricle, which may be expanded by firm grey growth with a papillary surface. Infiltration of the cerebellum or expansion of the upper cervical spinal cord can occur; occasionally the mass of growth protrudes through a foramen of Luschka into the cerebellopontine angle. In these examples cysts are not seen, but the cerebral types originating from the wall of a lateral ventricle

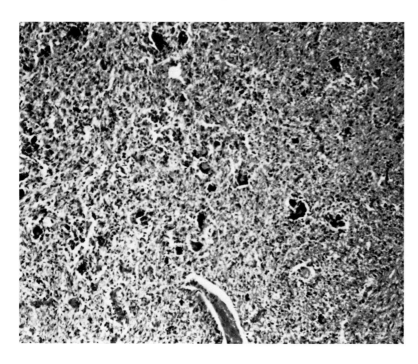

Fig. 5.73. Glioblastoma multiforme. (H and E; 100 ×)

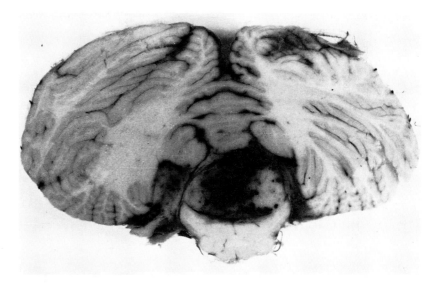

Fig. 5.74. Ependymoma of fourth ventricle extending out through foramen of Luschka.

and infiltrating cerebral tissue are often partly cystic and fairly well circumscribed. Calcified foci may be present in both types. Microscopic examination shows a variable mixture of polygonal or columnar cells and astrocytes. The former are sometimes arranged around a central lumen of variable size, forming a true rosette (Fig. 5.75). The tapering ends of these cells are more frequently aggregated around blood vessels to form perivascular pseudorosettes (Fig. 5.76). Those examples in which fibrillary astrocytes are more conspicuous than ependymal cells are often referred to as subependymomas, with the implication of an origin from the subependymal glia; they are rare in children.

Diagnosis is not difficult as a rule, but may sometimes be clinched by the demonstration of blephoroplasts, a point made by F.B. Mallory in 1902. These cytoplasmic bodies are more constantly found than the cilia which arise from them. They are less than 0.5 μm in diameter and are best identified with the phosphotungstic haematoxylin stain and an oil-immersion objective. In biopsy material, however, their separation from mitochondria is often impossible. For those with limited experience a comparison of the cells of the tumour with islands of ependymal inclusions adjacent to the normal ventricular wall at the tip of a horn of the lateral ventricle may facilitate diagnosis. Most ependymal tumours are histologically benign and mitoses are very infrequent. Rubinstein (1970) has reviewed the use of the term ependymoblastoma and suggested limiting it to a rare tumour composed of primitive cells, resembling spongioblasts with areas of differentiation to typical ependymal rosettes, as well as evidence of rapid growth and infiltration. The two cases he reported were in young children and in one there was extensive metastasis in the leptomeninges of the brain and cord.

Choroid plexus neoplasms are an interesting and clinically important group in children; the great majority are papillomas arising from the choroid plexus in the fourth ventricle or that in the vestibule of a lateral ventricle, usually the left. The common clinical presentation is with hydrocephalus, owing to obstruction in fourth-ventricle tumours and overproduction of cerebrospinal fluid in the case of lateral ventricle papillomas. Production of hydrocephalus by these papillomas was thought to be unlikely for many years but seems to have been demonstrated unequivocally in those examples in

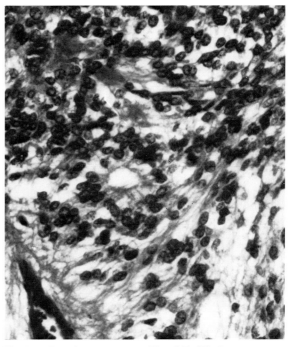

Fig. 5.75. Ependymoma rosette. (H and E; 400 ×)

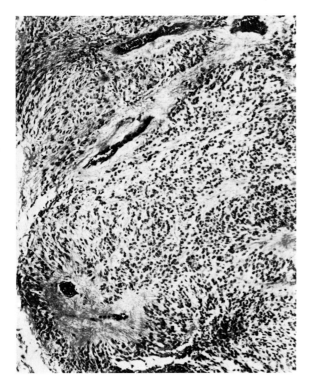

Fig. 5.76. Ependymoma pseudorosette. (H and E; 100 ×)

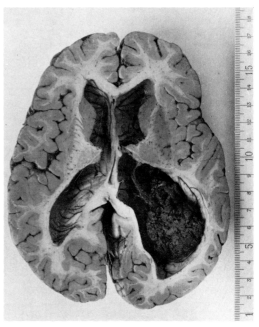

Fig. 5.77. Choroid plexus papilloma.

which cure of hydrocephalus was produced by operative removal of the tumour (Kahn and Luros 1952; Matson 1953). Occasionally a chronic ependymitis is produced by bleeding or secretion from the tumour mass (Smith 1955).

The papillomas are vascular papillary masses which can reach a considerable size (Fig. 5.77), but do not infiltrate brain tissue; fourth-ventricle lesions may protrude through the lateral recess. Microscopical examination shows a structure essentially similar to that of normal choroid plexus with cubical or columnar cells on a vascular connective tissue framework, but the aggregation of papillae may produce a pseudoadenomatous architecture. The connective tissue distinguishes them from ependymomas, in which there is a glia element seen in the stroma. Seedlings from papillomas are often found at various sites in the leptomeninges but they do not proliferate. The rare malignant tumours are adenocarcinomas of the cerebral choroid plexus, which may infiltrate through the wall of the ventricle into the cerebral tissue; microscopically the cells are large, with atypical nuclei and some mitotic activity.

Teratomas and pineal neoplasms: Most intracranial teratomas occur in the region of the pineal, a few in the region of the pituitary stalk and other sites. These are often cystic neoplasms composed of 'multiple tissues foreign to the part', in which epithelial tubules, connective tissue stroma, squamous epithelium, muscle, and cartilage may be identified. They usually occur in males before the age of 20.

The most common pineal neoplasm is the one that Russell now calls a germinoma and has repeatedly identified as a form of teratoma (although others have referred to it as a pinealoma). Its main histological constituent is a sheet of large polygonal cells mixed with small cells like lymphocytes (Fig. 5.78), mimicking exactly the appearance of a seminoma of the testis or dysgerminoma of the ovary. Areas of columnar epithelial tubules and smooth muscle are less frequent and conspicuous. This tumour occurs a decade or so later than the more typical teratoma considered in the previous paragraph. 'Ectopic forms' found in the floor of the third ventricle and tuber cinereum are often mistakenly referred to as ectopic pinealomas: they are germinomas found as usual in a mid-line position.

True pinealomas in which silver impregnation methods demonstrate cells with club-shaped processes similar to those of the normal pinealocytes are very rare, but have been described in children as well as adults. Pinealoblastomas are as rare, but are more frequent in children than in adults. Their histological pattern is similar to that of medulloblastomas of the undifferentiated type.

Medulloepithelioma: The existence of this tumour was disputed for many years but has been accepted since the case reported by Treip (1957). In a more recent article Deck (1969) recorded a further case with maturation into ependymal and ganglion cells and in his review accepted five other recorded examples. They occur in young children and may be congenital. The essential histological feature is the presence of columnar epithelial tubules with internal and external cell membranes and an absence of cilia and blephoroplasts.

Neuroblastoma, ganglioneuroma, and ganglioglioma are all rare in the brain. Examples of the first two are usually only found in children and may be congenital. The neuroblastoma is a tumour occurring in the cerebral hemispheres, which is similar histologically and in its behaviour to the medulloblastoma. The cells are polygonal, occur mostly in solid masses but with some orientation about vessels, and show, in some examples, grouping together of their tapering processes to form rosettes. The Bielschovsky method allows impregnation of neurofibrillary processes can be achieved. Russell and Rubinstein (1977) mention that a reticulin and collagenous stroma can be very abundant in some cases and suggest that this feature, which is not seen in neuroglial tumours, indicates an unusual capacity of these primitive tumour cells for stroma induction. They may grow rapidly to a large size and involve both hemispheres; the cut surface is usually grey with occasional gelatinous and haemorrhagic areas.

Ganglioneuromas and gangliogliomas can occur anywhere in the CNS, but a favoured site is the floor of the third ventricle, with consequent hypothalamic disturbances. The histological diagnosis of the tumours of ganglion cells is usually straightforward: The cells are obviously neuronal, with demonstrable Nissl substance and neurofibrils in mature and aberrant forms. An interesting case reported by Robertson et al. (1964) in a 15-year-old girl showed particles in the cytoplasm of the neurones with the electron microscope, which were comparable to the secretory granules found in the adrenal medulla and sympathetic ganglia. The authors suggested that the tumour had perhaps originated from hamartomatous ectopic sympathetic nervous tissue. The diagnosis of gangliogliomas is more difficult. It is necessary to demonstrate that the apparently neuronal cells really are neuronal, namely by demonstrating that Nissl substance and neurofibrils are present within them and that they are neoplastic. The latter is suggested by unusual aggregations and the presence of binucleate or giant cells.

Craniopharyngioma is the commonest supratentorial neoplasm in children and is usually a partially cystic tumour. It is thought to arise from remnants of the stomatodeal component of the pituitary because of its predominant squamous epithelial component and its relationship to the pituitary. It may be both in the sella and above it, but is more frequent above it. The cystic types above the sella are often referred to as suprasellar cysts. They come into intimate relationship with the chiasma, the floor of the third ventricle (which is displaced upwards), and the hypothalamus (Fig. 5.79). Microscopically keratinizing squamous epithelium is common, and is associated with keratin flakes and cholesterol in the cyst contents (Fig. 5.80), which sometimes have an oily consistency. The connective-tissue stroma is often abundant. In the solid areas loose stroma may separate columns of basal type epithelium simulating the so-called adamantinoma arising in the jaw. There is no evidence, however, that any of the craniopharyngiomas arise from ameloblasts. Because of the intimate relationship of the lateral walls of the tumour to the hypothalamus, successful surgical removal is almost impossible. Surgical treatment is therefore usually confined to aspiration of cyst content and establishment of a by-pass to relieve hydrocephalus.

Epidermoid and dermoid cysts are ascribed to deficiency or abnormality of closure of the primitive

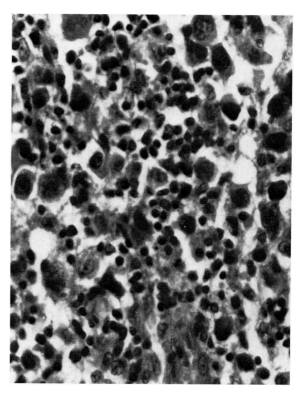

Fig. 5.78. Germinoma of pineal. (H and E; 400 ×)

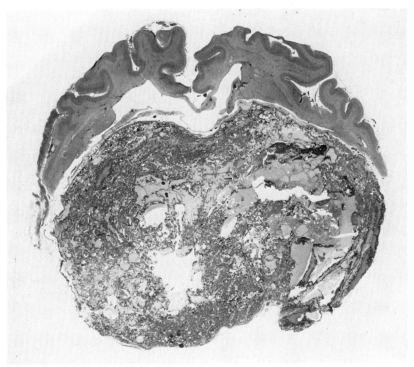

Fig. 5.79. Craniopharyngioma invading up into brain, from a stillborn infant. Courtesy of Prof. E. Wildi.

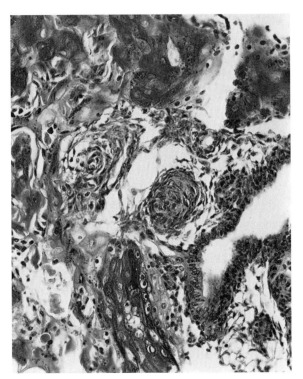

Fig. 5.80. Squamous epithelial islands in craniopharyngioma.

neural groove when they are found in the mid-line, or of secondary cerebral vesicles when they are lateral. They can thus be found within the dura or outside it in the bone or in both situations, and are often associated with a dimple or sinus in the skin. In epidermoid forms the cyst is lined with squamous epithelium and the content is keratin only, whereas in those designated as dermoid cysts there are appendages such as sebaceous and sweat glands attached to the epithelium and a more varied content. Tytus and Pennybacker (1956) group them together as 'pearly tumours'. Clinically they may be significant, because they compress brain or spinal cord or occasionally rupture, giving rise to a chronic meningitis through dispersal of the content, which has an irritative effect. Clinical manifestations of epidermoid forms are more common in adults and those of dermoids in children.

Matson (1969) classified 12 of his 750 intracranial tumours and 14 of 134 spinal tumours as dermoid cysts.

Vascular tumours and hamartomas include cavernous haemangiomas and those telangiectases that are found most commonly in the pons. These are not of significance in children, and Matson had no example of a haemangioblastoma of the cerebellum in his series. Haemangioblastoma of the cerebellum is rare, but is reported in children as part of the Von Hippel–Lindau syndrome (Zulch 1965).

Arteriovenous malformations, of which the cirsoid angioma or aneurysm is one variety, are of importance in children as a cause of subarachnoid or intracerebral haemorrhage; rarely they present as cases of congestive heart failure because of shunting effects. In adults these anomalies are most common in or around the Sylvian fissure within the middle cerebral area, but sites such as the frontal and parieto-occipital lobes and the region of the vein of Galen are more significant in children. In rare cases communication between the vein of Galen and a posterior cerebral artery may form a tortuous mass of vessels or a localized aneurysm, pressure from which on the aqueduct can cause hydrocephalus. Bleeding from small malformations may result in such destruction of tissue that their identification is difficult; they have been called cryptic by Crawford and Russell (1956). The haemorrhage may be fatal but in patients subjected to surgery Matson stresses the necessity of evacuating intracerebral clot and examining the margins of the cavity carefully, so that any tissue suspected or harbouring a vascular malformation is removed. However, the lesions may be very small, as seen in Fig. 5.81, which shows the small surface abnormality that may be the only indication of a lesion. In this example the surface lesions were not noted at post-mortem but became apparent after fixation. Beneath it was a collection of vessels extending to the margin of a haematoma, which had ruptured into the ventricular system at the vestibule.

Meningeal tumours: A malignant tumour infiltrating the meninges diffusely or occasionally forming a localized mass is more common in children than in adults; it may cause hydrocephalus. Histologically this tumour is fibroblastic with mitoses, reticulin formation, occasional areas of necrosis but no features of a preceding meningioma. The term meningeal sarcoma or fibrosarcoma is apt.

Benign meningiomas are so rare in children that they are not described here.

Tumours of the spinal cord are less common in children than adults, and much less common than intracranial tumours in children. Matson had 134 spinal tumours in his series in the same period that 750 intracranial tumour were encountered.

In Matson's series the gliomas were the commonest group, accounting for a quarter, followed by neuroblastomas and extradural lymphomas, while dermoid cysts and teratomas occurred in appreciable numbers, particularly in the younger age group. The maximal incidence as regards site was the thoracic region, with a higher incidence at the upper and lower ends of the spinal canal in the younger age groups, when the tumours of developmental origin are encountered more frequently. A maximal incidence in the thoracic region was reported in the analysis of Haft et al. (1959), whose paper gives a summary of the several large series of these neoplasms in the literature. About a third of the lesions are intramedullary and the remainder extramedullary with either an extra- or an intradural location.

Leukaemia: In fatal cases of acute leukaemia there is infiltration of the meninges or the perivascular tissue within the brain in 30 % of cases (Moore et al. 1960). Thus some neurological disturbance is not uncommon in the terminal illness.

Of greater clinical interest is the fact that some patients may present initially as a result of leukaemic involvement of the nervous system or that such involvement may interrupt a remission of the disease. The two pictures that are especially important are presentation with raised intracranial pressure and with cord involvement. In the former the combination of meningeal and perivascular infiltration and rarely infiltration of the nervous tissue itself may lead to cerebral swelling or meningeal infiltration may cause obstructive hydrocephalus. Haemorrhage into the brain, the subarachnoid, or the subdural space is a further hazard. Infiltration of the spinal meninges and nerve roots is usually the reason for spinal lesions rather than direct infiltration of the cord. Sometimes leukaemic plaques are found in the extrathecal region, although this is more frequently seen in lymphoma.

Lymphoma and microgliomatosis: 'Lymphoma' is used to cover those neoplastic conditions of the

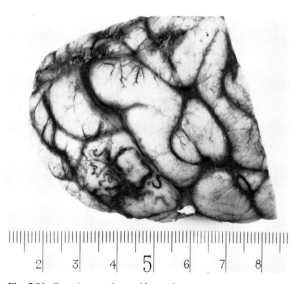

Fig. 5.81. Cryptic vascular malformation.

lymphoid tissue, such as Hodgkin's disease and lymphosarcoma, in which the lesions are situated predominantly in lymph nodes, spleen, and other extracranial sites and in which the nervous system is occasionally involved. Such involvement is rare in children and is likely to be secondary to skull lesions extending into the dura if the brain is affected or to extrathecal plaques in the event of spinal involvement. The only condition of this nature that is restricted to childhood is the involvement of the brain in Letterer–Siwe disease (histiocytosis X). Rube et al. (1967) described three cases in which scattered foci of proliferating histiocytic cells were found in the meninges and perivascular areas, but only in one was there clinical evidence of brain involvement.

Microgliomatosis is a term logically reserved for neoplastic proliferation of similar nature to that in lymphomas but arising within the CNS and composed of cells, some of which have histological similarities to the microglia cells. (The origin of these cells is discussed on p. 151). Characteristic features of the tumour cells according to Russell et al. (1948) were the lobed, twisted nuclei in some cells and spheroidal nuclei in others, and the cytoplasmic impregnation of a particular population of cells by the Weil-Davenport method. Initially such tumours were reported in adults but in recent years they have been reported in immune-deficiency syndromes and as a complication of successful organ transplantation. Brand and Marinkovich (1969) reported a

case in the Wiskott–Aldrich syndrome and used the term 'primary malignant reticulosis of the brain' rather than microgliomatosis, possibly because the cells did not impregnate with microglial methods. They emphasized the possibility of origin from perivascular reticulum cells. In a personally observed case of the Wiskott–Aldrich syndrome in which death occurred with subdural haemorrhage and meningitis there were foci of tumour proliferation in the mid-brain and adjacent to the posterior end of the third ventricle. The cellular picture was pleomorphic, with may pale reticulum cells (Fig. 5.82), others that impregnated as microglia (Fig. 5.83), and a few binucleate forms similar to but not typical for Reed–Sternberg cells.

Schneck and Penn (1971) reported that of 24 mesenchymal neoplasms that had occurred following renal transplantation, 11 involved the brain and eight were restricted to that organ. Nine of the 11 were categorized as reticulum-cell sarcomas and two as microgliomas. They discuss the reasons for cerebral localization of the neoplastic process.

Tumours of the peripheral nervous system: Neuroblastoma, ganglioneuroblastoma, and ganglioneuroma are described on p. 197. Neurilemmoma or schwannoma is the name given to the firm, grey, circumscribed neoplasm composed of neural sheath cells in which palisading is characteristic (Fig. 5.84). This is sometimes referred to as Antoni type A tissue,

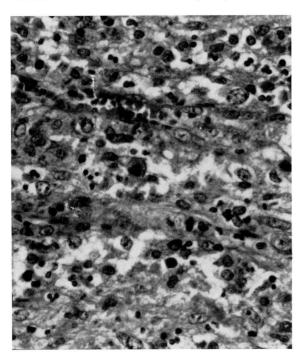

Fig. 5.82. Area of microgliomatosis in Wiskett–Aldrich syndrome. Some of the cells with pale nuclei and prominent nuclei impregnate as microglia. (H and E; 400 ×)

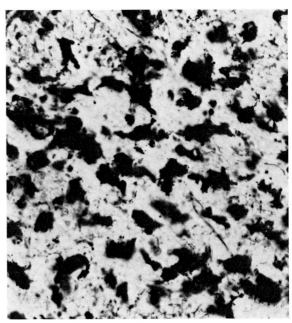

Fig. 5.83. Weil–Davenport impregnation of tumour shown in Fig. 5.80. (400 ×)

and may be intermingled with looser, less cellular myxomatous areas, namely Antoni type B tissue. The latter is probably the origin of the cystic areas sometimes present on section of the mass. In children they may occur intrathecally in the spinal canal or occasionally in relation to a peripheral nerve. Another favoured site is the posterior mediastinum, in which the tumour may be related to the intercostal nerve or be a dumbbell extension through the intervertebral foramen from a spinal root neoplasm. The tumours that arise from spinal roots are benign, and malignancy is a rare feature of those on peripheral nerves. Both may be solitary or multiple and a feature of von Recklinghausen's disease (neurofibromatosis), in which neurofibromas are more characteristic; in these there is an intimate mixture of nerve fibrils, neural sheath cells, and collagen. Malignant change in such neurofibromas is also exceptional in children.

11. Hydrocephalus

Hydrocephalus is a dilatation of the whole or part of the ventricular system within the brain resulting from an oversection of, obstruction to the flow of, or impaired absorption of the cerebrospinal fluid (CSF). The dilatation of the ventricular system that can occur following atrophy or destruction of cerebral tissue will not be considered here.

The importance of hydrocephalus has been emphasized by the development of effective shunt therapy, and in particular the use of the Spitz–Holter valve. This has led to survival of many who would otherwise have died soon after birth. In the population of Great Britain it was estimated that about 1000 shunt operations were performed annually during the immediate post-valve decade. Most of these were on infants with congenital hydrocephalus or hydrocephalus manifest during the first few weeks of life. Our knowledge of the pathology of some of the latter types is still incomplete despite the contribution of Russell (1949), who summarized her extensive observations with the thesis that hydrocephalus is caused by some form of obstruction to the flow of CSF, with the rare exception of overproduction of fluid by choroid plexus neoplasms (p. 195). Obstruction is by far the more important, and can occur at any point within the ventricular pathway of CSF flow, at the exits to the fourth ventricle, in the meninges at the base of the brain, in particular at the cisterna ambiens, and through occlusion of the venous sinuses. The term communicating hydrocephalus indicates that the obstruction is outside the ventricular system so that there is communication between intra- and extra-cerebral spinal fluid.

The obstruction may be due to malformations, inflammations or neoplasms. Malformations include stenosis and forking of the aqueduct, the Arnold–Chiari malformation, and the Dandy–Walker syndrome (see p. 158).

11.1. Caused by Malformations

Russell described aqueduct stenosis in which the transverse area of the passage was reduced but the histology was normal. She separated it from forking, in which the aqueduct was formed of two or more distinct and compressed channels. Two constrictions are normally found in the aqueduct, one beneath the middle of the superior quadrigemina and another at the commencement of the inferior. Woollam and Millen (1953) have provided figures for normal variations in size of the aqueduct showing that these can be wide, from 0.2 mm^2 to 1.8 mm^2 in the dilatation between the constrictions. Alvord (1961) emphasized that other factors than area, e.g., length, course, viscosity of fluid, and pressure differences are important in determining whether hydrocephalus is likely to follow a narrowing of the passage. His experiments suggest that in normal individuals an

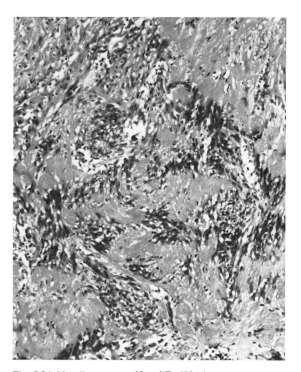

Fig. 5.84. Neurilemmoma. (H and E; 400 ×)

increase in the load of fluid presented to the aqueduct is not likely to be followed by hydrocephalus, whereas in stenosis the rise in intraventricular pressure may be precipitous if the amount of fluid presented to the aqueduct increases. This may explain why symptoms, and possibly hydrocephalus, sometimes only present in adult life. Possibly a temporary oversecretion of fluid may precipitate them. Although aqueduct stenosis is rare, a hereditary variety described by Bickers and Adams (1949) and Edwards et al. (1961) has been recognized more frequently in recent years, and is sometimes diagnosed before birth with the help of ultrasound. When the aqueduct is represented by two channels, lined with normal ependyma, and separated by normal neural tissue through part of its course, the term forking is appropriate. The ventral channel is often a compressed slit, the dorsal one branched with small groups of adjacent ependymal cells. One of these channels unites the third and fourth ventricles, while the other dwindles or disappears or unites with the main passage. Whether hydrocephalus develops or not depends upon the size of the patent channel.

The Chiari type II (Figs. 5.85 and 5.20) is the important subtype of the Arnold-Chiari malformation in the newborn. In this a myelomeningocele is present, together with an elongation of the medulla and downward protrusion of the cerebellar vermis through the foramen magnum. The medulla may show a dorsal kink or S-shaped bend at the

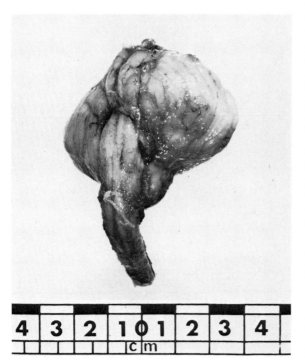

Fig. 5.85. Elongated medulla covered posteriorly by cerebellar tonsils in Arnold–Chiari malformation. (See also Fig. 5.20.)

junction with the cervical spinal cord so that a portion of it lies dorsal to the cord. In this segment the cervical nerves run rostrally from cord to exits; in the thoracic region they have a normal direction but in the lumbar segment a rostral path is sometimes seen. The cerebellum is usually smaller than normal although it may extend on to the ventral surface of the pons to obscure the basilar artery (Daniel and Strich 1958). The tentorium is attached close to the foramen magnum and the posterior fossa is small. Cameron (1957) described and indicated the incidence of other features in what could be called the Arnold–Chiari constellation, e.g., clefts in the cerebellum that communicate with the fourth ventricle, some degree of hydromyelia, microgyria of the cerebral cortex, the occasional presence of ectopic nodules of grey matter in the ependyma of the lateral ventricles, thickening of the interthalamic vermis, hypoplasia of the falx, and partial obliteration of the great longitudinal cerebral fissure. His analysis of the changes in the aqueduct are more detailed than many reported. It was abnormally narrow in 13 of 26 cases, which was attributable to postinflammatory gliosis in eight, to simple stenosis in one, and to forking without gliosis in two.

The degree of hydrocephalus varies considerably. Russell and Donald (1935) attributed it to downward displacement of the exits of the fourth ventricle below the foramen of Magnum so that CSF was unable to circulate about the block at this level caused by the displaced cerebellum and medulla, which being matted together by fibrous adhesions fill the hole. This concept is supported by the results of injecting coloured particulate matter into the lateral ventricles, which reaches the myelomeningocele but not the surface of the cerebellum or cerebrum, and by the fact that an ascending infection from the lumbar region is more likely to be complicated by a purulent ependymitis than by a basal meningitis. The narrowing of the aqueduct may also play a part in causing or increasing the hydrocephalus. There is no satisfactory explanation at present for all the possible lesions and the associated skeletal malformations. They are not easily explained in detail by a determining influence of brain size and shape on skull.

The Chiari I malformation is a deformity of the cerebellum in which an ectopia protrudes into the foramen magnum and may be associated with a bony abnormality such as platybasia.

11.2. Postinflammatory

Hydrocephalus resulting from inflammation is attributable to obstruction of the circulation of CSF at any stage in the process. Thus there may be a purulent exudate occluding the lumen of the aqueduct or a fibrosis of the leptomeninges in a strategic site such as the cisterna ambiens, which allows free circulation of the CSF in and out of the ventricular system but interferes with circulation in the subarachnoid space. In addition to infection, an important cause of inflammatory obstructive tissue is haemorrhage, evidence of which is often found histologically.

Gliosis of the aqueduct is often considered to be postinflammatory. It is distinguished from stenosis of the aqueduct by the fact that the residual pathway is surrounded by gliosis instead of normal neural tissue. Remnants of the original ependymal lining persist near the edge of the gliosis (Fig. 5.86). The histological picture suggests that some agent has damaged the ependymal and subependymal tissue in the aqueduct and that the reaction has led to considerable narrowing. It is rare, although more common than stenosis or forking. In her series Russell reported eight cases, seven of which were in infants or children. The onset is usually insidious, without clinical evidence of infection and without inflammatory cells in the region of the gliotic aqueduct or in the patches of subependymal gliosis that are sometimes present elsewhere in the ventricular system. Such subependymal gliosis can complicate the late stages of bacterial meningitis, as noted by Russell and others. Dennis and Alvord (1961) reported hydrocephalus resulting from aqueduct gliosis in a case of congenital toxoplasmosis,

and it may be a consequence of intraventricular haemorrhage in late fetal life. Such a lesion was described by Smith (1974) as a cause of the hydrocephalus present in neonatal thrombocytopenic purpura (Fig. 6.87); consideration of the clinical and pathological features revealed that some of the bleeding and the reaction to it in the aqueduct had occurred before birth. The possibility that such gliosis can result from viral infection is supported by the experimental production of lesions with myxoviruses, paramyxoviruses and reovirus type 1 (Johnson and Johnson 1969) as well as the record of a human nonfatal case developing some months after mumps (Timmons and Johnson, 1970).

Mechanical obstruction of the aqueduct lumen by old red cells and nuclear debris was reported by Larroche (1964) as a cause of hydrocephalus following intraventricular haemorrhage in the premature neonate. This usually arises from rupture of a subependymal plate haematoma (p. 170). However, in most cases of hydrocephalus complicating haemorrhage, whether intraventricular (Fig. 5.88) or primary subarachnoid, the cause is fibrosis in the meninges in which the haemorrhage has arisen or to which it has passed from the ventricles with the cerebrospinal fluid (Fig. 5.89). If the fibrosis leads to occlusion of the exits from the fourth ventricle the hydrocephalus is non-communicating; if it obstructs the cerebrospinal fluid through adhesions in the basal meninges it is communicating. Other rare causes of such communicating hydrocephalus fol-

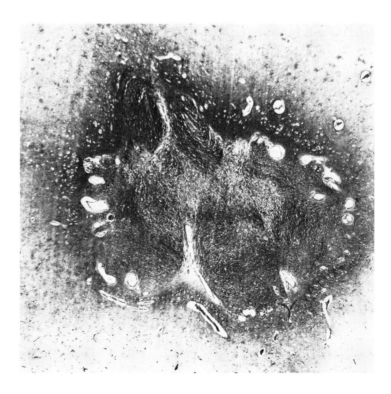

Fig. 5.86. Gliosis of the aqueduct. (Holzer; 40×)

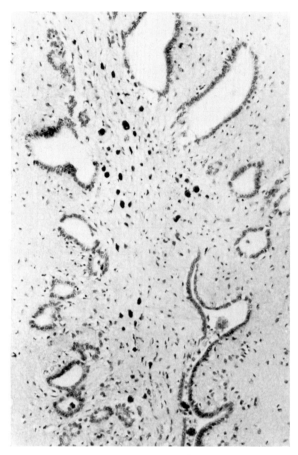

Fig. 5.87. Gliosis of the aqueduct following intraventricular bleeding in fetal life in a case of congenital thrombocytopenic purpura. (PAS; 100×)

lowing haemorrhage are subdural haemorrhage from tentorial tears in birth trauma and delayed haemorrhage into the cisterns of the transverse cerebral fissure in infants (Lourie and Berne 1965).

Hydrocephalus during a prolonged acute bacterial meningitis or as a consequence of healing or of granulomatous meningitis has already been mentioned. In the late stages of an acute bacterial meningitis exudate may block the exits from the fourth ventricle or the aqueduct or the subarachnoid space. Organization of such exudate may lead to permanent obstruction. This picture was not infrequent in the pre-antibiotic area but it is now less common and is mainly seen as a sequel to neonatal meningitis or tuberculous meningitis. The latter is particularly likely to cause obstruction in the subarachnoid space at the cisterna ambiens if vigorous therapy is not undertaken early in the disease.

Hydrocephalus with marked dilatation of the whole of the ventricular system and patchy fibrosis of the leptomeninges at such strategic sites as the foramina of Luschka or the cisterna ambiens made up an important group in Russell's series, accounting for 23 of her cases, 11 of whom were under 6 years of age. Although it was possible to demonstrate clear evidence of an infective cause in only a few, the fact that the pathological changes showed a sequence in the inflammatory process from cellular reactions to collagenous scars led to the classification of all of them as postmeningitic hydrocephalus. Her emphasis of the importance of meningitis in early life as a cause has been confirmed by more recent investigations, some of which have been discussed earlier. The condition is now infrequent in necropsies at general hospitals; it may

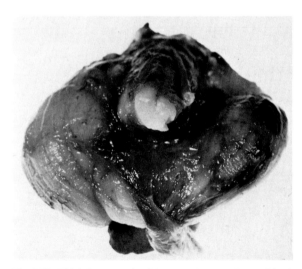

Fig. 5.88. Hydrocephalus in a 28-day premature baby due to bleeding from subependymal plate haemorrhage, residua of which are on the left of the lateral ventricle.

Fig. 5.89. Thick brown-stained leptomeninges at base of brain obstructing CSF circulation in a case of subependymal plate haemorrhage.

account for a number of those cases of communicating hydrocephalus in which the best results of shunt therapy are obtained. Thus Guthkelch and Riley (1969), in reviewing 166 cases of hydrocephalus with ventriculo-atrial drainage, reported that the best prognosis was achieved with 'the noninfective communicating' type. It is difficult to be sure that all such cases are noninfective. Some are probably the sequel of infection as discussed above, some the sequel of haemorrhage, while perhaps the majority are examples of congenital communicating hydrocephalus.

Russell also described hydrocephalus as a feature of gargoylism, the meninges showing fibrous thickening and mild inflammation consequent to lipid accumulation in the arachnoid cells.

The occurrence of hydrocephalus because of interference with reabsorption is now rare, as venous sinus thrombosis has almost disappeared.

Hydrocephalus in children caused by neoplasms is usually due to a block of the intraventricular flow of CSF as when an astrocytoma of the third ventricle obstructs the foramina of Monro (Fig. 5.70), a glioma of the brain stem obstructs the fourth ventricle or the aqueduct, or a medulloblastoma of the cerebellum obstructs the fourth ventricle or its exits—these examples are illustrative rather than complete. Compression of the ventricular system from without is seen when craniopharyngiomas deform the third ventricle or pineal tumours compress or deform the aqueduct. Infiltration of the leptomeninges by a metastasizing medulloblastoma is likely to be from a tumour already obstructing the fourth ventricle or its exits. This makes the assessment of such infiltration as a contributory element to interference with CSF circulation difficult. However, that meningeal growth can interfere with the third circulation in much the same way as chronic meningitis is exemplified by the rare diffuse sarcomas of the meninges seen in children. Russell suggested that many astrocytomas of the brain stem and other tumours in the posterior fossa produce hydrocephalus by extension, obstructing the basal cisterns and tentorial opening. De Lange and Vlieger (1970) have reported a case in a 16-year-old girl in whom removal of an extracranial arteriovenous malformation with transverse sinus connections was followed by diminution of a communicating hydrocephalus. Observations at operation showed a diminution of the pressure in the jugular foramen with the removal of the tumour.

11.3. Complications

Severe hydrocephalus may be complicated by hypothalamic disturbances but there are no detailed structural studies available to indicate changes. The use of shunts has decreased the incidence of mechanical effects such as enlargement of the head, erosion of bones of the skull, and spontaneous ventriculostomy, but has led to other problems. These include infection, thrombotic and embolic episodes, sudden acute blockage, endocarditis, cardiac tamponade from perforation of the heart, craniostenosis and shunt nephritis. Forrest and Cooper (1968) reported a 17% mortality (78 of 455 cases), sepsis and valve blockage being the two main causes of death.

However, shunts may not only arrest the progression of hydrocephalus, but lead to improvement of cerebral function. This suggests that the tissue damage caused by increased ventricular pressure is to some extent reversible. Possible mechanisms for this are discussed by Zwetnow (1970) and Granholm and Siesjo (1970).

References

Abrahamowicz A (1964) The pathogenesis of experimental periventricular cerebral necrosis and its possible relationship to the periventricular leucomalacia of birth trauma. J Neurol Neurosurg Psychiatry 27: 85

Ackerman BD, Dyer GY, Leydorff MM (1970) Hyperbilirubinemia and kernicterus in small premature infants. Pediatrics 45: 918

Adams JH (1976) In: Greenfield's Neuropathology, 3rd edn. Arnold, London, p 300

Adams RD, Kubik CS, Bunner FJ (1948) The clinical and pathological aspected of influenzal meningitis. Arch Paediatr 65: 354 and 408

Aguilar MJ, Rasmussen T (1960) Role of encephalitis in pathogenesis of epilepsy. Arch Neurol 2: 663

Aleu FP, Katzman R, Terry RD (1963) Fine structure and electrolyte analysis of cerebral edema induced by alkyl tin intoxication. J Neuropathol Exp Neurol 22: 403

Alexander GL, Norman RM (1960) The Sturge–Weber syndrome. Wright, Bristol

Alpers BJ (1931) Diffuse progressive degeneration of the grey matter of the cerebrum. Arch Neurol Psychiat 25: 469

Alvord EC (1961) The pathology of hydrocephalus. In: Fields WS, Desmond MM (eds) Disorders of the developing nervous system. Thomas, Springfield, p 343

Anderson JM, Milner RDG, Strich SJ (1967) Effects of neonatal hypoglycaemia on the nervous system: a pathological study. J Neurol Neurosurg Psychiatry 30: 295

Aronson GM, Volk BW, Epstein N (1955) Morphologic evolution of amaurotic family idiocy. Am J Pathol 31: 609

Banker BQ (1961) Cerebral vascular disease in infancy and childhood. J Neuropathol Exp Neurol 20: 127

Banker BQ (1967) Neuropathological effects of anoxia and hypoglycemia in newborn. Dev Med Child Neurol 9: 544

Banker BQ, Larroche J-C (1962) Periventricular leukomalacia of infancy. Arch Neurol 7: 386

Berman PH, Banker BQ (1966) Neonatal meningitis. A clinical and pathological study of 29 cases. Pediatrics 38: 6

Bertrand J, Bargeton E (1955) In: Proceedings of the Second International Congress of Neuropathology, London, Part II. Excerpta Medica, Amsterdam, p 519

Bertrong M, Sabiston DC (1951) Cerebral lesions in congenital heart disease. A review of autopsies on 162 cases. Bull Johns Hopkins Hosp 89: 384

Bickers DS, Adams RD (1949) Hereditary stenosis of the aqueduct of Sylvius as a cause of congenital hydrocephalus. Brain 72: 246

Billing BH, Lathe GH (1956) The excretion of bilirubin as an ester glucuronide, giving the direct van den Berg reaction. Biochem J 63: 6

Borberg A (1951) Clinical and genetic investigations into tuberous sclerosis and Recklinghausen's neurofibromatosis. Acta Psychiatr Neurol [Suppl] 71: 3

Bourneville DM (1880) Contribution à l'étude de l'idiotie. Arch Neurol (Paris) 1: 69

Bouteille M, Fontaine C, Vedvenne C, Delarue J (1965) Sur un cas d'encéphalite subaiguë à inclusions. Etude anatomo-clinique et ultrastructurale. Rev Neurol 113: 454

Brand MM, Marinkovich VA (1969) Primary malignant reticulosis of the brain in Wiskett–Aldrich syndrome. Arch Dis Child 44: 536

Brierley JB (1971) The neuropathological sequelae of profound hypoxia. In: Brierley JB, Meldrum BS (eds) Brain hypoxia. Heinemann Medical, London, p 147 (Spastics International Medical Publications. Clinics in Developmental Medicine 39/40)

Brown AW (1977) Structural abnormalities in neurones. J Clin Pathol [Suppl 30] 11: 155

Brust JCM, Mosel RH, Rosenberg RN (1968) Glia tumor metastases through a ventriculopleural shunt. Arch Neurol 18: 649

Buchan GC, Alvord EC (1969) Diffuse necrosis of subcortical white matter associated with bacterial meningitis. Neurology 19: 1

Burnet FM (1970) Immunological surveillance. Pergamon, Oxford, p 43

Butler NR, Bonham DG (1963) Perinatal mortality. The first report of the British Perinatal Mortality Survey. Livingstone, Edinburgh, p 203

Cameron AH (1956) The spinal cord lesions in spina bifida cystica. Lancet 2: 171

Cameron AH (1957) The Arnold–Chiari and other neuro-anatomical malformations associated with spina bifida. J Pathol Bacteriol 73: 195

Carmichael EA (1966) The current status of hemispherectomy for infantile hemiplegia. Clinical Proceedings of the Children's Hospital, Washington 22: 285

Cavanagh JB (1970) Reactions of neuroglia cells to injury. In: Williams D (ed) Modern trends in neurology. Butterworths, London, Chap 8

Chen HC, Lien IM, Lu TC (1965) Kernicterus in newborn rabbits. Am J Pathol 46: 331

Chen HC, Lin CS, Lein IN (1966) Ultrastructural studies in experimental kernicterus. Am J Pathol 48: 683

Corsellis JAN, Meldrum BS (1976) Epilepsy. In: Greenfield's Neuropathology, 3rd edn. Arnold, London, Chap 8

Courville CB (1953) Cerebral anoxia. San Lucan, Los Angeles

Crawford JV, Russell DS (1956) Cryptic arteriovenous and venous hamartomas of brain. J Neurol Neurosurg Psychiatry 19: 1

Crome L (1955) Morphological nervous changes in survivors of severe jaundice of the newborn. J Neurol Neurosurg Psychiatry 18: 17

Crome L (1962) A case of galactosaemia with the pathological and neuropathological findings. Arch Dis Child 37: 415

Daniel PM, Strich SJ (1958) Some observations on the congenital deformity of the central nervous system known as the Arnold–Chiari malformation. J Neuropathol Exp Neurol 17: 255

Deck JHN (1969) Cerebral medulloepithelioma with maturation into ependymal cells and ganglion cells. J Neuropathol Exp Neurol 28: 442

Degen R, Elbel U (1966) Die angeborene Toxoplasmose und ihre Prognose. Monatsschr Kinderheilkd 114: 110

de Lange SA, de Vlieger M (1970) Hydrocephalus associated with raised venous pressures. Dev Med Child Neurol 12: [Suppl 22] 28

Dennis JP, Alvord EC (1961) Microcephaly with intracerebral calcification and subependymal ossification, radiologic and clinicopathologic correlation. J Neuropathol Exp Neurol 20: 412

Desmonts G Couvreur J (1974) Toxoplasmosis in pregnancy and its transmission to the foetus. Bull NY Acad Med 50: 140

Dickerson WW (1955) Nature of certain osseous lesions in tuberous sclerosis. Arch Neurol Psychiatry 73: 525

Druckrey H, Ivankovic S, Preussmann R (1966) Teratogenic and carcinogenic effects in the offspring after single injection of ethylnitrosourea to pregnant rats. Nature 210: 1378

Earle KM, Baldwin M, Penfield W (1953) Incisural sclerosis and temporal lobe seizures produced by hippocampal herniation at birth. Arch Neurol 69: 27

Earnest F, Kenohan JW, Craig WMcK (1950) Oligodendrogliomas (Review of 200 cases). Arch Neurol 63: 964

Edwards JH, Norman RM, Roberts JM (1961) Sex-linked hydrocephalus. Arch Dis Child 36: 481

Emery JL, Kalhan SC (1970) The pathology of exencephalus. Dev Med Child Neurol [Suppl] 22: 51

Falconer MA, McFarlan AM, Russell DS (1943) Experimental brain abscess in the rabbit. Br J Surg 30: 245

Fitzgerald GM, Greenfield JG, Kounine B (1939) Neurological sequelae of kernicterus. Brain 62: 292

Forrest DM, Cooper DGW (1968) Complications of ventriculoatrial shunts. A review of 455 cases. J Neurosurg 29: 506

Fossard (1968) Cerebral tumors in infancy. Am J Dis Child 115: 302

Gardner WA, Konigsmark BW (1969) Familial nonhemolytic jaundice: Bilirubinosis and encephalopathy. Pediatrics 43: 365

Gartner LM, Synder RN, Chabon RS, Bernstein J (1970) Kernicterus: High incidence in premature infants with low serum bilirubin concentrations. Pediatrics 45: 906

Gastaut H, Poirer F, Payan H, et al. (1960) H.H.E. syndrome: Hemiconvulsions, hemiplegia, epilepsy. Epilepsia 1: 418

Gastaut H, Toga M, Roger J, Gibson WC (1959) A correlation of clinical, electroencephalographic and anatomical findings in nine autopsied cases of 'temporal lobe epilepsy'. Epilepsia 1: 56

Granholm L, Siesjö BK (1960) Signs of tissue hypoxia in infantile hydrocephalus. Dev Med Child Neurol 12: [Suppl 22] 73

Gunther M, Penrose LS (1935) Genetics of epiloia. J Genetics 31: 413

Guthkelch AN, Riley NA (1969) Influence of aetiology on prognosis in surgically treated infantile hydrocephalus. Arch Dis Child 44: 29

Haft H, Ransohoff J, Carter S (1959) Spinal cord tumors in children. Pediatrics 23: 1152

Hambleton G, Wigglesworth JS (1976) Origin of intraventricular haemorrhage in the preterm infant. Arch Dis Child 51: 651

Harrison VC, Heese H de V, Klein M (1968) Intracranial haemorrhage associated with hyaline membrane disease. Arch Dis Child 43: 116

Hart MN, Malamud N, Ellis WG (1972) The Dandy–Walker syndrome: A clinicopathological study based on 28 cases. Neurology 22: 771

Horta Barbosa L, Fuccillo DA, Sever JL (1969) Subacute sclerosing panencephalitis: Isolation of measles virus from a brain biopsy. Nature 221: 974

Ingraham TD, Matson DD (1944) Subdural hematoma in infancy. J Pediatr 24: 1

Johnson RT, Johnson KP (1969) Hydrocephalus as a sequela of experimental myxovirus infections. Exp Mol Pathol 10: 68

Kahn EA, Luros JT (1952) Hydrocephalus from overproduction of cerebrospinal fluid. J Neurosurg 9: 59

Keiller VH (1922) A contribution to the anatomy of spina bifida. Brain 45: 31

Larroche J-C (1964) Les hémorrhagies cérébrales intraventriculaires chez le prémature. Biol Neonate 7: 26

Larroche J-C (1972) Post haemorrhagic hydrocephalus in infancy. Anatomical study. Biol Neonate 20: 287

Larroche JC (1977) Developmental pathology of the neonate. Excerpta Medica, Amsterdam, p 325

Leigh D (1951) Subacute necrotizing encephalomyelopathy in an infant. J Neurol Neurosurg Psychiatry 14: 216

Lindenberg R (1955) Compression of brain arteries as pathogenetic factor for tissue necroses and their areas of predilection. J Neuropathol Exp Neurol 14: 223

Lindenberg R (1963) Patterns of CNS vulnerability in acute hypoxaemia, including anaesthesia accidents. In: Schade JP, McMenemy WH (eds) Selective vulnerability of the brain in hypoxaemia. Blackwell, Oxford, p 189

Lindenberg R, Swanson PD (1969) Infantile hydrancephaly—a report of five cases of infarction of both cerebral hemispheres in infancy. Brain 90: 839

Little WJ (1861) The influence of abnormal presentation, difficult labors, premature birth, asphyxia neonatorum on the mental and general condition of the child, especially in relation to deformity. Transactions of the Obstetric Society of London 3: 344

Louis-Bar D (1941) Sur un syndrome progressif comprenant des telangiectasies capillaires cutanées et conjonctivale symetriques: à disposition naevoïde et des troubles cérébelleux. Confin Neurol 4: 32

Lourie H, Berne AS (1965) A contribution on the aetiology and pathogenesis of congenital communicating hydrocephalus. The syndrome of delayed haemorrhage into the cisterns of the transverse cerebral fissure of infants. Neurology 15: 815

Lucey JF, Hibbard E, Behrman RE, Esquire de Gallardo FO, Windle WF (1964) Kernicterus in asphyxiated newborn rhesus monkeys. Exp Neurol 9: 43

Lyon G, Dodge PR, Adams RD (1961) The acute encephalopathies of obscure origin in infants and children. Brain 84: 680

Marin-Padilla M (1965) Study of the skull in human cranioschisis. Acta Anat (Basel) 62: 1

Marin-Padilla M (1972) Structural abnormalities of the cerebral cortex in human chromosomal aberration: a Golgi study. Brain Res 44: 625

Marin-Padilla M (1978) Congenital malformations of the spine and spinal cord. In: Vinker PJ, Bruyn GW (eds) Handbook of clinical neurology, vol 32. North-Holland, Amsterdam

Matson DD (1953) Hydrocephalus in a premature infant caused by a papilloma of the choroid plexus, with a report of the surgical treatment. J Neurosurg 10: 416

Matson DD (1969) Neurosurgery of infancy and childhood. Thomas, Springfield, p 403

Meyer JE (1949) Zur Ätiologie und Pathogenese des fetalen und frühkindlichen Cerebralschadens. Z Kinderheilkd 67: 123

Moore EW, Thomas LB, Shaw RK, Freireich EJ (1960) The central nervous system in acute leukaemia. Arch Intern Med 105: 451

Myers RE (1972) Two patterns of perinatal brain damage and their conditions of occurrence. Am J Obstet Gynecol 112: 246

Nellhaus G, Haberland C, Hill BJ (1967) Sturge–Weber disease with bilateral intracranial calcifications at birth and unusual pathologic findings. Acta Neurol Scand 43: 314

Norman RM (1963) In: Greenfield's Neuropathology, 2nd edn. Arnold, London, p 405

Norman RM (1964) The neuropathology of status epilepticus. Med Sci Law 4: 46

Norman RM, Urich H (1957) Dissecting aneurysm of the middle cerebral artery as a cause of acute infantile hemiplegia. J Pathol Bacteriol 73: 580

Oppenheimer J, Sullivan MP, Drewinko B, et al. (1973) Disseminated histoplasmosis complicating acute leukaemia of childhood. Clin Pediatr (Phila) 12: 306

Orth J (1875) Ueber das Vorkommen von Bilirubin-Krystallen bei neugeborenen Kindern. Virchows Arch [Pathol Anat] 63: 447

Padget D (1970) Neuroschisis and human embryonic development. J Neuropathol Exp Neurol 29: 192

Paulson GW, Lyle CB (1966) Tuberous sclerosis. Dev Med Child Neurol 8: 571

Pearson, HA, Shulman NR, Marder VJ, et al. (1964) Immune neonatal thrombocytopenic purpura. Blood 23: 154

Penrose LS (1963) The biology of mental defect. Sidgwick & Jackson, London, pp 172

Rabe EF, Flynn RE, Dodge PR (1962) A study of subdural effusions in an infant. Neurology 12: 79

Rakic P (1972) Mode of cell migration to the superficial layers of foetal monkey isocortex. J Comp Neurol 145: 61

Rakic P, Sidman RL (1968) Supravital DNA synthesis in the developing human and mouse brain. J Neuropathol Exp Neurol 27: 246

Ranck JB, Windle WF (1959) Brain damage in the monkey, *Macaca mulatta*, by asphyxia neonatorum. Exp Neurol 1: 130

Reye RDK, Morgan G, Baral J (1963) Encephalopathy and fatty degeneration of the viscera. Lancet 2: 749

Rich AR, McCordock HA (1933) The pathogenesis of tuberculous meningitis. Bull Johns Hopkins Hosp 52: 5

Richman DP, Stewart RH, Caviness VS Jr (1973) Microgyria, lissencephaly and neuron migration to the cerebral cortex, an architectonic approach. Neurology 23: 413

Richman DP, Stewart RH, Caviness VS Jr (1974) Cerebral microgyria in a 27 week foetus: an architectonic and topographic analysis. J Neuropathol Exp Neurol 33: 374

Robertson DM, Hendry WS, Vogel FS (1964) Central ganglioneuroma. A case study using electron microscopy. J Neuropathol Exp Neurol 23: 692

Rozdilsky B, Olszewski J (1961) Experimental study of the toxicity of bilirubin in newborn animals. J Neuropathol Exp Neurol 20: 193

Rubé J, de la Pava S, Pickren JW (1967) Histiocytosis X with involvement of the brain. Cancer 20: 486

Rubinstein LJ (1967) Development of extracranial metastases from a malignant astrocytoma in the absence of previous craniotomy. J Neurosurg 26: 542

Rubinstein LJ (1970) The definition of the ependymoblastoma. Arch Pathol 90: 35

Rubinstein LJ (1972) Tumors of the central nervous system. AFIP, Washington (Atlas of tumor pathology, 2nd series)

Russell DS (1949) Observations on the pathology of hydrocephalus. HMSO, London

Russell DS, Donald C (1935) The mechanism of internal hydrocephalus in spina bifida. Brain 58: 203

Russell DS, Rubinstein LJ (1977) Pathology of tumors of the nervous system, 4th edn. Arnold, London, p 6

Russell DS, Marshall AHE, Smith FB (1948) Microgliomatosis. Brain 71: 1

Schmorl G (1904) Zur Kenntnis des Ikterus neonatorum. Verh Dtsch Ges Pathol 6: 109

Schneck SA, Penn I (1971) De-novo brain tumours in renal-transplant recipients. Lancet 1: 983

Schwarz P (1961) Birth injuries of the newborn: morphology, pathogenesis, clinical pathology and prevention. Hafner, New York

Shapiro JL, Lux JJ, Sprofkin BE (1955) Histoplasmosis of the central nervous system. Am J Pathol 31: 319

Sherwood A, Hopp A, Smith JF (1978) Cellular reactions to subependymal plate haemorrhage in the human neonate.

Neuropathol Appl Neurobiol 4: 245

Shuster J (1966) Ataxia telangiectasia with cerebellar tumor. Pediatrics 37: 976

Silverman WA, Anderson H, Blanc WA, Crozier DN (1956) A difference in mortality rate and incidence of kernicterus among premature infants allotted to two prophylactic antibacterial regimens. Pediatrics 18: 614

Smith HV, Norman RM, Urich H (1957) The late sequelae of pneumococcal meningitis. J Neurol Neurosurg Psychiatry 20: 250

Smith JF (1955) Hydrocephalus associated with choroid plexus papillomas. J Neuropathol Exp Neurol 14: 442

Smith JF (1974) In: Pediatric Neuropathology. McGraw-Hill, New York, p 241

Smith JF, Landing BH (1960) Mechanisms of brain damage in *H. influenzae* meningitis. J Neuropathol Exp Neurol 19: 248

Smith JF, Rodeck C (1976) Multiple cystic and focal encephalomalacia in infancy and childhood with brain stem damage. J Neurol Sci 25: 377

Smith JF, McLaurin RL, Nichols JB, Asbury A (1960) Studies in cerebral oedema and cerebral swelling. The changes in lead encephalopathy in children compared with those in alkyl tin poisoning in animals. Brain 83: 411

Smith JF, Reynolds EOR, Taghizadeh A (1974) Brain maturation and damage in infants dying from chronic pulmonary insufficiency in the postnatal period. Arch Dis Child 49: 359

Strich S (1966) Pathological findings in three cases of ataxia-telangiectasia. J Neurol Neurosurg Psychiatry 29: 489

Tanaka T (1934) So-called breast milk intoxication. Am J Dis Child 47: 1286

Thieffry S, Arthuis M, Faure C, Lyon G (1961) Sturge–Weber angiomatosis. Bibl Paediatr 76: 315

Timmons GD, Johnson KP (1970) Aqueductal stenosis and hydrocephalus after mumps encephalitis. N Engl J Med 283: 1505

Treip CS (1957) A congenital medulloepithelioma of the midbrain. J Pathol Bacteriol 74: 357

Ts'o MOM, Fine BS, Zimmerman LE (1969) The Flexner–Wintersteiner rosettes in retinoblastoma. Arch Pathol 88: 664

Turnbull HM, McIntosh J (1926) Encephalomyelitis following vaccination. Br J Exp. Pathol 7: 181

Tytus JS, Pennybacker J (1956) Pearly tumors in relation to the central nervous system. J Neurol Neurosurg Psychiatry 19: 241

Wernicke C (1881–1883) Lehrbuch der Gehirnkrankheiten, Bd. 2. Fischer, Kassel Berlin

Wilson PJE (1970) Cerebral hemispherectomy for infantile hemiplegia. Brain 93: 147

Wolf A, Cowen D (1956) The cerebral atrophies and encephalomalacias of infancy and childhood. Proc Assoc Nerv Ment Dis 34: 199

Woollam DHM, Millen JW (1953) Anatomical considerations in the pathology of stenosis of the cerebral aqueduct. Brain 76: 104

Wright RL, Ballantyne HT (1967) Management of brain abscesses in children and adolescents. Am J Dis Child 114: 113

Yakovlev PI, Lecours AR (1967) The myelogenetic cycles of regional maturation of the brain. In: Minkowski A (ed) Regional development of the brain in early life. Blackwell, Oxford, p 3

Yakovlev PI, Wadsworth RC (1946) Schizencephalies; study of congenital clefts in cerebral mantle clefts with fused lips. J Neuropathol Exp Neurol 5: 169

Zulch KJ (1965) brain tumours. Their biology and pathology, 2nd American edn. Heinemann Medical, London, p 214

Zwetnow NN (1970) Effects of increased cerebrospinal fluid pressure on the blood flow and on the energy metabolism of the brain. An experimental study. Acta Physiol Scand [Suppl] 339: 1

Chapter 6

Gastrointestinal System

Colin L. Berry and Jean W. Keeling

Malformations of the gastrointestinal tract are an important cause of morbidity in early life. In this field, as in cardiovascular disease, effective surgical intervention is often practicable and requires prompt diagnosis and action. Massive irreparable defects are happily rare.

A brief account of the embryology of the entire tract will first be given; some further details are included in the text when relevant.

1. Embryology

After the separation of the primitive endoderm from the blastodisc at about day 14 the cells of this layer form the primitive yolk sac. At around the 20th day of development, the yolk sac becomes tucked under the head fold, thus forming the *fore-gut* (see Fig. 6.1). Initially, the notochord is embedded in its roof, its cranial extremity is separated from the stomatodaeum by the buccopharyngeal membrane, and it is surrounded by mesoderm. More caudally situated are the pleuropericardial canals, which later become the pleural cavities. The primitive heart lies ventrally.

Formation of the tail-fold a little later defines the *hind-gut* in a comparable way. The *mid-gut* communicates directly with the extra-embryonic part of the yolk sac via a broad stalk. The endoderm of all these regions gives rise to the gut epithelium and the mesoderm to the muscular, fibrous, and peritoneal coats. The intra-embryonic coelum on each side of the mid-gut forms the peritoneal cavity.

The endodermal part of the mouth and much of the pharynx arises from the cranial portion of the fore-gut. The branchial arches develop in the mesoderm alongside the fore-gut, and pouch-like extensions of the endoderm occur between them— ultimately giving rise to such structures as the middle ear cavity and the parathyroid and thymus glands (see Figs. 6.2–6.4).

At about the 10 mm stage nasal pits are seen, and at this time the stomatodaeum is bounded by the nasal folds and the mandibular and maxillary processes (Fig. 6.5). The maxillary processes then grow forward and join the medial nasal folds, forming primitive anterior and posterior nares. The primitive palate is formed from the lower deep aspect of the frontonasal process. Masses of maxillary mesoderm grow medially as the nasal septum develops, forming the palatal processes. These processes fuse with the posterior edge of the primitive palate, and then with each other and with the lower edge of the nasal septum. The tongue projects upwards between the maxillary palatal processes for a short time and is squeezed down as these processes fuse from the front backwards (Fig. 6.6).

The ventral diverticulum that will give rise to the larynx, trachea and lungs is seen at about 3 mm. After this the caudal part of the fore-gut lengthens rapidly as the primitive oesophagus, and a longitudinal ridge develops on each side, eventually fusing and separating the respiratory diverticulum from the oesophagus. If fusion of these ridges is incomplete, abnormal communications may be formed (see p. 218). As the embryo grows and the heart descends the oesophagus elongates rapidly. The stomach is visible as a small swelling at around 7 mm; by the 15 mm stage its form is well established, following extensive dorsal expansion, and the biliary system and pancreas are all in almost adult inter-relationships. The duodenum grows rapidly, its lumen becoming obliterated for a time. At about this stage the development of the liver and primitive kidney, together with elongation of the gut, results in

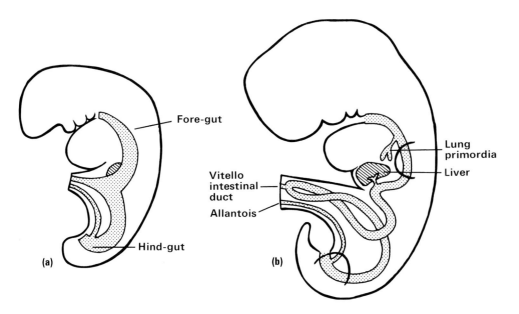

Fig. 6.1. a and **b** Early development of gastrointestinal tract showing the mid-gut loop at 3.5-mm (approx. 28-day) stage (**a**) and at the 7-mm (approx. 35-day) stage (**b**).

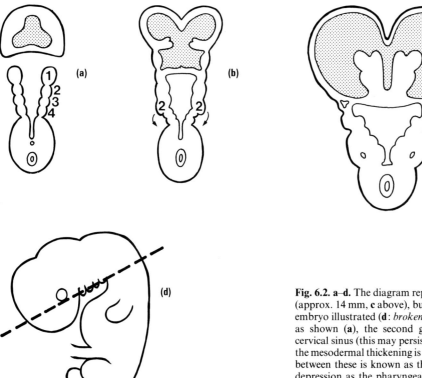

Fig. 6.2. a–d. The diagram represents an advanced embryo below (approx. 14 mm, **c** above), but the section plane is similar in each embryo illustrated (**d**: *broken line*). The branchial arches develop as shown (**a**), the second growing backwards to enclose the cervical sinus (this may persist as a pharyngeal fistula). Note that the mesodermal thickening is the branchial arch; the external cleft between these is known as the pharyngeal cleft and the interior depression as the pharyngeal pouch. These structures are transient and the first two are disappearing as the latter ones form. The structures derived from them are shown in Figs. 6.3. and 6.4.

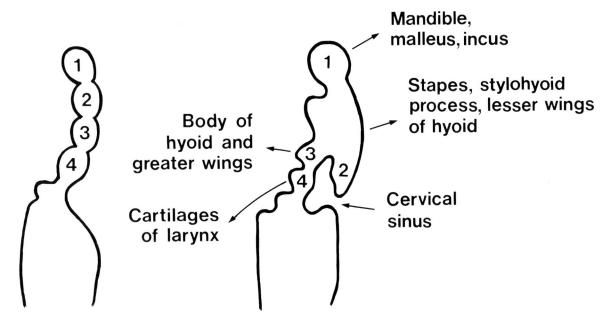

Fig. 6.3. Bony derivative of branchial arches.

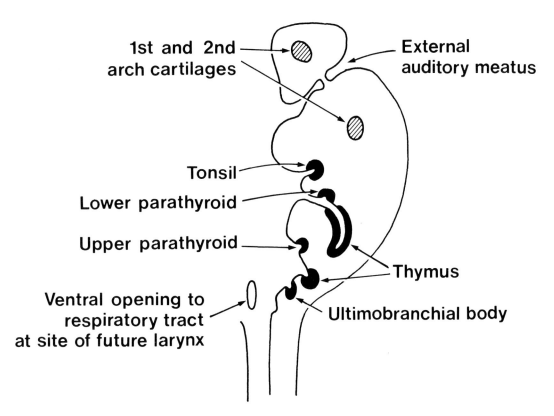

Fig. 6.4. Other derivatives of branchial arches. The only definitive structure formed from the pharyngeal pouches are the Eustachian tube and the tympanic cavity. This slice is from a later embryo.

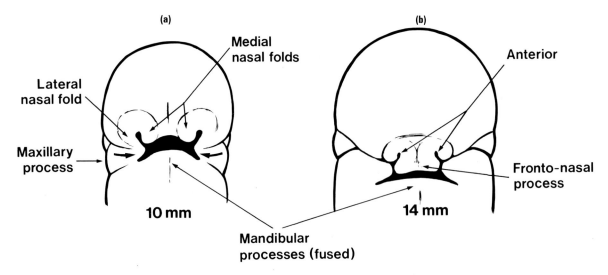

Fig. 6.5. a and **b** Formation of the main components of the nose and mouth in a 10-mm (**a**) and a 14-mm embryo.

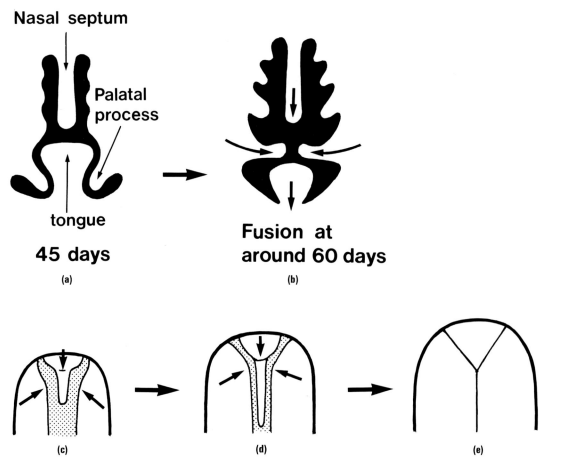

Fig. 6.6. a–e Formation of nasal septum and palate. **a** and **b** The various movements that accompany this; **c, d,** and **e** the ventral aspect of the palate at different stages of closure. **c** Shows the situation at approximately 60 days (29–32 mm).

a volume of tissue that cannot be contained within the intra-embryonic coelom. The gut herniates into the extra-embryonic coelom as a U-shaped loop, 'based' on the superior mesenteric artery. The cranial part of the loop, from the duodenal attachment, forms the jejunum and greater part of the ileum. This limb increases markedly in size. The remaining caudal loop forms the terminal ileum, caecum and appendix, ascending colon, and much of the transverse colon. The whole herniated loop rotates anticlockwise through 180° whilst herniated.

The distal part of the hind-gut is divided into the urogenital sinus and the rectum by a process analogous to that dividing oesophageal and respiratory primordia. More proximally, the left third of the transverse colon, the descending and the pelvic colon are formed from the caudal loop of the mid-gut U. At about the 10th week (42–48 mm) the region of the junction of the mid-gut loop and the hind-gut moves to the left and the small intestinal loops return to the abdomen, having rotated through a further 90°. The duodenal loop moves right and the caecum comes to lie in the right iliac fossa, having previously been below the right lobe of the liver after its return to the abdominal cavity. The ascending and descending mesocolons then fuse with the parietal peritoneum, and only transverse and sigmoid mesocolons remain as mesenteries into post-uterine life.

2. Facial and Oral Abnormalities

Massive disturbance of the formation of the anterior part of the embryo is usually incompatible with life. A few anomalies of very early development (formation of the facial swellings—say 2.5 mm stage) are compatible with life.

The defects may be classified as follows:

1. Failure of the major facial processes

  A. Agenesis of the frontomaxillary process

    i) Cyclopia (incompatible with life)

    ii) Arrhinencephaly

      a) *with medial harelip.* A true harelip, which resembles the normal condition in rabbits and which may be associated with notching of the alveolar process and a median tooth gap. In this group the pre-maxilla may be absent; there is a single nasal cavity and a cleft of the hard and soft palates

      b) *with lateral cleft lip and palate.* The maxillary process fails to move medially and there is a failure of fusion of the maxillary and palative bones, with palatal clefts in addition to lip abnormalities

  B. Abnormalities of the mandibular and maxillary swellings. A complex group including many syndromes often discussed under the heading of branchial arch anomalies, including:

    i) *Pierre–Robin syndrome.* Micrognathia with glossoptosis, hypoplasia of the mandible, usually with palatal clefts and visceral anomalies (congenital heart disease etc.)

    ii) *Treacher–Collin's syndrome.* Mandibulofacial dyostosis, hypoplasia of the facial bones, malformation of the internal and external ear, and oblique palpebral fissures sloping in an anti-mongoloid direction

    iii) Unilateral mandibulofacial dyostosis (Weyers)

2. Abnormalities of growth and fusion of the facial processes. These lesions form the commonest group, some forms occurring in approximately 1 in 1000 births

  A. Failure of fusion between the lateral nasal and maxillary swellings. An oblique fissure connecting the inner canthus with the upper lip without affecting the nose

  B. Defective growth of the mandibular and maxillary swellings

  C. Macrostomia. Failure of coordinated growth and fusion between the frontonasal and maxillary processes

    i) Simple cleft lip—may extend to the nostril and involve the alveolus (Fig. 6.7).

    ii) Cleft lip and palate (Fig. 6.8).

    iii) Isolated cleft palate (Fig. 6.9).

    Minor types are always posterior; complete types never extend beyond the incisive foramen.

These defects are not a single entity (see also p. 73). The anomalies are commoner in males (65% male, 35% female) and occur on the left more frequently than the right. The high incidence in the Japanese (1.71%) is probably related to facial shape (see discussion on polygenically determined anomalies: p. 69). Approximately two-thirds of children have cleft lip and palate, one-third having cleft lip alone.

Cleft lip can exist as a unilateral or bilateral notch in the lip, or extend into the nostril and involve the bony part of the maxilla. If the cleft is bilateral the portion of the maxilla bearing the upper incisors projects upwards and outwards and gives rise to a deformity which is difficult to correct.

Cleft palate results from failure of fusion of the palatine shelves. This can affect any part of the septum and varies in severity from bifid uvula to

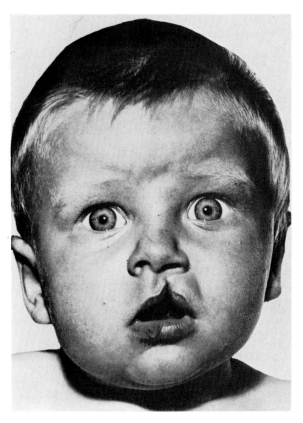

Fig. 6.7. Isolated cleft lip. Distortion of the nostril is evident.

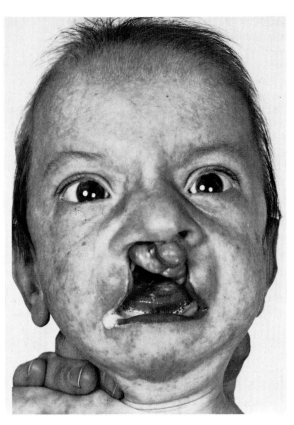

Fig. 6.8. Bilateral cleft lip and palate, with elevation and prominence of the mid-line structures.

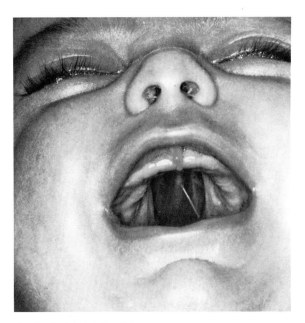

Fig. 6.9. Isolated cleft palate.

complete absence of the palate with the nasal cavity opening into the mouth. A unilateral defect may occur with one side of the nasal cavity opening into the mouth. The soft palate alone may be cleft but the hard palate is never cleft when the soft palate is found to be intact.

To illustrate the complexity of the interpretations of the pathogenesis of malformation in this area and to emphasize the occurrence of many atypical anomalies, Fig. 6.10 shows a child with macroglossia, unilateral accessory auricles, and some facial asymmetry. Underlying bones were normal; this is not a branchial arch syndrome of the conventional type.

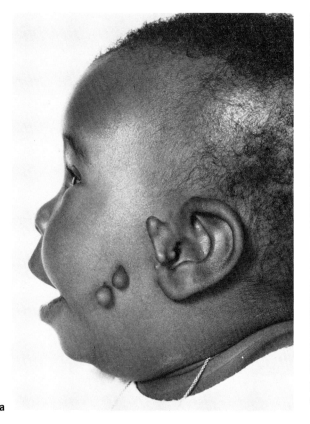

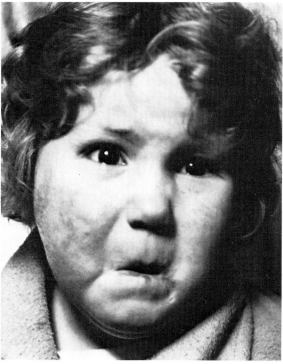

Fig. 6.11. Microstomia. Irregularity of the vermillion margin is common.

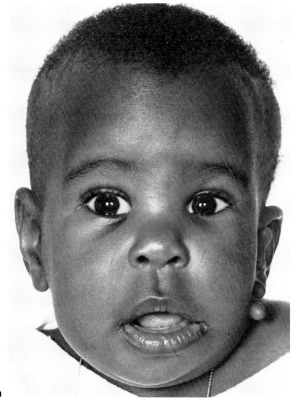

Fig. 6.10. a and **b** Atypical development of the face.

2.1. Other Abnormalities of the Mouth

2.1.1. Microstomia

Microstomia (Fig. 6.11) has been observed in certain families and is associated with trisomy 18. The mandible is hypoplastic and association with other skeletal anomalies is documented. The mouth is often small in Down's syndrome.

2.1.2. Macrostomia

Massive enlargement of the mouth occurs in association with other anomalies, including absence of the tongue. The mouth may literally extend from ear to ear, and the defect is due to incomplete growth and fusion of the maxillary process with the frontonasal process.

2.1.3. Dentition

Apart from minor forms associated with cleft lip and palate, abnormalities of the dentition are uncommon. The two central incisors of the lower jaw may be present at birth and are then usually poorly formed.

Anodontia occurs in two forms, partial (Fig. 6.12) and complete, and is inherited as a Mendelian dominant.

Amelogenesis imperfecta also occurs in two forms, *hereditary enamel hypoplasia*, in which the teeth are abnormally shaped with sharp-pointed cusps, resulting in excessive wear, and *hereditary enamel hypocalcification*, where the soft enamel is also readily worn away. In this latter group the wear is so severe that the teeth may be eroded to gum level, and the enamel is apparently porous, being readily stained. Both deciduous and permanent dentition may be affected.

In odontogenesis imperfecta the teeth are also susceptible to injury; the pulp canal of their stumpy roots is obliterated by bony proliferation and they may also become discoloured (Fig. 6.13). This lesion resembles, and may form part of, the syndrome of osteogenesis imperfecta.

Discoloration of teeth also occurs after tetracycline treatment during pregnancy, usually after prolonged or regular administration. The drug is incorporated into newly growing bone and dentine and there produces fluorescence seen under ultra-iolet light. Brownish-yellow tooth discoloration may occur after kernicterus.

In Down's syndrome growth arrest lines may be found in the teeth.

In hypophosphatasia there is early loss of deciduous teeth through bone resorption. This condition is inherited as a simple recessive characteristic.

The well-defined incisor and molar abnormalities in congenital syphilis may be related to the presence of *T. pallidum* in the developing tooth germ (Bradlaw 1953).

2.1.4. Tongue

The tongue may be fixed or tied by a short frenum, but it is doubtful whether this is of clinical significance except in very gross examples. The frenum may also be congenitally absent. Macroglossia can be associated with hypothyroidism, Down's syndrome (where the mouth may also be small), glycogen storage disease, and lymphangiectasia.

Granular cell myoblastoma, neurofibroma, lingual thyroid tissue, and haemangiomas may all form localized lingual swellings in infancy.

2.1.5. Cyst in the Mouth

Ranulae—retention cysts of the salivary gland ducts—are not uncommon. The cysts are unilocular, mucus-filled, and lined with a pale secreting epithelium. They may disappear spontaneously in neonates but often require surgical removal.

Cysts lined with a respiratory type of epithelium may occur along the line of fusion of the maxillary and frontonasal process.

2.1.6. Infections of the Oropharynx

Bacterial. Vincent's angina is an acute inflammatory process affecting the mouth, from which many

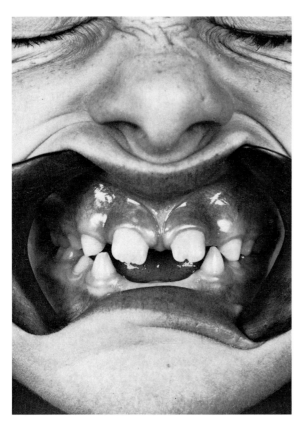

Fig. 6.12. Partial anodontia—absence of all lower and the lateral upper incisors.

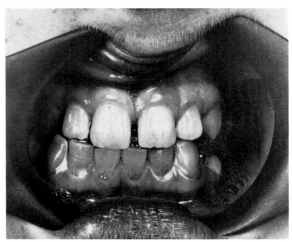

Fig. 6.13. Odontogenesis imperfecta. Discoloured lower teeth.

organisms, including anaerobic streptococci and spirochaetes, may be isolated. A necrotizing inflammatory process (noma) develops in debilitated individuals and may result in considerable perioral destruction of tissues.

Virus infections are common and have been divided by Dudgeon (1962) into infections in which:

A.The predominant lesion is oropharyngeal (Fig. 6.14):
 1) Herpes simplex stomatitis
 2) Coxsackie virus pharyngitis
 3) Adenovirus infections

B.Oropharyngeal lesions occur as part of a disseminated process:
 1) Acute exanthemas
 2) ECHOvirus infections
 3) Accidental infections (vaccinia, cowpox).

A further group of ulcerative lesions of uncertain aetiology may occur in childhood (e.g., recurrent aphthae, Stevens–Johnson syndrome, Bechet's disease).

Most viral infections are manifest as small vesicles, often containing some leucocytes and epithelial cells, which rupture, leaving discrete ulcers with punched-out edges. In herpetic infections multinucleate cells may be seen in buccal smears.

Fungal infections are almost entirely caused by *Candida* sp. with budding yeast-like forms and pseudomycelium present in infected tissues. The oral lesions consist of flat white plaques, which when scraped leave a flat surface with small discrete bleeding points. There is a mixed polymorph and lymphocyte infiltrate in the underlying tissues; in debilitated individuals or those with immune defects there may be very little tissue response.

2.1.7. Tumours of the Mouth

The term epulis is used to describe tumours on the gum (Fig. 6.15). These may be giant-celled fibromas or granular cell myoblastomas, the latter tumour occasionally being present at birth. Overlying epithelial hyperplasia is seen over almost all benign gum tumours.

Malignant tumours are very rare. Kissane and Smith (1967) describe a well-differentiated squamous carcinoma in a 12-year-old boy. Nasopharyngeal lymphomas may present as mouth swellings, but the commonest oral tumour in childhood is the lymphoepithelioma, an epidermal tumour with a conspicuous lymphoid infiltrate.

3. Salivary Glands

3.1. Heterotopias

In an article on the histogenesis of branchial cysts, Little and Rickles (1967) have discussed the frequently observed occurrence of lymphoid tissue in salivary glands and of salivary tissue in lymph nodes. Salivary gland tissue may also occur in the middle ear (Taylor and Martin 1961).

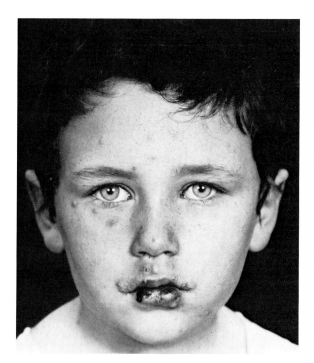

Fig. 6.14. Viral stomatitis, probably due to herpes simplex.

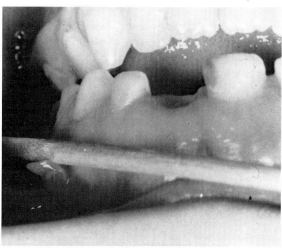

Fig. 6.15. Small fibrous tumour on gum.

3.2. Inflammatory Disorders

Bacterial infection is uncommon and occurs in dehydrated febrile individuals or following trauma to major salivary ducts. Mumps virus sialadentitis is accompanied by areas of focal necrosis, loss of epithelium, and lymphocytic infiltration. Desquamated cells may be seen in ducts. Local lymph nodes may contain giant Warthin–Finkeldey cells during the prodromal period.

Cytomegalovirus is commonly found in salivary gland epithelium—usually ductal. Its frequency of occurrence varies widely and is apparently higher in Eastern Europe.

3.3. Tumours

In our experience the commonest neoplastic lesions occurring in salivary glands in childhood are deposits from leukaemia. Salivary neoplasms excluding haemangioma, usually of the parotid gland, are distinctly rare. An excellent review is that of Kauffmann and Stout (1963), who described pleomorphic adenomas, Warthins tumour, mucoepiderdermoid carcinoma, and adenoid cystic carcinoma in children. More recently Nagao et al. (1980) have described the experience of their large registry, with comparable results.

4. Oesophagus

Absence. Bizarre monsters may have no structure resembling an oesophagus, but otherwise this structure is always present in some form.
Double oesophagus. The oesophagus may be doubled from pharynx to cardia. Gjørup (1934)

reported a case in which a double oesophagus and partial duplication of the stomach was present; further cases of this type have since been described.
Atresia. In about 95% of cases, oesophageal atresia is associated with a fistula into the trachea. This defect has been classified by many authors but there is agreement that type I in the diagram (Fig. 6.16) comprises around 90% of defects in all large series. Type II is the next commonest type (around 5%–8% in different studies), and all other varieties are rare. The straight-through trachea with virtual absence of the oesophagus is rarest of all.

The pathogenesis of the defect is generally considered to be a failure of the ventral diverticulum of the fore-gut, which will form the trachea, to separate from the oesophagus. This diverticulum appears as a longitudinal groove in the fore-gut at the 2.5 mm (4-week) stage, with caudal swellings that represent the future lung buds. The groove is then 'pinched off' from the oesophagus, resulting in an over-and-under double-barrelled shot gun appearance (at around 4 mm) with progressive separation of the two barrels by a caudocephalad gradient. It will be realized that partial failure of the processes of septation or separation may give rise to fistula. The rapid growth of the trachea that follows the 4–5 mm stage may cause displacement of developing oesophageal tissue and is a possible cause of atretic segments. Vascular pathogenetic factors related to the effects of obstruction due to persistence of the primitive right dorsal aorta have been considered by some to be important in the genesis of the oesophageal atresia.

In the commonest form of the defect the upper oesophageal pouch ends at about the level of the second thoracic vertebra. It is often rather thick-walled, and tends to be dilated (Fig. 6.17). The fistula is often narrowed at its site of entry into the trachea, usually just above and to the left of the posterior aspect of the carina. The fistula is generally

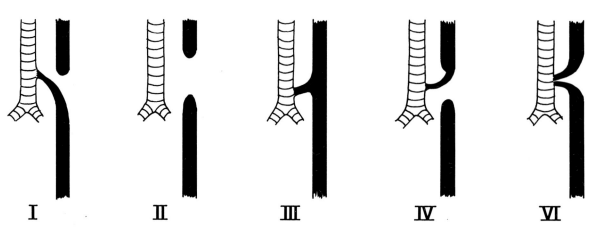

I   II   III   IV   VI

Fig. 6.16. Types of oesophageal atresia with associated tracheo-oesophageal fistula.

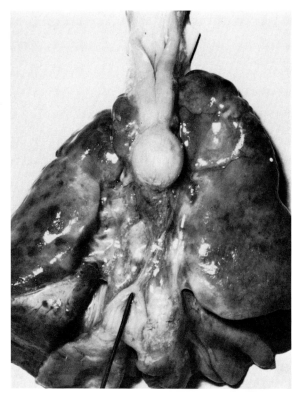

Fig. 6.17. Typical atresia with a cyst at the end of the upper pouch and area of atresia (type II).

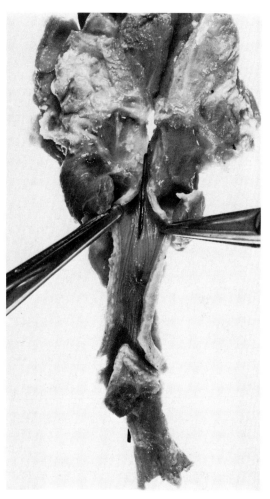

Fig. 6.18. Two fistulas into the trachea are seen, the upper containing a probe.

described as being lined with squamous epithelium, but in our experience of cases dying soon after birth respiratory epithelium may be found to extend well into the tract, suggesting that later appearances may be evidence of metaplasia. Rosenthal (1931) has described how squamous metaplasia may extend up to the larynx in some instances. A detailed review is that of Holder and Ashcraft (1970). Two fistulae may be present in 1%–8% of cases (Fig. 6.18) and may account for failure of an apparently successful repair (Hays et al. 1966).

4.1. Associated Anomalies

Polyhydramnios is a common feature of pregnancies resulting in infants with oesophageal atresia, and occurs in about 30% of cases. Associated anomalies include Down's syndrome, and an increased incidence of congenital heart disease and anorectal anomalies is found. The prognosis is greatly affected by the presence of additional malformations.

Recent reports suggest that abnormalities of oesophageal motility are common in survivors of repair procedures (Lancet 1978).

4.2. Stenosis

Stenosis occurs in the distal third of the viscus. It is usually due to fibrosis following peptic ulceration; ectopic gastric mucosa is not uncommon in the oesophagus. Stenosis may also follow surgery for fistula or atresia, ulceration, and fibrosis after ingestion of toxic or corrosive fluids, a common event in childhood (Fig. 6.19).

It is often difficult to establish that oesophageal stenosis is an independently occurring congenital anomaly. However, the cases described by Kumar (1963) and Paulino et al. (1963), in which cartilage rings were present outside the oesophageal wall, causing stenosis, are apparently true congenital defects. Obstruction of the lower oesophagus by membranes has also been described by Schwartz (1962).

Muscular obstruction of the oesophagus may occur in the distal third as a result of the thickening and hypertrophy of the muscularis, a condition

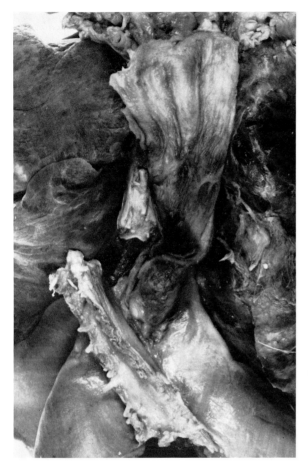

Fig. 6.19. Scarring and stenosis of the oesophagus following ingestion of strong alkali solution.

resembling hypertrophic pyloric stenosis. The autonomic innervation of this segment is apparently normal in these cases; in rare cases the whole oesophagus can be involved (Blank and Michael 1963).

4.3. Diverticula

Oesophageal diverticula are rare in childhood. They occur at three sites.

1) *Upper oesophageal/hypopharyngeal pouches* occur between cricopharyngeus and the superior oesophageal constrictor, as in adults. They have been found to have an entire muscular wall, unlike those found in adult life, and are, therefore, true congenital anomalies. Frequently the lesion is confused clinically with the upper pouch of an atretic oesophagus.

2) *Mid-oesophageal pouches* are thought to represent incomplete varieties of tracheo-oesophageal fistulae. They are generally small and lined with squamous epithelium.

There is an apparent connection with the so-called *oesophageal cysts*, reviewed by Cornell et al. (1950). These are found in the muscular part of the wall and bulge into the lumen. They are lined with ciliated epithelium and cartilage may be found in their walls. It seems likely that these lesions are in fact abortive attempts to bud off accessory respiratory diverticula early in development.

3) *Lower oesophageal diverticula* are very rare, and may be lined in part with gastric epithelium and contain pancreas in their wall. They probably represent fore-gut duplication rather than true diverticula (Mendl and Evans 1962). Postinflammatory traction diverticula, formerly common and usually due to tuberculosis, are now rare.

4.4. Inflammatory Disease

Herpetic infection and moniliasis may cause oesophageal ulceration in infants, but mucosal loss in the lower third of the viscus is most commonly found after death associated with protracted vomiting, anoxia or indwelling feeding tubes. The reddened mucosa shows linear ulcers, often apparently undermined. Histologically there is often little reaction but the picture is confused by autolytic changes (see Fig. 6.20).

4.5. Achalasia

Achalasia of the oesophagus is present in early life in about 5 % of cases, and some cases require surgery in childhood (Swenson and Oeconomopoulos 1961). The pathology of this condition in childhood differs in no way from that in adults (Fig. 6.21).

4.6. Rupture

Rupture of the oesophagus may occur, usually posteriorly and to the left, in the lower third where the unsupported area abuts on the pleural cavity. It commonly follows episodes of repeated vomiting (Wiseman et al. 1959). Apart from this, most perforations occur as a result of surgical trauma.

4.7. Foreign Bodies

Foreign bodies in the oesophagus are usually arrested at the level of cricopharyngeus, the left main-stem bronchus, or at the cardia. They are generally easily removed, but sharp objects may perforate the wall.

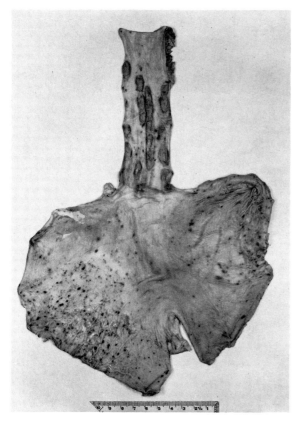

Fig. 6.20. Ulcers in the oesophagus of a leukaemic child. The stomach shows numerous petechial haemorrhages.

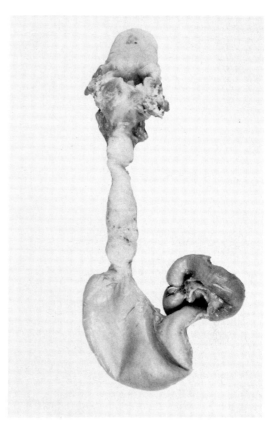

Fig. 6.21. Achalasia of the oesophagus in a child. The oesophagus is thick-walled and dilated.

4.8. Oesophageal Varices

Children with portal hypertension can develop oesophageal varices. Portal vein thrombosis (Fig. 6.22) is the most frequent cause of portal hypertension, but it may occur in later life following hepatic changes in cystic disease. Congenitally dilated veins may also be found in the lower oesophagus (Jorup 1948).

4.9. Neoplasms

Primary oesophageal neoplasms are rare in childhood, and we have seen only leiomyomas. The oesophagus is commonly involved by spread of mediastinal neoplasms or nodal metastases. Squamous carcinoma, rhabdomyosarcoma, and neurofibroma have all been reported in childhood.

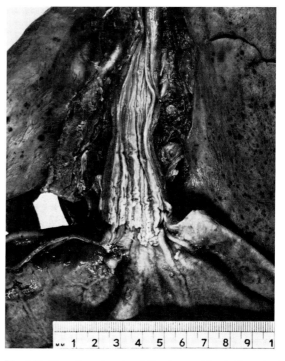

Fig. 6.22. Oesophageal varices following portal vein thrombosis in a 9-year-old child.

5. Stomach

Congenital anomalies of the stomach are rare. Absence is noted in acardiac monsters, and occasionally the organ remains as a simple tube-like structure owing to failure of the later rapid growth of the greater curve. Under these circumstances the duodenum is generally found to be mobile and in the mid-line.

Membranous atresia of the stomach may occur at the pylorus, and it is usually diagnosed as pyloric stenosis or, if the membrane prolapses down the duodenum, as duodenal atresia. We have seen an example of gastric atresia in which the continuity of the stomach was interrupted and a fibrous cord joined the duodenum. The stomach was vastly distended. However, gastric atresias account for less than 1% of all cases of gut atresia (Parrish et al. 1968).

In the many varieties of visceral transposition the stomach may be involved (see p. 139). Isolated gastric inversion has been recorded (Lieber and Rosenbaum 1965). In cases in which a left-sided diaphragmatic defect occurs the stomach is usually found in the thorax.

5.1. Hypertrophic Pyloric Stenosis (see also p. 69)

There is some doubt as to whether hypertrophic pyloric stenosis should really be considered a congenital defect, since it has not been reported in stillbirths and rarely presents in the first 24 h of life. However, the disease is apparently polygenically determined, with a well-defined pattern of inheritance. Marked variation in racial incidence is found (see Table 6.1). There is a marked male preponderance (around 5:1) and a pronounced tendency for first-born children to be affected.

At operation, usually at around 3 weeks of age, a fusiform mass of firm pale muscle up to 3–5 cm long is found at the pylorus (Fig. 6.23), with an abrupt return to normal gut wall distally (Fig. 6.24). The muscle mass is derived largely from the outer

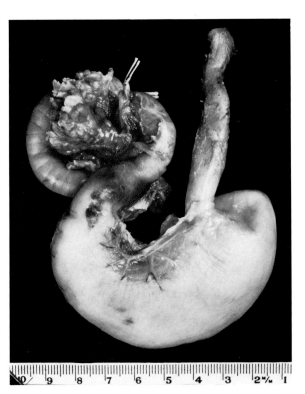

Fig. 6.23. From a case of pyloric stenosis dying at the age of 6 weeks in 1949. The stomach wall is thickened and the pylorus is seen as a discrete mass.

circular muscle coat, but all layers are involved. Secondary mucosal changes (oedema and ulceration) may occur in cases with a prolonged history. There have been extensive studies on the changes in autonomic innervation in the duodenum in this condition, and delayed maturation, secondary destruction, and 'overstimulation' of nervous tissue have all been discussed. In an extensive series of observations on serially sectioned pyloric tumours, Bodian found no evidence to support any of these hypotheses, most neuronal changes appearing to be secondary in character. It is apparent from an examination of his material that the changes in the muscle are mainly hypertrophic in character.

If the disease is not treated promptly ulceration of the mucosa of the distended stomach may occur, and hypertrophy of its muscle coats may also be found.

5.2. Diverticula

'Congenital diverticula' of the stomach are rare and consist of small pouches that may intussuscept and perforate. Descriptions of these lesions suggest that many are examples of reduplications (Ogur and Kolarsick 1951).

Table 6.1. Incidence of pyloric stenosis per 100 000 births in Hawaii (Morton 1970)

Source	Incidence
Caucasian	159
Japanese	68
Caucasian–Japanese F_1	54
Hawaiian	5
Filipino	14

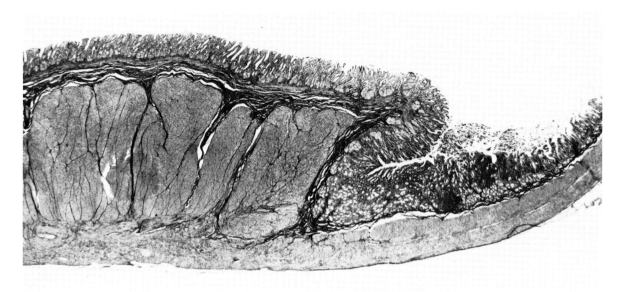

Fig. 6.24. Abrupt transition between pyrloric and duodenal musculature in an untreated case of pyloric stenosis.

5.3. Duplications

The precise nature of enteric duplications has been obscured by a number of reports of various cystic lesions. Kissane and Smith (1967) have suggested that the term *gastric* reduplications should be reserved to describe 'cystic or tubular lesions intimately connected with the stomach whether or not they are lined by gastric mucosa and whether or not they communicate with the definitive stomach'. This definition excludes many so-called gastric duplications in older reports (a good review is that of Lewis et al. 1961). Abrami and Dennison (1961) have reported on 39 duplications. These massess occur along the greater curve of the stomach (see Fig. 6.25). They are lined with gastric mucosa in over 50 % of cases, and pancreatic tissue is occasionally found in the wall.

5.4. Gastric Perforations

Since Herbut (1943) described areas of muscular deficiency in the stomach, this finding has been considered to be a major cause of 'spontaneous' gastric performation. Although some authors find frequent muscular abnormalities in cases of this type (Purcell 1962), we have not been impressed with their frequency. Potter (1961), however, illustrates such a defect.

Overdistention of the stomach with gases during resuscitation and perforation by catheters (misplaced on feeding) are the commonest cause of perforation of the stomach without previous ulceration. Dilatation due to untreated intestinal obstruction may result in necrosis and perforation due to impairment of the blood supply, which can also occur following gastric volvulus.

5.5. Gastric Heterotopias

Pancreatic tissue is not infrequently found in the gastric wall and has been discussed by Berant et al. (1965). We have seen a number of cases with intramural pancreatic tissue in the stomach and are under the impression that the frequency of this anomaly varies directly with the assiduity with which it is sought. It appears to be more common in children than in adults, which may represent a sampling problem or disappearance of the tissue with age.

5.6. Foreign Bodies

Many objects may be found in the stomach of children. The well-known trichobezar (Fig. 6.26) from hair chewing is now less common than formerly, small wheels from plastic vehicles being more frequently found. Most objects that reach the stomach pass through it and are voided. Figure 6.27 shows an assortment of nuts, pieces of plastic, seeds, beads, and leaves from the stomach of a 7-year-old boy with intestinal obstruction.

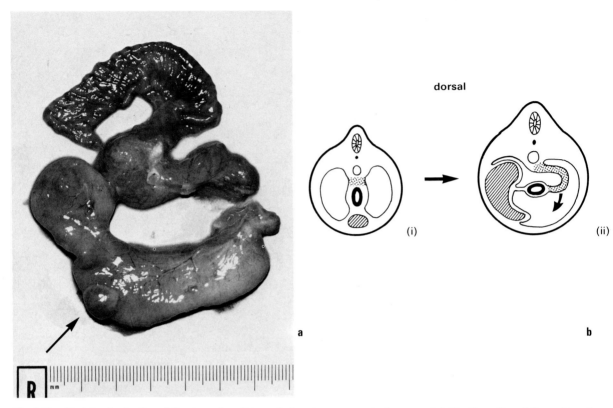

a

dorsal

(i)   (ii)

b

Fig. 6.25. a Nodular duplication of the stomach wall (*arrow*). Annular pancreas is also present. **b** The formation of the peritoneal reflections of the stomach from the dorsal mesogastrium (*stipple*) explains the presence of true gastric duplications only on the greater curve of the stomach. The *hatched area* is the hepatic primordium. (See also p. 230).

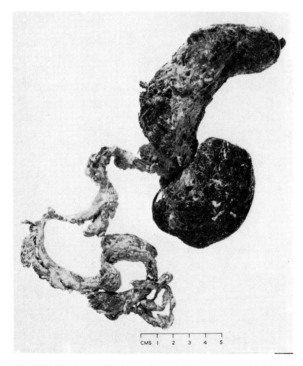

Fig. 6.26. Typical trichobezar from a 12-year-old girl with trichotillomania. Occasionally complete gastric casts are formed.

5.7. Peptic Ulceration

Although rare, the presence of peptic ulcers in infants and children is well documented. Up to the age of 6 years they are almost invariably acute, with haemorrhage a major presenting feature. In older children, as in adults, males are more frequently affected and duodenal lesions are commoner than gastric. A greater awareness of the presence of this type of ulcer in childhood has led to an increased frequency of obtaining typical histories of postprandial pain, and an earlier supposition that bleeding was a particularly common form of presentation in *this* age group (25%–50% in various series) is probably not justified. A family history is found in about half the cases seen (Habbick et al. 1968). More important is the presence of the Zollinger–Ellison syndrome in approximately 5% of these children (Ellison and Wilson 1964).

In infants and neonates peptic ulceration occurs acutely, often associated with severe systemic illness, and presents with haemorrhage or perforation. Fibrosis and reactive vascular changes are not seen.

Ulceration may also occur with space-occupying intracranial lesions in association with steroid therapy (Rosenlund and Koop 1970).

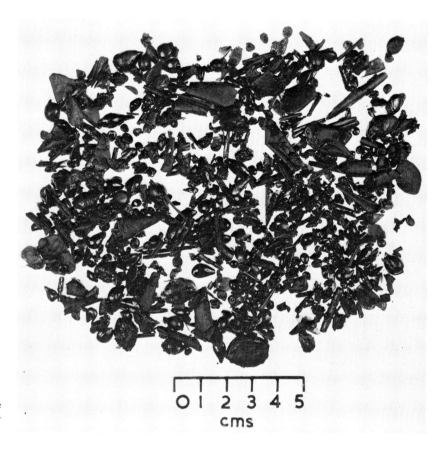

Fig. 6.27. Objects removed from the stomach at operation on a 7-year-old boy.

5.8. Inflammation

Accidental ingestion of medicines, which is un-happily common in children, may cause severe inflammation and ulceration of the stomach, sal-icylates and ferrous sulphate (Fig. 6.28) being particularly likely to cause this type of injury. Perforation and haemorrhage may occur.

Haemorrhage into the mucosa may occur in blood dyscrasias (Fig. 6.29).

5.9. Eosinophilic Gastritis

Eosinophilic gastritis can occur in childhood, sometimes as part of a diffuse involvement of the bowel. There is, typically, thickening of the pyloric or small intentinal mucosa but single or multiple foci of infiltration by oedema and a predominantly eosinophilic inflammatory cell mass. Blood eosin-ophilia is common, and malabsorption is some-times found. Polypoid lesions may cause intus-susception. A further case report of a 2-year-old child with diffuse disease and ileus is given by Konrad and Meister (1979), who review the litera-ture.

5.10. Tumours

Gastric polyps occur in the Peutz–Jeghers syndrome and are hamartomatous, as elsewhere in the gut. Achord and Proctor (1963) described a case in which death occurred from gastric carcinoma associated with the syndrome, but there is no clear evidence as to whether the tumour arose from a polyp. Williams and Knudson (1965), in reporting such a case in an adult duodenal polyp, concluded that there was very little risk of malignancy in this syndrome.

Gastric polyps may occur in some cases of familial colonic polyposis.

Neurofibromatosis may affect the stomach, and we have seen two examples of the rare gastric teratoma. True hamartomata also occur (Bogo-moletz and Cox 1975) (Fig. 6.30a and b).

Leiomyomas occur in children, and leiomyosar-comas have been described (Giberson et al. 1954).

However, malignant tumours are very rare, a total of about 50 cases having been reported in the world literature. Most have been carcinoma and lympho-sarcoma; carcinoid tumours have been reported. J. N. Cox (personal communication) has observed a leiomyoblastoma of the stomach in a 14-year-old girl (Fig. 6.31) (see also Stout 1962).

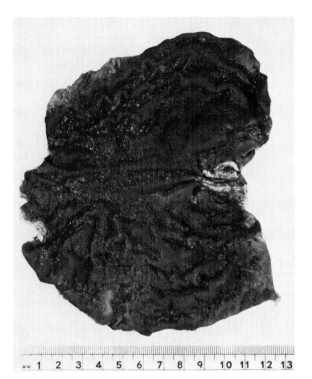

Fig. 6.28. Haemorrhagic gastritis following ingestion of FeSO₄ in a 4-year-old boy. Same case as in Fig. 8.22.

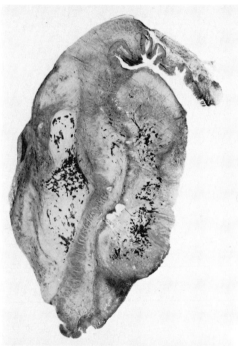

a

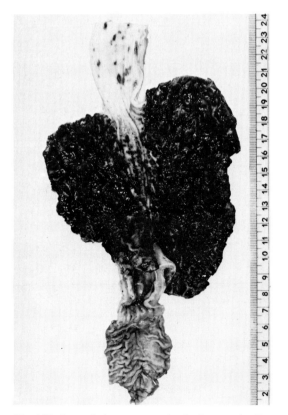

Fig. 6.29. Stomach from a case of aplastic anaemia. Haemorrhagic gastritis and some oesophageal ulceration is seen.

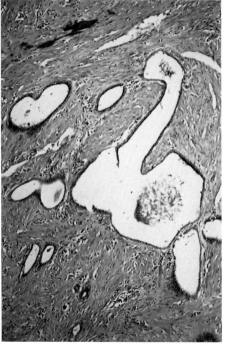

b

Fig. 6.30. a A hamartoma on the mucosal and serosal aspect of the muscularis propria. **b** Cystic dilation of glands in the submucosa, surrounded by fibrous tissue and smooth muscle.

6. Duodenum

6.1. Congenital Abnormalities

In patients with malrotation of the mid-gut loop, peritoneal bands, notably those running across from the right upper quadrant of the abdomen to the caecum, which lies in the epigastrium in this syndrome, may constrict the second part of the duodenum. The condition is cured by cutting the band and completing gut rotation.

6.2 Duplications (see p. 230)

6.2 Duplications (see p. 230)

Duplications in this area are extremely rare, and present as submucosal cysts bulging into the lumen, which they may ultimately obstruct.

6.3. Atresia and Stenosis

Duodenal atresia is usually membranous, a thin diaphragm variably covered by epithelium, stretching across the gut at the junction between the second and third parts. There may be a small hole in the membrane, but the distinction between stenosis and atresia is clinically of little significance. Down's syndrome and other gastrointestinal atresias may accompany this malformation: in two large series Down's syndrome was present in 21% and 30% of cases (Fonkalstrud et al. 1968; Young and Wilkinson 1968).

7. Pancreas

Figure 6.32 shows, in diagrammatic form, how the pancreas develops from two rudiments. These appear at week 4 (3 mm), and the adult form is arrived at by week 16. Many pancreatic abnormalities are explicable in terms of failure of the normal embryological processes.

7.1. Congenital Abnormalities

If the dorsal component of the pancreas fails to develop, the gland consists of an ovoid mass in the hollow of the duodenum. In rare cases failure of fusion of the two parts of the gland may occur, in varying degrees. Nodules of ectopic pancreas are common throughout the gastrointestinal tract.

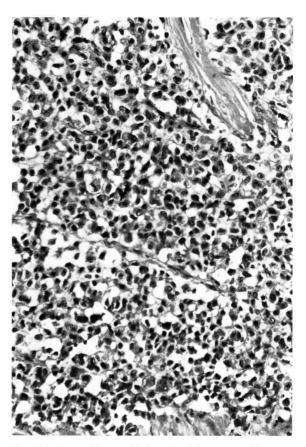

Fig. 6.31. From a 14-year-old girl with a left hypochondrial mass deforming the stomach on barium examination. A large cystic mass (5–6 cm) and two separate masses (2–3 cm) were found in the pyloric region. Large regular vacuolated cells are seen. Reproduced by permission of Dr. J. N. Cox. H and E; 240 ×).

7.2. Annular Pancreas

The second part of the duodenum may be completely surrounded by pancreas when the ventral part of the gland persists. The anomaly is seldom simple, and the pancreas may be found to have 'filled the gap' left by an atretic or stenotic duodenum. The relationship of this lesion to duodenal obstruction is unclear, although it is often cited as a cause of upper-gastrointestinal obstruction in neonates. However, associated gut anomalies—mainly duodenal—may be more important (Elliot et al. 1968; Young and Wilkinson 1968; Fonkalstrad et al. 1969).

7.3. Cystic Fibrosis

The generalized metabolic disease of cystic fibrosis of the pancreas is genetically determined, apparently as an autosomal recessive characteristic. The gene is estimated to occur in around 5% of the population, heterozygotes generally being asympto-

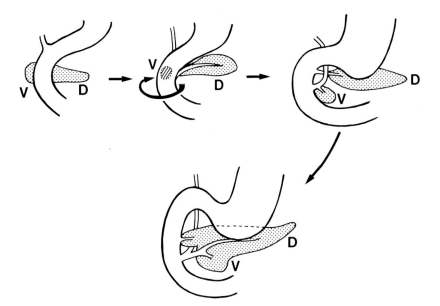

Fig. 6.32. Formation of the pancreas. The dorsal bud forms the upper part of the head, the isthmus, body, tail, the pancreatic duct proper, and the accessory duct of Santorini.

matic. The patients show a characteristic hypersecretion of sodium and chloride in sweat (and other secretions), the basis of a diagnostic test. Measurement of sweat electrolytes may give results above the population mean in siblings of affected individuals.

No discrete metabolic abnormality is known, but the production of a viscid and abnormal mucus at many sites is characteristic. Gastrointestinal (see below), pulmonary (p. 365), and hepatobiliary lesions (p. 288) occur, and in recent years it has become evident that obstructive lesions in the duct system of the testis render males infertile. Pregnancy in affected females is difficult to manage, because of pulmonary changes.

7.3.1. Pancreatic Changes

In infants dying in early life the pancreas may be macroscopically normal, but it is usually firm to the touch. A distinctly lobular feel is characteristic, and in those dying between 2 and about 10 years of age the gland feels as if it were composed of closely interrelated hard triangles of tissue. Later fibrosis, cystic change, focal necroses, and fatty infiltration blur the gross outline of the pancreas.

Histologically there is mucus plugging of distended ducts, with varying degrees of ectasia, fibrosis, and calcification correlating with the severity of the disease rather than the age of the patient. Acinar destruction occurs and the islet tissue appears unduly prominent (Fig. 6.33). Stones may form in the dilated ducts. Trypsin is absent from the stools of affected individuals.

7.3.2. Meconium Ileus

Meconium ileus accounts for about 15% of cases of neonatal intestinal obstruction (Donnison et al. 1966) and is the mode of presentation of 13% of new cases of mucoviscidosis (McParblin et al. 1972).

Macroscopically there is a progressive dilatation of loops of small intestine by tenacious greenish meconium, which is less marked proximally and maximal in the mid-ileum, where the wall is thickened due to muscular hypertrophy. The terminal ileum is narrowed and contains hard greyish calcium-flecked pellets of meconium, while the colon is collapsed and empty (Figs. 6.34 and 6.35).

Histologically the villi are distorted by the meconium in the lumen and the mucosal glands are distended by inspissated secretions. Epithelial cells are flattened and show secondary atrophic changes.

Mortality from meconium ileus has decreased dramatically since the introduction of the Bishop–Koop anastomosis in the management of the disease. Volvulus, perforation, small intestinal atresia, meconium peritonitis, and gangrene may complicate meconium ileus, and these complications are associated with a higher mortality. Meconium peritonitis, which can occur in utero, is manifest histologically as a serosal foreign-body reaction, often with calcification.

An association with hypertrophic pyloric stenosis is reported (McParblin et al. 1972). Peptic ulceration is more common in mucoviscidosis.

Oppenheimer and Esterley (1962) have reported meconium ileus without pancreatic disease.

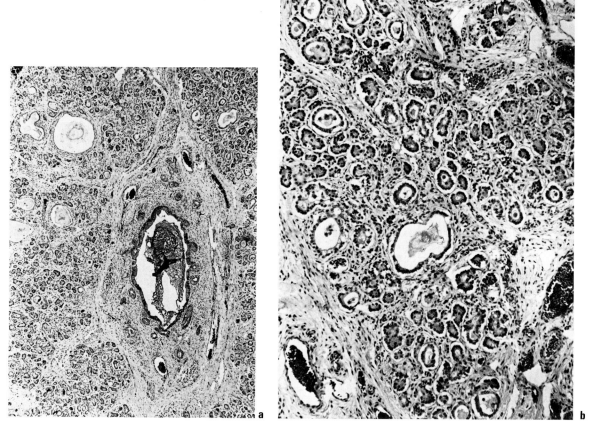

Fig. 6.33. a and **b** Ectactic mucus-filled ducts with separation of acini by fibrous tissue (**a**: H and E; 40 ×) and fibrosis within lobules, with distention of smaller ducts (**b**: H and E; 120 ×)

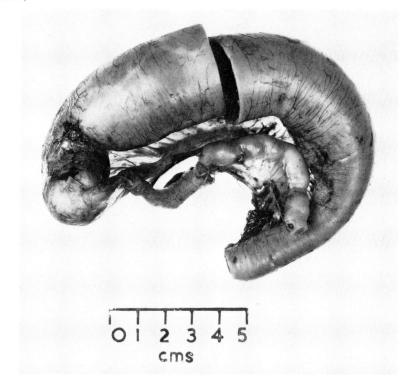

Fig. 6.34. Loop of ileum, distended by meconium, with grossly narrowed segment distally.

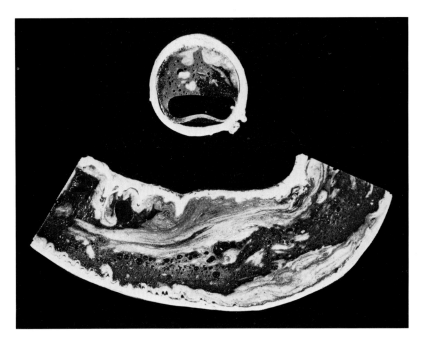

Fig. 6.35. Cut surface of fixed ileum, mucus plugging with mucosal and other debris present in the lumen.

7.4. Pseudocyst

Pseudocysts of the pancreas occur as a result of trauma. This may be an isolated phenomenon (Fraser 1969) or only one of the sequelae of generalized injury. Bongiovi and Logosso (1969) report a case as part of the battered child syndrome (see p. 678). The wall of the pseudocyst is composed of fibrinous tissue and usually contains clear fluid; anatomically it fills the lesser peritoneal sac.

Clinical symptoms are usually of vague abdominal discomfort with an ill-defined epigastric mass. Janudice may occasionally occur.

7.5. Exocrine Atrophy

The combination of exocrine atrophy of the pancreas, pancytopenia and skeletal (metaphyseal) abnormalities has been reported in approximately 100 cases (Lebenthal and Shwachman 1977).

The pancreas is replaced by fat, with prominent islets persisting. The skeleton shows irregular rarefaction and condensation, notably in the femoral necks. Bone marrow abnormalities appear in the form of neutropenia, but pancytopenia has been described, as has complicating leukaemia.

7.6. Pancreatitis

Haemorrhagic pancreatitis is rare in infancy, although it may occur in leukaemia following chemotherapy or after steroid therapy. Alcoholic children are rare, although pancreatitis in an alcoholic child has been reported by Schmidt et al. (1964).

Inflammation of the pancreas occurs in mumps and in toxoplasmosis, and when the ducts are infested by roundworms. Surgical intervention to remove worms from the biliary tract is seldom useful, the duct usually being rapidly repopulated unless infestation is cleared and recurrence can be prevented. Those with experience of this problem suggest that the ducts are seldom completely obstructed by the worms present in them (D. Uys, personal communication).

Injury to the upper abdomen may also cause pancreatitis, often developing 24–36 h after injury.

8. Small Bowel

8.1. Congenital Abnormalities

8.1.1. Enteric Duplications

'Enteric duplication' is the term applied to anomalies that arise early in development dorsal to the developing gut and are usually situated in a position indicating this site of origin. Thus, in parts of the gut with a persistent mesentery they are always found between its leaves. Duplications, with the exception of duodenal lesions, generally have well-defined muscle coats, in which peristalsis may be seen to occur. The lining epithelium may resemble that of the adjacent gut, but gastric mucosa is often present. The lumen may or may not communicate with the gut at one or more sites. In a large review Dohn and

Povlsen (1951) found that the vast majority of lesions were related to the small intestine, with an intrathoracic mass the next most common site (see Fig. 6.36). Sites of occurrence, in descending order of frequency, are ileum, ileocaecal region, oesophagus, jejunum, and stomach.

Enteric duplications probably have their origin in the trapping of endodermal cells in the mid-dorsal area of the fore-gut, with subsequent adherence to the notochord and eventual dorsal displacement. The frequency of abnormal vertebrae is greatly elevated in children with intrathoracic reduplications, and the entire topic has been discussed by Smith (1968), who clarified the nomenclature of these lesions, and by Bentley and Smith (1960). Figure 6.37 illustrates this concept of their pathogenesis. The intrathoracic enteric diverticula are discussed in detail by Goldberg and Johnson (1963), and the 'split notochord syndrome' of Bentley and Smith is a useful concept in the consideration of associated lesions, which are common. In rare instances, splitting of the notochord, with posterior gut herniation is present at birth (Denes et al. 1967). Figure 38 shows a postvertebral enteric cyst removed from an adult.

Lubolt (1968), in reviewing the literature, found that recurrent internal bleeding occurred in 20%–30% of cases of intestinal duplication. Intestinal obstruction and perforation may also occur.

8.1.2. Atresia and Stenosis

For many years it was assumed that during development the gut went through a stage where cell proliferation filled the lumen before recannalization established the definitive lumen. Moutsouris (1966) re-examined this hypothesis in human embryos, and found that complete obliteration of the lumen only occurred in the duodenum. This suggestion apparently afforded a less satisfactory explanation of atresia of the gut than had been thought in the past.

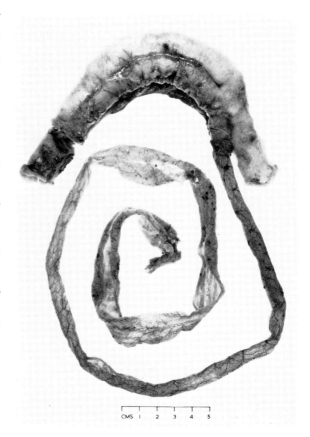

Fig. 6.36. Intestinal duplication. Part of the normal ileum is seen above an extensive, mainly thin-walled, duplication.

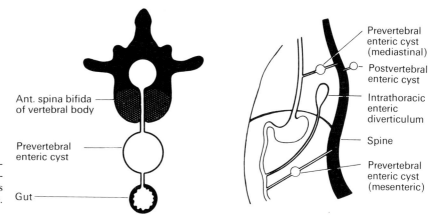

Fig. 6.37. Diagram showing developmental posterior enteric remnants and spinal malformations in the split notochord syndrome. Bentley and Smith 1960.

Ant. spina bifida of vertebral body

Prevertebral enteric cyst

Gut

Prevertebral enteric cyst (mediastinal)

Postvertebral enteric cyst

Intrathoracic enteric diverticulum

Spine

Prevertebral enteric cyst (mesenteric)

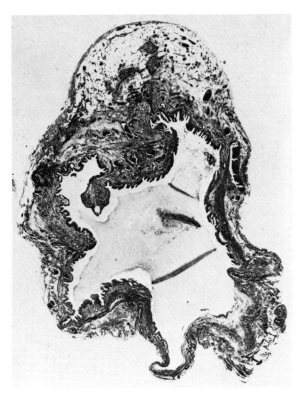

However, experiments involving intrauterine surgery have shown that jejunal atresia accompanied by agenesis of the dorsal mesentery results from intrauterine occlusion of the superior mesenteric artery proximal to its jejunal branches. For this reason vascular changes are now propounded as a probable cause of small-bowel atresia in man (see Louw and Barnard 1955; Abrams 1968).

Atretic and stenotic lesions of the bowel were first classified by Bland-Sutton (1889) into three types: type I, in which a 'diaphragm' was formed across the gut, often involving the muscularis mucosae but not deeper layers (Figs. 6.38 and 6.39); type II, in which there was an interruption in the continuity of the gut, with a fibrous cord connecting the two 'blind ends' (Figs. 6.40–6.42); and type III, in which a segment of gut and the fibrous cord were missing and in which there was, in addition, a V-shaped defect in the mesentery at the site of the atresia. Types II and III are more common than type I, but mixed types are found.

In a special form, the so-called apple-peel deformity, a proximal jejunal or distal duodenal atresia of type III is associated with distal small intestine,

Fig. 6.38. Postvertebral enteric cyst. This lesion was removed from within the dura of a 21-year-old male with progressive propaplegia. Courtesy of Dr M Squier. (H and E; 9 ×).

Fig. 6.39. (*below*) **a** Distended jejunum with membranous atresia with a pinhole communication. Resected at 10 months. In this time massive hypertrophy and dilatation of the proximal bowel has occurred. **b** The pinhole from below.

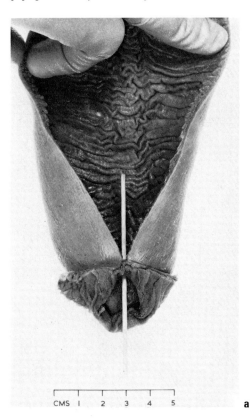

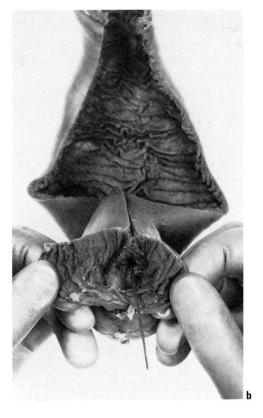

a

b

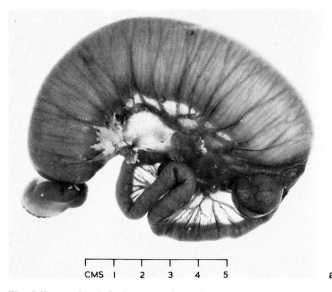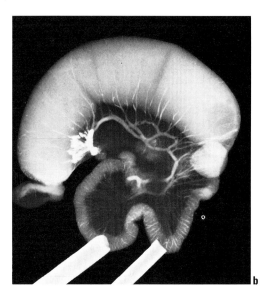

a

b

Fig. 6.40. a and **b** A further case of atresia, with membranous atresia in which postresection angiograms were performed. The membrane is at the site of the cystic dilatation. X-rays emphasize that vascular changes presumed to be important in the pathogenesis of complete atresias are not evident post-partum in the membranous form.

which coils around the marginal artery and receives its arterial supply distally. The mesentery is not fixed to the posterior abdominal wall (Fig. 6.43).

Duodenal atresia is more commonly associated with other congenital anomalies than are ileal or jejunal lesions. There is a male predominance in all types.

Atresia of the large bowel is very rare (Fig. 6.44). Evans (1951), in a review of 1948 reported cases of atresia, found only six of atresia in the colon. Coryllos and Simpson (1962) reviewed 20 cases and added two to the literature, and Hartman et al. (1963) reported a further 12. Benson et al. (1968) reviewed 209 instances of atresia or stenosis of the bowel, and found 22 in the colon, six being of Bland-Sutton's type I, seven of type II, and eight of type III. One case of stenosis in the sigmoid was recorded. Atresia of the colon has twice been reported in association with Hirschsprung's disease (Haffner and Schistad 1969; Hyde and De Lorimier 1968). This is of some interest, as ischaemic injury has been suggested as a cause of aganglionosis.

8.1.3. Malrotation

Malrotation occurs in complete or incomplete forms. In the latter, the caecum lies across the stomach and duodenum and may cause high intestinal obstruction by external pressure. This abnormality is often accompanied by volvulus, and less commonly by intussusception. Where the bowel

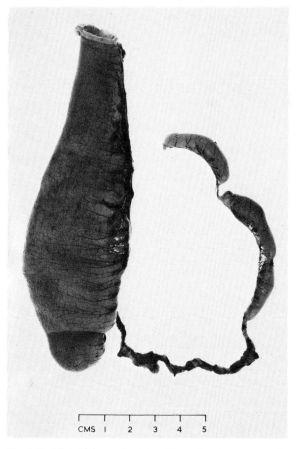

Fig. 6.41. Dilated jejunum leads to a fibrous band and eventually to two further patent segments separated by bands.

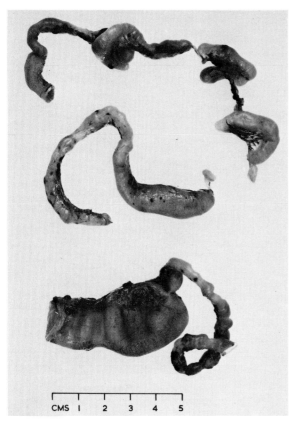

Fig. 6.42. Resections of gut from a case of multiple atresias showing blind ends and fibrous cords connecting patent bowel. A membranous atresia was present in the lowest (proximal) specimen.

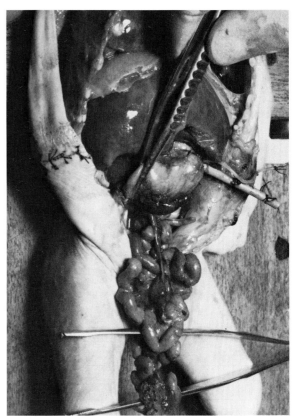

Fig. 6.43. Apple peel or maypole bowel. The intestines coil around the marginal artery, in this case the superior mesenteric.

remains on a single unfixed mesentery rotation around the superior mesenteric artery may occur with volvulus—the 'maypole' bowel syndrome (Fig. 6.43).

8.1.4. Meckel's Diverticulum

Meckel's diverticulum represents a partial persistence of the vitellointestinal duct and is usually found on the antimesenteric border of the ileum, about 1 metre proximal to the ileocaecal valve. It represents a failure of obliteration of the duct when the mid-gut loop returns to the abdomen at 10 weeks' gestation. Other anomalies of duct obliteration are shown in Fig. 6.45; all except Meckel's diverticulum are very rare. Meckel's diverticulum is commoner in males and is a true diverticulum. The lumen is lined with epithelium similar to that of the bowel from which it arises, but areas of gastric mucosa are found in up to 50% of cases, and gastrin-producing cells may be demonstrable (Capron et al. 1977). Most diverticula are symptomless but they may form the apex of an intussusception or be the site of peptic ulceration. Seagram et al. (1968)

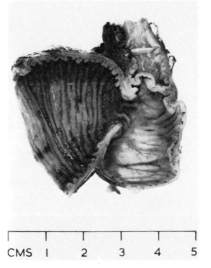

Fig. 6.44. A rare membranous atresia in the large bowel. Ileum to the left, caecum below and right; a membrane obstructs the proximal ascending colon.

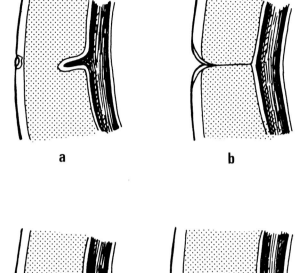

Fig. 6.45. a–d Abnormalities of the vitello-intestinal duct. **a** Meckel's diverticulum; **b** vitelline cord with umbilical sinus; **c** omphalomesenteric cyst; **d** vitelline fistula.

reviewed 218 patients, 81 of whom underwent surgery for complications. Gastric mucosa was found in 64%, pancreatic tissue in 4%, and colonic mucosa in 6%. The diverticulum usually lies free, but it may be attached to the umbilicus by a fibrous cord, in which case volvulus of the small intestine around the cord is an additional hazard.

8.1.5. Segmental Absence of Intestinal Musculature

In segmental absence of intestinal musculature there is an abrupt change from normal bowel wall to complete absence of both muscle coats for a few centimetres. The wall is very thin and the lumen collapsed. It is an uncommon cause of intestinal obstruction in the neonate.

8.1.6. Short Intestine

Congenitally short intestines, usually accompanied by malrotation, have been reported (see Yutani et al. 1973). These cases have no other morphological abnormality; the gut measures 30–45 cm and the affected individuals present with vomiting, diarrhoea, and failure to thrive.

The intestine may be shortened by massive resection, and is reported to be short in mucoviscidosis.

8.2. Malabsorption Syndromes

Malabsorption syndromes in infants and children may be divided into two broad groups: enteropathies of the small intestine, which are disorders characterized by mucosal morphological abnormalities (Table 6.2), and those in which the intestinal mucosa is histologically normal (Table 6.3).

Table 6.2. Causes of malabsorption with histological abnormality of the small intestine

Coeliac disease	
Postenteritic malabsorption	
Giardiasis	
Immunologic deficiency states	
Crohn's disease	(Chrispin and Tempany 1967)
Tropical sprue	(Mathan et al. 1969)
Cows' milk protein intolerance	
Soy protein intolerance	
Histiocytosis	
Dermatitis herpetiformis	
Whipple's disease	(Aust and Smith 1962)
A-β-Lipoproteinaemia	(Lloyd 1972)

Small-intestinal enteropathy sometimes present
Malnutrition
Iron-deficiency anaemia

Table 6.3. Causes of malabsorption without intestinal mucosal abnormality

Fibrocystic disease		
Short intestine:	Post-resection	
	Congenital	
Enzyme defects		(Holzel 1967)
Emotional deprivation		(Patten and Gardner 1962)
Malrotation		(Burke and Anderson 1966)
Pancreatic achylia and neutropenia		(Shmerling et al. 1969)
Endocrine:	Ganglioneuroma	(Rosenstein and Engelman 1963)
	Hypoparathyroidism	(Stickler et al. 1965)

8.2.1. Normal Intestinal Appearances

The villous pattern of the small intestine in infants and children differs from that in adults. This was first described by Chacko et al. (1960) in Indian children, but is probably a universal finding. In infants short ridges and leaf-like villi are commonplace (Fig. 6.46) but are covered by normal columnar epithelium, and in children a mixture of leaf-like and finger-like villi is usually present, with occasional short ridges (Fig. 6.47), in marked contrast to the mucosal appearance of the adult where finger-like villi predominate. The immature sterological appearance is reflected in the reduced surface: volume ratio of the mucosa in infants (Risdon and Keeling 1974). This normal variation in villous pattern in children may be responsible for some of the 'abnormalities' of the small intestine described in conditions such as iron-deficiency anaemia and malnutrition, particularly where minor abnormalities are described.

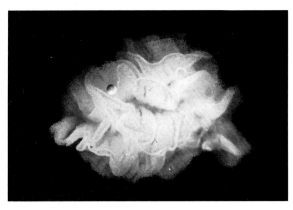

Fig. 6.46. Jejunal biopsy from an 18-month-old infant presenting with failure to thrive. Leaf-like villi and short ridges predominate but are narrow in cross-section. The epithelium was entirely normal.

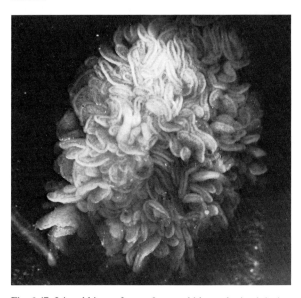

Fig. 6.47. Jejunal biopsy from a 9-year-old boy, obtained during the investigation of short stature; normal surface epithelium.

Jejunal biopsies are fragile and easily distorted during processing, and will repay very careful handling. If possible they should be brought to the laboratory in the biopsy capsule and removed from it by the pathologist with a needle or ophthalmic forceps. Orientation during blocking-out is easier if the biopsy is placed mucosal surface upwards on a piece of stiff paper or card. It will adhere firmly in seconds. Black French art paper is particularly suitable, as it provides good contrast for both dissecting microscopic examination and photography and its rough surface makes detachment during fixation less likely. The villous pattern is often easier to see if the biopsy is examined under fluid. Formol–saline is suitable for routine purposes and prevents autolysis of the specimen if dissecting microscopic examination is prolonged, although normal saline can be substituted if the part of the specimen is required for enzyme assay. It is not necessary to immerse the specimen and its mount in a large quantity of fluid; pipetting fluid dropwise onto the biopsy to form a large blob can provide sufficient fluid to float out the villi.

After fixation, a large biopsy can be bisected with a scapel but still left attached to the paper during processing, as this aids orientation at the blocking-out stage. Biopsies are sectioned at right angles to the luminal surface. It is convenient to have a short ribbon of sections mounted on the same slide and stained with haematoxylin/eosin and periodic acid Schiff with a nuclear stain. Common artifacts in jejunal biopsies are oblique cutting, which will produce spurious shortening of villi and stretching of the biopsy prior to fixation—particularly easy to do if the biopsy is superficial and does not include the muscularis mucosae for most of the length of the biopsy, as often happens when an 'infant' biopsy capsule is used. When this happens the villi are usually triangular in cross section, often with a tapering apical portion.

Siting of the biopsy is important, as duodenal villi are shorter than those of the jejunum, and minor villous shortening in a biopsy obtained without fluoroscopical monitoring should be viewed with caution.

The presence of lymphoid aggregates within the mucosa may give rise to local loss of villous pattern, whose cause is readily apparent in the section, and may produce an abnormality on dissecting microscopic examination (Fig. 6.48).

8.2.2. Coeliac Disease

Coeliac disease is a permanent intolerance to dietary gluten, producing a proximal small-intestinal enteropathy leading to malabsorption, with clinical

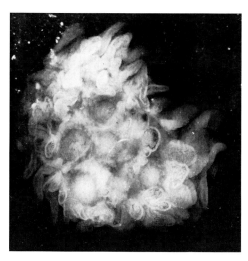

Fig. 6.48. Biopsy from a 5-year-old boy. The group of circles seen in the biopsy is produced by localized loss of villi where the mucosa is stretched over lymphoid aggregates in the submucosa.

and biochemical abnormalities; gluten withdrawal results in complete clinical remission and a histologically normal small-intestine mucosa.

This condition was first described in children by Samuel Gee (1888), but it was not until 1950 that Dicke identified gluten, the germ protein of wheat, rye, and other cereals, as the causal agent and demonstrated that its exclusion from the diet resulted in clinical remission. Subsequent investigations have shown that the most toxic component is a polypeptide with a molecular weight less than 15 000 in the α-gliadin fraction of gluten (Dissanayake et al. 1974).

Despite the precise identification of the toxic factor, the mechanism by which it produces mucosal damage is not certain. It has been suggested that a specific mucosal peptidase deficiency results in the intracellular accumulation of a toxic peptide, leading to epithelial cell damage and mucosal abnormality. Although dipeptidase deficiency has been demonstrated in coeliac disease with return to normal after the institution of a gluten-free diet (Douglas and Peters (1970), this may be the result rather than the cause of epithelial abnormality, and a parallel may be drawn with the mucosal disaccharidase deficiency demonstrable in untreated coeliac disease.

More recently, a variety of immunological abnormalities have been demonstrated in patients with coeliac disease, including elevated levels of immunoglobulins to dietary proteins and reticulin with elevations of IgA and reduction in IgC and IgM

levels (Kendrick and Walker-Smith 1970). Increased numbers of immunoglobulin-containing cells have been demonstrated in the lamina propria of the small intestine in untreated coeliac disease (Lancaster-Smith et al. 1974) and immune complexes in the basement membrane and lamina propria of the small intestine (Shiner and Ballard 1973). Doe et al. (1974) have demonstrated immune complexes in the serum following gluten challenge in treated coeliacs, and Carswell and Logan (1973) found low levels of β 1c and β 1a globulin in untreated coeliacs. They suggest that an Arthus-type reaction occurs in the lamina propria.

It is not clear whether the immunological abnormalities described are the result of the primary abnormality or whether they represent a secondary reaction to the toxic α-gliadin fraction.

Coeliac disease occurs in all areas where gluten is ingested. Its prevalence is unclear, particularly with the demonstration of symptomless cases in family studies where intestinal biopsies have been performed. Incidence estimates in the British Isles vary from 1:3000 births in England (Carter et al. 1957) to 1:1100 in Glasgow (McNeish et al. 1973) and 1:300 (Myotte et al. 1973) in West Ireland.

The familial occurrence of coeliac disease is well recognized, but the discordance of monozygotic twins for coeliac disease argues against a simple Mendelian inheritance (McNeish and Nelson 1974). A positive correlation between coeliac disease and the possession of histocompatibility antigens H-La1 and 8l) has been demonstrated (McNeish et al. 1973). These findings make a polygenic basis for susceptibility to environmental factors more likely. The HLA status may explain the correlation between coeliac disease and diabetes.

The small-intestine mucosal abnormality in coeliac disease has been demonstrated at laparotomy (Paulley 1954) and confirmed by peroral biopsy (Sakula and Shiner 1957). Dissecting microscopy shows replacement of normal villi (Fig. 6.49) by a 'cobblestone' appearance of the mucosa in which the mouths of crypts are seen (Fig. 6.50). Histological examination shows a 'flat' biopsy (Fig. 6.51). The surface epithelium is abnormal. The normal columnar epithelium, with its nuclei arranged at the base of the cell adjacent to the basement membrane, has been lost and is replaced by cuboidal epithelium with haphazard nuclear arrangement, often accompanied by infiltration of the epithelium by small, darkly staining, round cells, and patchy thickening of the basement membrane may be demonstrated by PAS staining. There is an increase in round cells, particularly plasma cells, in the lamina propria.

It was thought initially that this appearance was pathognomonic for coeliac disease, but it has since been shown that the same appearance may be

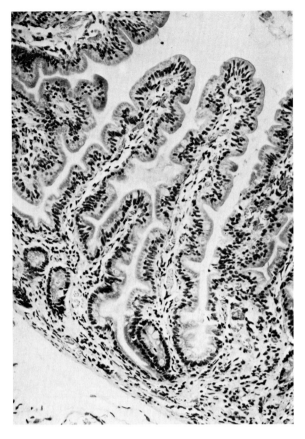

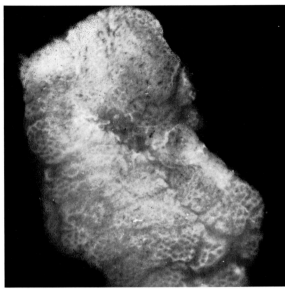

Fig. 6.50. (*top*) Jejunal biopsy from a 5-year-old boy who presented with bulky, offensive stools, anorexia, and poor weight gain. Villi are absent and the mouths of the crypts and the cobblestone appearance of the mucosa are seen.

Fig. 6.49. (*left*) Normal jejunal mucosa. Slender, tapering villi are covered by columnar epithelium with the nuclei of the epithelial cells arranged regularly along the basement membrane. A few round cells are seen in the lamina propria.

produced in infants by infective enteritis (Barnes and Townley 1973), and less commonly by cow's milk protein or soy protein intolerance and tropical sprue.

The diagnosis of coeliac disease, with its implication of permanent gluten intolerance requiring life-long adherence to a gluten-free diet, must leave no room for doubt. This is particularly important following the suggestion that a gluten-free diet may reduce the risk of intestinal neoplasia, to which untreated coeliacs are susceptible (Holmes et al. 1976), and because the return to a normal diet in older children or adults may not be accompanied by clinical symptoms or signs although the small intestinal mucosa becomes abnormal. After confirming the diagnosis by intestinal biopsy and the institution of a gluten-free diet for at least 2 years, or perhaps longer in very young children, a further biopsy should be obtained whilst the individual is on a gluten-free diet (Fig. 6.52a and b). Gluten should then be reintroduced (either as food or as pure, powdered gluten) into the diet. A further biopsy should be obtained after 3 months, unless symptoms precipitate the need to biopsy sooner. Most children with coeliac disease will have mucosal abnormalities (Fig. 6.53) but will not necessarily yield a flat biopsy

at this time (Packer et al. 1978). If the biopsy is normal, then a further biopsy should be obtained after 2 years on a gluten-containing diet. Children who still have a normal biopsy at this time are unlikely to have coeliac disease, although an occasional child may take longer than this to produce mucosal abnormalities (Egan-Mitchell et al. 1977).

Children with coeliac disease always have a flat biopsy at presentation provided that dietary manipulations have not been instituted before the biopsy is taken. The finding of less severe biopsy changes (degrees of partial villous atrophy) is so uncharacteristic in childhood that one should consider an alternative diagnosis.

Most children present at under 2 years of age, and although the interval between the introduction of cereals and development of symptoms is variable, most are symptomatic within 6 months. Because of the practice of very early introduction of cereals into the diet some infants present before 4 months; this group develop symptoms faster and may have an acute onset with diarrhoea and vomiting and be severely ill (Burke et al. 1965). The classic picture is of a miserable, anorexic toddler with distended abdomen, wasted buttocks, and abnormal bulky stools. Older children present with short stature and iron-deficiency anaemia; they may have no gastro-intestinal symptoms.

8.3. Infective Enteritis

Both bacterial and viral enteritis produce mucosal changes in the small intestine. These have been demonstrated by peroral biopsy in the acute stage, in a study (Barnes and Townley 1973) in which abnormalities were found in 25 of 31 infants. In five cases the biopsy was flat, and the others showed minor abnormalities and cellular infiltration of the lamina propria. The intestinal abnormalities, according to the findings of necropsy studies, are usually confined to the duodenum and jejunum, but the whole of the small intestine may be involved; there is often patchy involvement of the mucosa (Walker-Smith 1972).

Diarrhoea is often prolonged following infective enteritis in infancy, because of disaccharidase deficiency induced by mucosal damage. The mucosal abnormalities may also persist for many months and may be indistinguishable from those of coeliac disease. This has probably contributed to the concept that coeliac disease can be a self-limiting condition and makes gluten challenge mandatory in the diagnosis of coeliac disease.

8.4. Cow's Milk Protein Intolerance

Intolerance of cow's milk is an uncommon cause of diarrhoea and vomiting in infancy, and usually resolves spontaneously at around 2 years of age. It is important to the pathologist only in that histological abnormalities of the small intestine have been recorded in a few instances in this condition. Freir and Kletter (1972) have described shortening of villi with inflammatory cell infiltration and surface epithelial changes, but the mucosa is rarely completely flat.

8.5. Soy Protein Intolerance

Intolerance to soy protein, with small-intestine biopsy evidence of an enteropathy indistinguishable from coeliac disease, has been described by Ament and Rubin (1972). This may become more common with the increasing use of soy protein-based infant foods.

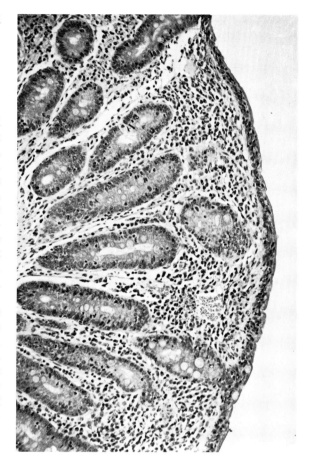

Fig. 6.51. Flat small intestinal biopsy. Villi have disappeared and the surface epithelium is no longer normal. The epithelial cell height is reduced and nuclei are irregularly sited within the cell. There is an apparent increase of inflammatory cells within the lamina propria.

8.6. Giardiasis

Gut infestation with *Giardia lamblia* can produce a variety of symptoms, from mild diarrhoea to a frank malabsorptive picture. Poor social conditions, institutionalization, a recent holiday abroad, or symptoms referable to immunological deficiency may be useful pointers in the history of such children.

Diagnosis is usually made by the demonstration of cysts in the stools or motile forms of the organism in duodenal juice, but parasites may be demonstrable in small-intestinal biopsies.

The histological features of the biopsy are shortening of the villi (occasionally a completely flat mucosa is seen but usually less severe degrees of villous atrophy are present [Fig. 6.54]), in-flammatory cell infiltration of the lamina propria,

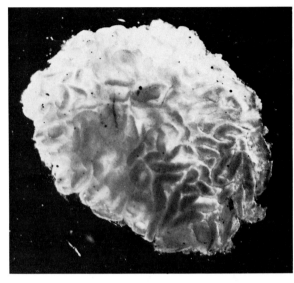

Fig. 6.53. Biopsy from an 11-year-old girl, on GFD for 10 years, after 9 weeks on a normal diet. Thick ridges are seen throughout the biopsy; mild irregularities of surface epithelium were seen on histological examination. A biopsy taken after a further 5 weeks was completely flat.

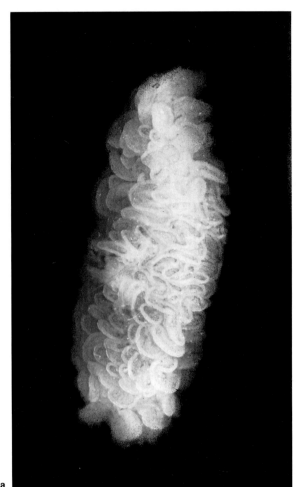

a

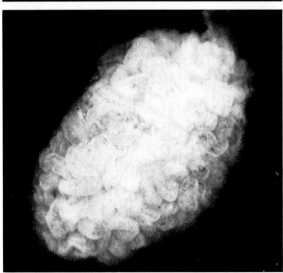

b

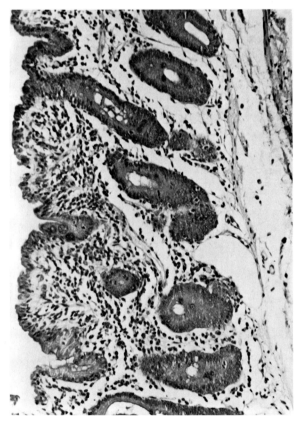

Fig. 6.52. a and **b** Biopsies from a 5-year-old girl who had been on a gluten-free diet (GFD) for 4 years. **a** Jejunal biopsy whilst on GFD; surface epithelium appeared normal; **b** Biopsy performed after 10 weeks on a diet containing at least 10 g natural gluten per day; the patient became anorexic and miserable. Short, thick ridges predominate. The surface epithelium was irregular.

Fig. 6.54. Gardiasis. Biopsy from a 7-year-old institutionalized boy with Down's syndrome, being investigated for diarrhoea. Villi are reduced in height and much thicker than normal. There is increased cellularity of the lamina propria. (H/PAS; 240 ×)

and shortening and irregularity of the surface epithelium (Fig. 6.55).

Infestation with *Giardia lamblia* is common in immune-deficiency states (Zinnemann and Kaplan 1972), and may be the cause of intestinal abnormalities reported as complications of immune-deficiency disorders. It has also been demonstrated in 24% of 58 coeliac patients by Carswell et al. (1973), but we have not encountered such a high rate of infestation in coeliac disease.

8.7. Histiocytosis X

Diarrhoea has been reported complicating histiocytosis X. Infiltration of the lamina propria and submucosa by abnormal histiocytes, including multinucleate forms, has been described. The infiltration is usually confined to the ileum, although duodenum and jejunum may be involved (Keeling and Harris 1973); in this case the normal villous pattern is lost (Fig. 6.56), although the surface epithelium remains normal. It seems likely that the diarrhoea is due to a combination of loss of absorptive area and interference with lymphatic drainage by the neoplastic proliferation.

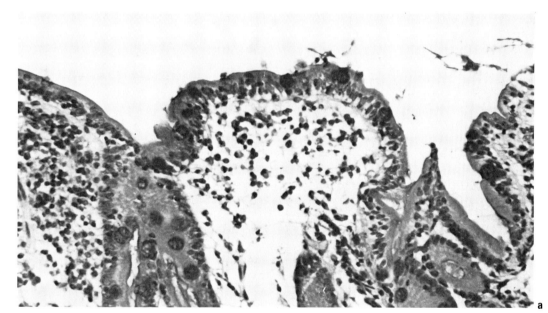

a

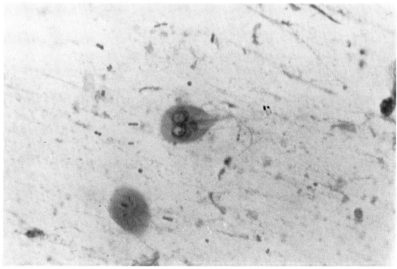

b

Fig. 6.55. a Same case as in Fig. 7.9. The surface epithelium is abnormal. *Giardia lamblia* are attached to the surface epithelium and lying free in the lumen. (H/PAS; 400 ×) **b** *Giardia lamblia* in duodenal aspirate. (Papanicolou; 1500 ×)

8.8. Iron-deficiency Anaemia

There is considerable variation in the severity of functional and histological abnormalities of the small intestine that are attributed to iron deficiency. Reports from Britain describe mild or equivocal histological changes (Doniach and Shier 1957; Cameron et al. 1962). Other authors report more severe abnormalities of villous pattern (Naiman et al. 1964; Berkel et al. 1970), with normal surface epithelium. Flat biopsies have been reported in iron deficiency in Indian children (Guga et al. 1968). Intestinal parasitic infestation was excluded by three stool examinations and a concentration procedure, and although clinical improvement was recorded in response to iron therapy, follow-up biopsies were not obtained. In the authors' experience of British children, those with iron-deficiency anaemia and a flat biopsy have responded to a gluten-free diet and not required iron supplements.

8.9. Malnutrition

Intestinal mucosal abnormalities, varying from minor abnormalities of the villous pattern accompanied by a normal surface epithelium to severe partial or subtotal villous atrophy, have been reported in kwashiorkor (Stanfield et al. 1965). These authors report persistence of mucosal abnormalities despite a return to normal nutritional status, a finding that might cast doubt on the implied causal relationship. The frequency of infective diarrhoea in areas where severe malnutrition is most common should not be overlooked.

8.10. Resection of Small Intestine

The common causes of massive resection of small intestine in infancy are volvulus complicating malrotation or some other congenital anomaly, or multiple small intestinal atresias. Successful adaptation of the remaining intestine depends on the extent and site of the resection. Hypertrophy of villi in residual ileum in animals has been described after jejunal resection, but little change occurred in the jejunum when the ileum was removed (Dowling and Booth 1967). Resection of large amounts of ileum may interrupt the enteropathic circulation of bile salts and so influence absorption. Resection of the ileocaecal valve may result in bacterial contamination of the small intestine resulting in a 'blind loop' syndrome. Valman (1976) followed up children who had undergone extensive intestinal resection in the neonatal period and found that they were shorter than their siblings, but of appropriate weight for their own height, a result of prolonged postoperative malnutrition that did not persist into later life. However, Valman and Roberts (1974) demonstrated vitamin B_{12} malabsorption following ileal resection in infancy, and showed that although serum levels of the vitamin remained normal in the face of malabsorption for some years, puberty was a critical time when supplementation might be required.

8.11. Necrotizing Enterocolitis

The 1960s saw publication of a number of reports of intestinal perforation, usually colonic, complicating

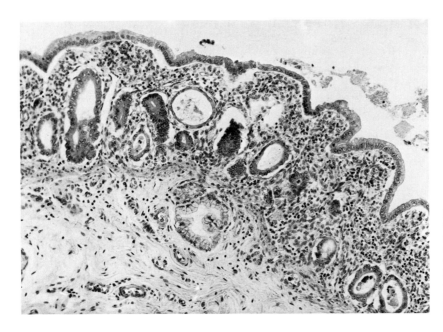

Fig. 6.56. Small intestine of infant with skin rash, hepatosplenomegaly, lymphadenopathy, and diarrhoea. She died aged 15 weeks with disseminated histiocytosis X. Small intestine shows loss of villi with infiltration of the lamina propria by abnormal histiocytes. The surface epithelium is normal.

exchange transfusion for rhesus incompatibility or umbilical venous catheterization for other reasons (Corkery et al. 1968; Orme and Eades 1968). Since then, with the marked decrease in the number of exchange transfusions performed in neonatal nurseries, necrotizing enterocolitis is usually seen in the very small, sick, preterm neonate, and both small and large intestine are involved. More recently, necrotizing enterocolitis has been described in term neonates after cardiac catheterization and angiography during investigation for congenital heart disease and the use of hypertonic contrast medium has been implicated in its pathogenesis (Cooke et al. 1980). Epidemics of necrotizing enterocolitis in full-term neonates associated with the isolation of Salmonella sp. (Stein et al. 1972) and *Clostridium butyricum* (Howard et al. 1977) have been reported, but most cases are sporadic and only normal gut flora are cultured from the stools.

The syndrome is a major cause of death in premature and newborn infants. Three general aetiological factors have been implicated: mucosal ischaemia; a gut flora that contains organisms which invade the damaged area; and feeding that enhances bacterial growth (Book et al. 1976).

Prophylaxis with kanamycin alters bacterial flora, but does not prevent the disease (Boyle et al. 1978), which may also follow ampicillin therapy in childhood (Auritt et al. 1978). Vascular factors may be of the greater significance in aetiology, and it has been suggested that the various factors that predispose to the condition (birth asphyxia, birth trauma, cyanotic heart disease, exchange transfusion, disseminated intravascular coagulation, etc.) all produce a selective ischaemia of the gut, which develops as a 'protective' mechanism for the rest of the circulation, e.g., brain or heart (Lloyd 1969).

The disease usually presents with ileus and abdominal distention after a period of bloody diarrhoea. Circulatory collapse is common (Fig. 6.57). The length of bowel involved is variable but the terminal ileum and ascending colon are almost always involved. The affected portion of bowel is distended and plum-coloured, with a friable wall. When it is opened, the often green-stained mucosa can be wiped off the muscularis. Perforation may occur.

The pathological findings are related to the age of the lesions. The earliest findings are irregularly shaped and sized areas of haemorrhagic infarction of the mucosa and submucosa, with variable deep extension to involve the muscularis propria and serosa (Fig. 6.58). They are usually between 0.5 and 2 cm in diameter and frequently multiple; it is rare for them to be circumferential.

The central part of the lesion may become necrotic, grey in colour with a surrounding hyperaemic halo (Fig. 6.59). The necrotic portion of the bowel may bulge above the serosal surface and perforation may occur. Generalized peritonitis with fibrin deposition on the serosal surface of dilated loops of bowel and free pus in the peritoneal cavity may then supervene or may be localized, depending on the site of perforation.

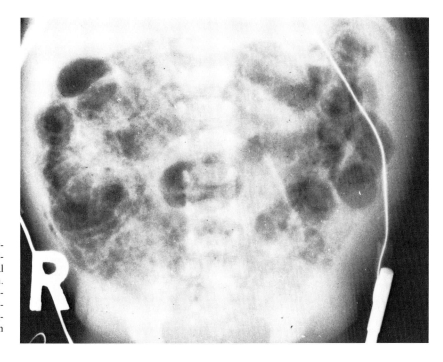

Fig. 6.57. X-ray picture of 5-day-old infant born at 36 weeks' gestation by emergency LSCS for fetal distress; asphyxiated at birth. Bloody stools and abdominal distension at 4 days. X-ray shows abdominal distention and double contour of intestinal wall due to gas in the submucosa.

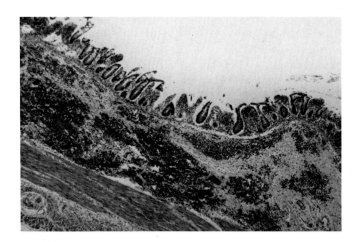

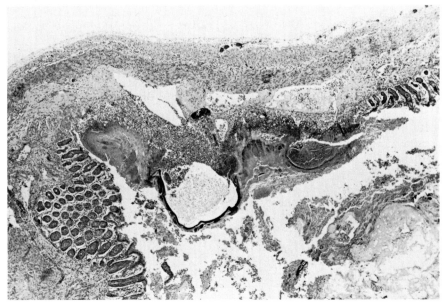

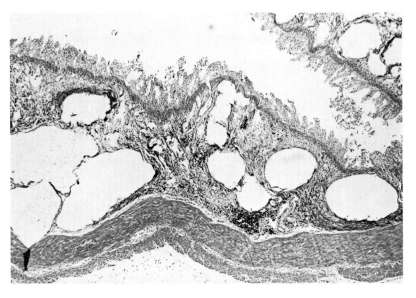

Fig. 6.58. (*top*) Early stages of enterocolitis with haemorrhage and infarction of mucosa. (H and E; 40 ×)

Fig. 6.59. (*centre*) Patchy infarction has been followed by gas formation and calcification. (H and E; 40 ×)

Fig. 6.60. (*bottom*) Typical multiple gas bubbles in enterocolitis. (H and E; 36 ×)

Once necrosis of the mucosa has occurred, gas may enter the bowel wall and it often spreads in the loose-textured submucosa (Fig. 6.60) but may be present beneath the serosa. Hepatic necrosis with gas-filled cyst formation may occasionally occur. As a late sequel stricture-producing obstruction and even atresia of the intestine may occur (see also p. 252).

8.12. Massive Intestinal Infarction

Massive infarction of the intestine may occasionally follow umbilical arterial catheterization in the neonate when complicated by aortic thrombosis. This complication usually occurs in very small, preterm infants whose condition necessitates prolonged catheterization, but this is not always the case.

8.13. Hirschsprung's Disease

Around 3% of the cases of Hirschsprung's disease seen at the Hospital for Sick Children, Great Ormond Street, have involved the ileum, while in 1% the disease has extended proximally to the duodenum. The extensive intestinal resection necessary in these children can prove fatal or interfere with normal growth and nutrition.

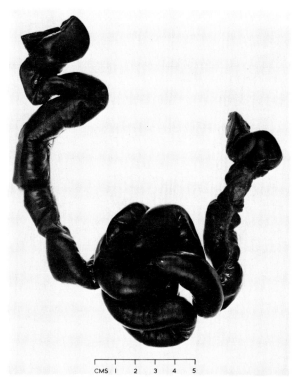

Fig. 6.61. Extensive resection of small bowel following volvulus in an infant. This was followed by malabsorption.

8.14. Volvulus

Intestinal volvulus occurs less commonly in the small intestine than in the colon, and usually affects the ileum. Abnormalities of mesenteric attachment, or of gut rotation, are important predisposing causes, as are enteric duplications (Howaniety et al. 1968). Extensive resection may lead to malabsorption (Fig. 6.61). Volvulus of the small intestine due to massive loading with Ascaris lumbricoides has been reported (Manhani and Sing 1967).

8.15. Perforation

Spontaneous perforation of the small intestine in infancy is rare, and usually complicates infarction of the bowel from any cause, or occurs in association with meconium ileus.

In recent years perforation has been associated with exchange transfusion and prolonged parenteral therapy via the umbilical veins, often appearing as part of the syndrome of enterocolitis.

8.16. Polypi

Solitary hamartomatous polypi are seen occasionally in the jejunum. They have a delicate branching structure with smooth muscle in the stroma and are covered by normal epithelium. They may occur as part of the Peutz–Jeghers syndrome (Figs. 6.62 and 6.63).

Such polypi can cause haemorrhage or intussusception; they are hamartomas and not adenomatous polypi. They do not undergo malignant change, although isolated reports of this complication exist.

8.17. Tuberculosis

Tuberculosis of the gastrointestinal tract has become progressively less common in Europe following the introduction of effective cattle control methods and treatment of milk. It is still seen commonly in the Indian subcontinent and in Africa.

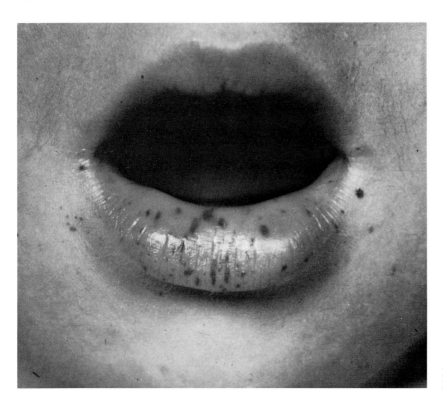

Fig. 6.62. Pigmentation around the lips in the Peutz–Jeghers syndrome.

8.18. Intussusception

Intussusception is the invagination of one portion of bowel into another. Once the invagination has started, it is carried further along the bowel lumen by peristalsis. The effects of intussusception are obstruction of the intestinal lumen, vascular occlusion resulting in gangrene, perforation, peritonitis, and adhesions between the two serosal surfaces, which are in apposition. Between 60% and 85% of intussusceptions occur in the first 2 years of life, and in most of these no definite cause for the intussusception can be found. Most are ileocaecal, the ileocaecal valve having its abundant lymphoid tissue at the apex; thus lymphoid hypertrophy is often advanced as a causative factor. Boys outnumber girls by 2:1 (Bjarnason and Petterson 1968).

In older children a predisposing cause is usually present, a Meckel's diverticulum, a polyp, or a tumour being found at the apex of the intussusceptum. We have seen lymphosarcoma of the small intestine presenting as an irreducible intussusception; Riker and Goldstein (1968) report a similar experience.

Stevenson et al. (1967) and McGovern and Gross (1968) reported intussusception in the postoperative period as a complication of a variety of operative procedures, the majority of which were intra-abdominal.

8.19. Haemangiomas

Haemorrhage from intestinal vascular abnormalities may be a cause of severe anaemia and ill health in childhood. Kaijser (1936) has classified these lesions into four groups:

1) Multiple phlebectasia. Varicose lesions—dilated veins in the submucosa. These are probably acquired and do not occur in childhood.

2) Cavernous haemangiomas, which may be diffuse or circumscribed

3) Capillary haemangiomas

4) Gastrointestinal haemangiomas associated with cutaneous lesions.

Haemangiomas of the small intestine are often multiple and may accompany angiomas in other organs. They are associated with thrombocytopenia as part of the Kippel–Trenaunay syndrome (Kuffer et al. 1968). The angiomas are usually confined to the submucosa and present as recurrent intestinal bleeding (Nader and Morgolin 1966), but may extend through to the peritoneal surface, causing intestinal obstruction following multiple adhesions. Useful reports are those of Rissier (1960) and Nader and Morgolin (1966).

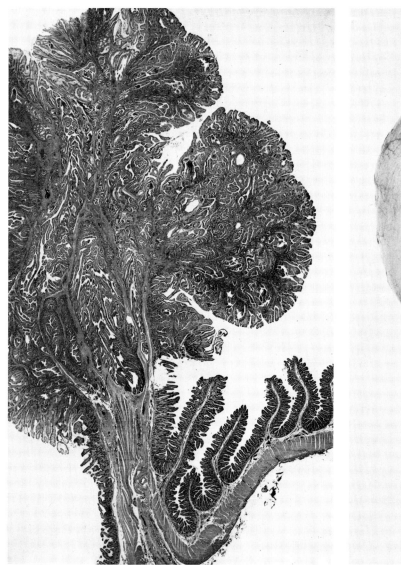

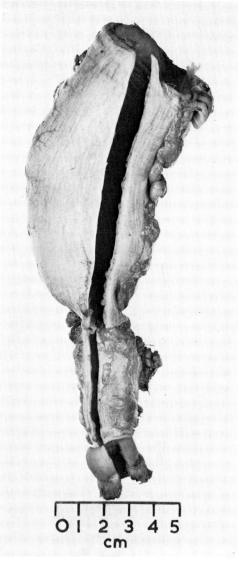

Fig. 6.63. Hamartomatous polyp in the Peutz–Jeghers syndrome. Smooth muscle is seen in the branching stroma.

Fig. 6.64. Short-segment Hirschsprung's disease with dilated segment, cone and narrowed zone. (Male child aged 2 years.)

9. Hirschsprung's Disease

Hirschsprung's disease is named after Hirschsprung, although as with many other eponymously named diseases there are a number of reports that antedate his report of 1887, which described two patients with magacolon. Although aganglionosis in the distal segment of the bowel was recorded only 14 years later by Tittel (1901), it was not until the work of Swenson and Bill in 1948 and Bodian et al. (1949) that the surgical and pathological findings in the disease were widely understood.

The disease develops as a result of failure of the normal craniocaudal migration of neuroblasts forming the myenteric plexus down the gut in weeks 5–12 of gestation. The submucus plexus is formed by migration of cells from the myenteric plexus and is also defective (Okamota and Vea 1967). Hirschsprung's disease occurs at a rate of around 1:2000 live births in England and Wales.

Of 220 cases reviewed by Bodian and Carter (1963), 82% involved the rectum and sigmoid colon (short segment) and 18%, the more proximal portion of the bowel (long segment). Two cases of total aganglionosis of the small bowel were seen; further examples of this form have since been reported (see Walker et al. [1966] for bibliography to that date). In short-segment cases there is a marked proponderance of males (8:1), which is present but less marked in long-segment disease. The proportion of affected siblings in short-segment index cases is in the order of 1 in 20 for brothers and 1 in 100 or lower for sisters. The proportion of affected siblings in long-segment index patients is in the order of 1 in 10 irrespective of sex (Bodian and Carter 1963). There is a marked association with Down's syndrome. Graivier and Sieber (1966) found that 3.4% of reported cases of Hirschsprung's disease occurred in mongols.

The disease generally presents in the neonatal period with intestinal obstruction, although other presentations are seen (Ajayi et al. 1969). There is no association with prematurity or anomalies other than Down's syndrome (Madsen 1964). The mortality rate in infants with this disease has varied from 6% to 43% in various series (see Erenpries 1967), and is related to age at diagnosis (Atwell 1968). In neonates the extent of disease also affects prognosis;

Fraser and Wilkinson (1967) found a mortality of 67% in long-segment disease, compared with 24% in the short segment type.

Pathological appearances vary with the length of the segment and the duration of the disease. Typically there is a dilated hypertrophied segment, a cone, and a narrowed zone (Figs. 6.64 and 6.65). The basic abnormality is the complete absence of ganglion cells from the myenteric, submucosal, and intramucosal plexuses in the affected segment. In the area of the myenteric and submucous plexuses large nonmedullated nerves can be seen (Fig. 6.66). A short transitional zone containing scanty ganglion cells and nerve trunks is generally formed in the junctional area between collapsed and dilated and hypertrophied segments of the bowel. This zone does not correlate with the cone often seen macroscopically. There is no satisfactory explanation as to why the abnormal segment of bowel in Hirschsprung's

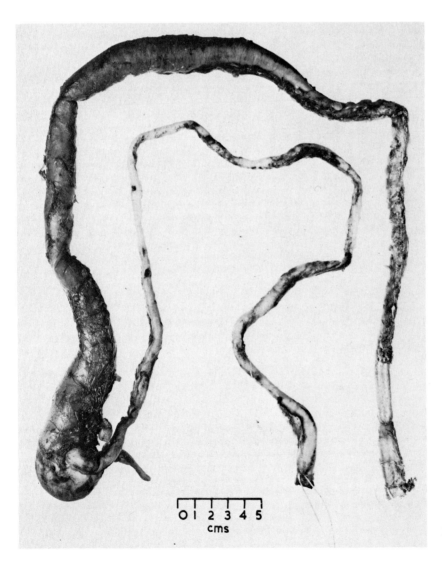

O 1 2 3 4 5
cms

Fig. 6.65. Long-segment disease where the zonation is not marked.

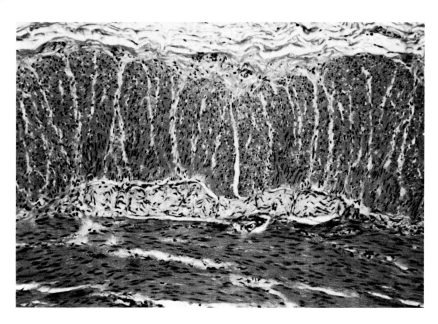

Fig. 6.66. Large nerve trunks in the myenteric plexus in Hirschsprung's disease.

disease is contracted. Absence of ganglion cells should leave the adrenergic system unopposed, with relaxation of the affected segment. The disease can exist in the presence of demonstrable adrenergic innervation. Peptidergic hormones have recently been suggested as a possible cause of contraction.

'Skip' segments, i.e., patchy loss of ganglion cells, were not found in over 300 resected specimens seen at Great Ormond Street, but there are several reports of this form of the disease in the literature (Tiffin et al. 1940; Keefer and Mokrohisky 1954; Perrot and Danon 1935; Lawrence and Van Warner 1961; Chenoweth 1969; Lee 1955; Sprinz et al. 1961). In several of these cases inflammatory changes and fibrosis have been described in the area of the myenteric plexus, suggesting that they may represent an acquired disease. In some reports detailed accounts of blocking techniques are not given, and the present authors remain sceptical about the existence of true skip lesions.

At present the diagnosis of Hirschsprung's disease is made on a combination of symptomatology, colon radiography, rectomanometry, and histological and histochemical findings in rectal biopsies. The abnormalities of formation of the nerve supply of the gut described above are accompanied by a proliferation of parasympathetic nerves (S2 to S4) with many thick acetylcholinesterase-positive fibres in the lamina propria where few fibres are normally found (Fig. 6.67a–c). This forms the basis of a histochemical method that can be used to establish the diagnosis on suction biopsies of the gut (Dobbins and Bill 1965). However, whilst this method is attractive, in the present authors' view it is valuable only if the result is confirmed at operation by full-thickness biopsy demonstrating aganglionosis dur-

ing definitive surgery; unhappily, normal bowel has been resected on the basis of histochemical findings alone.

Histologically the diagnosis depends on the demonstration of an aganglionic segment (see Claireaux 1969). The diagnosis from full-thickness biopsy of the wall, by cryostat or processed-tissue sections, presents little difficulty when longitudinal sections are examined. Rectal submucosal biopsies require careful interpretation because of potential sources of error dependent on the normal anatomy. Hofman and Orestano (1967) and Aldridge and Campbell (1968) have described the normal innervation of the anal canal and rectum in neonates, and Smith (1968), its maturation. It must be remembered that a 'transitional' zone, with scattered ganglion cells and nerve trunks, is seen at about the level of the internal sphincter, and that below this the gut is aganglionic. An area of up to about 1–1.5 cm above the anal valves may contain a few ganglion cells in the myenteric plexus in normal children, and a slightly more distal extension exists in the submucous plexus. In general, a biopsy extending to the inner muscle coat will be satisfactory if taken from at least 1 cm above the anal valves. Such biopsies should be sectioned serially and examined at 10-μm intervals. For suction biopsies a specimen at least 2 mm long from 3 cm above the pectinate line is necessary (Campbell and Noblett 1969).

9.1. Complications

9.1.1. Enterocolitis

Enterocolitis can affect both ileum and colon and is manifest as infarction and necrosis of geographical

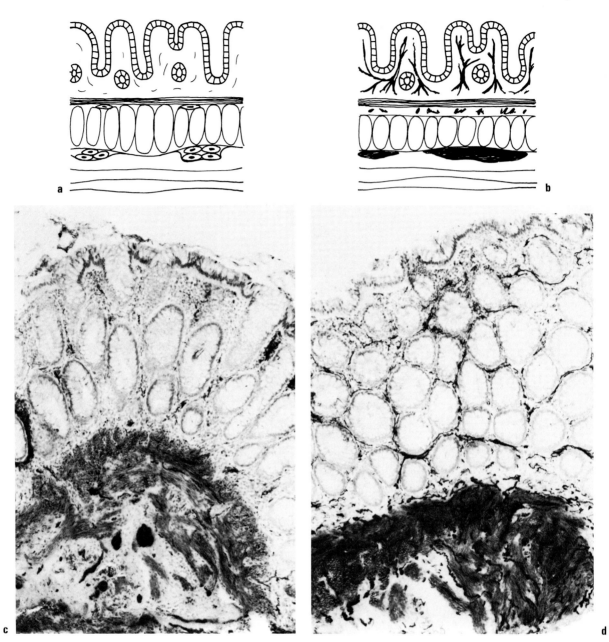

Fig. 6.67. a, b Diagram of the results of acetylcholinesterase staining in normal (**a**) and aganglionic (Hirschsprung's disease; (**b**) bowel.
c Suction rectal biopsy, normal, stained to show acetylcholinesterase activity. Note there are few nerve fibres in the lamina propria and muscularis mucosae. Ganglion cells are clearly shown in the submucosa. (125 ×) **d** Suction rectal biopsy, Hirschsprung's disease, stained to show acetylcholinesterase activity. Note the increased number of nerve fibres in the lamina propria and muscularis mucosae. (125 ×)

areas of mucosa (Figs. 6.68 and 6.69). During life strips of infarcted mucosa may be shed with the stool. Resolution is incomplete and the ulcerated areas are covered with a simple cuboidal epithelium with islets of normal mucosa remaining, giving a pseudopolypoid appearance (Fig. 6.70) (see Berry 1969). This lack of resolution may be accompanied by persistent clinical symptoms and recurrent acute episodes.

Enterocolitis is the most serious single complication of Hirschsprung's disease. Its incidence is apparently related to the length of time elapsing before treatment (Fraser and Berry 1967). The pathogenesis is obscure. The disease is not related to the presence of particular pathogens in the gut, and an allergic vasculitis has been suggested as a possible cause (Berry and Fraser 1968).

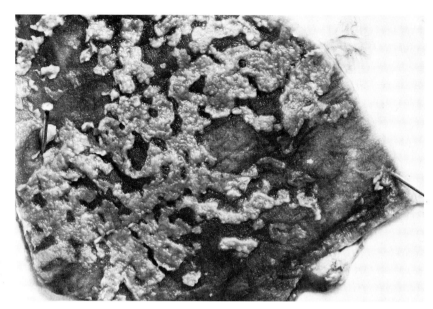

Fig. 6.68. Ileal lesions in entero-colitis associated with Hirsch-sprung's disease. 'Geographical' surviving areas of mucosa are seen.

9.1.2. Perforation

Modern treatment has greatly diminished the incidence of the serious complication of perforation, which can follow stercoral ulceration or local manipulation of inspissated faeces.

9.2. Conditions that may be Confused with Hirschsprung's Disease

In pathological terms, diseases likely to be confused with Hirschsprung's disease are uncommon. 'Ischaemic atrophy' of ganglion cells may occur, and they may be destroyed by Chagas disease (Ehrenpreis et al. 1966). At autopsy, collapsed large bowel below a dilated, apparently obstructed zone may be seen in the 'meconium plug' syndrome (Brennan et al. 1967; Vanheeuwan et al. 1967), and 'microcolon'—a collapse of the large bowel similar to that seen in long-segment disease—may occur in lower-small-bowel atresias. In all these instances histopathological examination resolves the difficulty in diagnosis.

More recently, however, non-Hirschsprung causes of constipation in childhood have been considered by some to form distinct disease entities. It may be that better understanding of local developmental anatomy and a combination of good histological and histochemical studies (see Toorman et al. 1977) will confirm that there are other entities in the diagnostic gap between Hirschsprung's disease and normality, but most studies in which pathological abnormalities are suggested indicate a failure to understand normal development and anatomy rather than Hirschsprung's *forme fruste*. Decreased mobility of the colon may be found

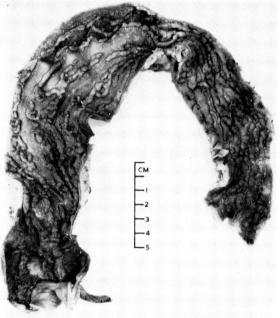

d

Fig. 6.69. Colonic lesion. Death 10 days after onset with some regeneration of surviving mucosa.

in association with gastrointestinal neurofibromatosis as part of the multiple endocrine neoplasia syndrome (Schimke et al. 1968). In some instances, the symptoms mimic Hirschsprung's disease, and the gross findings of megacolon with a cone in the sigmoid have been mistakenly interpreted as signs of this disease, resulting in bowel resection. It cannot be emphasized too strongly that, in the present authors' view, pathological examination by frozen section is necessary in all definitive surgical procedures.

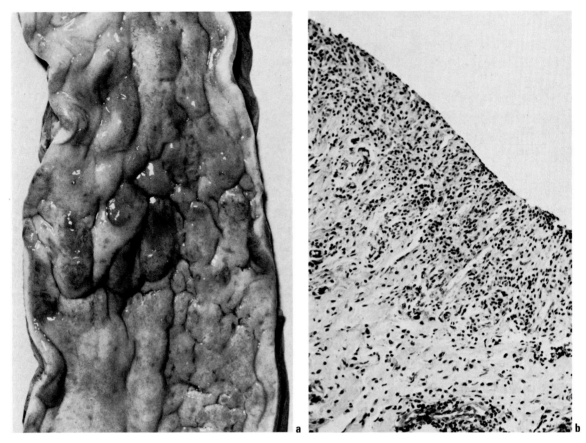

Fig. 6.70. a 'Healed' enterocolitis with irregular mucosa and linear fissuring. **b** Section showing persistent ulcertaion and granulation tissue.

10. Malformations of the Anus and Rectum

Collectively, congenital anal and rectal defects occur with a frequency of around 1 in 5000 live births. They seem to be slightly more common in males, and Weinstein (1965) has described families in which the disease is apparently sex-linked. Cozzi and Wilkinson (1968), examining the records of 133 cases of anorectal anomalies seen at Great Ormond Street, found two instances of the disease in monogygotic twins, three affected siblings, and three surviving unaffected dizygotic twins. Seven index patients had at least one sibling or other relative affected. In six of these the primary lesion was an anal stenosis, although only 16.6% of the defects were of this type. However, other studies have shown poor concordance (see Tünte 1969), and it seems likely that genetic factors are of relatively little significance.

Defects of the region have their origin in events taking place during days 50–60 of development

(Fig. 6.71), and older classifications, e.g., that of Ladd and Cross (1934) were based on a mechanistic interpretation of proposed developmental failures. Thus incomplete disappearance of the anal membrane gives rise to *congenital anal stenosis* (type I); *membranous imperforate anus* (type II) results from persistence of this membrane; and more severe types where the rectum ends blindly above an *imperforate anus* (type III) or the *bulbus analis* fails to develop (type IV), with a blind-ending rectum, were thought to be due to abnormalities of disappearance of the hind-gut or to epidermal/mesodermal induction failures, respectively. In all instances the mesodermally derived external anal sphincter was normal. Relatively recent studies have suggested that this classification is not entirely satisfactory. The work of Bill and Johnson (1953) demonstrated that in the absence of a normal anal orifice the rectum generally communicates with the genitourinary tract or perineum (in 64 of their 70 cases of this type). The mucosal lining of such fistulas and their muscular walls suggest that 'ectopic anus' would be a better descriptive term for these defects, and that they arise

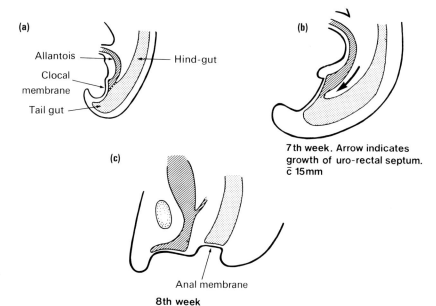

Fig. 6.71. a–c Formation of the urogenital region during the critical stages of development. The urorectal septum fuses with the cloacal membrane at around 16 mm; the anal membrane disappears at approximately 12 weeks' gestation. **a** Week 5 of gestation, approx. 5 mm; **b** Week 7 of gestation, approx. 15 mm. *Arrow* shows growth of urorectal septum; **c** Week 8 of gestation.

through a more complex process than simple failure of a major component of distal gut development: differential anterior perineal growth and altered migration of tissues are also important.

Alternative classifications to that of Ladd and Cross have been reported by Browne (1955) and Partridge and Gough (1961). It is difficult to give accurate figures for the type of defect found in various series, as they are described under different titles. Of 507 anomalies described by Cross (1953) 29 were of type I (congenital anal stenosis), 14 of type II (membranous imperforate anus), 443 of type III, and 21 of type IV. Eighty per cent of the type III anomalies had associated 'fistulas' to the genitourinary tract or perineum, as Bill and Johnson have noted. Partridge and Gough (1961) found 94 cases of types I and II defects, 212 of type III and 5 of type IV. Type III was divided broadly into cases with anorectal agenesis (114) and the so-called ectopic anus (98). Of the 114 cases of anorectal agenesis in this series, 62.3% had multiple congenital abnormalities, but only one of the five cases of type IV defect was accompanied by another defect. Of the 192 cases of 'low' anomaly, 25% had associated malformations.

These findings are of practical importance. In the presence of 'high' defects, other atresias, congenital heart disease and associated genitourinary abnormalities are likely to be found; these have been considered by Smith (1968) and Berdon et al. (1966). Vertebral abnormalities, including sacral agenesis, are also common. Fig. 6.72 illustrates a high agenesis with multiple associated defects.

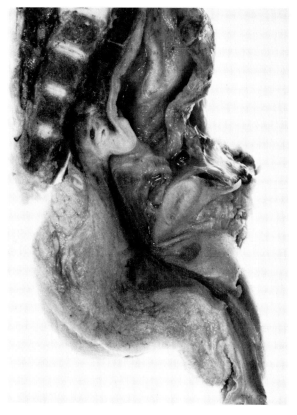

Fig. 6.72. Rectal agenesis. There was associated rectourethral fistula, oesophageal atresia with tracheo-oesophageal fistula, bilateral hydronephrosis and hydroureter, and dextrocardia with patent ductus arteriosus.

A detailed account of the more modern classification (see Table 6.4) may be found in the paper by Santulli et al. (1970), where the various defects are illustrated by line drawings.

10.1. Rectal Prolapse

Rectal prolapse can occur in otherwise normal children during episodes of violent diarrhoea. A distinction is generally made between true prolapse—to which the short, straight, relatively unsupported rectum of children predisposes—and mucosal prolapse, a result of redundancy of the rectal mucosa.

11. Polypoid Lesions of the Large Bowel

Polypoid lesions of the large bowel are not uncommon in childhood. Louw (1968) reviewed 194 cases, the majority of which were single (155) and of the juvenile type. 'Scattered multiple' polyps occurred in 25 cases and in a further 14 instances there was diffuse involvement of the gut by many tumours. Thirteen polyps in the Louw series were inflammatory and four were hamartomatous, being associated with Osler–Weber disease, neurofibromatosis, or the Peutz–Jeghers syndrome. There were

Table. 6.4. Classification of anorectal anomalies

Male	Female
A. Low (translevator)	
1. *At normal anal site*	1. *At normal anal site*
a) Anal stenosis	a) Anal stenosis
b) Covered anus, complete	b) Covered anus, complete
2. *At perineal site*	2. *At perineal site*
a) Anocutaneous fistula (covered anus, incomplete)	a) Anocutaneous fistula (covered anus, incomplete)
b) Anterior perineal anus	b) Anterior perineal anus
	3. *At vulvar site*
	a) Anovulvar fistula
	b) Anovestibular fistula
	c) Vestibular anus
B. Intermediate	
1. *Anal agenesis*	1. *Anal agenesis*
a) Without fistula	a) Without fistula
b) With rectobulbar fistula	b) With fistula
	1) Rectovestibula
	2) Rectovaginal, low
2. *Anorectal stenosis*	2. *Anorectal stenosis*
C. High (supralevator)	
1. *Anorectal agenesis*	1. *Anorectal agenesis*
a) Without fistula	a) Without fistula
b) With fistula	b) With fistula
1) Rectourethral	1) Rectovaginal, high
2) Rectovesical	2) Rectocloacal
	3) Rectovesical
2. *Rectal atresia*	2. *Rectal atresia*
D. Miscellaneous	
Imperforate anal membrane	
Cloacal exstrophy	

five lymphoid polyps. This pattern of lesions is typical of most large series (see also Shapiro 1950).

Presentation occurs most frequently between the ages of 3 and 6 years, usually with painless rectal bleeding, occasionally with passage of the polyp. When diffuse bowel involvement is excluded more than 80% of polyps are found to be in the sigmoid colon or rectum, and prolapse of the mass per rectum occurs in a significant number of cases.

The majority of childhood colonic polyps are of the *juvenile type*. These are usually single, although two or three lesions may be present. They are roughly spherical and appear reddened when compared with surrounding mucosa. They are usually about 1–2 cm in diameter, pedunculated, and smooth-surfaced, and show a distinctly cystic cut surface.

Microscopically there is a single layer of epithelium overlying an abundant, often lymphocyte-infiltrated, stromal core. Glands extend into this and are often obstructed, with the formation of large mucus lakes (Fig. 6.73). The muscularis mucosa is not included in the tumour, which may facilitate their autoamputation. Other secondary changes include ulceration of the thin epithelium with infection of the core.

The lesions may occur in a multiple form as juvenile polyposis coli in families in which adenomatous polyposis also occurs. Veale et al. (1966) have suggested that these probably hamartomatous polyps occur within the adenomatous polyposis genotype, its action being modified by a gene from a normal parent. There is no evidence that juvenile polyposis coli is associated with later colonic malignancy.

11.1. Adenomatous Polyps

Adenomatous lesions probably begin as areas of proliferation in the crypts of the large-bowel mucosa. The upward movement of the mass so formed pulls a number of mucosal components with it, often resulting in a poorly defined or absent stalk.

The surface is often lobulated, with intercommunicating cracks separating the lobules (Fig. 6.74). The tubules of hyperplastic epithelium are closely packed; there is no increase in interstitial tissue and no tendency to cyst formation. Few goblet cells are seen, and there may be nuclear hyperchromatism in epithelial cells. The stroma may contain a few smooth muscle cells.

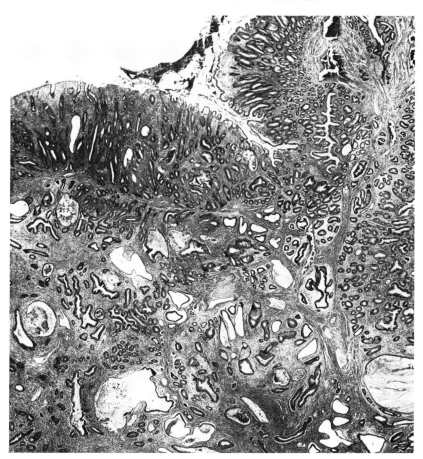

Fig. 6.73. Adenomatous colonic polyp. (H and E; 20 ×)

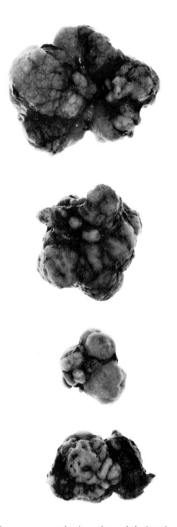

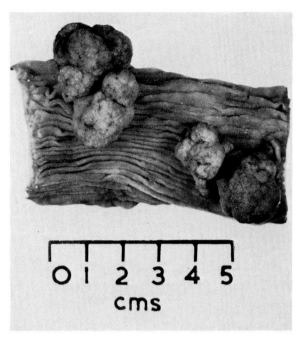

Fig. 6.75. Adenomatous polyps in segment of colon from a 7-year-old boy.

Fig. 6.74. Adenomatous colonic polyps; lobulated surfaces are clearly seen. (2 ×)

These lesions are rare as isolated findings in infancy, but are found in familial polyposis coli. In this disease, although tumours may appear in younger individuals (Fig. 6.75), most develop after the age of 15 years (Fig. 6.76), with death from associated adenocarcinoma of the large bowel occurring at around 40 years of age. However, juvenile forms are reported and adenocarcinoma of the rectum has occurred in a 12-year-old girl with this disease (Gross 1953).

From a number of studies it is apparent that the disease can be attributed to an autosomal dominant gene with high penetrance and variable expression (i.e., early- and late-onset polyposis coli, juvenile polyposis coli). Other associated connective tissue tumours may occur: osteomas, fibromas, dermoid tumours, lipomas, and leiomyomas have all been described (see Gardner and Richards 1953; Gardner 1962).

The polyps often present with blood loss as the major clinical problem, although other gastrointestinal complaints are common. However, the greatest danger to the individual is the premature development of adenocarcinoma of the colon, which may arise in the mucosa away from the polyps, and is frequently multicentric.

The important early studies of this disease from St Marks Hospital were reported by Dukes (1958).

11.2. Hamartomatous Polyps

Polyps associated with the Peutz–Jeghers syndrome commonly occur in the colon as well as the small bowel (p. 245). Although adenocarcinoma of the bowel has been reported in this condition some doubts remain about diagnosis since no patient has died of the disease.

11.3. Lymphoid Polyps

Corne (1961) reported on a series of 100 lymphoid polyps, six of which occurred in the first decade, with a further ten occurring in the second. A case of apparently familial lymphoid polyposis has also been recorded (Cosens 1958).

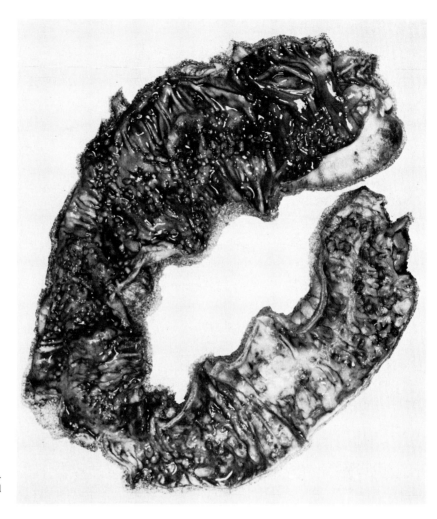

Fig. 6.76. Colon from a case of familial polyposis coli in a 12-year-old boy. Numerous polyps are seen.

12. Appendix

12.1. Congenital anomalies

12.1.1. Absence

Absence of the appendix is a rare anomaly, some 80 cases having been reported in the world literature. It is obviously compatible with a long and healthy existence: Manoil (1957) reported a case in a 90-year-old man. In the case reported by Robinson (1951) a 12×10 mm patch of lymphoid tissue was present in the caecal wall at the customary site of the appendiceal orifice.

12.1.2. Duplication

Duplication of the appendix was classified by Cave (1936) as partial duplication of the appendix alone, two separate appendices arising from a single caecum and duplication of both caecum and appendix. Watt (1959) has reviewed the many varieties of these types that have been reported.

In cases in which the caecum is duplicated there is in addition extensive duplication of the large bowel in many cases (Ravitch 1953).

12.2. Diverticula

It seems probable that reported diverticula of the appendix represent partial duplication in most instances, and not true diverticula (see Edwards 1934). However, Kissane and Smith (1967) have illustrated a true diverticulum.

12.3. Polyps

Adenomatous and juvenile polyps can occur in the appendix as in the colon.

12.4. Appendicitis

It is not proposed to discuss the aetiology of appendicitis in detail, since this has been dealt with elsewhere (see Morson 1966). There is some evidence to suggest that obstruction of the lumen is of greater practical importance in children than in adults. Hindmarsh (1954) found this to be present in 74 of 101 cases in childhood. Searches for virus in excised appendices have not been fruitful (Jackson et al. 1966). Pinworm infestation is commonly found in childhood, and there is little evidence that such infestation is a cause of appendicitis.

Pledger and Buchan (1969) have pointed out that about 40 children a year die of acute appendicitis in England and Wales. There is an eightfold greater mortality in those less than 5 years old than in the 5–14 year age group, a fact of some importance since 20%–25% of all cases occur at this time of life. Fields and Cole (1967) presented 30 cases of appendicitis in children less than 3 years old, adding these to their previous experience of 38 cases at the Los Angeles County Hospital. They pointed out that perforation is often seen in the young, being found in 76% of their cases.

13. Ulcerative Colitis

Ulcerative colitis commonly begins in childhood (around 10% of cases), and two large series of childhood cases have been reported, with 427 cases (Michener et al. 1961) and 134 cases (Langercrantz 1949), respectively. The bulk of these present at over 10 years of age, but ulcerative colitis is not rare before this; there are reports of 37 cases of the disease presenting in the first year of life. There is an excess of males, although this is probably less than 2:1.

Of the 401 cases in Michener's series in which the course of the disease was known 112 had died, 40 from colonic carcinoma, which had been found in 46 cases in all. He calculated the risk of developing carcinoma of the colon in this disease, presenting in childhood, as 556 times that in the normal population. The tendency to develop carcinoma was more pronounced with earlier onset; the mean duration of the disease before death from carcinoma occurred was 14.8 years. In 134 cases in individuals less than 15 years of age at the onset of the disease Korelitz et al. (1962) found eight carcinomas, seven of which had killed the patient. Three carcinomas were seen in the 18 cases described by Tumen et al. (1968).

The risk of carcinoma in ulcerative colitis and its prognosis when present have been discussed by Morson (1966). Onset of the disease early in life gives a greater potential time at risk of this complication and influences the management of the disease. Surgery is used more readily in therapy in childhood, owing both to this risk and to the systemic effects of the disease or therapy on growth and development (Hanley and Ray 1968).

The pathology of the disease, its complications, and the extraintestinal effects found do not differ from those in cases presenting during adult life.

14. Crohn's Disease

Crohn's disease (Fig. 6.77) presents no distinctive pathological findings in infancy and childhood, and the incidence of arthritis and arthralgia, erythema nososum, etc. is at least as great as that in adults. Growth retardation represents a distinctive systemic complication of this age group.

Crohn's disease of the large bowel presents in individuals less than 20 years old in one-third to one-half of reported cases (Lockart-Mummary and Morson 1964; Lindner et al. 1963). Korelitz et al. (1968) reported 25 cases aged 7–15 years of age, 16 in females and 9 in males. In six cases the disease was

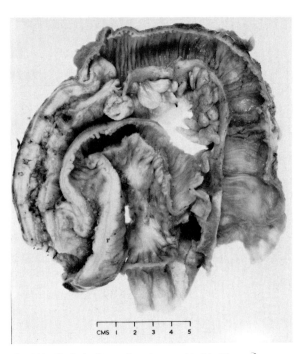

Fig. 6.77. Crohn's disease in a 9-year-old girl. The appearances are identical with those seen in adults.

initially confined to the colon; the rectum was spared in all. McGovern and Coulston (1968) also reported colon involvement in this disease and found sparing of the rectum in 24 cases.

15. Perforation of the Large Bowel

It is uncommon for perforation of the large bowel to occur in infancy and childhood, and this event generally represents a complication of ulcerative, granulomatous, or necrotizing colitis. Unfortunately, a number of iatrogenic causes are known. The rectum may be performated by a thermometer. Such performations occur in the anterior rectal wall just above the peritoneal reflection and are caused by insertion of the thermometer parallel with the floor of the cot, rather than with regard to rectal anatomy (Young 1965). Originally reported in 1957 by Segnitz, this injury has been reported several times since then (Miller 1962; Canby 1963; Warwich and Gikas 1959). More recent reports (Greenbaum et al. 1969) have emphasized the high mortality. Perforation may also occur during preparation of the bowel for surgery in Hirschsprung's disease. This complication is more frequent if the gut is affected by enterocolitis (Fraser and Berry 1967). Finally, perforation may occur in the enterocolitis following exchange transfusion (see p. 000). Such cases most often involve the large bowel, although the small bowel may be affected.

16. Hernias

16.1. Umbilical Hernias

There are two types of umbilical hernia, hernia into the cord through the anatomical site of the return of the mid-gut loop and omphalocele. The former group is less commonly associated with serious malformation than the latter. Young (1969) found that a hernia into the cord generally contained the mid-gut loop but no other viscus, whereas an omphalocoele often contained the liver, which was itself abnormally lobulated. In major omphaloceles the bulk of the abdominal viscera are in the sac and the abdomen appears scaphoid. The umbilical cord arises from the apex of the sac. Logan et al. (1965) have described the congenital abnormalities associated with omphalocele, but imperfect rotation of the gut is common.

16.2. Diaphragmatic Hernias

Diaphragmatic hernias occur mainly on the left-hand side, are frequently associated with other major defects, and usually occur posterolaterally. True oesophageal hiatus hernia is very uncommon in childhood.

Eventration of the diaphram may occur through the dome, or less commonly, retrosternally. Hypoplasia of the lung on the affected side is common.

16.3. Inguinal Hernias

Inguinal hernias occur with a frequency of 1.2/1000 live births (Knox 1959) and in a sex ratio of 10.3 male: 1 female. In reviewing 362 patients operated on under the age of 15 years, Gunnlaughsson et al. (1967) found when contralateral surgical exploration was performed at the time of operation that 60% of cases were bilateral. Although the lesion is much less common in females, Atwell (1962) was able to report 262 cases from The Hospital for Sick Children, Great Ormond Street. Of these cases, 60% were right-sided, 24.4% left-sided, and only 15% bilateral. Forty-two of the hernias contained viscera at operation, and the frequency with which the ovary was present in the sac was commented on by the author.

Inguinal hernia was found in 18 of 50 cases of the Hunter–Hurler syndrome by Coran and Eraklis (1967); other conditions in which visceromegaly occurs in early life also predispose to this condition.

17. Pneumatosis Intestinalis

Pneumatosis intestinalis is an uncommon condition, which can affect the large or small bowel of infants and children. Gas is said to be more often submucosal in infants and subserosal in adults, but in our experience either site may be involved in the young (Fig. 6.78). The gas fills cystic spaces in connective tissue and may be found in lymphatics and blood vessels; although gas-producing organisms have been suggested as a cause of the lesion, they have seldom been isolated at autopsy. Analysis of the gas does not support a microbiological origin.

The disease usually complicates some other illness, often with proximal intestinal obstruction. It is possible that gas is forced into the root of the mesentery from the stomach and then dissects distally, reaching the mucosa via the transmuscular arterial planes.

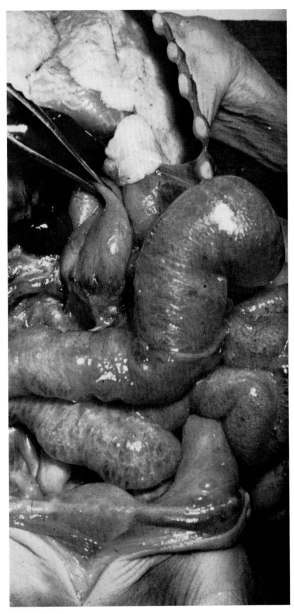

Fig. 6.78. Subserosal gas in the bowel and parietes of a female infant dying after operation for duodenal atresia.

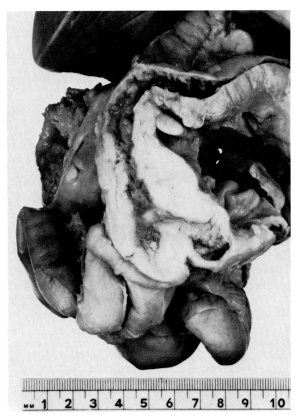

Fig. 6.79. Ileocaecal lymphosarcoma. Diffuse thickening of ileal and caecal walls with mucosal ulceration is commonly found in this condition.

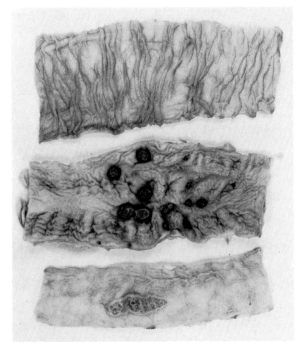

Fig. 6.80. Acute leukaemia, with deposits in ileal submucosa causing ulceration.

18. Malignant Tumours

Malignant gastrointestinal tumours are undoubtedly rare in childhood. As in adults *lymphosarcomas* are the commonest, and several large series describe the frequency of ileocaecal distribution (Fig. 6.79) and male predominance (Berry and Keeling 1970). Carcinoid tumours are uncommon in the first two decades of life, although isolated reports exist. Although adenocarcinomas have been described they have many unusual features and histories are sometimes atypical. Ungar (1949) reported three apparently typical tumours in an Israeli family, where the lesions resulted in death in the second decade.

Recently carcinoma of the jejunum has been reported in a 7-year-old boy (Büsing et al. 1977). Although the lesion was invasive but not metastatic, pulse cytophotometic investigation following DNA labelling suggested a malignant lesion. More studies of this kind might resolve the difficulties expressed about the so-called carcinomas that have been reported in association with Peutz–Jeghers syndrome.

Secondary tumours are also rare, although deposits of leukaemia may appear in the small bowel, some at the site of Peyer's patches (Fig. 6.80).

References

Abrami G, Dennison WM (1961) Duplications of the stomach. Surgery 49: 794

Abrams JS (1968) Intestinal atresia. Surgery 64: 185

Achord JL, Proctor HD (1963) Malignant degeneration and metastasis in Peutz–Jeghers syndrome. Arch Intern Med 111: 498

Ajayi OOA, Solanke TF, Seriki O, Bohrer SP (1969) Hirschsprung's disease in the neonate presenting as caecal performation. Paediatrics 43: 102

Aldridge RT, Campbell PE (1968) Ganglion cell distribution in the normal rectum and anal canal. J Pediatr Surg 3: 475

Ament ME, Rubin CE (1972) Soy protein—another cause of the flat intestinal lesion. Gastroenterology 62: 227

Atwell JD (1962) Inguinal hernia in female infants and children. Br J Surg 1: 294

Atwell JD (1968) The early diagnosis and surgical treatment of Hirschsprung's disease in infancy. Proc R Soc Med 61: 339

Auritt WA, Hervada AR, Fendrick F (1978) Fatal pseudomembranous entero-colitis following oral ampicillin therapy. J Pediatr 93: 882

Aust CS, Smith B (1962) Whipple's disease in a 3 months old infant with involvement of the bone marrow. Am J Clin Pathol 37: 66

Barnes CL, Townley RRW (1973) Duodenal mucosal damage in thirty-one infants with gastroenteritis. Arch Dis Child 48: 343

Benson CD, Lofti MW, Brough LAJ (1968) Congenital atresia and stenosis of the colon. J Pediatr Surg 3: 253

Bentley JFE, Smith JR (1960) Developmental posterior enteric remnants and spinal malformations. Arch Dis Child 35: 76

Berant M, Anead I, Jacobs J (1965) Heterotopic duodenal mucosa in the stomach. Am J Dis Child 110: 556

Berdon WE, Hochbert B, Baker D, Grossman H, Santulli TV (1966) The association of lumbosacral spine and genitourinary anomalies with imperforate anus. Am J Roentgenol 98: 181

Berkel I, Say B, Kiran O (1970) Intestinal mucosa in children with geophagia and iron deficiency anaemia. Scand J Haematol 7: 18

Berry CL (1969) Persistent changes in the large bowel following the enterocolitis associated with Hirschsprung's disease. J Pathol 97: 731

Berry CL, Fraser GC (1968) The experimental production of colitis in the rabbit; with particular reference to Hirschsprung's disease. J Pediatr Surg 3: 36

Berry CL, Keeling JW (1970) Gastrointestinal lymphomas in childhood. J Clin Pathol 23: 459

Bill AH Jr, Johnson RJ (1953) Failure of migration of the rectal opening as a cause for most cases of imperforate anus. Surg Gynecol Obstet 106: 643

Bjarnason G, Pettersson G (1968) The treatment of intussusception: thirty years experience at Gothenburg's Children's Hospital. J Pediatr Surg 3: 19

Bland-Sutton JD (1889) Imperforate ileum. Am J Med Sci 98: 457

Blank E, Michael TD (1963) Muscular hypertrophy of the esophagus; report of a case with involvement of the entire esophagus. Pediatrics 32: 595

Bodian M, Carter CO (1963) A family study of Hirschsprung's disease. Ann Hum Genet 26: 261

Bodian M, Stephens FD, Ward BCH (1949) Hirschsprung's disease and idiopathic megacolon. Lancet 1: 6

Bogomolitz WV, Cox JN (1975) Hamartoma of the stomach in childhood. Case report and review of the literature. Virchows Arch [Pathol Anat] 369: 69

Bongiovi J, Logosso RD (1969) Pancreatic pseudocyst occurring in the battered child syndrome. J Pediatr Surg 4: 220

Book LS, Herbst JJ, Jung AL (1976) Comparison of fast and slow feeding rate schedules to the development of necrotizing enteroliths. J Pediatr 89: 463

Boyle R, Nelson JS, Stonestreet BS, Peter G, Oh W (1978) Alterations in stool flora resulting from oral kanamycin prophylaxis of necrotizing enterocolitis. J Pediatr 93: 857

Bradlaw RV (1953) The dental stigmata of prenatal syphilis. Oral Surg 6: 147

Brennan LP, Weitzman JJ, Swenson O (1967) Pitfalls in the management of Hirschsprung's disease. J Pediatr Surg 2: 1

Browne D (1955) Congenital deformities of anus and rectum. Arch Dis Child 30: 42

Burke V, Anderson CM (1966) Chronic volvulus as a cause of hypoproteinaemia, oedema and tetany. Aust Paediatr J 2: 219

Burke V, Kerry KR, Anderson CM (1965) The relationship of dietary lactose to refractory diarrhoea in infancy. Aust Paediatr J 1: 147

Büsing CM, Haag D, Geiger H, Tschahargane C (1977) Microscopic and pulse cytophotometric investigation of a carcinoma of the jejunum in a seven year old child. Virchows Arch [Pathol Anat] 375: 115

Cameron AH, Astley R, Hallewell M, Rawson, AM, Miller CG, French JM, Hubble DV (1962) Duodeno-jejunal biopsy in the investigation of children with coeliac disease. Q J Med 31: 125

Canby JP (1963) Rectal perforation: a hazard of rectal temperatures. Clin Pediatr (Phila) 2: 233

Campbell PE, Noblett HR (1969) Experience with rectal suction biopsy in the diagnosis of Hirschsprung's disease. J Pediatr Surg 4: 410

Capron JP, Dupas JL, Marti R, Descombes P, Potet F (1977) Gastrin cells in Meckel's diverticulum (Letter). N Engl J Med 297: 1126

Carswell F, Logan RW (1973) Plasma B, C & B, A globulins and immunoglobulins in coeliac disease. Arch Dis Child 48: 587

Carswell F, Gibson AAM, McAlister IA (1973) Giardiasis and coeliac disease. Arch Dis Child 48: 414

Carter C, Sheldon W, Walker C (1957) The inheritance of coeliac disease. Ann Hum Genet 23: 266

Cave AJE (1936) Appendix vermiformis duplex. J Anat 70: 283

Chacko CJG, Paulson KA, Mathan VI, Baker SJ (1960) The villous architecture of the small intestine in the tropics: a necropsy study. J Pathol 98: 146

Chenoweth AI (1959) Intestinal obstruction in the neonatal period due to agenesis of the myenteric plexus. Ann Surg 149: 799

Chrispin AR, Tempany E (1967) Crohn's disease of the jejunum in children. Arch Dis Child 42: 631

Claireaux AE (1969) Histological techniques in the diagnosis of Hirschsprung's disease. In: Wilkinson AW (ed) Recent advances in paediatric surgery. Churchill-Livingstone, London

Cooke RWI, Meradji M, De Villeneuve VH (1980) Necrotising enterocolitis after cardiac catheterisation in infants. Arch Dis Child 55: 66

Coran AG, Eraklis AJ (1967) Inguinal hernia in the Hurler–Hunter syndrome. Surgery 61: 302

Corkery JJ, Dubowitz V, Lister J, Mossa A (1968) Colonic perforation after exchange transfusion. Br Med J iv: 335

Corne JS (1961) Multiple lymphomatous polyposis of the gastrointestinal tract. Cancer 14: 249

Cornell A, Blumberg ML, Sarot IA (1950) Cysts of the esophagus; case report and review of the literature. Gastroenterology 15: 260

Coryllos F, Simpson J (1962) Congenital atresia of the colon, review of the literature and report of two cases. Dis Colon Rectum 5: 37

Cosens CG (1958) Gastrointestinal pseudoleukaemia: a case report. Ann Surg 148: 129

Cozzi F, Wilkinson AW (1968) Familial incidence of congenital anorectal anomalies. Surgery 64: 669

Denes J, Jonh J, Leb J (1967) Dorsal herniation of the gut: a rare manifestation of the split notochord syndrome. J Pediatr Surg 2: 359

Dicke WK (1950) Coeliakia een onderzoek naar de nadelige invoeed van sommige graansoorten op de lÿder aan coeliakia. MD thesis, Utrecht

Dissanayake AS, Jerrome DW, Offerd RE, Truelove SC, Whitehead R (1974) Identifying toxic fractions of wheat gluten and their effect on the jejunal mucosa in coeliac disease. Gut 15: 931

Dobbins WO, Bill AH (1965) Diagnosis of Hirschsprung's disease excluded by rectal suction biopsy. N Engl J Med 272: 990

Doe WF, Henry K, Booth CC (1974) Complement in coeliac disease. In: Hekkens W, Pena A (eds) Coeliac disease. Proceedings of the Second International Coeliac Symposium. Stenfert Kroese, Leiden, p 189

Dohn K, Povlsen O (1951) Enterocystomas: report of six cases. Acta Chir Scand 102: 21

Doniach I, Shier M (1957) Duodenal and jejunal biopsies. II. Histology. Gastroenterology 33: 71

Donnison AB, Schwachman H, Gross RE (1966) A review of 164 children with meconium ileus seen at the Children's Hospital Medical Center, Boston. Pediatrics 37: 833

Douglas AP, Peters TJJ (1970) Peptide hydrolase activity of human intestinal mucosa in adult coeliac disease. Gut 11: 15

Dowling RG, Booth CC (1967) Structural and functional changes following small intestinal resection in the rat. Clin Sci Mol Med 32: 139

Dudgeon JA (1962) Oral pathology in the child: virus infections. In: Oral pathology in the child. International Academy of Oral Pathology, New York

Dukes CL (1958) Cancer control in familial polyposis of the colon. Dis Colon Rectum 1: 413

Edwards HC (1934) Diverticula of the vermiform appendix. Br J Surg 22: 88

Egan-Mitchell B, Fottrell PF, McNichol B (1977) Prolonged gluten tolerance in treated coeliac disease. In: McNicholl B, McCarthy CF, Fottrell PF (eds) Perspectives in coeliac disease. MTP Press, Lancaster p 251

Ehrenpreis J, Bentley JFR, Nixon HH (1966) Seminar on pseudo-Hirschsprung's disease and related disorders. Arch Dis Child 41: 143

Elliott GB, Kliman MR, Elliott KA (1968) Pancreatic annulus: a sign or a cause of duodenal obstruction? Can J Surg 11: 357

Ellison EH, Wilson SD (1964) The Zollinger–Ellison syndrome: Re-appraisal and evaluation of 260 registered cases. Ann Surg 160: 512

Erenpries T (1967) Mortality in Hirschsprung's disease in infancy. J Pediatr Surg 2: 569

Evans CH (1951) Atresias of the gastrointestinal tract. Int Abstr Surg 92: 1

Fields IA, Cole NM (1967) Acute appendicitis in infants thirty-six months of age or younger. Am J Surg 113: 269

Fonkalsrud EW, DeLaurimier AA, Hays DM (1968) Congenital atresia and stenosis of the duodenum. A review compiled from the members of the Surgical Section of the American Academy of Pediatrics. Pediatrics 43: 79

Fraser GC, Berry CL (1967) Mortality in neonatal Hirschsprung's disease with particular reference to entercolitis. J Pediatr Surg 2: 205

Fraser GC, Wilkinson AW (1967) Neonatal Hirschsprung's disease. Br Med J 3: 7

Freir S, Kletter B (1972) Clinical and immunological aspects of milk protein intolerance. Aust Paediatr J 8: 140

Gardner EJ (1962) Follow-up study of a family group exhibiting dominant inheritance for a syndrome including intestinal polyps, osteomas, fibromas, and epidermal cysts. Am J Hum Genet 14: 376

Gardner EJ, Richards RC (1953) Multiple cutaneous and subcutaneous lesions occurring simultaneously with hereditary polyposis and osteomatosis. Am J Hum Genet 5: 139

Gee S (1888) On the coeliac affection. St Bartholomew's Hospital Reports 24: 17

Giberson RG, Dockerty MB, Gray HK (1954) Leiomyoma of the stomach. Surg Gynecol Obstet 98: 186

Gjørup E (1934) Un cas d'oesophage double et estomac double. Acta Paediatr Scand 15: 90

Goldberg HM, Johnson TP (1963) Posterior abdomino-thoracic enteric duplication. Br J Surg 50: 445

Graivier L, Sieber WK (1966) Hirschsprung's disease and mongolism. Surgery 60: 458

Greenbaum EI, Carson M, Kincannon WN (1969) Rectal thermometer-induced pneumoperitoneum in the newborn. Report of two cases. Pediatrics 44: 539

Gross RE (1953) The surgery of infancy and childhood. Saunders, Philadelphia

Guga DK, Walia BNS, Tandon BN, Deo MG, Ghai OP (1968) Small bowel changes in iron-deficiency anaemia of childhood. Arch Dis Child 43: 239

Gunnlaughsson GH, Dawson B, Lynn HB (1967) Inguinal hernia in infants and children. Mayo Clin Proc 42: 129

Habbick BF, Melrose AG, Grant JL (1968) Duodenal ulcer in childhood. A study of predisposing factors. Arch Dis Child 43: 23

Haffner JF, Schistad G (1969) Atresia of the colon combined with Hirschsprung's disease. J Pediatr Surg 4: 560

Hanley PH, Ray JE (1968) Ulcerative colitis in children. South Med J 1231

Hartman SW, Kincannon WN, Greaney EM (1963) Congenital atresia of the colon. Am Surg 29: 699

Hays DM, Wooley MM, Snyder WH (1966) Two oesophageal

fistulae. J Pediatr Surg 1: 240

Herbut PA (1943) Congenital defect in the musculature of the stomach with rupture in a newborn infant. Arch Pathol 36: 91

Hindmarsh FD (1954) Acute appendicitis in childhood. Br Med J ii: 388

Hofman S, Orestano F (1967) Histology of myenteric plexus in relation to rectal biopsy. J Pediatr Surg 2: 575

Holder TM, Ashcraft KW (1970) Esophageal atresia and tracheo-esophageal fistula. Ann Thorac Surg 9: 445

Holmes GKT, Stokes PL, Sorahan TM, Prior P, Waterhouse HAH, Cooke WT (1976) Coeliac disease, gluten-free diet and malignancy. Gut 17: 612

Holzel A (1967) Sugar malabsorption due to deficiencies of disaccharidase activity and monosaccharide transport. Arch Dis Child 42: 341

Howaniety L, Lackmann D, Remes L (1968) Volvulus as a rare early complication of an enterogenous cyst of the newborn. Z Klin Chir 6: 48

Howard FM, Flynn DM, Bradley JM, Noone PE, Sjawatkowski M (1977) Outbreak of necrotising enterocolitis caused by clostridium butyricum. Lancet 2: 1099

Hyde GA, De Lorimier AA (1968) Colon atresia and Hirschsprung's disease. Surgery 64: 976

Jackson RH, Gardner PS, Kennedy J, McQuillin H (1966) Viruses in the etiology of acute appendicitis. Lancet 2: 711

Jorup S (1948) Congenital varices of the esophagus. Acta Paediatr Scand 35: 247

Kaijser R (1936) Über Hämangiome des Tractus gastrointestinalis. Arch Klin Chir 187: 351

Kauffmann SL, Stout AP (1963) Tumors of the salivary glands in children. Cancer 16: 1317

Keefer GP, Mokrohisky JF (1954) Congenital megacolon (Hirschsprung's disease). Radiology 63: 157

Keeling JW, Harris JT (1973) Intestinal malabsorption in infants with histiocytosis X. Arch Dis Child 48: 350

Kendrick KG, Walker-Smith JA (1970) Immunoglobulins and dietary protein antibodies in childhood coeliac disease. Gut 11: 635

Kissane JM, Smith MG (1967) Pathology of infancy and childhood. Mosby, St Louis

Knox G (1959) The incidence of inguinal hernia in Newcastle children. Arch Dis Child 34: 482

Konrad EA, Meister P (1979) Fatal eosinophilic gastroenterocolitis in a two year old child. Virchows Arch [Pathol Anat] 382: 347

Korelitz BI, Gribetz D, Danziger I (1962) The prognosis of ulcerative colitis with onset in childhood. I. The pre-steroid era. Ann Intern Med 57: 582

Korelitz BI, Gribetz D, Kopel FB (1968) Granulomatous colitis in children: a study of 25 cases and comparison with ulcerative colitis. Pediatrics 42: 446

Kuffer FR, Starzynsk EC, Girolam A, Murphy L, Grabstald H (1968) The Klippel–Trenaunay syndrome, visceral anteriomatosis thrombocytopenia. J Pediatr Surg 3: 65

Kumar R (1963) A case of congenital oesophageal stricture due to a cartilaginous ring. Br J Surg 49: 533

Ladd WE, Gross RE (1934) Congenital malformations of anus and rectum. Am J Surg 23: 167

Lancaster-Smith M, Kumar P, Clark ML (1974) Immunological phenomena following luten challenge in the jejunum of patients with adult coeliac disease and dermatitis herpetiformis. In: Hekken W, Pena A (eds) Coeliac disease. Proceedings of the Second International Coeliac Symposium. Stenfer Kroese, Leiden, p 173

Lancet (1978) Oesophageal troubles after repairs in infancy. Lancet 1: 700

Langercrantz R (1949) Ulcerative colitis in children. Nord Med 41: 258

Lawrence AG, Van Warner DE (1961) Intussusception due to

segmental aganglionosis. JAMA 175: 909

Lebenthal E, Shwachman H (1977) The pancreas; development, adaptation and malfunction in infancy and childhood. Clin Gastroenterol 6: 397

Lee CMU Jr (1955) Megacolon with particular reference to Hirschsprung's disease. Surgery 37: 762

Lewis PL, Holder T, Feldman M (1961) Duplication of the stomach; report of a case and review of the English literature. Arch Surg 82: 634

Lieber A, Rosenbaum HD (1965) Situs inversus of all organs except stomach. Am J Roentgenol 94: 353

Lindner AE, Marshak RH, Wolf BS, Janowitz HD (1963) Granulomatous colitis. N Engl J Med 269: 379

Little JW, Rickles NH (1967) The histiogenesis of the branchial cyst. Am J Pathol 50: 533

Lloyd JK (1972) Hypolipoproteinaemia. J Clin Pathol [Suppl] 5: 53

Lloyd JR (1969) The etiology of gastrointestinal perforations in the newborn. J Pediatr 4: 77

Lockart-Mummary HE, Morson BC (1964) Crohn's disease of the large intestine. Gut 5: 493

Logan WD, Crispin RH, Patterson JH, Abbot OA (1965) Ectopia cordis: report of a case and discussion of surgical management. Surgery 57: 898

Louw JH (1968) Polypoid lesions of the large bowel in children with particular reference to benign lymphoid polyposis. J Pediatr Surg 3: 195

Louw JH, Barnard CN (1955) Congenital intestinal atresia. Lancet 2: 1065

Lubolt W (1958) Duplication of the intestine as a cause of recurring intestinal bleeding in childhood. Paediatr Prax 7: 449

McGovern JB, Gross RE (1968) Intussusception as a post-operative complication. Surgery 63: 507

McGovern VJ, Coulston SJM (1968) Crohn's disease of the colon. Gut 9: 164

McNeish AS, Anderson CU (1974) Coeliac disease in childhood. Clin Gastroenterol 3: 127

McNeish AS, Nelson R (1974) Coeliac disease in one of monozygotic twins. Clin Gastroenterol 3: 143

McNeish AS, Nelson R, Macintosh P (1973) H-LA 1 and 8 in childhood coeliac disease. Lancet 1: 668

McParblin JF, Dickson JAS, Swain VAJ (1972) Meconium ileus: immediate and long-term survival. Arch Dis Child 47: 207

Madsen CM (1964) Hirschsprung's disease. Munksgaard, Copenhagen

Manhani Sing A (1967) Volvulus of the small intestine due to Ascaris. Indian J Surg 29: 328

Manoil C (1957) Congenital absence of the appendix. Am J Surg 93: 1040

Mathan VI, Joseph S, Baker SJ (1969) Tropical sprue in children. A syndrome of idiopathic malabsorption. Gastroenterology 56: 556

Mendl K, Evans CJ (1962) Congenital and acquired epiphrenic diverticula of the oesophagus. Br J Radiol 35: 53

Michener WM, Gage RP, Sauer WG, Stickler GB (1961) The prognosis of chronic ulcerative colitis in children. N Engl J Med 265: 1076

Miller JA (1962) The 'football sign' in neonatal perforated viscus. Am J Dis Child 104: 311

Morson BC (1966) Cancer in ulcerative colitis. Gut 7: 425

Morton NE (1970) Birth defects in racial crosses. In: Clarke Fraser F, McKusick VA (eds) Congenital Malformations. Excerpta Medica, Amsterdam New York, p 264

Moutsouris C (1966) 'Solid' stage and congenital intestinal atresia. Pediatr Surg 1: 446

Myotte M, Egan-Mitchell B, McCarthy CF, McNicholl B (1973) Incidence of coeliac disease in the West of Ireland. Br Med J i: 703

Nader PR, Margolin F (1966) Haemangioma causing gastrointestinal bleeding. Am J Dis Child 111: 215

Nagao K, Matsuzaki O, Saiga H, Sugano I, Kaneko T, Katoh T, Kitamura T (1980) Histopathological studies on parotid gland tumors in Japanese children. Virchows Arch [Pathol Anat] 388: 263

Naiman JL, Oski FA, Diamond LK, Vawter GF, Schwachman H (1964) The gastro-intestinal effects of iron-deficiency anaemia. Pediatrics 33: 83

Ogur GL, Kolarsick AJ (1951) Gastric diverticula in infancy. J Pediatr 39: 723

Okamota E, Vea T (1967) Embryogenesis of intramural ganglia of the gut and its relation to Hirschsprung's disease. J Pediatr Surg 2: 437

Oppenheimer EH, Esterley JR (1962) Observations in cystic fibrosis of the pancreas. II. Neonatal intestinal obstruction. Bull Johns Hopkins Hosp 111: 1

Orme RL'E, Eades SM (1968) Perforation of the bowel in the newborn as a complication of exchange transfusion. Br Med J iv: 349

Packer SM, Charlton V, Keeling JW, Risdon RA, Osilure D, Rowlatt RJ, Larcher VF, Harris JT (1978) Gluten challenge in treated coeliac disease. Arch Dis Child 53: 449

Parrish RA, Kanavage CB, Wells JA, Moretz WH (1968) Congenital antral membrane. Surg Gynecol Obstet 127: 999

Partridge JP, Gough MH (1961) Congenital abnormalities of the anus and rectum. Br J Surg 49: 37

Patten RG, Gardner LI (1962) Influence of family environment on growth syndrome (maternal deprivation). Paediatrics 30: 957

Paulino F, Roselli A, Aprigliano F (1963) Congenital esophageal stricture due to tracheobranchial remnants. Surgery 53: 547

Paulley JW (1954) Observation on the aetiology of idiopathic steatorrhoea; jejunal and lymph node biopsies. Br Med J ii: 1318

Perrot A, Danon L (1935) Obstruction intestinale de cause rare, chez un nourrisson. Ann Anat Pathol (Paris) 12: 157

Pledger HG, Buchan R (1969) Deaths in children with appendicitis. Br Med J iv: 466

Potter E (1961) Pathology of the fetus and newborn. Year Book Publishers, Chicago, p 296

Purcell WR (1962) Perforation of the stomach in a newborn infant. Am J Dis Child 103: 66

Ravitch MM (1953) Hind-gut duplication—doubling of colon and genital urinary tracts. Ann Surg 137: 588

Riker WL, Goldstein RI (1968) Malignant tumours of childhood masquerading as acute surgical conditions. J Pediatr Surg 3: 580

Risdon RA, Keeling JW (1974) Quantitation of the histological changes found in small intestinal biopsy specimens from children with suspected coeliac disease. Gut 15: 9

Rissier HL (1960) Haemangiomatosis of the intestine. Discussion, review of the literature and report of two cases. Gastroenterologia (Basel) 93: 357

Robinson JO (1951) Congenital absence of the vermiform appendix. Br J Surg 39: 344

Rosenlund ML, Koop CE (1970) Duodenal ulcer in childhood. Pediatrics 45: 283

Rosenstein BJ, Engelman K (1963) Diarrhoea in a child with a catecholamine-secreting ganglioneuroma. J Pediatr 63: 217

Rosenthal AH (1931) Congenital atresia of the esophagus with trache-esophageal fistula. Report of eight cases. Arch Pathol 12: 756

Sakula J, Shiner M (1957) Coeliac disease with atrophy of the small intestine mucosa. Lancet 2: 876

Santulli TV, Kiesewetter WB, Bill AH Jr (1970) Anorectal anomalies: a suggested international classification. J Pediatr Surg 5: 281

Schimke RM, Hartmann WH, Thaddeus MD, Prout TE, Rimoin DL (1968) Syndrome of bilateral pheochromocytoma, medul-

lary thyroid carcinoma and multiple neuromas. A possible regulatory defect in the differentiation of chromaffin tissue. N Engl J Med 279: 1

Schmidt EJ, Barros Barreto AP, Barbante PJ, Ramos OL, Concone MCMP, Queiroz AS, Carvalho AA (1964) Pancreatic lithiasis due to malnutrition and alcoholism in a child. J Pediatr 65: 613

Schwartz SI (1962) Congenital membranous obstruction of esophagus. Arch Surg 85: 480

Seagram CGF, Louch RE, Stephens CA, Wentworth P (1968) Meckel's divericulum: a 10-year review of 218 cases. Can J Surg 11: 369

Segnitz RG (1957) Accidental transanal perforation of the rectum. Am J Dis Child 93: 255

Shapiro S (1950) Occurrence of proctologic disorders in infancy and childhood; statistical review of 2700 cases. Gastroenterology 15: 653

Shiner R, Ballard J (1973) Mucosal secretory IgA and secretory piece in adult coeliac disease. Gut 14: 778

Shmerling DH, Prader A, Hitzig WH, Giedion A, Hadorn B, Kuhni M (1969) The syndrome of exocrine pancreatic insufficiency, neutropenia, metaphyseal exostosis and dwarfism. Helv Paediatr Acta 24: 547

Smith ED (1968) Urinary anomalies and complications in imperforate anus and rectum. J Pediatr Surg 3: 337

Smith J (1968) Pre- and post-natal development of the ganglion cells of the rectum and its surgical implications. J Pediatr Surg 3: 386

Sprinz H, Cohen A, Heaton JD (1961) Hirschsprung's disease with skip area. Ann Surg 153: 143

Stanfield JP, Hutt MSR, Tunnicliffe R (1965) Intestinal biopsy in kwashiorkor. Lancet 2: 519

Stevenson EO, Hays DM, Snyder WH Jr (1967) Post-operative intussusception in infants and children. Am J Surg 113: 562

Stickler GB, Peyla TL, Dower JC, Sloof JP (1963) Moniliasis, steatorrhoea, diabetes mellitus, cirrhosis, gallstones and hypoparathyroidism in a 10 year old boy. Clin Pediatr 4: 276

Stein H, Beck J, Solomon A, Schmaman A (1972) Gastroenteritis with necrotising enterocolitis in premature babies. Br Med J ii: 616

Stout AP (1962) Bizarre smooth muscle tumours of the stomach. Cancer 15: 400

Swenson O, Bill AH Jr (1948) Resection of rectum and rectosigmoid with preservation of the sphincter for benign spastic lesions producing megacolon. Surgery 24: 212

Swenson O, Oeconomopoulos C (1961) Acholasia of the esophagus in children. J Thorac Cardiovasc Surg 41: 49

Taylor GD, Martin HF (1961) Salivary gland tissue in the middle ear. A rare tumour. Arch Otolaryng 73: 651

Tiffin ME, Chandler LR, Faber HK (1940) Localized absence of the ganglion cells of the myenteric plexus in congenital megacolon. Am J Dis Child 59: 1071

Tittel K (1901) Ueber eine angeborene Missbildung des Dickdarmes. Wien Klin Wochenscher 14: 903

Toorman J, Bots TAM, Vio PMA (1977) Acetylcholinesterase activity in rectal mucosa of children with obstipation. Virchows Arch [Pathol Anat] 376: 159

Tumen HJ, Valdes-Dapena A, Haddad H (1968) Indications for surgical intervention in ulcerative colitis in children. Am J Dis Child 116: 641

Tünte W (1969) Analatresie bei Zwillingen. Z Kinderheilkd 105: 21

Ungar H (1949) Familial carcinoma of the duodenum in adolescence. Br J Cancer 3: 321

Valman HB (1976) Diet and growth after resection of ileum in childhood. J Pediatr 88: 41

Valman HB, Roberts PD (1974) Vitamin B12 absorption after resection of ileum in childhood. Arch Dis Child 49: 932

Vanheeuwan G, Riley WC, Glen L, Woodruff C (1967) Meconium plug syndrome with aganglionosis. Pediatrics 40: 665

Veale AMO, McColl I, Bursey HJR, Morson BC (1966) Juvenile polyposis coli. J Med Genet 3: 5

Walker AW, Kempson RL, Ternberg JL (1966) Aganglionosis of the small intestine. Surgery 60: 449

Walker-Smith JA (1972) Uniformity of dissecting microscope appearances in proximal small intestine. Gut 13: 17

Warwich WJ, Gilkas PW (1959) Neonatal transanal perforation of the rectum. Am J Dis Child 97: 869

Watt JK (1959) Appendix duplex. Br J Surg 46: 472

Weinstein ED (1965) Sex-linked imperforate anus. Pediatrics 35: 715

Williams JP, Knudson A (1965) Peutz–Jeghers syndrome with metastasizing duodenal carcinoma. Gut 6: 179

Wiseman JH, Celano ER, Hester FC (1959) Spontaneous rupture of the esophagus in a newborn infant. J Pediatr 55: 207

Young DG (1965) 'Spontaneous' rupture of the rectum. Proc R Soc Med 58: 615

Young DG (1969) Anterior abdominal wall defects. In: Wilkinson AW (ed) Recent advances in paediatric surgery. Churchill-Livingstone, London, p 153

Young DG, Wilkinson AW (1968) Abnormalities associated with neonatal duodenal obstruction. Surgery 63: 832

Yutani C, Sakurai M, Miyaji T, Okuno M (1973) Congenital short intestine; a case report and review of the literature. Arch Pathol 96: 81

Zinnemann HH, Kaplan AP (1972) The association of giardiasis with reduced intestinal secretory immunoglobulin A. Digestive Dis 17: 793

Chapter 7

Liver and Gallbladder

Colin L. Berry and Jean W. Keeling

1. Embryology

The liver forms initially as a diverticulum from the endoderm of the mid-gut around the 25th day of gestation. It develops by dichotomous branching after giving off an unpaired diverticulum, the future gallbladder. Extending into the mesenchyme of the septum transversum, which gives rise to the interstitial tissues and capsule, the irregularly arranged cords of liver cells are mixed with capillary loops, which eventually form sinusoids. The arrangement of definitive liver lobules arises from a series of right-angled branches arising from the primary cell cords, and from these branches a further series of radiating branches develops. These give rise to lobules and the axial cells from which the branches arise differentiate into the branch of the hepatic duct system that drains the lobule.

The major part of the bile duct system is derived from the cells of the hepatic cords and develops in situ; 'invasion' of the liver by developing ducts does not occur.

The vascular pattern of the mature liver is established after disruption of the vitelline veins by growth of the hepatic cords in the septum transversum. Ultimately the right vitelline vein alone remains to form the hepatic vein.

The umbilical veins, which enter the lateral aspect of the sinus venosus, are engulfed in the expanding liver, which provides direct venous return to the heart. The right umbilical vein and the post-hepatic left vein then disappear, leaving the remnant of the left-sided vein to form the ductus venosus by fusion with a vascular pathway formed in the developing sinusoids connecting with the common hepatic vein.

The portal vein develops following selective atrophy of parts of three transverse anastomotic channels between the vitelline veins. These complex patterns of venous change have been well illustrated by Hamilton et al. (1972).

In later pregnancy, the left lobe of the liver is supplied by umbilical vein blood predominantly and the right by portal venous blood. This probably accounts for the differing relative sizes of the two lobes seen between infant and adult, and for other variations in histological appearances. Haematopoietic tissue is more prominent in the right lobe.

2. Anomalies of Position, Form, and Size

In situs inversus totalis or situs inversus abdominis, the liver lies in the left upper quadrant and the left lobe is larger than the right. In the asplenia syndrome (see p. 139) (Ivemark 1955) the liver is symmetrical, the left lobe being increased in size and occupying the left hypochondrium.

Increase in size occurs in diaphragmatic hernia, probably because the liver is not constrained by the usual intra-abdominal pressures. If part of the liver lies in a hemithorax the shape of the liver is also abnormal, and there may be a fissure at the level of the diaphragm caused by localized pressure (Fig. 7.1). Infants with exomphalos usually have an enlarged liver for similar reasons. If part or all of the liver is contained in the exomphalos sac, then abnormal symmetry of the organ is evident (Fig. 7.2). Supernumerary lobes are not uncommon and are without functional or clinical significance, although Reidel's lobe may be palpated on abdominal examination.

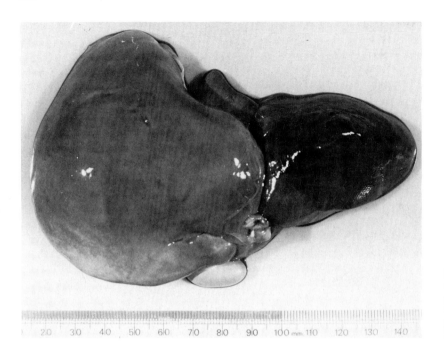

Fig. 7.1. The liver from an infant with a left-sided diaphragmatic hernia. The congested left lobe lay in the left hemithorax. The vertical groove was made by the margin of the incomplete diaphragm.

3. Physiological Neonatal Jaundice

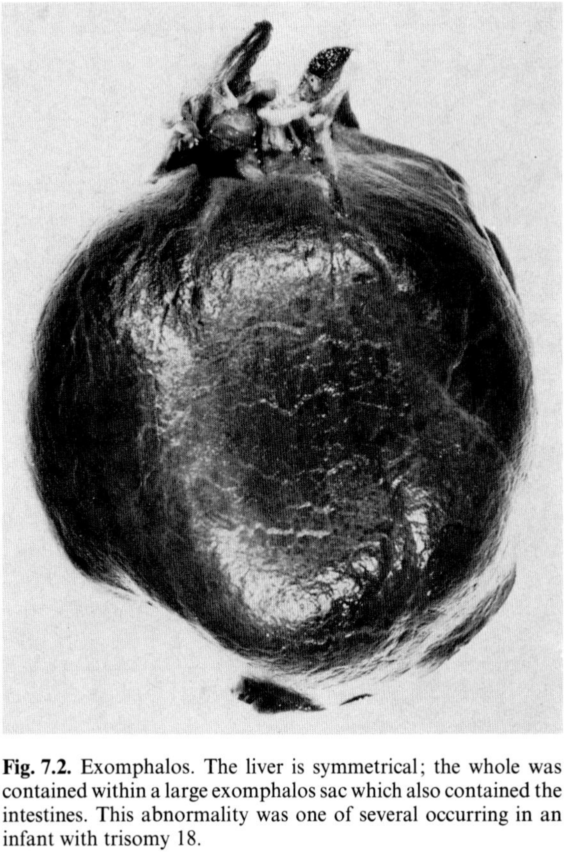

Jaundice with unconjugated hyperbilirubinaemia occurs in 90% of full-term infants. Maximum levels occur between the 2nd and 4th days of life and seldom exceed 6 mg/100 ml (102 mmol/litre). In preterm infants higher serum levels of unconjugated bilirubin are common, and often levels of 12–14 mg/100 ml (204–238 μmol/litre) are present. Maximum levels occur later in the preterm infant, usually from the 5th to the 7th day; a rise in bilirubin may persist until the 10th day of life.

Hyperbilirubinaemia is present in the neonate when serum levels exceed 15 mg% (255 mmol/litre) in the term baby and 12 mg% (204 mmol/litre) in the preterm infant. It is important to recognize, investigate, and treat unconjugated hyperbilirubinaemia in the neonate so that kernicterus can be prevented (cf. Chap. 5, Section 5).

Physiological hyperbilirubinaemia in the neonate is the result of a number of ill-understood factors (Lathe 1974). Increased bilirubin production occurs because of decreased erythrocyte survival, ineffective haematopoiesis, and increased turnover of haem-containing enzymes. There is reduced liver cell uptake of bilirubin as a result of poor hepatic perfusion resulting from continuing patency of the ductus venosus and the other haemodynamic changes that occur at birth. Poor liver cell uptake of bilirubin also occurs as a result both of the relative

Fig. 7.2. Exomphalos. The liver is symmetrical; the whole was contained within a large exomphalos sac which also contained the intestines. This abnormality was one of several occurring in an infant with trisomy 18.

immaturity of cell membrane transport systems and of cytoplasmic binding and glucuronidation—the major conjugation mechanism. Saturation of the excretion process may occur. Another important contributory factor is the reabsorption of unconjugated bilirubin from meconium in the gut lumen, particularly if gut emptying is slow. Poor bacterial breakdown of bilirubin in the gut is related to incomplete colonization.

4. Erythroblastosis Fetalis

In blood group incompatabilities between mother and fetus that cause severe haemolysis in utero (usually rhesus incompatability) there is hepatosplenomegaly with extensive haematopoiesis in the hepatic sinusoids and within portal tracts (Fig. 7.3). An excess of iron is present in hepatocytes (Fig. 7.4). In some cases, evidence of cholestasis may be present.

5. Metabolic Defects

5.1. Bilirubin Metabolism

Several defects along the degradation pathway of the haem molecule are described and are due to enzyme defects, not all of which have been specifically characterized. They give rise to jaundice in infancy and childhood. Causes of neonatal unconjugated hyperbilirubinaemia are shown in Table 7.1.

5.1.1. Gilbert's Syndrome

Gilbert's syndrome is a benign, autosomally recessive familial disorder with mild unconjugated bilirubinaemia, often without overt jaundice. It is thought that there is defective uptake of bilirubin by hepatocytes. Children are usually asymptomatic although nausea, fatigue, and upper abdominal discomfort are described in adults and are precipitated by alcohol, infection, or strenuous exercise

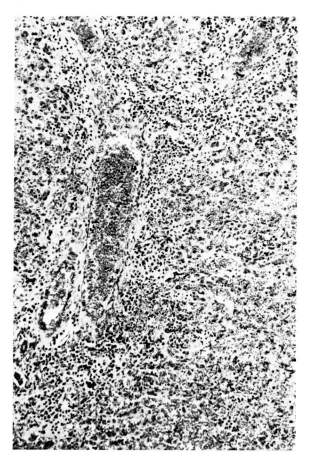

Fig. 7.3. Erythroblastosis fetalis. Within the liver of this infant with rhesus haemolytic disease, there is excessive erythropoiesis both in portal areas and within sinusoids. (H and E; 120×)

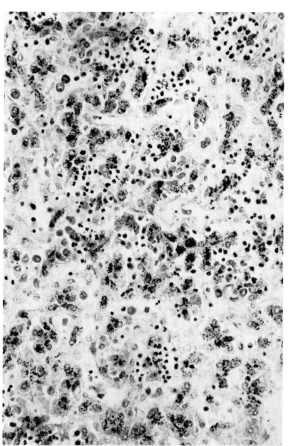

Fig. 7.4. Erythroblastosis fetalis. Much iron pigment is present within hepatocytes. Erythropoiesis is seen within sinusoids. (Pearle's reaction; 300×)

Table 7.1. Causes of neonatal unconjugated hyperbilirubinaemia[a]

Physiological jaundice of newborn
Haemolytic anaemia
   Hereditary spherocytosis, ovalocytosis
   Infantile pyknocytosis
   Pyruvate kinase deficiency
   Glucose-6-phosphate dehydrogenase deficiency
   Sickle-cell disease
   Isoimmunization (Rh, ABO)
   Drugs
   Infection
Polycythemia
   Twin-to-twin transfusion
   Delayed cord clamping
Dehydration
Maternal diabetes mellitus
Congenital adrenal hyperplasia
Neonatal thyrotoxicosis
Hypothyroidism
Down's syndrome
Galactosaemia
Weideman–Beckwith syndrome
Haematomata
Conjugation defects
   Reduction in glucuronyl transferase
      Type 1, autosomal recessive (Crigler–Najjar)
      Type 11, autosomal dominant
   Inhibition of glycuronyl transferase
      Drugs (novobiocin)
      Breast milk
      Familial transient hyperbilirubinaemia
Intestinal obstruction
Idiopathic indirect hyperbilirubinaemia

---

[a] After Lanzkowsky 1975.

(Gilbert and Lereboullet 1901; Berk et al. 1970).
   The liver is histologically normal.

5.1.2. Crigler–Najjar Syndrome

There are two disorders of bilirubin metabolism associated with uridine diphosphate glucuronyl transferase deficiency (Crigler–Najjar syndrome). Type I is rare and severe, with unconjugated hyperbilirubinaemia arising in the neonatal period and persisting throughout life. Severe neurological defects occur.

In type II the hyperbilirubinaemia is less severe and kernicterus does not occur.

The two types of disorder appear to be genetically distinct but both are probably inherited as autosomal recessive conditions (Crigler and Najjar 1952).

5.1.3. Dubin–Johnson Syndrome

In the Dubin–Johnson syndrome there is defective excretion of conjugated bilirubin from the hepatocytes into the bile canaliculi. There is mild fluctuating jaundice in childhood, which may become more severe in later life. Nausea, malaise, anorexia, and hepatomegaly occur, but infrequently. The diseases is inherited as an autosomal recessive condition. The prognosis is good.

The liver is greenish black on naked-eye examination, and hepatocytes contain lipochrome pigment within lysosomes. The pigment is apparently a melanin. The liver architecture is normal (Dubin and Johnson 1954).

5.1.4. Rotor's Syndrome

Clinically and biochemically Rotor's syndrome resembles the Dubin–Johnson syndrome, but without the accumulation of pigment in hepatocytes (Rotor et al. 1948).

5.2. Wilson's Disease

Hepatolenticular degeneration is a rare inherited (autosomal recessive) disorder of copper metabolism in which copper is deposited in the liver, brain, cornea, and kidneys. When the disease presents in childhood, the symptoms are usually manifestations of liver damage. Jaundice and portal hypertension with oesophageal varices and hypersplenism may occur. Biochemical abnormalities of liver function may be demonstrated, and depend on the degree of liver damage. Serum copper and caeruloplasmin levels are low and urinary copper increased. There is sometimes copper deposition in the cornea in older children. Treatment with oral penicillamine effectively removes copper from the body and produces clinical improvement when started early in the disease.

Histological abnormalities produced in the liver in Wilson's disease are cirrhosis, an increase in fibrous tissue, and striking vacuolation of hepatocyte nuclei caused by glycogen accumulation (Walshe 1962).

5.3. Galactosaemia (see also p. 163)

Galactosaemia is an inherited disorder of carbohydrate metabolism resulting from deficiency of the enzyme galactose-l-phosphate uridyl transferase. It is inherited in an autosomal recessive fashion. There is defective conversion of galactose to glucose, with accumulation of galactose-1-phosphate and galactosuria.

The infants are well at birth and symptoms are precipitated by milk feeding. There is usually vomiting, failure to thrive, jaundice, and hepatomegaly. If the disorder is not recognized and glactose ingestion continues, cirrhosis develops, with liver failure and signs of portal hypertension. Cataracts usually form and untreated infants seem to be susceptible to severe infection. Treatment is by restriction of lactose ingestion; most untreated infants die in infancy.

The earliest hepatic lesion is portal fibrosis. There is rapid liver cell damage with replacement fibrosis leading to cirrhosis (Fig. 7.5).

6. Cystic Disease

6.1. Solitary Cysts

Solitary cysts of the liver are rare and are usually an incidental finding at necropsy. Occasionally sufficient fluid may accumulate within them to give rise to an abdominal mass. They are lined by a single layer of biliary epithelium and presumably arise as a result of localized obstruction of the biliary tree. They have no effect on liver function.

6.2. Multiple Cysts

Multiple cysts of the liver in children are also uncommon. In about half the cases reported they are associated with polycystic disease of the kidneys of the adult type (Montgomery 1940; Blyth and Ockenden 1971). They rarely achieve a sufficiently large size to distort the normal contours of the liver, varying between one millimetre and several centimentres in diameter.

6.3. Infantile Polycystic Disease and Congenital Hepatic Fibrosis

The disorders of the liver characterized by proliferation, dilatation, and excessive branching of the intrahepatic bile ducts without concomitant abnormality of the hepatic parenchyma have many histological similarities. On these grounds they might be considered different expressions of the basic disorder, from Von Meyenburg's complexes to infantile polycystic disease, embracing both congenital hepatic fibrosis and Caroli's disease. However, the responses of tissues to injury are not infinite and similarly of appearance cannot always be equated with common aetiology.

Kerr et al. (1961) described 13 children with 'congenital hepatic fibrosis' who presented between the ages of 2.5 and 16 years (more than half before 6 years of age) with complications of portal hypertension. One of three children who died had typical infantile polycystic renal disease. They reviewed 24 cases from the literature which they considered to be examples of congenital hepatic fibrosis: 15 of these had polycystic kidneys, although case 2 of

Parker (1956) seems to be an example of Meckel's syndrome. Three of the 15 cases with liver and kidney involvement were siblings. The authors stated that the presence of renal disease made the diagnosis of congenital hepatic fibrosis certain. Familial cases of congenital hepatic fibrosis have also been described by Lorimer et al. (1967), who report their findings in two sisters presenting at 30 and 34 years of age with portal hypertension. Two other siblings from this family were also thought to have the same disorder. The kidneys were of normal size but were not biopsied.

Blyth and Ockenden (1971) described a spectrum of disease in children presenting from birth to 5 years, all having cystic disease of both liver and kidneys. In their two younger groups, i.e., infants in whom the disease was obvious at birth or who presented in the first month of life, presenting signs and symptoms related to the renal abnormality, with the perinatal group dying as a result of respiratory insufficiency caused by concomitant pulmonary hypoplasia and the neonatal group from progressive renal failure. All cases had diffuse liver disease.

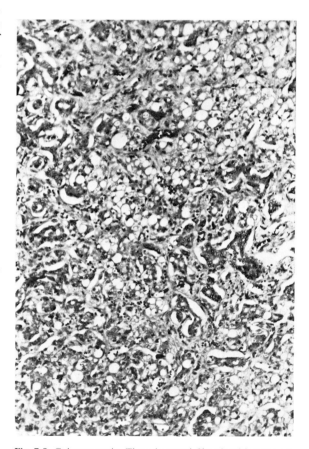

Fig. 7.5. Galactosaemia. There is portal fibrosis with some apparent bile duct reduplication and ductular change in degenerating hepatocyte. Marked fatty degeneration of hepatocytes is present.

These authors also described two further subgroups of patients, presenting at 3–6 months of age, the infantile group, and between 1 and 5 years. In the infantile group, patients presented with either chronic renal failure or increasing portal hypertension. In all cases, cystic changes were present in both liver and kidneys, but the renal disease was not as extreme as in the younger patients. Children in the juvenile group all had signs referable to portal hypertension. In this group renal tubular dilatation was minor (less than 10% of tubules involved) and portal fibrosis was more severe in these cases. Thus, although all cases had spectacular bile duct abnormalities throughout the liver, clinical signs or symptoms due to the hepatic lesion were present only in those infants who survived at least several months. Time seems to be an important factor in the development of portal hypertension; whether this is the result of increasing fibrosis in the portal tracts or is merely a reflection of the time taken for the complications of portal hypertension to occur is not clear. The authors found other affected family members in several cases and suggested an autosomal recessive mode of inheritance. Their conclusion was that their cases were a spectrum of expression of the same basic disorder.

Lieberman et al. (1971) described infantile polycystic disease in 14 patients, including three from one family; five other patients had affected siblings. Seven presented before 1 month of age, the rest at up to 7 months. Five died within the first 7 months of life from respiratory or renal problems. The surviving patients were hypertensive and it was noted that kidney size decreased over a period of time. Some had hepatomegaly; there was portal hypertension in two, and splenomegaly in one other case. All had the typical histology of infantile polycystic disease. The same authors described four patients with congenital hepatic fibrosis presenting between 7 weeks and 11 years 3 months, three being siblings, all with signs and symptoms of portal hypertension. The three familial cases had cystic kidneys, the cystic change being of a minor degree, as well as diffuse cystic abnormalities of the liver, while in the fourth case the renal biopsy seemed to be inadequate. These authors feel that congenital hepatic fibrosis is a different disorder from infantile polycystic disease, but do not advance a very good case in support of this view.

Using quantitative methods of assessment of liver sections from patients with cystic bile duct abnormalities, Landing et al. (1980) found that the perinatal, neonatal, and infantile forms of infantile polycystic disease were indistinguishable, and concluded that they represented differing presentations of the same condition. The juvenile group of polycystic disease of Blyth and Ockendon (1971) was indistinguishable from congenital hepatic fibrosis.

Following three-dimensional reconstruction of the biliary system in cystic liver disease in neonates, Jorgensen (1971, 1972) demonstrated that the abnormal biliary system was in the form of curved plates. He concluded that the basic defect was a failure of resorption of most of the fetal duct plate system of the embryo. The intrahepatic portal venous system was normal, but the amount of fibrous tissue in portal areas varied from case to case. These studies support the concept of a single basic anomaly in infantile cystic liver disease.

In infantile polycystic disease the liver is enlarged and firm with expanded portal tracts visible through the capsule. The cut surface may show cystic dilatation of large bile ducts (Fig. 7.6), but this is probably present in a minority of cases. The portal areas are pale and prominent. Histologically there is spectacular dilation and branching of the bile ducts,

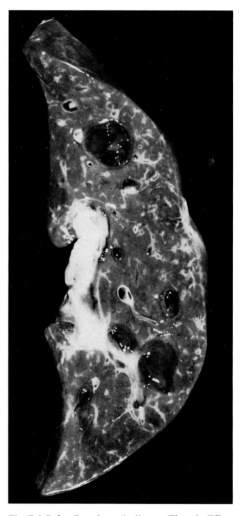

Fig. 7.6. Infantile polycystic disease. There is diffuse expansion of portal tracts by fibrous tissue. Localized dilatation of large ducts is seen.

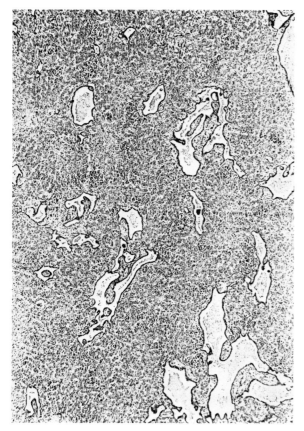

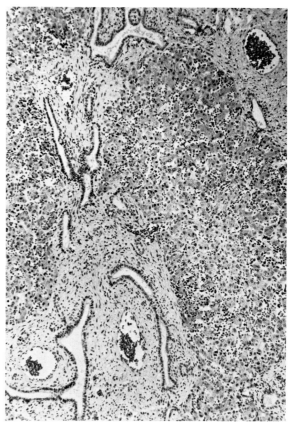

Fig. 7.7. Infantile polycystic disease in a neonate. There is irregular cystic dilatation of bile ducts in all portal areas. (H and E; 60 ×)

Fig. 7.8. Infantile polycystic disease. Female died aged 4 with respiratory insufficiency. The bile ducts are irregularly dilated, there is marked portal fibrosis. The hepatic parenchyma appears normal. The kidneys in this case were typical of infantile polycystic disease. (H and E; 108 ×)

but there is no abnormality of the hepatic parenchyma; in particular, no intrahepatic bile retention or bile plugging are seen (Figs. 7.7 and 7.8).

In older children in whom portal hypertension is present, portal fibrosis is often more severe and the dilatation of the ducts is not as prominent as it is in neonates.

6.4. Meckel's Syndrome

Meckel's syndrome is characterized by cerebral abnormality (usually an encephalocele), cystic kidneys, cleft palate, congenital heart disease, postaxial polydactyly, and eye and other abnormalities (Opitz and Howe 1969). It is thought to be inherited in an autosomal recessive fashion (Crawfurd et al. 1978).

Cystic change in the liver is frequently present, but the organ presents a spectrum of abnormalities ranging from hepatic enlargement with cysts visible through the capsule or readily recognizable on slicing, to a reduction in size with portal fibrosis. Histological examination may reveal diffuse cystic dilatation of bile ducts in all portal areas (Fig. 7.9) in addition to any macroscopic cysts. The absence of cysts on naked-eye inspection and failure to undertake adequate histological examination of the fetus may account for the liver's being described as normal in some cases.

6.5. Trisomy 17–18

Diffuse dilatation of the bile ducts without parenchymal damage or biliary obstruction may occur as part of the spectrum of hepatobiliary anomalies in the trisomy 17–18 syndrome (see pp. 76, 279).

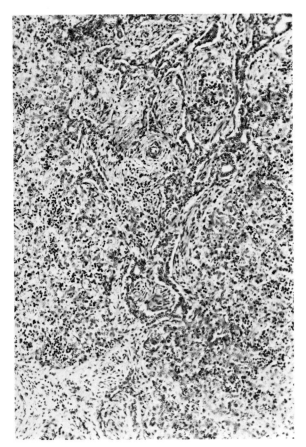

Fig. 7.9. Meckel's syndrome. Infant died aged 1 day with occipital encephalocoele and bilateral renal enlargement with diffuse cystic change. Excessively branching undilated bile ducts are seen throughout the liver. (H and E; 144 ×)

7. Liver Disease with Giant-cell Transformation and Cholestasis

7.1. Intrahepatic Cholestasis

'Giant cell hepatitis' is a term that has fallen into disrepute, particularly with clinicians. However, one can find fault with the synonyms 'neonatal hepatitis' and 'neonatal hepatitis syndrome' for the same reasons; all these terms appear to insist on an infective aetiology when in practice none is found in most cases. The commonest predisposing factor in one large series was an inherited defect of protein transport, presumably an enzyme defect (Mowat et al. 1976). 'Obstructive cholangiopathy of infancy' seems etymologically correct and all-embracing, but rather clumsy. 'Giant cell hepatitis', however, has two distinct advantages—it draws attention to a spectacular histological feature that is exclusive to the diseased neonatal liver and, because of long usage, it is widely understood.

Giant cell hepatitis and extrahepatic biliary atresia were for many years regarded as distinct entities, and although it has long been recognized that giant cell transformation in the neonatal liver can have many aetiologies, not all of them inflammatory, biliary atresia was regarded as a congenital anomaly. It is now recognized that in biliary atresia the bile ducts develop normally and the atresia is a secondary phenomenon, usually developing during intrauterine life, although in some cases the damage probably occurs postnatally. Most atresias, particularly where there is widespread obliteration of the duct lumen, have an infective aetiology (Landing 1974). In others, particularly those with localized lesions, it is likely that an ischaemic episode in utero is responsible (a parallel may be drawn with multiple localized atresias of the jejunum and ileum). Some workers think that the same aetiological factors may be responsible for both extrahepatic biliary atresia and neonatal hepatitis, the factors determining the type of damage produced being the severity of the infection, the stage of pregnancy at which it occurred, and the type of response the fetus is able to mount (Landing 1974; Mowat et al. 1976). This view is not universally accepted; Danks et al. (1977a), whilst accepting that the majority of cases of neonatal hepatitis are attributable to unidentified intrauterine infective agents, think that the agents responsible for extrahepatic biliary atresia are different, although similarly operative in utero. Although it seems that giant cell hepatitis and biliary atresia may be two ends of the same spectrum, it is still important for the clinician to be able to distinguish between these disorders. With new surgical techniques, increasing numbers of infants with biliary atresia can be treated (Kasai 1975), although subsequent reports on the outcome have not been so optimistic (Howard and Mowat 1977). Routine tests of biliary function are poor discriminants in this situation, but Mowat et al. (1976) have found the combination of percutaneous needle liver biopsy and the rose bengal secretion test to be completely reliable. It has been suggested that laparotomy should be avoided in infants with giant cell hepatitis, as this predisposes to cirrhosis (Boggs and Lawson 1974). However, such a causal relationship is by no means established, as 5 of 14 cases in this report were familial, which would, of itself, give an unfavourable prognosis (Danks et al. 1977a).

The causes of conjugated hyperbilirubinaemia in the neonate are given in Table 7.2. The frequency of aetiological factors in the hepatitis syndrome of infancy found in two large published series of cases, together with the cases of extrahepatic and intrahepatic biliary atresia seen over the same periods of time, are given in Table 7.3.

The histological features are giant cell transformation of hepatocytes, which can involve only part of a lobule or be very extensive, with few mononuclear forms remaining (Fig. 7.10). Similarly, hepatocyte necrosis may be minimal, and seen clearly only on sections stained for reticulin, or may be widespread with fibrous replacement of liver cells. There is inflammatory cell infiltration of both hepatic lobule and portal tracts, and in many cases, particularly those with an infective aetiology, haematopoiesis persists. Intracellular bile retention and bile plugging may be present. In only a small proportion of cases is it possible to visualize the aetiological agent, e.g., cytomegalovirus (CMV), herpes virus, varicella zoster virus, or perhaps *Toxoplasma gondii* and *Treponema pallidum*. Virus

Table 7.2. Causes of conjugated hyperbilirubinaemia in the neonate[a]

Primary hepatocellular dysfunction

    Idiopathic neonatal hepatitis
    Specific neonatal hepatitis
    Hepatitis B virus, Cytomegalovirus infection,
      Herpes simplex, rubella, Coxsackie virus,
      Echo virus 11
    Escherichia coli, Listeria
    Toxoplasma
    Syphilis
    Galactosaemia
    α_1-Antitrypsin deficiency
    Dubin–Johnson and Rotor's syndromes
    Transient direct hyperbilirubinaemia in haemolytic
      disease of the newborn
    Intravenous alimentation

Extrahepatic biliary obstruction

    Extrahepatic biliary atresia
    Choledochal cyst
    Mucoviscidosis

---

[a] After Lanzkowsky 1975.

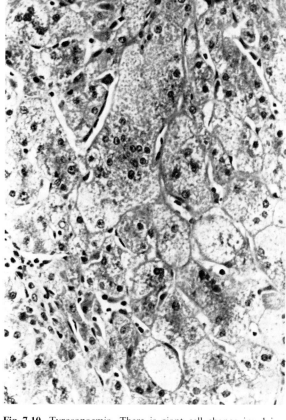

Fig. 7.10. Tyrosanaemia. There is giant cell change involving hepatocytes throughout the lobule. (H and E; 360 ×)

Table 7.3. Causes of neonatal conjugated hyperbilirubinaemia

	Mowat et al. 1976		Danks et al. 1977a
Extrahepatic biliary atresia		32	55
Intrahepatic biliary atresia		1	11
Choledochal cyst		2	
Neonatal hepatitis		102	105
Idiopathic	70		69
α_1-Antitrypsin deficiency	24		8
Galactosaemia	1		6
Tyrosinaemia	1		–
Cytomegalovirus	1		13
Hepatitis B virus	2		1
Rubella virus	2		2
Toxoplasmosis	1		2
Coxsackie B_2 virus	–		1
Coxsackie B_4 virus	–		1
Parainfluenza 3 virus	–		1
Syphilis	–		1
	137		161

cultures, serological techniques, and observation of
extrahepatic disease may enable a definite diagnosis
to be made in other cases. Some infants with
neonatal hepatitis make a full recovery, about a third
develop cirrhosis (Fig. 7.11) and succumb to its
various complications, and in 10%–20% of cases the
disease runs a fulminant course in the neonatal
period. When so little is known about the underlying
abnormality in many cases an accurate assessment of
the prognosis is difficult. Danks et al. (1977a) found
that the prognosis was poor amongst infants with
persistent jaundice and acholic stools. The presence
of a second disease (Table 7.4) had serious implications. In two groups, infants with transient
jaundice and minimal obstructive picture and those
in whom CMV infection was the underlying problem, there was a relatively good prognosis. A
positive family history of neonatal liver disease was a
poor prognostic sign (Danks et al. 1977b).

7.2. Alpha₁-antitrypsin Deficiency

Alpha₁-antitrypsin is a polymorphic glycoprotein
(mol. wt. 45000) synthesized in the liver. It migrates
as an α^2-globulin on paper electrophoresis. It has in
vitro protease-inhibitor activity, but its function in
vivo is unknown (trypsin, collagenase, elastase
thrombin, and plasmin are all inhibited).

The production of this glycoprotein is governed
by a pair of completely penetrant co-dominant
autosomal alleles with 13 variant alleles (or more)
known as the Pi (protease inhibitor) system. The
subtypes are designated by letter according to their
electrophoretic mobility: PiF (fast), PiM (medium),
PiS (slow), and PiZ (ultraslow). Most people are of

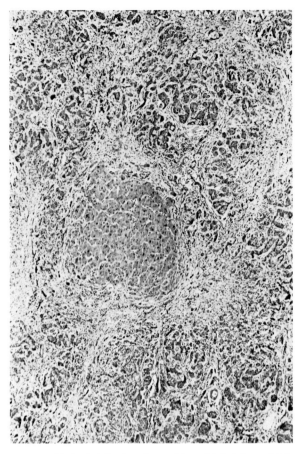

Fig. 7.11. Cirrhosis following giant cell hepatitis in infancy. Male aged 5 years, hepatitis in infancy, chronic liver damage apparent from 16 months of age. Giant cell transformation is present in the central regenerative nodule (H and E; 57×)

Table 7.4. Other diseases seen in infants with idiopathic neonatal intrahepatic cholestasis

	Mowat et al. 1976	Danks et al. 1977a
Total no. with idiopathic NNH[a]	70	59
No. with other disease	9	24
Rh incompatibility	–	6
Down's syndrome	4	4
Chondrodysplasia punctata	–	3
Sepsis	3	–
Cystic fibrosis	2	2
Fibromatosis	–	2
Cystenosis	–	1
Niemann–Pick disease	–	1
Hepatic haemangioendothelioma	–	1
Polycystic kidneys	–	1
Hydrocephalus	–	1
Congenital heart disease	–	1
Multiple congenital abnormalities	–	1

[a] Neonatal hepatitis.

the genotype PiMM, and PiZZ corresponds to the clinical homozygous deficiency state. The frequency of the PiZZ phenotype is said to be 1 in 3460 in Britain, so that about 230 alpha$_1$-antitrypsin-deficient infants are born in England and Wales each year (Cook 1974). Probably 10%–15% of these infants will develop liver disease. It was formerly thought that hepatitis-associated antigen might be the additional triggering factor required to produce liver disease in deficient infants (Porter et al. 1972), but this has been discounted. Alpha$_1$-antitrypsin deficiency was described in association with infantile cirrhosis (Sharp et al. 1968) and shortly afterwards in four infants with neonatal hepatitis, which in two children progressed to cirrhosis (Johnson and Alper 1970). Subsequently, a relationship between alpha$_1$-antitrypsin deficiency and some cases of adult liver disease was also demonstrated (Berg and Eriksson 1972). An association between pulmonary emphysema in young adults and low serum alpha$_1$-antitrypsin levels was noted by Laurell and Eriksson (1963).

It was considered formerly that individuals with low alpha$_1$-antitrypsin levels might be healthy or develop liver or lung disease, but not both types. This view has subsequently been shown to be erroneous in both children (Glasgow et al. 1971; legend to Fig. 7.13) and adults (Cohen et al. 1973).

The relationship between Pi phenotype and the development of liver disease is complex, but a proportion of PiZZ individuals present with conjugated hyperbilirubinaemia in the neonatal period and these have been shown to have intrahepatic cholestasis with giant cell transformation of hepatocytes on liver biopsy. A characteristic appearance of the liver in these infants is the presence of PAS-positive, diastase-resistant globules in the cytoplasm of hepatocytes, particularly those adjacent to portal areas (Fig. 7.12). These globules seem to be a precursor of alpha$_1$-antitrypsin not excreted by the hepatocytes. Peptide mapping has shown that this molecule differs from that of PiMM individuals in that a glutamic acid molecule in the normal is replaced by lysine in the PiZZ individual. That this material is antigenically similar to alpha$_1$-antitrypsin can be demonstrated by immunohistochemical methods based on fluorescein- or peroxidase-labelled antihuman alpha$_1$-antitrypsin: the lobules are said not to be present in infants under 12 weeks of age (Talbot and Mowat 1975). Cottrall et al. (1974) found alpha$_1$-antitrypsin deficiency to be as common as extrahepatic biliary atresia in conjugated hyperbilirubinaemia in infancy in a study in southeast England.

Intrahepatic cholestasis of infancy in alpha$_1$-antitrypsin deficiency can progress to cirrhosis (Fig. 7.13). The deficiency may be found in individuals with cirrhosis with no history of jaundice in the neonatal period (Cottrall et al. 1974), although anicteric liver damage beginning in early life cannot be ruled out. Aagenaes et al. (1974) suggest that in alpha$_1$-antitrypsin deficiency liver disease may be present in utero, and suggest that the low birth weight in infants with neonatal hepatitis and alpha$_1$-antitrypsin deficiency compared with apparently normal infants with low serum alpha$_1$-antitrypsin levels is evidence for prenatal damage. They also describe a slow but definite deterioration towards

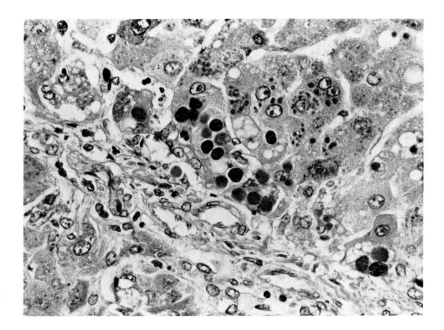

Fig. 7.12. Alpha$_1$-antitrypsin deficiency. Diastase-resistant PAS,-positive globules are seen in the cytoplasm of periportal hepatocytes. (PAS; 576 ×)

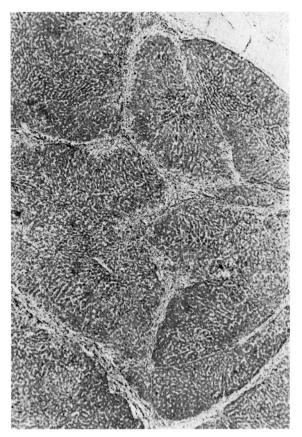

Fig. 7.13. Cirrhosis is alpha$_1$-antitrypsin deficiency. Female aged 12 years. Giant cell hepatitis in infancy. Portal fibrosis by 16 months. Cirrhosis by 3 years of age. Death from respiratory insufficiency due to emphysema (H and E; 36 ×)

cirrhosis in all their patients, despite initial improvement in liver function tests and apparent well-being. Cottrall et al. (1974) found that the prognosis in neonatal intrahepatic cholestasis was worse in patients with alpha$_1$-antitrypsin deficiency than in the rest of the group.

A recent review covering the biochemical and clinical aspects of alpha$_1$-antitrypsin deficiency is given by Morse (1978a, b).

7.3. Obstructive Jaundice

7.3.1. Intrahepatic Biliary Atresia

Atresia of the intrahepatic bile ducts is an uncommon cause of obstructive jaundice in childhood, being found in only 1 of 137 cases prospectively studied by Mowat et al. (1976), and its very existence as a primary pathological abnormality might be challenged. Two cases of intrahepatic biliary hypoplasia described by Longmire (1964) were in older

children with concomitant extrahepatic biliary obstruction and may represent secondary atrophy of intrahepatic bile ducts following prolonged obstruction. In the cases described by Sass-Kortsak et al. (1956) and Rosenthal et al. (1961, bile ducts were uniformly absent from portal areas throughout the liver, and bile plugging of periportal bile canaliculi was present. Inflammatory cell infiltration of portal areas was absent, as was hepatic parenchymal necrosis. The extrahepatic biliary system was normal.

Some infants in whom the intrahepatic bile ducts are said to be absent have many cutaneous xanthomas, which may appear before 1 year of age and are always associated with prolonged elevation of serum cholesterol levels (Rosenthal et al. 1961). Danks et al. (1977a) found intrahepatic biliary atresia in 11 of 171 babies with neonatal jaundice in a comprehensive study of neonatal jaundice in Victoria over an 11-year period. All the affected infants had odd facies. Eight had pulmonary valve stenosis or atresia. Two of the infants were brother and sister. The presence of similar extrahepatic abnormalities in all cases gives weight to the existence of intrahepatic biliary atresia as a separate entity. Alagille et al. (1975) have reported similar cases with a peculiar facies and cardiovascular anomalies. Danks et al. (1977a) suggest that the intrahepatic bile ducts in these cases are susceptible to injury, perhaps by a variety of agents, atresia being the end-result. A biochemical defect in bile elimination may be the primary disorder and ductular atrophy a secondary phenomenon (Harris and Anderson 1960).

7.3.2. Extrahepatic Biliary Obstruction

Extrahepatic biliary obstruction usually presents with conjugated hyperbilirubinaemia and acholic stools from birth, although in a small number of cases the infant is initially normal and obstructive jaundice starts in early postnatal life. The commonest cause of extrahepatic biliary obstruction is extrahepatic biliary atresia, affecting all or part of the extrahepatic biliary system (Fig. 7.14). In a few cases, obstruction of the extrahepatic bile ducts is caused by a choledochal cyst (see p. 295), a situation that can be remedied surgically and should be sought actively in every case. Where biliary obstruction is localized, it may be possible to effect satisfactory bile drainage by anastomosing part of the duct system or the gallbladder to the small intestine. Where there is widespread extrahepatic biliary atresia clearance of the fibrosed ducts and fibrous tissue from the porta hepatis to the intestine by way of a Roux-en-Y procedure may relieve the obstruction (Kasai et al. 1975), although ascending cholangitis may be a

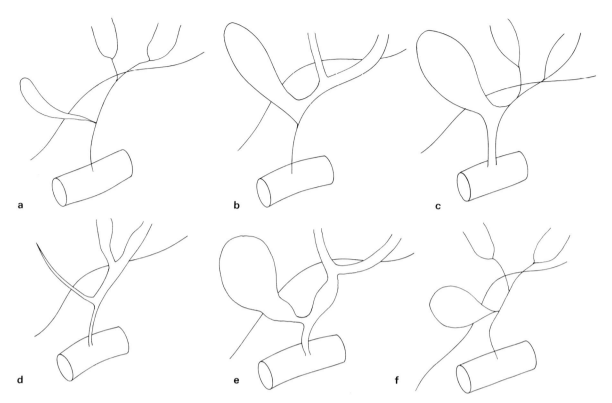

Fig. 7.14. a–f. Biliary atresia. Severity of the extrahepatic obstruction from complete atresia of the extrahepatic biliary tree with hypoplasia of the gallbladder (**a**), localized atresia (**b** and **c**) hypoplasia of the extrahepatic biliary system (**d**), or localized narrowing at the distal end of the common bile duct (**e**). A gallbladder of normal size may be found in the presence of atresia of the whole of the extrahepatic biliary system (**f**).

problem in some cases. Occasionally, extrahepatic biliary obstruction is produced by inspissated mucus in the biliary tree in mucoviscidosis or by bile plugs or sludging in the extrahepatic ducts.

Histologically there is expansion of the portal areas by fibrous tissue and proliferation of interlobular bile ducts and small ductules at the periphery of portal areas (Fig. 7.15). These ducts often contain bile, and bile duct plugging within the hepatic lobule is frequently seen. There may be inflammatory cell infiltration in the portal areas; this is not a florid change and the inflammatory cells are not usually seen in the parenchyma. Giant cell transformation of hepatocytes may be present, being usually focal in distribution and rarely conspicuous (Fig. 7.16).

If the obstruction is not relieved portal fibrosis progresses to biliary cirrhosis and death results from hepatic failure or intercurrent infection. In the late stages of the disease bile duct proliferation is not as florid as at the outset.

A liver biopsy exhibiting the changes caused by extrahepatic biliary obstruction does not usually present any diagnostic problem; any giant cell transformation of hepatocytes is usually minor in degree and inflammatory infiltration is confined to the portal areas, being absent in the lobule, whilst bile duct proliferation is marked and uniform throughout the biopsy. When errors are made, the problem seems to be that of over-interpreting the patchy and usually minor ductular proliferation in hepatitis, with the changes being interpreted as those of extra-hepatic obstruction (Brough and Bernstein 1974). Ductular proliferation may be widespread in alpha$_1$-antitrypsin deficiency, but the absence of interlobular duct proliferation and the presence of diastase-resistant, PAS-positive globules in the cytoplasm of periportal hepatocytes indicate the correct diagnosis. Brough and Bernstein (1974) counsel against assessment of possible bile duct proliferation on sections stained by trichrome methods as this tends to accentuate small bile radicles. In their hands it has contributed to over-interpretation of minor degrees of ductular proliferation.

7.4. Trisomy 17–18 Syndrome

A spectrum of liver abnormalities may occur in the trisomy 17–18 syndrome. Weichsel and Luggatti (1965) described extrahepatic biliary atresia in an

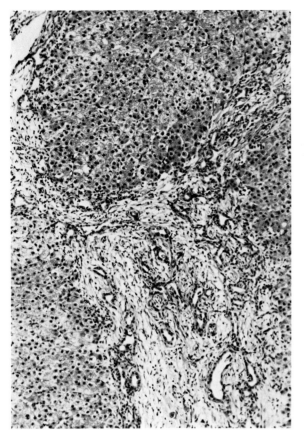

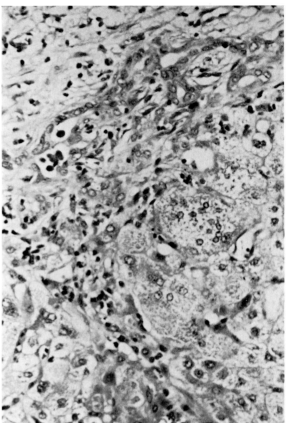

Fig. 7.15. Biliary atresia. Expansion of the portal area by fibrous tissue within which many small bile ducts are present (H and E; 57 ×)

Fig. 7.16. Biliary atresia. A minor degree of giant cell transformation of hepatocytes may be present. Note absence of inflammation within the lobule. (H and E; 360 ×)

infant with 17–18 trisomy. In the cases described by Alpert et al. (1969), three of ten infants with cytogenetically proven 17–18 trisomy had hepatitis with giant cell transformation, bile stasis and hepatocellular necrosis. They also described hepatitis in four of nine phenotypic cases and biliary atresia in two others (Figs 7.17 and 7.18). A personally observed case had cystically dilated intrahepatic bile ducts with no inflammation, giant cell transformation of hepatocytes, or bile plugging (Fig. 7.19). There was a patent extrahepatic biliary system.

8. Intravenous Alimentation

It has long been recognized that intravenous administration of fat (e.g., Intralipid) as part of a total parenteral nutritional regime results in its uptake by reticuloendothelial cells throughout the body. The material can be demonstrated by fat stains in spleen, lymph nodes, and thymus and in the Kupffer cells. On routine staining the Kupffer cells

are distended and easily seen within the sinusoids (Fig. 7.20). The cytoplasm has a foamy appearance because of the accumulation of fat globules (Fig. 7.21).

Jaundice complicating parenteral nutrition was first recognized by Peden et al. (1971), and there have been several subsequent reports. Bernstein et al. (1977) included liver biopsy in the investigation of their cases. Hepatic immaturity seems to be an important factor, and although all Bernstein's (1977) cases had necrotizing enterocolitis, this had occurred as a complication of prematurity rather than an aetiological factor in disturbing liver function. Cholestatic jaundice develops after several weeks of intravenous alimentation, and maximum serum bilirubin levels are seen at 7–15 weeks from the onset of treatment. Recovery occurs after cessation of intravenous feeding.

The histological appearance of the liver is that of cholestasis with bile plugging and intracellular bile retention (Fig. 7.20). Some of the intracellular brown pigment is lipofuscin (Fig. 7.22). Giant cell transformation of hepatocytes is often present and may be widespread. Patchy liver cell necrosis is present in some cases. There is no accompanying inflammatory cell infiltration, but haematopoiesis is seen in portal areas and is an indication of the immaturity of the patient.

Electron microscopic examination of the liver reveals matrix-rich giant mitochondria, mitochondrial heterogeneity, and damage to microsomal membranes. These findings are nonspecific indicators of hepatocellular injury.

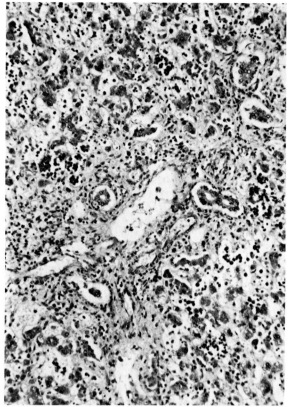

Fig. 7.18.

Fig. 7.17. (*bottom left*) Trisomy 18. Female died 1 day. Multiple congenital abnormalities. The common bile duct is hypoplastic. (H and E; 60 ×)

Fig. 7.18. (*right*) Same case as in Fig. 8.18. Portal areas are expanded. There is some proliferation of bile ducts and loss of hepatocytes with fibrous replacement within the lobule. (H and E; 156 ×)

Fig. 7.19. (*bottom right*) Trisomy 18. Expansion of portal areas. Bile ducts are excessively branching and somewhat dilated. Some contain bile plugs. The extrahepatic biliary tree was patent. (H and E; 108 ×)

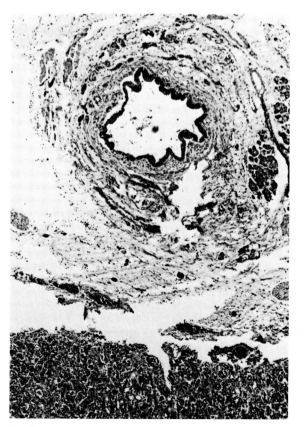

Fig. 7.17.

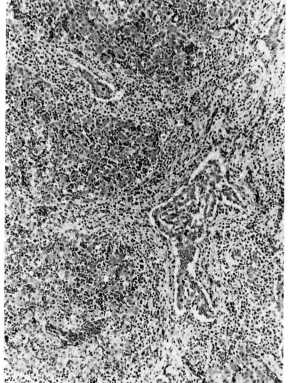

Fig. 7.19.

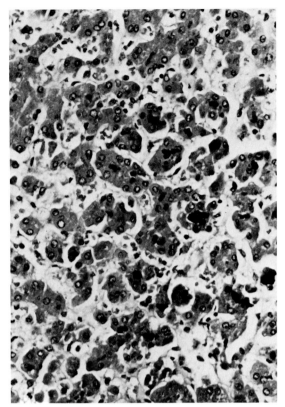

Fig. 7.20.

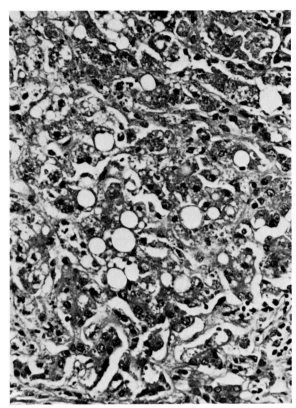

Fig. 7.22.

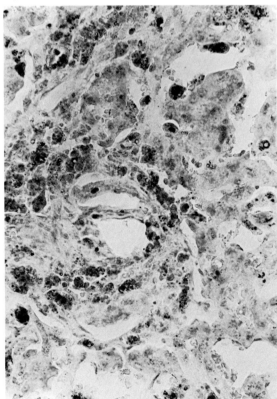

Fig. 7.21.

Fig. 7.20. (*top left*) Intravenous alimentation. The sinusoids are distended and Kupffer cells are prominent; their cytoplasm is foamy. Bile plugs are prominent. (H and E; 360 ×)

Fig. 7.21. (*left*) Intravenous alimentation. Fat droplets are seen within Kupffer cells. (Oil Red O; 144 ×)

Fig. 7.22. (*top right*) Intravenous alimentation. Pigment retention and fatty change are seen within hepatocytes. (H and E; 144 ×)

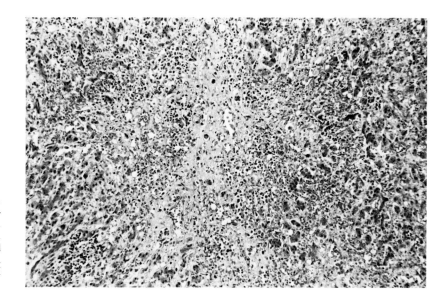

Fig. 7.23. Congenital syphilis. Fresh stillbirth at 34 weeks gestation. Maternal W.R.-positive. Treated 2 weeks before delivery. There is marked fibrosis of portal tracts which extends into the lobule. Extensive hepatocyte necrosis. (H and E; 120×)

9. Infections

9.1. Listeriosis

The liver is usually involved in perinatal infection with *Listeria monocytogenes*. The infection is acquired from the maternal genital tract in the few weeks before delivery. Miliary creamy-white necrotic granulomas are visible through the liver capsule. Gram-positive bacilli can be demonstrated within the necrotic foci in histological sections.

9.2. Syphilis

Intrauterine syphilitic infection of the fetus produces hepatomegaly and examination of the neonatal liver reveals extensive replacement of hepatic parenchyma by fibrous tissue, which begins as an expansion of portal areas (Fig. 7.23) and extends to produce cirrhosis. Giant cell transformation of hepatocytes occurs and in severe cases isolated multinucleate cells surrounded by fibrous tissue are seen (Fig. 7.24).

9.3. Viral Hepatitis

9.3.1. Type A

Viral hepatitis type A is of worldwide distribution and is endemic in many areas. Transmission is usually by the faecal/oral route, so that crowded conditions and poor standards of hygiene facilitate spread. In these conditions infection in childhood is likely.

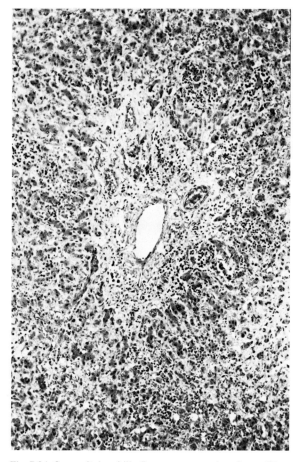

Fig. 7.24. Congenital syphilis. Same case as previous figure. Giant cell transformation of hepatocytes and extensive fibrosis. (H and E; 120×)

In children, the disease is frequently mild and jaundice does not necessarily occur, particularly in infants. In rare cases the infection is fulminant, with rapidly deepening jaundice. If death occurs at this stage the histological picture is that of extensive hepatic necrosis, as in adults. Although most patients seem to recover completely, postnecrotic cirrhosis develops in some cases.

9.3.2. *Type B*

Viral hepatitis type B is not a common problem in paediatric practice in Britain. There are, however, particular circumstances in which this type of hepatitis may occur.

Infection may occur in the perinatal period and the infant's limited immune competence at this time may be a contributory factor. Most of the infants who have developed hepatitis B in the perinatal period have been born to mothers with clinical hepatitis in the last trimester of pregnancy, and it is probable that infections occurs intrapartum by contamination with maternal blood or ingestion of bloody liquor (Cossart 1974). Neonatal infection with type B hepatitis may progress to cirrhosis (Wright et al. 1970).

A small proportion of infants born to mothers who are carriers of hepatitis B surface antigen also become HBs Ag-positive. The susceptibility to vertical transmission of hepatitis B surface antigen may be genetically determined; a recent survey in London seems to indicate an increased susceptibility amongst the offspring of Chinese mothers (Woo et al. 1979). None of these infants developed signs of biochemical abnormalities suggestive of liver disease.

Perinatal hepatitis type B infection may follow the transfusion of blood that is HBA-positive (Dupuy et al. 1975). This can readily be prevented by using only screened donor blood or blood products, but chronic, often subclinical, liver disease remains a problem in some countries with a high incidence of hepatitis amongst children requiring repeated blood transfusion, e.g., those with thalassaemia (Masera et al. 1980). Children with malignant disease and who may be receiving immunosuppressive therapy and at the same time require many transfusions with blood or blood products are particularly vulnerable.

Institutionalized children form another group at risk for hepatitis type B infection, particularly the mentally handicapped, amongst whom adequate standards of hygiene may be difficult to maintain. Children with Down's syndrome, who are particularly susceptible to infections, constitute a very vulnerable group.

9.4. Cytomegalovirus Infection

Cytomegalovirus (CMV) infection of the liver in the neonate may be part of a generalized infection acquired in utero and manifest at birth, or may be acquired just before or during delivery. Infection may also result from blood transfusion in utero or in the neonatal period, and may be subsequently transmitted to the nonimmune mother by her infant (Tobin et al. 1975). It occurs in older children who are treated with immunosuppressive drugs and who require frequent blood transfusion.

In the neonate, CMV infection is often histologically manifest as a neonatal hepatitis syndrome; giant cell transformation of hepatocytes and inflammatory cell infiltration of the parenchyma occur and an occasional typical intranuclear viral inclusion may be seen in bile duct epithelium or in a periportal hepatocyte (Fig. 7.25).

Cytomegalovirus infection may, however, produce severe acute hepatic disease as part of a generalized infection, the hepatitis resembling that

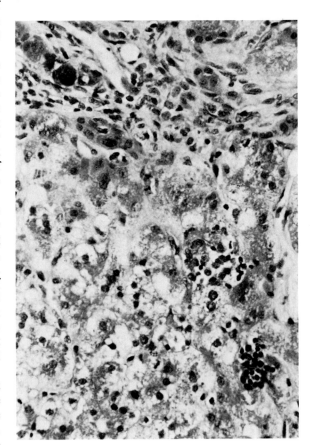

Fig. 7.25. Cytomegalovirus infection producing "giant-cell hepatitis". There is giant cell transformation of hepatocytes. Haematopoiesis persists with in the lobule. An intranuclear viral inclusion is seen in biliary epithelium within the portal tract (*top right*). (H and E; 576 ×)

produced by Herpes simplex (CMVs are members of the same group). Areas of necrosis may be seen throughout the liver and intranuclear viral inclusions are readily apparent, usually at the perimeter of the necrotic focus (7.26 and 7.27).

9.5. Herpes Simplex

The neonate is usually protected from Herpes simplex infection by maternal antibody, so infection rarely occurs. Severe, generalized infection can occur in the infant of a nonimmune mother (*Br Med J* 1969). The disease has a high mortality rate, and hepatitis is usually present.

The characteristic features are focal necrosis and intranuclear viral inclusions.

9.6. Echovirus Infection

Infants and children seem to be susceptible to infection by Echovirus 11. Neonatal meningitis and renal haemorrhage with small-vessel thrombosis of kidneys and adrenals were found in an outbreak in a special care baby unit (Nagington et al. 1978). Hepatitis may occur, with sudden collapse, jaundice, and haemorrhage. There is widespread necrosis of the hepatic parenchyma, which is largely centrilobular in distribution with mixed inflammatory cell infiltration (Figs. 7.28 and 7.29).

10. Fatty Degeneration

The infant liver readily undergoes fatty change, particularly in response to malnutrition, anoxaemia, or sepsis. Fat accumulates in the cytoplasm of the hepatocytes in fine droplets rather than in the solitary globule so commonly seen in the adult liver. For this reason it is easily overlooked in haematoxylin-, eosin-, or trichochrome-stained sections, but is readily demonstrable by specific fat stains.

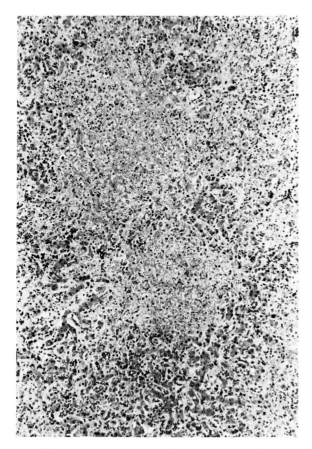

Fig. 7.26. Cytomegalovirus hepatitis. Infant born at 26 weeks gestation. Died aged 63 days with disseminated cytomegalovirus infection. Focal necrosis seen within the liver. (H and E; 144×)

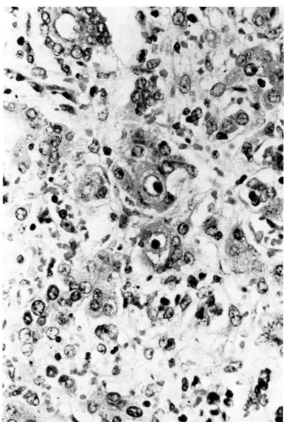

Fig. 7.27. Same case as in Fig. 7.25. Intranuclear viral inclusions are present in hepatocytes at the periphery of a necrotic focus. There is marked inflammatory cell infiltration within the lobule. (H and E; 576×)

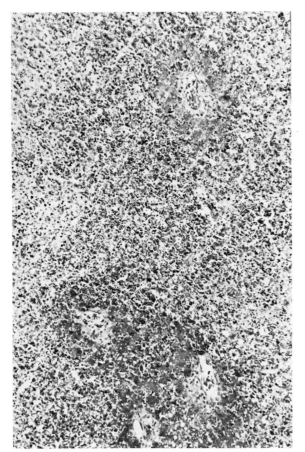

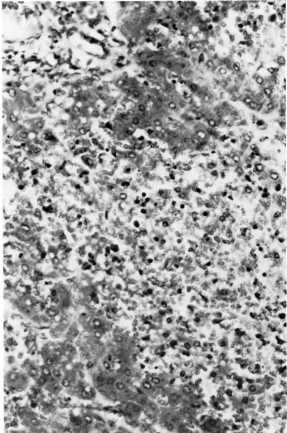

Fig. 7.28. Echo 11 hepatitis. Term male infant. Sudden deterioration on day 6 with pallor, hypothermia and hepatomegaly. Generalized bleeding tendency and jaundice and convulsions at age 8 days. Extensive parenchymal necrosis is present. Hepatocytes survive only in periportal areas. (H and E; 144 ×)

Fig. 7.29. Echo 11 hepatitis. Focal necrosis with diffuse inflammatory cell infiltration (H and E; 360 ×)

11. Reye's Syndrome

The association of acute encephalopathy and fatty degeneration of the viscera was described by Reye et al. in 1963, and must be considered in the differential diagnosis of convulsions or altered consciousness, particularly if accompanied by severe vomiting proceeding rapidly to coma, in a child who has been previously well. There may be evidence of a mild infective illness. Papilloedema is commonly found, but there are no localizing CNS signs. There may be mild to moderate hepatomegaly and hypoglycaemia is usual, as are reduced prothrombin activity and a markedly raised aspartate aminotransferase level. The blood ammonia level may also be elevated. A liver biopsy demonstrating severe, panlobular, fatty change confirms the diagnosis but is rarely done, either because the clinician does not consider the

diagnosis of Reyes' syndrome or because of reluctance to undertake such a procedure in the face of reduced prothrombin activity.

The necropsy findings are those of severe cerebral oedema in the absence of any inflammatory cell infiltration of brain or meninges, hepatomegaly with severe panlobular fatty degeneration and accumulation of lipid in renal tubules.

A variety of toxic and infective processes have been linked with Reye's syndrome. Virus infection has been suggested as a cause, in particular by influenza B, although influenza A, parainfluenza, adenovirus, and varicella zoster viruses (Linneman et al. 1975), and more recently respiratory syncytial virus (Griffin et al. 1979), have also been implicated. Aflatoxin ingestion has been incriminated in Thailand (Hogan et al. 1978) and ingestion of a variety of drugs and chemicals has been thought to be causal (Glasgow and Ferris 1968; Shield et al. 1977). One outbreak has been associated with agricultural spraying with insecticide, and similar changes were produced in mice following a combination of exposure to the insecticide and virus infection

(Crocker et al. 1974). An apparent association with salicylate ingestion may be related to the frequency of a prodromal illness, although in one report, several children were taking high doses of salicylates (Linneman et al. 1975). There is no common molecular configuration amongst the drugs and chemicals whose use has been associated with Reye's syndrome, nor do the histological abnormalities suggest that viral invasion of the brain or liver occurs.

12. Kwashiorkor

Severe fatty degeneration of the liver is almost universal in kwashiorkor, when up to 50% wet weight of liver may be fat (Waterlow 1948). This is probably a reflection of abnormal triglyceride transport secondary to reduced plasma lipoprotein levels.

Histological appearances are those of panlobular accumulation of fat in small vacuoles distending the hepatocytes (Fig. 7.30). Hepatic architecture is not disturbed, but periportal round-cell infiltration may be present. Focal hepatocellular necrosis is occasionally present. The liver returns to normal following resumption of normal nutritional status (Cook and Hutt 1967).

13. Cirrhosis

Cirrhosis of the liver in childhood is uncommon. In comparison with adults, a much greater proportion of cases complicate a recognized liver disease or metabolic abnormality involving the liver. The majority of cases follow the hepatitis syndrome of infancy (Fig. 7.12), particularly when this is a manifestation of alpha$_1$-antitrypsin deficiency (Fig. 7.14) and biliary atresia (Fig. 7.15). Cirrhosis is a rare complication of viral hepatitis, but is common in galactosaemia and may occur in Wilson's disease and the mucopolysaccharidoses. It is a late complication of thalassaemia major (see below).

Hepatocellular carcinoma is a rare but well-recognized sequel of cirrhosis in childhood. As in adults, its occurrence is probably related to the length of survival and not to any specific underlying abnormality (Keeling 1971).

Cirrhosis in mucoviscidosis is uncommon. Its special features are described below.

Indian childhood cirrhosis, a liver disorder that is almost universally fatal, usually affects children in the first 5 years of life, and is virtually limited to the Indian subcontinent. Its aetiology is unknown.

The histological picture varies from massive hepatic necrosis in the acute stage to portal cirrhosis. The presence of cytoplasmic hyaline degeneration indistinguishable from Mallory's alcoholic hyaline degeneration by histological stains and histochemical methods (Nayak et al. 1969) is unique amongst the childhood cirrhoses, and has been interpreted as an index of toxic injury to the hepatocyte.

14. Thalassaemia

In thalassaemia major, as a result of transfusion overload, there is progressive iron deposition within the the liver with increasing age. Iron accumulates within hepatocytes and also within macrophages in portal areas. There is a gradual increase in portal fibrous tissue (Fig. 7.31) with progression to cirrhosis in individuals who survive

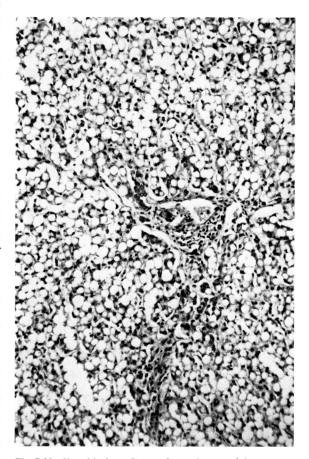

Fig. 7.30. Kwashiorkor. Severe fatty change of hepatocytes throughout the lobule. There is periportal round-cell infiltration. Liver architecture is normal. (H and E; ×150×)

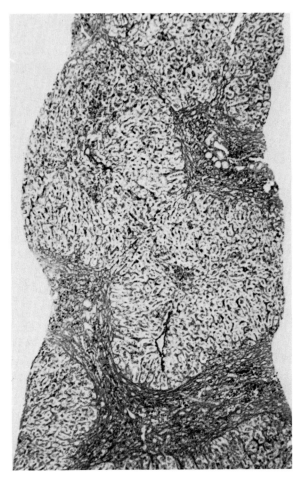

Fig. 7.31. Thalassaemia. Cirrhosis present in a needle liver biopsy.

15. Mucoviscidosis

There is some liver involvement in most children with cystic fibrosis, although the majority are asymptomatic. The pathogenetic mechanism of the liver disease is similar to that producing pathological changes in other organs, namely the production of viscid secretions by mucus-producing cells in the biliary tract, which obstruct bile flow and give rise to a localized cholangitis and portal fibrosis. On the whole, the severity of liver involvement in cystic fibrosis is related to length of survival, but one may find minimal liver damage in adolescents who have very extensive lung damage and complete fatty replacement of the pancreas.

15.1. Focal Portal Fibrosis

Focal portal fibrosis or focal biliary cirrhosis is the commonest hepatic lesion in mucoviscidosis, and is usually discovered as an incidental finding at laparotomy or necropsy.

Fibrosis often occurs just beneath the capsule of the liver (Fig. 7.32). Portal tracts are irregularly expanded by fibrous tissue, and fibrous bands run between adjacent portal areas. The involved portal tracts contain elevated numbers of bile ducts. Mucus is sometimes seen within the ducts or duct epithelial cells but concretions are rare.

15.2. Biliary Cirrhosis

Some children with cystic fibrosis develop biliary cirrhosis during childhood. Jaundice is uncommon and biochemical tests of liver function usually yield normal results, the signs and complications of portal hypertension being the presenting features (Di Sant'Agnese and Blanc 1956).

The liver has an irregular nodularity; the fibrous scars may produce fissuring resembling the 'hepar lobatum' of congenital syphilis (Craig et al. 1957).

There is marked portal fibrosis and within the fibrous tissue there are very many dilated bile ducts filled with inspissated material (Fig. 7.33), an appearance pathognomic of cystic fibrosis. There is bile plugging within the lobules in many cases; regenerative nodules are not conspicuous. Fatty change of the parenchyma is variable and probably reflects the general nutritional status of the patient.

into their second or third decade. Risdon et al. (1975) found a linear relationship between the extent of fibrosis and the age of the patients and an exponential relationship between both the rate and extent of hepatic fibrosis and the amount of iron deposited in the liver. They concluded that the reduction in liver iron concentration produced by chelation therapy produced a considerable reduction in the rate of fibrosis within the liver.

Reports from Italy (De Virgiliis 1980; Masera 1980) suggest that chronic active or chronic persistent hepatitis following hepatitis B infection may contribute to deterioration in liver function in patients with thalassaemia. Acute infection was largely subclinical but the incidence of subsequent chronic liver disease was higher amongst patients with thalassaemia than amongst non-thalassaemic individuals. It has been suggested that interaction between low-dose infection and iron overload might play a part in perpetuating chronic liver disease in thalassaemic subjects (De Virgiliis 1980).

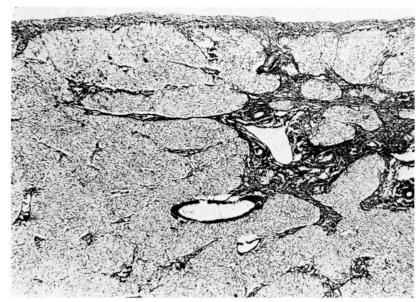

Fig. 7.32. Mucoviscidosis. Male died age 12 with bronchiectasis and bronchopneumonia. Patchy portal fibrosis seen beneath the liver capsule. (Gordon's and Sweet's reticulin stain; 36 ×)

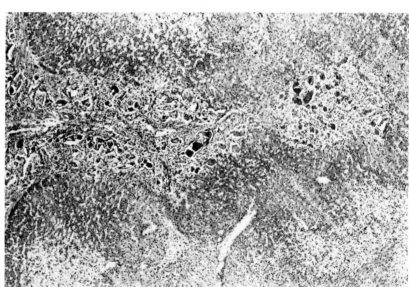

Fig. 7.33. Mucoviscidosis. There is marked bile duct proliferation and dilatation within portal areas. Many ducts are filled with inspissated material. (H and E; 36 ×)

15.3. Neonatal Jaundice

In a small number of patients with cystic fibrosis, obstructive jaundice in the neonatal period may be the mode of presentation, but it is more commonly seen at this age in infants presenting with meconium ileus or ileal atresia (Oppenheimer and Esterly 1975). The jaundice may be persistent (Valman et al. 1971).

The histological appearance of the liver at this time is typical of extrahepatic biliary obstruction with proliferation of small bile radicles in portal areas, bile plugging, and perhaps some minor degree of giant cell transformation of hepatocytes in the presence of a demonstrably patent extrahepatic biliary tree. Mucus in the bile ducts around the porta hepatis may produce marked localized dilatation of the ducts, which is usually transient (Oppenheimer and Esterly 1975). The jaundice may be persistent (Valman et al. 1971).

The histological appearance of the liver at this time is typical of extrahepatic biliary obstruction with proliferation of small bile radicles in portal areas, bile plugging, and perhaps some minor degree of giant cell transformation of hepatocytes in the presence of a demonstrably patent extrahepatic biliary tree. Mucus in the bile ducts around the porta hepatis may produce marked localized dilatation of the ducts, which is usually transient (Oppenheimer and Esterly 1975).

16. Budd-Chiari Syndrome

The clinical course and appearances of the liver are similar in childhood to those seen in the adult. Occasional causes of Budd–Chiari syndrome in children are congenital anomalies, such as stenosis of a hepatic vein and anomalous valves and sphincters. More commonly it complicates other diseases, such as tumours or leukaemia, sickle-cell disease, polycythaemia, and allergic vasculitis.

17. Trauma

The liver of infants and children is more liable to trauma than that of the adult because of its relatively large size and the poor protection offered by the developing rib cage.

The liver may be damaged during delivery, and subcapsular haematomas with or without haemoperitoneum are not uncommon, particularly in preterm infants. Liver damage may follow vigorous external cardiac massage in the neonate, when a linear haematoma along the costal margin or extensive haemorrhage beneath the capsule of the right lobe may be produced (Fig. 7.34).

In older children, laceration of the liver may be the result of nonpenetrating injuries to the abdomen, usually as a result of road traffic accidents, but falls and nonaccidental injury can also produce liver damage.

The mortality from laceration of the liver is high, often because of failure of diagnosis, although prompt surgical intervention may be successful (Sparkman 1954).

18. Tumours

18.1. Hepatoblastoma (see p. 660)

18.2. Hamartoma

Hamartomas of the liver are of two basic types, angiomas, which form the larger group, and those composed of liver and fibrous tissue.

Angiomas are tumours of infancy. They are often large at the time of birth and may rupture during delivery, causing death by exsanguination (Claireaux 1960). Some are the cause of cardiac failure in the neonatal period because of shunting (Figs. 7.35–7.37) (Bamford et al. 1980) with a high cardiac output (Linderkamp et al. 1976), and others are palpated as an abdominal mass which is often rapidly enlarging. Resection of a single large tumour and the surrounding liver may be necessary to control heart failure, but ligation of its supply vessels

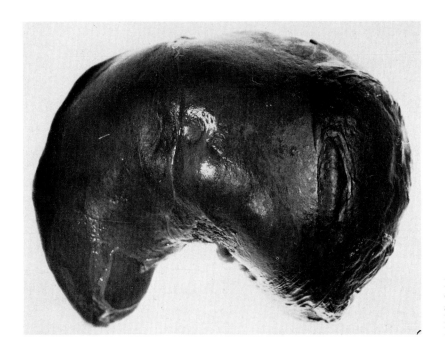

Fig. 7.34. Subcapsular haematoma of liver. Male born at 28 weeks, died aged 2 days. Large subcapsular haematoma of the right lobe of liver.

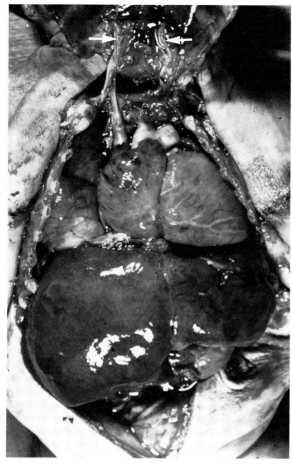

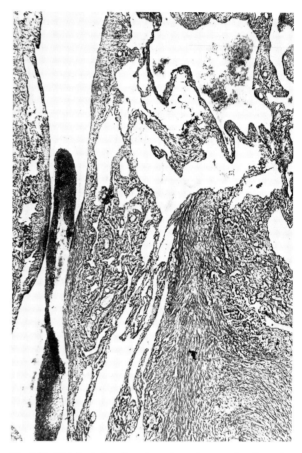

Fig. 7.37. Histological section shows irregular vascular channels. (Gordon's and Sweet's reticulin method; 81 ×)

Fig. 7.35. Female born at 36 weeks. Hepatomegaly with prominent left lobe at 2 h. Cardiomegaly. Left ventricular angiocardiogram showed enormously dilated internal mammary arteries supplying an AV malformation of the left lobe of the liver. Died aged 3 days with disseminated intravascular coagulation despite ligation of feeding vessels. There is marked hepatomegaly with irregular contour to the left lobe and cardiomegaly. Both internal mammary arteris (*arrows*) are dilated and tortuous.

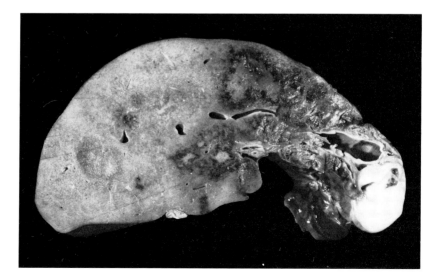

Fig. 7.36. Arteriovenous malformation. Slice of liver shows left lobe of liver replaced by irregular vascular channels. Areas of infarction present in right lobe.

may be possible. The lesions may be accompanied by a consumptive coagulopathy due to clotting within the angioma or an isolated thrombocytopenia occurring as a result of increased mechanical destruction of platelets in the abnormal vessels. There may be jaundice, which in some cases is obstructive in type. Angiomas are frequently single, but may be multiple (Balazs 1978). They may be capillary, cavernous, or mixed.

The fibrous type of hamartoma presents as an abdominal mass, which may enlarge rapidly as cystically dilated duct elements filled with fluid (Fig. 7.38).

Other malformations reported as accompanying hepatic hamartomas include tracheo-oesophageal fistula and annular pancreas (Keeling 1971), atrial septal defect, patent ductus arteriosus, meningo-myelocele, renal agenesis, hypoplastic mandible, and cutaneous angiomas (cited by Linderkamp et al. 1976). All are commonly occurring malformations and there seems to be no specific association.

Regression following steroid therapy has been documented (Goldberg and Fonkalstrued 1969) and flattening of endothelial cells, with loss of capillary buds and increased stromal fibrosis followed steroids and radiotherapy in the case described by Balazs et al. (1978).

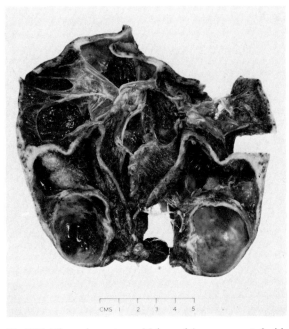

Fig. 7.38. Fibrous hamartoma. Male aged 4 years presented with abdominal enlargement. The mass is composed of epithelial lined cysts. These are surrounded by fibrous tissue and there are many focal haemorrhages. Reproduced by kind permission of the Editor (JT Harries), and Publishers of *Essentials of Paediatric Gastroenterology*.

18.3. Hepatocellular Carcinoma

Hepatocellular carcinoma occurs in the older child, usually presenting after the age of 6 years. The symptoms are vomiting, abdominal pain, loss of weight, and abdominal distension; jaundice occurs late in the disease. The liver is usually palpably enlarged and a liver scan may demonstrate the site of the tumour. Liver function tests are usually normal, although the serum alpha-fetoprotein level may be raised.

Hepatocellular carcinomas can arise in a previously normal liver or in one with pre-existing disease. Cirrhosis, itself the sequel to extrahepatic biliary atresia or hepatitis in infancy, may predispose to the development of carcinoma in some cases. Hepatocellular carcinoma has been found in children with a variety of metabolic disorders, including glycogen storage disease, Niemann–Pick disease, and hereditary tubular dysplasia (de Toni–Fanconi disease) (Keeling 1971).

Within the liver there may be a solitary tumour mass (Fig. 7.39) or multiple tumour nodules throughout the organ. There are lobulated, yellow/tan in colour, and appear to be encapsulated. Histologically and at the ultrastructural level the liver cell carcinoma of older children is identical with that found in the adult (Fig. 7.40), and quite distinct from hepatoblastoma of the infant liver, which may differentiate along a largely hepatocellular line (Misugi et al. 1967); Ito and Johnson 1969). At present treatment of these tumours does not have any long-term success, irrespective of the presence or absence of pre-existing liver disease.

18.4. Rhabdomyosarcoma

Rhabdomyosarcoma also occurs in the liver of the older child. It is thought to arise from the muscle in the wall of the intrahepatic bile ducts. Symptoms include jaundice, which may be severe, anorexia, abdominal pain, and swelling.

A single mass, often in the vicinity of a large bile duct, may be present, or there may be multiple widely separated tumour nodules throughout the liver (Fig. 7.41). The tumour is cream in colour, and firm; translucent polypoid nodules may protrude into the lumen of an adjacent bile duct (Fig. 7.42). In some tumours, cystic degeneration is a prominent feature.

Histologically, the tumour is composed of large mesenchymal cells with large pale-staining nuclei exhibiting considerable pleomorphism (Fig. 7.43). The cytoplasm of the cells may be densely eosinophilic or foamy. 'Tadpole' or elongated 'strap' cells are often present, but cytoplasmic striations are

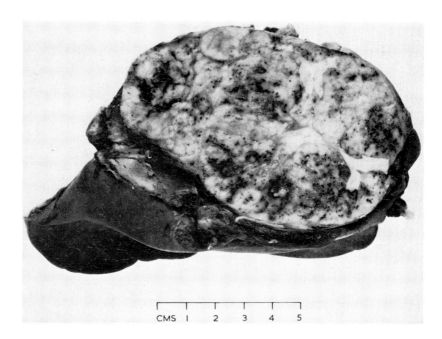

Fig. 7.39. Hepatocellular carcinoma. Lobulated tumour with multiple small haemorrhages scattered throughout. (Keeling 1971, by courtesy of the Editor of the *Journal of Pathology*.)

not seen in these tumours as commonly as in rhabdomyosarcomas arising in the urogenital tract.

These tumours metastasize to lymph nodes in the porta hepatis. Haematogenous spread to the lungs may occur early in the disease.

18.5. Malignant Mesenchymal Tumour

Malignant mesenchymal tumour also occurs in older children, presenting as an abdominal mass, often with fever and pain (Stanley et al. 1973). Arteriography reveals poor perfusion, and on resection the tumours are seen as large, partly cystic, mucoid masses. Histologically they are poorly differentiated. Bizarre giant cells are seen in a myxoid stroma, with many spindle cells forming a background of varying density (Fig. 7.44).

18.6. Teratoma

True teratomas of the liver are very rare, and must be distinguished from hepatoblastoma with squamous metaplasia and osteoid formation. Both benign (Yarborough and Evashnick 1956) and malignant tumours (Misugi and Reiner 1965) have been described.

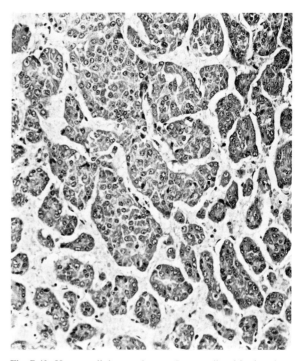

Fig. 7.40. Hepatocellular carcinoma. Large cells with abundant cytoplasm having a trabecular configuration. (H and E; 100×)

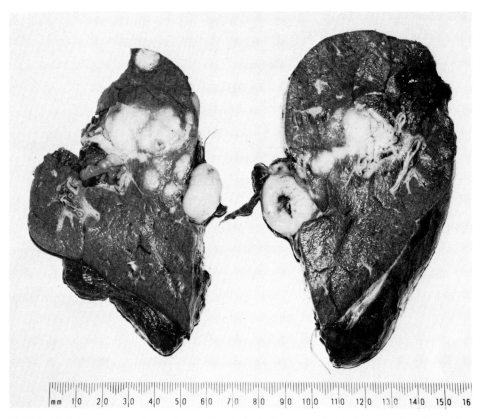

Fig. 7.41. Rhabdomyosarcoma from a 6-year-old male child who presented with obstructive jaundice and hepatomegaly. The cut surface of the liver shows multiple tumour nodules.

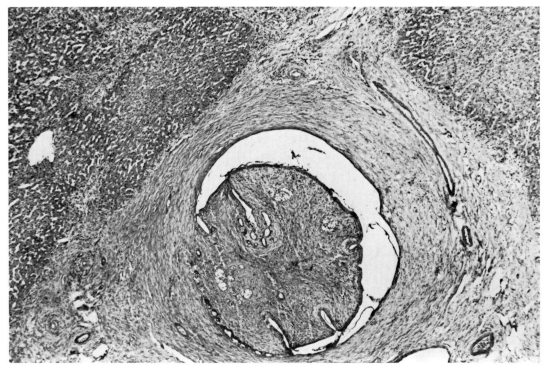

Fig. 7.42. Rhabdomyosarcoma. An epithelial covered tumour nodule protrudes into a dilated bile duct. (H and E; 48 ×)

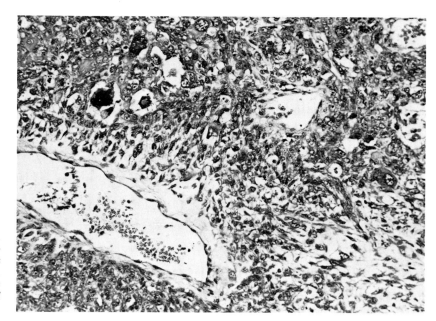

Fig. 7.43. Rhabdomyosarcoma. There is marked cellular and nuclear pleomorphism. Cytoplasmic degeneration is seen at lower right. (H and E; 100 ×). (Keeling 1971, by courtesy of the Editor of the *Journal of Pathololgy*.)

19. Gallbladder

19.1. Congenital Anomalies

Congenital abnormalities of the gallbladder are very rare and take the form of septation and duplication. Complete duplication of the gallbladder may occur, each having its own spiral valve and cystic duct, which may empty into the common bile duct or directly into the duodenum. It is usually of no consequence in infancy but may give rise to problems in the presence of acquired disease.

An externally normal gallbladder may be divided internally by an intraluminal septum composed of muscle and covered by biliary epithelium. A diverticulum may arise from the gallbladder or from the cystic duct. It is distinguished from an Aschoff–Rokitansky sinus by the presence of a muscular wall.

19.2. Choledochal Cysts

A choledochal cyst is a focal dilatation of the common bile duct, which may take the form of a fusiform or eccentric saccular dilatation or may be pedunculated. There is enormous variation in size, from those having a volume of only a few millilitres to enormous cysts containing several litres of bile-stained fluid. Large cysts may be palpable *per*

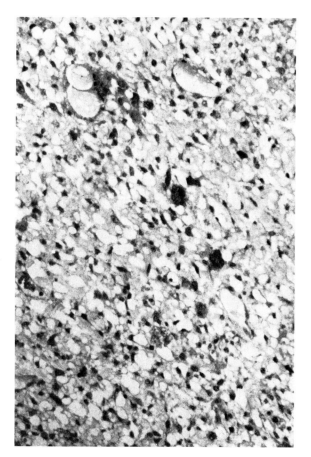

Fig. 7.44. Malignant mesenchymal tumour from a 12-year-old girl presenting with shoulder-tip pain. Death occured 6 months later after two resections. Myxoid tissue, with bizarre large cells. (H and E; 240 ×)

abdomen or visualized by ultrasound or radiological techniques. They are thought to arise at points of weakness in the muscle of the duct wall following obstruction of the bile flow caused by a mucosal flap, or a prolonged oblique course of the duct through the duodenal wall (Fig. 7.45). Presenting symptoms include obstructive jaundice, particularly in the neonate, upper abdominal pain, or a mass in the right hypochondrium. Radiological examination may aid preoperative diagnosis and the cyst may displace the right kidney downwards or the duodenum anteriorly and medially.

The cysts are lined with biliary epithelium but this is frequently disrupted by inflammation. The wall consists of smooth muscle and fibrous tissue.

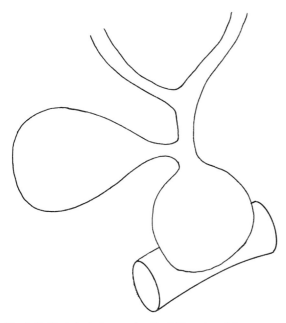

Fig. 7.45. Choledochal cyst: a localized dilatation of the common bile duct, which may be palpable through the abdominal wall.

19.3. Cholecystitis

Cholecystitis is extremely rare in infancy and childhood and resembles acute inflammation of this viscus in the adult.

19.4. Cholelithiasis

Cholelithiasis in children usually occurs as a complication of haemolytic anaemia or sickle-cell disease.

Spontaneous perforation of the common bile duct is an occasional neonatal surgical emergency (Howard et al. 1976).

References

Aagenaes O, Fagerhol M, Elgjo K, Munthe E, Hovig T (1974) Pathology and pathogenesis of liver disease in alpha-1-antitrypsin deficient individuals. Postgrad Med J 50: 365

Alagille D, Odievre M, Gautier M, Dommergnes JP (1975) Hepatic ductular hypoplasia associated with characteristic facies, vertebral malformations, retarded physical, mental and sexual development, and cardiac murmur. J Pediatr 86: 63

Alpert LI, Strauss L, Hirschhorn K (1969) Neonatal hepatitis and biliary atresia associated with trisomy 17–18 syndrome. N Engl J Med 280: 16

Balazs Marta, Denes J, Lukacs VF (1978) Fine structure of multiple neonatal haemangioendothelioma of the liver. Virchows Arch [A] 379: 157–168

Bamford MFM, de Bono D, Pickering D, Keeling JW (1980) An arteriovenous malformation of the liver giving rise to persistent transitional (fetal) circulation. Arch Dis Child 55: 244

Berg NO, Eriksson S (1972) Liver disease in adults with alpha-1-antitrypsin deficiency. N Engl J Med 287: 1264

Berk PD, Bloomer JR, Howe RB, Berlin NI (1970) Constitutional hepatic dysfunction (Gilbert's syndrome). A new definition based on kinetic studies with unconjugated radiobilirubin. Am J Med 49: 296

Bernstein J, Chang CH, Brough AJ, Heidelberger KP (1977) Conjugated hyperbilirubinaemia in infancy associated with parenteral alimentation. J Pediatr 90: 361

Blyth H, Ockenden BG (1971) Polycystic disease of kidneys and liver presenting in childhood. J Med Genet 8: 257

Boggs JD, Lawson EE (1974) Long-term follow up of neonatal hepatitis: Safety and value of surgical exploration. Paediatrics 53: 650

Brough AJ, Bernstein J (1974) Conjugated hyperbilirubinemia in early infancy. A reassessment of liver biopsy. Hum Pathol 5: 507

Claireaux AE (1960) Neonatal hyper-bilirubinaemia. Br Med J i: 1528

Cohen KL, Rubin PE, Echevarria RA, Sharp HL, Teague PO (1973) Alpha-1-antitrypsin deficiency, emphysema and cirrhosis in an adult. Ann Intern Med 78: 227

Cook PJL (1974) Genetic aspects of the Pi system. Postgrad Med J 50: 362

Cook GC Hutt MSR (1967) The liver after Kwashiorkor. Br Med J iii: 454

Cossart YE (1974) Acquisition of hepatitis B antigen in the newborn period. Postgrad Med J 50: 334

Cottrall K, Cook PJL, Mowat AP (1974) Neonatal hepatitis syndrome and alpha-1-antitrypsin deficiency: An epidemiological study in south-east England. Postgrad Med J 50: 376

Craig JM, Haddad H, Shwachman H (1957) The pathological changes in the liver in cystic fibrosis of the pancreas. Am J Dis Child 93: 357

Crawfurd M d'A, Jackson P, Kohler HG (1978) Case report: Meckel's syndrome (dysencephalia splanchnocystica) in two Pakistani sibs. J Med Genet 15: 242

Crigler JF, Najjar VA (1952) Congenital familial non-haemolytic jaundice with kernicterus. Paediatrics 10: 169

Crocker J, Royce K, Ogere R (1974) Insecticide and viral interaction as a cause of fatty visceral changes and encephalopathy in the mouse. Lancet 2: 22

Danks DM, Campbell PE, Jack I, Rogers J, Smith AL (1977a) Studies of the aetiology of neonatal hepatitis and biliary atresia. Arch Dis Child 52: 360

Danks DM, Campbell PE, Smith AL, Rogers J (1977b) Prognosis of babies with neonatal hepatitis. Arch Dis Child 52: 368

De Virgiliis S, Fiorelli G, Gargion S, Gornacchia G, Sanna G, Cossu P, Murgia V, Cao A (1980) Chronic liver disease in transfusion-dependent thalassaemia: hepatitis B virus marker studies. J Clin Pathol 33: 949

di Sant' Agnese PA, Blanc WA (1956) Distinctive type of biliary cirrhosis of the liver associated with cystic fibrosis of the pancreas. recognition through signs of portal hypertension. Pediatrics 15: 387

Dubin IN, Johnson FB (1954) Chronic idiopathic jaundice with unidentified pigment in liver cells. Medicine 33: 155

Dupuy JM, Frommmel D, Alagille D (1975) Severe viral hepatitis type B in infancy. Lancet 1: 191

Gilbert A, Lereboullet P (1901) La cholémie simple familiale. Sein Med (Paris) 21: 241

Glasgow JFT, Ferris JAJ (1968) Encephalopathy and visceral fatty infiltration of probable toxic aetiology. Lancet 1: 451

Glasgow JFT, Hercz A, Levison H, Lynch MJ, Sass-Kortsak A (1971) Alpha-1-antitryspin (AT) deficiency with both cirrhosis and chronic obstructive lung disease in two sibs. Pediatr Res 5: 427

Goldberg SJ, Fonkalsrud E (1969) Successful treatment of hepatic hemangioma with corticosteroids. JAMA 208: 2473

Griffin N, Keeling JW, Tomlinson AH (1979) Reye's syndrome associated with respiratory syncytial virus infection. Arch Dis Child 54: 74

Hamilton WJ, Boyd JD, Mossman HW (1972) Human embryology. Heffer, Cambridge, p 342

Harries JT (ed) (1977) Essentials of paediatric gastroenterology. Churchill Livingstone, Edinburgh London New York, p 327

Harris RC, Anderson DH (1960) Intrahepatic bile duct atresia, paper presented at the Annual Meeting of the American Pediatric Society, May 5, 1960

Hogan GR, Ryan NJ, Hayes AW (1968) Aflatoxin B and Reye's syndrome. Lancet 1: 561

Howard ER, Johnston DI, Mowat AP (1976) Spontaneous perforation of common bile duct in infants. Arch Dis Child 51: 883

Howard ER, Mowat AP (1977) Extrahepatic biliary atresia: recent developments in management. Arch Dis Child 52: 825

Ito J, Johnson WW (1969) Hepatoblastoma and hepatoma in infancy and childhood. Light and electron microscopic studies. Arch Pathol Lab Med 87: 259

Ivemark BI (1955) Implications of the agenesis of the spleen on pathogenesis of cono-truncal anomalies in childhood. Acta Paediatr Scand 44: [Suppl 104] 1

Johnson AM, Alper CA (1970) Deficiency in childhood liver disease. Pediatrics 46: 921

Jorgensen M (1971) A case of abnormal intrahepatic bile duct arrangement submitted to three-dimensional reconstruction. Acta Pathol Microbiol Scand [A] 79: 303

Jorgensen M (1972) Three-dimensional reconstruction of intrahepatic bile ducts in a case of polycystic disease of the liver in an infant. Acta Pathol Microbiol Scand [A] 80: 201

Kasai M, Watanabe J, Ohi R (1972) Follow-up studies of long-term survivors after hepatic portoenterostomy for 'non-correctable' biliary atresia. J Pediatr Surg 10: 173

Keeling JW (1971) Liver tumours in infancy and childhood. J Pathol 103: 69

Keer DNS, Harrison CV, Sherlock S, Milnes Walker R (1961) Congenital hepatic fibrosis. J Med N S XXX 117: 91

Landing BH (1974) Considerations of the pathogenesis of neonatal hepatitis, biliary atresia and choledochal cysts: the conception of infantile obstructive cholangiopathy. Prog Paediatr Surg 6: 113

Landing BH, Wells, TR, Claireaux AE (1980) Morphometric analysis of liver lesions in cystic disease of childhood. Hum Pathol 2: Suppl 549

Lanzkowsky P (1975) The jaundiced neonate: Causes and importance. Mead Johnson Laboratory, Evansville Ind

(Hematological diseases in children: Micrograph series, no. 2)

Lathe GH (1974) Newborn jaundice: bile pigment metabolism in the fetus and newborn infant. In: Davis GA, Dobbing J (eds). In: Scientific foundation of paediatrics. Heinemann, London, p 105

Laurell CB, Eriksson S (1963) The electrophoretic alpha-1-globulin pattern of serum in alpha-1-antitrypsin deficiency. Scand J Clin Lab Invest 15: 132

Leading article (1969) Med J ii: 204

Lieberman E, Salinas-Madrigal L, Gwinn JL, Brennan LP, Fine RN, Landing BH (1971) Infantile polycystic disease of the kidneys and liver. Medicine 50: 277

Linderkamp O, Hopner F, Klose H, Riegel KC, Hecker W (1976) Solitary hepatic hemangioma in a newborn infant complicated by cardiac failure, consumption coagulopathy, microangiopathic hemolytic anemia, and obstructive jaundice. Eur J Pediatr 124: 23

Linneman CC, Shea L, Partin JC, Schubert WK, Schiff GM (1975) Reye's syndrome: Epidemilogical and viral studies, 1963–1974. Am J Epidemiol 101: 517

Longmire WP (1964) Congenital biliary hypoplasia. Am Surg 159: 335

Lorimer AR, McGee J, McAlpine SG (1967) Congenital hepatic fibrosis. Postgrad Med J 43: 770

Masera G, Jean G, Conter V, Terzoli S, Mauri RA, Cazzaniga M (1980) Sequential study of liver biopsy in thalassaemia. Arch Dis Child 55: 800

Misugi K, Okajima H, Misugi N, Newton WA Jr (1967) Classification of primary malignant tumors of liver in infancy and childhood. Cancer 20: 1760

Misugi K, Reinger CB (1965) A malignant true teratoma of liver in childhood. Arch Pathol 80: 409

Montgomery AH (1940) Solitary nonparasitic cysts of the liver in children. Arch Surg 41: 422

Morse JO (1978) Alpha$_1$-antitrypsin deficiency. I. N Engl J Med 299: 1045

Morse JO (1978) Alpha$_1$-antitrypsin deficiency. II. N Engl J Med 299: 1099

Mowat AP, Psacharopoulos HT, Williams R (1976) Extrahepatic biliary atresia versus neonatal hepatitis. Review of 137 prospectively investigated infants. Arch Dis Child 51: 763

Nagington J, Wreghitt TG, Gandy G, Robertson NCR, Berry PJ (1978) Fatal echovirus 11 infections in outbreak in a special care baby unit. Lancet 2: 725

Nayak NC, Sagreiya K, Ramalingaswami V (1969) Indian childhood cirrhosis. Arch Pathol 88: 631

Opitz JM, Howe JJ (1969) The Meckel syndrome (dysencephalia splanchnocystica, the Gruber Syndrome). Birth Defects 5: 167

Oppenheimer EH, Esterly JR (1975) Hepatic changes in young infants with cystic fibrosis: Possible relation to focal biliary cirrhosis. J Pediatr 5: 683

Parker RGF (1956) Fibrosis of the liver as congenital anomaly. J Pathol 71: 359

Peden VH, Witgleben CL, Skelton MA (1971) Total parenteral nutrition. J Pediatr 78: 180

Porter CA, Mowat AP, Cook PJL, Haynes DWG, Shilkin KB, Williams R (1972) Alpha-1-antitrypsin deficiency and neonatal hepatitis. Br Med J ii: 435

Reye RDK, Morgan G, Baral J (1963) Encephalopathy and fatty degeneration of the viscera: a disease entity in children. Lancet 2: 749

Risdon RA, Barry M, Flynn DM (1975) Transfusional iron overload: the relationship between tissue iron concentration and hepatic fibrosis in thalassaemia. J Pathol 116: 83

Rosenthal IM, Spellberg MA, McGrew EA, Rozenfeld IH (1961) Absence of interlobular bile ducts. Report of a case of probable intrahepatic bile duct agenesis with severe hypercheolsterolemia, xanthomatosis, and glomerular lipid deposition. Am J Dis Child 101: 228

Rotor AB, Manahan L, Florentin A (1948) Familial non-hemolytic jaundice with direct van der Bergh reaction. Acta Medica Philippina 5: 37

Sass-Kortsak A, Bowden DH, Brown RJK (1956) Congenital intrahepatic biliary atresia. Pediatrics 17: 383

Sharp H, Freier E, Bridges R (1968) Alpha-1-globulin deficiency in a familial infant liver disease. Pediatr Res 2: 298

Shield LK, Coleman TL, Markesbery WR (1977) Methyl bromide intoxication: neurologica features, including simulation of Reye's syndrome. Neurology (Minneap) 27: 959

Sparkman RS (1954) Hepatic rupture: report of 8 cases with survival. Am Surg 139: 690

Stanley RJ, Dehner LP, Hesker AE (1973) Primary malignant mesenchymal tumours (mesenchymoma) of the liver in childhood. Cancer 32: 973

Talbot IC, Mowat AP (1975) Liver disease in infancy: histological features and relationship to alpha-1-antitrypsin phenotype. J Clin Pathol 28: 559

Tobin JO'H, Macdonald H, Brachey M, Macauley D (1975) Cytomegalovirus infection and exchange transfusion. Br Med J iv: 404

Valman HB, France NE, Wallis PG (1971) Prolonged neonatal jaundice in cystic fibrosis. Arch Dis Child 46: 805

Walshe JM (1962) Wilson's disease: The presenting symptoms. Arch Dis Child 37: 253

Waterlow JC (1948) Fatty liver disease in infants in the British West Indies. HMSO, London (Medical Research Council special report series, no. 263)

Weichsel ME, Luggatti L (1965) Trisomy 17–18 syndrome with congenital extrahepatic biliary atresia and congenital amputation of the left foot. J Pediatr 67: 324

Woo D, Cummins M, Davies PA, Harvey DR, Hurley R, Waterson AP (1979) Vertical transmission of hepatitis B surface antigen in carrier mothers in two west London hospitals. Arch Dis Child 54: 670

Wright R, Perkins JR, Bower BD, Jerrome DW (1970) Cirrhosis associated with the Australia antigen in an infant who acquired hepatitis from her mother. Br Med J iv: 719

Yarborough SM, Evashnick G (1956) Case of teratoma of the liver with 14 years post-operative survival. Cancer 9: 848

Chapter 8

Respiratory System

Jerry N. Cox

In the industrialized world there have been considerable changes in the pathology of the respiratory system in infants and children during the last two decades. This is largely due to the newer methods for establishing early diagnosis, associated with prompt and more aggressive treatment and with the wide range of antibiotics at our disposal for treating most acute problems. Some of these improvements, however, bring adverse effects with them, and have a distinct morbidity. In contrast, in most parts of the developing world many of the pathological conditions that were commonly observed during the early part of this century are still prevalent, and are often associated with lesions now peculiar to those areas.

1. Development

The respiratory system comprises the nose, nasopharynx, larynx, trachea, bronchi, and lungs.

The development of the face and nasopharynx has been dealt with on p. 212.

1.1. Larynx

Between the 3rd and 4th weeks of gestation (about 3 mm) the respiratory primordia, including the tracheo-bronchial groove, make their appearance caudal to the hypobronchial eminence. At the end of the 4th week the epithelial component of the larynx develops rapidly with the appearance of the hypopharyngeal eminences on either side, indicating the site of the right and left arytenoid swellings, forming the primitive laryngeal aditus.

Towards the end of the 5th week and during the 6th week, the *epiglottis* makes its appearance as a midventral prominence at the base of the third and fourth arches, cephalic to the glottis. The arytenoid swellings continue to grow toward the base of the tongue, enfolding the epiglottis during the process. At this stage of development, actively proliferating epithelium temporarily obliterates the entrance to the larynx. In the ensuing weeks, the growth of the larynx proceeds rapidly, and the lumen is re-established. However, the entrance becomes ovoid, and there is a persistent interarytenoid notch in the saggital plane. By the 10th week, the essential elements of the larynx are established, and the vocal cords appear on either side of the laryngeal lumen. The larynx now grows much more slowly, and it is not until the last trimester of intrauterine life that it attains its definitive form.

1.2. Trachea

The tracheo-bronchial groove appears early during the 4th week of gestation. At this stage, it has a blunted caudal end but an extensive communication with the ventro-caudal part of the pharynx. The future trachea, represented by the distal portion of the groove, lies ventral to and parallel with the oesophagus from which it is separated by the tracheo-oesophageal septum. The blunted end forms the *primary bronchial (lung) buds*. Tracheo-oesophageal separation occurs during the 4th and 5th weeks.

The endodermal outgrowth from the pharynx gives rise to the epithelial lining and glands of the trachea, while the cartilage, muscle, and connective tissue investing the organ are derived from the surrounding mesenchyme.

Cartilage rings are identifiable during the 10th week. The epithelial glands are not apparent until about the 4th month, and during subsequent weeks they assume their final characteristics. By the 5th month, the main anatomical features of the trachea are established.

1.3. Lungs

The *pulmonary primordia* or *lung buds* appear towards the end of the 3rd and beginning of the 4th week of gestation at the caudal end of the tracheo-bronchial groove. They are generally asymmetrical, inclining to the right, and are made up of two lobes, a large right and a smaller left lobe, separated by a shallow sulcus. During the following weeks and up to the 7th week, by a series of monopodial and irregular dichotomous branchings, the principal bronchi appear, establishing the basic organization of the mature lung into lobar and segmental units. At this stage there are ten principal branches on the right and eight on the left. Between the 10th and 14th weeks, there is active division and ramification of the bronchi, producing about 70% of the bronchial generations. By the 16th week, the bronchial tree is fully developed and the lung has a glandular appearance. Capillaries rapidly penetrate the epithelium, and the glandular appearance becomes canalicular. The number of bronchial generations is now complete and is actually in excess of the final number found in adults; by a process of alveolarization some of the nonrespiratory bronchioles are transformed into respiratory bronchioles, finally leaving some 27 generations.

The bronchial tree is now represented by the two main bronchi; these are subdivided into lobar bronchi, segmental bronchi, lobular bronchi and alveolar ducts. The first 19 of these form the conducting airway, whose main role is to convey air to and from the lungs, and which does not take part in gas exchange. The first seven divisions are cartilaginous in type, while the remaining twelve are membranous, nonrespiratory bronchioles and terminal bronchioles. The following four (generations 20–23) are respiratory bronchioles and, like the remaining four (generations 24–27), which form the alveolar ducts, participate in gas exchange.

At birth, the respiratory unit is the primitive alveolus or 'saccule', of which there are about 25 million; further development continues, increasing in rate at about 2 months after birth, resulting in the maximum number of alveoli (about 300 millions) at the age of 8 years (Fig. 8.1.).

As the pulmonary primordia appear, and subsequently divide and proliferate, the bronchi invade the mass of mesenchymal tissue along the mid-line and thus create the future mediastinum. Growth continues into the developing pleural cavities, and eventually the surface becomes covered by mesothelial cells which are continuous with those of the pleura.

The mesenchymal tissues encircling the bronchi gives rise to the cartilaginous elements, smooth muscle layers, and the supporting connective tissue. This connective tissue becomes very scanty as one approaches the periphery of the bronchial tree. The cartilaginous elements make their appearance about the 7th week, and are fully established by the 25th week.

Mucus-secreting structures are recognizable by the 13th week of intrauterine life, when goblet cells are observed in the epithelium of the trachea, and the proximal and intrasegmental bronchi. They seem to grow most rapidly between the 14th and 28th weeks; at birth they are not found distal to the bronchi.

The blood supply to the respiratory primordium appears about the 5th week (5 mm) as a capillary network arising from the sixth arch. These vessels take up position next to the branches of the bronchial system, and remain interrelated throughout development. These are the pulmonary artery branches, which are referred to as conventional branches. Besides these arteries, there are additional vessels—supernumerary or accessory arteries—which appear about the 12th week and arise from the hilum. Both systems are complete by the 16th week.

The blood supply to the developing lungs drains into a venous plexus, forming a single pulmonary vein that empties into the heart. This vein finally becomes incorporated into the future left atrium, and its main branches on each side form the superior and inferior pulmonary veins.

The pseudostratified columnar epithelium of the large airways is made up of various types of cells. The most common is the ciliated cell, which continues into the respiratory bronchioles where it is somewhat flatter or cuboidal. These cells are covered by cilia (Fig. 8.2), which are partly anchored by dynein arms and contractile elements to the apical portion of the cell (Fig. 8.3). Contractile elements are also present within cilia. Ciliary movements play an important role in the defence mechanism of the respiratory system, and its absence is associated with certain disease entities.

Between isolated or small groups of ciliated cells are the goblet cells, which empty their secretion on the epithelial surface. Against the basal membrane and between the basal portions of the two previous cell types mentioned are the basal cells, which are reserve cells capable of replacing either the ciliated or goblet cells as may be necessary.

Two other cell types, which are less common, are also encountered. The Kulchitsky (argyrophil) cell, which is more prevalent in fetuses and newborns, contains granules (kinins) in its cytoplasm. These

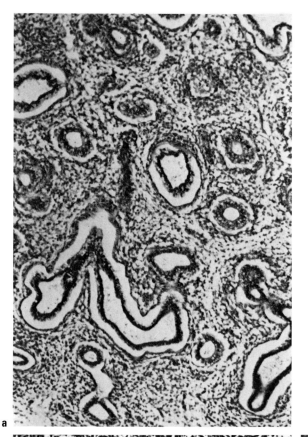

cells are considered to be precursors of bronchial carcinoids and have been associated with oat-cell carcinomas. Brush cells are even more rare, and are covered by microvilli. Their function is unknown.

The epithelial layer of the respiratory bronchioles is cuboidal in shape and lined principally by two types of cells; ciliated epithelial cells resembling those described above and the more conspicuous, nonciliated clara cells (Fig. 8.4).

Fig. 8.1. a–c Fetal lung: **a** The bronchial tree presents a glandular pattern and is lined by columnar epithelial cells. A loose mensenchymal tissue separates the branches. Gestational age 11 weeks, length 6 cm, 5.3 g. (H and E; 160 ×) **b** Extensive branching of the bronchial tree (canalicular phase) and formation of a lobular pattern. Gestational age about 18 weeks, 20.8 cm, 192 g. (H and E; 25 ×) **c** Formation of a alveolar saccules. Gestational age 36 weeks, 2860 g. (H and E; 25 ×)

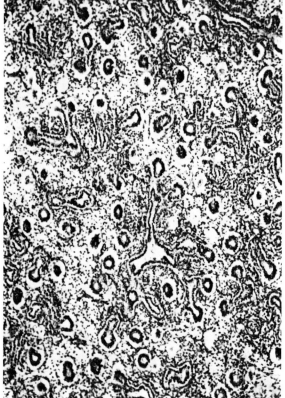

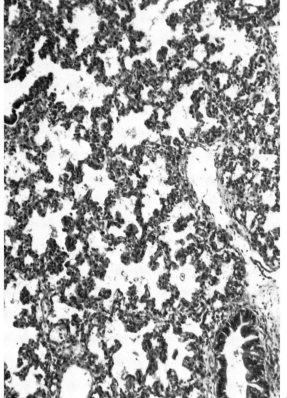

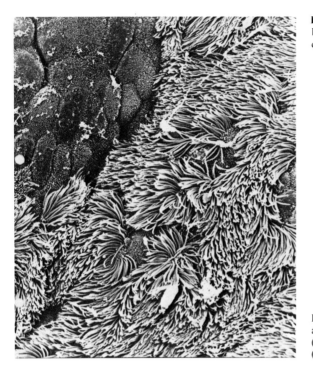

Fig. 8.2. Scanning electron microphotograph showing cilia of bronchiolar epithelial surface. Clara cell surface upper left hand corner. Courtesy of Dr. Y. Kapanci (2500 ×)

Fig. 8.3. a (*below*) Electron micrograph showing basal bodies (*B*) and basal feet (*bf*) of cilia. Microfilaments and microtubules (*arrow*) can be seen radiating from the basal feet. Mitochondria (*m*) are also present. (28 000 ×).

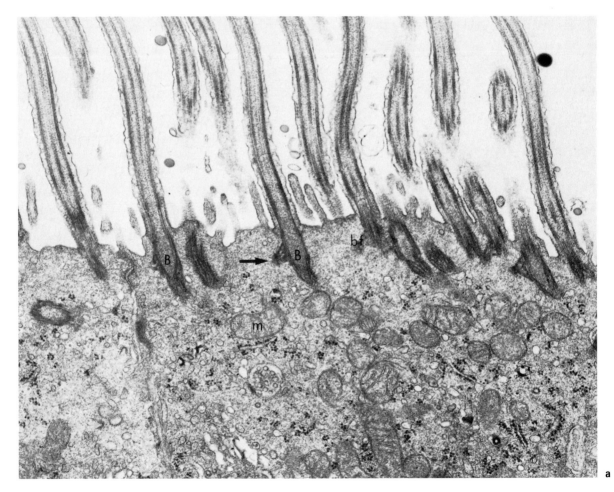

a

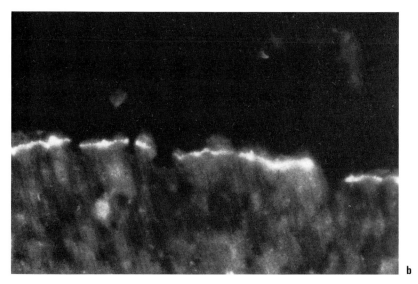

Fig. 8.3. b Immunofluorescent staining of human bronchial epithelium with AAA serum showing a subciliary fluorescent band of actin. (400 ×) Courtesy of Dr Y. Kapanci.

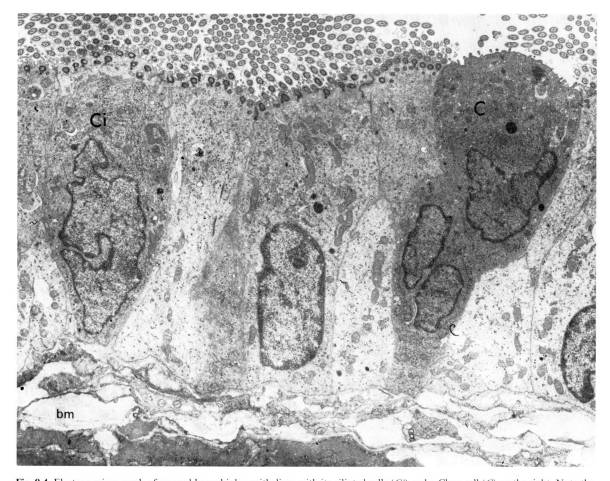

Fig. 8.4. Electron micrograph of normal bronchiolar epithelium with its ciliated cells (*Ci*) and a Clara cell (*C*) on the right. Note the basal membrane (*bm*). Courtesy of Dr Y. Kapanci. (6300 ×)

At this point, it is necessary to describe briefly the terminal respiratory unit and the interalveolar septum. The terminal respiratory unit consists of those structures that are distal to the terminal bronchiole. Each terminal bronchiole gives off two to five orders of respiratory bronchioles. The last respiratory bronchiole leads into the first alveolar ducts, which vary in number between two and five. Each alveolar duct opens into as many as 10–16 alveoli. The alveoli are separated by an interalveolar septum made up of three parts: the alveolar epithelium, capillary and interstitial tissue.

Alveolar epithelium is made up of two cell types: Type I cells or squamous pneumocytes have a broad thin cytoplasmic sheet and nuclei that often protrude above the epithelial surface. These cells cover about 90% of the alveolar surface. Type II cells, or granular pneumocytes, are more numerous than type I cells, but because of their configuration—round or cuboidal—they occupy only about 5% of

the alveolar surface. They are characterized by surface microvilli and the presence of cytoplasmic osmiophilic lamellar bodies, suggesting a secretory function. These bodies, which appear in the cells at about the 25th week of gestation, are associated with the production of surface active material (surfactant), a substance that plays an important role in lung expansion. Type II pneumocytes are also considered to play an important role in epithelial regeneration. Both cell types are attached to a continuous basement membrane.

The alveolar septa are provided with a single capillary network. The capillary has a basement membrane, which is covered by a single layer of endothelial cells; pericytes are present in the capillary wall (Fig. 8.5).

The interstitial tissue contains some collagen and elastic fibres among which are found contractile interstitial cells or myofibroblasts (Fig. 8.6). There are also some macrophages in varying numbers

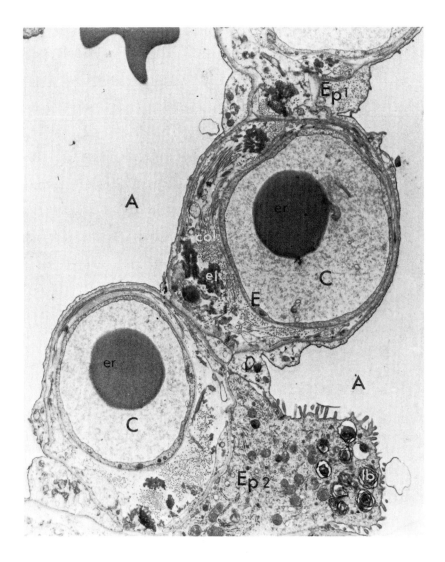

Fig. 8.5. Electron microphotograph of human alveolar septum. The alveolar spaces (*A*) are lined with type II (*Ep 1*) and type II (*Ep 2*) epithelial cells, the latter containing lamellated bodies (*lb*). Capillaries (*C*) contain erythrocytes (*er*) and are lined with endothelial cells (*E*). Collagen fibres (*col*) and elastic fibres (*el*) are conspicuous. Courtesy of Dr Y. Kapanci. (5700 ×)

within the interstitium (Boyden 1969; Charnock and Doershuk 1973; Emery and Wilcock 1966; Gehr et al. 1978; Huang 1978; Kapanci et al. 1979; McDougall 1978; Murray 1976; O'Rahlly and Tucker 1973; Patten 1968; Reid 1967; Reverdin 1975; Yoneda 1977).

Pathology

The respiratory system can be divided into two parts: (A) the upper respiratory system, comprising the nose, nasopharynx, larynx and trachea; (B) the lower respiratory system, comprising the bronchi and lungs.

2. Nose and Nasopharynx

2.1. Congenital Abnormalities of the Nose

Illustrations of various malformations of the nose have been documented by Patten (1968) and Potter (1962) (Fig. 8.7). *Congenital absence* of the nose and anterior nasopharynx is a rare condition. Gifford et al. (1972) described two cases and reviewed the literature on the subject. In *cyclopia*, another rare condition, in which there is fusion of the eyes, there is a proboscis-like cylindrical fleshy mass hanging from the nasal region or the forehead in place of the nose. Sometimes this bears a single central orifice representing a nostril, but in other instances there is no external opening. In most cases there is no communication with the nasopharynx (Landing 1957; Potter 1962). Recently Rontal and Duritz (1977) described a case in which a lateral proboscis replaced one of the nostrils. Cyclops have also been described in association with chromosomal abnormalities, and principally with trisomies (Arakaki and Waxman 1969). In a somewhat milder form of cyclopedia, *cebocephaly*, there is hypoplasia of the maxillary bones and nose associated with a lissencephalic brain with fusion of the cerebran hemispheres and internal hydrocephaly. *Frontonasal dysplasia*, another relatively rare condition, may or may not be associated with cleft lip and cleft palate. The condition appears to be a developmental defect not necessarily related to chromosomal abnormalities (Sedano et al. 1970). *Aplasia* of the alae nasi is rare and is often associated with other abnormalities including deafness and abnormal endocrine function (Johanson and Blizzard 1971). Cleft lip and palate are discussed on p. 213.

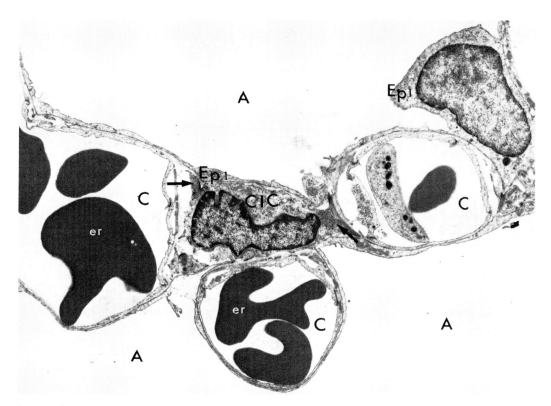

Fig. 8.6. Septal contractile interstitial cell (*CIC*) containing bundles of microfilaments (*arrows*). Capillaries (*C*) containing erythrocytes (*er*) separate the alveolar spaces (*A*). Type I epithelial cell (*ep*). Courtesy of Dr Y. Kapanci. (5600 ×)

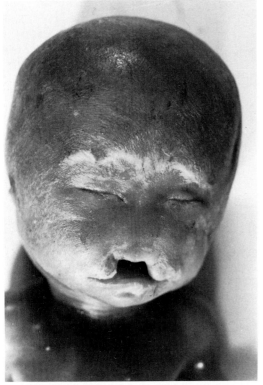

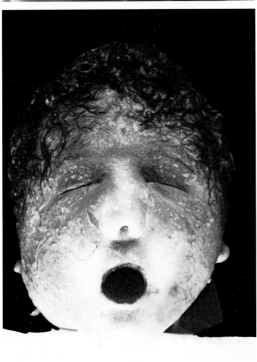

b

Fig. 8.7. a Absence of the nose of a polymalformed female fetus of 22 weeks' gestation with trisomy 13; b Male fetus of 36 weeks' gestation with malformed nose and a central dimple but no nasal openings.

Choanal atresia can be divided into two main types, depending on location. Anterior atresias are found when the epithelial plugs between the developing medial and lateral nasal placodes are not absorbed in the embryo. Posterior (choanal) atresia, by far the most common form although still a rare anomaly, is usually situated at the level of the sphenoid, vertical vomer and palatine bones adjacent to the nasopharynx. It is an important cause of neonatal asphyxia; it can be relieved by a simple surgical procedure or by prompt medical management (Carpenter and Neel 1977; Evans and MacLachlan 1971; Winther 1978).

The anomaly occurs as a result of bony overgrowth, an excess of hyperplastic cartilage, or membranous proliferations, or results from combinations of these factors. It is most commonly unilateral, with a right-sided predominance, but may be bilateral, complete or incomplete. It has been known to be inherited as a dominant trait in certain families. Choanal atresia has a female predominance (estimated at 2:1), and is often associated with other congenital anomalies, mainly of the cardiovascular system, face, and, in rare instances, the kidney (Buckfield et al. 1971; Carpenter and Neel 1977; Ransome 1964; Trail et al. 1973).

Cysts. Dermoid cysts of the nose are rare. They may be the cause of a widened nasal septum, septal deviation or duplication (Hoshaw and Walike 1971; Szalay and Bledsoe 1972; Taylor and Erich 1967), and are classified according to location into: (a) *superficial*, found mainly in the perpendicular plate of the ethmoid bone or the quadrangular cartilage; (b) *deep or septal*, found within the columella and the vomer. They may also be observed in Jacobson's organ or the nasopalatine region of the floor of the nose (Pratt 1965; Sing and Pahor 1977). Some communicate with the dermis by a fistulous tract opening in the mid-line of the nasal bridge or by a small dimple in the skin (Nydell and Masson 1959; Pratt 1965; Sing and Pahor 1977). Macroscopically, they are round or oval, firm or rubbery masses which, on histological examination, show a cavity lined with stratified squamous epithelium (Fig. 8.8).

2.2. Acquired Disease

In infants and children, the majority of acquired pathological conditions are associated with infections or trauma. Chemical irritants or obstructions of the nares by foreign bodies are also important in this age group. In infections, bacterial or virological studies of secretions or scrapings will often indicate the pathogenic agent responsible. Both tuberculosis and congenital syphilis of the nose have become rare entities, at least in industrialized countries. The nasal lesions formerly encountered in yaws in the developing countries have been almost completely eliminated; however, leprosy still remains a problem, and the diagnosis can often be established from nasal scrapings (Barton and Davey 1976; Olson et al. 1979).

Hypertrophic or 'hyperplastic' rhinitis is a relatively common condition among adolescents, and has been considered to be associated with chronic infection of the nose or the paranasal sinuses. However, there is evidence that it might be related to a hypersensitivity reaction and that hormonal factors may be important (Cowan 1968; Davison 1963; Williams and Williams 1968).

Excised mucosa shows squamous metaplasia of the epithelium together with glandular atrophy. There is marked submucosal oedema with some fibrosis and a varying degree of chronic inflammation.

Rhinoscleroma is a chronic granulomatous disease, often beginning as a bilateral lesion in the nose with nasopharyngeal extension. In some instances the larynx and trachea are involved (Holinger et al. 1977; Tolsdorff 1973).

Though endemic in Eastern Europe, Central and South America, Africa and the Far East, it can be encountered in any region of the globe and can affect either sex of any race at any age. The disease affects the mucous membranes, causing hyperplasia and hypertrophy of the surface epithelium. As it progresses, an atrophic rhinitis develops, with the formation of nodular granulation tissue, which, in most cases, obstructs and destroys the narines. Destruction of the surrounding tissues including the bony skeleton follows (Fisher and Dimling 1964; Holinger et al. 1977).

Histologically there is granulation tissue with numerous plasma cells. In the mixed inflammatory cell infiltrate are large histiocytes or foam cells (Mikulicz cells) with a central nucleus and a clear, vacuolated cytoplasm. Some of these histiocytes contain several gram-positive bacilli (*Klebsiella rhinoscleromatis* or Frisch bacilli), which are considered to be the cause of the disease. The bacilli, although apparent in gram-stained tissue, are more distinct in sections stained by silver impregnation techniques, and are readily observed on electron microscopy. The tissue is variably fibrotic, depending on the stage of the disease. The surface epithelium may be atrophic, but in most cases it is hyperplastic or shows a pseudoepitheliomatous hyperplasia (Gaafar and Harada 1976; Hoffmann et al. 1973; Levine et al. 1974).

Rhinoscleroma must be distinguished histo-

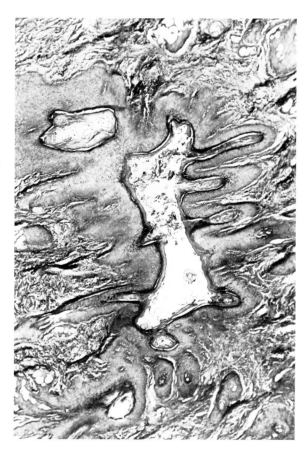

Fig. 8.8. Fistulous tract of nasal dermoid cyst lined with stratified squamous epithelium in an 8-year-old boy. (H and E; 35 ×)

logically from *benign sinus histiocytosis*, another condition that sometimes involves the nasopharynx, which is usually accompanied by massive lymphadenopathy, principally in the cervical region. Sinus histiocytosis appears to be more common in developing countries, and is observed mainly among children. Histologically, the tissue is infiltrated by large histiocytes with a clear cytoplasm and large indented nuclei with prominent nucleoli (Fig. 8.9). The cytoplasm is PAS-positive, vacuolated, and contains pigment granules. Some of the cells may be very large and show evidence of phagocytosis of erythrocytes and lymphocytes. An occasional atypical histiocyte resembling the Reed–Sternberg cell has been described. Serum from patients with this condition usually present a high antibody titre for the Epstein–Barr virus (Lober et al. 1973; Nezelof et al. 1978; Rosai and Dorfman 1972).

Lethal mid-line granuloma or 'nonhealing mid-line granuloma' is described as a rare inflammatory disease affecting the nasal cavity, and it has been reported in children. However, recent studies suggest that this condition is a clinical entity that may be pathologically caused by a range of conditions that

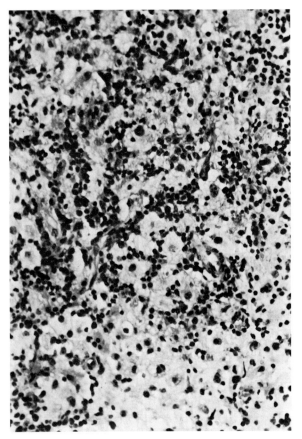

Fig. 8.9. Sinus histiocytosis in a 9-year-old-boy, presenting as polypoid nasal masses with extensive involvement of the surrounding tissues and destruction of the adjacent bony structures. (H and E; 160 ×)

are not necessarily inflammatory in nature. The condition usually begins as superficial ulceration of the nasal cavity. The ulcers progress rapidly, with necrosis of the mucous membranes and surrounding tissues including cartilage and bone, and eventually reach the superficial tissues. The nasal cavity, sinuses, orbits, and buccal cavity may be extensively involved (Fechner and Lamppin 1972; Kassel et al. 1969; McGuirt and Rose 1976). The lesions may be the result of collagen disease or a neoplasm of the lymphoma group. The histological picture is therefore quite variable. The correct diagnosis is only possible if numerous histological sections from outside the necrotic areas are examined (DeRemee et al. 1978; Fauci and Wolff 1973; Kassel et al. 1969; McGuirt and Rose 1976; Michaels and Gregory 1977).

Fu and Perzin (1979), Kassel et al. (1969), and Michaels and Gregory (1977), after careful histological studies of cases occurring mainly in adults, have concluded that in the majority of cases a malignant neoplasm of histiocytic lymphoma type is the most frequent underlying pathological condition. How-

ever, it is necessary in all cases to exclude the possibility of *Wegener's granuloma*, which often presents clinically in this way. Baliga et al. (1978) collected eight childhood cases of Wegener's granuloma from the literature, and three of these were of the generalized type. Moorthy et al. (1977) were able to collect seven cases of the generalized type and added two of their own. Recently, Nespoli et al. (1979) described another case in a 27-month-old girl, the youngest on record.

2.3. Tumours

Neoplasms of the nose and nasopharynx in infancy and childhood are rare: however, tumours of the surrounding tissue (brain, meninges, bony skeleton) may protrude into the nasal cavity or nasopharynx symptoms, mainly obstruction.

Nasal polyps are not true neoplasms but are associated with chronic nasal inflammation or repeated allergic reactions within the nasal cavity. They may also be associated with vascular disturbances in the mucosa or be the result of mechanical obstruction. They are frequently encountered in certain systemic diseases, the principal of which is fibrocystic disease of the pancreas (mucoviscidosis) (Berman and Colman 1977). These last authors, among others, have suggested that one should always look for cystic fibrosis in children presenting with nasal polyps. Tos et al. (1977) could not find differences between nasal polyps from cases of cystic fibrosis and those of other origins; however, Oppenheimer and Rosenstein (1979) have shown histochemical differences between polyps in cystic fibrosis and those of atopic patients.

Polyposis forms an integral part of Kartagener's syndrome (Siewert–Kartagener), a hereditary condition in which patients present with situs inversus, chronic bronchitis with bronchiectasis (bilateral), rhinosinusitis, nasal polyposis, and chronic and recurrent otitis media, with absence or underdevelopment of the frontal sinuses and infertility in males due to spermatozoal immotility. In this syndrome, there is partial or complete lack of ciliary motility of the epithelial cells lining the upper and lower respiratory system and the middle ear as well as the tails of spermatozoa. Ciliary dysfunction is considered to be the cause of the disease, and is due to the absence of or abnormalities in the ciliary dynein arms (normally rich in ATPase) and an abnormal internal structural arrangement of the microtubular doublets within the cilia (Rott 1978; Sturgess et al. 1979). Kartagener's syndrome is now considered to be part of the more general 'immotile cilia syndrome', in which there is absence of or diminished cilial motility, various structural abnormalities of cilia associated with chronic infection of the upper and lower respiratory system, and male infertility, irrespective of situs inversus. Some authors have separated another group from the immotile cilia syndrome, for which they have coined the term 'ciliary dyskinesis'. In these cases some ciliary motility was present; however, there were distinctive ultrastructural cilia abnormalities (Fox et al. 1980; Jahrsdoerfer et al. 1979; Pederson and Mygind 1980; Veerman et al. 1980). Forrest et al. (1979) have shown that the administration of exogenous ATPase could induce cilial motility in cases with Kartagener's syndrome, thus suggesting the possibility of a membrane permeability defect rather than a deficiency of the dynein arms of the cilia in this condition.

Most polyps arise from the mucosa of the ethmoidal cells at the level of the middle meatus or in the paranasal sinuses. They may be single or multiple, uni- or bilateral, and either sessile or pedunculated. They are often the source of nasal bleeding or obstruction, and may cause displacement and even destruction of the bones limiting the nasal cavity (Winestock et al. 1978). On gross inspection, they present as smooth round or oval myxomatous masses, yellowish in colour. Histologically there is hypertrophy of the mucous membrane covered by columnar ciliated epithelium, sometimes with squamous metaplasia. The stroma is very loose, fibrillar and oedematous. There is stromal atypia in some cases, which may be falsely interpreted as sarcoma (Compagno et al. 1976). The vessels are dilated, and there are scattered aggregates of lymphocytes and plasma cells with eosinophils (Fig. 8.10). The submucosal glands are generally hyperplastic, but may be atrophic in some areas.

Choanal polyps are a different clinical entity. They generally arise from the mucosa of the maxillary sinuses and project towards the posterior choanae. Their histology is very similar to that of other nasal polyps.

In tropical and subtropical countries, many mycotic infections of the nose in children can present as nasal polyps (Engzell and Jones 1973). Histological examination often reveals granulation tissue, sometimes with granulomas and/or foci of necrosis. Special staining techniques (silver impregnation or PAS) are often necessary for identifying the particular fungus. Cultures may be necessary in establishing the diagnosis.

Epithelial tumours of the nasal cavity are rare in the paediatric age group. *Papillomas* are occasionally observed in which the epithelium is hyperplastic and well differentiated; there are varying degrees of dyskeratosis and some hyperkeratotic areas (Fig. 8.11). Inverted papillomas may also be seen, and Synder and Perzin (1972) have

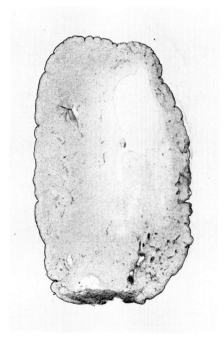

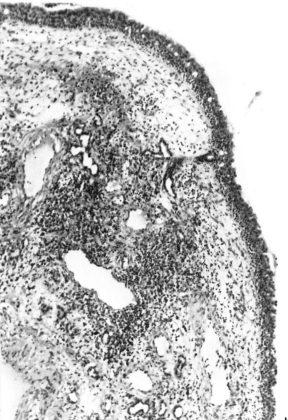

Fig. 8.10. a Nasal polyp from a 12-year-old boy with cystic fibrosis; **b** Nasal polyp in a child with chronic sinusitis. (H and E; 90×)

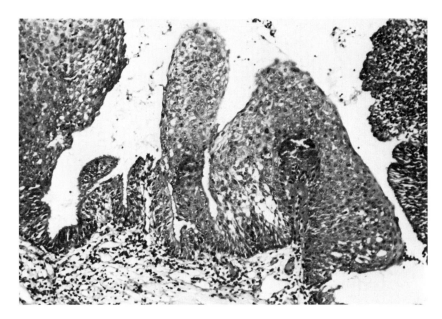

Fig. 8.11. Nasal papilloma in a 14-year-old girl with papillomatosis of the laryngotracheal tree discovered at age 3. (H and E; 160 ×)

listed the many synonyms by which the *inverted papilloma* is known. The tumour is usually unilateral, can be localized or diffuse, and can occur in any region of the nasal cavity. Histologically, there is a marked proliferation of basal cells, which replace ciliated cells in some areas. This hyperplastic epithelium produces invaginations within the fibrous stroma. There are relatively few mitotic figures, and nucleic atypia is rare (Synder and Perzin 1972). Many of these tumours appear to be histologically benign but are locally aggressive. Clinically they behave as malignant tumours, and inadequate removal is followed by local recurrences (Clairmont et al. 1975; Fechner and Sessions 1977; Lesser et al. 1976; Vrabec 1975).

Squamous-cell carcinoma of the nasal cavity is very rare in childhood. We have observed a case in a 9-year-old boy who presented with a large polypoid necrotic mass obstructing the right nostril and causing extensive destruction of the corresponding maxilla (Fig. 8.12). Carcinoma of the nasopharynx, on the other hand, is more prevalent, even though Jaffé (1973a) recorded only three cases in his review of 178 tumours of the head and neck in children.

In childhood, *carcinomas of the nasopharynx* are more common in the Far and Middle East, and especially in Africa, where they may represent about 15% of all nasopharyngeal carcinomas. These tumours do occur in other areas but are rare; they cause nasal obstruction, deafness, cranial nerve palsy, and protosis. There is a male predominance and a high incidence of distant metastases. Patients with these tumours have high antibody titres to Epstein–Barr virus.

Carcinomas of the nasopharynx vary in histological appearance. The well-differentiated epidermoid carcinoma is more often encountered in the adult, while in childhood the tumours are generally poorly differentiated, resembling transitional cell carcinoma. The cells are large with an almost inconspicuous cytoplasm, and sometimes they have a syncytial appearance. Their nuclei are quite large, round or oval with prominent nucleoli. Some cases may have the appearance of a lymphoepithelial carcinoma of the *Schmincke–Regaud* type, while others may be anaplastic in character (Deutsch et al. 1978; Fernandez et al. 1976; LeMaigre et al. 1977; Pick et al. 1974; Shanmugaratnam et al. 1980).

Intranasal mixed tumours (*pleomorphic adenomas*) have also been reported in children. The histology is similar to that of pleomorphic tumours of the major salivary glands, but they have a relatively lower rate of recurrence (Compagno and Wong 1977).

The majority of nasopharyngeal tumours (benign or malignant) in childhood are derived from the supporting tissues and from neighbouring structures.

Vascular tumours. Haemangiomas of the nose and nasopharynx are occasionally encountered in infancy and childhood. They can arise anywhere in the nasal cavity but have a predilection for the anterior nasal septum, and are a frequent cause of bleeding. They may present as extremely vascular sessile or pedunculated polyps. *Benign haemangioendothelioma* has also been described in children. In these highly cellular tumours the capillaries are lined with prominent but uniform endothelial cells (Fu and Perzin 1974a).

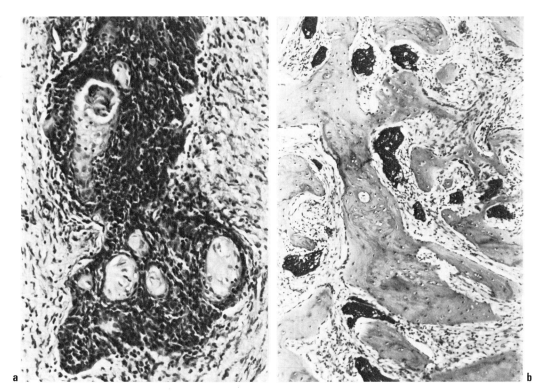

Fig. 8.12. a Squamous-cell carcinoma of the nasal cavity in an 11-year-old boy. (H and E; 225 ×) **b** Infiltration and destruction of the adjacent bones. (H and E; 60 ×)

Juvenile nasopharyngeal angiofibroma is a rare haemangiomatous tumour occurring principally in adolescent males. It occasionally appears before puberty, but grows rapidly during this period and may regress in later years, undergoing hyalinization and fibrosis. These clinical features have suggested hormonal dependence even though the tumour has been reported in adults and in females (Conley et al. 1968; Fu and Perzin 1974a; Hicks and Nelson 1973).

The pathology of this lesion has been described in detail (Arnold and Huth 1978; Taxy 1977a). It generally develops as a solitary, sessile, somewhat lobulated mass in the region of the sphenoethmoidal recess or the choana, from where it may protrude into the nasal cavity, producing obstruction. It can extend into neighbouring structures. Histologically, the angiofibroma is covered by normal naso-pharyngeal epithelium and is composed of numerous distended vessels lined with a flattened endothelium in a relatively dense fibrous stroma. The vessel walls are devoid of elastic fibres, and their muscular coats are irregular, incomplete, or even absent in smaller vessels. The stroma is fibrocytic in appearance with little elastic fibre, but it sometimes contains scattered smooth-muscle elements (Fig. 8.13). Arnold and Huth (1978) and Taxy (1977)

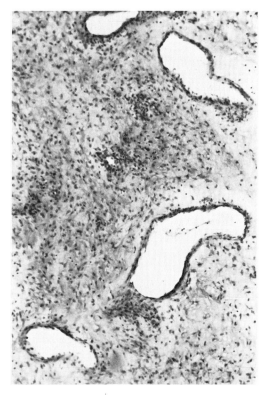

Fig. 8.13. Juvenile nasopharyngeal angiofibroma in a 13-year-old boy. Note the fibrocytic stroma with the stellate cells and the scattered vessels devoid of muscular layers. (H and E; 160 ×)

have recently described the ultrastructure of these tumours. Angiofibromas create many therapeutic problems due to bleeding, local extension, and a high rate of local recurrence (Boles and Dedo 1976; Krekorian and Kato 1977; Pletcher et al. 1975). Androgen receptors have been demonstrated in these tumours (Lee et al. 1980), suggesting that they may be androgen-dependent.

Lymphangioma of the nasal cavity is extremely rare but may sometimes be seen in adolescents. It presents as a polypoid mass covered by normal respiratory epithelium; in a fibrous stroma there are numerous dilated lymphatic vessels lined with flattened endothelial cells (Fig. 8.14).

Haemangiopericytoma has also been recorded in the nasal cavity (Fu and Perzin 1974a). Benveniste and Harris (1973) reviewed the literature and found ten cases, one of which was in a 4-year-old girl. They added one case of their own, which occurred in a newborn. Compagno (1978) has reviewed the subject of haemangiopericytomas of the nasal cavity, and found that although they do occur in childhood they are more common among adults.

Fibrous tumours are exceedingly rare in children.

Fu and Perzin (1976b) did not find any cases of *fibroma* in the paediatric age group in their material, but observed three cases of *fibromatosis*. Townsend et al. (1973) described a case of what they referred to as an histiocytoma in a 3-year-old boy, while Rice et al. (1973) recorded a case in a 13-year-old girl. Jaffe (1973a) has reported a case of *malignant histiocytoma* of the nose in an infant. The histological picture usually shows fibroblast-like cells with a histiocytic component presenting a wide range of morphologic changes (Perzin and Fu 1980).

Fibrosarcoma is also very rare. Fu and Perzin (1976b) found only one case below 15 years of age among their 13 patients, and made reference to two others in children (Fig. 8.15).

Muscular tumours. Smooth-muscle tumours (*leiomyoma* and *leiomyosarcoma*) of the nasal cavity are rare. There were no cases in children in the series of Fu and Perzin (1975). Striated-muscle tumours are more common. Fu and Perzin (1976a) described one case of *rhabdomyoma* and found another in the literature; Canalis et al. (1978) have reviewed the

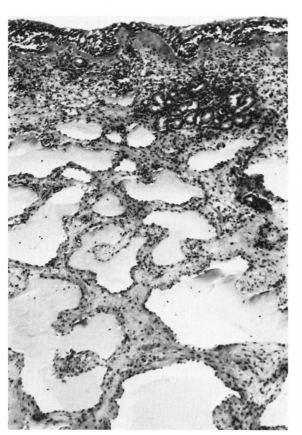

Fig. 8.14. Lymphangioma in a 15-year-old boy. (H and E; 60 ×)

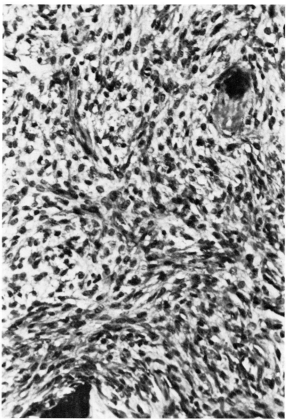

Fig. 8.15. Slow-growing fibrosarcoma of the nasal cavity in a 13-year-old boy. (H and E; 225 ×)

literature on *rhabdomyosarcoma* in this region and found 96 recorded cases, 56 of which were well documented, and added four of their own. Rhabdomyosarcomas can occur in the nose or nasopharynx, and often present as polypoid masses (Jaffe 1973a; Fu and Perzin 1976a), often with a history of repeated local resection. The predominant histological pattern encountered is of the embryonal type. The tumours infiltrate the surrounding structures extensively, making resection difficult, if not impossible, in most cases (Donaldson et al. 1973; Liebner 1976).

Tumours of cartilaginous and osseous nature are uncommon in the nasal cavity in children. *Chondromas* have been mentioned in the literature (Fu and Perzin 1974c) and are usually found in the nasal septum as a polypoid mass. Histologically, it is difficult to determine whether these lesions are neoplasms or merely hypertrophic areas of the cartilaginous septum or heterotopic islets of cartilage. *Chondrosarcoma* was observed in four children by Fu and Perzin (1974c), who collected 25 documented cases from the literature, including some children. *Chordomas* are uncommon in the nasopharynx, and even more so in childhood. Although the histology is characteristic in most cases (Fig. 8.16), it can present difficulty, especially when mixed with other tissue components, mainly cartilaginous foci (Heffelfinger et al. 1973).

Both *fibrous dysplasia* and *ossifying fibroma* are extremely rare. Fu and Perzin (1974b) reported eight cases of these two conditions presenting in the first two decades. Ossifying fibroma, although a benign tumour, provokes extensive local bone destruction. The tumour is made up of bony trabeculae separated by abundant fibrous tissue (Dehner 1973). This tissue is quite cellular, containing numerous spindle-shaped fibroblasts sometimes arranged in whorls.

There are occasional rare mitotic figures. Other types of benign osseous tumours, and *osteosarcomas* and *myxomas*, have been encountered in childhood (Fu and Perzin 1974b, 1977).

Other tumours. Tumours derived from nervous tissue are sometimes found in the nasal cavity. *Heterotopic nervous tissue* (Fig. 8.17) can be found in the nasopharynx, but *gliomas* appear to be much more common (Feroldi et al. 1974; Enfors and Herngren 1974). Karma et al. (1977) have reviewed

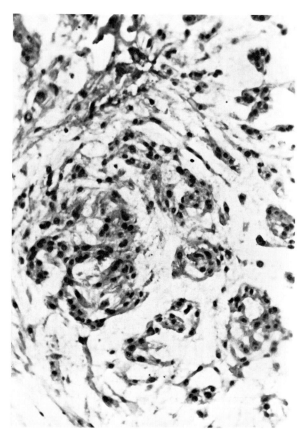

Fig. 8.16. Chordoma of the paranasal sinuses Courtesy of Dr C. Bozic (H and E; 225 ×)

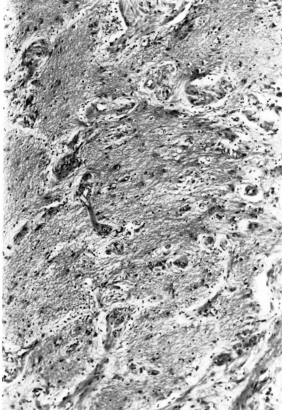

Fig. 8.17. Heterotopic glial tissue at the bridge of the nose in a 17-month-old boy. Courtesy of Dr C. Bozic. (H and E; 120 ×)

the literature on the subject and collected 136 cases, adding two of their own. Most cases were observed in children, and 30 % of these had arisen in the nasal cavity. These tumours appear as polypoid, firm masses covered by normal respiratory epithelium. Histologically, they are formed from astrocytic neuroglial cells, sometimes having a fibrillar appearance, embedded in a vascular, fibrous stroma (Fig. 8.18). Primary menangioma of the nasal cavities and sinuses is rare. Ho (1980) found seven cases (with approximately equal sex distribution) described in children among the nineteen reported in the literature.

Olfactory neuroblastoma, or aesthesioneuroblastoma, has also been described in children. Bailey and Barton (1975) presented a case in a 6-year-old boy and reviewed the literature. They found 25 cases occurring before the age of 20 years, three in the first decade and 22 in the second. These tumours appear to arise from the basal layer of the olfactory sensory epithelium in the upper nasal cavity above the middle turbinate and are of neural crest origin. Even though they may be related to the childhood neuroblastoma of other regions, they are quite distinct biologically although arginine vasopressin has recently been recovered from such a tumour (Chaudry et al. 1979; Elkon et al. 1979; Singh et al. 1980). Histologically the tumour consists of groups or nests of neuroblasts, which have a lymphocytoid appearance. The cells have a round or oval nucleus with coarse or thin chromatin; the cytoplasm is scanty, the stroma is fibrillary, and there may be pseudo-

rosettes around some fibrillar elements (Fig. 8.19). These tumours extend into the adjacent paranasal sinuses but rarely metastasize (Kahn 1974; Oberman and Rice 1976; Taxy and Hidvegi 1977).

Teratomas of the nasopharynx are rare and can be the cause of neonatal asphyxia: sometimes they are not noticed and present symptoms during childhood (Badrawy et al. 1973; Charles 1960; Chattopadhyay and Dasgupta 1976; Kesson 1954; Nikol'skaia 1968). These tumours are generally of the adult type, but other types have also been described.

Malignant lymphomas (non-Hodgkin's) are not uncommon on childhood and occasionally affect the nasopharynx, presenting in either a nodular or a diffuse form (Wollner et al. 1976). In Africa, however, lymphoblastic lymphona (*Burkitt's lymphona*) is quite prevalent in the paediatric age group, and may first present as a simple isolated mass or multiple tumours in the jaw, maxilla, nasal cavity, or nasopharynx, with distortion and destruction of the bones (Burkitt 1970). The histological, cytological and ultrastructural features of this fascinating tumour, together with the environmental factor(s) that may play a role in its aetiology, have all been fully documented (Epstein and Achong 1970; Wright 1970). The histology is characteristic, with sheets of immature lymphoblasts among which are scattered large histiocytes, giving the tumour the characteristic 'starry sky' appearance. The histocytes have an abundant, clear vesicular cytoplasm containing phagocytosed cellular elements (Fig. 8.20).

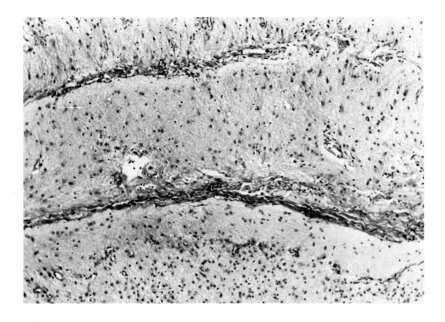

Fig. 8.18. Glioma of the nasal cavity in a 2-month-old male infant. Courtesy of Dr C. Bozic. (H and E; 120 ×)

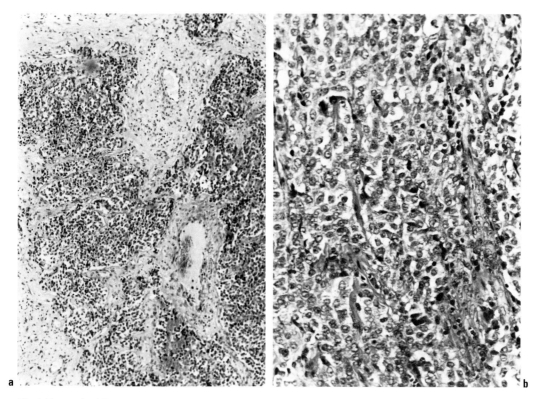

Fig. 8.19. a and **b** Ofactory neuroblastoma (aesthesioneuroblastoma) in a 11-year-old boy. Courtesy of Dr C. Bozic. (H and E; **a** 40 ×, **b** 120 ×)

3. Larynx and Trachea

3.1. Congenital Malformations

Congenital laryngeal atresia is an extremely rare condition; few cases have been recorded in the literature, and these have often presented in association with other congenital anomalies (Fox 1964; Smith and Bain 1965; Vargas and Patron 1971). The atretic zone can be localized in the glottic, supraglottic, or subglottic region, or it can affect the entire larynx. The cricoid cartilage may form a diaphragm across the stenosed larynx. We have seen a case in which this diaphragm was pierced by a small hole. The condition results from the failure of resorption of epithelium during the 7th and beginning of the 8th week of intrauterine life. Partial resorption of the lamina may lead to *stenosis*, which usually occurs in the subglottic region with narrowing of the inferior margin of the inferior margin of the cricoid cartilage. Two main histological variants can be observed, cartilaginous and soft-tissue anomalies. This abnormality is more frequently encountered than atresia (Landing and Dixon 1979; Robin and Dalton 1974; Tucker et al. 1979). This abnormality is more frequently encountered than atresia (Robin and Dalton 1974). Malformation of the epiglottis may be associated with these and other anomalies (Healy et al. 1976).

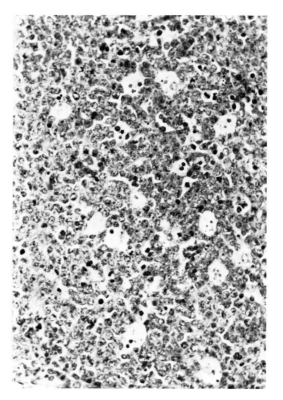

Fig. 8.20. Burkitt's lymphoma, with its starry-sky appearance, in a 9-year-old African boy. (H and E; 120 ×)

Laryngeal webs are much more common than atresias, but may be considered to be lesser degrees of the same lesion. They, like atresia or stenosis, are causes of cyanosis, stridor, or other signs of respiratory distress in the newborn. Webs are usually thin bands situated at the anterior portion of the vocal cords, partially obstructing the laryngeal orifice. They result from failure of normal separation of the two vocal cords. Occasionally they are observed on the posterior portion (Landing 1957a; Holinger and Brown 1967). Histologically these webs are made up of dense connective tissue, sometimes containing skeletal muscle and numerous capillaries. The proximal surface is covered with squamous epithelium and the distal surface, with respiratory epithelium.

There have been occasional case reports or reviews of the relatively rare condition of *cleft larynx*, but the abnormality may be more prevalent than the literature suggests. The length of the cleft varies quite widely. In some cases it presents as a slit in the posterior mid-line of the cricoid cartilage, resulting in a communication between the larynx and the superior portion of the (often atretic) oesophagus. In other cases, it extends to the level of the trachea as far as the carina, resulting in an oesophagotrachea. This abnormality is known to run in families; it affects mostly girls and has been reported in siblings. The clinical symptoms (stridor, feeding difficulties, recurrent aspiration) generally appear shortly after birth, but can go unnoticed until childhood. In severe cases, prompt treatment is needed. Surgical repairs have been attempted with some success (Beazer et al. 1973; Berkovits et al. 1974; Cohen 1975; Novoselac et al. 1974; Phelan et al. 1973; Pillsbury and Fisher 1977; Pracy and Stell 1974).

Laryngeal cysts (mucocele), like *laryngoceles* (aerocele), are generally located at the level of the laryngeal ventricle, and there is often some confusion between the two conditions. Cysts are closed cavities and do not have an outlet into the laryngeal lumen, in contrast to laryngoceles. These abnormalities can protrude into the lumen or be situated within the wall of the larynx. Less commonly they are found at any level in the neck; they attain a considerable size, displacing adjacent organs. Stell and Maran (1975) reviewed the literature on laryngocele and found some 139 cases described in both children and adults. Cysts may increase in diameter as their mucus content increases, and laryngoceles can also vary in size, depending on the quantity of air trapped inside them (Bachman 1978; Holinger et al. 1978). Histologically both cysts and laryngoceles are lined with respiratory epithelium.

Tracheal agenesis. Total or partial absence of the trachea is a rare abnormality (Altman et al.

1972; Hong et al. 1973; Hopkinson 1972; Joshi 1969; McNie and Pryse-Davis 1970). Hong et al. (1973) found 21 documented cases of total tracheal agenesis, and all but two had communications between the oesophagus and the bronchi. Usually in this abnormality, the trachea is absent throughout its entire length, and the larynx opens at the level of the cricoid cartilage, into the oesophagus. The main bronchi arise from the lower oesophagus. Tracheal atresia can be divided into three anatomical types, based on the chronology of the development and separation of the trachea from the oesophagus during intrauterine life. In type I the upper trachea is atretic but the lower trachea, bronchi, and lungs are normal; in type II the whole trachea is absent and the bronchi join in the mid-line (the majority of cases fall in this category); in type III, the bronchi arise separately from the oesophagus (Ashley 1972; Landing and Dixon 1979). Oesophageal atresia and other congenital anomalies have been described in association with this abnormality (Lyons and Bruce 1968; McCracken et al. 1964).

Tracheal stenosis occurs in several forms and is often associated with abnormalities of the main stem bronchi or other congenital malformations (Greene 1976; Landing and Wells 1973; Lesbros et al. 1979). The condition may present as one or several continuous complete or solid tracheal rings at any level of the tracheal tree, with narrowing of the segment involved. In rare instances, the trachea is completely cartilaginous, and the lungs have been found to be abnormal in some cases. Tracheal stenosis may also be the result of compression by an abnormal adjacent vessel (vascular rings and anomalous left pulmonary artery).

Tracheomalacia and *bronchomalacia* are conditions in which the tracheobronchial tree shows abnormal flaccidity and softness of the cartilaginous framework (defective calcium deposits), with a tendency to collapse during respiration (Landing and Wells 1973). When the anomaly affects the larynx it is known as *laryngomalacia*. Hypercellularity with staining abnormalities of the cartilaginous matrix have been noted (Shulman et al. 1976) in a familial case of laryngomalacia.

Tracheo-oesophageal fistula is a relatively common congenital malformation, with various anatomical presentations that may or may not be associated with oesophageal atresia. Tracheal abnormalities are not uncommon and include cartilage deficiency with an increase in the length of the muscle in the membranous part of the tracheal ring (Holden and Wooler 1970; La Salle et al. 1979; Sunder et al. 1975; Wailoo and Emery 1979). Emery and Haddadin (1971) and Maeta et al. (1977) have shown that there is extensive squamous metaplasia of the tracheal epithelium, especially in cases with associated oesophageal atresia (see also p. 219). This condition is often associated with other malformations involving various systems, thus giving rise to complex patterns.

3.2. Acquired Lesions

3.2.1. Traumatic.

Various *foreign bodies* can lodge in the larynx or trachea in children and provoke symptoms of obstruction.

Lesions induced by *endotracheal intubation* are common in infants treated in intensive care units for the respiratory distress syndrome or for other neonatal respiratory difficulty. The lesions may be localized in the larynx at the level of the vocal cords, but are more often observed in the subglottic region or in the trachea. Less severe lesions consist of erosion of the mucosa; in the more severe forms the submucosa is ulcerated and infiltrated by inflammatory cells. The cartilage may be severely eroded in areas (Fig. 8.21) (Duc et al. 1974; Hawkins 1978; Joshi et al. 1972), and perforation can occur (Schild et al. 1976; Serlin and Daily 1975). These lesions are becoming less frequent owing to better techniques and modifications of the materials used in tube manufacture; however, healed lesions may cause severe scarring and subglottic or tracheal stenosis (Strong and Passay 1977; Weber and Grillo 1978a).

Corrosive agents (acids and alkalis) ingested accidentally and vomited may subsequently be aspirated, causing oedema and necrosis of the laryngeal and tracheal mucosa (Fig. 8.22). Lysol and kerosene cause similar lesions, the latter especially in developing countries. In rare instances, toxic gases may be the cause of irritation of the mucosa with oedema, congestion, and a secondary inflammatory reaction (Greene and Stark 1978).

3.2.2. Infections. *Laryngo–tracheo–Bronchitis*.

Acute infections of the larynx and trachea, including the epiglottis, may be life-threatening and require

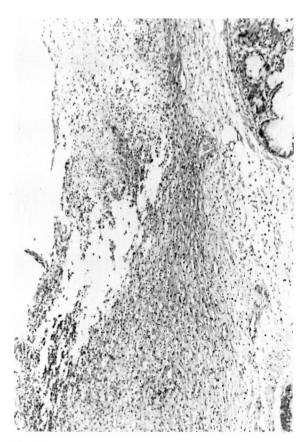

Fig. 8.21. Ulceration and necrosis of the tracheal mucosa and cartilage induced by endotracheal intubation for respiratory distress in a premature baby. (H and E; $60 \times$)

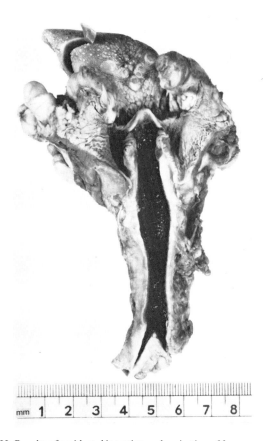

Fig. 8.22. Results of accidental ingestion and aspiration of ferrous sulphate.

prompt medical or surgical attention (Bass et al. 1974; Cantrell et al. 1978; Cohen and Chai 1978; Scheidemandel and Page 1975). Various micro-organisms have been recovered, the most common organisms being *haemophilus influenzae*, α-haemo/lytic streptococci, β-haemolytic streptococci group A, *staphylococcus aureus*, pneumococci and neisseria. In many developing countries, *Coryne-bacterium diphtheriae* still plays an important role in infections of this region.

Anatomically, changes in the epiglottis are the most striking: however, both the larynx and the trachea are usually also involved. The epiglottis is markedly swollen, oedematous, and congested. Its edges are rounded, and there is partial stenosis of the laryngeal orifice as a result of this. The larynx is also oedematous, and the vocal cords may touch in the middle. Histologically there is marked oedema of the submucosal tissues of the epiglottis and larynx, extending into the trachea. A diffuse polymorpho-nuclear infiltration extending into the deeper layers may be seen, usually sparing the cartilaginous structures. The lesions are nonspecific (Fig. 8.23). With *C. diphtheriae* infection there is necrosis of the mucosa and a pseudomembrane, composed of a fibrin network in which there are leukocytes and numerous bacteria, is present.

Virus infections usually affect the subglottic region and are characterized by oedema with marked congestion and some round-cell infiltration; associated bacterial infection is common.

The larynx and trachea may be the site of

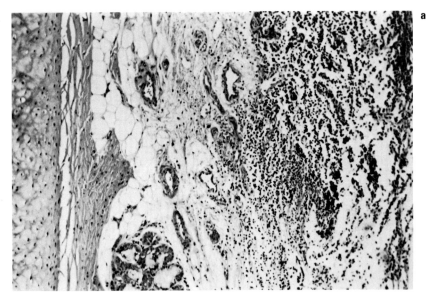

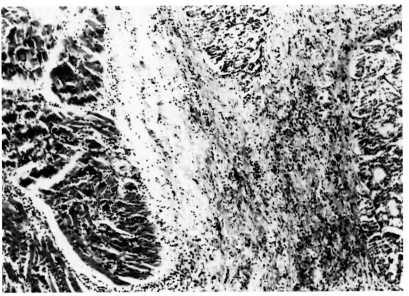

Fig. 8.23. a and **b** Acute epiglottis in an 8-month-old boy. (H and E; 90×) **a** Acute inflammation with ulceration and oedema of the epi-glottic mucosa; **b** Inflammation of the subglottic region with extension into the deep muscle layers.

nonspecific granulomas in cases of acute and chronic infections. In the developing world tuberculosis of the region may be encountered and the lesions usually present as mucosal ulcerations with the characteristic appearance. Mycotic infections are not infrequent in severely ill or debilitated infants in those countries. Cohen et al. (1978) have described a case of Wegener's granulomatosis of the larynx in a 12-year-old girl with the diffuse systemic form of the disease.

3.2.3. Tumours

Tumours of the larynx and trachea are quite uncommon among infants and children.

Papilloma is by far the most common tumour of this area and is more appropriately referred to as juvenile laryngotracheal papillomatosis, since multiple lesions are the rule. These tumours occur more frequently among children whose mothers present with condyloma acuminata during pregnancy, and in recent years evidence has accumulated that a papova virus may be responsible for the lesion. Papillomatosis often begins as a single wart on the vocal cords and spreads along the mucosa of the larynx to reach the trachea and even the main stem bronchi. The warts may disappear spontaneously at puberty, but are frequently recurrent despite repeated excisions (Bone et al. 1976; Boyle et al. 1973; Gross and Hubbard 1974; Quick et al. 1978; Spoendlin and Kistler 1978). Recent reports suggest that carcinoma may develop after many years (Fechner et al. 1974; Lundquist et al. 1975; Runckel and Kessler 1980; Siegel et al. 1979; Shapiro et al. 1976).

Histologically there is marked hyperplasia of the squamous epithelium with some degree of keratosis and parakeratosis but no hyperkeratosis (Fig. 8.24). The hyperplastic epithelium is thrown into folds about a thin stalk of connective tissue containing few capillaries and a few chronic inflammatory cells.

Squamous-cell carcinoma of the larynx in children is extremely rare. Large national surveys of tumours in children have failed to show up this tumour; however, there are some cases in the literature (Askin 1975; Jaffé 1973b; Jones and Gabriel 1969; Orton 1947). In a review of the recorded cases, Gindhart et al. (1980) collected 54 cases and added one of their own. The origin is often in the vocal cords and there is a male predominance (3:2). X-ray irradiation for juvenile papillomas may be a predisposing factor. There have also been reports indicating that carcinomas in the supraglottic area in adults have developed in laryngoceles (Micheau et al. 1976). The histological appearance of this tumour is similar to that of other squamous cell carcinomas. Weber and Grillo (1978b) treated a case of squa-

mous cell carcinoma of the trachea in a 13-year-old girl.

Briselli et al. (1978) in a review of the literature on tracheal *carcinoids* found one reported case in a 13-year-old adolescent girl.

Vascular tumours. Haemangiomas of the larynx and trachea, although uncommon, are important lesions because of the diagnostic problems they present and the high mortality among infants with these lesions. They may be observed at birth or shortly thereafter, grow progressively with age, and usually present some months after birth. They are occasionally associated with cutaneous haemangiomas. Spontaneous regression after the first year of life has been observed. They are almost always localized in the subglottic region and appear as sessile, flat, pinkish or bluish masses in the mucosa. Biopsy is not recommended because of the haemorrhage that may result (Benjamin 1978; Ferguson and Flake 1961; Feuerstein 1973; Holborow and Mott 1973).

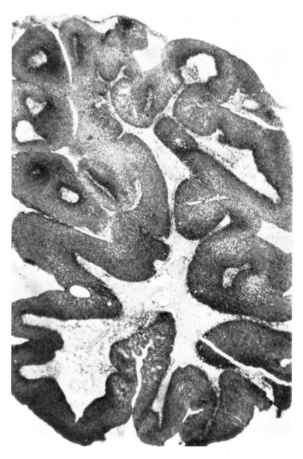

Fig. 8.24. Laryngeal papilloma. In this 11-year-old girl papillomas extend from the larynx into the main stem bronchi. (H and E: 35×)

Jaffé (1973b) described a case of *lymphangioma* in the larynx of a 2½-month-old boy. The same author also observed an *haemangiopericytoma* in a 3-month-old boy.

Tumours of nervous origin. Neurofibromas of the larynx may occur and are sometimes associated with neurofibromatosis (von Recklinghausen's disease). In recent reviews of this subject (Jafek and Stern 1973; Maisel and Ogura 1974) there were four recorded cases in the paediatric age group, one of which occurred in a 3-month-old boy.

Tumours of muscular origin. Granular cell myoblastoma of the larynx has been reported in children by Booth and Osborn (1970), Nasser et al. (1970), and Thawley and Osborn (1974).

Leiomyoma of the trachea is extremely rare, and Kitamura et al. (1969) could only find nine published cases, one of which was in a 15-year-old patient presented by Unger (1952). *Rhabdomyosarcoma*, although an uncommon tumour, is perhaps more prevalent than most other soft-tissue tumours of these parts. There have been reports of this tumour occurring in the larynx of children by Canalis et al. (1976), Frugoni and Ferlito (1976), Fu and Perzin (1976), and Wayoff and Labaeye (1973).

Cartilaginous tumours (chondroma, chondrosarcoma) of the larynx and trachea have been recorded in adults but are exceptional in childhood.

Chemodectomas (non-chromaffin paraganglia) of possible Kultschitzky cell origin sometimes occur in the larynx. Hohbach and Mootz (1978) found 23 recorded cases in the literature, one of which occurred in a 14-year-old boy, and added one of their own. Cohen et al. (1978a) described a case of a primary *lymphosarcoma* of the larynx in a girl aged 4 years 7 months, and also reported on a *solitary plasmocytoma* affecting the larynx and upper trachea in a 15-year-old girl treated for systemic lupus erythematosus (Cohen et al. 1978b).

Other tumours. Gilbert et al. (1953), in their review of tracheal tumours, found nine cases of *fibromas* among children. Cohen et al. (1978a) described a case of *fibrous histiocytoma* in the trachea of a 2½-year-old girl, and Sandstrom et al. (1978), in their review, found one case in a 15-year-old girl. Witwer and Tampas (1973) described a case of a tracheal *fibroxanthoma* in a 5-year-old boy, and discovered a second case in the literature. Recently Som et al. (1979) described the case of a benign pleomorphic adenoma of the larynx in a 15-year-old boy.

4. Lungs

4.1. Congenital Abnormalities

Congenital abnormalities of the lungs are varied and often complex. They may be isolated to the lungs but it is not uncommon to find such abnormalities associated with other organ or system malformation.

Pulmonary agenesis. There is no general agreement on the classification of this condition. Schneider (1912) first attempted to divide the abnormality into three groups: (a) agenesis, in which there is complete absence of bronchi, alveolar tissue, and their blood supply; (b) a group in which a rudimentary bronchus arose from the trachea with no pulmonary tissue investing its tips; and (c) a group with a poorly developed main bronchus invested by a fleshy mass of ill-developed pulmonary tissue. This classification was subsequently modified by Boyden (1955), who recommended a system based on the degree of developmental arrest. There were also three categories: (a) complete absence of one or both lungs (agenesis); (b) suppression of all but a rudimentary bronchus (aplasia), and (c) abortive growth (hypoplasia). Recently Spencer (1977a, b) has proposed yet another classification, based on the categories of anomalies: (1) bilateral complete agenesis; (2) unilateral agenesis, which is further subdivided into three groups, which are identical with Schneider's three groups; and (3) lobar agenesis and other lesser forms of congenital abnormalities.

We shall follow this last general classification.

Bilateral or complete pulmonary agenesis is a very rare condition, and there are few recorded cases. The laryngotracheal tree may terminate blindly at the level of the larynx, or trachea, or even at the main stem bronchi. The pulmonary artery normally takes its origin from the right ventricle, but terminates in the thoracic aorta by way of the ductus arteriosus. The bronchial arteries and pulmonary veins are usually absent, and there are other associated abnormalities affecting the oesophagus, the cardiovascular system and the face. An accessory spleen has been reported, as has asplenia (De Buse and Morris, 1973; Östör et al. 1978).

Unilateral pulmonary agenesis is much more common than complete agenesis, and is not compatible with normal life. This condition has been referred to by several names in the numerous case reports or reviews on the subject. According to Spencer's (1977a, b) classification there are three subgroups, each of which corresponds to one of Schneider's (1912) three groups, described above. There may be other associated abnormalities involving the cardiovascular system, the gastrointestinal tract, the ipsilateral facial bones, vertebral column and upper limbs and their associated muscles, and the urogenital system. The life expectancy of these patients depends on the severity of the associated malformations and the problem of infections in the existing lung (Booth and Berry 1967; Bretagne et al. 1972; Jimenez-Martinez et al. 1965; Maltz and Nadas 1968; McCormick and Kuhns 1979; Paillie et al. 1967; Samaan 1970). Ryland and Reid (1971) and Hislop et al. (1979) have further shown that in existing lung tissue there is bronchial reduction with an increase in alveolar density. The pulmonary artery in their case also showed a reduction in both the conventional and the supernumerary branches, which was more marked for the former group of vessels.

Minor abnormalities. Abnormal lobulation is not an uncommon finding in post-mortem material, and is often the result of lobar fusions or accessory fissures. It is generally associated with other congenital malformations, usually cardiovascular, e.g., Ivemark's syndrome, Fallot's tetralogy, polysplenia, and situs inversus (Landing and Wells 1973). The bronchial tree of these abnormal lungs also shows variations from the normal bronchial pattern, and it must be emphasized that many accessory lobes (azygos, cardiac, left middle) are variations of normal lobulation.

There is a very uncommon condition in which the lungs are fused in the mid-line behind the heart, giving them a *horse-shoe* appearance. Cipriano et al. (1975) described a case in a 7-month-old girl and referred to two other cases from the literature. In their own case there was dextrocardia associated with other congenital malformations.

Pulmonary hypoplasia. A decrease in lung volume and weight is referred to as pulmonary hypoplasia. This abnormality is divided into two groups, *primary* and *secondary*, by certain authors (Bates 1965; Mendelsohn and Hutchins 1977). In the view of these authors, primary hypoplasia involves both lungs and is usually associated with oligo-hydramnios and renal agenesis (Potter's syndrome) and hydramnios. Secondary hypoplasia is generally associated with a reduction of the intrathoracic volume and may be unilateral or bilateral (Fig. 8.25). In either case, the lung or lungs may appear normal on gross inspection but there is a marked reduction in volume and weight compared with those of other fetuses of comparable gestational age or newborns. This reduction may be to as little as 25 % of normal.

Among the common causes of pulmonary hypoplasia are: congenital diaphragmatic hernia (by far the most frequent cause), pleural effusion (hydrops fetalis), polycystic renal disease, idiopathic cardiac hypertrophy, anencephaly, thoracic or other

skeletal dystrophy or dysplasia, tracheal compression, and certain pulmonary vascular anomalies (Hislop et al. 1973; Mendelsohn and Hutchins 1977; Muller et al. 1978; Oberklaid et al. 1977; Pena and Shokeir 1974; Perlman and Levin 1974; Punnett et al. 1974; Thomas and Smith 1974; Ponté et al. 1974; Swischuk et al. 1979).

Areechon and Reid (1963) have studied the lungs in congenital diaphragmatic hernia and have shown that there is a reduction of bronchial and bronchiolar development in both lungs, but that this is much more marked in the hypoplastic lung. This reduction is greater in the bronchiolar than in the bronchial region, and there is a reduction in the size, rather than the number, of alveoli. These results explain the histologic picture of the hypoplastic lung in which the bronchi appear numerous, being relatively close to each other, and extend to the periphery. The alveoli and alveolar ducts are markedly reduced (Fig. 8.26).

Boyden (1972b), employing a wax construction method, has confirmed the findings of Areechon and Reid (1963). Kitagawa et al. (1971) have further

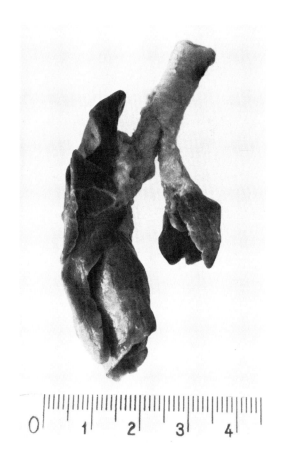

Fig. 8.25. Pulmonary hypoplasia of left lung in a patient presenting with a large left diaphragmatic hernia. Courtesy of Dr C. Bozic.

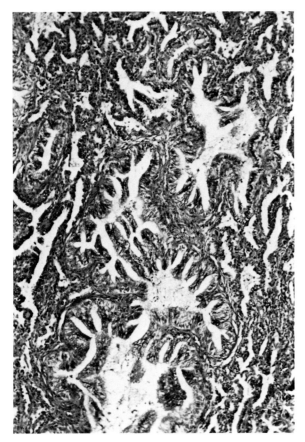

Fig. 8.26. Pulmonary hypoplasia showing grouping of the reduced bronchial and bronchiolar branches. Courtesy of Dr C. Bozic. (H and E; 35 ×)

shown that the number of alveoli per acinus is proportionally less reduced than the total number of alveoli in the lung. This suggests that alveolar multiplication is regulated by acinar rather than the total alveolar number, and that as a result the lung may grow after surgical correction of the hernia. Since then, other authors (Finegold et al. 1971; Hislop et al. 1979; Reale and Esterly 1973) have employed other methods, including morphometry, to evaluate the extent of pulmonary hypoplasia in congenital diaphragmatic hernia and other conditions resulting in hypoplasia, and have shown that there is no essential difference between the various types.

4.2. Accessory Lungs and Pulmonary Sequestration

Müller (1918) defined *accessory lung* as an organ-like mass of pulmonary tissue with its own pleura, separated from the rest of the lung. The accessory lung may connect with either the tracheobronchial

tree or the fore-gut. *Pulmonary sequestration*, on the other hand, describes a piece of lung which, although lying within the same pleura as the normal lung, is not connected to its bronchial system or derivatives. The sequestrated tissue receives its blood supply from a systemic artery. Sequestered lung may be located within the main lung (*intralobar sequestration*) or separate from it (*extralobar sequestration*). It is possible, from these broad definitions, to separate four main pathological entities without considering minor variations or combined abnormalities. These are: (1) accessory lung with connections to the tracheobronchial tree; (2) accessory lung with bronchi arising from foregut derivatives; (3) extralobar pulmonary sequestration; and (4) intralobar pulmonary sequestration.

These various lesions used to be considered rare abnormalities, and were usually accidental findings at post mortem. They were sometimes discovered during treatment of a repeated pulmonary infection, or during the course of certain radiographic procedures. As radiographic procedures and techniques improve, the lesions are discovered more frequently, and have been reported at all ages. Pulmonary sequestration is sometimes associated with funnel chest deformity and other anomalies (Accard et al. 1970; Dutau et al. 1973; Felson 1972; Gerle et al. 1968; Iwa and Watanabe 1979; Jaubert de Beaujeu et al. 1973; Savic et al. 1979).

1) *Accessory lung with connections to the tracheobronchial tree:* The accessory bronchus takes its origin from the normal tracheobronchial tree and terminates in a mass of poorly defined pulmonary tissue. The latter may be cystic or may resemble a hamartoma. Examples of this type of abnormality have been described by Cotton et al. (1962) and Herxheimer (1901).

2) *Accessory lung with bronchi arising from foregut derivatives:* The accessory bronchus originates from fore-gut derivatives, usually the lower (occasionally upper) portion of the oesophagus or the stomach. The tissue lies outside and separate from the lung proper. Histologically it is made up of tubular structures lined by ciliated respiratory-type epithelium. The bronchus leading to the accessory lung may be lined by squamous epithelium similar to that of the oesophagus or by gastric-type mucosa, depending on its origin. The artery supplying the accessory lung generally arises from the aorta (Boyden et al. 1962; Gerle et al. 1968; Grans and Potts 1951; Kobler and Ammann 1977; Pai et al. 1971).

3) *Extralobar pulmonary sequestration:* These masses consist of bronchial and alveolar structures, often lying behind the lung. They may be located at any level from the neck to the diaphragm. The majority have been found on the left, and they are

frequently associated with diaphragmatic hernia or some other congenital malformation. The arterial supply to the sequestrated tissue is usually by a number of small branches from the thoracic or abdominal aorta, but occasionally from the subclavian or intercostal arteries. The venous drainage is by way of the azygos system (Accard et al. 1970; Bliek and Mulholland 1971; Jaubert de Beaujeu et al. 1970; Merlier et al. 1970; Stocker and Kagan-Hallet 1979).

4) *Intralobar pulmonary sequestration:* This is a relatively common abnormality. The sequestrated pulmonary tissue does not communicate with the tracheobronchial tree, and is contained within the pleura of the normal lung. It is usually situated in the lower lobes and mostly on the left, although other lobes may contain the lesions. The posterior basal segment is most frequently involved. This abnormality is rarely associated with other malformations.

The sequestrated tissue frequently consists of a single cystic cavity or a group of interconnecting cysts. Less commonly, a solid mass of tissue is found, which is not separable from the surrounding normal lung. This mass contains dilated bronchus-like spaces lined with respiratory-type epithelium whose walls sometimes contain cartilage plates. Alveolus-like structures are also observed.

The artery supplying the sequestrated tissue is usually quite prominent, taking its origin from the thoracic or abdominal aorta, or occasionally from the intercostal arteries. The supplying artery is generally short, of large diameter, and has an elastic structure similar to that of the pulmonary artery. The venous drainage is by way of the pulmonary venous system (Buchanan 1959; Dutau et al. 1973; Pryce 1946; Pryce et al. 1947; Zelefsky et al. 1971).

The embryogenesis and pathogenesis of these abnormalities are still a matter of debate and there are many theories on their formation (Delarue et al. 1959; Gebauer and Mason 1959; Gerle et al. 1968; Pryce et al. 1947; Kyllonen 1964).

4.3. Cysts

Lung cysts remain a controversial subject with no satisfactory classification available, although several have been proposed. They can be divided into two main groups, congenital and acquired, the latter being by far the most common. There is still some difficulty in deciding whether a cyst is congenital or acquired, especially when it is discovered after the neonatal period. One can only be sure that a cyst is congenital if it is discovered in a fetus or newborn, since acquired cysts can occur in the first months of life after pulmonary infection, particularly staphylococcal or viral infections. In older children the distinction between the two becomes almost impossible. They can affect only a portion of the lung or of a lobe, and can be single or multiple. Either sex may be affected (Bale 1979; Boyden 1958; Moffat 1960; Rogers and Osmer 1964; Welchert et al. 1970).

Spencer (1977b) has presented a temporary classification based on pathology. His groups are: (A) Congenital, further subdivided into four types: (1) central and peripheral; (2) lymphangiomatous; (3) cystic change in an intralobular sequestrated or accessory lung, and enterogenous cysts; (4) congenital cystic adenomatoid malformation; (B) Acquired cysts. There are also four large subgroups of this class, which will not be discussed further here.

Central cysts are often referred to as bronchogenic. They are usually observed in the mediastinum, near the hilum or a main bronchus, and appear to have been derived from a large bronchus. Less commonly they occur in the wall of the oesophagus or in the subcutaneous tissue of the chest wall or neck. They are most often single cysts, variable in size, and do not necessarily communicate with the tracheobronchial tree but may simply be attached by a fibrous band. Histologically the cysts are lined by a pseudostratified columnar epithelium, the wall consisting of smooth muscle bundles, cartilage plates, and abundant elastic fibres. There are also numerous subepithelial glands, which explain the presence of mucus in the lumen (Fig. 8.27). The changes caused by infection may be superadded.

Peripheral cysts probably develop as a result of disturbance in the growth of the bronchial tree at a late stage of intrauterine life or even after birth. They are usually multiple, and may affect both lungs, a lobe or part of a lobe, or even an entire lung. Microscopically they may communicate with a parent bronchus, and they are a form of honeycomb lung of infancy. Histologically, they are lined with ciliated or cuboidal respiratory epithelium. Their wall consists of connective tissue in which there are many elastic fibres and a few small cartilage plates but practically no smooth muscle fibres. Subepithelial mucus glands are usually absent (Fig. 8.28).

Cystic adenomatoid malformation is a relatively rare condition, and has often been included with congenital cystic disease of the lung or pulmonary sequestration or cited as a hamartoma. Congenital adenomatoid malformation is known to be associated with anasarca, maternal hydramnios, and congenital malformations. The abnormality is usually unilateral, affecting one or more lobes, usually the lower lobe (Aslam et al. 1970; Dempster 1969; Gille et al. 1973; Kohler and Rymer 1973; Merenstein 1969; Michalsen 1974; Moncrieff et al. 1969; Spector et al. 1960; Weber et al. 1978). Ch'In and Tang (1949) cited Sternberg as the only author to have described bilateral lesions. Tumours are known to develop in or in association with this malformation (Stephanopoulos and Catsaras 1963; Ueda et al. 1977).

Kwittken and Reiner (1962) were among the first to attempt to define the condition histologically, and included the following characteristics: it shows an increase of terminal respiratory structures with intercommunicating cysts of various sizes lined with respiratory-type or cuboidal epithelium, with a polypoid formation of the mucosa and an increased amount of elastic fibres in the wall beneath the epithelium. There was usually absence of cartilage and there were no inflammatory cells.

In 1973, Van Dijk and Wagenvoort described three cases of this condition and proposed a new classification into cystic, intermediate, and solid types. Stocker et al. (1977) reviewed 38 cases and

proposed a different classification. These authors also grouped their cases into three distinct categories, based on clinical, gross, and histological criteria: *type I* lesions presented only a few large, thick-walled cysts containing air or fluid. These cysts were lined with ciliated pseudostratified columnar epithelium with numerous polypoid projections in the lumen. The wall contained smooth-muscle fibres and elastic tissue, but very few cartilage plates. There were smaller cysts adjacent to the larger ones, and large alveolus-like structures were observed between the cysts. Sometimes these alveolus-like structures communicated with the smaller cysts. The blood vessels were normal. *Type II* lesions presented as numerous, evenly spaced cysts, generally less than 1 cm in diameter. They communicated with the normal bronchial tree. The cysts were lined with

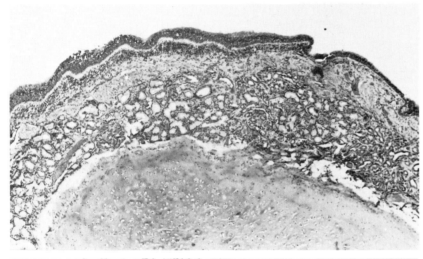

Fig. 8.27. Wall of central bronchial cyst from a 15-year-old girl. It resembles that of the normal bronchial wall. (H and E; 25 ×)

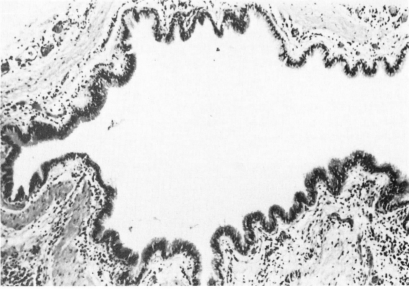

Fig. 8.28. Wall of peripheral bronchogenic cyst from a 4-year-old boy. Courtesy of Dr C. Bozic. (H and E; 35 ×)

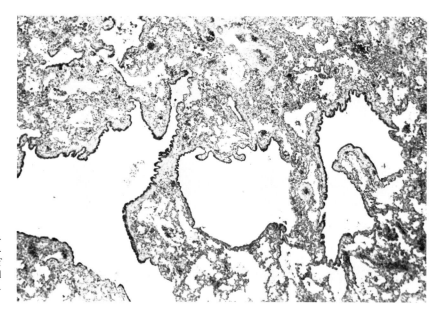

Fig. 8.29. Congenital cystic adenomatoid malformation, corresponding to type II lesions of Stocker et al., from a 3-day-old baby girl. Courtesy of Dr C. Bozic. (H and E; 25×)

cuboidal or tall columnar ciliated epithelium, with rare areas of pseudostratification (Fig. 8.29). The wall consisted of a thin layer of loose connective tissue, and in this there were dense concentrations of elastic tissue beneath the epithelium, as well as irregular bundles of striated muscles fibres. Cartilage was observed only as a normal component of the bronchi. *Type III* lesions were less numerous and presented as bulky and firm masses of pulmonary tissue occupying almost the entire lobe or lobes and containing very small visible cysts (less than 0.5 cm). The cysts were similar to bronchioles in size and distribution, and were lined in areas with ciliated cuboidal epithelium or, in most places, with non-ciliated cuboidal epithelium (Fig. 8.30). Electron microscopic studies of these cells (Olson and Mendelsohn 1978) have shown that they are composed primarily of granular pneumocytes (type II) and few type I pneumocytes. They resembled the glandular structure of the developing lung and were separated by a loose connective-tissue stroma with a few elastic fibres and occasional smooth-muscle fibres. Cartilage was absent.

In their series, Stocker et al. (1977) found that type I and type II lesions were by far the most frequently observed. They also noted that type I lesions were larger, involving almost the entire lobe or lobes with no adjacent normal pulmonary tissue. Furthermore, type I lesions were more commonly associated with other congenital malformations.

Östör and Fortune (1978) consider congenital cystic adenomatoid malformation to be a distinct

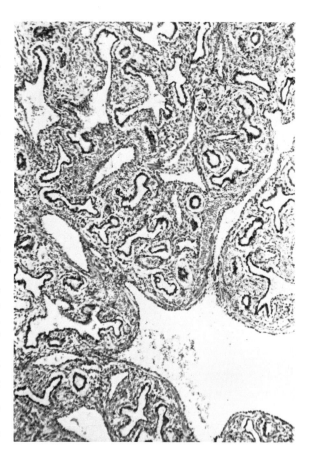

Fig. 8.30. Type III lesion of congenital cystic adenomatoid malformation after Stocker et al., from a premature baby boy. (H and E; 60×)

pathological entity within the general group of congenital cystic diseases of the lung, and believe that the types I and II lesions of Stocker et al. (1977) fall in this category. These authors consider only the type III lesions as truly adenomatoid.

Pulmonary lymphangiectasis is not uncommon. Clinically it presents as respiratory distress in the neonate. Infants with this anomaly rarely survive beyond 24 h; however, cases have been recorded of survival for some weeks. Males seem to be more frequently affected than females. The abnormality has been described in association with other congenital malformations, although no specific associations occur.

The aetiology is obscure, and various theories are proposed as to its pathogenesis, including obstruction of the pulmonary venous flow, obstruction of the pulmonary lymphatics, and anomalous pulmonary development with failure or regression of the developing lymphatic network (Bankl and Wimmer 1972; Esterly and Oppenheimer 1970; Felman et al. 1972; France and Brown 1971; Laurence 1959; Le Tan Vinh et al. 1977).

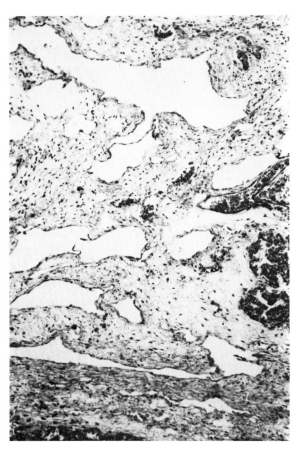

Fig. 8.31. Congenital pulmonary lymphangiectasia in a 34 weeks premature femal infant with hypoplastic left ventricle. Courtesy of Dr J. Pryse-Davies. (H and E; 160 ×)

Macroscopically both lungs are generally involved, although there are a few reported cases in which only one lung has been involved. The lungs are large and firm, with a grossly lobulated or nodular surface. Between the lobules, one can observe the lymphatic network, with multiple round or ovoid cystic cavities lying beneath the pleura and containing fluid. The cut surface may appear relatively normal or show a honeycomb appearance with thickening of the intralobular septa, which may contain numerous cysts, resembling interstitial emphysema. Histologically the septa are thickened throughout the lung, and they contain a lace-like network of distended lymphatic vessels of variable sizes extending into the intrapleural space (Fig. 8.31). The lymphatics are thin-walled, lined with a single layer of endothelial cells, and do not have valves. Muscles fibres are absent from the thickened septa, and there is no lymphoid tissue present.

4.4. Heterotopic Tissue in the Lungs

There are a few recorded cases of ectopic tissue within the pulmonary parenchyma. Brain has been observed in the lungs in cases of anencephaly or in other cerebral malformations (Charles 1960; Gonzalez-Crussi et al. 1980; Kanbour et al. 1979; Odeka 1978; Valdes-Dapena and Arey 1967). Masses of striated muscle have also been reported (Aterman and Patel 1970; Remberger and Hübner 1974), as has ectopic adrenal cortical tissue (Bozic 1974).

4.5. Lobar Emphysema

Lobar emphysema is also referred to in the literature as regional infantile emphysema or congenital obstructive emphysema, and the condition is due to air-trapping by a check-valve. The lesion can involve one or several segments, one or multiple lobes, or even an entire lung; the upper lobes are most often affected, with a slight predominance on the left. In rare cases both lungs have been involved. The condition is observed principally in neonates and infants. Clinically it manifests itself as a rapidly progressive respiratory distress syndrome, with dyspnoea and cyanosis leading to cardiorespiratory failure. On X-ray pictures the affected area is hyperlucent, and there is compression atelectasis of the adjacent pulmonary parenchyma with displacement of the mediastinum toward the opposite side. A relatively high incidence of associated malformations, including cystic adenomatoid malformation, is recorded in these patients (Lincoln et al. 1971; Strunge 1972; Sulayman et al. 1975; Young et al. 1978; Moyland and Shannon 1979).

Although the underlying mechanism causing this

condition is not always clear, obstruction of the bronchus leading to the involved segment, lobe, or lung is an important cause. Extrinsic factors that can obstruct the bronchus include anomalous mediastinal blood vessels, enlarged lymph nodes, bronchogenic mediastinal cysts, and enteric duplications (Desvignes et al. 1974; Gerami et al. 1969; Powell and Elliot 1977; Schapiro and Evans 1972). Intrinsic causes include mucus plugs or redundant bronchial mucosal folds. More common, however, are structural defects in the bronchial wall, which may be overlooked unless careful histological studies of the main bronchus leading to the involved emphysematous zone are performed. The bronchus may be atretic or stenosed, or it may have abnormal cartilages, with cartilage present as hypoplastic or fragmented cartilage plates affecting either a localized area or several bronchi. The hypoplasia may be partial or total. Bronchomalacia may be included among the defects causing lobar emphysema (Chang et al. 1968; Desvignes et al. 1974; Hendren and McKee 1966; Lacquet et al. 1971; Powell and Elliott 1977; Lincoln et al. 1971; Lynch 1970; MacMahon and Ruggieri 1969), as may rotation of a lobe (Hislop and Reid 1971).

By quantitative analyses of lungs with congenital lobar emphysema or 'apparent' emphysema, Hislop and Reid (1970, 1971) and Henderson et al. (1971) were able to illustrate other causes. These various authors were able to separate combinations of anatomical lesions that may be associated with congenital lobar emphysema. They described the *polyalveolar* lobe (*acinus giantism*), in which there was an increase in alveolar number, and further showed that unilateral congenital emphysema can be present in a hypoplastic lung with contralateral compensatory emphysema.

4.6. Neonatal Pathological Conditions

It is impossible to overemphasize the importance of an X-ray examination of the body or the thorax before post mortem to enable the pathologist to exclude certain abnormalities within the thoracic cavity. The need to test the pleural spaces for pneumothorax is evident in view of the widespread use of assisted ventilation, and since useful information can be gained from bacteriological and virological studies, material from the trachea, bronchi, lungs, and blood from the heart may be cultured. These examinations often supply valuable information and are often helpful in cases where the gross pathology is uninformative.

Amniotic fluid and meconium aspiration. It is well established that the fetal lung secretes a liquid that occupies the terminal air spaces and airways and whose composition and viscosity are different from those of the plasma and amniotic fluid (Adams 1966; Adamson et al. 1969a). There has been considerable controversy as to whether there are spontaneous fetal respiratory movements in utero, with mixing of the amniotic fluid with that of the fetal lung. Recent studies using various methods (mainly ultrasonic monitoring) have shown that fetal breathing movements in utero occur both in experimental animals and in man. These movements, which are associated with contractions of both the diaphragmatic and the intercostal muscles, have been detected early in gestation and they become more regular with advancing gestational age. Because of the high viscosity of lung fluid and the short duration of inspiration, normal breathing is insufficient to clear the tracheal dead space, and therefore the tidal volume is very small. It is mainly during 'gasping', under various adverse conditions, that relatively large volumes of amniotic fluid may be inspired by the fetus (Adamson et al. 1980; Biggs et al. 1974; Boddy and Dawes 1975; Dawes 1973; Fox and Hohler 1977; Patrick et al. 1976; Patrick et al. 1980). The amniotic fluid may sometimes be stained with meconium, suggesting fetal distress. However, Miller et al. (1975) and Seppälä and Aho (1975) have suggested that the passage of meconium is not always a result of hypoxia or fetal distress, but may be a spontaneous or even a physiological phenomenon. Whatever the determining factors may be, the amount of meconium released and the quantity of meconium-stained amniotic fluid aspirated by the fetus depends largely on the duration and intensity of the stimulating factor.

Aspiration of amniotic fluid or meconium-stained fluid occurs mainly in mature or postmature infants, but can also be observed in the premature. It is generally associated with fetal anoxia, which may in turn to be related to cerebral haemorrhage, vagal reflex, intrauterine pneumonia, congenital heart disease or other malformation, or drugs administered to the mother during pregnancy or at delivery. Aspiration may result in intrauterine death or the meconium aspiration syndrome of the newborn (Boddy and Dawes 1975; Eskes 1971; Fujikura and Klionsky 1975; Gunn et al. 1970; King et al. 1978; Meis et al. 1978; Naeye 1978; Vidyasagar et al. 1975). The lung may show little on gross examination; however, the presence of meconium on the perianal region, within the external ear, or on other parts of the body and the placenta is an indication that intrauterine fetal distress or anoxia has occurred. The external ear should always be examined for meconium in a neonate; if the body has been washed postnatally, as often happens, traces can be discovered with a swab. The histological lesions are variable and include aspiration of amniotic fluid into the terminal airways, which are distended and contain fluid, a few squamous epithelial cells, and some cellular debris, and show congestion of surrounding capillaries. When such meconium is aspirated, the distal airways are distended, containing masses of meconium with some squamous epithelial cells; the trachea and large bronchi may contain large meconium plugs; the bronchioles and terminal airways are also distended and are partly or completely filled with squamous epithelial cells and a little meconium (Fig. 8.32). In both instances there is congestion of the capillaries.

When squames are observed in the distal airways of infants several weeks after birth, it is, of course, possible that there might have been a period of intrauterine fetal distress with aspiration of amniotic fluid.

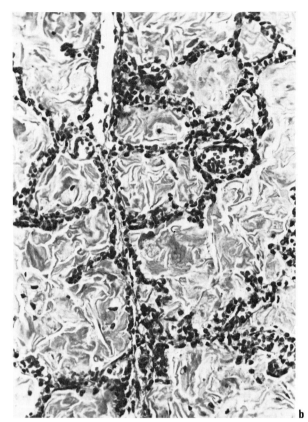

Fig. 8.32. a–c Lungs in neonatal asphyxia. (H and E; 225 ×) **a** Progressive respiratory distress in a full-term infant. Alveolar saccules are filled with amniotic fluid but contain little debris. **b** Severe respiratory distress with marked extension of alveolar saccules filled with squamous epithelial cells. **c** Prolonged respiratory distress. There is a giant cell reaction associated with secondary inflammation.

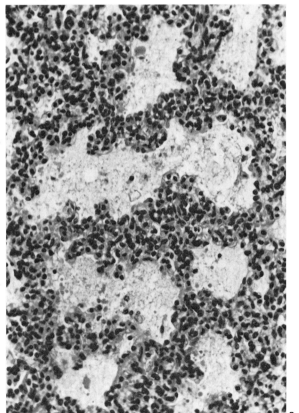

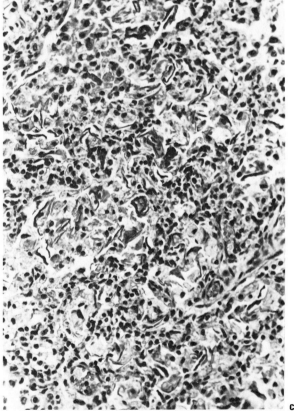

Perinatal pneumonia. Pneumonia in stillborn and newborn infants is a relatively common post-mortem finding. It is responsible for the deaths of 5%–20% of infants dying within the first 24–48 h of extrauterine life, and may be found in as many as 30% of stillbirths. Most authors refer to pneumonia occurring in those dying within 48 h of birth as intrauterine or congenital pneumonia, and associate it with aspiration of infected amniotic fluid in utero, maternal sepsis, or infection acquired during passage through the birth canal (intrapartal infection). The term *neonatal pneumonia* is reserved for pneumonia occurring during the first days or weeks after birth, but not after the first month of age. It is generally associated with infections acquired from the environment (delivery room and nursery).

In most infants dying in the immediate neonatal period, between 24 and 48 h of age, it is impossible to distinguish between the two groups (Fedrik and Butler 1971a; Gunn et al. 1970; Lauweryns et al. 1973; Naeye et al. 1971).

Most intrauterine pneumonia is the result of infection ascending from the birth canal into the amniotic sac. It is associated with premature rupture of the membranes and prolonged labour, conditions that favour chorioamnionitis, whose incidence increases significantly after 24 h. Congenital pneumonia has also been observed in prolonged labour with intact membranes or where there have been obstetric manoeuvres during labour. In the remaining cases, infection is transplacental and is often associated with clinical symptoms in the mother, e.g., pyelonephritis.

Premature infants appear to be more susceptible to intrauterine pneumonia (Gunn et al. 1970; Naeye et al. 1971; Scott and Henderson 1972).

The commonest causative organisms are: *Escherichia coli*, β-haemolytic streptococci group B, *Streptococcus faecalis*, *Staphylococcus aureus*, *Klebsiella–aerobacter* and *Pseudomonas aeruginosa*; less frequently *Haemophilus influenzae* and *Pneumococci* are responsible. Numerous other pathogens have been isolated occasionally, including viruses, fungi and mycoplasmas (Ablow et al. 1976; Bale and Watkins 1978; Barson 1971; Barter and Hudson 1974; Chabrolle et al. 1977; Gibson and Williams 1978; Gotoff and Behram 1970; Ho and Aterman 1970; Nicholls et al. 1975; O'Herlihy et al. 1976; Olding 1970).

Gross inspection of the lungs reveals nothing apart from occasional localized pleurisy. Histologically, the distal airways are filled wtih a polymorphonuclear rich inflammatory reaction, which may or may not contain squames. The most striking feature characterizing this type of pneumonia is the absence of fibrin, which has created doubt as to whether the histological picture is a true in-flammatory response to infection or caused by simple aspiration of amniotic elements containing polymorphonuclear leucocytes. The studies of Lauweryns et al. (1973) make the latter explanation unlikely. The alveolar septa, bronchioles, and bronchi are not involved. Bacteria are not usually observed in sections and if present, are few (Fig. 8.33). In neonatal pneumonia the exudate contains fibrin, and interstitial inflammatory changes with monocytic cell infiltration can be seen. The bronchi and bronchioles may be surrounded by or infiltrated with mononuclear cells. Necrosis is common but may occur with the formation of microabscesses, notably in staphylococcal infections.

Pulmonary haemorrhage. The real incidence of massive pulmonary haemorrhage in the newborn is not known; there are wide variations in the individual series studied. It is sometimes found in stillborn infants, but is most common among those dying in the first 48 h of life. Premature infants and those small for gestational age are the most often affected. Symptoms may appear immediately after or within a few hours of birth and resemble a severe respiratory distress syndrome.

Although fluid escaping from the nose and mouth may resemble blood, chemical analyses have shown it to be a mixture of plasma filtrate and a small quantity of blood, comparable to haemorrhagic oedema fluid (Adamson et al. 1969b; Cole et al. 1973; Fedrick and Butler 1971b).

Several aetiologies have been proposed for this condition. It has been described in association with prenatal and perinatal asphyxia or anoxia, bacterial or viral infection, cerebral oedema and/or intraventricular haemorrhage, hypothermia, cardiac anomalies (patent ductus arteriosus or ventricular septal defect), haemorrhagic disease of the newborn, hyaline membrane disease, and hyperammonaemia (Adamson et al. 1969b; Chessels and Wigglesworth 1971; Cole et al. 1973; Esterly and Oppenheimer 1966; Fedrick and Butler 1971b; Sheffield et al. 1976). The recent studies of Cole et al. (1973) and those of Trompeter et al. (1975) suggest that massive pulmonary haemorrhage in the neonate covers a spectrum of conditions that may rapidly lead to acute left ventricular failure owing to asphyxia. This is followed by an increase in pulmonary capillary pressure and pulmonary haemorrhage.

On gross examination the lungs are heavy, fleshy, and of normal size. They may have one or several dark, haemorrhagic areas: in most instances an entire lobe or several lobes may be involved. The trachea and large bronchi often contain blood-stained fluid. Histologically, the distended distal airways, bronchioles, and some bronchi are filled with erythrocytes. The alveolar septa are markedly

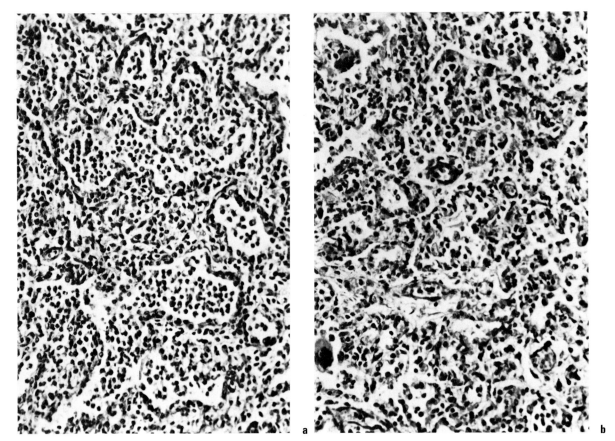

Fig. 8.33. a Intrauterine pneumonia in a stillborn fetus. The alveolar saccules are distended and filled with polymorphonuclear leucocytes. Conspicuous absence of fibrin. **b** Intrauterine pneumonia with giant cells, probably of viral origin, in a 2-day-old infant whose mother presented with a temperature of unknown origin. No bacteria present. (H and E; 225 ×)

congested and show zones of interstitial haemorrhage (Fig. 8.34). Hyaline membranes, squames, and mild inflammatory reactions have all been observed in association with this condition.

Idiopathic respiratory distress syndrome (hyaline membrane disease) used to be the most frequent cause of death among neonates, especially the premature, and it was estimated that the condition was responsible for approximately 12 000 deaths each year in the United States, representing roughly 20 % of all neonatal deaths. The figure varies between 25 % and 75 % in other countries. Due to the enormous progress that has been made in neonatal care during the last decade the death rate due to this disorder has fallen considerably over the last few years, and in most large centres there are relatively few cases of infants dying with hyaline membrane disease alone. Such deaths show a male preponderance; in addition the second-born of twins appears to be at greater risk than the first-born. There have been reports of a familial predisposition

(Farrell and Avery 1975; Farrell and Wood 1976; Machin 1975; Manniello and Farrell 1977; Nelson 1970).

Prenatal identification of infants at risk and the standardization of treatment in most centres have resulted in the more favourable outcome. Most patients who now succumb usually present with associated pathological conditions or complications of therapy (Banerjee et al. 1972; Farrell and Avery 1975; Northway et al. 1967; Taghizadeh and Reynolds 1976).

It is generally accepted that there are three main predisposing factors among infants who present with the respiratory distress syndrome: (1) *Prematurity* or *immaturity*. Infants of low birth weights (800–1500 g) appear to be more susceptible to this disorder than infants born at or near term. It should be noted that the condition has seldom been recorded in fetuses below 800 g and has not been seen in stillborn infants; (2) *Caesarean section.* There is still much controversy as to whether Caesarean section per se predisposes to hyaline membrane

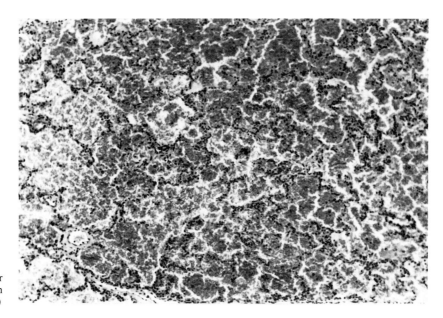

Fig. 8.34. Diffuse intra-alveolar haemorrhage of unknown origin in a newborn infant. (H and E; 90 ×)

disease; the evidence suggests that it does, and that this is more apparent following certain indications for section (fetal distress, maternal bleeding, and placenta praevia); (3) *Maternal diabetes*. Here again, hyaline membrane disease alone does not seem to be directly related to maternal diabetes, but may simply be the reflection of the high rate of premature delivery and Caesarean section among this group of infants. The severity of the disease in the mother may be related to the disorder (Brazy et al. 1978; Cohen et al. 1960; Farrell and Avery 1975; Fedrick and Butler 1970; Leviton et al. 1977; O'Neill et al. 1978; Robert et al. 1976; Usher et al. 1971).

Histopathology. Hyaline membranes do not occur in stillborn infants. An infant must breathe for a short period before the clinical manifestations of the syndrome begin, or hyaline membranes develop. On gross inspection, the lungs are airless, reddish grey in colour, and rubbery in consistency, but there is no change in weight and size.

Infants who succumb within the first 2 h after birth present diffuse bilateral atelectasis. The terminal air spaces are occasionally recognizable, and may contain oedema fluid. The interstitial tissues are also oedematous, and the capillaries are congested while the lymphatics appear dilated. There is destruction and desquamation of epithelial cells of the terminal air spaces and some necrosis of the bronchiolar epithelium. The denuded basement membrane is swollen and covered by small patches of hyaline membranes in places. McAdams et al. (1973) have noted membranes after 8 min of breathing, while Gandy et al. (1970) observed them at 30 min; however, they are not conspicuous in

histological sections at this stage. Interstitial haemorrhages may also be seen.

After about 12 h the lesions are more extensive; dilated distal bronchioles and terminal airways are more conspicuous and alternate in an irregular fashion with atelectatic zones. The membranes are now quite conspicuous, extensive, and confluent, and may be observed in atelectatic areas. They appear as homogeneous eosinophilic bands on the denuded, thickened basal membrane, or epithelial cells of the distal bronchioles and terminal air spaces are seen below, containing epithelial cellular debris and pyknotic nuclei (Fig. 8.35).

Interstitial and intraluminal haemorrhages are common findings. Arterioles appear contracted while the veins are congested. Lymphatics are usually dilated. In infants dying after 12 h the lesions are even more widespread, and the hyaline membranes are extensive, thicker, and well defined.

Beyond 36 h of life the first signs of repair appear. Epithelial cells begin to regenerate at the margins of denuded areas and beneath the hyaline membranes; by the 3rd day these changes are well defined. The membranes become fragmented and resorption takes place (phagocytosis by macrophages). There is active interstitial fibroblast proliferation, and this, with epithelial cell growth, seems to incorporate the membranes into the alveolar wall, leading to fibrosis of varying degree. Meanwhile the oedema has diminished considerably (Finlay-Jones et al. 1973; Gandy et al. 1970; Lauweryns 1969, 1970; Lauweryns et al. 1971; Nilsson et al. 1978).

The chemical composition of hyaline membranes has been extensively documented. They are weakly PAS-positive and rich in fibrin deposits, being most readily identified by fluorescent or electron microscopy. Conventional stains for fibrin (Mallory phosphotungstic acid haematoxylin) are often disappointing. Hyaline membranes have also been shown to contain high quantities of tyrosine, α_1-antitrypsin, and C_3 fractions of complement (Benatre et al. 1978; Berezin 1969; Demarquez et al. 1976; Gitlin and Craig 1956; Lauweryns 1970; Singer et al. 1976).

The pathogenesis of hyaline membrane disease is probably variable. Hyaline membranes have been described in association with or complicated by the aspiration of amniotic fluid, premature rupture of the membranes, neonatal asphyxia with acute anoxia and acidosis, hypothermia, intrauterine infection, congenital heart disease leading to rapid heart failure, pulmonary hypoperfusion, birth injury, erythroblastosis fetalis, and deficient lung fibrinolytic activity (plasminogen activator). Immunological factors and neuroendocrine disorders have also been incriminated (Ambrus et al. 1974; Berkowitz et al. 1978; Farrell and Avery 1975; Fedrick and Butler 1970a; Kenny et al. 1976; Lieberman 1969).

However, the most important single contributory factor in the pathogenesis of the respiratory distress syndrome is the absence of *surfactant* (*surface-active materials*). The role of surfactant in the normal lung

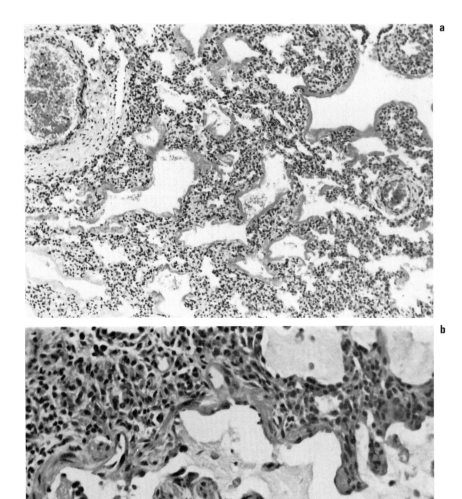

Fig. 8.35. a and **b** Lungs in respiratory distress syndrome. **a** Some alveolar saccules are lined with hyaline membranes, while others are collapsed. (H and E; 90×) **b** Organization of hyaline membranes invested by fibroblasts. (H and E; 120×)

is well established. The terminal air spaces in the normal newborn infant, like the alveoli in adults, are lined with a surface-active complex (surfactant) (Fig. 8.36), which maintains their stability by lowering surface tension at the air–liquid interface, thus preventing alveolar collapse during pulmonary expansion. It has been noted that the lungs of newborn infants dying with hyaline membrane disease are consistently lacking in surfactant, which is normally secreted by the granular pneumocytes. Between the 20th and 24th weeks of gestation, the granular pneumocytes (type II alveolar cells) make their appearance in the terminal air spaces of the developing lung. Soon afterwards, osmiophilic lamellar inclusion bodies appear within their cytoplasm, representing the first morphological expression of the secretory activity of these cells. About the same period, surface-active materials, mainly phospholipids, can be recovered from the pulmonary fluid of the fetus or from the amniotic fluid in small quantities. From then on, the number of granular pneumocytes increases rapidly, and by the 30th week they are producing large quantities of surfactant, which attain their maximum levels at about the 35th week of gestation (Fig. 8.37). The most active component of surfactant is dipalmitoyl phosphatidylcholine (saturated lecithin). This substance can already be detected in very small quantities between the 18th and 20th weeks of gestation, and increases in amount with advancing gestational age. As a result, the determination of this phospholipid in amniotic fluid is now widely used to evaluate fetal lung maturity and predict which infants are at risk. Its value is expressed as a ratio of lecithin to sphingomyelin (L/S) (Adams et al. 1970; Elrad et al. 1978; Gluck et al. 1971, 1972; Goerke 1974; Kapanci et al. 1972; Lemons and Jaffé 1973; Rosenthal et al. 1974).

The regulation of lung phospholipid biosynthesis depends on certain enzymes, principally phosphatidic acid phosphohydrolase, within the granular pneumocytes. This enzyme can also be detected in the lung and amniotic fluids; its level increases with gestational age. Its concentration in amniotic fluid

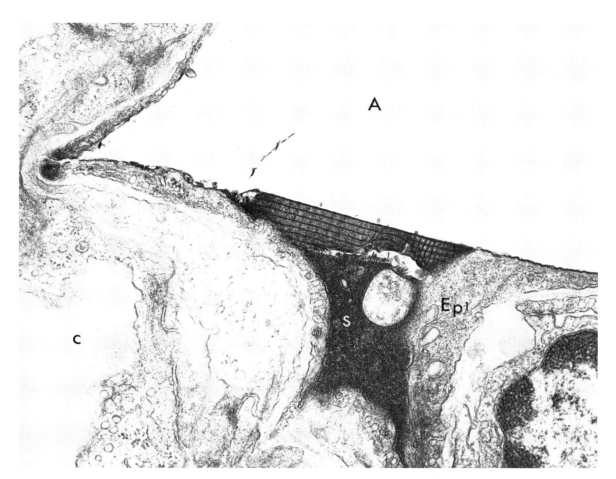

Fig. 8.36. Electron microphotograph of surfactant (*S*) lining the alveolar surface. *A*, alveolus; *C*, capillary; *EP₁*, epithelial cell type I. Courtesy of Dr Y. Kapanci. (41 000 ×)

can also be used as an indicator of lung maturity as it rises in parallel with the L/S ratio (Doran et al. 1979; Herbert et al. 1978; Jimenez et al. 1975; Jimenez and Johnston 1976; Mavis et al. 1978).

Besides the active phospholipid component (dipalmitoyl phosphatidylcholine), surfactant also contains variable amounts of proteins and carbohydrates. Smaller amounts of phosphatidylethanolamines, phosphatidylglycerol, and sphingomyelins are also present, and neutral lipids, mainly cholesterol, have been obtained in small quantities (Gluck et al. 1972; Goerke 1974; King 1974; Maguire et al. 1977).

In recent years it has been demonstrated that glucocorticoids may accelerate lung maturation in the fetus, activating the synthesis and secretion of pulmonary surfactant. It has also been shown that the antepartum administration of glucocorticoids to mothers of premature infants at risk significantly lowers the incidence of the respiratory distress syndrome. The glucocorticoids, mainly cortisol, seem to have a direct effect on metabolism within the type II pneumocytes. It is of interest that lung cells have been shown to have the highest levels of cortisol-specific receptors in the body (Ballard and Ballard 1974; Ekelund et al. 1976; Giannopoulos 1974; Liggins and Howie 1972; Spellacy et al. 1973). More recently, thyroid hormone has been shown to accelerate fetal lung maturity and to reduce the incidence of the respiratory distress syndrome (Mashiach et al. 1978). Bergman and Hedner (1978) have also demonstrated that the prepartum administration of terbutaline (a β_2-receptor stimulating drug) may also lower the incidence of hyaline membrane disease among premature infants.

It is generally accepted that pulmonary surfactant is deficient in infants presenting with hyaline membrane disease; however, it is not certain what factor(s) may be responsible for its absence from the lungs. Absence may be the result of inadequate production and secretion or of delayed synthesis in the immature lung.

Various lesions are found in association with hyaline membrane disease. *Pulmonary infection* is common in infants dying with this condition. The pulmonary infiltration may be mild or may involve

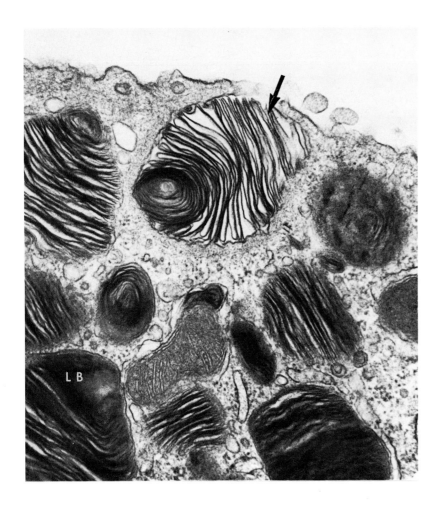

Fig. 8.37. Electron microphotograph of granular pneumocyte (type II cell), showing numerous lamellated bodies (LB), one of which (*arrow*) is undergoing exocytosis. Courtesy of Dr Y. Kapanci. (68 000 ×)

large areas of several lobes or the entire lung. Squamous debris may be observed in the terminal air spaces, suggesting the aspiration of amniotic fluid. *Pulmonary haemorrhage*, although less common, can also be associated with hyaline membrane disease. The haemorrhage can be focal, but occasionally presents as massive lesions. Pulmonary infection and haemorrhage can co-exist with hyaline membranes (Fedrick and Butler 1970a).

Intraventricular haemorrhage is commonly associated with hyaline membrane disease. It is observed mainly among premature infants, especially among those weighing less than 1500 g. When associated with hyaline membrane disease, intraventricular haemorrhage is often the cause of death among infants dying early in the course of the illness, usually within the first 24 h of life (Anderson et al. 1976; Fedrick and Butler 1970b; Leviton et al. 1977; Machin 1975; Wigglesworth et al. 1976). *Tentorial tears* occur with elevated frequency in infants with hyaline membrane disease, mostly among infants of advanced gestational age, at or near term. Many of these cases have presented obstetric difficulties at the time of delivery (Barson 1978).

Complications associated with therapy. The administration of oxygen in the treatment of hyaline membrane disease has resulted in a significant decrease in mortality and improved survival rates. This mode of therapy is not without its hazards, and various complications have been described in association with it. A diffuse type of pulmonary fibrosis, generally referred to as *pulmonary fibroplasia* or *bronchopulmonary dysplasia*, is perhaps the most significant lesion in those receiving oxygen and artificial ventilation for long periods. A high oxygen concentration, the precise method of ventilation, and the duration of treatment appear to be the main determinants in the production of the pulmonary lesions (Berg et al. 1975; Gupta et al. 1974; Philip 1975; Roloff et al. 1973; Schneegans et al. 1975; Stahlman et al. 1973; Truog et al. 1978). The changes are variable and affect all components of lung tissue. Macroscopically the lungs are dark red in colour, and larger and heavier than normal. The cut surface shows enphysematous zones alternating with collapsed areas, manifest histologically as distended terminal air spaces alternating with atelectatic zones. In the early stages there is interstitial oedema, with necrosis of the epithelial cells lining the distal bronchi, bronchioles, and terminal air spaces. The arteriolar walls are oedematous with capillary damage and intraluminal or interstitial haemorrhages. At later stages the interstitial oedema has regressed, but it leaves marked thickening following fibroblastic proliferation (Fig. 8.38). The bronchiolar epithelium shows re-

generative changes with some degree of hyperplasia and squamous metaplasia. Severe cases show an obliterative bronchitis and bronchiolitis. The bronchiolar muscular layer becomes thickened, and there is peribronchiolar fibrosis. Hyperplasia and hypertrophy of the media of the pulmonary arterioles are not uncommon findings, while the lymphatics may be somewhat distended and surrounded by fibrous tissue. Foci of chronic inflammatory cells may be observed within the interstitium and/or around the thickened bronchioles and vessels (Anderson et al. 1973; Banerjee et al. 1972; Bonikos et al. 1976a; Edwards et al. 1977; Rosan 1975; Taghizadeh and Reynolds 1976.

It has been accepted that oxygen toxicity is mainly responsible for these anatomical changes; however, some authors (Stocks et al. 1978; Taghizadeh and Reynolds 1976) have suggested that a mode of ventilation resulting in mechanical trauma to the airways may be a more important factor in the pathogenesis of the lesions. Recently Ehrenkranz et al. (1978) have shown that the administration of vitamin E during the early phase of therapy decreases the oxygen injury to the lung and modifies the development of bronchopulmonary dysplasia.

Other complications due to artificial ventilation include pneumothorax, interstitial pulmonary emphysema, pneumatosis pulmonalis and pneumomediastinum with pneumopericardium (Aranda et al. 1972; Brewer et al. 1979; Campbell and Hoffman 1974; Fletcher et al. 1970). Gas embolism has also been described (Gregory and Tooley 1970).

In recent years, a variant of hyaline membrane disease, *yellow pulmonary hyaline membrane disease*, has been observed in hyperbilirubinaemic premature infants with the respiratory distress syndrome treated with positive pressure-assisted ventilation and relatively high levels of oxygen. In all cases, treatment had been administered for long periods and bilirubinaemia was never very high.

On gross inspection the lungs are lemon or bright yellow in colour. Histologically they show areas of atelectasis, and other zones with dilated terminal air spaces and bronchioles, often lined with yellow hyaline membranes. In some instances the membranes line the denuded surfaces, while in others they cover eosinophilic membranes or are mixed with the latter. Yellow hyaline membranes stain positively for bile and never occur without eosinophilic membranes. Other histological changes in the lung are consistent with bronchopulmonary dysplasia. The liver has shown severe cholestasis in almost all cases.

It has been suggested that these yellow membranes are produced as a result of increased permeability of the air–blood barrier in the lung to a serum protein–bilirubin complex, and that the prolonged survival

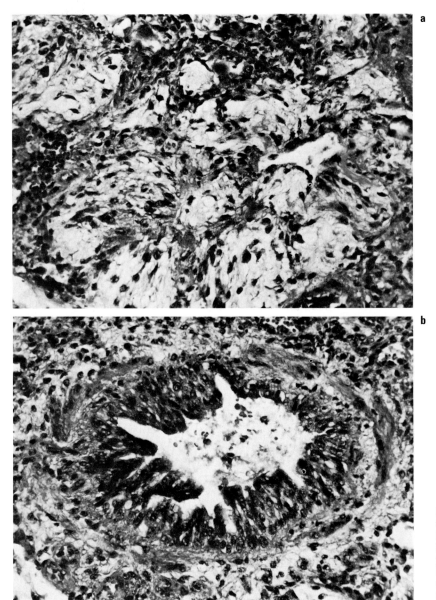

Fig. 8.38. a and b Bronchopulmonary dysplasia in a premature infant as a complication of prolonged oxygen therapy for the respiratory distress syndrome. (H and E; 225×) a Alveolar saccules are obliterated by a proliferating fibroblastic tissue. b Metaplasia of the bronchial epithelium.

time in these infants is a contributory factor in their development (Blanc 1976; Cho and Sastre 1976; Valdes-Dapena et al. 1976b).

Wilson–Mikity Syndrome. Wilson and Mikity (1960) described a pulmonary dysmaturity syndrome in small premature infants with respiratory distress at birth or during the course of the 1st week of life. The infants usually have a prolonged illness lasting several weeks, the clinical, radiological, and pathophysiologic features of which have been well documented. However, the pathological lesions are nonspecific and are often confused with those of bronchopulmonary dysplasia (Coates et al. 1978; Cooperman 1969; Dette and Gathmann 1974;

Hodgmann et al. 1969; Krauss et al. 1970; Wang et al. 1971). A few cases have also been recorded in full-term infants (Keidel and Feingold 1971).

Gross examination of the lung reveals areas of hyperinflation alternating with atelectatic areas. Histologically, there are areas of distended terminal air spaces, which alternate with collapsed areas showing septal thickening (Cooperman 1969; Hodgmann et al. 1969). These changes are not pathognomonic. The interstitial fibrosis, the bronchiolar changes, and the vascular modifications characteristic of bronchopulmonary dysplasia are absent, but the effects of therapy for respiratory distress could account for most of the changes seen.

4.7. Common Infections

4.7.1. Bacterial. The antibiotic era has dramatically modified the morphological appearances of inflammation of the pulmonary parenchyma. This is especially true in the industrialized nations, where both mortality and morbidity have been significantly reduced. In many developing nations, however, these modifications are less spectacular and classic pathological lesions can still be encountered among infants and children and the aged, principally because of inadequate medical services and poor handling of antibiotics. Inflammation of the lung in infants and children is by far the most common pathological lesion observed at post mortem, and may be the primary cause of death or a terminal episode accompanying other pathological conditions.

In lobar *pneumonia*, a lobe, an entire lung, or both lungs may be involved at any one time. The lesions usually begin in the terminal air spaces or alveoli, and spread to adjacent tissue. The involved lobes show lesions at the same stage of evolution. In the case of *bronchopneumonia*, the primary inflammatory reaction begins in the distal respiratory tract, extending into the surrounding parenchyma; lesions are generally at various stages of evolution. It is not necessary to describe the typical pathological features of pneumonia with its characteristic four stages, but certain specific features should be considered.

Streptococcal infections are an important cause of pulmonary infections among infants and children. *Streptococcus pneumoniae* is the principal cause of lobar pneumonia in this age group, especially after the first year of life, when over 90% of cases of pneumonia are related to this organism. Bacteria can be demonstrated in the lung in large numbers in the early stages of the disease. Pneumococcal pneumonia may be found to be associated with viral or other infectious agents when infants are carefully investigated. Lung abscesses and empyaema are significant complications (Asmar et al. 1978a; Klein 1969a; Rhodes et al. 1975; Siegel et al. 1978).

Other types of streptococcal infections (*β*-haemolytic) can occasionally cause lobar pneumonia, but are more often the cause of bronchopneumonia. The involved drug is oedematous but the inflammatory response is moderate, with only scattered aggregates of polymorphonuclear leucocytes. Interstitial haemorrhages are common, and typical and atypical hyaline membranes may form. Gram-positive cocci are identifiable (Ablow et al. 1976; Cayeux 1972; Franciosi et al. 1973; Slack and Mayon-White 1978).

Staphylococcal infections usually produce bronchopneumonia. The great majority of cases occur within the first year of life, and may occur in small epidemics, especially among children in hospital. Staphylococcal infection is commonly associated with cystic fibrosis.

The affected lung is consolidated and shows focal haemorrhagic areas. The pleura may be covered by a fibrinous exudate, and empyaema is not rare. The alveoli are usually filled with erythrocytes, oedema fluid, and a few polymorphonuclear leucocytes. Sometimes macrophages are abundant, containing numerous micro-organisms. Necrosis, often leading to abscess formation, is common. Interstitial emphysema and pneumatoceles are frequent complications of staphylococcal infections, and may cause pneumothorax (Boisset 1972; Gooch and Britt 1978; Klein 1969; Oliver et al. 1959).

Haemophilus influenzae (Pfeiffer's bacillus) infection of the lung is increasing in frequency in the paediatric age group. It may be a cause of the respiratory distress syndrome in the neonate (Speer et al. 1978). The bacillus is a common inhabitant of the nasopharynx, and often causes acute laryngo–tracheo–bronchitis and bronchopneumonia. All lobes of the lungs can be involved, but the lower lobes are most often affected. Well-defined nodules around bronchi and bronchioles filled with pus are seen, with destruction of the bronchiolar epithelium and a mucopurulent exudate in the lumen. The bronchial and bronchiolar walls are infiltrated by mononuclear cells, chiefly lymphocytes, and some polymorphonuclear leucocytes. The inflammatory reaction extends into the surrounding alveoli, where oedema and interstitial haemorrhage may be found. Thrombosis of small vessels occurs in the acute phase of infection, while long-standing infections may produce obstruction of the bronchioles (Asmar et al. 1978b; Bale and Watkins 1978; Lilien et al. 1978; Nicholls et al. 1975).

Escherichia coli is an important cause of gastro-intestinal infections and septicaemia in the newborn period, and such infections are usually accompanied by neonatal (intrauterine) pneumonia. *E. coli* pneumonia is common after the 4th week of life. It can occasionally cause a pneumatocele (Klein 1969, Kuhn and Lee 1973).

Klebsiella pneumoniae (Friedländer's bacillus) occasionally causes bronchopneumonia in infants and children. It is often associated with other bacterial or viral infections and is important in children with immunodeficiency states or in those receiving cytotoxic drugs for the treatment of malignancy. The lung in these cases shows many consolidated nodules of variable sizes disseminated in one or more lobes of both lungs. In the acute phase there is marked oedema extending into the inter-lobar spaces, alveolar destruction, and a polymorphonuclear leucocyte infiltration. Klebsiella bacilli are numerous in gram-stained sections. These lesions often lead on to abcess formation, and pneumatoceles may be encountered (Barter and Hudson 1974; Papageorgiou et al. 1973).

Pseudomonas aeruginosa (*Bacillus pyocyaneus*) affects premature infants and may be the cause of epidemics in nurseries. It is often found in children treated with broad-spectrum antibiotics, steroids, or cytotoxic drugs. The lungs show firm, irregular nodules, greenish-yellow in colour, scattered throughout the parenchyma, which is oedematous. The pleural cavities may contain a haemorrhagic pleural effusion. Histologically, the nodules often show a central necrotic zone and a polymorphonuclear leucocytic infiltrate surrounded by haemorrhagic areas. The distal arteries contain fibrinous thrombi, and organisms are frequently observed in the vessel walls.

Listeria monocytogenes is a gram-positive, motile bacillus, which has been associated with epidemics of abortion and encephalitis in animals. It was only during World War II that this pathogen was recognized in man, and since then numerous cases of listeriosis have been recorded. The exact distribution of the disease is not known, and its prevalence seems to be much higher in continental Europe than in Great Britain, the United States, and Canada. Human infection is supposedly contracted by contact with infected animals, although proof of this means of transmission has not often been established.

The disease can affect both infants and adults, and presents in various clinical forms. In paediatrics, it is most common in the perinatal period, presenting either in a generalized form (*granulomatosis infantiseptica*) or as meningitis. Infection usually occurs during the second half of pregnancy and may be the cause of premature delivery, stillbirth or repeated abortions. Intrauterine infection can be acquired transplacentally, resulting in widespread lesions of various organs, or via the membranes, when the lung and gastrointestinal tract are mainly involved, probably as a result of aspiration and ingestion of infected amniotic fluid. Infection may also be acquired during delivery as the infant passes through the birth canal. Such infants usually present with meningitis in the first 10 days of life (Ahlfors et al. 1977; Albritton et al. 1976; Giraud and Denis 1973; Giraud et al. 1973; Humbert et al. 1977a, b; Jacobs et al. 1978; Moore and Zehmer 1973; Rappaport et al. 1960; Robertson 1977; Voigt et al. 1971).

In cases of listerial infection the lung may be normal in appearance, or it may be heavy and firm, with numerous minute whitish nodules on both the pleural and the cut surfaces. Haemorrhagic areas may also be observed. Similar lesions may be seen on the skin, where they present as a purpuric rash, and in other organs and the placenta.

Microscopically, the nodules are focal areas of necrosis or small granulomas, occasionally surrounded by congested vessels or haemorrhagic zones. The bronchi may be ulcerated or involved in the granulomatous process (Fig. 8.39). The necrotic tissue contains cellular debris and pyknotic nuclei and some mononuclear leucocytes. Gram staining reveals numerous gram-positive bacilli; some of the rods may appear gram-negative, and some take the shape of a comma. The vessel wall may be involved in the necrotic process, resulting in focal haemorrhages.

Pneumonia caused by *Legionnaires' disease* bacterium, *Legionella pneumophila*, has recently been recognized, and it is seen at all ages. It is known to occur in epidemics or sporadically. The aetiological agent is a gram-negative bacterium, which has special staining qualities in tissues and requires special media for its culture. The lungs show areas of consolidation and resemble lungs affected by confluent bronchopneumonia or lobar pneumonia, often with a fibrinous pleuritis. Pleural effusion is common. The alveoli contain an exudate that is rich in polynuclear leucocytes, macrophages, and fibrin. Extensive lysis of the exudate, in areas, is a common feature. The oedematous and congested alveolar septa show areas of necrosis and an inflammatory reaction. Hyaline membranes may be associated with the lesions. Bronchial necrosis is common in affected areas. Legionnaires' disease bacterium can be demonstrated in the cells of the inflammatory exudate and cytoplasmic debris by the Dieterle silver stain. The majority of fatal cases have so far been diagnosed in adults, and patients receiving corticotherapy or cytotoxic drugs are particularly susceptible to the disease (Blackmon et al. 1978; Blackmon et al. 1979; Sanford 1979; Vella 1978; Winn et al. 1978).

Chlamydial pneumonia, another recently described condition, chiefly affects infants less than 6 months of age, with a peak incidence between the 2nd and 3rd months of life. It can cause severe respiratory distress and apnoea in children. The disease is caused by *Chlamydia trachomatis*, and is often associated with viral infections (cytomegalovirus, respiratory syncytial virus, adenovirus). The organism may be found in respiratory tract secretions or shed epithelial cells from the nasopharynx. Biopsy material has shown interstitial and alveolar infiltrations of monocytes and neutrophils (Frommell et al. 1977; Harrison et al. 1979; Tipple et al. 1979).

4.7.2. Viral. Viral infections of the respiratory system are very common among infants and children. The viruses involved are varied, and new strains are isolated and identified each year. They usually

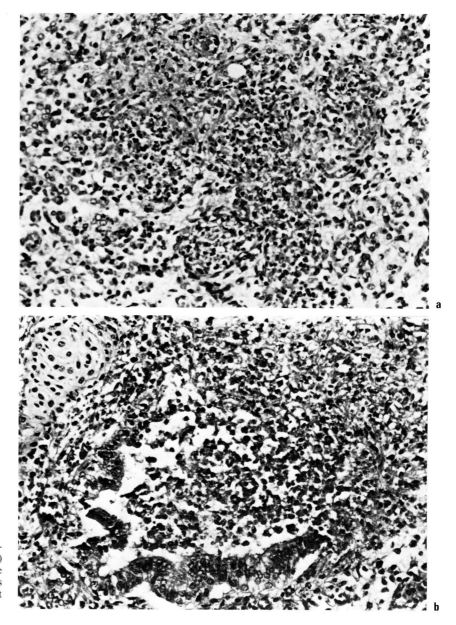

Fig. 8.39. a and **b** Listeriosis in a 3-day-old baby girl. (H and E; 120 ×) **a** Confluent microabscesses in the pulmonary parenchyma. **b** Necrosis of the bronchial wall and adjacent tissue.

affect the entire respiratory system and can cause severe damage to the lung parenchyma. The lesions produced by many viruses are histologically similar, and as a result one cannot rely solely on histological changes to establish a diagnosis with certainty. Furthermore, viral infections of the lung are not infrequently associated with one or more bacterial infections.

In all cases where a viral infection is suspected, tissue should be taken for culture and for immunological and ultrastructural studies if adequate facilities exist. Serum should also be preserved for appropriate examination. It is only by the isolation or identification of the virus that a definitive diagnosis can be established.

Cytomegalovirus (DNA virus) is a member of the Herpes virus group. It has a worldwide distribution and appears to be more prevalent among the lower socioeconomic group. Infection by the virus in childhood may be acquired (a) in utero (congenital), (b) perinatally, or (c) postnatally.

(a) *Congenital infection*. Intrauterine cytomegalovirus infection may occur in as many as 1%–2% of all newborns. Severe intrauterine infection, especially in the early part of the first half of pregnancy, may be the cause of death of the fetus in utero owing to disseminated disease. However, only a small proportion of infected infants present with the major clinical manifestations of the disease at birth. Most affected infants, especially those that acquire the disease during the second half of pregnancy, are asymptomatic, but they may have viraemia and/or excrete the virus in their saliva for some months or even years after birth. Many of these infants will go on to present with various neurological symptoms as a result of brain damage of varying degrees. The disease has also been reported in siblings from consecutive pregnancies.

(b) *Perinatal infection* is believed to be acquired during delivery, probably from the cervix, as the infant passes through the birth canal. Infants infected in this way are usually asymptomatic; however, virus can be recovered from the urine and saliva for long periods after birth.

(c) *Postnatal infection* is considered to be quite common, and is generally asymptomatic. The mode of transmission is varied. Among the most frequently incriminated is blood transfusion, in which case the patient may present with a syndrome referred to as *cytomegalovirus mononucleosis*. This has clinical and haematological features resembling those of infectious mononucleosis, but there is a negative Paul–Bunnell reaction. Infection by the virus is also prevalent among infants receiving chemotherapy for malignant diseases in immunodeficiency states, in those with monoclonal macroglobulinaemia, and in those with renal allografts treated with immunosuppressive agents. Many of these patients present with interstitial pneumonitis.

Cytomegalovirus infection of the lung has also been observed with other pulmonary conditions, such as hyaline membrane disease, congenital syphilis, bacterial or viral pneumonias, and pneumocystis carinii (Ahlfors et al. 1978; Benirschke et al. 1974; Boué and Cabau 1978; Cox and Hughes 1975; Davis et al. 1971; Fiala et al. 1975; Granström et al. 1977; Kibrick and Loria 1974; Reynolds et al. 1978; Rola-Pleszezynski et al. 1977; Schopfer et al. 1978; Smith et al. 1977; Umetsu et al. 1975; Weinberg et al. 1973; Yeager et al. 1977).

On gross examination the lungs may show little change unless affected by some other condition. Histologically the diagnosis may go unnoticed if one is not attentive. The presence of the characteristic viral inclusion with its clear halo (owl's eye) in some other organ (kidney, liver, pancreas, salivary gland, etc.) may draw the pathologist's attention to possible pulmonary involvement. Careful examination will reveal an occasional grossly hyperplastic alveolar cell with its intranuclear inclusion. In severe disseminated pulmonary disease the virus is observed in the nuclei or cytoplasm of the enlarged alveolar lining cells and is sometimes seen free in the alveoli (Fig. 8.40). In the early stages, the intranuclear inclusions are acidophilic, but they become basophilic with time. The acidophilic intranuclear inclusion body stains purple with Masson's trichrome, while the intracytoplasmic inclusions stain intensely with the PAS stain or Giemsa. The cytoplasm of the infected cell is basophilic and granular. There is no inflammatory reaction unless secondary infection occurs. Bronchial and bronchiolar epithelial cells may be infected in addition to the epithelial cells of the peribronchial glands. Viral inclusions are occasionally observed in endothelial cells of blood vessels.

Measles (rubeola) pneumonia. Measles is due to an RNA virus of the myxovirus group. The disease is still quite common in developing countries and countries without immunization programmes, and it occurs in epidemics. In developing countries, pulmonary complications are common and mortality is high, especially among children suffering from various types of malnutrition. Secondary bacterial infection is common and is responsible for the high mortality in many series. Fatal cases have been described in apparently healthy children and in adults or patients with immunological disorders, including those receiving cytotoxic or immunosuppressive treatments for malignancies. The majority of these cases do not present the exanthema characteristic of the disease, and have not necessarily had previous contact with patients suffering form the disease.

Atypical measles pulmonary lesions are known to occur and persist in individuals receiving killed measles vaccine, and fatal cases of measles pneumonia have been recorded after the administration of live measles vaccine to infants with immunodeficiency disorders (Mihatsch et al. 1972).

The main feature of the pulmonary lesion is the multinucleated syncytial giant cell, which should be distinguished from the pathognomonic giant (Warthin–Finkeldey) cell observed in the lymphoid tissues during the prodromal stage of the disease or in the very early phase of the rash in these patients. Hecht's giant-cell pneumonia was formerly considered to be a separate entity; however, recent studies have shown that the virus responsible for this condition is identical with that observed in cases of measles pneumonia, and therefore it is now generally admitted that the two conditions are in fact the same (Archibald et al. 1971; Barkin 1975; Becroft and Osborne 1980; Dover et al. 1975; Guillozet 1979; Haram and Jacobsen 1973; Joliet et al. 1973; Laptook et al. 1978; Lewis et al. 1978; Lightwood et al. 1970; Olson and Hodges 1975; Sobonya et al. 1978).

Macroscopically the lungs are heavier than normal. They show homogeneous, firm, greyish-white consolidated areas, variable in size, sometimes occupying an entire lobe or lung. The lesions are generally bilateral.

Microscopically there is interstitial pneumonia with oedema of the interstitium and alveolar wall.

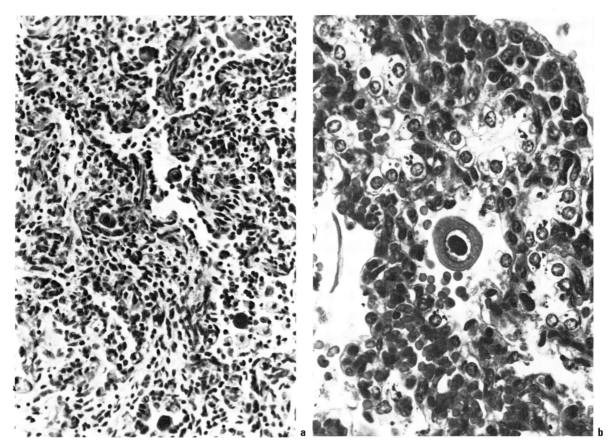

Fig. 8.40. a Cytomegalovirus inclusion disease in a 2-day-old premature infant (H and E; 90 ×); **b** Characteristic owl's eye appearance. Absence of inflammatory reaction. (H and E; 300 ×)

The inflammatory infiltrate consists mainly of mononuclear cells. The numerous multinucleated syncytial giant cells have a crescentic shape and are found lining the alveolar wall, the alveolar ducts, and the distal bronchioles. These giant cells may contain 10–50, or even 100 nuclei. Intranuclear and intracytoplasmic eosinophilic bodies are conspicuous, and stain with the Phloxine–tartrazine stain. The alveolar spaces are rich in oedema fluid mixed with fibrin. Hyaline membranes may be present (Fig. 8.41). The bronchial and bronchiolar epithelia show degenerative changes in places, and in other areas there is marked epithelial hyperplasia with loss of ciliated epithelium. Squamous metaplasia may be prominent. There is a peribronchial mononuclear infiltration with hyperplasia of the lymphoid tissue. It is not unusual to observe endothelial hyperplasia of the small vessels with some degree of stenosis.

Influenza pneumonia. Influenza can occur sporadically, but often occurs in epidemics. During these outbreaks fatal cases may occur in children, in particular in the immunosuppressed. Several types of virus are known to be responsible for infection of the respiratory system, and new strains and subgroups are isolated each year. The virus provokes an interstitial pneumonitis, which can progress to an haemorrhagic pneumonia and death. Pneumonia due to superimposed bacterial infection is the main cause of death (Aherne et al. 1970; Foy et al. 1979; Hers and Mulder 1961; Joshi et al. 1973; Lindsay et al. 1970; Laraya-Cuasay et al. 1974; Sabin 1977; Zinserling 1972).

Macroscopic examination of the lungs may reveal nothing in the early phase of the disease, while in the full-blown disease they are heavy, reddish, and markedly haemorrhagic, with abundant oedema. The bronchi and bronchioles are quite congested, and the epithelium of the main bronchi may be ulcerated. Their lumen may be filled with a thick, yellow, blood-stained exudate. Histologically congestion of the capillaries is a prominent feature. The capillaries are extremely dilated; the septa are oedematous and thickened and contain mononuclear inflammatory cells. There are areas of focal necrosis with interstitial haemorrhage. Hyperplasia of the alveolar lining cells is conspicuous, and there is some desquamation into the alveolar spaces, where

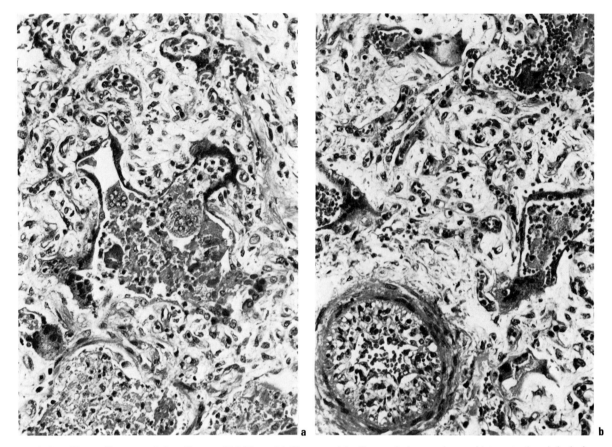

Fig. 8.41. a Giant-cell pneumonia in a 12-year-old African girl. The syncytial cells contain intranuclear and intracytoplasmic inclusion bodies consistent with those of measles. **b** Arteritis and endothelial proliferation associated with giant-cell pneumonia. (H and E; 225 ×)

fibrin, erythrocytes, macrophages, and mononuclear cells may be seen. Hyaline membranes are also present. In some areas the alveolar epithelium regenerates. The bronchi and bronchioles show marked congestion, with areas of mucosal necrosis, oedema of their wall, and a diffuse mononuclear infiltrate. Squamous metaplasia of the bronchial epithelium is an indication of regeneration; simultaneously there is epithelial hyperplasia of the bronchioles and alveolar ducts. Healing of the lesions may lead to alveolar fibrosis. Delage et al. (1979) described a giant cell pneumonia due to parainfluenza type 3 virus in infants with immunodeficiency diseases, which histologically resembled measles pneumonia.

Rhinoviruses are often the cause of an influenza-like infection of the upper respiratory tract in infants and children. Neonates and premature babies are particularly subject to infection. The disease often runs a benign course, but fatal cases can occur. The viruses may cause an interstitial pneumonia or bronchopneumonia affecting one or more lobes or an entire lung, and the involvement is often bilateral

(Fig. 8.42). Rhinoviruses have been associated with the sudden infant death syndrome.

Adenovirus infection of the respiratory system is relatively common among infants and children and in young adults; however, the disease is hardly ever fatal, although it may cause severe chronic lung damage, including pulmonary fibrosis, bronchiectasis, and bronchiolitis obliterans of the small bronchi and bronchioles. The disease appears to be more common in developing countries, and especially among children suffering from severe malnutrition or other debilitating conditions. It has also been described in association with measles. Numerous strains of adenovirus have been isolated and identified, and although several types are known to cause respiratory disease in man, only a few have been recorded as being responsible for fatal diseases in children (Herbert et al. 1977; Loker et al. 1974; Schonland et al. 1976; Scott et al. 1978; Wright et al. 1964; Zahradnik et al. 1980; Zinserling 1972).

Macroscopically the lungs are heavy and firm, with bilateral grey consolidated zones mainly occupying the posterior lower lobes. The parenchyma is markedly oedematous, and the trachea and large bronchi are hyperaemic and ulcerated in places. Their lumen is often filled with thick mucoid material that is rich in fibrin. Histologically there is extensive denudation of the epithelium lining the bronchi and bronchioles, with occasional vesicles in the residual mucosa. In other areas, there is widespread eosinophilic necrosis of the mucosa, which may form a pseudomembranous layer in places. The inflammatory reaction in the wall may be mild or moderate, and it consists in lymphocytes, plasma cells, and some histiocytes. The alveolar ducts and alveoli are filled with eosinophilic material containing oedema fluid mixed with fibrin and dense hyaline membranes. Parenchymal necrosis may be focal or widespread, with little or no inflammatory reaction. The alveoli contain hyperplastic alveolar cells (histiocytes) whose nuclei occasionally show basophilic nuclear inclusion bodies, often surrounded by a hollow rim. The inclusion bodies (Giemsa- and Feulgen-positive) may also be observed within the nuclei of desquamated bronchial and bronchiolar epithelial cells and in the regenerating hyperplastic epithelium.

Respiratory syncytial virus is known to have a worldwide distribution and is one of the most important causes of acute respiratory disease among infants and children, especially the premature and those less than 6 months of age. Although it is not often fatal it can cause a diffuse interstitial-type

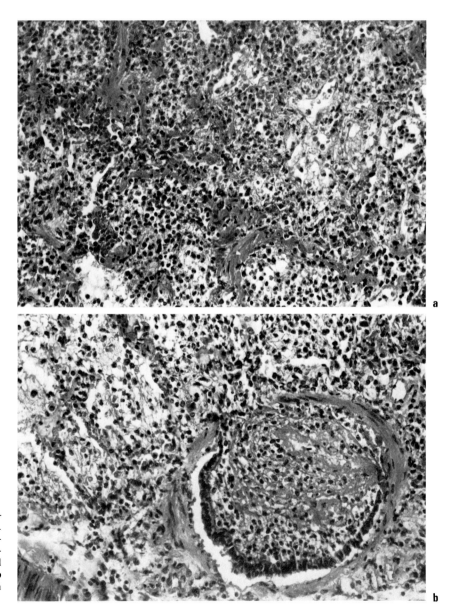

Fig. 8.42. a and **b** Rhinovirus pneumonia in a 4-year-old African girl. (H and E; 120 ×) **a** Extensive necrosis of the alveolar wall with distension of the alveolar spaces filled mainly with mononuclear cells; **b** Necrosis of bronchial wall with bronchiolitis obliterans.

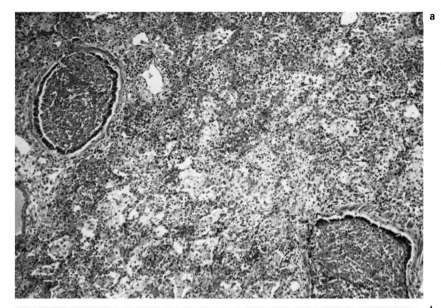

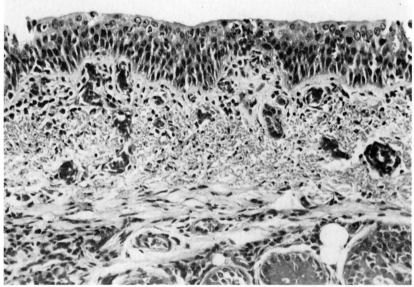

Fig. 8.43. a and b Respiratory syncytial virus pneumonia in a 22-
month-old boy with Reye's syndrome. Courtesy of Dr J.W. Keeling.
a Bronchitis and bronchiolitis obliterans with pneumonitis. (H and E;
35 ×) b Squamous-cell metaplasia
of the tracheal epithelium. (H and
E; 225 ×)

bronchopneumonia or pneumonia. Very often
infection with this virus is asymptomatic, and it has
been described in association with the sudden infant
death syndrome and Reye's syndrome (Bruhn and
Yeager 1977; Bruhn et al. 1977; Griffin et al. 1979;
Hall et al. 1979; Henderson et al. 1979; Kaul et al.
1978; Martin et al. 1978; Scott et al. 1978). Only a
few fatal cases have been documented in the
literature, and most of these have occurred in the
neonatal period (Aherne et al. 1970; Zinserling
1972).

Macroscopically the lungs show focal areas of
consolidation indistinguishable from those seen in
most other conditions. Histologically there is hyperplasia of the epithelium lining the medium-sized
bronchi and bronchioles, with desquamation in

places (Fig. 8.43). The wall is sometimes infiltrated
by mononuclear cells, with some polymorphonuclear leucocytes. There is also marked shedding of
the epithelial cells lining the alveoli, into a lumen
filled with dense oedematous fluid. Occasionally
inclusion bodies may be observed within cytoplasmic vacuoles in the alveolar and bronchiolar
epithelial cells. Areas of necrosis may be prominent,
and the septa are infiltrated with lymphocytes,
histiocytes, and plasma cells.

Varicella (chickenpox) pneumonia. Varicella is a
common childhood infection, which is seldom fatal.
It is estimated that the mortality rate among infants
and children is 1%, whereas it is probably between
10% and 50% among adults. Varicella pneumonia,

which may manifest itself a few days after the rash, is considered to be the most serious complication among adults and pregnant women, and it can be accompanied by secondary bacterial infection. In both children and adults the disease may run a fatal course in patients who are receiving steroids or cytotoxic drug therapy for malignancies.

Virus can be transmitted to the fetus in utero and can result in congenital varicella (fatalities occur owing to pneumonia). Newborns who develop the rash 5 days or more after birth have a higher mortality than those who develop the rash within the first 4 days (Glick et al. 1972; Jones and Cameron 1969; McKendry and Bailey 1973; Meyers 1974; Nisenbaum et al. 1969; Selleger 1978; Triebwasser et al. 1967).

Macroscopically the lungs are often oedematous, enlarged, and rose-coloured with firm dark-red areas. The bronchi contain abundant blood-stained mucus. Histologically the thickened oedematous alveolar septa show areas of necrosis in places, while in others the alveolar spaces are filled by a dense eosinophilic serous fluid mixed with fibrin and numerous desquamated hyperplastic alveolar epithelial cells with occasional multinucleated giant cells (Fig. 8.44). The bronchi, bronchioles, and blood vessels in the involved areas are often necrotic. Intranuclear acidophilic inclusion bodies can be seen in the hypertrophied alveolar cells and in the tracheal and bronchial epithelium. The inflammatory reaction is moderate and is comprised chiefly of mononuclear cells. Healing of the necrotic areas may leave calcified nodules within the pulmonary parenchyma.

Herpes simplex virus. There are two antigenically different types of herpes simplex virus known to affect man (type I and type 2). Herpes type 2 virus appears to be venereally transmitted, and as a result is responsible for most congenital herpes virus infection. Fetuses and neonates infected by the virus in utero may present with a fatal, disseminated form of the disease involving the brain, liver and adrenals, and sometimes the lungs. Children in developing countries may present with the generalized disease, and the majority of fatal cases have been recorded among children suffering from various forms of malnutrition. Bronchopneumonia is a common complication (Chalhub et al. 1977; Jones and Cameron 1969; Pettay et al. 1972; Templeton 1970).

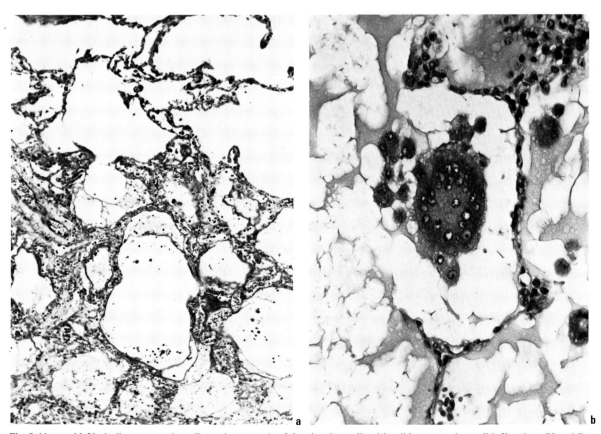

Fig. 8.44. a and **b** Varicella pneumonia: **a** Extensive necrosis of the alveolar walls with mild mononuclear cell infiltration. (H and E; 35 ×) **b** interstitial giant-cell pneumonitis with intranuclear inclusion bodies. (H and E; 225 ×)

Macroscopically the lungs can appear normal; however, in some cases the cut surface shows some miliary whitish nodules. Microscopically there are multiple round or oval foci of necrosis. Inflammatory cells may be absent or may occasionally be found at the periphery of the involved zone. The exudate is made up principally of mononuclear inflammatory cells. Bronchioles in the area may undergo necrosis, while in other areas of the lung the bronchial and bronchiolar epithelium are hyperplastic. Focal areas of squamous metaplasia can also be seen. Eosinophilic intranuclear bodies are sometimes seen in the hyperplastic epithelial cells or in the necrotic cells at the periphery of the lesions. In patients who survive, calcification of the necrotic area may occur.

Mycoplasma pneumoniae. Mycoplasmas are members of the class Mollicutes, family *Mycoplasmataccae*, sharing common properties with both bacteria and viruses. There are many strains. *Mycoplasma pneumoniae* infection is endemic; it occurs in epidemics and has a worldwide distribution. It affects mainly the respiratory system, especially in children and young adults, but can cause many nonrespiratory infections. Pulmonary infection can be mild or severe, causing bronchopneumonia or pneumonia (primary atypical pneumonia). Atelectasis, bullous emphysema, pulmonary abcesses, and pleuritis with pleural effusion are associated complications. Meningoencephalitis is a common complication of Mycoplasma infection, and myocarditis with pericarditis and pancreatitis have also been described. Fatal cases have been documented, many of them in patients with immunodeficiency states or sickle-cell anaemia. Transplacental infection has been reported (Halal et al. 1977; Harwick et al. 1970; Jansson 1978; Levine and Lerner 1978; Stevens et al. 1978; Zinserling 1972).

Macroscopically the lungs are markedly oedematous, reddish, and heavy. Focal zones of intrapulmonary haemorrhage can be seen, sometimes associated with areas of bronchopneumonia. The bronchi and bronchioles are congested, and the distal branches can be partially obliterated by a thick oedematous fluid rich in mucus and mucopus. Microscopically the lesions are often indistinguishable from those of viral pneumonias, hence the term 'atypical viral pneumonia'. The alveolar septa are markedly thickened by a dense oedematous fluid and are infiltrated by lymphocytes, plasma cells, and macrophages. The alveolar spaces contain numerous hyperplastic desquamated alveolar cells mixed with erythrocytes, macrophages, and fibrin. Lysis of the desquamated alveolar cells is prominent in places, and hyaline membranes are observed in some

areas. Single or grouped organisms may be recognized in the nuclei of the modified alveolar epithelial cells or those of the bronchial mucosa. Bronchiolitis is prominent and widespread. There is marked congestion of the vessels, some of which may contain fibrinous thrombi or show necrosis of their walls.

4.7.3. Fungal. Mycotic infections of the lung in childhood are uncommon, and the majority of such infections encountered are secondary or opportunist infections. However, a few cases of congenital infection have been described with some species of fungus. In most instances the particular mycotic infection is observed in association with children receiving antibiotic or steroid treatment or in those suffering from some form of chronic debilitating disease. In recent years there has been an increasing number of reports among children treated with immunosuppressive drugs or cytotoxic agents for malignancies. These infections are more common in tropical and subtropical zones, where certain species of fungus are prevalent. Special stains (gram, PAS, Grocott's silver methenamine) may be necessary to identify the organisms in sections, while culture and immunological studies are essential in determining the exact species involved.

Moniliasis (Candida). Several species of Candida can affect man but *Candida albicans* is usually responsible for pulmonary lesions in the paediatric age group. Both congenital and neonatal pulmonary moniliasis have been described. In childhood the lesions may be localized in the tracheo-bronchial tree, where the fungus may produce ulceration of the mucosa, or in the pulmonary parenchyma, with the formation of microabcesses. In severe cases, there is diffuse pulmonary and sometimes vascular involvement. Associated bacterial infection is common, and in these cases an inflammatory infiltrate is often pronounced. In the newborn period moniliasis may be associated with prolonged umbilical vein catheterization and it is seen in older children who have had other intravenous catheters in place for long periods (Dvorak and Gavaller 1966; Emanuel et al. 1962; Linhartova and Chung 1963; Schirar et al. 1974).

Pulmonary aspergillosis is also uncommon in children, and it has been observed mainly as an opportunistic infection. It can be a complication of tuberculosis, pneumatocele, and/or an infected bronchogenic cyst. Eosinophilia is a common feature of the condition.

As in the adult, the disease may present in several forms: (a) allergic bronchopneumonia, which is extremely rare; (b) aspergilloma, a relatively more common entity; and (c) disseminated or septicaemic pulmonary aspergillosis. The morphological features are identical with those observed in adult cases (Beauvais et al. 1975; Berger et al. 1972; Gonzalez-Crussi et al. 1979a; Slavin et al. 1970).

Pulmonary thrombi containing fungal hyphae, sometimes associated with infarction, are the most striking features (Fig. 8.45). There is sometimes necrosis of the vessel wall with secondary infection of the surrounding tissue in disseminated infection.

Two forms of *histoplasmosis* are thought to exist: (1) *Histoplasma capsulatum* (North American form); and (2) *Histoplasma Duboisii* (African form).

The North American form of *Histoplasma capsulatum* has a worldwide distribution and is known to be endemic in certain regions. The clinical and radiological features are nonspecific and can resemble those of a viral lung infection or, in some instances, tuberculosis. The disease is common in children and can cause death in endemic areas. It presents as (a) an acute influenza-like illness with a variable outcome (usually the infection is benign); (b) a chronic pulmonary infection with one or more pulmonary cavities, resembling tuberculosis, in which secondary calcification is frequently observed; or (c) disseminated histoplasmosis, with widespread dissemination by the bloodstream. This last form of the disease generally affects younger children, and is often rapidly fatal (Dumont and Piché 1969; Salfelder et al. 1970).

African histoplasmosis or *Histoplasma Duboisii* is more restricted to the tropical and subtropical belt of Africa. The organisms may occasionally produce pulmonary lesions, which are mainly granulomatous: in rare instances cavities develop (Williams et al. 1971).

Other mycoses (blastomycosis, mucormycosis, nocardiosis, etc.) may be responsible for pulmonary lesions in infants and children; however, they are unusual (Powell and Schuit 1979).

4.7.4. Parasitic. The lung is commonly affected by parasitic disease, and in many tropical countries parasites or their eggs can be observed in the lung parenchyma. The extent of pulmonary involvement is variable.

Pulmonary Pneumocystis carinii (interstitial plasma cell pneumonia). Pneumocystis carinii is a parasite of uncertain taxonomic position, presently considered to be a protozoon, a member of the *Sporozoae.* It has a worldwide distribution and

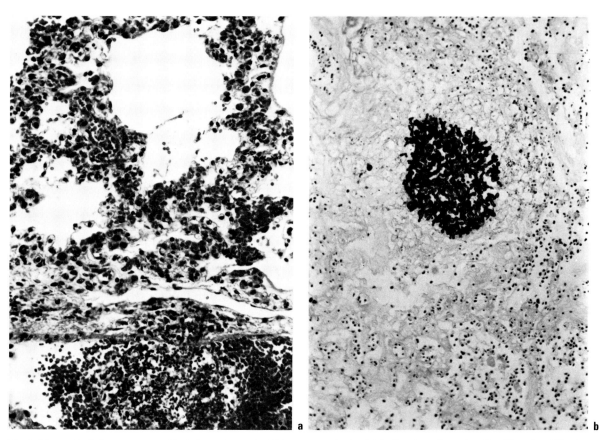

Fig. 8.45. a and **b** Pulmonary aspergillosis in an 8-month-old boy. Thrombosis with infiltration of vessel wall. **a** (H and E; 225 ×) **b** silver stain to illustrate fungi. (Grocott; 200 ×)

appears to be a saprophyte in the lungs of several domestic animals as well as in man. Its mode of transmission is still unknown; however, it is generally accepted that the organisms reach the lungs by inhalation. The disease is known to be endemic in some areas, and it is not uncommon among the inmates of institutions. Epidemics have been described, principally in Central Europe. The lung is the organ most often affected, but the organisms have been observed in the regional lymph nodes and, in severe disseminated cases, in the spleen, liver, and bone marrow.

The condition has been described among premature babies and debilitated infants, especially those with congenital immunological abnormalities, recurrent infections, or severe malnutrition. The disease has been severe and rapidly progressive, with a high mortality rate, in most cases reported. Penumocystis carinii has been reported in siblings, and transplacental transmission has been documented. Effective therapy has now greatly modified the course of the disease.

At present, Pneumocystis carinii is most commonly encountered as an opportunistic infection in immunodeficient subjects and after prolonged antibiotic therapy. It has also been described in association with congenital heart disease, severe aplastic anaemia, and Letterer–Siwe disease. The organisms have also been reported in association with various bacterial infections, cytomegalovirus infection, and infection by Candida albicans.

The clinical and radiological features are nonspecific. Serological and immunological studies may be helpful in establishing the diagnosis (Arnaud et al. 1976; Chusid and Heyrman 1978; Dutz 1970; Gentry and Remington 1970; Henderson et al. 1974; Hughes et al. 1973; Le Golvan and Heidelberger 1972; Le Tan Vinh et al. 1969b; Pifer et al. 1978; Price and Hughes 1974; Rahimi 1974; Wang et al. 1970; Weber et al. 1977).

Macroscopically the lungs are heavier than normal, and they may show focal greyish areas of consolidation. In severe cases the lesions may be diffuse, involving one or more lobes or the entire lung, but there are numerous variations between the two extremes.

Histologically there is some degree of hyperplasia of the alveolar lining cells, with desquamation into the alveolar space in the early stages or in mild infection. The parasites can be observed in the alveolar cells when stained with appropriate stains (PAS, Grocott, and specific immunofluorescent sera). The interstitial inflammatory reaction is usually mild and is composed chiefly of lymphocytes, plasma cells, and a few histiocytes. In the severe form, the alveoli are distended and filled with an exudate of foamy material mixed with de-

squamated cells and some macrophages. The organisms are seen in large numbers within the cells but occur mainly in the amorphous cellular debris (Fig. 8.46). The alveolar wall is thickened, cellular, and diffusely infiltrated by lymphocytes, many plasma cells and some histiocytes, which may contain parasites. Giant cells and noncaseating granulomas have been observed, and calcification has been recorded in these lesions. Survivors may show pulmonary fibrosis of varying degrees.

Toxoplasmosis of the lung. Toxoplasma gondii is a protozoon, a member of the *Sporozoa* group. The parasite has a worldwide distribution and infects many animal species and man. In man it has a wide spectrum of manifestations, varying from a subclinical or mild infection to a severe generalized disease. Although the mode of transmission is not fully understood, the organisms may be acquired in utero or during childhood, and various surveys have shown that over 90% of some populations, notably those living in hot humid climates, have antibodies to the parasite.

Infection of the mother during pregnancy may result in intrauterine death, stillbirth, or neonatal death in about 10% of cases. Should the parasite be acquired during the first 6 months of gestation transplacental transmission is infrequent, but the lesions are severe in the fetuses and infants who do acquire the disease. After the 6th month there is a much higher rate of transplacental transmission, and the infection is more often benign or asymptomatic in the offspring. A few reports have suggested that persistent maternal infection results in repeated abortion in successive pregnancies, but this has not been substantiated. Congenital toxoplasmosis may cause perinatal death, serious abnormalities of the central nervous system and the eyes (chorioretinitis), or latent disease. Over 60% of infants born to mothers who have the disease during pregnancy show no evidence of infection. Infants may acquire the disease during passage through the birth canal or in childhood. Toxoplasma infection is not uncommon among patients with malignant disease or other conditions requiring corticosteroid drugs and/or cytotoxic or immunosuppressive agents. In these patients the disease often runs a fatal course if not treated adequately (Alford et al. 1974; Bamatter 1971; Couvreur 1971; Feldman 1974; Frenkel 1974a, b; Jacobs 1974; Neu 1971; Roth et al. 1971).

Macroscopically the lungs can appear normal or show reddish, firm, sometimes confluent nodules. Areas of consolidation have been observed in the diffused neonatal form of the disease. Microscopically the alveolar spaces are filled with desquamated epithelial lining cells and macrophages. The alveolar wall is thickened, containing numerous

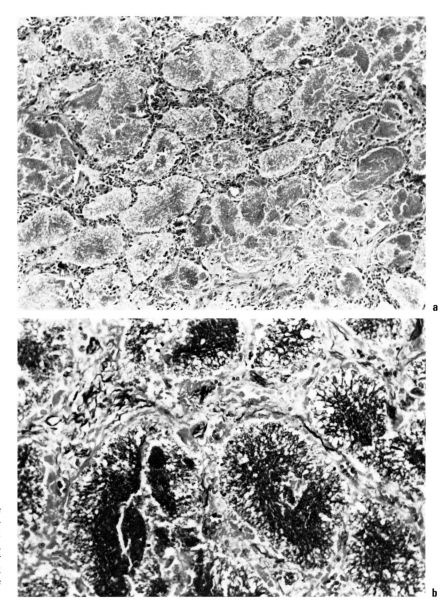

Fig. 8.46. a and **b** *Pneumocystis carinii* pneumonia in a case of treated leukaemia. Courtesy of Dr C. Bozic. **a** The alveoli are distended, and full of foam cells and cellular debris. (H and E; 35 ×) **b** Abundant *P. carinii* in intra-alveolar exudate (Grocott's stain; 225 ×)

macrophages with many plasma cells and lymphocytes, and few eosinophils and polymorphonuclear leucocytes. Toxoplasma pseudocysts may be seen free in the alveolar spaces, but occur principally in the cytoplasm of the desquamated alveolar cells and macrophages. Sometimes they can be seen in the cytoplasm of the swollen endothelial cell.

Amoebic Lung Abscesses. The protozoon *Entameoba histolytica* (class *Rhizopoda*, genus *Entamoeba*) is endemic in tropical and subtropical countries. It is also known to exist in certain temperate countries, and in recent times has been encountered more frequently than before, as a result of rapid air travel and the shifting of populations.

The parasite attacks principally the colon, but can spread to the liver by way of the portal system, and can eventually reach the lung and brain. The disease has been observed at all ages but there are no figures for its true incidence. Intestinal infection in children is not altogether uncommon, but secondary spread to the liver with formation of liver abscesses is rare, and pulmonary involvement even less common. The lung is infected from an amoebic liver abscess. The liver capsule overlying the abscess may adhere to the diaphragm, and eventually the abscess ruptures into the thoracic cavity, extending into the pulmonary parenchyma. A bronchopulmonary fistula has been observed in certain instances. There is little or no secondary inflammatory reaction (Abioye and Edington 1972; Jessee et al. 1975; Shabot and Patterson 1978; Strauss and Bove 1975; Woodruff 1975).

Several other parasites can be observed in the lungs during childhood. The lung may be involved in the life cycle of some of these parasites or it may be infected secondarily by the eggs, larvae, or adult parasites.

Hydatid cystic disease (*E. granulosus*) is one of the most important of these. This parasite has a worldwide distribution, and there is a high morbidity in areas where the disease is endemic. *E. multilocularis*, another species, is limited to certain parts of Europe, including Switzerland. The larval form of *E. granulosus* is responsible for the classic hydatid cyst, while *E. multilocularis* is associated with the alveolar (multilocular) hydatid cyst (Poole and Marcial-Rojas 1971).

Four types of *schistosomes* are known to affect man: *S. mansoni, S. haematobium, S. japonicum,* and *S. intercalatum*.

Eggs of *S. mansoni* and *S. haematobium*, and to a lesser extent of *S. japonicum*, have been described in the lungs of patients harbouring the parasites in endemic zones. In some cases the eggs lodge in the alveolar wall of the interstitial tissue with little or no reaction, while in others they may produce a

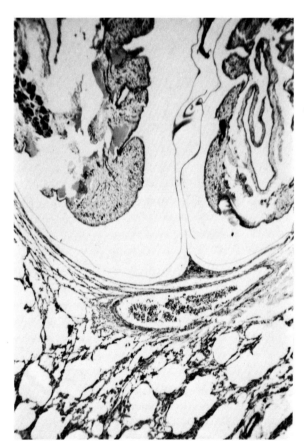

Fig. 8.47. Pulmonary pentastomiasis in a 6-year-old African girl with fatal disseminated infestation. (H and E; 25 ×)

granulomatous reaction with marked septal fibrosis. Embolism of the eggs in the pulmonary circulation is one cause of pulmonary hypertension. The adult worms can occasionally be observed in the lumen of the pulmonary vessels with little or no reaction of the endothelial cells (Berthoud 1972; Cowper 1973; Pettersson et al. 1974).

The larvae of *Strongyloides stercoralis* have been reported in the lungs of infants and children in association with hyperinfection, especially among those who are suffering from severe malnutrition or those who are receiving treatment with cytotoxic or immunosuppressive agents (Boyd et al. 1978; Burke 1978; Scowden et al. 1978).

Larvae of *Ascaris lumbricoides* can be observed in the lungs in children infested with this parasite. The larvae reach the lung by way of the blood vessels and can be seen in the capillaries or free in the alveolar wall, where there is sometimes an inflammatory reaction with numerous eosinophils. The larvae of *A. lumbricoides* must be distinguished histologically from those of *S. stercoralis* (Arean and Crandall 1971).

In endemic zones where *filariasis* is a major problem, microfilariae can be identified in the lung. The organisms are often free in the alveolar wall or in the capillaries. Occasionally there is a secondary inflammatory reaction around the microfilariae. Filiarasis of the lung is often associated with pulmonary eosinophilia (Meyers et al. 1977; Webb et al. 1960).

There are several types of *pentastomiasis*, and the causative parasites are known to inhabit the nasopharynx of birds and mammals in various parts of the world. Man may become infected secondarily, and the second-stage larva may be found in several organs, including the lung (Fig. 8.47) (Self 1969).

Recently a case of *capillariasis* (*Capillaria acrophila*) was described in a child in Iran by Aftandelians et al. (1977). Pulmonary paragonimiasis may be encountered in children coming from the Far East (Mayer 1979).

4.7.5. Diffuse Fibrosing Aleolitis (Desquamative Interstitial Pneumonia). Several synonyms for diffuse fibrosing alveolitis are found in the literature, including Hamman–Rich syndrome, fibrotic lung disease, interstitial pneumonia, interstitial pulmonary fibrosis, fibrocystic dysplasia, and idiopathic pulmonary fibrosis. We prefer the term *diffuse fibrosing alveolitis*. The terminology is complex, and those interested in its derivation should examine the work of Carrington et al. (1978), Dreisin et al. (1978), Eisenberg et al. (1977), Fishman (1978), Liebow et al. (1965), Patchefsky et al. (1973), Reynolds et al. (1977), and Scadding and Hinson (1967).

Fibrosing alveolitis has been described in association with pathological changes in other organs in a certain number of cases, especially in patients suffering from collagen or autoimmune diseases such as rheumatoid arthritis, lupus erythematous, Sjögren's syndrome, chronic active hepatitis, Hashimoto's thyroiditis, and ulcerative colitis. The disease affects all ages, and the clinical presentation is variable. It has been described in families, and in most of such cases it seems to have an autosomal dominant mode of inheritance. The radiological appearances are in no way specific for the condition. Histological patterns are often indistinguishable from those produced by drugs, allergic reactions, and certain viral pneumonias. Intranuclear inclusions have been observed in a number of cases, but they do not appear to be of viral origin. Calcification and ossification have been reported in some instances (Bolens et al. 1970; Crystal et al. 1978; Kawanami et al. 1979; Scadding 1974, 1978; Solliday et al. 1973; Stillwell et al. 1980; Tubbs et al. 1977).

Hewitt et al. (1977) reviewed the literature on cases of fibrosing alveolitis occurring in childhood. All pertinent features of the disease in the paediatric age group were evaluated, and a comparison of fibrosing alveolitis in children and adults was made.

Macroscopically the lungs are heavier than normal, firm, noncrepitant, and airless. They are greyish in colour and in the late stages present a honeycomb appearance. Microscopically, in the early phase, the air spaces are distended, filled with desquamated, PAS-positive, granular pneumocytes (type II cells) and some macrophages, which may contain haemosiderin pigment. The alveoli are lined with hyperplastic alveolar cells, some of which show cuboidal metaplasia. The alveolar wall is thickened and infiltrated by a mononuclear exudate but there are no polymorphonuclear leucocytes (Fig. 8.48). There is no necrosis, and hyaline membranes are not found. Lymphoid aggregates may be conspicuous, and follicles with prominent germinal centres are frequently observed, especially in the cryptogenic phase.

During the late stages, the alveolar wall shows varying degrees of thickness and fibrosis. The extent of these changes depends on the evolution and duration of the disease. Reticulin and collagen fibres are increased, while elastic fibres are numerous and thickened. There is an active proliferation of smooth-muscle cells. Some alveoli may become obliterated by the process, while others become cyst-like, leading to the typical honeycomb appearance. The bronchiolar epithelium may show metaplasia, and the bronchial wall is usually thickened as a result of muscular hyperplasia. The bronchi and bronchioles are often surrounded by lymphoid follicles.

Platelet aggregates have been observed in capillaries in the early phase. In general, vessel walls are thickened due to muscular hyperplasia with moderate to severe fibrosis. In the late stages, the large and medium-sized vessels are thickened and fibrosed.

4.7.6. Extrinsic Allergic Alveolitis (Hypersensitivity Pneumonitis). Extrinsic allergic alveolitis is an inflammatory reaction of the distal airways to various inhaled antigenic materials. A variety of agents, including proteins of animal and avian origin, fungi, and thermophilic organisms, have been incriminated as responsible for the lesions, and new aetiological agents continue to be identified. Extrinsic allergic alveolitis is often an occupational hazard; however, social and environmental factors are also contributory elements. Although the majority of cases have been reported in adults, infants and children are also affected.

Extrinsic allergic alveolitis is mainly associated with type III immune reaction, and the pathogenesis is believed to involve both immune-complex disease

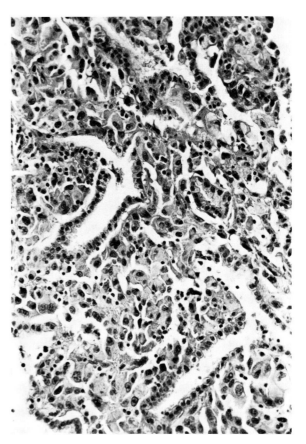

Fig. 8.48. Desquamative interstitial pneumonia in a 7-month-old boy, which progressed to diffuse pulmonary fibrosis by the 20th month. (H and E; 225 ×)

and cellular hypersensitivity (cell-mediated) reactions in the terminal air spaces in association with complement (C_3). Genetic and environmental factors seem to play an important role and may determine the host's response to the particular antigenic insult. HLA antigens and antibodies to the P_1-erythrocyte antigen also appear to be of some importance, at least in some cases, in determining the response of the host. Antigen, immunoglobulins (mainly IgG with smaller quantities of IgA and IgM), and complement (C_3) can be detected in the lungs of patients suffering from the disease. Their identification depends partly on the sensitivity of the tests, and in particular on the time of evolution of the disease process. They are more frequently found in the early stage of the disease, before extensive phagocytic infiltration or fibrosis has occurred.

Pathologically it is not possible to distinguish between immune complex disease and cellular hypersensitivity lesions in the lung. Furthermore, in the late stages of the disorder, it is not possible to differentiate between extrinsic allergic alveolitis and fibrosing alveolitis.

Diagnosis is made on the basis of the clinical and immunological findings in susceptible individuals. The radiological findings are nonspecific. The presence of specific antigens in the serum is of prime importance, and the analysis of cells and proteins from broncho–alveolar lavage may be helpful. Skin tests, in general, have been of no value (Hinson 1970; Roberts and Moore 1977; Salvaggio and Karr 1979; Bureau et al. 1979).

Macroscopically the lungs present features similar to those of fibrosing alveolitis. However, in most cases, lung tissue is obtained by biopsy for histological and immunological studies during the course of the disease. Microscopically there is a wide variability in the lesions, depending on the stage of the disease. In the early stages there is oedema of the alveolar wall, which is thickened and infiltrated by aggregates of lymphocytes, some plasma cells, and many histiocytes with a foamy cytoplasm. The alveolar spaces and bronchiolar lumen may contain few desquamated epithelial cells with some histiocytes (Fig. 8.49). At a later stage the inflammatory reaction is more prominent, histiocytes are more numerous, and there are well-developed lymph follicles, sometimes with well-defined germinal centres. Epithelioid-cell granulomas with foreign body-type giant cells are now conspicuous. Some giant cells may also be seen in the alveolar spaces among the few histiocytes and desquamated epithelial cells. Schauman bodies may occasionally be present. The small bronchi and bronchioles are also involved in the inflammatory process. Their walls are thickened and infiltrated by mononuclear cells and histiocytes, and bronchiolitis obliterans may

occur as the disease progresses. Small vessels may also participate in the reaction, and arteritis with eventual thickening and fibrosis of the vessel wall is sometimes observed.

In the late stages, there is moderate to severe thickening of the alveolar wall, which is rich in collagen and reticulin fibres. The inflammatory reaction is now patchy or almost absent, and granulomas are no longer present. Remodelling of the parenchyma and formation of cystic spaces gives rise to the honeycomb appearance, which is indistinguishable from that seen in fibrosing alveolitis.

4.7.7. Eosinophilic Pneumonias. Eosinophilic pneumonias are a group of allergic inflammatory reactions in the lung, characterized by a marked eosinophilic exudate in the lung parenchyma; they can occur with or without blood eosinophilia. The clinical and radiological manifestations are quite variable and are often nonspecific. Löffler's syndrome describes a particular clinical presentation.

The eosinophilic pneumonias occur in childhood. They are generally associated with certain drug reactions, fungi, or parasitic diseases, but there are other instances where the aetiology remains unknown or uncertain. Various drugs, including penicillin, sulphonamides, and p-aminosalicylic acid, have been described in association with this entity, and among the fungi *Aspergillus fumigatus* appears to be the most important offender. Numerous parasites known to cause blood eosinophilia (tropical eosinophilia) are associated with the condition; among the most common are microfilariae and the larvae of *A. lumbricoides*, *S. stercoralis*, *A. duodenale*, *T. canis*, and *T. cati*.

The pulmonary lesions may be caused by a local immunological type I or type III reaction. There is a diffuse inflammation in the pulmonary parenchyma. Eosinophils usually predominate, and histiocytes are also present. Focal areas of necrosis can be observed and granulomas are not uncommon. The most striking feature in many cases is fibrinoid necrosis of the peripheral arteries and arterioles in and about the lesions. In parasitic infections, sections of microfilariae or larvae can sometimes be identified within the granulomas (Carrington et al. 1969; Katzenstein et al. 1975; Lancet 1969; Pearson and Rosenow 1978; Rao et al. 1975; Webb et al. 1960).

4.7.8. Wegener's Granulomatosis. A relative uncommon condition of unknown aetiology, Wegener's granulomatosis has been described in children (Baliga et al. 1978; Moorthy et al. 1977). The disease can be limited to the lung (Carrington and Liebow 1966), showing areas of necrosis

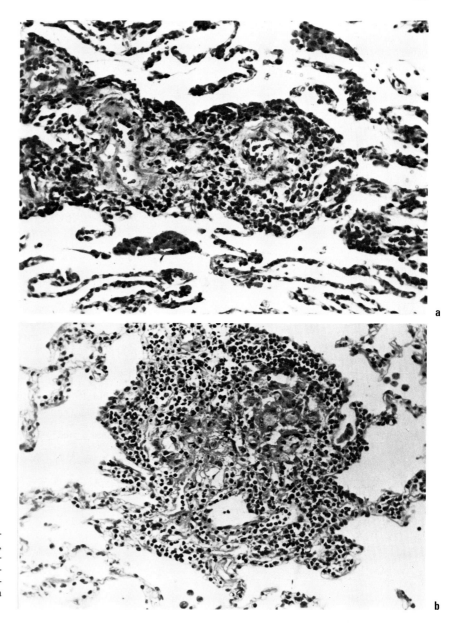

Fig. 8.49. a Hypersensitivity pneumonitis associated with animal furs, principally horsehair, in an 11-year-old girl. **b** Hypersensitivity pneumonitis associated with pigeon proteins (pigeon fancier's lung) in a 13-year-old girl. (H and E; 180 ×)

resembling infarcts but with little haemorrhage. There is necrotizing, granulomatous bronchitis and angiitis affecting both arteries and veins. In the disseminated or generalized form, the disease shows widespread necrotizing and granulomatous vasculitis of arteries and veins of the upper and lower respiratory tracts, the kidneys, and to a lesser extent of the skin, joints, and peripheral nervous systems. In the lung, the large necrotic areas usually contain aggregates of chronic inflammatory cells. Giant cells of the foreign-body type may be seen on the periphery of the lesions. The limited form of this condition must be distinguished from *lymphatoid granulomatosis*, which has also been reported in childhood. Lymphatoid granulomatosis is charac-

terized by an infiltrative process of the lung by small lymphocytes, plasma cells, histiocytes, and atypical lymphoreticular cells associated with necrotizing angiocentric and angiodestructive lesions. Extrapulmonary involvement, especially of the skin and brain, is not uncommon. Although the disease appears to have features in common with both classic Wegener's granulomatosis and lymphoma, it is possible that they represent a spectrum of the same disease process (Katzenstein et al. 1979c; Wall et al. 1979).

4.7.9. Asthma. Bronchial asthma is considered one of the most important chronic respiratory diseases in childhood; however, death from the condition in this age group is uncommon, and is usually due to status asthmaticus.

The clinical, radiological, and pathophysiological aspects of this disease entity have been fully documented, but the pathogenesis of the pulmonary lesions is still unknown. The pulmonary lesions often resemble those of eosinophilic pneumonia, and it is almost impossible in some cases to differentiate between the two conditions on morphological grounds. Some lesions may simulate Wegener's granulomatosis (Cooper et al. 1977; Cutz et al. 1978; Dunnill 1960; Scadding 1971).

Macroscopically the lungs are very large and emphysematous, but they are not heavy unless superadded infection has occurred. Microscopically the lesions are nonspecific and largely confined to the medium-sized and small bronchi. The distal airways are markedly distended, partially or totally obliterated by a thick, tenacious mucus (mucoid impaction) plug containing macrophages, desquamated epithelial cells, and eosinophils. There is a marked increase in goblet cells of the distal bronchial and bronchiolar epithelium, with hypersecretion of mucus. The basement membrane appears to be thickened, but is in fact supported by a hyaline-like collagen deposit containing reticulin but no elastic fibres. The role of this deposit is not fully understood, and several hypotheses have been proposed (deposition of immunoglobulins, trapping of proteins). The smooth muscle of the bronchial wall shows varying degrees of hypertrophy, and aggregates of chronic inflammatory cells accompanied by eosinophils are observed in the wall (Fig. 8.50).

The alveoli in the immediate vicinity of the bronchial lesions are generally thickened and are infiltrated by lymphocytes, plasma cells, and some eosinophils. The majority are usually distended.

The large bronchi also show goblet-cell hyperplasia, and there can be some degree of squamous metaplasia. The peribronchial glands are also hyperplastic.

4.7.10   Idiopathic   Pulmonary   Haemosiderosis (Ceelen's Disease). Idiopathic pulmonary haemosiderosis is an uncommon disorder of unknown aetiology. It has been reported mainly in infants and children and among young adults. The disease is characterized by repeated widespread intrapulmonary haemorrhages leading to respiratory distress, haemoptysis, and severe iron-deficiency anaemia.

In children the majority of cases occur before the age of 10 years, and the incidence is about equal in both sexes; among adults there is a male predominance. The clinical symptoms are variable but the severity may increase, leading to marked disability and eventually to a fatal outcome. Some

cases are asymptomatic. The radiological appearance is not diagnostic for the condition. The prognosis is unpredictable, and in the chronic stages pulmonary fibrosis may result. The condition has been described in association with myocarditis, and some cases have presented with diabetes. Chromosomal abnormalities and familial cases have been reported.

The diagnosis is usually made by elimination, since other conditions (mitral stenosis, pulmonary hypertension, veno-occlusive disease, etc.) can be accompanied by pulmonary haemosiderosis. The pathogenesis is unknown; however, some authors have proposed an immunological mechanism at the level of the basal membrane of the alveolar capillaries. This would suggest a mechanism similar to that occurring in Goodpasture's syndrome; however, immunoglobulins and complement have not been demonstrated on the basal membranes in idiopathic pulmonary haemosiderosis. Other authors have envisaged a connective tissue abnormality limited to the elastic tissue in the lung, and principally at the level of the small vessels. Cow's milk proteins acting as allergens on the capillary wall have been suggested as causative agents by a few, but there is no conclusive evidence to support this theory (Byrd and Gracey 1973; Donald et al. 1975; Foulon et al. 1974; Gilman and Zinkham 1969; Gonzalez-Crussi et al. 1976; Thaell et al. 1978).

Macroscopically the lungs are firm, somewhat nodular, and reddish brown in colour. The hilar lymph nodes are enlarged and brown. Microscopically the changes depend on the stage of the disease. Initially the distended alveolar spaces are filled with numerous macrophages laden with haemosiderin. Macrophages are accompanied by erythrocytes, indicating recent haemorrhages, which are also observed in the bronchiolar wall. Intraalveolar fibrin deposits can be demonstrated by means of special stains or immunofluorescence. The alveolar wall is oedematous and somewhat thickened, and it contains iron-filled histiocytes. This thickening is accentuated by the hyperplasia of the alveolar epithelial cells (mainly type II cells), which appear cuboidal. The capillary basement membrane shows some degree of thickening. There is no tissue necrosis or vasculitis. During the later stages, the thickening of the alveolar wall is more apparent, and fibrosis may be marked. There is an increase in collagen and reticulin fibres, accompanied by thick fragmented elastic fibres. Intra- and interalveolar haemorrhages may be widespread. Haemosiderin pigment deposits are abundant at this point, diffuse, and also observed in the interlobular spaces. Fibrotic nodules, some of which are siderotic, can be identified, and elastic tissue fragments are also impregnated by the pigment. Foreign-body giant

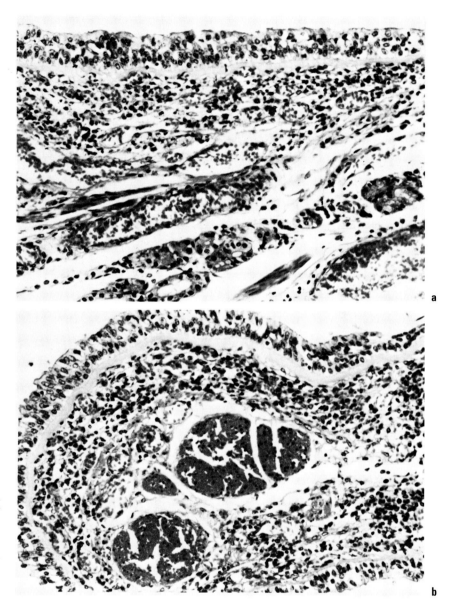

Fig. 8.50. a and **b** A 17-year-old female patient, hospitalized for asthma on many occasions since the age of 3. (H and E; 225 ×) **a** Hyperplasia of goblet cells and marked thickening of the basement membrane; **b** similar changes in main stem bronchus. Note marked muscular hypertrophy.

cells containing elastic fragments are seen in the alveolar spaces and elsewhere in the parenchyma.

There are few inflammatory cells, and they are observed in the alveolar wall of the peribronchial and perivascular spaces, often associated with histiocytes containing haemosiderin pigment.

4.7.11. Goodpasture's Syndrome. Goodpasture's syndrome is a rare condition characterized by pulmonary haemorrhages and acute glomerulonephritis. The disease has a predilection for young adults, and males are predominantly affected. The condition has also been recorded in infants and children.

The clinical symptoms closely resemble those of idiopathic pulmonary haemosiderosis, but in addition, the patients present with proteinuria and haematuria, indicating renal involvement. An influenza-like infection often precedes the symptoms. The course of the disease is variable and it often has a rapidly fatal outcome. The disease has been described in children with sickle-cell disease (Chambers et al. 1871; Loughlin et al. 1978; Martinez and Kohler 1971; Whitworth et al. 1974).

Macroscopically the lungs are heavy and there are subpleural haemorrhages in the acute stages, but later reddish brown, firm areas are found. The cut surface shows numerous old and recent haemorrhages scattered throughout the lung. Microscopically the alveolar spaces are distended, filled with erythrocytes and macrophages laden with haemosiderin pigment. Fibrin strands can be identified by special stains or immunofluorescence. The alveolar wall is oedematous, generally thickened, and may be infiltrated in some cases by few inflammatory cells, mainly lymphocytes with few plasma cells and histiocytes. Polymorphonuclear leucocytes are rare. The alveolar epithelial cells are hyperplastic, cuboidal or even multi-layered. Scattered foci of alveolar wall necrosis are occasionally observed and vasculitis has been reported. Arteritis, when present, may be suggestive of periarteritis nodosa or some form of hypersensitivity reaction, and thus make diagnosis difficult. Immunofluorescent staining for immunoglobulins reveals the presence of extensive fluorescence for IgG and β_{1C} on the alveolar basement membrane and capillary basement membrane as a linear, almost continuous pattern. Similar patterns are also observed on the glomerular basement membrane and portions of Bowmans capsule (see p. 413).

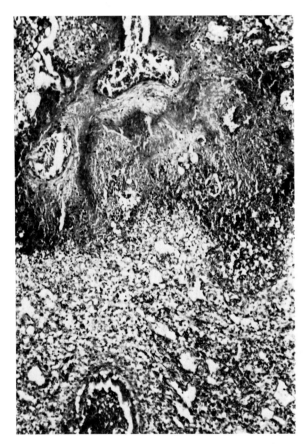

Fig. 8.51. Aspiration pneumonia due to aspiration of gastric juice, causing necrosis of the pulmonary parenchyma (*left*). (H and E; 60 ×)

4.7.12. Aspiration Pneumonia.

Although considered a rare condition, aspiration pneumonia may be more prevalent than is readily admitted. The condition may often go unrecognized and be incorrectly diagnosed as some other disease. The pulmonary lesions depend largely on the material inhaled, the quantity, and the time elapsing between the episode(s) and medical examination.

Gastric secretions or contents may be inhaled accidentally into the lungs and may be the cause of severe respiratory insufficiency, occasionally resulting in death of the patient. Inhalation of gastric contents in infants and children is more likely to occur among those who suffer with dysphagia, diaphragmatic hernias, or pyloric or oesophageal stenosis; in mentally retarded, in wasted, and debilitated children; in certain comatose states and during or after general anaesthesia; and in any condition associated with repeated vomiting.

When pure gastric secretion, with its high hydrochloric acid content, is inhaled into the lung, oedema results immediately with stasis, followed by widespread haemorrhages. Destruction of the tracheobronchial mucosa ensues, and within hours a diffuse inflammatory reaction occurs in the pulmonary parenchyma. The lesions contain few or no bacteria and are caused by the action of the hydrochloric acid on the lung tissue (Fig. 8.51).

In mild cases there is usually consolidation, which finally resolves, leaving mild pulmonary fibrosis, while in severe cases there may be abscess formation. The lungs may eventually become fibrosed with significant changes in pulmonary function.

In instances in which the gastric secretions are mixed with foreign material (partially digested food), the pulmonary lesions depend largely on the quantity of foreign material aspirated and on whether the process is acute or chronic. In the acute stage the lesions are nonspecific, and the only indication of the pathogenesis is the presence of food particles (vegetables, meat, etc.) identifiable in histological sections. In chronic aspiration, there is often a foreign body giant cell reaction, some cells containing particles of foreign material.

Numerous micro-organisms (including saprophytic anaerobes) are commonly associated with aspiration of foreign material. Abscesses are quite common in the lungs of these patients. The right lung is most often involved, and principally the lower segment of the right upper lobe and superior segment of the right lower lobe. The presence of saprophytic organisms can cause putrefaction of the lung tissue, giving it a characteristic foul odour (Awe et al. 1966; Bartlett et al. 1974a; Cameron et al. 1967; Kaplan et al. 1978; Moran et al. 1955; Sladen et al. 1971).

Milk inhalation pneumonia results from repeated

inhalation by infants of milk or milk products into the tracheobronchial tree, sometimes resulting in bronchopneumonia. The condition is usually associated with tracheo-oesophageal fistula, cleft palate, or posterior laryngeal cleft.

The inhalation of milk causes severe respiratory distress and can result in severe pneumonia, depending on the age of the patient, the duration of the condition, the amount of material inhaled and the frequency, and any secondary infections that may accompany the disease. Chest X-rays are of little value in diagnosis, but examination of bronchial secretions will reveal macrophages laden with fat droplets and also free fat globules.

The pulmonary lesions are variable and cover a wide spectrum of histological patterns, varying from mild acute bronchitis to pulmonary fibrosis. In the acute stages there is oedema and stasis together with pulmonary haemorrhages, followed by an acute inflammatory reaction in the lung parenchyma. Secondary infection is very common and results in confluent bronchopneumonia and sometimes empyema. The alveoli contain some desquamated epithelial cells among the many polymorphonuclear leucocytes, and few lymphocytes and plasmocytes. However, the most striking feature of the lesion is the presence of numerous macrophages in the alveolar spaces and alveolar wall laden with fat droplets (oil red O, Sudan black B-positive). Within a few days many giant cells are observed, also containing fat droplets. Lung abscesses are not uncommon. Bronchiectasis is common in these infants.

As the condition becomes chronic there is thickening of the alveolar wall, and bronchiolitis obliterans occurs. In some cases, localized consolidation is observed, with central accumulation of fat-laden macrophages and free fat globules surrounded by a dense fibrous tissue. In the late stages there is progressive pulmonary fibrosis, which is often indistinguishable from other cases of the 'mural' type of fibrosing alveolitis (Moran 1953; Olson 1970; Williams 1973; Williams and Freeman 1973). Parental nutrition with Intralipid infusions or other fat emulsions in very immature, low-birth-weight babies may be responsible for intravascular fat accumulation in the lungs resulting in ventilation/perfusion disturbances and even infarcts in some instances (Levene et al. 1980).

Lipid pneumonia is the result of the accumulation of lipids in the distal airways. The origin of the fatty substances can be either endogenous or exogenous. Endogenous lipid pneumonia is believed to result from a pneumonic lesion with obstructed bronchi and liberation of cellular lipids; these are phagocytosed by alveolar macrophages, which accumulate in the alveolar spaces and alveolar wall. The endogenous form may also result from disorders of fat metabolism. Exogenous lipid pneumonia is more frequent, and occurs when oily substances of different chemical natures are inhaled into the lower respiratory system. The oily substance may be of vegetable, animal, or mineral origin, and the tissue reaction produced will vary according to the lipids involved. Vegetable oils generally produce little or no pulmonary reaction, while animal oils, which are rapidly hydrolysed to give fatty acids, produce necrosis of the tissue with a severe inflammatory reaction. Mineral oils, which are not hydrolysed but emulsified, produce little or no necrosis but do lead to extensive fibrosis.

Lipid pneumonia is more common among infants and old people. In childhood the disease is usually associated with the intake of cod liver oil, oily nasal sprays or drops, and mineral oils used as laxatives, to name but a few. The condition is relatively more common in debilitated or mentally retarded infants.

The pulmonary lesions are described as diffused (infantile type) and localized (adult type), often as paraffinomas, mostly in adults. The lesions are generally located in the lower segment of the upper right lobe and/or the apical segments of the lower right lobe. However, both lungs may be involved to varying degrees.

The clinical manifestations are often misleading and the radiological patterns are nondiagnostic. Lipophages or free lipids may be recovered from the sputum, and macrophages laden with lipid droplets may be seen in material from bronchial washings (Borrie and Gwynne 1973; Heckers et al. 1978; Hutchins and Boitnott 1978; Salm and Hughes 1970).

Macroscopically the area involved is fairly well delimited, heavy, and firm. It is often yellowish in colour, and enlarged hilar lymph nodes may also be yellow. Microscopically the lesions are variable, depending on the oily substance involved. The alveoli may be distended and filled with macrophages with a clear cytoplasm (foam cells). The alveolar wall can be thickened, somewhat congested, and oedematous. The inflammatory reaction is also quite variable. When there is secondary bacterial infection, both the alveolar spaces and alveolar walls contain polymorphonuclear leucocytes and lymphocytes, with few plasma cells. When the pneumonitis is due to animal or mineral oils the inflammatory reaction is more intense and there is active remodelling of the alveolar walls, which show varying degrees of thickening. In the chronic stages there is diffuse fibrosis associated with emphysematous blebs. The lesions usually progress to the mural stage of fibrosing alveolitis. Foreign-body giant cells can be observed in the chronic stages.

The lipids may be stained by one of the fat stains

(oil red O, Sudan, or Scharlach R).

Paraffinoma is usually associated with a long period of inhalation of oily substances, and is characterized by one or several localized masses, which may resemble tuberculomas, neoplasms, or fungal infections. Histologically the lesion contains masses of macrophages laden with fat droplets and free lipids surrounded by a dense fibrous network. Some of the fat globules are bordered with multinucleated foreign-body giant cells. There are scattered aggregates of lymphocytes and often well-developed lymphoid follicles with prominent germinal centres. The distal bronchi may contain fat-laden macrophages, and their walls are infiltrated by mononuclear cells. The distal arteries often show various degrees of endarteritis obliterans.

Kerosene pneumonia. Kerosene is a by-product of petroleum and is the cause of a significant form of pneumonitis in childhood. Kerosene is widely used for fuel and lighting in many developing countries or areas not supplied with gas or electricity. Infants and children may inadvertently swallow the substance, which causes severe irritation of the stomach followed by severe vomiting and regurgitation. Under these circumstances the substance can be inhaled and reach the distal airways, producing a diffuse necrotizing pneumonitis. Death may follow due to pulmonary, gastrointestinal, or central nervous system effects.

In the respiratory system there is an immediate, marked, diffuse oedema with congestion of the lungs. This is followed by widespread necrosis of the pulmonary parenchyma, with a severe inflammatory response. The exudate is rich in fibrin and polymorphonuclear leucocytes, and fibrin may line the alveolar ducts and bronchioles. The lesions are generally bilateral, but are more frequently located in the right lung than in the left. There is extensive necrosis of the bronchial and bronchiolar epithelium, accompanied by infiltration of the walls by mononuclear cells and polymorphs. Necrosis of the peripheral vessels with haemorrhages is common, and in the healing stages the vessel walls are usually markedly thickened and sclerosed. Patients who survive show extensive pulmonary fibrosis (Nouri and Al-Rahim 1970; Press et al. 1962).

Powder aspiration can occasionally cause respiratory distress in infants under 2 years of age; a relatively high mortality is associated with this condition. The accidental aspiration of talcum powder (rich in zinc oxide) causes bronchial obstruction, and after a relatively long latent period produces massive bronchitis with bronchiolitis. Oedema and congestion of the lungs may precede the inflammatory reaction. When there is complete obstruction of the bronchial lumen atelectasis

ensues, and if death does not occur compensatory emphysema follows (Motomatsu et al. 1979; Pfenninger and D'Apuzzo 1977).

Dain et al. (1970) have described the presence of *starch granules in the lungs* of newborns treated with positive pressure ventilation for the respiratory distress syndrome, chiefly hyaline membrane disease. They suggested that the source of the starch was the sterile gloves used in handling the endotracheal catheter. The substance was not usually recognizable with routine haematoxylin–eosin stains, but exhibited the characteristic maltese crosses when observed under polarized light. The starch granules may be free in the alveolar spaces or intermingled with the bronchial and alveolar exudate in the early stages. After a few days they are found in macrophages or in foreign-body giant cells within the alveoli.

4.7.13. Paraquat Lung. Paraquat (1, l'dimethyl-4, 4'-bipyridylium dichloride) is an herbicide. When ingested by man, it causes a rapid onset of diffuse pulmonary fibrosis, with severe respiratory failure and death within weeks of intake. The substance may be swallowed accidentally by children, and it can be taken up through the skin.

Paraquat causes ulceration of the mouth and upper gastrointestinal tract, with vomiting and diarrhoea. These symptoms are accompanied by acute renal failure, jaundice, and increasingly severe dyspnoea with cyanosis, leading to marked pulmonary insufficiency within days. Cerebral symptoms may also be present. Paraquat is poorly absorbed by the intestine, and is excreted in the urine. The substance is metabolized in the liver and reaches the lungs from the circulation. It causes hepatic necrosis and damage to the adrenals, myocardium, and renal tubules. It accumulates in the lungs and muscles.

The pulmonary lesions and the prognosis in general seem to depend on the concentration of the active substance ingested. In general, pulmonary fibrosis occurs over a variable period. Surfactant is lacking, following destruction of the type II cells or granular pneumocytes (Campbell 1968; Gaultier et al. 1973; McDonagh and Martin 1970; Rebello and Mason 1978; Robertson et al. 1976; Smith et al. 1974; Smith and Heath 1974a, b).

Macroscopically the appearance depends on the time lapse after the intake of the substance, since little if any of the substance reaches the lungs by way of the bronchial tree. Within the first 4 days the lungs are heavy, congested, and oedematous. Later they show areas of consolidation, or appear solid with a somewhat rubbery consistency, and within weeks they take on a honeycomb appearance.

Microscopically, in the first few days of the condition there is congestion with marked oedema of the alveolar wall. Inter- and intra-alveolar haemorrhages are conspicuous. The alveolar spaces are filled with a fibrinous exudate containing desquamated alveolar lining cells (some of which are undergoing degeneration) and numerous macrophages and erythrocytes. Polymorphonuclear leucocytes and aggregates of lymphocytes and plasma cells may be seen. Hyaline membranes are prominent, lining both the alveolar spaces and the distal airways. There is destruction of the epithelial lining of the distal bronchi and bronchioles. Some of these lesions may be due to oxygen therapy. In later stages of the disease there is a very active, but variable, organization of the intra-alveolar exudate. The alveolar spaces are invaded by an active fibroblastic proliferation resembling the pattern of growth seen in a tissue culture. These cells have been referred to as 'profibroblasts' and are probably myofibroblasts. Finally the alveolar space is obliterated by a fibrous process with collagen, reticulin fibres, and a few elastic fibres. There is also a rich capillary network, and a few foci of chronic inflammatory cells are present. Simultaneously a similar process takes place in the alveolar wall, and eventually it is impossible to distinguish the alveolar wall from the alveolar space. As the lesion progresses there is diffuse pulmonary fibrosis, with an increase in collagen and reticulin fibres, and finally honeycombing.

The bronchial and bronchiolar walls are also affected by the fibrotic process, and can be obliterated. Bronchiectasis may occur, and other bronchi and bronchioles may show epithelial proliferation and hyperplasia. Small pulmonary arteries show thickening and fibrosis of their walls. Arterioles show distinct muscular hyperplasia.

4.7.14. Lung Abscesses. There are many possible causes of lung abscesses in childhood, including bronchial obstruction by an inhaled foreign body, by an inspissated mucus plug, or by infected material associated with some surgical procedure in the mouth or oropharynx. The majority of abscesses are located in the lower segments of the upper lobes or the upper segments of the lower lobes, and they are more often found on the right side. Whatever the source, the material is generally accompanied by a mixture of both anaerobic and aerobic micro-organisms. Necrosis of the bronchial wall takes place at the site of obstruction, with active bacterial proliferation and a marked inflammatory exudate. The related distal airways collapse and become necrotic, and a purulent inflammatory reaction develops. The centre of the lesion undergoes liquefaction, and partial drainage may take place by way of the eroded bronchus.

In chronic cases the wall of the abscess is surrounded by a dense fibrous layer bordered by granulation tissue. The cavity may be lined with a squamous epithelial lining in continuity with the epithelial lining of the bronchus.

Lung abscesses may also be associated with bacterial pneumonia or bronchopneumonia. *Staphylococcus aureus*, which is known to cause extensive tissue destruction, is by far the most common offender. Other micro-organisms commonly responsible for such lesions are *Klebsiella pneumoniae*, *Pneumococcus* and *Pseudomonas*.

Septic emboli may affect the lung in septicaemia, and in childhood an important cause is thrombophlebitis around an indwelling catheter. *Staphylococcus aureus* is most often associated with these abscesses (Bartlett et al. 1974b; Brook and Finegold 1979; Mark and Turner 1968; Pryce 1948).

4.7.15. Granulomatous Lesions. Numerous agents are known to produce granulomatous lesions in the lung (Ulbright and Katzenstein 1980). In certain instances special staining techniques make it possible to identify the agent responsible for the lesions within the granulomas, and infectious causes including *Mycobacterium tuberculosis*, coccidioidomycosis, aspergillosis, blastomycosis, and histoplasmosis are discussed elsewhere.

4.7.16. Sarcoidosis (Boeck's Sarcoid, Besnier-Boeck-Schaumann's Disease). Sarcoidosis has a worldwide distribution, the incidence varying from one area to another, and even within the same region. The clinical and radiological features of the condition have been extensively documented. The disease usually presents as a slowly progressive chronic inflammatory reaction affecting the skin (erythema nodosum), lungs, lymph nodes, and uveal tract. Spontaneous healing may occur after a long period. Less frequently, the disease also affects many other organs or systems (heart, kidney, skeletal muscles, central nervous system, bone and joints—arthralgia). The symptoms are often quite variable and may go unnoticed; in many instances the disease is an accidental finding on routine chest radiographs or at post-mortem.

A female predominance has been indicated by some authors, while others claim that there is an equal male-to-female ratio. The disease has been reported in families, and there are strong indications that it is more common among negroes. Sarcoidosis is not common in childhood; it is prevalent among children in their teens and rare in infants below 5 years of age.

Descriptions of the disease in childhood show no features distinguishing it from the condition seen in adults (Fig. 8.52) (Carrington et al. 1976; Daniele et al. 1978; Harris and Spock 1978; Mitchell et al. 1977; Rosen et al. 1977, 1978; Studdy et al. 1978; Turiaf et al. 1974, 1978).

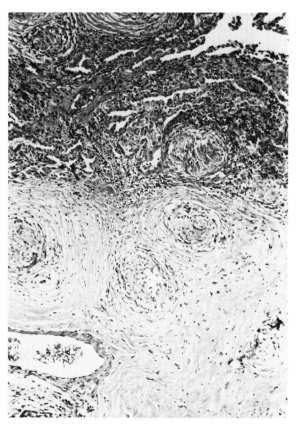

Fig. 8.52. Pulmonary sarcoidosis showing numerous confluent granulomas (on the *left*) with marked hyalinization. (H and E; 60×)

4.7.18. BCG Granulomas. Generalized BCG in-granulomatous disease is characterized by severe, chronic, and recurrent infections, usually involving the skin, lung, liver, bone, and lymph nodes, but any organ can be involved. The first clinical symptoms generally appear during the first year of life, and the disease may run a fatal course before the age of 10 if inadequately treated.

The condition occurs in a number of forms with variable modes of inheritance but a recessive mode of transmission is most commonly found (see p. 546).

In the lung, pneumonia or bronchopneumonia with abscess formation may be present. There may also be numerous noncaseating granulomas with foreign-body giant cells, together with many histiocytes containing lipid pigments. On the periphery of the lesions are lymphocytes, and occasionally central necrosis can be identified containing few poly-morphonuclear leucocytes (Dilworth and Mandell 1977; Holmes et al. 1966; Landing and Shirkey 1957; Schlegel 1974; Thompson and Soothill 1970).

4.7.18. BCG Granulomas. Generalized BCG infection is a rare complication of BCG vaccination in childhood. It has been reported to have a fatal outcome in some instances, mainly among infants with some form of immune abnormality. Inadequate preparation of the vaccine may be responsible for the condition. The lung, and often the intestine and other organs, are the site of numerous granulomas in these cases. The lesions are typical granulomas and may show caseation. Groups of acid-fast bacilli can be observed in the epitheloid cells and/or in the necrotic areas (Genin et al. 1977; Passwell et al. 1976; Torriani et al. 1979).

4.7.19. Rheumatic Pneumonitis. There is still no unanimity as to whether the pulmonary lesions observed during the course of acute rheumatic fever are specific for the condition, although they are generally referred to as rheumatic pneumonitis.

The radiological images of diffuse pulmonary consolidation are in no way specific, and the morphological features may resemble those seen in a number of other conditions. Associations with the clinical aspects of the disease are the only guiding factors. The lesions are generally observed in cases presenting with severe valvular involvement or fulminant pancarditis (Grunow and Esterly 1972; Massumi and Legier 1966).

Macroscopically the lungs are quite oedematous, large, and heavy. They are often reddish in colour and rubbery in consistency. Microscopically the lesions are widespread. The alveolar spaces are filled with a thick fibrinous exudate, which is haemorrhagic in some areas. There are fibrin strands and a few desquamated alveolar cells with some macrophages containing pigment granules. Scattered groups of inflammatory cells, chiefly mononuclear cells, are often present. Some of the alveolar spaces and alveolar ducts are lined with thick bands of hyaline membranes. The alveolar walls are thickened, oedematous and congested. Intraseptal and intra-alveolar haemorrhages are constant findings. Alveolar wall necrosis has been observed in a number of cases, and in many of these fibrinoid necrosis of the wall of the distal branches of the pulmonary artery is present (Fig. 8.53). In advanced stages there are signs of organization of the intra-alveolar exudate, characterized by the penetration of fibroblasts. The epithelium of the distal bronchi and bronchioles may show evidence of necrosis, and their walls may be infiltrated by a few mononuclear cells or surrounded by peribronchial lymphoid tissue. During regeneration there is metaplasia of the bronchial epithelium.

These lesions are in no way specific, and there is still some doubt as to whether they are primary lesions. Aschoff nodules are not identified with this pneumonitis.

4.7.20. Pulmonary Alveolar Proteinosis (Idiopathic Alveolar Lipoproteinosis). The rare condition of pulmonary alveolar proteinosis is characterized by the accumulation in the alveolar spaces and bronchioles of large amounts of an amorphous material rich in lipids and proteins, leading to severe respiratory insufficiency. There are reports of 30–40 childhood cases, with a significant male preponderance.

The symptoms of pulmonary alveolar proteinosis (PAP) are nonspecific and variable. They may regress spontaneously or proceed to progressive pulmonary insufficiency, and sometimes death if not adequately treated. The radiological pattern is not diagnostic for the condition, and pulmonary function tests are suggestive of a restrictive type of disease.

The aetiology of PAP is unknown. The disease was often considered as a form of lung response to a variety of agents, often related to an occupation. There have been reports of PAP in association with tuberculosis and neoplasms in the lung and with a number of mycotic infections, *Nocardiosis* being by far the most prevalent of these. *Aspergillosis crypto-coccosis, Mucormycosis, Candidosis* and *Cytomegalic inclusion disease* have all also been reported, but less frequently. In childhood the condition is very often associated with some form of immune abnormality or haematological disorders.

Extensive research on the amorphous material in the alveolar spaces has shown that it is composed of insoluble lipids and proteins with large quantities of cellular debris, macrophages, and granular pneumocytes (type II). The lipid concentration is several times that observed in normal lungs or in other pathological conditions, and is composed principally of phospholipids (palmitoyl lecithin or surfactant). These lipids differ from circulating lipids. The proteins are immunoproteins from the serum and they appear to be selective (albumin, α_1-antitrypsin, α_1-acid glycoprotein, and pre-albumin). The other constituents are disintegrating granular pneumocytes and macrophages with various types of inclusion bodies, including lamellar structures and myelin bodies.

The excessive production of surfactant or its accumulation as a result of impaired removal or a combination of both abnormalities may be implicated in the pathogenesis of the disease (Béal et al. 1974; Bell and Hook 1979; Coleman et al. 1980; Heppleston and Young 1971; Hook et al. 1978; Kuhn et al. 1966; Rosen et al. 1958; Sunderland et al. 1972).

Macroscopically the lungs are enlarged and firm with consolidated areas. The cut surface is moist, revealing yellowish grey zones alternating with dark red areas. Microscopically the alveolar spaces and

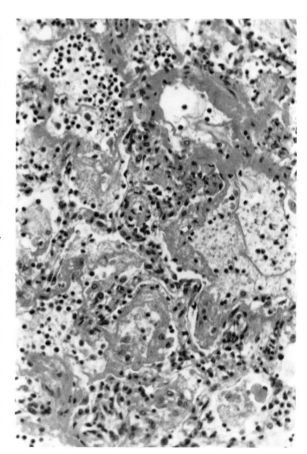

Fig. 8.53. Rheumatic pneumonitis in a 12-year-old boy with extensive pancarditis and severe valvular lesions. (H and E; 120×)

bronchioles are distended with an abundant quantity of amorphous, eosinophilic, granular material in which cellular debris is associated with varying numbers of granular pneumocytes at different stages of disintegration and some macrophages (Fig. 8.54). The alveolar wall is not altered and shows no inflammatory reaction. It is mainly lined with flattened epithelial cells.

The intra-alveolar granular material is strongly PAS-positive even after amylase digestion, and is metachromatic when stained with toludine blue. It is slightly positive with fat stains, principally Sudan black B. When viewed under polarized light, large numbers of doubly refractile crystals are visible (mostly cholesterol). The macrophages also contain large quantities of this lipoproteinous material in their cytoplasm, as shown by special stains and ultrastructural studies. In chronic stages of the disease pulmonary fibrosis ensues.

4.7.21. Pulmonary Alveolar Microlithiasis. Pulmonary alveolar microlithiasis is a relatively rare pulmonary condition of unknown aetiology. The disease has a worldwide distribution and has been described in all races. All ages are affected, and it has been documented at birth. It was formerly thought that principally adults were affected, but the disease seems to be more prevalent among children in Japan. It has an equal distribution between the sexes or perhaps a slight male predominance. There is a familial tendency, suggesting that some genetically determined disturbance of metabolism may be present, although there are no abnormalities of the metabolism of calcium and phosphorus in these patients. The disease is often asymptomatic, and may be discovered at routine chest radiography or when dyspnoea of unknown origin is investigated. Surveys in families may reveal new cases. There is generally a significant discrepancy between the severe radiographic changes and the absent or mild clinical symptoms. Pulmonary function tests give variable results, depending largely on the stage of the disease, its distribution, and the extent of the lesions. Evolution is also quite varied, extending over a period of a few months or years or even several decades as the pulmonary function deteriorates.

There is no satisfactory treatment (Caffrey and Altman 1965; Clark and Johnson 1961; Fuleihan et al. 1969; Kino et al. 1972; Onadeka et al. 1977; Sears et al. 1971).

Macroscopically the lungs are much heavier than normal, very hard in consistency, and reddish in colour. The lesions may predominate in the lower lobes, but all lobes can be affected. Microscopically the lesions vary with the stage of evolution. In the early stages the alveolar spaces are filled with psammoma-like bodies, which are darker in their centres. These bodies are strongly PAS-positive, and stain intensely for calcium with the von Kossa stain. They are known as calcospherites, and are different from the *corpora amylacea* associated with chronic congestive heart failure or pulmonary fibrosis. The alveolar wall shows little or no histological modification at this stage (Fig. 8.55). Later the calcospherites not only appear as laminated bodies with radial striations, but also show extensive calcification, with ossification occurring at the periphery. The alveolar walls are thickened, fibrosed, disrupted in places, and infiltrated by mononuclear cells

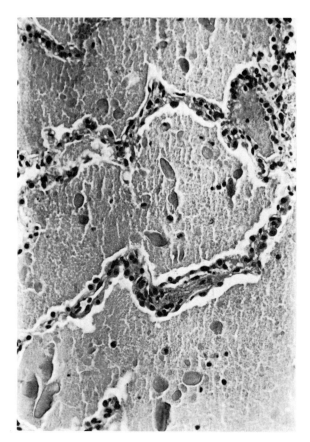

Fig. 8.54. Alveolar lipoproteinosis with distended alveoli full of an eosinophilic proteineous material. Absence of inflammatory reaction. Courtesy of Dr C. Bozic (H and E; 225 ×)

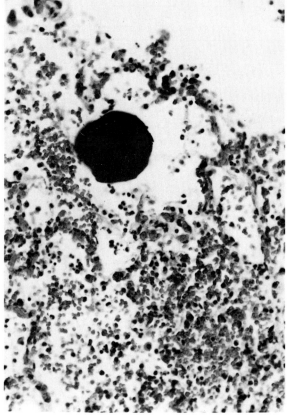

Fig. 8.55. Pulmonary microlithiasis in a girl of 2 years 5 months. Courtesy of Dr C. Bozic. (H and E; 180 ×)

(chiefly monocytes and lymphocytes). Giant cells may be observed in some instances, and calcospherites may be incorporated within the thickened alveolar wall or situated in the proximity of small vessels.

Chemical analyses have shown that calcospherites are composed mainly of calcium phosphates with small quantities of iron and fat.

5. Bronchial Lesions

5.1. Intrauterine (Congenital) Bronchiolitis Obliterans

Bronchiolitis obliterans is not uncommon. It has been described in numerous conditions and is associated mainly with various inflammatory reactions of the respiratory tract. Bacterial and viral infections are chiefly responsible for the lesions, and all age groups can be affected.

Intrauterine bronchiolitis obliterans is rare, and only a few reports are recorded. The aetiology is not known; however, it is generally accepted that intrauterine infection may be responsible for the lesions (Nezelof et al. 1970; Rosen and Gaton 1975; Sir 1962; Sueishi et al. 1974).

Macroscopically the lesions are observed in premature infants or in the immediate neonatal period. The lungs are diffusely consolidated and heavy, and appear dark red with some haemorrhagic areas. Microscopically there are areas of intrauterine pneumonia. Some of the alveoli are filled with squames accompanied by polymorphonuclear leucocytes. Occasional giant cells with vacuolated cytoplasm may be present. The distal bronchi and

bronchioles are obliterated by polypoid masses consisting of granulation tissue projecting into the lumen from an area of damaged wall. Some of the lesions show various degrees of organization, fibroblasts, collagen fibres, and hyalinization being present. Vascular penetration from the base of insertion of the polyp may be apparent (Fig. 8.56).

The bronchial epithelium shows signs of regeneration, sometimes with squamous metaplasia, while in other areas there is evidence of hypersecretion. The bronchial wall and surrounding tissues are infiltrated with polymorphonuclear leucocytes and some lymphocytes.

5.2. Bronchitis and Bronchiolitis

Inflammation of the lower respiratory tract is extremely common in infants and children, and all levels of the bronchial tree are liable to injury by the agent or agents responsible. Bacterial infections have been considered to be responsible for most of the lesions; however, it is now well established that viral infections are the major cause of bronchitis and bronchiolitis in childhood and the principal cause in infancy. Secondary bacterial infections may be associated with viral infection.

The development of better tissue culture techniques and specific serological tests have resulted in the isolation and identification of the various viruses responsible for the lesions. Direct and indirect immunofluorescence antibody techniques have proved to be useful tools in the diagnosis of viral infections.

Respiratory syncytial virus infection is the commonest in infants during the first 2 years of life. Other viruses known to cause these illnesses include

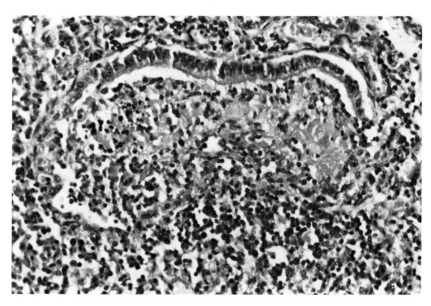

Fig. 8.56. Intrauterine bronchiolitis obliterans in a newborn infant who lived for 12 h. (H and E; 180 ×)

adenovirus, *parainfluenza viruses*, *influenza A and B viruses* and *measles virus*. Other organisms, e.g., *pertussis* and *Mycoplasma pneumoniae* can produce severe infections. Physical, chemical, or gaseous injury to the distal airway may be responsible for similar lesions.

The clinical symptoms are in no way specific for any one virus. There is generally an upper respiratory tract infection with a catarrhal reaction, raised temperature, cough, dyspnoea, and wheezing. Diffuse interstitial pneumonia is sometimes present, and hyperventilation may be observed. The radiological patterns are nonspecific.

Although mortality is relatively low in many of these infections, morbidity can be high and repeated infections may be responsible for significant abnormalities of lung function. The physiopathological features of the condition have been well documented and it has been shown that the respiratory difficulties are related principally to the obstruction of the distal bronchi and bronchioles. The severity of the lesions in infancy depends largely on the anatomical

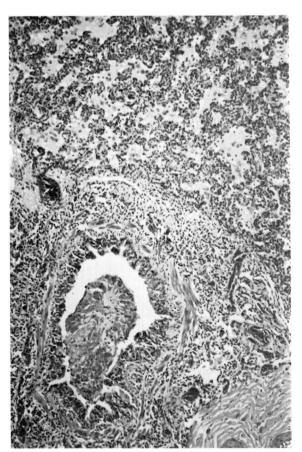

Fig. 8.57. Acute bronchitis and bronchiolitis with dense mononuclear cell infiltration extending into the pulmonary parenchyma. (H and E; 35 ×)

structure of the lung at that age. Other factors, including immunological ones, may also be important (Aherne et al. 1970; Becroft 1971; Gardner et al. 1973; Kaul et al. 1978; Simpson et al. 1974; Wohl and Chernick 1978).

Microscopically the bronchial and bronchiolar mucosa show patchy or widespread ulceration with necrosis of the epithelium. Signs of regeneration are characterized by the proliferation of epithelial cells, which become cuboidal. The walls of the distal airways are congested, oedematous, and infiltrated by mononuclear cells. The lumen may be partially or completely obliterated by an exudate composed of cellular debris, fibrin, some mucus, and a large number of inflammatory, principally mononuclear, cells. Patchy atelectatic foci may be present when obstruction is complete. There is also peribronchial and peribronchiolar inflammatory infiltration extending from the walls of the affected airways into the surrounding pulmonary parenchyma, resulting in localized zones of pneumonia (Fig. 8.57).

These lesions are common to the majority of viruses involved; however some viruses (adenovirus, influenza A virus) may produce severe residual lung damage with extensive destruction of the distal bronchi and bronchioles and obliteration of the lumen. In chronic disease there is organization of the intraluminal material, resulting in bronchiolitis obliterans. In this case there is vascular granulation tissue initially, which progresses to fibrous scarring with partial or complete obliteration of the affected distal bronchi and bronchioles.

5.3. Bronchiectasis

Bronchiectasis is not uncommon in infants and children, and it is often associated with chronic and frequent repeated lung infections. There is much controversy and debate on the aetiology and pathogenesis. Some authors maintain that there are two forms of the disease (a) *congenital*, related to malformations in the bronchial wall as a result of absent or deficient cartilage plates; and (b) *acquired*, associated with acute respiratory infection resulting in severe pulmonary damage with sequelae. Most authors consider the lesions to be acquired in most cases, with only a very small percentage attributable to congenitally determined defects. In support of this hypothesis, it is true to say that bronchiectasis has never been observed at birth or in the neonatal period. In almost all cases, including most of those described as congenital, the condition has developed after a period of acute bronchitis or pneumonia during infancy (generally within the first 2 years of life). Obstruction (extrinsic or intrinsic) of a bronchus or of bronchi may also be associated with the development of bronchiectasis.

The disease begins in infancy, often during the first or second year of life, after an attack of what is generally referred to as bronchitis or pneumonia. In well-documented cases, the association of the development of bronchiectasis with syncytial virus, adenovirus, influenza virus, measles, pertussis or *Mycoplasma pneumoniae* infections has been established.

Bronchiectasis may affect only a small percentage of infants or children after viral epidemics, and is not apparent immediately after infection. Host as well as immunological factors probably play an important role in the development of the lesions. The stage of lung development may be an additional factor.

The disease may be progressive, with a high incidence of chronic and frequent recurrent infections of the respiratory tract. Cough is often associated with wheezing. Haemoptysis is a variable finding. In the chronic stages of the disease, dyspnoea occurs on exercise, and finger clubbing may be seen. Radiography, and principally bronchography, is important in establishing the diagnosis, and repeated examinations may be necessary to follow its evolution.

Bronchiectasis has been observed in association with certain syndromes, notably the unilateral hyperlucent lung (Swyer–James syndrome or MacLeod's syndrome), a clinical and radiological entity that was once thought to be congenital but is now recognized as being a sequela of various insults to the lung, including viral infections, *tuberculosis*, *Mycoplasma pneumoniae*, foreign-body aspiration, ingestion of hydrocarbons, and radiotherapy. It is also an integral part of Kartagener's syndrome, in which bronchiectasis is associated with situs inversus and chronic paranasal sinusitis. This syndrome has a familial tendency.

Bronchiectasis is associated with small-airway disease, with obstruction of the involved airways and bronchiolitis obliterans. Atelectasis of the parenchyma distal to the obstruction is often encountered. There is hypersecretion of mucus distal to the occlusion, with subsequent infection leading to abscess formation and foci of pneumonia. Destruction and weakening of the bronchial walls occur proximal to the lesions, with profound remodelling of the surrounding tissue as a result of chronic inflammation. Subsequently there is dilatation of these bronchi, owing in part to the negative intrathoracic pressure and to the traction exerted by the surrounding fibrous tissue. The basic physiopathological problem in bronchiectasis is one of perfusion/ventilation associated with air-trapping (Aherne et al. 1970; Becroft 1971; Cho et al. 1973; Clark 1963; Herbert et al. 1977; Kogutt et al. 1973; Matsuba and Thurlbeck 1973; Mitchell and Bury 1975; Ranga and Kleinerman 1978; Stokes et al.

1978; Williams and Campbell 1960; Williams et al. 1972; Wohl and Chernick 1978).

Macroscopically, dilated bronchi may be cylindrical in form or show saccular dilatation, or both. The changes are often severe and widespread. They may be unilateral or bilateral, and may affect one or more lobes or segments. The left lower lobes, the lingula, the right middle lobe, and the posterior basal segments are most frequently involved (Fig. 8.58). Microscopically there is marked dilatation of the bronchi, and mucus with an inflammatory exudate may occupy the lumen. The bronchial epithelium is variable from one area to another, being generally hyperplastic and lined with tall columnar cells whose cytoplasm contains large amounts of mucus. In other areas squamous metaplasia may be conspicuous. The wall is infiltrated by a dense mononuclear infiltrate, which is more prominent in the submucosa. In some instances the inflammatory reaction is overwhelming and consists of lymphocytes extending into the surrounding parenchyma. Well-developed lymphoid follicles with prominent germinal centres can be seen in this infiltration (Fig. 8.59). The submucosal glands are usually atrophic but some glands may be dilated, containing large quantities of mucus englobing inflammatory cells. The bronchial muscular layer is hypertrophied in some places and atrophied in others. Fibrous bands may encircle, dissect, or completely replace the muscle bundles. The peribronchial elastic fibres are fragmented and disorganized. In some instances, especially in areas where the dilatation is saccular, the bronchial wall is completely destroyed and the regenerated epithelium, which may show squamous metaplasia, covers a layer of granulation tissue with no other supporting structures.

The bronchial arteries show extensive hypertrophy of their walls, while the pulmonary arteries in the neighbourhood may have been destroyed in the inflammatory process or may show severe endarteritis. As a result there is shunting of blood by bronchopulmonary anastomoses, leading to pulmonary hypertension.

In cases of congenital bronchiectasis there is hypoplasia of the involved lung. The inflammatory reaction is scanty and the cartilage plates are poorly developed. The most striking feature is marked hypertrophy of the bronchial muscle, which appears disorganized. Lymphangiectasis may be an associated abnormality.

5.4. *Cystic Fibrosis of the Pancreas (Mucoviscidosis)*

Inherited as an autosomal recessive trait, mucoviscidosis is characterized by pancreatic deficiency, chronic pulmonary infection, steatorrhoea, and

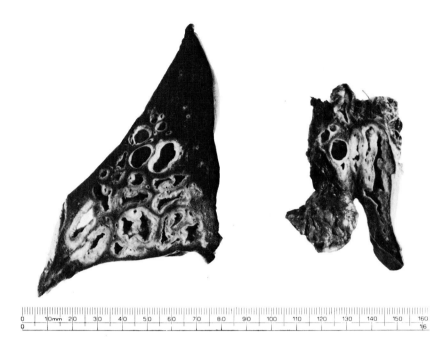

Fig. 8.58. Significant bronchiectasis in an 18-month-old infant. Courtesy of Dr C. Bozic.

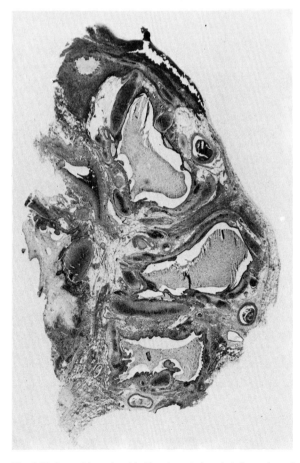

Fig. 8.59. Bronchiectasis with fibrosis and chronic inflamation of the wall containing lymphoid follicles. (H and E; 25 ×)

markedly increased sodium and chloride levels in the patients' sweat, among other clinical manifestations. Caucasian races are much the most susceptible to the disease, and the incidence in negroes and orientals is low.

The disease may be manifest at birth as intestinal obstruction resulting from meconium ileus (see p. 228). However, pulmonary involvement is by far the most serious complication of the disease, and is responsible for the high morbidity and mortality. Pulmonary manifestations may be recognized during early infancy but may go unnoticed until adolescence or adult life.

The patients usually present with repeated chronic pulmonary infections, which become progressively more severe. Areas of bronchopneumonia may never resolve as other areas are affected. These chest infections are often accompanied by severe pansinusitis, with or without nasal polyp formation. *Staphylococcus aureus* has been considered to be responsible for most infections, but recently it has been appreciated that other organisms are more important as the patients grow older. *Pseudomonas aeruginosa* is the organism most often incriminated in these cases, and *Haemophilus influenzae* is also known to play an important role. It has been shown that the *Pseudomonas aeruginosa* (mucoid type) antigen forms antigen–antibody complexes, which can be localized in many tissues in these patients, including the lung, and it is considered that some of the pulmonary damage may result from these complexes.

The frequent, repeated, and chronic pulmonary infections are the result of obstruction of the bronchial tree, in particular the distal airways, by a thick, viscoid mucus or mucopurulent secretion. Subsequently bronchopneumonia, bronchiectasis and bronchiolectasis, loss of lung elasticity, and diffuse emphysema with modifications in pulmonary function tests develop. Pulmonary hypertension follows, leading to right ventricular hypertrophy. In most cases hypertrophy of the carotid bodies is found. Pneumothorax may be a troublesome complication (Anderson 1962; Boat et al. 1969; Høiby et al. 1977; Kollberg et al. 1978; Lack 1977; Landau et al. 1979; McCrae and Raeburn 1974; Oppenheimer and Rosenstein 1979; Oppenheimer and Esterly 1974; Schiøtz et al. 1977; Schwachman et al. 1977; Stern et al. 1976, 1977; Zelkowitz and Giammona 1969). The ultrastructure of cilia in both nasal and bronchial epithelium in patients with cystic fibrosis may show various anomalies, including compound cilia, excessive cytoplasmic matrix, abnormal number and arrangement of microtubular doublets and rippled ciliary contour, abnormalities which have also been described in chronic inflammation of the respiratory tract (Howell et al. 1980; Katz and Holsclaw 1980).

Macroscopically the entire lung is involved. It is large, reddish, and emphysematous, especially at the anterior margin, while the posteriorly sited lobes may show areas of atelectasis. There are areas of consolidation, and the bronchi and bronchioles are dilated, containing abundant viscous mucus (Fig. 8.60). Abscesses are sometimes present. Microscopically the most striking feature is diffuse bronchial and bronchiolar dilatation, with the lumen completely obliterated by adherent mucus plugs. The inspissated mucus secretions contain numerous inflammatory cells, chiefly polymorphonuclear leucocytes, but including eosinophils, lymphocytes, and some plasma cells. Bacteria can be identified by gram staining.

The lesions involve the distal bronchi and bronchioles initially. These become obliterated, causing atelectasis of some of the pulmonary parenchyma distal to the obstruction. The larger bronchi are then affected, and as a result of repeated episodes of chronic inflammation there is partial destruction of the bronchial wall with cylindrical dilatation of the involved segments. These changes may involve one or more lobes, or the entire lung (Fig. 8.61).

The bronchial mucosa is covered by hypertrophic and hyperplastic mucus-secreting cells whose cytoplasm is filled with a strongly PAS- and Alcian blue-positive mucus. The bronchial wall is generally fibrous and thinned, but isolated areas show signs of muscular hypertrophy. Chronic inflammatory cells are abundant.

Areas of bronchopneumonia are found, and resolution of these zones leaves alveolar wall scarring. Abscesses are sometimes observed in the vicinity of affected airways or within the parenchyma. Most of the lung outside these areas is markedly emphysematous. Pulmonary arteries show the changes associated with moderate pulmonary hypertension.

6. Lung Involvement in Metabolic Diseases

The lung is known to be involved in Gaucher's disease. Pulmonary lesions are much more common in the infantile form (type II), but when the lesions occur in the adult form (type I) they may be widespread and cause the death of the patient. In both types the lungs show large areas of consolidation, and an entire lobe or lung may be involved. Histologically there is a diffuse infiltration of the alveolar spaces by Gaucher cells and numerous histiocytes. Alveolar walls are also infiltrated

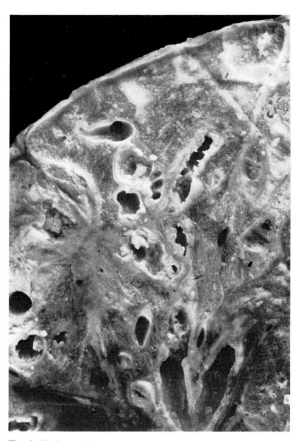

Fig. 8.60. Bronchiectasis and pulmonary consolidation in a 14-year-old boy with cystic fibrosis.

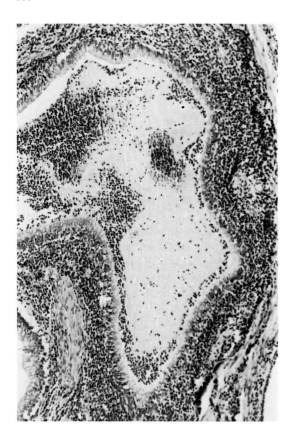

◁ **Fig. 8.61.** Bronchiectasis in cystic fibrosis. Increased number of goblet cells and mucopus obliterating the lumen. The inflammatory exudate contains numerous polymorphonuclear leucocytes. (H and E; 35 ×)

or angiomas of the lungs in infants and children are congenital developmental defects of the pulmonary vasculature, which are referred to under several synonyms: *pulmonary arteriovenous fistulas* or *aneurysms, congenital arteriovenous varix,* and *pulmonary angiomatosis.*

A significant proportion of patients with these lesions present with co-existing vascular anomalies in other organs (mucous membranes, skin, brain), forming part of a more generalized syndrome of hereditary telangiectasia of the Rendu–Osler–Weber type. Familial occurrence has been recorded.

Vascular anomalies are generally located in the periphery of the lung or in the subpleural zones. They are more common in the lower lobes, may present as localized structures, single or multiple, and are often bilateral. An elevated incidence of cerebral abscesses has been reported among patients with these lesions (Arnett and Patton 1976; Shirakusa 1978; Utzon and Bandrup 1973; Wagenvoort et al. 1978).

Microscopically the lesions may resemble capillary or cavernous angiomas, the latter becoming distended as a result of large arteriovenous anastomoses (Fig. 8.63). These abnormal vessels are lined with flattened endothelial cells, while the structure of their walls varies, being arterial and venous in different areas.

Sclerosing haemangioma of the lung (Liebow and Hubbell 1956) is a circumscribed pulmonary lesion described in the literature under several synonyms (histiocytoma, fibroxanthoma, alveolar angioblastoma, mast-cell granuloma), depending on the histological patterns which the lesion may exhibit.

These lesions have been reported in children. They are often described in the lower lobes, but can be located in any lobe and occur mainly in the periphery of the lung. Most patients are asymptomatic and the tumours are discovered on routine chest radiography. Haemoptyses have been recorded as the most common clinical symptom.

The pathogenesis of the lesions is unknown and their aetiology remains obscure. Some authors regard them as pseudoinflammatory reactions, while others consider them to be vascular lesions in various stages of sclerosis with secondary epithelial proliferation. Others, in turn, regard them as a proliferation of undifferentiated pulmonary epithelial mesenchymal tissue with secondary vascular changes (Katzenstein and Maurer 1979; Katzenstein

by histiocytes and some Gaucher cells (Fig. 8.62). Some of the distal bronchi and bronchioles may also contain these cells (Schneider et al. 1977) (p. 623).

In other forms of sphingolipidosis (Niemann–Pick), pulmonary involvement is more common, however, and it has also been seen in Fabry's disease (Bartimmo et al. 1973; Martin et al. 1972). The pulmonary parenchyma shows consolidated areas in which the alveoli are filled with foam cells. Lung involvement has also been recorded in cases of gangliosidosis (Volk et al. 1975) and mucopolysaccharidosis (de Montis et al. 1972). Recently, pulmonary vascular obstruction has been described in association with cholesterylester storage disease in a 15-year-old girl (Michels et al. 1979).

7. Tumours

Although primary lung tumours are uncommon in infancy and childhood, both benign and malignant tumours have been described in this age group. Metastatic tumours are more prevalent.

7.1. Benign

Vascular. Haemangiomas of the lung are extremely rare. Most of the lesions described as haemangiomas

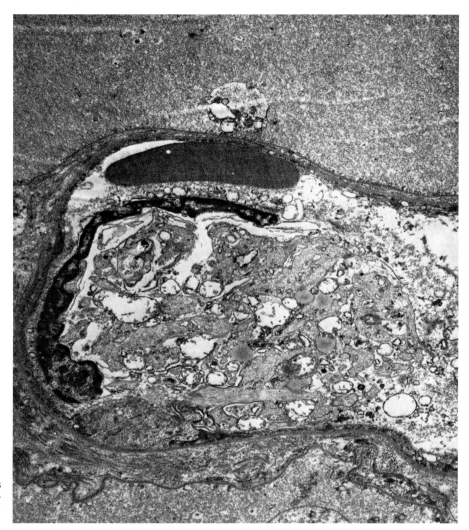

Fig. 8.62. Lung in Gaucher's disease. Gaucher cell electron photomicrograph. (15 000 ×)

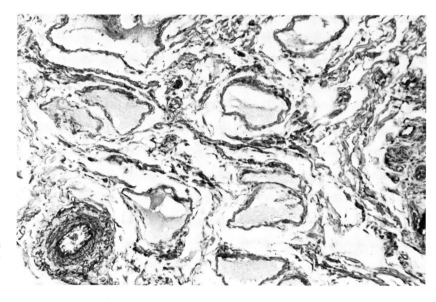

Fig. 8.63. Pulmonary arteriovenous shunt (pulmonary varix) in a newborn with cardiac malformation. (VG–Elastin; 120 ×)

et al. 1980; Lago et al. 1976; Nair et al. 1974). Ultrastructural studies have not helped to resolve the problem. Haas et al. (1972) concluded from their observations that the lesions were primarily angiomatous in nature, but Hill and Eggleston (1972) considered the primary lesions to be predominantly epithelial, with the other changes secondary phenomena.

Macroscopically, sclerosing haemangiomas are solitary, circumscribed, round or oval masses, firm or rubbery in consistency, yellow in colour, with tan or haemorrhagic areas. Calcification and even ossification have been observed in some cases.

Microscopically there may be papillary structures lined with alveolus-like mesenchymal cells, cuboidal and/or columnar in appearance, mainly at the periphery of the lesions. The supporting stroma is fibroblastic with some histiocytes, and contains many irregular dilated capillaries. In other areas the stroma is composed of numerous spindle cells separated by large bands of collagen. Hyalinization may occur in other regions, where the vessels may be seen as slit-like openings. Mitotic figures are few, and there is no cellular atypia. Evidence of both recent and old haemorrhage is seen. Plasma cells, lymphocytes, and mast cells have been observed scattered throughout lesions of this type.

Plasma-cell granuloma, although a relatively uncommon tumour, is perhaps the most common benign tumour of the lung in childhood. The lesion, in which plasma cells predominate, must be distinguished from its malignant counterpart, the pulmonary plasmacytoma. Plasma-cell granuloma has been considered to be a postinflammatory pseudotumour, and some authors use the term 'plasma-cell pseudo-tumour' when referring to the lesion. It has also been mistakenly called a fibroxanthoma, because of the presence of numerous fat-laden histiocytes, and has further been confused with sclerosing haemangioma.

The majority of plasma cell granulomas have been reported in children, and there is a female predominance. The aetiology is unknown. Clinically the condition is asymptomatic unless it produces obstruction of bronchi, causing dyspnoea. It is often discovered during routine chest radiography, and presents as a solitary, circumscribed parenchymal mass or coin lesion. The prognosis is generally good, and surgery is the treatment of choice (Bahadori and Liebow 1973; Pearl and Woolley 1973).

Macroscopically the lesions are firm or rubbery in consistency, round or oval, and yellowish-white or grey in colour. They may appear brownish owing to haemorrhages, and occasionally show central necrotic zones. They may also contain fine granular calcification. The lesions are usually peripheral and intraparenchymatous but may sometimes involve bronchi, causing obstruction.

Microscopically the tumour is made up of mature plasma cells with some lymphocytes and mononuclear cells. Russell bodies may be conspicuous. Polymorphonuclear leucocytes are occasionally observed. Histiocytes may be prominent, grouped together and located among fibroblasts arranged in whorls and supported by dense collagen bundles. Many of the histiocytes are laden with fat globules, giving the lesion a xanthomatous pattern. Mast cells are scattered throughout the tumour and some eosinophils may be present. Lymphoid follicles with germinal centres are sometimes visible.

Lymphangioleiomyomatosis (lymphangiomyomatosis) is a fairly common clinicopathological entity, with a worldwide distribution. The disease has been described exclusively in females, mainly of childbearing age, and it is not inherited. Cases have been described before the age of 20 and the clinical symptoms often begin during childhood. The lesions are not confined to the lung, but involve extrapulmonary structures, mainly the lymph nodes and lymphatics. The condition has been reported in association with tuberous sclerosis but there is some controversy as to whether the two conditions are really interrelated.

The clinical symptoms may go unrecognized for some time. The patients present with breathlessness, recurrent pneumothorax, and sometimes haemoptyses. Chylothorax is not an uncommon finding in this condition, and may be associated with chylous ascites. Pulmonary haemorrhages have also been recorded. The disease follows a relentlessly progressive course, with death from respiratory failure. The period over which this occurs is variable. Most patients affected die within 10 years of discovery; however, some have survived for more than 20 years.

Extensive hypertrophy and proliferation of smooth muscle in the wall of lymphatic vessels are the principal histological characteristics of the abnormality, but recently some authors have suggested that the proliferating cells in the lung may be derived from immature pluripotent myoid stromal cells or myofibroblasts (Bradley et al. 1980; Carrington et al. 1977e; Corrin et al. 1975; Kane et al. 1978; Kreisman et al. 1978; Monteforte and Kohnen 1974).

Macroscopically the most characteristic picture is one of honeycombing of the entire lung, with enlarged hilar lymph nodes. The pleura is thickened and the lymphatics are prominent and well defined. Microscopically the alveolar septa are diffusely thickened by proliferation and hyperplasia of smooth-muscle cells along the lymphatic channels (Fig. 8.64). Sometimes these cells form nodules about myoid stromal cells. The lesions may surround the lymphatics in the interlobular spaces, in the bronchial wall, and in the walls of the pulmonary veins, where venous obstruction may result. Intra-alveolar haemorrhages may follow, and numerous macrophages containing haemosiderin pigment are present in the alveolar spaces.

Muscular. Smooth- or striated-muscular tumours of the lung are exceedingly rare. Taylor and Miller (1969) found 21 cases of solitary *leiomyomas* described in the literature, and added one of their own. Four of these were in children and both sexes were affected, but overall there was a significant female predominance. The tumour may be situated in the periphery of the lung parenchyma (most cases) or related to a bronchus. It is possible that these tumours originate from the smooth muscles of small bronchioles or ultimately from the wall of pulmonary vessels.

Multiple congenital leiomyomas have also been described in association with multiple congenital mesenchymal tumours or fibromatosis. About 20 such cases had been reported up to 1971 (Lin and Svoboda 1971). These are multiple yellow tumour masses of variable size, distributed throughout the lung. Similar lesions are also seen in various other organs, including the skin, muscle, bone, and viscera. Most cases have been discovered shortly after birth or within the first 6 weeks of life; few cases have occurred in infancy. There is a strong male predominance and the condition is not inherited. The tumours are located adjacent to bronchioles and blood vessels, and may show central necrosis and even calcification.

These leiomyomas must be distinguished from the multiple pulmonary leiomyomatous 'hamartomas' observed in adult women, which are associated with leiomyoma of the uterus or similar subcutaneous lesions (Becker et al. 1976; Kaplan et al. 1973; Silverman and Kay 1976).

Granular cell myoblastoma is a very rare benign tumour of the respiratory tract. The tumour has been reported in childhood; the histology is similar to that described for other sites (Ostermiller et al. 1970; Suzuki et al. 1971).

Pulmonary tumours of *nervous origin* are really very rare, even though those arising in the mediastinum are common in childhood. Isolated cases of intrapulmonary tumours of nervous origin have been recorded in infancy and childhood. They include neurofibromas (often associated with generalized neurofibromatosis), neurilemmoma, and benign schwannoma (Bartley and Arean 1965; Gay and Bonmati 1954; Massero et al. 1965; Neilson 1958).

Others. Fibromas of the lung are very rare, and when present may be located peripherally in the pul-

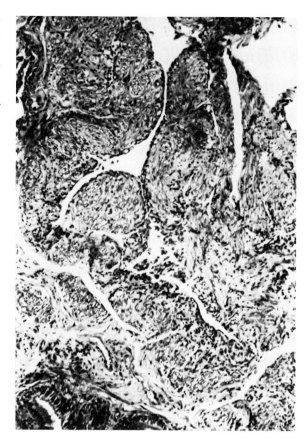

Fig. 8.64. Lymphangioleiomyomatosis from a female patient presenting with symptoms from the age of 11 years, with chylus effusion. (H and E; 225 ×)

monary parenchyma or the bronchial wall. The tumour has been reported in children. It is composed mainly of fibrocytes supported by collagen fibres, with some myxomatous areas (Roenspies et al. 1978).

Chondromas are benign, well-differentiated, hyaline cartilage outgrowths arising from the cartilaginous plates of bronchi, and are often lined with bronchial epithelium. They have been observed in childhood and present as polypoid or lobulated masses, projecting into the bronchial lumen and causing stenosis or bronchial obstruction.

Chondromas must be distinguished from chondromatous hamartomas, benign lesions made up largely of cartilage. They are considered to be hamartomas, although they continue to grow after body growth ceases. Their histogenesis is still unsettled. The lesions are relatively common and are most frequently described in adults, with a peak incidence between the fourth and sixth decades; nevertheless they do sometimes present in childhood.

Chondromatous hamartoma has been described by several synonyms (chondromas, fibroadenoma, lipochondroadenoma, adenochondroma), depending on the predominant tissue in the lesion. They are most commonly located in the lung parenchyma towards the periphery (intrapulmonary), and less frequently in the bronchial wall (endobronchial). The lesions are usually single and either lung may be affected. There is a male preponderance. Multiple tumours have also been described but they are less common, often bilateral, and are observed almost exclusively in females.

The clinical features are nonspecific and depend largely on the size and localization of the tumour. Radiography is usually of no help in establishing the diagnosis (Bateson 1965, 1970, 1973; Koutras et al. 1971; Minasian 1977).

Macroscopically the tumour is variable in size and is generally made up of a round or oval mass with a smooth surface, often lobulated. It is whitish in colour, somewhat translucent, firm in consistency, well circumscribed, and separated from the surrounding parenchyma by a pseudocapsule. Microscopically the greater portion is composed of lobules of well-differentiated hyaline cartilage interrupted by cleft-like spaces lined by cuboidal or columnar

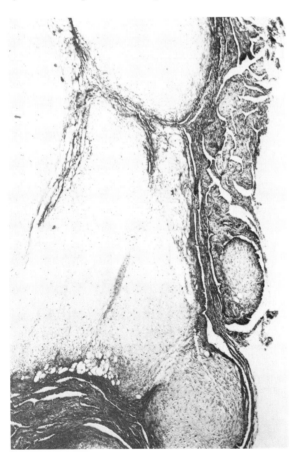

Fig. 8.65. Chondroma of the right main bronchus in a 16-year-old male (H and E; 100 ×)

epithelium resembling that of the respiratory tract (Fig. 8.65). The remainder of the tumour is made up of an admixture of various amounts of fibrous tissue, fat tissue, muscle bundles (striated and smooth), and occasionally metaplastic bone and aggregates of lymphocytes. Calcification may occur occasionally.

Recent ultrastructural studies by Stone and Churg (1977) have shown that the epithelial component of the chondromatous hamartoma is made up of cells resembling those lining the distal bronchioles and alveoli of adult lung.

Intrapulmonary teratomas are rare. Day and Taylor (1975) found only 19 recorded cases of intrapulmonary teratoma in the literature, and added one of their own. In their review they reported one malignant teratoma in an infant: the ages of the other cases ranged from 16 to 66 years. The left upper lobe was most commonly involved, and of the 16 cases for whom adequate histological descriptions are provided, nine tumours were benign and seven malignant.

Teratomas in the lung are usually large masses of greyish white, fleshy tissue, sometimes surrounding cystic cavities of variable diameter. Tissue derivatives of the three embryonic germ layers may be identified histologically. In a case described by Day and Taylor (1975) the tumour seems to have developed in ectopic thymic tissue within the lung. Another case has recently been described by Holt et al. (1978).

7.2. Malignant

7.2.1. Primary. *Haemangiopericytoma* of the lung is exceedingly rare and most of the published reports have dealt with adults. Meade et al. (1974) collected 24 cases of this tumour in the literature, and added four of their own. Three cases of the total were in children, all male. There was an overall female predominance in the total group. Babashev (cited in Ueda et al. 1977) also described a case in a 13-year-old patient with cystic lung disease. Prognosis is variable and surgery appears to be the treatment of choice.

Fibrosarcoma of soft tissues is not uncommon in childhood, but it is very rare in the lung. In a review, Webb and Hare (1961) found ten documented cases and added one of their own. Five of these were in children and the distribution between the sexes was about equal. Other cases have been described by Curry and Fuchs (1950) and Rienhoff and Broyles (1934). Guccion and Rosen (1972) did not find any cases of this lesion in the paediatric age group among the 13 cases they studied.

Primary *leiomyosarcoma* of the lung is also very rare. Ownby et al. (1976) reviewed the published cases of this tumour in childhood and found five cases (2 boys and 3 girls). They added one further case occurring in a 14-month-old boy. Two other cases have been studied by Guccion and Rosen (1972).

The tumours may take their origin in the bronchial wall or, more commonly, in the lung parenchyma. Histologically, it is important to differentiate this tumour from fibrosarcoma and certain tumours of neurogenic origin. Special stains, tissue culture, and ultrastructural studies may be necessary to arrive at a correct diagnosis. Leiomyosarcoma tends to metastasize by way of the bloodstream; involvement of the lymphatic system appears to be infrequent.

Primary rhabdomyosarcoma of the lung in childhood is rare. Ueda et al. (1977) reported a case of an embryonal rhabdomyosarcoma in a $1\frac{1}{2}$-year-old girl. This developed in a congenital cystic adenomatoid malformation. An apparent case described by Stephanopoulos and Catsaras (1963) in a 2-year-old infant was also associated with a congenital cystic malformation, and was reported as a myxosarcoma. It seems probable that the case described by Boss (1961) was a similar tumour (embryonal rhabdomyosarcoma) developing in a teratoma. Fallon et al. (1971) described a case in a 6-year-old girl, where the tumour arose from the right main bronchus.

A peculiar lesion described as *'rhabdomyomatous dysplasia'* of the lung has also been reported by Remberger and Hübner (1974), with a review of the literature and a discussion of the possible histogenesis. This appears to be a benign lesion in which the alveolar septa and bronchiolar walls are thickened and contain bundles of striated muscle fibres.

A *primary pulmonary embryonal liposarcoma* has been described in a 9-year-old girl who presented with the adrenogenital syndrome (Wu et al. 1974).

Chondrosarcoma of the lung is rare and the cases reviewed by Daniels et al. (1967) included one in a 17-year-old girl.

The term *bronchial adenoma* is now generally used to include four distinct neoplasms arising in the bronchus. Each of these lesions forms a well-defined entity. A total of 58 cases have been reported in childhood (Wellons et al. 1976).

The four tumour types are: (1) mucous gland adenoma; (2) bronchial carcinoid; (3) cylindroma or adenoid cystic carcinoma; and (4) mucoepidermoid tumour.

Mucous gland adenoma is the only truly benign lesion of the group, and is also the rarest. Emory et al. (1973) only found 11 reported cases of this lesion and they added one case of their own, occurring in a 14-year-old boy. These tumours generally take their origin in the submucosal glands of the large bronchus, and involve both the glands and their ducts. They may cause obstruction of the

bronchial lumen or stenosis by compression.

Carcinoid tumours are most common among this group, representing 80%–85% of all bronchial adenomas. They take their origin from the Kulchitsky cells (APUD) in the bronchial mucosa and have been reported at all ages. Lawson et al. (1976) subdivided this tumour into three histological subgroups: typical (most common), atypical, and metastasizing. Carcinoids are known to be of low-grade malignancy, and may metastasize to neighbouring lymph nodes or other sites after a long period. The carcinoid syndrome has been reported in some cases (Ricci et al. 1973), and acromegaly has been associated with this tumour. Most go unnoticed as they infiltrate the bronchial wall and adjacent tissue or proliferate into the lumen until large enough to cause obstruction with atelectasis, infection, and bronchiectasis. Some undergo calcification or ossification. Haemoptysis is the most frequent clinical symptom and is associated with intraluminal growth.

Cylindroma is rare, accounting for about 12%–15% of all bronchial adenomas. They are derived from the mucus-secreting cells of the bronchial mucosa, mainly the large bronchi, and histologically they resemble tumours of the major salivary glands, having that characteristic histological pattern. The tumour, although of low-grade malignancy, may slowly infiltrate the surrounding tissues with metastases to the lymph nodes and other organs. It is considered that the cylindrinoma is the most aggressive of the three malignant types, followed by the carcinoid.

Mucoepidermoid carcinoma is the least common of these tumours (2%–3%), and also the least malignant. It originates from the mucus-secreting cells of the bronchial mucosa and has a glandular pattern with areas of squamous epithelium (Condon and Phillips 1962; Conlan et al. 1978; Johnson et al. 1974; Marks and Lamberty 1977; Mullins and Barnes 1978; de Paredes et al. 1970; Régy et al. 1970; Wellons et al. 1976).

Primary carcinoma of the lung is rare in childhood. Nittu et al. (1974) reviewed the literature, which included 39 cases, including their own in a boy of 15 years 7 months. The youngest patient in the Japanese series was 2 years 3 months old; the youngest reported case is in an infant of 5 months.

The condition is usually discovered during chest radiography for ill-defined clinical symptoms, and is often misinterpreted for long periods before the correct diagnosis is made with growth of the tumour. There is an equal distribution between the sexes. Undifferentiated carcinoma is the commonest histological type in Western countries, while in Japan adenocarcinoma has been prevalent, but it must be mentioned that in many Western reports the tumour was unclassified. Squamous-cell carcinoma was rare. Metastases to one or both lungs or to distant organs have been reported. It is important to emphasize that some of the cases described as adenocarcinomas might prove to be carcinoids if reviewed critically. Long periods of survival have been reported after surgery for localized tumours. Spencer et al. (1980), in a review of 21 cases of noninvasive bronchial epithelial tumours, found one case in a boy of 7. These tumours are usually undifferentiated neoplasms, and in the case of the boy described the peripheral tumour appeared to be composed of a complex papillary process covered by cuboidal, nonciliated columnar epithelial cells bearing a striking resemblance to Clare cells, with local invasion. Askin et al. (1979) have reported on a group of malignant small round cell tumours, probably of neural origin, occurring in the thoracopulmonary region of children and adolescents. They have a distinct histological picture, different from that of neuroblastoma, Ewing's sarcoma, and rhabdomyosarcoma.

Pulmonary blastoma is also a very rare primary lung tumour, approximately 40 cases having been documented in the literature. This tumour has been described in infants and children; the youngest case recorded appears to be that of a 2-month-old infant. There is a significant male predominance.

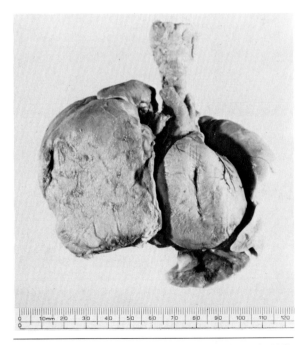

Fig. 8.66. Pulmonary blastoma occupying the inferior and middle lobes of the right lung in a 6-month-old boy. Courtesy of Dr C. Bozic.

The condition was initially described as an embryona of the lung, because of its resemblance to fetal lung. Either lung may be affected, but the lesions are located principally in the peripheral regions. The clinical symptoms and radiological features are those seen in tumours of the lung in general.

Blastomas are locally invasive and give rise to regional and distant metastases to brain, liver, adrenals, pancreas, and retroperitoneum. The size of the tumour and the extent of the metastases are important in determining the survival time. Cases with extensive metastases usually die within 2 years.

There is still much debate as to the histogenesis of this lesion. Some authors consider that the tumour is derived from pluripotent immature pulmonary blastoma; others believe that it may be a variant of carcinosarcoma. Ultrastructural studies have not been able to resolve this particular problem and the histogenesis remains uncertain (Fung et al. 1977; Jayet et al. 1977; Karcioglu and Someren 1974; Kennedy and Prior 1976; McCann et al. 1976; Valderrama et al. 1978).

Macroscopically the tumour is bulky, greyish white, fleshy and somewhat friable, occupying an entire lobe or lung. Small tumours have also been recorded. There may be large areas of necrosis and zones of old and recent haemorrhages (Fig. 8.66). Microscopically the tumour presents two distinct components, mesenchymatous and glandular (Fig. 8.67). The mesenchymatous component, which is by far the most prominent, is made up of nodules or sheets of spindle cells resembling undifferentiated sarcoma. The nuclei are round or oval, hyperchromatic, and may show pleomorphism. Nucleoli are often prominent. Mitotic figures are variable in number but not plentiful. Occasional giant cells may be present. The ground substance is myxomatous, and reticulin and collagen fibres are not abundant. Striated- or smooth-muscle elements have been noted in some cases, and chondromatous or osteoid structures have also been observed. The mesenchymatous nodules do not always surround the glandular component. This is made up of well-defined tubular structures, variable in size and number, lined with pseudostratified or stratified columnar epithelium whose cytoplasm is rich in glycogen.

Solitary pulmonary plasmacytoma is extremely rare. Recently, Baroni et al. (1977) reported a case in a 14-year-old boy, associated with an abnormal secretion of IgM. This was corrected after surgical resection of the tumour. Microscopically the tumour is made up of plasma cells at various stages of maturation. Lymphocytes may be present, occasionally forming well-defined lymphoid follicles.

Veliath et al. (1977) described a case of a *primary lymphosarcoma* of the lung in a 5-year-old girl in whom a diagnosis was made on tissue obtained by percutaneous needle biopsy of a right pulmonary mass. The child was well 1 year later, following radio- and chemotherapy. The 8½-year-old girl described by Liebow et al. (1972) with *lymphomatoid granulomatosis* of the lung was found, 2 years later, to have an eosinophilic granuloma of the skull. Furthermore, DeRemee et al. (1978) consider lymphomatoid granulomatosis to be identical pathologically with polymorphic reticulosis. It appears that one should be extremely cautious before making this diagnosis, which should be suggested only in the absence of other histological entities.

7.2.2. Metastases. The metastases of many childhood tumours are blood-borne, and they generally produce massive secondaries in the lung. These may be limited in number, or occasionally there is a diffuse dissemination of small lesions scattered throughout the parenchyma. Metastases to the lung are common in *Wilm's tumour, hepatoblastoma, osteosarcoma, Ewing's sarcoma*, and *sarcomas of soft tissues. Neuroblastoma* spreads to the lung less readily, but is a common tumour, so pulmonary deposits are frequently found (Exelby 1974; Harrison et al. 1974; Jenkin 1976; MacIntosh et al. 1975; Price et al. 1975; Roggli et al. 1980; Rosen et al. 1974).

In childhood *leukaemia* the vessels of the lung contain leukaemic cells, and these cells may be seen infiltrating the alveolar wall. Perivascular aggregates can be observed in severe cases. *Non-Hodgkin's lymphomas* may also be localized in the lung, either as a primary lesion or, more often, as a secondary infiltration. *Hodgkin's disease* in childhood may involve the lung and infiltrate the parenchyma, forming nodules, or produce peribronchial or bronchial infiltrations with bronchial stenosis (Jenkin et al. 1975; O'Conor 1961; Tan et al. 1975; Wood and Coltman 1973).

7.2.3. Histiocytosis X and Similar Conditions The group of diseases commonly classed under the heading of histiocytosis X frequently involve the lung. As stated elsewhere (see p. 554), histiocytosis X includes three clinical conditions: eosinophilic granuloma, Letterer–Siwe disease, and Hand–Schüller–Christian disease.

In Letterer–Siwe disease the pulmonary lesions are diffuse and bilateral; they often appear in successive crops and can be associated with pneumothorax. There may be numerous areas of necrosis with abscess formation. Microscopically there is a diffuse proliferation of histiocytes with large giant cells, containing a yellowish granular pigment in their cytoplasm. The inflammatory infiltrate may be

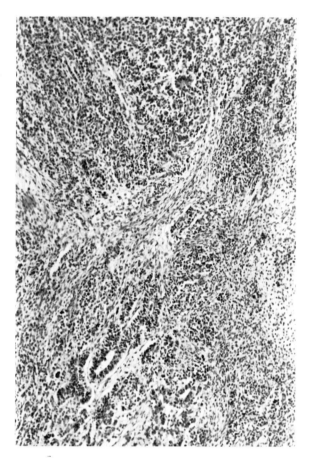

Fig. 8.67. Pulmonary blastoma with its epithelial nests in an abundant loose mesenchymal stroma. Courtesy of Dr C. Bozic. and E; 60×)

minimal away from areas of necrosis, but scattered polymorphonuclear eosinophils sometimes accompany the lesion.

Hand–Schüller–Christian disease commonly shows pulmonary involvement. The lesions are bilateral and diffuse, with formation of granulation tissue associated with active fibrosis and a chronic inflammatory infiltrate. The abnormal histiocytes often have a xanthomatous appearance.

Although eosinophilic granuloma is generally described in bones, it has long been recognized that it can occur as an isolated lesion in the lung. The majority of cases have been reported in adults, with a male preponderance. Radiography of the chest reveals disseminated nodules in both lung fields, which are more prominent in the hilar region. Sometimes cavities of variable sizes are apparent, and emphysema is not infrequent. During the late stages of the disease fibrosis with honeycombing may be conspicuous. Pneumothorax and pleural effusion have been recorded in a number of cases.

Macroscopically the lungs show numerous small cavities throughout the parenchyma. There is also nodular fibrosis with a classic honeycomb appearance in some cases. Microscopically there is marked fibrous thickening of the alveolar wall, with the presence of a granulomatous infiltration containing numerous large histiocytes having a foamy granular cytoplasm with pigment granules. The nuclei are large and folded; nucleoli are prominent. There is a moderate infiltration of lymphocytes and plasmocytes accompanied by varying quantities of eosinophils scattered throughout the granulation tissue. Fibroblastic proliferation is also evident. Distal bronchi and bronchioles and the vessels in adjacent areas are involved in the granulomatous process. Similar lesions are sometimes observed in the pleura.

Ultrastructural studies of histiocytes in histiocytosis X have shown that they contain specific cytoplasmic invaginations (X-bodies) characteristic of the group of diseases (Aftimos et al. 1974; Basset et al. 1978; Jacot-des-Combes and Kapanci 1977; Matlin et al. 1972; Nezelof et al. 1980; Smith et al. 1974; Vogel and Vogel 1972).

7.2.4. Pleural Tumours. Mesothelioma of the pleura is very rare in childhood. In a retrospective study,

Grundy and Miller (1972) were able to collect 13 well-documented cases of malignant mesothelioma in the United States. Eight of the patients were 16 years of age or less and the remaining five were 17 years old. The youngest patient was 4. There was a significant male predominance. Histologically the majority of tumours showed a fibrous pattern, which is often described in the literature in the paediatric age group (Fig. 8.68).

The tumour often progresses without clinical symptoms until late in the course of the disease, when the patient presents with thoracic pain, sometimes dyspnoea, and pleural effusion. Death usually takes place within 12 months of the initial symptoms. Although malignant mesothelioma in adults is often related to environmental factors, principally exposure to asbestos (Whitewell et al. 1977), no such relationship was found in the cases studied by Grundy and Miller (1972). Li (1977), in a review of second malignant tumours after treatment of malignancy in childhood, recorded mesothelioma arising 16 years after radiotherapy for Wilms' tumour.

The microscopical pattern is very often mixed

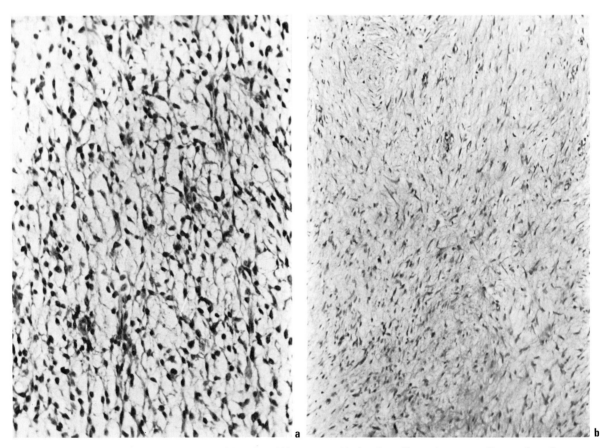

Fig. 8.68. a and **b** Mesothelioma in a 14-year-old girl: **a** Pleural biopsy at age 12, showing a fibrocytic tumour of low-grade malignancy. (H and E; 120 ×) **b** At post-mortem 1½ years later, numerous atypical cells and mitotic figures are present. (H and E; 160 ×)

(Klima and Gyorkey 1977), and ultrastructural studies have confirmed that these tumours are derived from both epithelial and fibroblastic components of the mesothelial layer (Osamura 1977).

Malignant mesenchymoma of the pleura has been described by Darling et al. (1967: cited in Holdsworth Mayer et al. 1974) in a 3-month-old girl. This tumour showed the histological patterns encountered in similar tumours in other sites.

Fibroma or *benign localized mesothelioma* of the pleura, although rare, has been recorded in childhood. The tumours can occur singly but are sometimes multiple and bilateral, and are known to evolve over very long periods. They may recur after excision (Scattini and Orsi 1973). Fibromas of the pleura are variable in size and usually nodular, firm, and yellowish white; they have been observed on both the visceral and parietal layers. Spontaneous regression has been recorded in some cases. Microscopically they are composed of proliferating fibroblasts supported by thick collagen bundles and reticulin fibres, sometimes set in a myxoid ground substance. Mitotic figures may be prominent but metastases do not occur and the prognosis is favourable, supporting the benign nature of these lesions.

General References: Development and Structure

Boyden EA (1969) The pattern of the terminal air spaces in a premature infant of 30–32 weeks that lived nineteen and a quarter hours. Am J Anat 126: 31

Charnock EL, Doershuk CF (1973) Developmental aspects of the human lung. Pediatr Clin North Am 20: 275

Emery JL, Wilcock PF (1966) The post-natal development of the lung. Acta Anat (Basel) 65: 10

Gehr P, Bachofen M, Weibel ER (1978) The normal human lung: Ultrastructure and morphometric estimation of diffusion capacity. Respir Physiol 32: 121

Huang TW (1978) Composite epithelial and endothelial basal laminas in human lung. Am J Pathol 93: 681

Kapanci Y, Mo Costabella P, Cerutti P, Assimacopoulos A (1979) Distribution and function of cytoskeletal proteins in lung cells with particular reference to 'contractile interstitial cells'. In: Jasmin G, Cantin M (eds) Methods and achievements in experimental pathology. Karger, Basel, p 147

McDougall J (1978) Endocrine-like cells in the terminal bronchioles and saccules of human fetal lung: an ultrastructural study. Thorax 33: 43

Murray JF (1976) The normal lung: the basis for diagnosis and treatment of pulmonary disease. Saunders, Philadelphia, p 1

O'Rahlly R, Tucker JA (1973) The early development of the larynx in staged human embryos. 1. Embryos of the first five weeks (to stage 15). Ann Otol Rhinol Laryngol 82 [Suppl]: 3

Patten BM (1968) Human embryology, 3rd edn. Blakiston Division of McGraw-Hill, NY, p 345 and p 395

Reid L (1967) The embryology of the lung. In : De Reuck AVS, Porter R (eds) Development of the lung. Little, Brown, Boston (Ciba Foundation Symposium, p 109)

Reverdin N, Gabbiani G, Kapanci Y (1975) Actin in tracheobronchial ciliated epithelial cells. Experientia 31: 1348

Yoneda K (1977) Pilocarpine stimulation of the bronchiolar Clara cell secretion. Lab Invest 37: 447

References

Abioye AA, Edington GM (1972) Prevalence of amoebiasis at autopsy in Ibadan. Trans R Soc Trop Med Hyg 66: 754

Ablow RC, Driscoll SG, Effmann EL, Gross I, Jolles CJ, Vaux R, Warshaw JB (1976) A comparison of early-onset group B streptococcal neonatal infection and the respiratory distress syndrome of the newborn. N Engl J Med 294: 65

Accard JL, Toty L, Personne C, Hertzog P (1970) Etude d'une série de 35 séquestrations avec référence aux formes particulières. Ann Chir Thorac Cardiovasc 9: 501

Adams FH (1966) Functional development of the fetal lung. J Pediatr 68: 794

Adams FH, Fujiwara T, Emmanouilides GC, Räihä N (1970) Lung phospholipids of human fetuses and infants with and without hyaline membrane disease. J Pediatr 77: 833

Adamson TM, Boyd BDH, Platt HS, Strang LB (1969a) Composition of alveolar liquid in the foetal lamb. J Physiol 204: 159

Adamson TM, Boyd RDH, Normand ICS, Reynolds EOR, Shaw JL (1969b) Haemorrhagic pulmonary oedema ('massive pulmonary haemorrhage') in the newborn. Lancet 1: 494

Adamson GD, Cousin AJ, Gare DJ (1980) Rhythmic fetal movements. J Obstet Gynecol 136: 239

Aftandelians R, Roafat F, Taffazoli M, Beaver PC (1977) Pulmonary capillariasis in a child in Iran. Am J Trop Med Hyg 26: 64

Aftimos S, Nassar V, Najjar S (1974) Primary pulmonary histiocytosis in an infant. Am J Dis Child 128: 851

Aherne W, Bird T, Court SDM, Gardner PS, McQuillin J (1970) Pathological changes in virus infections of the lower respiratory tract in children. J Clin Pathol 25: 7

Ahlfors CE, Goetzman BW, Halsted CC, Sherman MP, Wennberg RP (1977) Neonatal listeriosis. Am J Dis Child 131: 405

Ahlfors K, Ivarsson SA, Johnsson T, Svensson I (1978) Congenital and acquired cytomegalovirus infections. Virological and clinical studies on a Swedish infant population. Acta Paediatr Scand 67: 321

Albritton WL, Wiggins GL, Feeley JC (1976) Neonatal listeriosis: distribution of serotypes in relation to age at onset of disease. J Pediatr 88: 481

Alford CA Jr, Stagno S, Reynolds DW (1974) Congenital toxoplasmosis: clinical, laboratory and therapeutic considerations, with special reference to sub-clinical disease. Bull NY Acad Med 50: 160

Altman RP, Randolph JG, Shearin RB (1972) Tracheal agenesis: Recognition and management. J Pediatr Surg 7: 112

Ambrus CM, Weintraub DH, Choi TS, Eisenberg B, Staub HP, Courey NG, Foote RJ, Goplerud D, Moesch RV, Ray M, Bross IDJ, Jung OS, Mink IB, Ambrus JL (1974) Plasminogen in the prevention of hyaline membrane disease. Am J Dis Child 127: 189

Anderson DH (1962) Pathology of cystic fibrosis. Ann NY Acad Sci 93: 500

Anderson JM, Bain AD, Brown JK, Cockburn F, Forfar JO, Machin GA, Turner TL (1976) Hyaline-membrane disease, alkaline buffer treatment, and cerebral intraventricular haemorrhage. Lancet 1: 117

Anderson RW, Strickland MB, Tsai SH, Haglin JJ (1973) Light microscopic and ultrastructural study of the adverse effects of oxygentherapy on the neonate lung. Am J Pathol 73: 327

Arakaki DT, Waxman SH (1969) Trisomy D in a cyclops. J Pediatr 74: 620

Aranda JV, Stern L, Dunbar JS (1972) Pneumothorax with pneumoperitoneum in a newborn infant. Am J Dis Child 123: 163

Archibald RWR, Weller RO, Meadow SR (1971) Measles pneumonia and the nature of the inclusion-bearing giant cells: a light-and-electron microscope study. J Pathol 103: 27

Arean VM, Crandall CA (1971) Ascariasis. In: Marcial-Rojas PA (ed) Pathology of protozoal and helminthic disease with clinical correlation. Williams & Wilkins, Baltimore, p 769

Areechon W, Reid L (1963) Hypoplasia of lung with congenital diaphragmatic hernia. Br Med J i: 230

Arnaud JP, Prat JJ, Griscelli C, Gentilini M, Nezelof C (1976) Le diagnostic de la pneumonie à Pneumocystis carinii par l'immunofluorescence indirecte. Technique, intérêt et limites de la méthode. Nouv Presse Med 5: 2607

Arnett JC Jr, Patton RM (1976) Pulmonary varix. Thorax 31: 107

Arnold W, Huth F (1978) Electron microscope findings in four cases of nasopharyngeal fibroma. Virchows Arch [Pathol Anat] 379: 285

Ashley DJB (1972) A case of congenital tracheal obstruction with oesophageal atresia. J Pathol 108: 261

Askin FB (1975) Nose, nasopharynx, larynx and trachea. In Kissane JM (ed) Pathology of infancy and childhood. Mosby, St Louis, p 464

Askin FB, Rosai J, Sibley RK, Dehner LP, McAlister WH (1979) Malignant small cell tumor of the thoracopulmonary region in childhood. A distinctive clinicopathologic entity of uncertain histogenesis. Cancer 43: 2438

Aslam PA, Korones SB, Richardson RI Jr, Pate JW (1970) Congenital cystic adenomatoid malformation with anasarca. JAMA 212: 622

Asmar BI, Thirumoorthi MC, Dajani AS (1978a) Pneumococcal pneumonia with pneumatocele formation. Am J Dis Child 132: 1091

Asmar BI, Slovis TL, Reed JO, Dajani AS (1978b) Hemophilus influenzae type B pneumonia in 43 children. J Pediatr 93: 389

Aterman K, Patel S (1970) Striated muscle in the lung. Am J Anat 128: 341

Awe WC, Fletcher WS, Jacob SW (1966) The pathophysiology of aspiration pneumonitis. Surgery 60: 232

Bachman AL (1978) Benign, non-neoplastic conditions of the larynx and pharynx. Radiol Clin North Am 16: 273

Badrawy R, Fahmy SA, Taha AM (1973) Teratoid tumours of the nasopharynx. J Laryngol Otol 87: 795

Bahadori M, Liebow AA (1973) Plasma cell granulomas of the lung. Cancer 31: 191

Bailey BJ, Barton S (1975) Olfactory neuroblastoma—neuroblastoma—management and prognosis. Arch Otolaryngol 101: 1

Bale JF Jr, Watkins M (1978) Fulminant neonatal Hemophilus influenzae pneumonia and sepsis. J Pediatr 92: 233

Bale PM (1979) Congenital cystic malformation of the lung: A form of congenital bronchiolar ('adenomatoid') malformation. Am J Clin Pathol 71: 411

Baliga R, Chang CH, Bidani AK, Perrin EV, Fleischmann LE (1978) A case of generalized Wegener's granulomatosis in childhood: successful therapy with cyclophosphamide. Pediatrics 61: 286

Ballard PL, Ballard RA (1974) Cytoplasmic receptor for glucocorticoids in lung of the human fetus and neonate. J Clin

Invest 53: 477

Bamattar F (1971) Toxoplasmose et grossesse. Rev Med Liege 12: 463

Banerjee CK, Girling DJ, Wigglesworth JS (1972) Pulmonary fibroplasia in newborn babies treated with oxygen and artificial ventilation. Arch Dis Child 47: 509

Bankl H, Wimmer M (1972) Angeborene pulmonale Lymphangiektasien bei Linksherzhypoplasie mit Lungenvenenfehlmündung. Monatsschr Kinderheilkd 120: 152

Barkin RM (1975) Measles mortality. Am J Dis Child 129: 307

Baroni CD, Mineo TC, Ricci C, Guarino S, Mandelli F (1977) Solitary secretory plasma cytoma of the lung in a 14-year-old boy. Cancer 40: 2329

Barson AJ (1971) Fatal Pseudomonas aeruginosa bronchopneumonia in a children's hospital. Arch Dis Child 46: 55

Barson AJ (1978) Tentorial tears as a problem for the paediatrician. Paper presented at the Twenty-eighth meeting of the Paediatric Pathology Society, Bristol

Barter RA, Hudson JA (1974) Bacteriological findings in perinatal pneumonia. Pathology 6: 223

Bartimmo EE Jr, Guisan M, Moser KM (1972) Pulmonary involvement in Fabry's disease: a reappraisal. Follow-up of a San Diego kindred and review of the literature. Am J Med 53: 755

Bartlett JG, Gorbach SL, Finegold SM (1974a) The bacteriology of aspiration pneumonia. Am J Med 56: 202

Bartlett JG, Gorbach SL, Tally FP, Finegold SM (1974b) Bacteriology and treatment of primary lung abscess. Am Rev Respir Dis 109: 510

Bartley TD, Arean VM (1965) Intrapulmonary neurogenic tumors. J Thorac Cardiovasc Surg 50: 114

Barton RPE, Davey TF (1976) Early leprosy of the nose and throat. J Laryngol 90: 953

Bass JW, Steele RW, Wiebe RA (1974) Acute epiglottitis. A surgical emergency. JAMA 229: 671

Basset F, Corrin B, Spencer H, Lacronique J, Roth C, Soler P, Batteste JP, Georges R, Chrétien J (1978) Pulmonary histiocytosis X. Am Rev Resp Dis 118: 811

Bates HR Jr (1965) Fetal pulmonary hypoplasia and hydramnios. Am J Obstet Gynecol 91: 295

Bateson EM (1965) Relationship between intrapulmonary and endobronchial cartilage-containing tumours (so-called hamartomata). Thorax 20: 447

Bateson EM (1970) Histogenesis of intrapulmonary and endobronchial hamartomas and chondromas (cartilage-containing tumours). A hypothesis. J Pathol 101: 77

Bateson EM (1973) So-called hamartoma of the lung. A true neoplasm of fibrous connective tissue of the bronchi. Cancer 31: 1458

Béal G, Nezelof C, Meyer B, Paupe J, Vialatte J (1974) Protéinose alvéolaire pulmonaire. A propos d'un cas mortel chez un enfant de 3 ans. Ann Pediatr 21: 127

Beauvais P, Binet JP, Neel P, Braissaud HE (1975) Aspergillome bronchopulmonaire de l'enfant et kyste bronchogénique. Une nouvelle observation. Sem Hop Paris 51: 2775

Beazer R, DeSa DJ, Freeland AP, Roberton NRC (1973) Laryngo–tracheo–oesophageal cleft. Arch Dis Child 48: 912

Becker RM, Viloria J, Chiu CJ (1976) Multiple pulmonary leiomyomatous hamartomas in women. J Thorac Cardiovasc Surg 71: 631

Becroft DMO (1967) Histopathology of fatal adenovirus infection of the respiratory tract in young children. J Clin Pathol 20: 561

Becroft DMO (1971) Bronchiolitis obliterans, bronchiectasis and other sequelae of adenovirus type 21 infection in young children. J Clin Pathol 24: 72

Becroft DMO, Osborne DRS (1980) The lungs in fatal measles infection in childhood: Pathological, radiological and immunological correlations. Histopathology 4: 401

Bell DY, Hook GER (1979) Pulmonary alveolar proteinosis: Analysis of airway and alveolar proteins. Am Rev Respir Dis 119; 979

Benatre A, Laugier J, Grangeponte MC (1978) La maladie des membranes hyalines. Rôle du complément. Rev Fr Mal Respir 6: 67

Benirschke K, Mendoza GR, Bazeley PL (1974) Placental and fetal manifestations of cytomegalovirus infection. Virchows Arch [Cell Pathol] 16: 121

Benjamin B (1978) Treatment of infantile subglottic hemangioma with radioactive gold grain. Ann Otol 87: 18

Benveniste RJ, Harris HE (1973) Nasal hemangiopericytoma. Arch Otolaryngol 98: 358

Berezin A (1969) Histochemical study of the hyaline membrane of newborn infants and of that produced in guinea pigs. Biol Neonate 14: 90.

Berg TJ, Pagtakhan RD, Reed MH, Langston C, Chernick V (1975) Bronchopulmonary dysplasia and lung rupture in hyaline membrane disease: influence of continuous distending pressure. Pediatrics 55: 51

Berger I, Phillips WL, Shenker IR (1972) Pulmonary aspergillosis in childhood—A case report and discussion. Clin Pediatr 11: 178

Bergman B, Hedner T (1978) Antepartum administration of Terbutaline and the incidence of hyaline membrane disease in preterm infants. Acta Obstet Gynecol 57: 217

Berkovits RNP, Bos CE, Struben WH, Vervat D, Van Es HW (1974) Congenital laryngotracheoesophageal cleft. Arch Otolaryngol 100: 442

Berkowitz RL, Kantor RD, Beck GJ, Warshaw JB (1978) The relationship between premature rupture of the membranes and the respiratory distress syndrome. An update and plan of management. Am J Obstet Gynecol 131: 503

Berman JM, Colman BH (1977) Nasal aspects of cystic fibrosis in children. J Laryngol Otol 91: 133

Berthoud S (1972) Les multiples aspects de la bilharziose. A propos de quelques cas observés à Genève. Praxis 61: 809

Biggs JSG, Hemming J, McGeary H, Gaffney TJ (1974) Human amniotic and fetal neonatal pharyngeal fluids. J Obstet Gynaecol Br Cwlth 81: 70

Blackmon JA, Hicklin MD, Chandler FW (1978) Legionnaires' disease. Pathological and histological aspects of a 'new disease'. Arch Pathol Lab Med 102: 337

Blackmon JA, Chandler FW, Hicklin MD (1979), Legionnaire's disease: A review for pathologists. Pathol Annu 14: 383

Blanc WA (1976) Yellow lung in premature infants. J Pediatr 89: 131

Bliek AJ, Mulholland DJ (1971) Extralobal lung sequestration associated with fetal neonatal respiratory distress. Thorax 26: 125

Boat TF, di Sant'Agnese PA, Warwick WJ, Handwerger SA (1969) Pneumothorax in cystic fibrosis. JAMA 209: 1498

Boddy K, Dawes GS (1975) Fetal breathing. Br Med Bull 31: 3

Boisset G (1972) Subpleural emphysema complicating staphylococcal and other pneumonias. J Pediatr 81: 259

Bolens M, Mégevand A, Kapanci Y (1971) Evolution d'une pneumonie desquamative interstitielle en fibrose pulmonaire diffuse. Helv Paediatr Acta 26: 114

Boles R, Dedo H (1976) Nasopharyngeal angiofibroma. Laryngoscope 86: 364

Bone RC, Feren AP, Nahum AM, Winkelbake BG (1976) Laryngeal papillomatosis: immunologic and viral basis for therapy. Laryngoscope 86: 341

Bonikos DS, Bensch KG, Northway WH Jr (1976a) Oxygen toxicity in the newborn. The effect of chronic continuous 100 percent oxygen exposure on the lungs of newborn mice. Am J Pathol 85: 623

Bonikos DS, Bensch KG, Northway WH Jr, Edwards DK (1976b) Bronchopulmonary dysplasia, the pulmonary pathologic sequel of necrotizing bronchiolitis and pulmonary fibrosis. Hum Pathol 7: 643

Booth JB, Berry CL (1967) Unilateral pulmonary agenesis. Arch Dis Child 42: 361

Booth JB, Osborn DA (1970) Granular cell myoblastoma of the larynx. Acta Otolaryngol 70: 279

Borrie J, Gwynne JF (1973) Paraffinoma of lung: lipoid pneumonia. Thorax 28: 214

Boss JH (1962) Mixed embryonic tumor of the lung in a three-year-old girl. Am Rev Respir Dis 85: 735

Boué A, Cabau N (1978) Epidémiologie des infections par le cytomégalovirus. Nouv Presse Med 7: 3135

Boyd WP Jr, Campbell FW, Trudeau WL (1978) Strongyloides stercoralis. Hyperinfection. Am J Trop Med Hyg 27: 39

Boyden EA (1955) Developmental anatomy, physiology and pathology. Developmental anomalies of the lung. Am J Surg 80: 79

Boyden EA (1958) Bronchogenic cysts and the theory of intralobar sequestrations; new embryologic data. J Thorac Surg 35: 604

Boyden EA (1972) Structure of compressed lungs in congenital diaphragmatic hernia. Am J Anat 134: 497

Boyden EA, Bill AH Jr, Creighton SA (1962) Presumptive origin of a left lower accessory lung from an esophageal diverticulum. Surgery 52: 323

Boyle WF, Riggs JL, Oshiro LS, Lennette EH (1973) Electron microscopic identification of Papova virus in laryngeal papilloma. Laryngoscope 83: 1102

Bozic C (1974) Ectopic fetal adrenal cortex in the lung of a newborn. Virchows Arch [Pathol Anat] 363: 371

Bradley SL, Dines DE, Soule EH, Muhm JH (1980) Pulmonary lymphangiomyomatosis. Lung 158: 69

Brazy JA, Crenshaw MC, Brumley GE (1978) Amniotic fluid cortisol in normal and diabetic pregnant women and its relation to respiratory distress in the neonate. Am J Obstet Gynecol 132: 567

Bretagne MC, Hazeaux M, Deschamps JP, Pernot C, Werner J, Neimann N, Theheux A (1972) Diagnostic radiologique des agénésies et hypoplasies pulmonaires. A propos de 8 observations du C.H.U. de Nancy. J Radiol Electrol Med Nucl 53: 125

Brewer LL, Moskowitz PS, Carrington CB, Bensch KG (1979) Pneumatosis pulmonalis: A complication of the idiopathic respiratory distress. Am J Pathol 95: 171

Briselli M, Mark GJ, Grillo HC (1978) Tracheal carcinoids. Cancer 42: 2870

Brook I, Finegold SM (1979) Bacteriology and therapy of lung abscess in children. J Pediatr 94: 10

Bruhn FW, Yeager AS (1977) Respiratory syncytial virus in early infancy. Circulating antibody and the severity of infection. Am J Dis Child 131: 145

Bruhn FW, Mokrohisky ST, McIntosh K (1977) Apnea associated with respiratory syncytial virus infection in young infants. J Pediatr 90: 382

Buchanan MC (1959) Sequestration of the lung. Arch Dis Child 34: 137

Buckfield PM, Holdaway MD, Horowitz S, Kean MR (1971) Bilateral congenital choanal atresia associated with anomalies of the foregut. Aust Paediatr J 7: 37

Bureau MA, Fecteau C, Patriquin H, Rola-Pleszczynski H, Masse S, Begin R (1979) Farmer's lung in early childhood. Am Rev Respir Dis 119: 671

Burke JA (1978) Strongyloidiasis in childhood. Am J Dis Child 132: 1130

Burkitt DP (1970) General features and facial tumours. In: Burkitt DP, Wright D (eds) Burkitt's lymphoma. Livingstone, Edinburgh, p 6

Byrd RR, Gracey DR (1973) Immunosuppressive treatment of idiopathic pulmonary hemosiderosis. JAMA 226: 458

Caffrey PR, Altman RS (1965) Pulmonary alveolar microlithiasis occurring in premature twins. J Pediatr 66: 758

Cameron JL. Anderson RP, Zuidema GD (1967) Aspiration pneumonia. A clinical and experimental review. J Surg Res 7: 44

Campbell RE, Hoffman RR Jr (1974) Predictability of pneumothorax in hyaline membrane disease. Am J Roentgenol 120: 274

Campbell S (1968) Death from paraquat in a child. Lancet 1: 144

Canalis RF, Platz CE, Cohn AM (1976) Laryngeal rhabdomyosarcoma. Arch Otolaryngol 102: 104

Canalis RF, Jenkins HA, Hemenway WG, Lincoln C (1978) Nasopharyngeal rhabdomyosarcoma. A clinical perspective. Arch Otolaryngol 104: 122

Cantrell RW, Bell RA, Moricka WT (1978) Acute epiglottis—Intubation versus tracheostomy. Laryngoscope 88: 994

Carpenter RJ, Neel HB (1977) Correction of choanal atresia in children and adults. Laryngoscope 87: 1304

Carrington CB, Liebow AA (1966) Limited forms of angiitis and granulomatosis of Wegener's type. Am J Med 41: 497

Carrington CB, Addington WW, Goff AM, Madoff IM, Marks A, Schwaber JR, Gaensler EA (1969) Chronic eosinophilic pneumonia. N Engl J Med 280: 786

Carrington CB, Gaensler EA, Mikus JP, Schachter AW, Burke GW, Goff AM (1976) Structure and function of sarcoidosis. Ann NY Acad Sci 278: 265

Carrington CB, Cugell DW, Gaensler EA, Marks A, Reeding RA, Schaaf JT, Tomasian A (1977) Lymphangioleiomyomatosis: physiologic–pathologic–radiologic correlations. Am Rev Respir Dis 118: 977

Carrington CB, Gaensler EA, Coutu RE, Fitzgerald MX, Gupta RG (1978) Natural history and treated course of usual and desquamative interstitial pneumonia. N Engl J Med 298: 801

Cayeux P (1972) Infections néonatales à streptocoques du groupe B. Constatations étiologiques. A propos de 77 observations. Arch Fr Pediatr 29: 391

Chabrolle JP, Valleur D, Caldera R, Carnot JF, Denavit MF, Lesage B, de Montis G, Rossier A (1977) Essai d'évaluation objective de l'infection néonatale. Ann Pediatr 24: 23

Chalhub EG, Baenziger J, Feigen RD, Middlekamp JN, Shackelford GD (1977) Congenital herpes simplex type II infection with extensive hepatic calcification, bone lesions and cataracts: complete postmortem examination. Dev Med Child Neurol 19: 527

Chambers SR, Chambers CL, Baskin TW (1971) Pulmonary alveolar haemorrhage with glomerulonephritis and SA sicklemia. Goodpasture's syndrome in a Negro girl. Clin Pediatr 10: 351

Chang N, Hertzler JH, Gregg RH, Wael Lofti M, Brough AJ (1968) Congenital stenosis of the right mainstem bronchus: a case report. Pediatrics 41: 739

Charles D (1960) Fetal lung pathology and hydramnios. Obstet Gynecol 16: 495

Chattopadhyay AK, Dasgupta G (1976) Teratoid polyp of the nasopharynx. J Laryngol Otol 90: 1065

Chaudhry AP, Haar JG, Koul A, Nickerson PA (1979) Olfactory neuroblastoma (esthesioneuroblastoma). A light and ultrastructural study of two cases. Cancer 44: 564

Chessels JM, Wigglesworth JS (1971) Haemostatic failure in babies with rhesus isoimmunisation. Arch Dis Child 46: 38

Ch'In KY, Tang MY (1949) Congenital adenomatoid malformation of one lobe of a lung with general anasarca. Arch Pathol 48: 221

Cho CT, Hiatt WO, Behbehani AM (1973) Pneumonia and massive pleural effusion associated with adenovirus type 7. Am J Dis Child 126: 92

Cho SY, Sastre M (1976) Pulmonary yellow hyaline membrane disease. Arch Pathol Lab Med 100: 145

Chusid MJ, Heyrman KA (1978) An outbreak of *Pneumocystis*

carinii pneumonia at a pediatric hospital. Pediatrics 62: 1031

Cipriano P, Sweeney LJ, Hutchins GM, Rosenquist GC (1975) Horse-shoe lung in an infant with recurrent pulmonary infections. Am J Dis Child 129: 1343

Clairmont AA, Wright RE, Rooker DT, Butz WC (1975) Papillomas of the nasal and paranasal cavities. South Med J 68: 41

Clark NS (1963) Bronchiectasis in childhood. Br Med J i: 80

Clark RB III, Johnson FC (1961) Idiopathic pulmonary alveolar microlithiasis. A case report and brief review of the literature. Pediatrics 28: 650

Coates AL, Bergsteinsson H, Desmond K, Outerbridge EW, Beaudry PH (1978) Long-term pulmonary sequelae of the Wilson–Mikity syndrome. J Pediatr 92: 247

Cohen MM, Weintraub DH, Lilienfeld AM (1960) The relationship of pulmonary hyaline membrane to certain factors in pregnancy and delivery. Pediatrics 26: 42

Cohen SR (1975) Cleft larynx. A report of seven cases. Ann Otol 84: 747

Cohen SR, Chai J (1978) Epiglottis: twenty-year study with tracheotomy. Ann Otol 87: 461

Cohen SR, Landing BH, Isaacs H (1978a) Fibrous histiocytoma of the trachea. Ann Otol Rhinol Laryngol 87: 2

Cohen SR, Landing BH, Isaacs H, King KK, Hanson V (1978b) Solitary plasmacytoma of the larynx and upper trachea associated with systemic lupus erythematosus. Ann Otol Rhinol Laryngol 87: 11

Cohen SR, Landing BH, King KK, Isaacs H (1978c) Wegener's granulomatosis causing laryngeal and tracheobronchial obstruction in an adolescent girl. Ann Otol Rhinol Laryngol 87: 15

Cohen SR, Landing BH, Byrne WJ, Feig S, Isaacs H (1978d) Primary lymphosarcoma of the larynx in a child. Ann Otol Rhinol Laryngol 87: 20

Cole VA, Normand ICS, Reynolds EOR, Rivers RPA (1973) Pathogenesis of hemorrhagic pulmonary edema and massive pulmonary haemorrhage in the newborn. Pediatrics 51: 175

Coleman M, Dehner LP, Sibley RK, Burke BA, l'Heureux PR, Thompson TR (1980) Pulmonary alveolar proteinosis: An uncommon cause of chronic neonatal respiratory distress. Am Rev Respir Dis 121: 583

Collins HA, Guest JL, Daniel RA Jr (1964) Primary lung abscess. J Thorac Cardiovasc Surg 47: 383

Compagno J (1978) Hemangio-pericytoma-like tumors of the nasal cavity: a comparison with hemangiopericytoma of soft tissues. Laryngoscope 88: 460

Compagno J, Wong RT (1977) Intranasal mixed tumors (pleomorphic adenomas). A clinicopathologic study of 40 cases. Am J Clin Pathol 68: 213

Compagno J, Hyams VJ, Lepore ML (1976) Nasal polyposis with stromal atypia: review and follow-up study of 14 cases. Arch Pathol Lab Med 100: 244

Condon VR, Phillips EW (1962) Bronchial adenoma in children. A review of the literature and report of three cases. Am J Roentgenol 88: 543

Conlan AA, Payne WS, Woolner LB, Sanderson DR (1978) Adenoid cystis carcinoma (cylindroma) and muco-epidermoid carcinoma of the bronchus. J Thorac Cardiovasc Surg 76: 369

Conley J, Healey WV, Blaugrund SM, Perzin KH (1968) Nasopharyngeal angiofibroma in the juvenile. Surg Gynecol Obstet 126: 825

Cooper DM, Cutz E, Levison H (1977) Occult pulmonary abnormalities in asymptomatic asthmatic children. Chest 71: 361

Cooperman EM (1969) Wilson–Mikity syndrome (pulmonary dysmaturity syndrome). Can Med Ass J 100: 909

Corrin B, Liebow AA, Friedman PJ (1975) Pulmonary lymphangiomyomatosis. A review. Am J Pathol 79: 347

Cotton BH, Spaulding K, Penido JRF (1952) An accessory lung:

report of a case. J Thorac Surg 23: 508

Couvreur J (1971) Epidémiologie et fréquence de la toxoplasmose. Rev Med Liege 12: 407

Cowan DE (1968) The relationships of allergic and infectious conditions to the upper respiratory tract. Trans Am Acad Ophthal Otolaryngol 72: 943

Cowper SG (1973) Bilharziasis (schistosomiasis) in Nigeria. Trop Geogr Med 25: 105

Cox F, Hughes WT (1975) Cytomegaloviremia in children with acute lymphocytic leukemia. J Pediatr 87: 190

Crystal RG, Fulmer JD, Baum BJ, Bernardo J, Bradley KH, Bruel SD, Elson NA, Fells GA, Ferrans VJ, Gadek JE, Hunninghake GW, Kawanami O, Kelman JA, Line BR, McDonald JA, McLees BD, Roberts WC, Rosenberg DM, Tolstoshev P, Von Gal E, Weinberger SE (1978) Cells, collagen and idiopathic pulmonary fibrosis. Lung 155: 199

Curry JJ, Fuchs JE (1950) Expectoration of a fibrosarcoma: patient well four years later. J Thorac Surg 19: 135

Cutz E, Levison H, Cooper DM (1978) Ultrastructure of air ways in children with asthma. Histopathology 2: 407

Dain DW, Randall JL, Smith JW (1970) Starch in the lungs of newborns following positive-pressure ventilation. Am J Dis Child 119: 218

Daniele RP, McMillan LJ, Dauber JH, Roseman MD (1978) Immune complexes in sarcoidosis. A correlation with activity and duration of disease. Chest 74: 261

Daniels AC, Conner GH, Straus FH (1967) Primary chondrosarcoma of the tracheobronchial tree. Report of a unique case and brief review. Arch Pathol 84: 615

Davis LE, Tweed GV, Stewart JA, Bernstein MT, Miller GL, Gravelle CR, Chin TDY (1971) Cytomegalovirus mononucleosis in a first trimester pregnant female with transmission to the fetus. Pediatrics 48: 200

Davison FW (1963) Hyperplastic sinusitis: A five year study. Trans Am Laryngol Assem 84: 75

Dawes GS (1973) Revolutions and cyclical rhythms in prenatal life: fetal respiratory movements rediscovered. Pediatrics 51: 965

Day DW, Taylor SA (1975) An intrapulmonary teratoma associated with thymic tissue. Thorax 30: 582

DeBuse PJ, Morris G (1973) Bilateral pulmonary agenesis, oesophageal atresia and the first arch syndrome. Thorax 28: 526

Dehner LP (1973) Tumors of the mandible and maxilla in children. I. Clinicopathologic study of 46 benign lesions. Cancer 31: 364

Delage G, Brochu P, Pelletier M, Jasmin G, Lapointe N (1979) Giant-cell pneumonia caused by parainfluenza virus. J Pediatr 94: 426

Delarue J, Paillas J, Abelanet R, Chomette G (1959) Les bronchopneumopathies congénitales. Bronches 9: 114

Demarquez JL, Arsene-Henry-Fizet D, Babin JP, Allain D, Bentegeat J, Moulinier J, Martin C (1976) Alpha-1 antitrypsine et détresse respiratoire idiopathique du nouveau-né. Etude dans le sérum et dans les poumons. Arch Fr Pediatr 33: 359

Dempster AG (1969) Adenomatoid hamartoma of the lung in a neonate. J Clin Pathol 22: 401

DeRemee RA, Weiland LH, McDonald TJ (1978) Polymorphic reticulosis, lymphomatoid granulomatosis. Two diseases or one? Mayo Clin Proc 53: 634

Desvignes C, Hummel J, Jamet G, Levasseur P, Rojas-Miranda A, Verley J, Merlier M (1974) Emphysème pulmonaire et atrésie bronchique. A propos de quatre observations. Ann Chir Thorac Cardiovasc 13: 135

Dette GA, Gathmann HA (1974) Das Wilson–Mikity Syndrom. Klin Paediatr 186: 369

Deutsch M, Mercade R Jr, Parsons JA (1978) Cancer of the nasopharynx in children. Cancer 41: 1128

Dilworth JA, Mandell GL (1977) Adults with chronic granulomatous disease of 'childhood'. Am J Med 63: 233

Donald KJ, Edwards RL, McEvoy JDS (1975) Alveolar capillary basement membrane lesions in Goodpasture's syndrome and idiopathic pulmonary hemosiderosis. Am J Med 59: 642

Donaldson SS, Castro JR, Wilbur JR, Jesse RH Jr (1973) Rhabdomyosarcoma of head and neck in children. Combination treatment by surgery, irradiation and chemotherapy. Cancer 31: 26

Doran TA, Ford JA, Allen LC, Wong PY, Benzie RJ (1979) Amniotic fluid lecithin/sphingomyelin ratio, palmitic acid, palmitic acid/stearic acid ratio, total cortisol, creatinine and percentage of lipid-positive cells in assessment of fetal maturity and fetal pulmonary maturity: a comparison. Am J Obstet Gynecol 133: 302

Dover AS, Escobar JA, Duenas AL, Leal EC (1975) Pneumonia associated with measles. JAMA 234: 612

Dreisin RB, Schwarz MI, Theofilopoulos AN, Stanford RE (1978) Circulating immune complexes in the idiopathic interstitial pneumonias. N Engl J Med 298: 353

Duc TV, Vinh LT, Huault G, Thieffry S (1974) Lésions laryngotrachéales provoquées par l'intubation endotrachéale chez l'enfant. Etude anatomique de 53 observations. Nouv Presse Med 3: 365

Dumont A, Piché C (1969) Electron microscopic study of human histoplasmosis. Arch Pathol 87: 168

Dunnill MS (1960) The pathology of asthma with special references to changes in the bronchil mucosa. J Clin Pathol 13: 27

Dutau G, Rochiccioli P, Petel B, Fanic H, Fabre J, Dalous A (1973) Séquestration pulmonaire de l'enfant. A propos d'une observation avec étude bronchologique, angiographique et anatomique. Ann Pediatr 20: 373

Dutz W (1970) Pneumocystis carinii pneumonia. Pathol Annu 5: 309

Dvorak AM, Gavaller B (1966) Congenital systemic candidiasis. Report of a case. N Engl J Med 274: 540

Edwards DK, Dyer WM, Northway WH Jr (1977) Twelve years' experience with bronchopulmonary dysplasia. Pediatrics 59: 839

Ehrenkranz RA, Bonta BW, Ablow RC, Warshaw JB (1978) Amelioration of bronchopulmonary dysplasia after vitamin E administration. N Engl J Med 299: 564

Eisenbert H, Barnett E, Simmons H (1977) Diffuse pulmonary interstitial disease, an immune complex disease. Clin Res 25: 132 A

Ekelund L, Arvidson G, Ohrlander S, Ädstedt B (1976) Changes in amniotic fluid phospholipids at treatment with glucocorticoids to prevent respiratory distress syndrome. Acta Obstet Gynecol Scand 55: 413

Elkon D, Hightower SI, Lim ML, Cantrell RW, Constable WC (1979) Esthesioneuroblastoma. Cancer 44: 1087

Elrad H, Beydoun SN, Hagen JH, Cabalum MT, Aubry RH, Smith C (1978) Fetal pulmonary maturity as determined by fluorescent polarization of amniotic fluid. Am J Obstet Gynecol 132: 681

Emanuel B, Lieberman AD, Goldin M, Sanson J (1962) Pulmonary candidiasis in the neonatal period. J Pediatr 61: 44

Emery JL, Haddadin AJ (1971) Squamous epithelium in respiratory tract of children with tracheo-oesophageal fistula. Arch Dis Child 46: 236

Emory WB, Mitchell WT Jr, Hatch HB Jr (1973) Mucous gland adenoma of the bronchus. Am Rev Respir Dis 108: 1407

Enfors B, Herngren L (1975) Nasal glioma. J Laryngol Otol 89: 863

Engzell VCG, Jones AW (1973) Rhinosporidiosis in Uganda. J Laryngol Otol 87: 795

Epstein MA, Achong BG (1970) The fine structure of cultured Burkitt lymphoblasts of established in vitro stains. In: Burkitt DP, Wright D (eds) Burkitt's Lymphoma. Livingstone, Edinburgh, p 118

Eskes TKA (1971) Intrauterine pressure and the human foetus. In: Gevers RH, Ruys JH (eds) Physiology and pathology in the perinatal period. Leiden University Press, Leiden, p 28

Esterly JR, Oppenheimer EA (1966) Massive pulmonary haemorrhage in the newborn. I. Pathologic considerations. J Pediatr 69: 3

Esterly JR, Oppenheimer EA (1970) Lymphangiectasis and other pulmonary lesions in the asplenia syndrome. Arch Pathol 90: 553

Evans JNG, MacLachlan RF (1971) Choanal atresia. J Laryngol Otol 85: 903

Exelby PR (1974) Management of embryonal rhabdomyosarcoma in children. Surg Clin North Am 54: 849

Fallon G, Schiller M, Kilman JW (1971) Primary rhabdomyosarcoma of the bronchus. Ann Thorac Surg 12: 650

Farrell PM, Avery ME (1975) Hyaline membrane disease. Am Rev Respir Dis 111: 657

Farrell PM, Wood RE (1976) Epidemiology of hyaline membrane disease in the United States: Analysis of national mortality statistics. Pediatrics 58: 167

Fauci AS, Wolff SM (1973) Wegener's granulomatosis: Studies in eighteen patients and a review of the literature. Medicine 52: 535

Fechner RE, Lamppin DW (1972) Midline malignant reticulosis: A clinicopathologic entity. Arch Otolaryngol 95: 467

Fechner RE, Sessions RB (1977) Inverted papilloma of the lacrimal sac, the paranasal sinuses and the cervical region. Cancer 40: 2303

Fechner RE, Goepfert H, Alford BR (1974) Invasive laryngeal papillomatosis. Arch Otolaryngol 99: 147

Fedrick J, Butler NR (1970a) Certain causes of neonatal death. I. Hyaline membranes. Biol Neonate 15: 229

Fedrick J, Butler NR (1970b) Certain causes of neonatal death. II. Intraventricular haemorrhage. Biol Neonate 15: 257

Fedrick J, Butler NR (1971a) Certain causes of neonatal death. III. Pulmonary infection (a) Clinical factors. Biol Neonate 17: 458

Fedrick J, Butler NR (1971b) Certain causes of neonatal death. IV. Massive pulmonary haemorrhage. Biol Neonate 18: 243

Feldman HA (1974) Toxoplasmosis: an overview. Bull NY Acad Med 50: 110

Felman AH, Rhatigan RM, Pierson KK (1972) Pulmonary lymphangiectasis; observation in 17 patients and proposed classification. Am J Roentgenol 116: 548

Felson B (1972) The many faces of pulmonary sequestration. Semin Roentgenol 7: 3

Ferguson CF, Flake CG (1961) Subglottic hemangioma as a cause of respiratory obstruction in infants. Ann Otol Rhinol Laryngol 70: 1095

Fernandez CF, Cangir A, Samaan NA, Rivera R (1976) Nasopharyngeal carcinoma in children. Cancer 37: 2787

Feroldi J, Morgon A, Martin C (1974) A propos d'un cas de gliome des fosses nasales. J Fr Otorhinolaryngol 23: 889

Feuerstein SS (1973) Subglottic hemangioma in infants. Laryngoscope 83: 466

Fiala M, Payne JE, Berne TV, Moore TC, Henle W, Montgomerie JZ, Chatterjee SN, Guze LB (1975) Epidemiology of cytomegalovirus infection after transplantation and immunosuppression. J Infect Dis 132: 421

Finegold MJ, Katzew H, Genieser NB, Becker MH (1971) Lung structure in thoracic dystrophy. Am J Dis Child 122: 153

Finlay-Jones JM, Papadimitriou JM, Barter RA (1973) Pulmonary hyaline membrane: light and electron microscopic study of the early stage. J Pathol 112: 117

Fisher ER, Dimling C (1964) Rhinoscleroma. Light and electron microscopic studies. Arch Pathol 78: 501

Fishman AP (1978) UIP, DIP, and all that. N Engl J Med 298: 843

Fletcher BD, Outerbridge EW, Dunbar JS (1970) Pulmonary interstitial emphysema in newborn. J Can Assoc Radiol 21: 273

Forrest JB, Rossman CM, Newhouse MT, Ruffin R (1979) Activation of nasal cilia in immotile cilia syndrome. Am Rev Resp Dis 120: 511

Foulon E, Nogues C, Joron F, Charles J, Meyer B, Paupe J, Vialatte J (1974) Hémosidérose pulmonaire idiopathique de l'enfant. A propos de deux observations. Ann Pediatr 21: 145

Fox H (1964) Laryngeal atresia. Arch Dis Child 39: 641

Fox HE, Hohler CW (1977) Fetal evaluation by Real-time imaging. Obstet Gynecol 20: 339

Fox B, Bull TB, Arden GB (1980) Variations in the ultrastructure of human nasal cilia including abnormalities found in retinitis pigmentosa. J Clin Pathol 33: 327

Foy HM, Cooney MK, Allan I, Kenny GE (1979) Rates of pneumonia during influenza epidemics in Seattle, 1964 to 1975. JAMA 241: 253

France NW, Brown RJK (1971) Congenital pulmonary lymphangiectasis. Arch Dis Child 46: 528

Franciosi RA, Knostman JD, Zimmerman RA (1973) Group B streptococcal neonatal and infant infections. J Pediatr 82: 707

Frenkel JK (1974a) La toxoplasmose chez l'animal et chez l'homme. Med Hyg 32: 323

Frenkel JK (1974b) Breaking the transmission chain of toxoplasma: A program for the prevention of human toxoplasmosis. Bull NY Acad Med 50: 228

Frommell GT, Bruhn FW, Schwartzman JD (1977) Isolation of Chlamyelia trachomatis from infant lung tissue. N Engl J Med 296: 1150

Frugoni P, Ferlito A (1976) Pleomorphic rhabdomyosarcoma of the larynx. A case report and review of the literature. J Laryngol 90: 687

Fu YS, Perzin KH (1974a) Non-epithelial tumors of the nasal cavity, paranasal sinuses and nasopharynx: a clinicopathologic study. I. General features and vascular tumors. Cancer 33: 1275

Fu YS, Perzin KH (1974b) Non-epithelial tumors of the nasal cavity, paranasal sinuses and nasopharynx: a clinicopathologic study. II. Osseous and fibro-osseous lesions, including osteoma, giant cell tumor and osteoblastoma. Cancer 33: 1289

Fu YS, Perzin KH (1974c) Non-epithelial tumors of the nasal cavity, paranasal sinuses and nasopharynx: a clinicopathologic study. III. Cartilaginous tumors (chondroma, chondrosarcoma). Cancer 34: 453

Fu YS, Perzin KH (1975) Non-epithelial tumors of the nasal cavity, paranasal sinuses and nasopharynx: a clinicopathologic study. IV. Smooth muscle tumors (leiomyoma, leiomyosarcoma). Cancer 35: 1300

Fu YS, Perzin KH (1976a) Non-epithelial tumors of the nasal cavity, paranasal sinuses and nasopharynx: a clinicopathologic study. V. Skeletal muscle tumors (rhabdomyoma and rhabdomyosarcoma). Cancer 37: 364

Fu YS, Perzin KH (1976b) Non-epithelial tumors of the nasal cavity, paranasal sinuses and nasopharynx: a clinicopathologic study. VI. Fibrous tissue tumors (fibroma, fibromatosis, fibrosarcoma). Cancer 37: 2912

Fu YS, Perzin KH (1977) Non-epithelial tumors of the nasal cavity, paranasal sinuses and nasopharynx: a clinicopathologic study. VII. Myxomas. Cancer 39: 195

Fu YS, Perzin KH (1979) Nonepithelial tumors of the nasal cavity. Paranasal sinuses and nasopharynx. A clinicopathologic study. X. Malignant lymphomas. Cancer 43: 611

Fujikura T, Klionsky B (1975) The significance of meconium staining. Am J Obstet Gynecol 121: 45

Fuleihan FJD, Abboud RT, Balikian JP, Nucho KN (1969) Pulmonary alveolar micro-lithiasis. Lung function in cases. Thorax 24: 84

Fung CH, Lo JW, Yonan TN, Milloy FJ, Hakami MM, Changus GW (1977) Pulmonary blastoma: an ultrastructural study with a brief review of literature and a discussion of pathogenesis. Cancer 39: 153

Gaafar H, Harada Y (1976) Rhinoscleroma: a scanning electron-microscopic study. ORL 38: 350

Gandy G, Jacobson W, Gairdner D (1970) Hyaline membrane disease. I. Arch Dis Child 45: 241

Gardner PS, Court SDM, Brocklebank JT, Downham MAPS, Weightman D (1973) Virus gross-infection in paediatric wards. Br Med J ii: 571

Gaultier M, Bescol-Liversac J, Fréjaville JP, Leclerc JP, Guillam C (1973) Etude anatomo-clinique et expérimentale de l'intoxication par le Paraquat. Sem Hop Paris 49: 1972

Gay BB Jr, Bonmati J (1954) Primary neurogenic tumors of the lung and interlobar fissures: a review of clinical and radiologic findings in reported cases with addition of two new cases. Radiology 63: 43

Gebauer PW, Mason CB (1959) Intralobar pulmonary sequestration associated with anomalous pulmonary vessels: a non entity. Dis Chest 35: 282

Genin C, Touraine JL, Berger F, Bryon PA, Valancogne A, Philippe N, Monnet P (1977) BCGite généralisée dans un déficit immunitaire mixte et grave: évolution défavorable malgré une tentative de greffe de moelle osseuse. Arch Fr Pediatr 34: 639

Gentry LO, Remington JS (1970) Pneumocystis carinii pneumonia in siblings. J Pediatr 76: 769

Gerami S, Richardson R, Harrington B, Pate JW (1969) Obstructive emphysema due to bronchogenic cysts in infancy. J Thorac Cardiovasc Surg 58: 432

Gerle RD, Jaretzki A III, Ashley A, Berne AS (1968) Congenital broncho-pulmonary foregut malformation. N Engl J Med 278: 1413

Giannopoulos G (1974) Variations in the levels of cytoplasmic glucocorticoid receptors in lungs of various species at different developmental stages. Endocrinology 94: 450

Gibson M, Williams PP (1978) Haemophilus influenzae amnionitis associated with prematurity and premature membrane rupture. Obstet Gynecol 52: 70

Gifford GH Jr, Swanson L, MacCollum DW (1972) Congenital absence of the nose and anterior nasopharynx. Report of two cases. Plast Reconstr Surg 50: 5

Gilbert JG, Mazzarella LA, Feit LJ (1953) Primary tracheal tumors in the infant and adult. Arch Otolaryngol 58: 1

Gille P, Pageant G, Barbier G, Bauer J (1973) Malformation adénomateuse pulmonaire kystique congénitale. Présentation anatomoclinique d'une observation. Ann Chir Infant 14: 175

Gilman PA, Zinkham WH (1969) Severe idiopathic pulmonary hemosiderosis in the absence of clinical or radiologic evidence of pulmonary disease. J Pediatr 75: 118

Gindhart TD, Johnston WH, Chism SE, Dedo HH (1980) Carcinoma of the larynx in childhood. Cancer 46: 1683

Giraud JR, Denis F (1973) Listériose et grossesse. Nouv Presse Med 2: 211

Giraud JR, Denis F (1973) Listériose et grossesse. Nouv Presse Med 2: 211

Giraud JR, Denis F, Gargot F, Fizazi T, Babin P, de Rautlin de la Roy Y, Hoppeler A, Brisou J, de Tourris H (1973) La listériose—Incidence dans les interruptions spontanées de la grossesse. Nouv Presse Med 2: 215

Gitlin D, Craig JM (1956) The nature of the hyaline membrane in asphyxia of the newborn. Pediatrics 17: 64

Glick N, Levin S, Nelson K (1972) Recurrent pulmonary infarction in adult chickenpox pneumonia. JAMA 222: 173

Gluck L, Kulovich MV, Boere RC Jr, Brenner PH, Anderson GG, Spellacy WN (1971) The diagnosis of the respiratory distress syndrome (RDS) by amniocentesis. Am J Obstet Gynecol 109: 440

Gluck L, Kulovich MV, Eidelman AI, Cordero L, Khazin AF (1972) Biochemical development of surface activity in mammalian lung. IV. Pulmonary lecithin synthesis in the human fetus and newborn and etiology of the respiratory distress syndrome. Pediatr Res 6: 81

Goerke J (1974) Lung surfactant. Biochim Biophys Acta 344: 241

Gonzalez-Crussi F, Hull MT, Grosfield JL (1976) Idiopathic pulmonary hemosiderosis: evidence of capillary basement membrane abnormality. Am Rev Respir Dis 114: 689

Gonzalez-Crussi F, Mirkin LD, Wyllie RM, Escobedo M (1979) Acute disseminated aspergillosis during the neonatal period. Report of an instance in a 14-day-old infant. Clin Pediatr 18: 137

Gonzalez-Crussi F, Boggs JD, Raffensperger JG (1980) Brain heterotopia in the lungs. A rare cause of respiratory distress in the newborn. Am J Clin Pathol 73: 281–285

Gooch JJ, Britt EM (1978) Staphylococcus aureus colonization and infection in newborn nursery patients. Am J Dis Child 132: 893

Gotoff SP, Behrman RE (1970) Neonatal septicemia. J Pediatr 76: 143

Grans SL, Potts WJ (1951) Anomalous lobe of lung arising from the esophagus. J Thorac Surg 21: 313

Granström ML, Leinikki P, Santavuori P, Pettay O (1977) Perinatal cytomegalovirus infection in man. Arch Dis Child 52: 354

Greene DA (1976) Congenital complete tracheal rings—Report of a case. Arch Otolaryngol 102: 241

Greene R, Stark P (1978) Trauma of the larynx and trachea. Radiol Clin North Am 16: 309

Gregory GA, Tooley WH (1970) Gas embolism in hyaline membrane disease. N Engl J Med 282: 1141

Griffin N, Keeling JW, Tomlinson AH (1979) Reye's syndrome associated with respiratory syncytial virus infection. Arch Dis Child 54: 74

Gross CW, Hubbard R (1974) Management of juvenile papilloma: further observations. Laryngoscope 84: 1090

Grundy GW, Miller RW (1972) Malignant mesothelioma in childhood. Report of 13 cases. Cancer 30: 1216

Grunow WA, Esterly JR (1972) Rheumatic pneumonitis. Chest 61: 298

Guccion JG, Rosen SH (1972) Bronchopulmonary leiomyosarcoma and fibrosarcoma. A study of 32 cases and review of the literature. Cancer 30: 836

Guillozet N (1979) Measles in Africa: a deadly disease. Some personal comments. Clin Pediatr 18: 95

Gunn GC, Mishell DR Jr, Morton DG (1970) Premature rupture of the fetal membranes: a review. Am J Obstet Gynecol 106: 469

Gupta JM, Van Vliet PKJ, Vonwiller JB, Abrahams N, Fisk GC (1974) Positive airway pressure in respiratory distress syndrome. Med J Aust 1: 90

Haas JE, Yunis EJ, Totten RS (1972) Ultrsstructure of a sclerosing hemangioma of the lung. Cancer 30: 512

Halal F, Brochu P, Delage G, Lamarre A, Rivard G (1977) Severe disseminated lung disease and bronchiectasis probably due to Mycoplasma pneumoniae. Can Med Ass J 117: 1055

Hall CB, Kopelman AE, Douglas RG Jr, Geiman JM, Meagher MP (1979) Neonatal respiratory syncytial virus infection. N Engl J Med 300: 393

Haram K, Jacobsen K (1973) Measles and its relationship to giant cell pneumonia (Hecht pneumonia). Acta Pathol Microbiol Scand [A] 81: 761

Harris RO III, Spock A (1978) Pulmonary infiltrates as an early sign in a very young child. Clin Pediatr 17: 119

Harrison J, Myers M, Rowen M, Vermund H (1974) Results of combination chemotherapy, surgery and radiotherapy in children with neuroblastoma. Cancer 34: 485

Harrison HR, Alexander ER, Chiang WT, Giddens WE Jr, Boyce JT, Benjamin D, Gale JL (1979) Experimental nasopharyngitis and pneumonia caused by Chlamydia trachomatis in infant baboons: Histopathologic comparison with a case in a human infant. J Infect Dis 139: 141

Harwick H, Purcell RH, Iuppa JB, Fekety FR Jr (1970) Mycoplasma hominis and abortion. J Infect Dis 121: 260

Hawkins DB (1978) Hyaline membrane disease of the neonate prolonged intubation in management: effects on the larynx. Laryngoscope 88: 201

Healy GB, Holtand GP, Tucker JA (1976) Bifid epiglottis: a rare laryngeal anomaly. Laryngoscope 86: 1459

Heckers H, Melcher FW, Dittmar K, Knorpp K, Nekarda K (1978) Long-term course of mineral oil pneumonia. Lung 155: 101

Heffelfinger MJ, Dahlin DC, MacCarty CS, Beabout JW (1973) Chordomas and cartilaginous tumors at the skull base. Cancer 32: 410

Henderson DW, Humeniuk V, Meadows R, Forbes IJ (1974) *Pneumocystis carinii* pneumonia with vascular and lymph nodal involvement. Pathology 6: 235

Henderson FW, Collier AM, Clyde WA Jr, Denny FW (1979) Respiratory-syncytial-virus infections and immunity. A prospective longitudinal study in young children. N Engl J Med 300: 530

Henderson R, Hislop A, Reid L (1971) New pathological findings in emphysema of childhood. III. Unilateral congenital emphysema with hypoplasia and compensatory emphysema of contralateral lung. Thorax 26: 195

Hendren WH, McKee DM (1966) Lobar emphysema of infancy. J Pediatr Surg 1: 24

Heppleston AG, Young AE (1971) Alveolar lipo-proteinosis: an ultrastructural comparison of the experimental and human forms. J Pathol 107: 107

Herbert FA, Wilkinson D, Burchak E, Morgante O (1977) Adenovirus type 3 pneumonia causing lung damage in childhood. Can Med Ass J 116: 274

Herbert WNP, Johnson JM, MacDonald PC, Jimenez JM (1978) Human amniotic fluid phosphatidate phosphohydrolase activity through normal gestation and its relation to the lecithin/sphingomyelin ratio. Am J Obstet Gynecol 132: 373

Hers JFP, Mulder J (1961) Broad aspects of the pathology and pathogenesis of human influenza. Am Rev Respir Dis 83: 84

Herxheimer G (1901) Ueber einen Fall von echter Nebenlunge. Zentralbl Allg Pathol 12: 529

Hewitt CJ, Hull D, Keeling JW (1977) Fibrosing alveolitis in infants and childhood. Arch Dis Child 52: 22

Hicks JL, Nelson JF (1973) Juvenile nasopharyngeal angiofibroma. Oral Surg 35: 807

Hill GS, Eggleston JC (1972) Electron microscopic study of so-called pulmonary sclerosing hemangioma. Cancer 30: 1092

Hinson KFW (1970) Diffuse pulmonary fibrosis. Hum Pathol 1: 275

Hislop A, Reid L (1970) New pathological findings in emphysema of childhood. I. Polyalveolar lobe with emphysema. Thorax 25: 682

Hislop A, Reid L (1971) New pathological findings in emphysema of childhood. II. Overinflation of a normal lobe. Thorax 26: 190

Hislop A, Hey E, Reid L (1979) The lungs in congenital bilateral renal agenesis and dysplasia. Arch Dis Child 54: 32

Hislop A, Sanderson M, Reid L (1973) Unilateral congenital dysplasia of lung associated with vascular anomalies. Thorax 28: 435

Ho CY, Aterman K (1970) Infection of the fetus by Candida in a spontaneous abortion. Am J Obstet Gynecol 106: 705

Ho KL (1980) Primary meningioma of the nasal cavity and paranasal sinuses. Cancer 46: 1442

Hodgmann JE, Mikity VG, Tatter D, Cleland RS (1969) Chronic respiratory distress in the premature infant—Wilson–Mikity syndrome. Pediatrics 44: 179

Hoffmann EO, Loose LD, Harklin JC (1973) The Mikulicz cell in rhinoscleroma. Light, fluorescent and electron microscopic studies. Am J Pathol 73: 47

Hohbach C, Mootz W (1978) Chemodectoma of the larynx. A clinicopathological study. Virchows Arch [Pathol Anat] 378: 161

Høiby N, Flensborg EW, Beck B, Friis B, Jacobsen SV, Jacobsen L (1977) *Pseudomonas aeruginosa* infection in cystic fibrosis. Diagnostic and prognostic significance of *Pseudomonas aeruginosa* precipitins determined by means of crossed immunoelectrophoresis. Scand J Respir Dis 58: 65

Holborow CA, Mott TJ (1973) Subglottic hemangioma in infancy. J Laryngol Otol 87: 1013

Holden MP, Wooler GH (1970) Tracheo-oesophageal fistula and oesophageal atresia: results of 30 year's experience. Thorax 25: 406

Holdsworth Mayer CM, Favara BE, Holton CP, Rainer WG (1974) Malignant mesenchymoma in infants. Am J Dis Child 128: 847

Holinger LD, Barnes DR, Smid LJ, Holinger PH (1978) Laryngocele and saccular cysts. Ann Otol Rhinol Laryngol 87: 675

Holinger PH, Brown WT (1967) Congenital webs, cysts, laryngoceles and other anomalies of the larynx. Ann Otol Rhinol Laryngol 76: 744

Holinger PH, Gelman HK, Wolfe CK (1977) Rhinoscleroma of the lower respiratory tract. Laryngoscope 87: 1

Holmes B, Quie PG, Windhorst DB, Good RA (1966) Fatal granulomatous disease of childhood—an inborn abnormality of phagocytic function. Lancet 1: 1225

Holt S, Deverall PB, Boddy JE (1978) A teratoma of the lung containing thymic tissue. J Pathol 126: 85

Hong SW, Baran GM, Schnaufer L, Stool SE (1973) Tracheal agenesis with broncho-oesophageal fistula. Laryngoscope 83: 250

Hook GER, Bell D, Gilmore LB, Nadeau D, Reasor MJ, Talley FA (1978) Composition of bronchoalveolar lavage effluents from patients with pulmonary alveolar proteinosis. Lab Invest 30: 342

Hopkinson JM (1972) Congenital absence of the trachea. J Pathol 107: 63

Hoshaw JW, Walike TC (1971) Dermoid cysts of the nose. Arch Otolaryngol 93: 487

Howell JT, Schochet SS Jr, Goldman AS (1980) Ultrastructural defects of respiratory tract cilia associated with chronic infections. Arch Pathol Lab Med 104: 52

Hughes WT, Price RA, Kim HK, Coburn TP, Grigsby D, Feldman S (1973) *Pneumocystis carinii* pneumonitis in children with malignancies. J Pediatr 82: 404

Humbert G, Duval C, Fessard C, Meunier M, Ledoux A (1977a) Aspects actuels des listérioses en France (à propos d'une statistique de 824 cas). 1. Lyon Med 237: 275

Humbert G, Duval C, Fessard C, Meunier M, Ledoux A (1977b) Aspects actuels des listérioses en France (à propos d'une statistique de 824 cas). 2. Listériose de la femme enceinte et listérioses néonatales. Lyon Med 237: 455

Hutchins GM, Boitnott JK (1978) Atypical mycobacterial infection complicating mineral oil pneumonia. JAMA 240: 539

Iwa T, Watanabe Y (1979) Unusual combination of pulmonary sequestration and funnel chest. Chest 76: 314

Jacobs L (1974) Toxoplasma gondii: parasitology and transmission. Bull NY Acad Med 50: 128

Jacobs MR, Stein H, Buqwane A, Dubb A, Segal F, Rabinowitz L, Ellis U, Freiman I, Witcomb M, Vallabh V (1978) Epidemic listeriosis: report of 14 cases detected in 9 months. S Afr Med J 54: 189

Jacot-des-Combes E, Kapanci Y (1977) Granulome éosinophile du poumon. Utilité de l'étude ultrastructurale pour une approche étiologique. Rev Fr Mal Respir 5: 405

Jafek BW, Stern FA (1973) Neurofibroma of the larynx occurring with venereal disease: report of a case. Arch Otolaryngol 98: 77

Jaffe BF (1973a) Pediatric head and neck tumors: a study of 178 cases. Laryngoscope 83: 1644

Jaffe BF (1973b) Unusual laryngeal problems in children. Ann Otol 82: 637

Jahrsdoerfer R, Feldman PS, Rubel EW, Guerrant JL, Eggleston PA, Selden RF (1979) Otitis media and the immotile cilia syndrome. Laryngoscope 89: 769

Jansson E (1978) *Mycoplasma pneumoniae* infection. Scand J Respir Dis 59: 175

Jaubert de Beaujeu M, Mollard P, Campo-Paysan A (1970) Aspects particuliers des séquestrations pulmonaires. Chir Thorac Cardiovasc 9: 515

Jaubert de Beaujeu M, Chavrier Y, Korkmaz G (1973) Séquestrations pulmonaires chez l'enfant. Réflexions à propos de 10 observations. Ann Chir Infant 14: 341

Jayet A, Bozic C, Saegesser F (1977) Pneumoblastomes. A propos de deux observations. Schweiz Med Wochenschr 107: 349

Jenkin RDT (1976) The treatment of Wilms' tumor. Pediatr Clin North Am 23: 147

Jenkin RDT, Brown TC, Peters MV, Sonley M (1975) Hodgkin's disease in children. A retrospective analysis: 1958–1973. Cancer 35: 979

Jessee WF, Ryan JM, Fitzgerald JF, Grosfeld JL (1975) Amebic abscess in childhood. Clin Pediatr 14: 134

Jimenez JM, Johnston JM (1976) Fetal lung maturation. IV. The release of phosphatidic acid phosphohydrolase and phospholipids into the human amniotic fluid. Pediatr Res 10: 767

Jimenez JM, Schultz FM, Johnston JM (1975) Fetal lung maturation. III. Amniotic fluid phosphatidic acid phosphohydrolase (PAPase) and its relation to the lecithin/sphingomyelin ratio. Obstet Gynecol 46: 588

Jimenez-Martinez M, Perez-Alvarez JJ, Perez-Trevino G, Rubio-Alvarez V, De Rubiens J (1965) Agenesis of the lung with patient ductus arteriosus treated surgically. J Thorac Cardiovasc Surg 50: 59

Johanson A, Blizzard R (1971) A syndrome of congenital aplasia of the alae nasi, deafness, hypothyroidism, dwarfism, absent permanent teeth and malabsorption. J Pediatr 79: 982

Johnson S, Roberts CR II, Oxford B, Seidel J, Heaney JP (1974) An unusual case of bronchial adenoma in childhood. Arch Surg 109: 829

Joliat G, Abetel G, Schindler AM, Kapanci Y (1973) Measles giant cell pneumonia without rash in a case of lymphocytic lymphosarcoma. An electron microscopic study. Virchows Arch [Pathol Anat] 358: 215

Jones DG, Gabriel CE (1969) The incidence of carcinoma of the larynx in persons under twenty years of age. Laryngoscope 70: 251

Jones EL, Cameron AH (1969) Pulmonary calcification in viral pneumonia. J Clin Pathol 22: 361

Joshi VV (1969) Tracheal agenesis. Am J Dis Child 117: 341

Joshi VV, Mandavia SG, Stern L, Wiglesworth FW (1972) Acute lesions induced by endotracheal intubation. Occurrence in the upper respiratory tract of newborn infants with respiratory distress syndrome. Am J Dis Child 124: 646

Joshi VV, Escobar MR, Stewart L, Bates RD (1973) Fatal influenza A_2 viral pneumonia in a newborn infant. Am J Dis Child 126: 839

Kahn LB (1974) Esthesioneuroblastoma: a light and electron microscopic study. Hum Pathol 5: 364

Kanbour AI, Barmada MA, Klionsky B, Moossy J (1979) Anencephaly and heterotopic central nervous tissue in lungs. Arch Pathol Lab Med 103: 116

Kane PB, Lane BP, Cordice JWV, Greenberg GM (1978) Ultrastructure of the proliferating cells in pulmonary lymphangiomyomatosis. Arch Pathol Lab Med 102: 618

Kapanci Y, Tosco R, Eggermann J (1972) Demonstration of the extracellular alveolar lining layer (surfactant) in human lungs. An ultrastructural study. Virchows Arch [Cell Pathol] 10: 243

Kaplan C, Katoh A, Shamoto M, Rogow E, Scott JH, Cushing Wand Cooper J (1973) Multiple leiomyomas of the lung: benign or malignant. Am Rev Respir Dis 108: 656

Kaplan SL, Gnepp DR, Katzenstein ALA, Feigin RD (1978) Miliary pulmonary nodules due to aspirated vegetable particles. J Pediatr 92: 448

Karcioglu ZA, Someren AO (1974) Pulmonary blastoma. A case report and review of the literature. Am J Clin Pathol 61: 287

Karma P, Rasanen O, Karja J (1977) Nasal gliomas. A review and report of 2 cases. Laryngoscope 87: 1169

Kassel SH, Echevarria RA, Guzzo FP (1969) Midline malignant reticulosis (so-called lethal midline granuloma). Cancer 23: 920

Katz SM, Holsclaw DS Jr (1980) Ultrastructural features of respiratory cilia in cystic fibrosis. Am J Clin Pathol 73: 682

Katzenstein AL, Maurer J (1979) Benign histiocytic tumor of lung. A light and electron microscopic study. Am J Surg Pathol 3: 61

Katzenstein AL, Liebow AA, Friedman PJ (1975) Bronchocentric granulomatosis, mucoid impaction and hypersensitivity reactions of fungi. Am Rev Respir Dis 111: 497

Katzenstein ALA, Carrington CB, Liebow AA (1979) Lymphomatoid granulomatosis. A clinicopathologic study of 152 cases. Cancer 43: 360

Katzenstein ALA, Gmelich JT, Carrington CB (1980) Sclerosing hemangioma of the lung. A clinicopathologic study of 51 cases. Am J Surg Pathol 4: 343

Kaul A, Scott R, Gallagher M, Scott M, Clement J, Ogra PL (1978) Respiratory syncytial virus infection — rapid diagnosis in children by use of indirect immunofluorescence. Am J Dis Child 132: 1088

Kawanami O, Ferrans VJ, Fulmer JD, Crystal RG (1979) Nuclear inclusions in alveolar epithelium of patients with fibrotic lung disorders. Am J Pathol 94: 301

Keidel WN, Feingold LM (1971) Wilson–Mikity syndrome in a full-term male twin. Pediatrics 47: 779

Kennedy A, Prior AL (1976) Pulmonary blastoma: a report of two cases and a review of the literature. Thorax 31: 776

Kenny JD, Adams JM, Corbet AJS, Rudolph AJ (1976) The role of acidosis at birth in the development of hyaline membrane disease. Pediatrics 58: 184

Kesson CW (1954) Asphyxia neonatorum due to a nasopharyngeal teratoma. Arch Dis Child 29: 254

Kibrick S, Loria RM (1974) Rubella and cytomegalovirus. Current concepts of congenital and acquired infection. Pediatr Clin North Am 21: 513

King CR, Prescott G, Pernoll M (1978) Significance of meconium in midtrimester diagnostic amniocentesis. Am J Obstet Gynecol 132: 667

King RJ (1974) The surfactant system of the lung. Fed Proc 33: 2238

Kino T, Kohara Y, Tsuji S (1972) Pulmonary alveolar microlithiasis. A report of two young sisters. Am Rev Respir Dis 105: 105

Kitagawa M, Hislop A, Boyden EA, Reid L (1971) Lung hypoplasia in congenital diaphragmatic hernia. A quantitative study of airway, artery and alveolar development. Br J Surg 58: 342

Kitamura S, Maeda M, Kawashima Y, Masaoka A, Manabe H (1969) Leiomyoma of the intrathoracic trachea — Report of a case successfully treated by primary end-to-end anastomosis following circumferential resection of the trachea. J Thorac Cardiovasc Surg 57: 126

Klein JO (1969) Diagnostic lung puncture in the pneumonias of infants and children. Pediatrics 44: 486

Klein JO, Buckland D, Finland M (1969) Colonization of newborn infants by mycoplasmas. N Engl J Med 280: 1025

Klima M, Gyorkey F (1977) Benign pleural lesions and malignant mesothelioma. Virchows Arch [Pathol Anat] 376: 181

Kobler E, Ammann RW (1977) Accessory lung arising from the upper esophagus. A rare congenital anomaly in the adult. Respiration 34: 236

Kogutt MS, Swischuk LE, Goldblum R (1973) Swyer–James syndrome (unilateral hyperlucent lung) in children. Am J Dis

Child 125: 614

Kohler HG, Rymer BA (1973) Congenital cystic malformation of the lung and its relation to hydramnios. J Obstet Gynecol 80: 130

Kollberg H, Mossberg B, Afzelius BA, Philipson K, Camner P (1978) Cystic fibrosis compared with the immotile-cilia syndrome. A study of mucociliary clearance, ciliary ultrastructure, clinical picture and ventilatory function. Scand J Respir Dis 59: 297

Koutras P, Urschel HC Jr, Paulson DL (1971) Hamartoma of the lung. J Thorac Cardiovasc Surg 61: 768

Krauss AN, Levin AR, Grossman H, Auld PAM (1970) Physiologic studies on infants with Wilson–Mikity syndrome. J Pediatr 77: 27

Kreisman H, Robitaille Y, Dionne P, Palayew MJ (1978) Lymphangiomyomatosis syndrome with hyperparathyroidism. A case report. Cancer 42: 364

Krekorian EA, Kato RH (1977) Surgical management of nasopharyngeal angiofibroma with intracranial extension. Laryngoscope 87: 154

Kuhn C, Gyrokey F, Levine BE, Ramirez-Rivera J (1966) Pulmonary alveolar proteinosis. A study using enzyme histochemistry, electron microscopy and surface tension measurement. Lab Invest 15: 492

Kuhn JP, Lee SB (1973) Pneumatoceles associated with *Escherichia coli* pneumonias in the newborn. Pediatrics 51: 1008

Kwittken J, Reiner L (1962) Congenital cystic adenomatoid malformation of the lung. Pediatrics 30: 759

Kyllonen KEJ (1964) Intralobar pulmonary sequestration and theory as to its etiology. Acta Chir Scand 127: 307

Lack EE (1977) Carotid body hypertrophy in patients with cystic fibrosis and cyanotic congenital heart disease. Hum Pathol 8: 39

Lacquet LK, Fornhoff M, Dierickx R, Buyssens N (1971) Bronchial atresia with corresponding segmental pulmonary emphysema. Thorax 26: 68

Lago JV, Pujol JL, Reboiras SD, Larrauri J, Schacke de Miguel L (1976) Fibrous histiocytoma of the lung. Thorax 31: 475

Lancet (1969) The eosinophilic pneumonias. (Leading article). Lancet 2: 1237

Landau LI, Mellis CM, Phelan PD, Bristowe B, McLennan L (1979) 'Small airways disease' in children: no test is best. Thorax 34: 217

Landing BH (1957) Anomalies of the respiratory tract. Pediatr Clin North Am 4: 73

Landing BH, Dixon LG (1979) Congenital malformations and genetic disorders of the respiratory tract (larynx, trachea, bronchi, and lungs). Am Rev Respir Dis 120: 151

Landing BH, Shirkey HS (1957) A syndrome of recurrent infection and infiltration of viscera by pigmented lipid histiocytes. Pediatrics 20: 431

Landing BH, Wells TR (1973) Tracheobronchial anomalies in children. In: Rosenberg HS, Boland RP (eds) Perspectives in pediatric pathology. Year Book Medical Publishers, Chicago, p 1

Laptook A, Wind E, Nussbaum M, Shenker IR (1978) Pulmonary lesions in atypical measles. Pediatrics 62: 42

Laraya-Cuasay LR, Deforest A, Palmer J, Huff DS, Lischner HW, Huang NN (1974) Chronic pulmonary complications of early influenza virus infection. Am Rev Respir Dis 109: 703

Lasalle AJ, Andrassy RJ, Steeg KV, Ratner I (1979) Congenital tracheoesophageal fistula without esophageal atresia. J Thorac Cardiovasc Surg 78: 583

Laurence KM (1959) Congenital pulmonary lymphangiectasis. J Clin Pathol 12: 62

Lauweryns J, Deleersnyer M, Boussauw L (1971) A morphometrical study of the aeration of the pulmonary parenchyma in neonatal hyaline membrane diseases. Beitr Pathol 144: 344

Lauweryns J, Bernat R, Lerut A, Detournay G (1973) Intrauterine pneumonia—an experimental study. Biol Neonate 22: 301

Lauweryns JM (1969) The body lymphatics in neonatal hyaline membrane disease. Pediatrics 44: 126

Lauweryns JM (1970) 'Hyaline membrane disease' in newborn infants. Macroscopic, radiographic and light and electron microscopic studies. Hum Pathol 1: 175

Lawson RM, Ramanathan L, Hurley G, Hinson KW, Lennox SC (1976) Bronchial adenoma: review of an 18-year experience at the Brompton Hospital. Thorax 31: 245

Lee DA, Rao BR, Meyer JS, Prioleau PG, Bauer WC (1980) Hormonal receptor determination in juvenile nasopharyngeal angiofibromas. Cancer 46: 547

Le Golvan DP, Heidelberger KP (1973) Disseminated granulomatous *Pneumocystis carinii* pneumonia. Arch Pathol 95: 344

Le Maigre G, Diebold J, Temmim L, Arseniev L, Lecharpentier Y, Allouache A, Delaitre B, Abelanet R (1977) Carcinome du naso-pharynx chez le sujet jeune: étude clinique, anatomique et ultrastructurale de 50 cas observés dans l'Est algérien. Nouv Presse Med 6: 3509

Lemons JA, Jaffe RB (1973) Amniotic fluid lecithin/sphingomyelin ratio in the diagnosis of hyaline membrane disease. Am J Obstet Gynecol 115: 233

Lesbros D, Ferran JL, Rieu D, Jean R (1979) Sténose trachéale congénitale et bronche surnuméraire. Arch Fr Pediatr 36: 703

Lesser A, Rothfeld PR, Shapiro RS (1976) Epithelial papilloma and squamous cell carcinoma of the nasal cavity and paranasal sinuses. A clinico-pathological study. Cancer 38: 2503

Le Tan Vinh LT, Duc TV, Huault G, Thieffry S, Lelong M (1969) Association de la pneumonie à 'pneumocystis' avec une cytomégalie généralisée et intrapulmonaire. Etude de huit observations. Arch Fr Pediatr 26: 889

Le Tan Vinh LT, Tran Van Duc TV, Lallemand D, Huault G (1977) Lymphangiectasie pulmonaire congénitale. Une nouvelle observation avec blocage complet de la circulation veineuse pulmonaire de retour et important emphysème interstitiel. Nouv Presse Med 6: 1861

Levene MI, Wigglesworth JS, Desai R (1980) Pulmonary fat accumulation after intralipid infusion in the preterm infant. Lancet 2: 815

Levine DP, Lerner AM (1978) The clinical spectrum of *Mycoplasma pneumoniae* infections. Med Clin North Am 62: 961

Levine MG, Hoxt RE, Peter JE (1974) Scleroma. An etiological study. J Clin Invest 26: 281

Leviton A, Gilles F, Strassfeld R (1977) The influence of route of delivery and hyaline membranes on the risk of neonatal intracranial hemorrhages. Ann Neurol 2: 451

Lewis MJ, Cameron AH, Shah KJ, Purdham DR, Mann JR (1978) Giant-cell pneumonia caused by measles and methotrexate in childhood leukaemia in remission. Br Med J i: 330

Li FP (1977) Second malignant tumors after cancer in childhood. Cancer 40: 1899

Lieberman J (1969) Pulmonary plasminogen—Activator activity in hyaline membrane disease. Pediatr Res 3: 11

Liebner EJ (1976) Embryonal rhabdomyosarcoma of head and neck in children: correlation of stage, radiation dose, local control and survival. Cancer 37: 2777

Liebow AA, Hubbell DS (1956) Sclerosing hemangioma (histiocytoma, xanthoma of the lung). Cancer 9: 53

Liebow AA, Steer A, Billingsley JG (1965) Desquamative interstitial pneumonia. Am J Med 39: 369

Liebow AA, Carrington CRB, Friedman PJ (1972) Lymphomatoid granulomatosis. Hum Pathol 3: 457

Liggins GC, Howie RN (1972) N-A controlled trial of antepartum glucocorticoid treatment for prevention of the respiratory distress syndrome in premature infants. Pediatrics 50: 515

Lightwood R, Nolan R, Franco M, White AJS (1970) Epithelial giant cells in measles as an aid in diagnosis. J Pediatr 77: 59

Lilien LD, Yeh TF, Novak GM, Jacobs NM (1978) Early onset

Haemophilus sepsis in newborn infants: clinical, roentgeno-graphic and pathologic features. Pediatrics 62: 299

Lin JJ, Svoboda DJ (1971) Multiple congenital mesenchymal tumors. Multiple vascular leiomyomas in several organs of a newborn. Cancer 28: 1046

Lincoln JCR, Stark J, Subramanian S, Aberdeen E, Bonham-Carter RE, Berry CL, Waterston DJ (1971) Congenital lobar emphysema. Ann Surg 173: 55

Lindsay ML Jr, Hermann EC Jr, Morrow GW Jr, Brown AL Jr (1970) Hong Kong influenza. Clinical, microbiologic and pathologic features in 127 cases. JAMA 214: 1825

Linhartova A, Chung W (1963) Bronchopulmonary monialiasis in the newborn. J Clin Pathol 16: 56

Lober M, Rawlings W, Newell JR, Reed RJ (1973) Sinus histiocytosis with massive lymphadenopathy. Cancer 32: 421

Loker EF Jr, Hodges GR, Kelly DJ (1974) Fatal adenovirus pneumonia in a young adult associated with ADV-7 vaccine administered 15 days earlier. Chest 66: 197

Loughlin GM, Taussig LM, Murphy SA, Strunk RS, Kohnen PW (1978) Immune-complex-mediated glomerulonephritis and pulmonary hemorrhage simulating Goodpasture syndrome. J Pediatr 93: 181

Lundquist PG, Frithiof L, Wersall J (1975) Ultrastructural features of human juvenile laryngeal papillomas. Acta Otolaryngol 80: 137

Lynch JI (1970) Bronchomalacia in children—Considerations governing medical vs surgical treatment. Clin Pediatr 9: 279

Lyons SM, Bruce AEG (1968) Tracheal agenesis. A report of 2 cases. Anaesthesia 23: 98

Machin GA (1975) A perinatal mortality survey in south-east London, 1970–73: the pathological findings in 726 necropsies. J Clin Pathol 28: 428

MacIntosh DJ, Price CHG, Jeffree GM (1975) Ewing's tumour: a study of behaviour and treatment in forty-seven cases. J Bone Joint Surg [Br] 57: 331

MacMahon HE, Ruggieri J (1969) Congenital segmental broncho-malacia: report of a case. Am J Dis Child 118: 923

Maeta T, Fujiwara Y, Ohizumi T, Kato E, Kakizaki G, Ishidate T, Fujiwara T (1977) Pathological study of tracheal and pulmonary lesions in autopsy cases of congenital esophageal atresia. Tohoku J Exp Med 123: 23

Maguire JJ, Shelley SA, Paciga JE, Balis JU (1977) Isolation and characterization of proteins associated with the lung surfactant system. Prep Biochem 7: 415

Maisel RH, Ogura JH (1974) Neurofibromatosis with laryngeal involvement. Laryngoscope 84: 132

Maltz DL, Nadas AS (1968) Agenesis of the lung: presentation of eight new cases and review of the literature. Pediatrics 42: 175

Manniello RL, Farrell PM (1977) Analysis of United States neonatal mortality statistics from 1968 to 1974, with specific reference to changing trends in major causalities. Am J Obstet Gynecol 129: 667

Mark PH, Turner JAP (1968) Lung abscess in childhood. Thorax 23: 216

Marks C, Lamberty J (1977) The cellular structure of bronchial carcinoids. Postgrad Med J 53: 360

Martin AJ, Gardner PS, McQuillin J (1978) Epidemiology of respiratory viral infection among paediatric inpatients over a six-year period in North-East England. Lancet 2: 1035

Martin JJ, Philippart M, Van Hauwaert J, Callahan JW, Deberdt R (1972) Niemann–Pick disease (Crocker's group A)—Late-onset and pigmentary degeneration resembling Hallervorden–Spatz syndrome. Arch Neurol 27: 45

Martinez JS, Kohler PF (1971) Variant 'Goodpasture's syndrome'? The need for immunologic criteria in rapidly progressive glomerulonephritis and hemorrhagic pneumonitis. Ann Intern Med 75: 67

Mashiach S, Barkai G, Sack J, Stern E, Goldman B, Brish M, Serr DM (1978) Enhancement of fetal lung maturity by intra-amniotic administration of thyroid hormone. Am J Obstet Gynecol 130: 289

Massaro D, Kayz S, Matthews MJ, Higgins G (1965) Von Recklinghausen's neurofibromatosis associated with cystic lung disease. Am J Med 38: 233

Massumi RA, Legier JF (1966) Rheumatic pneumonitis. Circulation 33: 417

Mathis RK, Freier EF, Hunt CF, Krivit W, Sharp HL (1973) Alpha-1-antitrypsin in the respiratory distress syndrome. N Engl J Med 288: 59

Matlin AH, Young LW, Klemperer MR (1972) Pleural effusion in two children with histiocytosis X. Chest 61: 33

Matsuba K, Thurlbeck WM (1973) Disease of the small airways in chronic bronchitis. Am Rev Respir Dis 107: 552

Mavis RD, Finkelstein JN, Hall BP (1978) Pulmonary surfactant synthesis. A highly active microsomal phosphatidate phospho-hydrolase in the lung. J Lipid Res 19: 467

Mayer GJ (1979) Pulmonary paragonimiasis. J Pediatr 95: 75

McAdams AJ, Coen R, Kleinman LI, Tsang R, Sutherland J (1973) The experimental production of hyaline membranes in premature Rhesus monkeys. Am J Pathol 70: 277

McCann MP, Fu YS, Kay S (1976) Pulmonary blastoma. A light and electron microscopic study. Cancer 38: 789

McCormick TL, Kuhns LR (1979) Tracheal compression by a normal aorta associated with right lung agenesis. Pediatr Radiol 130: 659

McCracken AW, Flanagan N, Flanagan P (1964) Tracheal atresia associated with cor biloculare. Thorax 19: 530

McCrae WM, Raeburn JA (1974) The patterns of infection in cystic fibrosis. Scot Med J 19: 187

McDonagh BJ, Martin J (1970) Paraquat poisoning in children. Arch Dis Child 45: 425

McGavran MH, Sessions DG, Dorfman RF, Davis DO, Ogura JH (1969) Nasopharyngeal angiofibroma. Arch Otolaryngol 90: 68

McGuirt WF, Rose EF (1976) Lethal midline granuloma: a pathological spectrum. J Laryngol 90: 459

McKendry JBJ, Bailey JD (1973) Congenital varicella associated with multiple defects. Can Med Ass J 108: 66

McNie DJM, Pryse-Davies J (1970) Tracheal agenesis. Arch Dis Child 45: 143

Meade JB, Whitwell F, Bickford BJ, Waddington JKB (1974) Primary haemangiopericytoma of lung. Thorax 29: 1

Meis PJ, Hall M III, Marshall JR, Hobel CJ (1978) Meconium passage: a new classification for risk assessment during labour. Am J Obstet Gynecol 131: 509

Mendelsohn G, Hutchins GM (1977) Primary pulmonary hypoplasia: report of a case with polyhydramnios. Am J Dis Child 131: 1220

Merenstein GB (1969) Congenital cystic adenomatoid malformation of the lung. Report of a case and review of the literature. Am J Dis Child 118: 772

Merlier M, Rochainzanir A, Rojas-Miranda A, Levasseur P, Sulzer JD, Verley JM, Langlois J, Binet JP, LeBrigand H (1970) Les aspects anatomo-cliniques des séquestrations pulmonaires. A propos de 46 observations. Ann Chir Thorac Cardiovasc 9: 511

Meyers JD (1974) Congenital varicella in term infants: risk reconsidered. J Infect Dis 129: 215

Meyers WM, Neafie RC, Connor DH (1977) Onchocerciasis: invasion of deep organs by Onchocerca volvulus. Autopsy findings. Am J Trop Med Hyg 26: 650

Michaels L, Gregory MM (1977) Pathology of 'non-healing (midline) granuloma'. J Clin Pathol 30: 317

Michalsen H (1974) Congenital cystic adenomatoid malformation of the lung. A report of two cases. Acta Paediatr Scand 63: 793

Micheau C, Luboinski B, Sancho H, Cachin Y (1975) Modes of invasion of cancer of the larynx. A statistical, histological and radioclinical analysis of 120 cases. Cancer 38: 346

Michels VV, Driscoll DJ, Ferry GD, Duff DF, Beaudet AL (1979) Pulmonary vascular obstruction associated with cholesteryl ester storage disease. J Paediatr 94: 621

Mihatsch MJ, Ohnacker H, Just M, Nars PW (1972) Lethal measles giant cell pneumonia after live measles vaccination in a case of thymic alymphoplasia Gitlin. Helv Paediatr Acta 27: 143

Miller FC, Sacks DA, Yeh SY, Paul RH, Schifrin BS, Martin CB Jr, Hon EH (1975) Significance of meconium during labor. Am J Obstet Gynecol 122: 573

Minasian H (1977) Uncommon pulmonary hamartomas. Thorax 32: 360

Mitchell DN, Scadding JG, Heard BE, Hinson KFW (1977) Sarcoidosis: histopathological definition and clinical diagnosis. J Clin Pathol 30: 395

Mitchell RE, Bury RG (1975) Congenital bronchiectasis due to deficiency of cartilage (Williams–Campbell syndrome). J Pediatr 87: 230

Moffat AD (1960) Congenital cystic disease of the lung and its classification. J Pathol 79: 361

Moncrieff MW, Cameron AH, Astley R, Roberts KD, Abrams LD, Mann JR (1969) Congenital cystic adenomatoid malformation of the lung. Thorax 24: 476

Monteforte WJ Jr, Kohnen PW (1974) Angiomyolipomas in a case of lymphangiomyomatosis syndrome: relationships to tuberous sclerosis. Cancer 34: 317

Montis G de, Garnier P, Thomassin N, Job JC, Rossier A (1972) La mucolipidose type II (maladie des cellules à inclusion). Etude d'un cas et revue de la littérature. Ann Pediatr 19: 369

Moore RM, Zehmer RB (1973) Listeriosis in the United States. J Infect Dis 127: 610

Moorthy AV, Chesney RW, Segar WE, Groshong T (1977) Wegener granulomatosis in childhood: prolonged survival following cytotoxic therapy. J Pediatr 91: 616

Moran TJ (1953) Milk aspiration in human and animal subjects. Arch Pathol 55: 286

Moran TJ (1955) Experimental aspiration. IV. Inflammatory and reparative changes produced by introduction of autologous gastric juice and hydrochloric acid. Arch Pathol 60: 122

Motomatsu K, Adachi H, Uno T (1979) Two infant deaths after inhaling baby powder. Chest 75: 448

Moylan FMB, Shannon DC (1979) Preferential distribution of lobar emphysema and atelectasis in bronchopulmonary dysplasia. Pediatrics 63: 130

Müller H (1918) Ueber Lappungsanomalien der Lungen, insbesondere über einen Fall von trachealer Nebenlunge. Virchows Arch 225: 284

Müller WD, Wendler H, Becker H (1978) Beidseitige Aplasie des Zwerchfelles mit Hypoplasie beider Lungen. Klin Paediatr 190: 129

Mullins JD, Barnes RP (1979) Childhood bronchial mucoepidermoid tumors. A case report and review of the literature. Cancer 44: 315

Naeye RL (1978) Amniotic fluid infections, neonatal hyperbilirubinemia and psychomotor impairment. Pediatrics 62: 497

Naeye RL, Dellinger WS, Blanc WA (1971) Fetal and maternal features of antenatal bacterial infections. J Pediatr 79: 733

Nair S, Nair K, Weisbrot IM (1974) Fibrous histiocytoma of the lung (sclerosing hemangioma variant?). Chest 65: 465

Nasser WY, Keogh PF, Doshi R (1970) Myoblastoma of the larynx. J Laryngol 84: 751

Neilson DB (1958) Primary intrapulmonary neurogenic sarcoma. J Pathol 76: 419

Nelson NM (1970) On the etiology of hyaline membrane disease. Pediatr Clin North Am 17: 943

Nespoli L, Duse M, Vitiello MA, Perinotto G, Fiocca R, Giannetti A, Colombo A (1979) A rapid unfavorable outcome of Wegener's granulomatosis in early childhood. Eur J Pediatr 131: 277

Neu HC (1971) Toxoplasmose, complication des affections malignes. Rev Med 12: 487

Nezelof C, Meyer B, Dalloz JC, Joly P, Paupe J, Vialatte J (1970) La bronchiolite oblitérante: à propos de deux observations anatomocliniques infantiles. Ann Pediatr 17: 534

Nezelof C, Griscelli C, Jaubert F, Girot R, Lemaigre G, Khitri A, Benlatrache S (1978) L'histiocytose sinusale cytophagique adénomégalique. Etude morphologique et immunologique d'une observation. Arch Fr Pediatr 35: 118

Nezelof C, Frileux-Herbet F, Cronier-Sachot J (1979) Disseminated histiocytosis X. Analysis of prognostic factors based on a retrospective study of 50 cases. Cancer 44: 1824

Nicholls S, Yuille TD, Mitchell RG (1975) Perinatal infections caused by *Haemophilus influenzae*. Arch Dis Child 50: 739

Niitu Y, Kubota H, Hasegawa S, Horikawa M, Komatsu S, Suetake T, Fujimura S, Nagashima Y (1974) Lung cancer (squamous cell carcinoma) in adolescence. Am J Dis Child 127: 108

Nikol'skaia LP (1968) Teratoma in the right half of the nose and nasopharynx in the newborn. Vestn Otorinolaryng 28: 106

Nilsson R, Grossmann G, Robertson B (1978) Lung surfactant and the pathogenesis of neonatal bronchiolar lesions induced by artificial ventilation. Pediatr Res 12: 249

Nisenbaum C, Wallis K, Herczeg E (1969) Varicella pneumonia in children. Helv Paediatr Acta 24: 212

Northway WH Jr, Rosan RC, Porter DY (1967) Pulmonary disease following respirator therapy of hyaline-membrane disease. Bronchopulmonary dysplasia. N Engl J Med 276: 357

Nouri L, Al-Rahim K (1970) Kerosene poisoning in children. Postgrad Med J 46: 71

Novoselac M, Dangel P, Fisch V (1974) Laryngo-tracheo-esophageal cleft. A cast report. J Fr Otorhinolaryngol 23: 753

Nydell CC Jr, Masson JK (1959) Dermoid cysts of the nose: a review of 39 cases. Ann Surg 150: 1007

Oberklaid F, Danks DM, Mayne V, Campbell P (1977) Asphyxiating thoracic dysplasia: clinical, radiological and pathological information on 10 patients. Arch Dis Child 52: 758

Oberman HA, Rice DH (1976) Olfactory neuroblastomas: a clinico-pathologic study. Cancer 38: 2494

O'Conor GT (1961) Malignant lymphoma in African children. II. A pathological entity. Cancer 14: 270

O'Herlihy C, Gearty J, Troy P (1976) Congenital septicaemia and pneumonia due to group B streptococcus. Ir J Med Sci 145: 135

Okeda R (1978) Heterotopic brain tissue in the submandibular region and lung. Report of two cases and comments about pathogenesis. Acta Neuropathol 43: 217

Olding L (1970) Value of placentitis as a sign of intrauterine infection in human subjects. A morphological, bacteriological, clinical and statistical study. Acta Pathol Microbiol Scand 78: 256

Oliver TK Jr, Smith B, Clatworthy HW Jr (1959) Staphylococcal pneumonia, pleural and pulmonary complications. Pediatr Clin North Am 6: 1043

Olson JL, Mendelsohn G (1978) Congenital cystic adenomatoid malformation of the lung. Arch Pathol Lab Med 102: 248

Olson M (1970) Benign effects on rabbits' lungs of respiration of water as compared with 5% glucose or milk. Pediatrics 46: 538

Olson RW, Hodges GR (1975) Measles pneumonia—Bacterial suprainfection as a complicating factor. JAMA 232: 363

Olson KD, Carpenter RJ III, Kern EB (1979) Nasal septal trauma in children. Pediatrics 64: 32

Onadeko BO, Beetlestone CA, Cooke AR, Abioye AA, Adetuyibi A, Sofowora EO (1977) Pulmonary alveolar microlithiasis. Postgrad Med J 53: 165

O'Neil GJ Jr, Davies IJ, Siu J (1978) Palmitic/stearic ratio of amniotic fluid in diabetic and nondiabetic pregnancies and its relationship to development of respiratory distress syndrome. Am J Obstet Gynecol 132: 519

Oppenheimer EH, Esterly JR (1974) Medial mucoid lesions of the pulmonary artery in cystic fibrosis, pulmonary hypertension and other disorders. Lab Invest 30: 411

Oppenheimer EH, Rosenstein BJ (1979) Differential pathology of nasal polyps in cystic fibrosis and atopy. Lab Invest 40: 445

Orton HB (1947) Carcinoma of the larynx: clinical report of case—age 13½ years. Laryngoscope 57: 299

Osamura RY (1977) Ultrastructure of localized fibrous mesothelioma of the pleura. Report of a case with histogenetic considerations. Cancer 39: 139

Ostermiller WE, Comer TF, Barker WL (1970) Endobronchial granular cell myoblastoma. A report of three cases and review of the literature. Ann Thorac Surg 9: 143

Östör AG, Fortune DW (1978) Congenital cystic adenomatoid malformation of the lung. Am J Clin Pathol 70: 595

Östör AG, Stillwell R, Fortune DW (1978) Bilateral pulmonary agenesis. Pathology 10: 243

Ownby D, Lyon G, Spock A (1976) Primary leiomyosarcoma of the lung in childhood. Am J Dis Child 130: 1132

Pai SH, Cameron CTM, Lev R (1971) Accessory lung presenting as juxtagastric mass. Arch Pathol 91: 569

Pallie W, Alhady SMA, Din OB (1967) Agenesis of the right lung: an unusual presentation. Thorax 22: 368

Papageorgiou A, Bauer CR, Fletcher BD, Stern L (1973) Klebsiella pneumonia with pneumatocele formation in a newborn infant. Can Med Assoc J 109: 1217

Paredes CG de, Pierce WS, Groff DB, Waldhausen JA (1970) Bronchogenic tumors in children. Arch Surg 100: 574

Passwell J, Katz D, Frank Y, Spirer Z, Cohen BE, Ziprkowski M (1976) Fatal disseminated BCG infection. An investigation of the immuno-deficiency. Am J Dis Child 130: 433

Patchefsky AS, Israel LH, Hoch WS, Gordon G (1973) Desquamative interstitial pneumonia: relationship to interstitial fibrosis. Thorax 28: 680

Patrick JE, Dalton KJ, Dawes GS (1976) Breathing patterns before death in fetal lambs. Am J Obstet Gynecol 125: 73

Patrick J, Campbell K, Carmichael L, Natale R, Richardson B (1980) Patterns of human fetal breathing during the last 10 weeks of pregnancy. Obstet Gynecol 56: 24

Patten BM (1968) Human embryology, 3rd edn. McGraw-Hill, New York, p 358

Pearl M, Woolley MM (1973) Pulmonary xanthomatous postinflammatory pseudotumors in children. J Pediatr Surg 8: 255

Pearson DJ, Rosenow EC III (1978) Chronic eosinophilic pneumonia (Carrington's). A follow-up study. Mayo Clin Proc 53: 73

Pedersen M, Mygind N (1980) Ciliary motility in the 'immotile cilia syndrome'. First results of microphoto-oscillographic studies. Br J Dis Chest 74: 239

Pena SDJ, Shokeir MHK (1974) Syndrome of camptodactyly, multiple ankyloses, facial anomalies and pulmonary hypoplasia: a lethal condition. J Pediatr 85: 373

Perlman M, Levin M (1974) Fetal pulmonary hypoplasia, anuria and oligohydramnios: clinicopathologic observations and review of the literature. Am J Obstet Gynecol 118: 1119

Perzin KH, Fu YS (1980) Non-epithelial tumors of the nasal cavity, paranasal sinuses and nasopharynx. A clinicopathologic study. XI. Fibrous histiocytomas. Cancer 45: 2616

Pettay O, Leinikki P, Donner M, Lapinleimu K (1972) Herpes simplex virus infection in the newborn. Arch Dis Child 47: 97

Pettersson T, Stenström R, Kyrönseppa H (1974) Disseminated lung opacities and cavitation associated with *Strongyloides stercoralis* and *Schistosoma mansoni* infection. Am J Trop Med Hyg 23: 158

Pfenninger J, D'Apuzzo V (1977) Powder aspiration in children. Report of two cases. Arch Dis Child 52: 157

Phelan PD, Stocks JG, Williams HE, Danks DM (1973) Familial occurrence of congenital laryngeal clefts. Arch Dis Child 48: 275

Philip AGS (1975) Oxygen plus pressure plus time: the etiology of bronchopulmonary dysplasia. Pediatrics 55: 44

Pick T, Maurer HM, McWilliams NB (1974) Lymphoepithelioma in childhood. J Pediatr 84: 96

Pifer LL, Hughes WT, Stagno S, Woods D (1978) *Pneumocystis carinii* infection: evidence for high prevalence in normal and immunosuppressed children. Pediatrics 61: 35

Pillsbury HC, Fischer ND (1977) Laryngotracheoesophageal cleft. Diagnosis, management and presentation of a new diagnostic device. Arch Otolaryngol 103: 735

Pletcher JD, Newton TH, Dedo HH, Norman D (1975) Preoperative embolization of juvenile angiofibromas. Ann Otol 83: 740

Ponté C, Ribet M, Rémy J, Bonte C, Lequien P, Gosselin B (1974) Rétentions localisées du liquide alvéolaire foetal. Ann Pediatr 21: 343

Poole JB, Marcial-Rojas PA (1971) Echinococcosis. In: Marcial-Rojas PA (ed) Pathology of protozoal and helminthis diseases with clinical correlation. Williams & Wilkins, Baltimore, p 635

Potter EL (1962) Pathology of the fetus and infant, 2nd edn. Year Book Medical Publishers, Chicago, p 492

Powell DA, Schuit KE (1979) Acute pulmonary blastomycosis in children: clinical course and follow-up. Pediatrics 63: 736

Powell HC, Elliott ML (1977) Congenital lobar emphysema. Virchows Arch [Pathol Anat] 374: 197

Pracy R, Stell PM (1974) Laryngeal cleft: diagnosis and management. J Laryngol 88: 483

Pratt LW (1965) Midline cysts of the nasal dorsum: embryologic origin and treatment. Laryngoscope 75: 968

Press E, Adams WC, Chittenden RF, Christian JR, Grayson R, Stewart CC, Everist BW (1962) Co-operative kerosene poisoning study. Evaluation of gastric lavage and other factors in the treatment of accidental ingestion of petroleum distillate products. Pediatrics 29: 648

Price CHG, Zhuber K, Salzer-Kuntschik M, Salzer M, Willert HG, Immenkamp M, Groh P, Matejovsky Z, Keyl W (1975) Osteosarcoma in children. A study of 125 cases. J Bone Joint Surg [Br] 57: 341

Price RA, Hughes WT (1974) Histopathology of *Pneumocystis carinii* infestation and infection in malignant disease in childhood. Hum Pathol 5: 737

Pryce DM (1948) The lining of healed but persistent abscess cavities in the lung with epithelium of ciliated columnar type. J Pathol 60: 259

Pryce DM (1946) Lower accessory pulmonary artery with intralobar sequestration of lung: report of 7 cases. J Pathol Bacteriol 58: 457

Pryce DM, Sellors TM, Blair LG (1947) Intralobar sequestration of lung associated with an abnormal pulmonary artery. Br J Surg 35: 18

Punnett HH, Kistenmacher ML, Valdes-Dapena M, Ellison RT Jr (1974) Syndrome of ankylosis, facial anomalies and pulmonary hypoplasia. J Pediatr 85: 375

Quick CA, Faras A, Krzysek R (1978) The etiology of laryngeal papillomatosis. Laryngoscope 88: 1789

Rahimi SA (1974) Disseminated *Pneumocystis carinii* in thymic alymphoplasia. Arch Pathol 97: 162

Ranga V, Kleinerman J (1978) Structure and function of small airways in health and disease. Arch Pathol Lab Med 102: 609

Ransome J (1964) Familial incidence of posterior choanal atresia. J Laryngol Otol 78: 551

Rao M, Steiner P, Rose JS, Kassner EG, Kottmeier P, Steiner M (1975) Chronic eosinophilic pneumonia in a one-year-old child. Chest 68: 118

Rappaport F, Rabinowitz M, Toaff R, Krochik N (1960) Genital listeriosis as a cause of repeated abortion. Lancet 1: 1273

Reale FR, Esterly JR (1973) Pulmonary hypoplasia: a morphometric study of the lungs of infants with diaphragmatic hernia, anencephaly, and renal malformations. Pediatrics 51: 91

Rebello G, Mason JK (1978) Pulmonary histological appearances in fatal paraquat poisoning. Histopathology 2: 53

Régy JM, Fauchier C, Lamagnère JP, Combe P (1970) Tumeur carcinoïde bronchique chez une fille de 14 ans. Ann Pediatr 17: 882

Remberger K, Hübner G (1974) Rhabdomyomatous dysplasia of the lung. Virchows Arch [Pathol Anat] 363: 363

Reynolds DW, Stagno S, Alford CA (1978) Congenital cytomegalovirus infection. Teratology 17: 179

Reynolds HY, Fulmer JD, Kazmierowski JA, Roberts WC, Frank MM, Crystal RC (1977) Analysis of cellular and protein content of bronchoalveolar lavage fluid from patients with idiopathic pulmonary fibrosis and chronic hypersensitivity pneumonitis. J Clin Invest 59: 165

Rhodes PG, Burry VF, Hall RT, Cox R (1975) Pneumococcal septicemia and meningitis in the neonate. J Pediatr 86: 593

Ricci C, Patrassi N, Massa R, Benedetti-Valentini F Jr, Mineo TC (1973) Carcinoid syndrome in bronchial adenoma. Am J Surg 126: 671

Rice DH, Batsakis JG, Headington JT (1974) Fibrous histiocytomas of the nose and paranasal sinuses. Arch Otolaryngol 100: 398

Rienhoff WF, Broyles EN (1934) The surgical treatment of carcinoma of the bronchi and lungs. JAMA 103: 1121

Robert MF, Neff RK, Hubbell JP, Taeusch HW, Avery ME (1976) Association between maternal diabetes and respiratory distress syndrome in the newborn. N Engl J Med 294: 357

Roberts RC, Moore VL (1977) Immunopathogenesis of hypersensitivity pneumonitis. Am Rev Respir Dis 116: 1075

Robertson B, Grossmann G, Ivemark B (1976) The alveolar lung layer in experimental paraquat poisoning. Acta Pathol Microbiol Scand [A] 84: 40

Robertson MH (1977) Listeriosis. Postgrad Med J 53: 618

Robin PE, Dalton GA (1974) Subglottic stenosis in infants. Eight cases and their surgical and conservative management. J Laryngol Otol 88: 233

Roenspies U, Morin D, Gloor E, Hochstetter AR von, Saegesser F, Senning A (1978) Bronchopulmonale Hamartome, Chondrome, Fibrome und Myxome. Schweiz Med Wochenschr 108: 332

Rogers LF, Osmer JC (1964) Bronchogenic cyst: a review of 46 cases. Am J Roentgenol 91: 273

Roggli VL, Kim HS, Hawkins E (1980) Congenital generalized fibromatosis with visceral involvement. A case report. Cancer 45: 954

Rola-Pleszczynski M, Frenkel LD, Fuccillo DA, Hensen SA, Vincent MM, Reynolds DW, Stagno S, Bellanti JA (1977) Specific impairment of cell-mediated immunity in mothers of infants with congenital infection due to cytomegalovirus. J Infect Dis 135: 386

Roloff DW, Outerbridge EW, Stern L (1973) Combined positive and negative pressure ventilation in the management of severe respiratory distress syndrome in newborn infants. Biol Neonate 22: 325

Rontal M, Duritz G (1977) Proboscis lateralis—Case report and embryonic analysis. Laryngoscope 87: 996

Rosai J; Dorfman RF (1972) Sinus histiocytosis with massive lymphadenopathy: a pseudolymphomatous benign disorder. Cancer 30: 1174

Rosan RC (1975) Hyaline membrane disease and a related spectrum of neonatal pneumopathies. In: Rosenberg HS, Bolande RP (eds) Perspectives in pediatric pathology, vol 12. Year Book Medical Publishers, Chicago, p 15

Rosen G. Wollner N, Tan C, Wu SJ, Hajdu SI, Cham W, D'Angio GJ, Murphy ML (1974) Disease-free survival in children with Ewing's sarcoma treated with radiation therapy and adjuvant four-drug sequential chemotherapy. Cancer 33: 384

Rosen N, Gaton E (1975) Congenital bronchiolitis obliterans. Beitr Pathol 155: 309

Rosen SH, Castleman B, Liebow AA (1958) Pulmonary alveolar proteinosis. N Engl J Med 158: 1123

Rosen Y, Moon S, Huang CT, Gouring A, Lyons HA (1977) Granulomatous pulmonary angiitis in sarcoidosis. Arch Pathol Lab Med 101: 170

Rosen Y, Athanassiades TJ, Moon S, Lyons HA (1978) Nongranulomatous interstitial pneumonitis in sarcoidosis—Relationship to development of epitheloid granulomas. Chest 74: 122

Rosenthal AF, Vargas MG, Schiff SV (1974) Comparison of four indexes of fetal pulmonary maturity. Clin Chem 20: 486

Roth JA, Siegel SE, Levine AS, Berard CW (1971) Fatal recurrent toxoplasmosis in a patient initially infected via a leukocyte transfusion. Am J Clin Pathol 56: 601

Rott HD (1979) Kartagener's syndrome and the syndrome of immotile cilia. Hum Genet 46: 249

Runckel D, Kessler S (1980) Bronchogenic squamous carcinoma in non-irradiated juvenile laryngotracheal papillomatosis. Am J Surg Pathol 4: 293

Ryland D, Reid L (1971) Pulmonary aplasia—A quantitative analysis of the development of the single lung. Thorax 26: 602

Sabin AB (1977) Mortality from pneumonia and risk conditions during influenza epidemics. High influenza morbidity during nonepidemic years. JAMA 237: 2823

Salfelder K, Brass K, Doehnert G, Doehnert R, Sauerteig E (1970) Fatal disseminated histoplasmosis. Anatomic study of autopsy cases. Virchows Arch [Pathol Anat] 350: 300

Salm R, Hughes EW (1970) A case of chronic paraffin pneumonitis. Thorax 25: 762

Salvaggio JE, Karr RM (1979) Hypersensitivity pneumonitis: state of the art. Chest 75: 2705

Samaan HA (1970) Complete agenesis of the lung. Postgrad Med J 46: 578

Sandstrom RE, Proppe KH, Trelstad RL (1978) Fibrous histiocytoma of the trachea. Am J Clin Pathol 70: 429

Sanford JP (1979) Legionnaires' disease—the first thousand days. N Engl J Med 300: 654

Savic B, Birtel FJ, Tholen W, Funke HD, Knoche R (1979) Lung sequestration: report of seven cases and review of 540 published cases. Thorax 34: 96

Scadding JG (1971) Eosinophilic infiltrations of the lungs in asthmatics. Proc R Soc Med 64: 381

Scadding JG (1974) Diffuse pulmonary alveolar fibrosis. Thorax 29: 271

Scadding JG (1978) Talking clearly about diseases of the pulmonary acini. Br J Dis Chest 72: 1

Scadding JG, Hinson KFW (1967) Diffuse fibrosing alveolitis (diffuse interstitial fibrosis of the lungs). Correlation of histology at biopsy with prognosis. Thorax 22: 291

Scattini CM, Orsi A (1973) Multiple bilateral fibromas of the pleura. Thorax 28: 782

Schapiro RL, Evans ET (1972) Surgical disorders causing neonatal respiratory distress. Am J Roentgenol 114: 305

Scheidemandel HE, Page RS (1975) Special considerations in epiglottis in children. Laryngoscope 85: 1738

Schild JP, Wuilloud A, Kollberg H, Bossi E (1976) Tracheal perforation as a complication of nasotracheal intubation. J Pediatr 88: 631

Schiøtz PO, Høiby N, Juhl F, Permin H, Nielsen H, Svehag SE (1977) Immune complexes in cystic fibrosis. Acta Pathol Microbiol Scand [C] 85: 57

Schirar A, Rendu C, Vielh JP, Gautray JP (1974) Congenital mycosis (Candida albicans). Biol Neonate 24: 273

Schlegel RJ (1975) Chronic granulomatous disease 1974. JAMA 231: 615

Schneegans E, Burgun P, Peter JD, Cajuste G (1975) Traitement de la maladie des membranes hyalines par une méthode nouvelle de presion positive continue. Premiers résultats. Nouv Presse Med 4: 1629

Schneider EL, Epstein CJ, Kaback MJ, Brandes D (1977) Severe pulmonary involvement in adult Gaucher's disease. Report of three cases and review of the literature. Am J Med 63: 475

Schneider P (1912) Die Missbildungen der Atmungsorgane. In: Schwalbe E (ed) Die Morphologie der Missbildungen des Menschen und der Tiere, Bd III. Fischer, Jena, p 763

Schonland M, Strong ML, Wesley A (1976) Fatal adenovirus pneumonia—Clinical and pathological features. S Afr Med J 50: 1748

Schopfer K, Laurer E, Krech U (1978) Congenital cytomegalovirus infection in newborn infants of mothers infected before pregnancy. Arch Dis Child 53: 536

Scott DJ, Gardner PS, McQuillin J, Stanton AN, Downham MAPS (1978) Respiratory viruses and cot death. Br Med J ii: 12

Scott JM, Henderson A (1972) Acute villous inflammation in the placenta following intrauterine transfusion. J Clin Pathol 25: 872

Scowden EB, Schaffner W, Stone WJ (1978) Overwhelming strongyloidiasis: an unappreciated opportunistic infection. Medicine 57: 527

Sears MR, Chang AR, Taylor AJ (1971) Pulmonary alveolar microlithiasis. Thorax 26: 704

Sedano HO, Cohen MM Jr, Jirasek J, Gorlin RJ (1970) Frontonasal dysplasia. J Pediatr 76: 906

Self JT (1969) Biological relationships of the Pentastomida: a bibliography on the Pentastomida. Exp Parasitol 24: 63

Selleger C (1979) Pneumonie varicelleuse mortelle chez l'adulte—Rapport de deux, cas et revue de la littérature. Rev Fr Mal Respir 7: 9

Seppälä M, Aho I (1975) Physiological role of meconium during delivery. Acta Obstet Gynecol Scand 54: 209

Serlin SP, Daily WJR (1975) Tracheal perforation in the neonate: complication of endotracheal intubation. J Pediatr 86: 596

Shabot JM, Patterson M (1978) Amebic liver abscess: 1966–1976. Am J Dig Dis 23: 110

Shanklin DR (1959) Cardiovascular factors in development of pulmonary hyaline membrane. Arch Pathol 68: 49

Shanmugaratnam K, Chan SH, De The G, Goh JEH, Khort TN, Simons MJ, Tye CY (1979) Histopathology of nasopharyngeal carcinoma. Correlations with epidemiology, survival rates and other biological characteristics. Cancer 44: 1029

Shapiro RS, Marlowe FI, Butcher J (1976) Malignant degeneration of non-irradiated juvenile laryngeal papillomatosis. Ann Otol 85: 101

Sheffield LJ, Danks DM, Hammond JW, Hoogenradd NJ (1976) Massive pulmonary hemorrhage as a presenting feature in congenital hyperammonemia. J Pediatr 88: 450

Shirakusa T (1978) Long-term follow-up of two cases of pulmonary varicosity. Thorax 33: 653

Shulman JB, Hollister DW, Thibeault DW, Krugman ME (1976) Familial laryngomalacia: a case report. Laryngoscope 86: 84

Schwachman H, Kowalski M, Khaw KT (1977) Cystic fibrosis: a new outlook—70 patients above 25 years of age. Medicine 56: 129

Siegel JD, Gartner JC, Michaels RH (1978) Pneumococcal empyema in childhood. Am J Dis Child 132: 1094

Siegel SE, Cohen SR, Isaacs H Jr, Stanley P (1979) Malignant transformation of tracheobronchial juvenile papillomatosis without prior radiotherapy. Ann Otol 88: 192

Silverman JF, Kay S (1976) Multiple pulmonary leiomyomatous hamartomas. Report of a case with ultrastructure examination. Cancer 38: 1199

Simpson W, Hacking PM, Court SDM, Gardner PS (1974) The radiological findings in respiratory syncytial virus infection in children. II. The correlation of radiological categories with clinical and virological findings. Pediatr Radiol 2: 155

Sing KP, Pahor AL (1977) Congenital cyst of nasopharynx. J Laryngol Otol 91: 75

Sing W, Ramage C, Best P, Angus B (1980) Nasal neuroblastoma

secreting vasopressin. A case report. Cancer 45: 961

Singer AD, Thibeault DW, Hobel CJ, Heiner DC (1976) Alpha-1-antitrypsin in amniotic fluid and cord blood of preterm infants with the respiratory distress syndrome. Pediatrics 88: 87

Sir G (1962) Bronchiolitis obliterans connata. Zentralbl Allg Pathol 103: 129

Slack MPE, Mayon-White RT (1978) Group B streptococci in pharyngeal aspirates at birth and the early detection of neonatal sepsis. Arch Dis Child 53: 540

Sladen A, Zanca P, Hadnott WH (1971) Aspiration pneumonitis—The sequelae. Chest 59: 448

Slavin RG, Laird TS, Cherry JD (1970) Allergic bronchopulmonary aspergillosis in a child. J Pediatr 76: 416

Smith II, Bain AD (1965) Congenital atresia of the larynx, a report of nine cases. Ann Otol 74: 338

Smith M, McCormack LJ, Van Ordstrand HS, Mercer RD (1974) 'Primary' pulmonary histiocytosis X. Chest 65: 176

Smith P, Heath D (1974a) The ultrastructure and time sequence of the early stages of paraquat lung in rats. J Pathol 114: 177

Smith P, Heath D (1974b) Paraquat lung: a reappraisal. Thorax 29: 643

Smith P, Heath D, Kay JM (1974) The pathogenesis and structure of paraquat-induced pulmonary fibrosis in rats. J Pathol 114: 57

Smith SB, Schwartzman M, Mencia F, Blum EB, Krogstad D, Nitzkin J, Healy GR (1977) Fatal disseminated strongyloidiasis presenting as acute abdominal distress in an urban child. J Pediatr 91: 607

Smith SD, Cho CT, Brahmacupta N, Lenahan MF (1977) Pulmonary involvement with cytomegalovirus infections in children. Arch Dis Child 52: 441

Sobonya RE, Hiller C, Pingleton W, Watanabe I (1978) (Rubeola) pneumonia in adults. Arch Pathol Lab Med 102: 366

Solliday NH, Williams JA, Gaensler EA, Coutu RE, Carrington CB (1973) Familial chronic interstitial pneumonia. Am Rev Respir Dis 108: 193

Som PM, Nagel BD, Feuerstein SS, Strauss L (1979) Benign pleomorphic adenoma of the larynx. A case report. Ann Otol Rhinol Laryngol 88: 112

Spector RG, Claireaux AE, Williams ER (1960) Congenital adenomatoid malformation of lung with pneumothorax. Arch Dis Child 35: 475

Speer M, Rosan RC, Rudolph AJ (1978) Hemophilus influenzae infection in the neonate mimicking respiratory distress syndrome. J Pediatr 93: 295

Spellacy WN, Buhi WC, Rigall FC, Holsinger KL (1973) Human amniotic fluid lecithin sphingomyelin ratio changes with estrogen or glucocorticoid treatment. Am J Obstet Gynecol 115: 216

Spencer H (1977a) Congenital abnormalities of the lung, pulmonary vessels and lymphatics. In: Spencer H (ed) Pathology of the lung, vol I. Pergamon, Oxford, p 71

Spencer H (1977b) Congenital abnormalities of the lung, pulmonary vessels and lymphatics. In: Spencer H (ed) Pathology of the lung, vol. I. Pergamon, Oxford, p 87

Spencer H, Dail DH, Arneaud J (1980) Non-invasive bronchial epithelial papillary tumors. Cancer 45: 1486

Speondlin H, Kistler G (1978) Papova-virus in human laryngeal papillomas. Arch Otorhinolaryngol 218: 289

Stahlman M, Hedwall G, Dolanski F, Faxelius G, Burko H, Kirk V (1973) A six-year follow-up of clinical hyaline membrane disease. Pediatr Clin North Am 20: 433

Stell PM, Maran AGD (1975) Laryngocele. J Laryngol Otol 89: 915

Stephanopoulos C, Catsaras H (1963) Myxosarcoma complicating a cystic hamartoma of the lung. Thorax 18: 144

Stern RC, Boat TF, Doershuk CF, Tucker AS, Primiano FP Jr, Mathews LW (1976) Course of cystic fibrosis in 95 patients. J Pediatr 89: 406

Stern RC, Boat TF, Doershuk CF, Tucker AS, Miller RB, Matthews LW (1977) Cystic fibrosis diagnosed after age 13—Twenty-five teenage and adult patients including three asymptomatic men. Ann Intern Med 87: 188

Sternberg SS (1954) Pathology of juvenile nasopharyngeal angiofibroma—a lesion of adolescent males. Cancer 7: 15

Stevens D, Swift PGF, Johnston PGB, Kearney PJ, Corner BD, Burman D (1978) *Mycoplasma pneumoniae* infections in children. Arch Dis Child 53: 38

Stillwell PC, Norris DG, O'Connell EJ, Rosenow EC III, Weiland LH, Harrison EG Jr (1980) Desquamative interstitial pneumonitis in children. Chest 77: 165

Stocker JT, Kagan-Hallet K (1979) Extralobar pulmonary sequestration. Analysis of 15 cases. Am J Clin Pathol 72: 917

Stocker JT, Madewell JE, Drake RM (1977) Congenital cystic adenomatoid malformation of the lung. Classification and morphologic spectrum. Hum Pathol 8: 155

Stocks J, Godfrey S, Reynolds EOR (1978) Airway resistance in infants after various treatments for hyaline membrane disease: special emphasis on prolonged high levels of inspired oxygen. Pediatrics 61: 178

Stokes D, Sigler A, Khouri NF, Talamo RC (1978) Unilateral hyperlucent lung (Swyer–James syndrome) after severe *mycoplasma pneumoniae* infection. Am Rev Respir Dis 117: 145

Stone FJ, Churg AM (1977) The ultrastructure of pulmonary hamartoma. Cancer 39: 1064

Strauss RG, Bove KE (1975) Fever, shock and hepatomegaly in a 13-month-old boy. J Pediatr 87: 819

Strong RM, Passay V (1977) Endotracheal intubation: complications in neonates. Arch Otol 103: 329

Strunge P (1972) Infantile lobar emphysema with lobar agenesia and congenital heart disease. Acta Paediatr Scand 61: 209

Studdy P, Bird R, Geraint-James D, Sherlock S (1978) Serum angiotensin-converting enzyme (SACE) in sarcoidosis and other granulomatous disorders. Lancet 2: 1331

Sturges JM, Chao J, Turner JAP (1980) Transposition of ciliary microtubules. Another cause of impaired ciliary motility. Engl J Med 303: 318

Sturgess JM, Chao J, Wong J, Aspin N, Turner JAP (1979) Cilia with defective radial spokes. A cause of human respiratory disease. N Engl J Med 300: 53

Sueishi K, Watanabe T, Tanaka K, Shin H (1974) Intrauterine bronchiolitis obliterans: report of an autopsy case and review of the literature. Virchows Arch [Pathol Anat] 362: 223

Sulayman R, Thilenius O, Replogie R, Arcilla RA (1975) Unilateral emphysema in total anomalous pulmonary venous return. J Pediatr 87: 433

Sundar B, Guine EJ, O'Donnell M (1975) Congenital H-type tracheo-oesophageal fistula. Arch Dis Child 80: 862

Sunderland WA, Campbell RA, Edwards MJ (1972) Pulmonary alveolar proteinosis and pulmonary cryptococcosis in an adolescent boy. J Pediatr 80: 450

Suzuki C, Oshibe M, Nagashima Y (1971) Granular cell myoblastoma of the bronchus. Report of a case with treatment by upper lobectomy and sleeve resection of the stem bronchus. J Thorac Cardiovasc Surg 61: 271

Swischuk LE, Richardson CJ, Nichols MM, Ingman MJ (1979) Primary pulmonary hypoplasia in the neonate. J Pediatr 95: 573

Synder R, Perzin K (1972) Papillomatosis of the nasal cavity and paranasal sinuses (inverted papilloma, squamous papilloma). A clinico-pathologic study. Cancer 30: 668

Szalay GC, Bledsoe RC (1972) Congenital dermoid cyst and fistula of the nose. Am J Dis Child 124: 392

Taghizadeh A, Reynolds EOR (1976) Pathogenesis of bronchopulmonary dysplasia following hyaline membrane disease. Am J Pathol 82: 241

Tan C, D'Angio GJ, Exelby PR, Lieberman PH, Watson RC, Cham WC, Murphy ML (1975) The changing management of childhood Hodgkin's disease. Cancer 35: 808

Taxy JB (1977) Juvenile nasopharyngeal angiofibroma. An ultrastructural study. Cancer 39: 1044

Taxy JB, Hidvegi DF (1977) Olfactory neuroblastoma. An ultrastructural study. Cancer 39: 131

Taylor BW, Erich JB (1967) Dermoid cysts of the nose. Mayo Clin Proc 42: 488

Taylor TL, Miller DR (1969) Leiomyoma of the bronchus. J. Thorac Cardiovasc Surg 57: 284

Templeton AC (1970) Generalized herpes simplex in malnourished children. J Clin Pathol 23: 24

Thaell JF, Greipp PR, Stubbs SE, Siegal GP (1978) Idiopathic pulmonary hemosiderosis. Two cases in a family. Mayo Clin Proc 53: 113

Thawley SE, Osborn DA (1974) Granular cell myoblastoma of the larynx. Laryngoscope 84: 1545

Thomas IT, Smith DW (1974) Oligohydramnios, cause of the nonrenal features of Potter's syndrome, including pulmonary hypoplasia. J Pediatr 84: 811

Thompson EN, Soothill JF (1970) Chronic granulomatous disease: quantitative clinico-pathological relationships. Arch Dis Child 45: 24

Tipple MA, Beem MO, Saxon EM (1979) Clinical characteristics of the afebrile pneumonia associated with *Chlamydia trachomatis* infection in infants less than 6 months of age. Pediatrics 63: 192

Tolsdorff P (1973) Das Rhinosklerom—Klinik und Pathologie. Z Laryngol Rhinol 52: 486

Torriani R, Zimmermann A, Morell A (1979) Die BCG-Sepsis als letale Komplikation der BCG-Impfung. Schweiz Med Wochenschr 109: 708

Tos M, Mogensen C, Thomsen J (1977) Nasal polyps in cystic fibrosis. J Laryngol Otol 91: 827

Townsend GL, Neel HB III, Weiland LH, Devine KD, McBean JB (1973) Fibrous histiocytoma ofthe paranasal sinuses. Report of a case. Arch Otolaryngol 98: 51

Trail ML, Creely JJ Jr, Landrum CE (1973) Congenital choanal atresia. South Med J 66: 460

Triebwasser JH, Harris RE, Bryant RE, Rhoades ER (1967) Varicella pneumonia in adults. Report of seven cases and a review of literature. Medicine 46: 409

Trompeter R, Yu VYH, Aynsley-Green A, Roberton NRC (1975) Massive pulmonary haemorrhage in the newborn infant. Arch Dis Child 50: 123

Truog WE, Prueitt JL, Woodrum DE (1978) Unchanged incidence of bronchopulmonary dysplasia in survivors of hyaline membrane disease. J Pediatr 92: 261

Tubbs RR, Benjamin SP, Reich NE, McCormack LJ, Scott van Ordstrand H (1977) Desquamative interstitial pneumonitis. Cellular phase of fibrosing alveolitis. Chest 72: 159

Tucker GF, Ossoff RH, Newman AN, Holinger LD (1979) Histopathology of congenital subglottic stenosis. Laryngoscope 89: 866

Turiaf J, Battesti JP, Jeanjean Y, Fourestier V (1978) Sarcoïdose Nouv Presse Med 3: 1351

Turiaf J, Battesti JP, Jeanjean Y, Foursetier V (1978) Sarcoïose familiale. 26 cas dans 12 familles. Nouv Presse Med 7: 913

Ueda K, Gruppo R, Unger F, Martin L, Bove K (1974) Rhabdomyosarcoma of lung arising in congenital cystic adenomatoid malformation. Cancer 40: 383

Ulbright TM, Katzenstein ALA (1980) Solitary necrotizing granulomas of the lung. Differentiating features and etiology. Am J Surg Pathol 4: 13

Umetsu M, Chiba Y, Horino K, Chiba S, Nakao T (1975) Cytomegalo-virus-mononucleosis in a newborn infant. Arch Dis Child 50: 396

Unger L (1952) The recognition of nonallergic asthma. Dis Chest 22: 671

Usher RH, Allen AC, McLean FH (1971) Risk of respiratory

distress syndrome related to gestational age, route of delivery and maternal diabetes. Am J Obstet Gynecol 111: 826

Utzon F, Brandrup F (1973) Pulmonary arteriovenous fistulas in children. A review with special reference to the disperse telangiectatic type. Illustrated by a report of a case. Acta Paediatr Scand 62: 422

Valderrama E, Saluja G, Shende A, Lanzkowsky P, Berkman J (1978) Pulmonary blastoma. Report of two cases in children. Am J Surg Pathol 2: 415

Valdes-Dapena MA, Arey JB (1967) Pulmonary emboli of cerebral origin in the newborn: a report of two cases. Arch Pathol 84: 643

Valdes-Dapena MA, Nissim JE, Arey JB, Godleski J, Schaaf HD, Haust MD (1976) Yellow pulmonary hyaline membranes. J Pediatr 89: 128

Van Dijk C, Wagenvoort CA (1973) The various types of congenital adenomatoid malformation of the lung. J Pathol 110: 131

Vargas F, Patron M (1971) Un cas d'atrésie congénitale du larynx. Ann Chir Inf 12: 355

Veerman AJP, Van Delden L, Feenstra L, Leene W (1980) The immotile cilia syndrome: Phase contrast light microscopy, scanning and transmission electron microscopy. Pediatrics 65: 698

Veliath AJ, Khanna KK, Subhas BS, Ramakrishnan MR, Aurora AL (1977) Primary lymphosarcoma of the lung with unusual features. Thorax 32: 632

Vella EE (1978) Legionnaires' disease: a review. J R Soc Med 71: 361

Vidyasagar D, Yeh TF, Harris V, Pildes RS (1975) Assisted ventilation in infants with meconium aspiration syndrome. Pediatrics 56: 208

Vogel JM, Vogel P (1972) Idiopathic histiocytosis: a discussion of eosinophilic granuloma, the Hand–Schüller–Christian syndrome and the Letterer–Siwe syndrome. Semin Hematol 9: 349

Voigt JC, Claireaux AE, Hopper PK (1971) Perinatal listeriosis. J Obstet Gynecol Br Commonwlth 78: 570

Volk BW, Adachi M, Schneck L (1975) The gangliosidoses. Hum Pathol 6: 555

Vrabec DP (1975) The inverted schneiderian papilloma: a clinical and pathological study. Laryngoscope 85: 186

Wagenvoort CA, Beetstra A, Spijker J (1978) Capillary haemangiomatosis of the lungs. Histopathology 2: 401

Wailoo MP, Emery JL (1979) The trachea in children with tracheo-oesophageal fistula. Histopathology 3: 329

Wall CP, Goff AM, Carrington CB, Gaensler EA (1979) Lymphomatoid granulomatosis. Case report from the thoracic services. Boston University Medical School. Respiration 38: 332

Wang AH, Naiman JL, Kendall N, Kirkpatrick JA (1971) Wilson–Mikity syndrome followed by 'idiopathic' pulmonary hemosiderosis. J Pediatr 78: 503

Wang NS, Huang SN, Thurlbeck WM (1970) Combined Pneumocystis carinii and cytomegalovirus infection. Arch Pathol 90: 529

Wayoff M, Labaeye P (1973) Sarcome botryoide du larynx chez un garçon de 10 ans. J Fr Otorhinolaryngol 22: 349

Webb JK, Job CK, Gault EW (1960) Tropical eosinophilia: demonstration of microfilariae in lung, liver and lymph nodes. Lancet 1: 835

Webb WR, Hare WV (1961) Primary fibrosarcoma of the bronchus. Am Rev Respir Dis 84: 881

Weber AL, Grillo HC (1978a) Tracheal stenosis. Radiol Clin North Am 16: 291

Weber AL, Grillo HC (1978b) Tracheal tumors. A radiological, clinical and pathological evaluation of 84 cases. Radiol Clin North Am 16: 227

Weber ML, Rivard G, Perreault G (1978) Prune belly syndrome associated with congenital cystic adenomatoid malformation of the lung. Am J Dis Child 132: 315

Weber WR, Askin FB, Dehner LP (1977) Lung biopsy in Pneumocystis carinii pneumonia. A histopathologic study of typical and atypical features. Am J Clin Pathol 67: 11

Weichert RF III, Lindsey ES, Pearce CW, Waring WW (1970) Bronchogenic cyst with unilateral obstructive emphysema. J Thorac Cardiovasc Surg 59: 287

Weinberg AG, McCracken GH Jr, LoSpalluto J, Luby JP (1973) Monoclonal macroglobulinemia and cytomegalic inclusion disease. Pediatrics 51: 518

Weller MH (1973) The roentgenographic course and complications of hyaline membrane disease. Pediatr Clin North Am 20: 381

Wellons HA Jr, Eggleston P, Golden GT, Allen MS (1976) Bronchial adenoma in childhood. Two case reports and review of literature. Am J Dis Child 130: 301

Westerheide RL (1964) An unusual complication of a bronchogenic cyst. J Thorac Cardiovasc Surg 47: 389

Whitwell F, Scott J, Grimshaw M (1977) Relationship between occupations and asbestos-fibre content of the lungs in patients with pleural mesothelioma, lung cancer and other diseases. Thorax 32: 377

Whitworth JA, Lawrence JR, Meadows R (1974) Goodpasture's syndrome. A review of nine cases and an evaluation of therapy. Aust NZ J Med 4: 167

Wigglesworth JS, Keith IH, Girling DJ, Slade SA (1976) Hyaline membrane disease, alkali and intraventricular haemorrhage. Arch Dis Child 51: 755

Williams AO, Lawson EA, Lucas AO (1971) African histoplasmosis due to Histoplasma duboissii. Arch Pathol 92: 306

Williams HE (1973) Inhalation pneumonia. Aust Paediatr J 9: 279

Williams HE, Campbell P (1960) Generalized bronchiectasis associated with deficiency of cartilage in the bronchial type. Arch Dis Child 35: 182

Williams HE, Freeman M (1973) Milk inhalation pneumonia. The significance of fat filled macrophages in tracheal secretions. Aust Paediatr J 9: 286

Williams HE, Landau LI, Phelan PD (1972) Generalized bronchiectasis due to extensive deficiency of bronchial cartilage. Arch Dis Child 47: 423

Williams HL, Williams RI (1969) The therapeutic implications of the hypotheses of allergic hypersensitivity as a dysfunction of the intracellular immune mechanisms. Ann Allergol 27: 434

Williams RI (1960) Modern concepts in the clinical management of allergy in otolaryngology. Ann Otol 76: 1389

Wilson MG, Mikity VG (1960) A new form of respiratory disease in premature infants. Am J Dis Child 99: 489

Winstock DP, Burtlett PC, Sondheimer FK (1978) Benign nasal polyps causing bone destruction in the nasal cavity and paranasal sinuses. Laryngoscope 88: 675

Winn WC Jr, Glavin FL, Perl DP, Keller JL, Andres TL, Brown TM, Coffin CM, Sensecqua JE, Roman LN, Craighead JE (1978) The pathology of Legionnaires' disease. Fourteen fatal cases from the 1977 outbreak in Vermont. Arch Pathol Lab Med 102: 344

Winther LK (1978) Congenital choanal atresia. Anatomic, physiological and therapeutic aspects, especially the endonasal approach under endoscopic vision. Arch Otolaryngol 104: 72

Witwer JP, Tampas JP (1973) Tracheal fibroxanthoma in a child. Postgrad Med 54: 228

Wohl MEB, Chernick V (1978) Bronchiolitis. Am Rev Respir Dis 118: 759

Wollner N, Burchenal JH, Lieberman PH, Exelby PR, D'Angio GJ, Murphy ML (1975) Non-Hodgkin's lymphoma in children. Med Pediatr Oncol 1: 235

Wood NL, Coltman CA Jr (1973) Localized primary extranodal Hodgkin's disease. Ann Intern Med 78: 113

Woodruff AW (1975) Diseases of travel, with particular reference to tropical diseases. Postgrad Med J 51: 825

Wright DH (1970) Microscopic features, histochemistry, histogenesis and diagnosis. In: Burkitt DP, Wright D (eds) Burkitt's lymphoma. Livingstone, Edinburgh, p 82

Wright HT Jr, Beckwith JB, Gwinn JL (1964) A fatal case of inclusion body pneumonia in an infant infected with adenovirus type 3. J Pediatr 64: 528

Wu JP, Gilbert EF, Pellett JR (1974) Pulmonary liposarcoma in a child with adrenogenital syndrome. Am J Clin Pathol 62: 791

Yeager AS, Martin HP, Stewart JA (1977) Congenital cytomegalovirus infection outcome for the subsequent sibling. Clin Pediatr 16: 455

Young LW, Kim KS, Sproles ET III (1978) Radiological case of the month. Am J Dis Child 132: 311

Zahradnik JM, Spencer MJ, Porter DD (1980) Adenovirus infection in the immunocompromised patient. Am J Med 68: 725

Zelefsky MN, Janis M, Bernstein R, Blatt C, Lin A, Meng CH (1971) Intralobar bronchopulmonary sequestration with bronchial communication. Chest 59: 266

Zelkowitz PS, Giammona ST (1969) Cystic fibrosis—Pulmonary studies in children, adolescents and young adults. Am J Dis Child 117: 543

Zinserling A (1972) Pecularities of lesions in viral and mycoplasma infections of the respiratory tract. Virchows Arch [Pathol Anat] 356: 259

Chapter 9

Diseases of the Kidney and Lower Urinary Tract

R. Anthony Risdon

1. Embryology

The kidneys develop from an intermediate mass of mesoderm (the nephrogenic cord) situated on the posterior wall of the intraembryonic coelom between the dorsal somites and the lateral plate mesoderm. Three successive excretory organs develop in the early human embryo—the prenephros, the mesonephros, and the metanephros. These three 'kidneys' form sequentially and progressively and more caudally, but there is considerable overlap both chronologically and topographically. The pronephros and mesonephros are transient vestigial structures, and the definitive kidney forms from the metanephros. The mesonephric (or Wolffian) duct persists in male embryos as the duct of the epididymis, the vas deferens, and the ejaculatory duct.

The metanephros develops in two parts; the nephrons (glomeruli and tubules) from the nephrogenic cord caudal to the mesonephros (the metanephric blastema) and the excretory system (the ureter, pelvis, calyces, and collecting ducts) from the ureteric bud, which develops as a branch of the Wolffian duct near its distal end. During early development the ureteric bud grows cranially and impinges on the metanephric blastema, where it begins a process of rapid dichotomous branching. Our understanding of the differentiation of the metanephros has been greatly extended by the microdissection studies of human fetal kidneys by Osathanondh and Potter (1963a–c, 1966a, b). These authors recognized two parts of the ureteric bud and each of its branches:

1) The dilated tips, or ampullae, which are capable of dichotomous branching and the induction of nephron formation in the related metanephric blastema;

2) Tubular, or interstitial, portions behind the ampullae, which are capable of growth by elongation.

Rapid branching of the ureteric bud on reaching the metanephric blastema results in a large number of ampullae with short interstitial portions. Nephron formation and subsequent urine secretion causes their dilatation and coalescence to form the renal pelvis and calyces. The renal pelvis and major calyces are derived from the first three to five branches and the minor calyces from the next three to five branches of the ureteric bud. Urine production causes dilatation and coalescence of the generations of branches forming the minor calyces, but the differentiation of nephrons around the calyces limits the dilatation of adjoining calyces and results in the invagination of overlying parenchyma to produce the renal papillae surrounded by flask-shaped calyces.

During the early phase of nephron production branching of the ureteric bud continues. Condensations of metanephric blastema, from which the nephrons develop, become related to the ampullae. As the nephrons form they quickly become attached to the ampullae, which in turn develop into collecting ducts. This rapid attachment to the growing tips of the ureteric bud ensures that the nephrons are carried outwards as the ureteric bud grows and branches. Figure 9.1 illustrates the process of nephron formation. Subsequently (from about the 14th week of gestation onwards) branching of the ureteric bud ceases and each ampulla becomes capable of inducing the formation of a number of new nephrons. Each of these becomes attached in turn to the previously formed nephrons, to form a chain, or nephron arcade. The inner members of the arcade are formed first, and the innermost nephron in the chain is one of those formed during the first

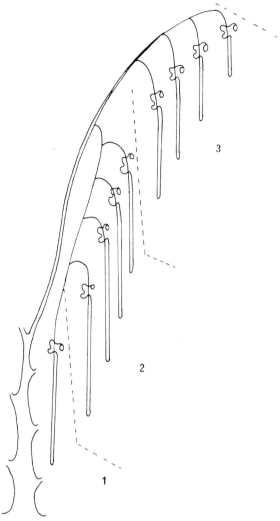

Fig. 9.1. Nephron formation (after Osthanondh and Potter 1963); 1, nephrons formed during initial phase of ureteric bud branching; 2, nephron arcade; 3, nephrons added singly till nephronogenesis ceases (32–36 weeks).

phase when the ureteric bud was branching.

After about the 22nd week of gestation the ampullae advance outwards beyond the point where nephron arcades are formed, and subsequently new nephrons are added singly. At this stage the nephrons become attached just behind the zone of active ampullary growth, and are not, therefore, carried outwards as the ampullae advance. By the 36th week of gestation ampullary growth and new nephron induction cease (Fig. 9.2).

Individual nephrons form from oval condensations of metanephric blastema, which rapidly develop a lumen that elongates and become S-shaped. The lumen of the developing nephron rapidly connects with the lumen of the ureteric bud. The proximal part of the S-shaped nephron becomes

concave around the capillaries that form the glomerular tuft, which are derived from capillary sprouts arising from arteriovenous shunts adjacent to the glomeruli. The wall of the proximal limb of the developing nephron become stretched over the tuft to form the epithelial cells covering the glomerular tuft capillaries (the podocytes) and the lining cells of Bowman's capsule, with the lumen between them forming the urinary space. The rest of the curved tubular portions of the developing nephron elongate and differentiate into the various parts of the nephronic tubules (proximal and distal convoluted tubules and the loop of Henle).

2. Congenital Anomalies

The commoner congenital abnormalities of the kidney can conveniently be divided into (1) anomalies of position and form; and (2) parenchymal maldevelopments.

2.1. Renal Ectopia

During its development, the metanephros ascends to its ultimate level (between the 12th thoracic and 3rd lumbar vertebrae). This apparent upward migration is largely due to differential growth of the caudal part of the embryo, and is accompanied by medial rotation of the kidney so that the hilum and renal pelvis, which are at first located anteriorly, come to lie on the anteromedial aspect. Interference with, or arrest of, this process results in an abnormal position and often in an abnormal shape of one or both kidneys, or to their fusion across the mid-line.

Ectopic kidneys are most commonly found at the pelvic brim or in the pelvic cavity. They are usually malrotated with the renal pelvis pointing forward, are rounded or lobulated rather than reniform, and have an ectopic blood supply. Commonly a number of small arteries supply the kidney rather than a single large renal artery; these arise from the aorta near the bifurcation, or from the iliac arteries. It is not uncommon for ectopic kidneys to exhibit parenchymal maldifferentiation (renal dysplasia), and distortion or kinking of the renal pelvis may cause hydronephrosis predisposing to renal infection. Ectopia may be unilateral or bilateral and its incidence is about 1:800; it is slightly commoner in females and on the left. Occasionally unilateral renal ectopia is associated with absence of the contralateral kidney (renal agenesis). Pelvic ectopia is sometimes associated with anorectal anomalies.

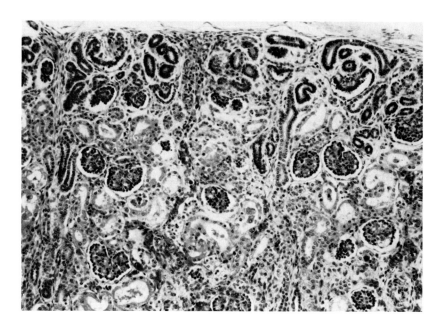

Fig. 9.2. Subcapsular 'nephrogenic zone' in the outer cortex of a premature infant. (H and E; 80 ×)

2.2. Crossed Ectopia

Occasionally ectopic kidneys occur on the opposite side to the ureteric orifice, the ureter crossing the mid-line. Both kidneys are thus located on the same side of the body and may be fused. This is a rare anomaly, with an incidence of approximately 1:8000. The displaced kidney may lie behind the aorta or vena cava.

2.3. 'Horseshoe' and 'Doughnut' Kidney

Fusion of the two kidneys across the mid-line can be regarded as a form of renal ectopia. Most commonly fusion of the lower poles occurs, to produce the horseshoe kidney; the incidence of this condition is about 1:600 (Fig. 9.3). Ring or doughnut kidneys fused at both poles are much rarer. The fused mass of renal tissue may be palpable as an apparently pulsatile mass owing to the underlying aorta, thus giving rise to a mistaken diagnosis of an aneurysm. There is an elevated incidence of renal fusion in Turner's syndrome and in association with other congenital urogenital anomalies.

2.4. Renal Agenesis

Complete absence of the kidney may be unilateral or bilateral. In the latter case the lesion is incompatible with life, although the affected infant may live for a few days after birth. Bilateral agenesis is associated with a syndrome of defects (Potter 1946), including pulmonary hypoplasia, bow legs, low-set ears,

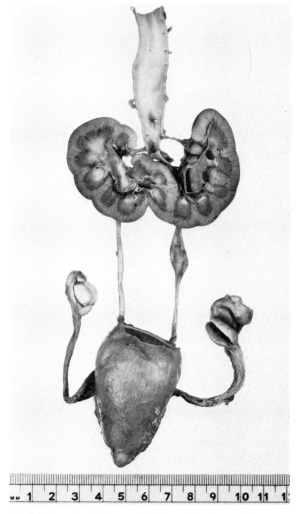

Fig. 9.3. Horseshoe kidney with fusion of the lower poles.

receding chin, and a beak-like nose (Fig. 9.4) attributed to the oligohydramnios associated with this condition (Fantel and Shepard (1975). The majority of patients with renal agenesis exhibit genital anomalies. In the male, the testis usually fails to descend and mesonephric duct derivatives (the vas deferens and seminal vesicles) are often absent. In the female, abnormalities or absence of paramesonephric-duct derivatives (Fallopian tubes, uterine horns, and upper vagina) are common (Fig. 9.5). Lower limb abnormalities, particularly sirenomelia (posterior limb bud fusion and absence of hind-gut, sacrum, bladder, urethra, and external genitalia) are often associated with bilateral agenesis. In a proportion of such cases, the bladder, urethra, and external genitalia fail to develop. The adrenals are disc-shaped because of the lack of moulding by the kidney, and in a small number of cases the gland fails to develop. Major anomalies of other systems are common, and in unilateral agenesis are the usual reason for clinical presentation.

Bilateral renal agenesis has an incidence of about 1:4000, while the incidence of unilateral agenesis is about 1:1000. The corresponding ureter and trigonal area of the bladder are usually absent, but occasionally a short stump of a lower ureter can be identified. Studies of arsenate-induced renal agenesis in the rat (Burk and Beaudoin 1977) indicate that the lesion is caused by failure of the mesonephric duct to give rise to the ureteric bud, with subsequent failure of induction of the metanephric blastema.

2.5. Supernumerary Kidneys

'Extra' kidneys are extremely rare, and precise diagnosis requires complete separation of two kidneys on the affected side of the body with separate pelvicalyceal systems. The draining ureters may fuse or join the bladder separately.

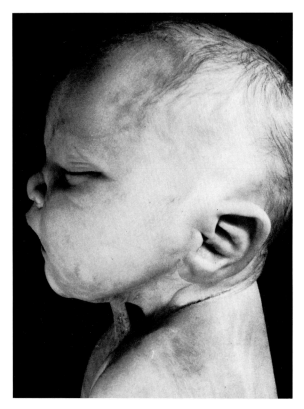

Fig. 9.4. Potter facies. Note the low-set ears, slightly receding chin, and beak-like nose.

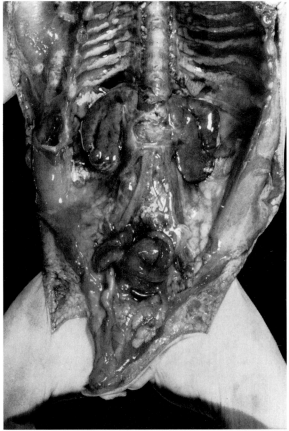

Fig. 9.5. Renal agenesis. Note the disc-shaped adrenals, absent kidneys and ureters and the anomaly of the femal genital tract (bicornuate uterus).

2.6. Renal Hypoplasia and Dysplasia

Normally renal growth is allometric, i.e., there is a close correlation between body size and renal weight. Table 9.1 shows the mean normal kidney weights at various ages up to 12 years, derived from the studies of Coppoletta and Wolbach (1933), whose findings are in striking agreement with those of Landing and Hughes (1962). Similar correlations exist between renal mass and body surface area (Risdon 1975).

Renal hypoplasia can thus be defined as a condition in which the kidney is congenitally small (i.e., its size is more than 2 SD below the expected mean). In practice, however, this definition may be very difficult to apply, since kidneys may be shrunken as a result of acquired disease, while conversely, congenitally small kidneys may themselves be prone to acquired injuries, such as pyelonephritis or hydronephrosis, masking the underlying developmental anomaly.

Table 9.1. Mean normal kidney weights at various ages from birth to 12 years[a]

Age	Renal weight (g)		
	Right	Left	Combined
Birth to 3days	13	14	27
3– 7 days	14	14	28
1– 3 weeks	15	15	30
3– 5 weeks	16	16	32
5– 7 weeks	19	18	37
7– 9 weeks	19	18	37
9–13 weeks	20	19	39
– 4 months	22	21	43
– 5 months	25	25	50
– 6 months	26	25	51
– 7 months	30	30	60
– 8 months	31	30	61
– 9 months	31	30	61
–10 months	32	31	63
–11 months	34	33	67
–12 months	36	35	71
–14 months	36	35	71
–16 months	39	39	78
–18 months	40	43	83
–20 months	43	44	87
–22 months	44	44	88
–24 months	47	46	93
– 3 years	48	49	97
– 4 years	58	56	114
– 5 years	65	64	129
– 6 years	68	67	135
– 7 years	69	70	139
– 8 years	74	75	149
– 9 years	82	83	165
–10 years	92	95	187
–11 years	95	96	189
–12 years	95	96	191

[a]Data of Coppoletta and Wolbach (1933)

The majority of congenitally small kidneys also show microscopic evidence of anomalous metanephric differentiation, often associated with cyst formation.

These are currently described as dysplastic kidneys. The term renal hypoplasia should thus be retained for cases where the kidney is abnormal only in terms of its overall size, number of nephrons, and perhaps its number of lobules (reniculi).

Simple hypoplasia of this type is very rare and is usually bilateral. Extreme degrees of bilateral renal hypoplasia are encountered in the condition *oligoméganéphronie* (oligonephronic hypoplasia) described by Royer et al. (1962). The kidneys are extremely small (with combined weights of as little as 20 g) and are usually uni- or birenicular. The number of nephrons in the kidneys is greatly reduced, and those present are enlarged and hypertrophied. Cross-sectional areas of glomeruli are increased some 12 times and microdissection studies show marked hypertrophy and hyperplasia of the proximal convoluted tubules, whose mean length is 4 times the normal length and whose mean volume is approximately 17 times normal (Fetterman and Habib 1969). Children with olignephronic hypoplasia suffer from impaired renal function with polyuria, polydipsia, dehydration, anaemia, and growth failure. The ureters and lower urinary tract are usually normal in reported cases, and familial incidence has not been observed.

Much less severe degrees of bilateral hypoplasia have been described in association with congenital anomalies or with long-standing disease of the central nervous system (Bernstein and Mayer 1964; Roosen-Runge 1949).

Unilateral simple hypoplasia (i.e., without evidence of dysplasia) is extremely rare, and one of the few acceptable cases in the literature is that described by Bernstein and Mayer (1972). However, ectopic kidneys may be smaller than expected even in the absence of dysplasia; this may be related to their abnormal blood supply.

2.6.1. Segmental Hypoplasia (Ask-Upmark Kidney)

The term 'segmental hypoplasia' refers to a particular type of small kidney associated with hypertension in childhood (Ask-Upmark 1929). The condition may be unilateral or bilateral, and it is characterized by reduced renal size and the presence of a transverse groove on the capsular surface, classically near the upper pole, overlying an area of marked parenchymal thinning and an elongated, calyx-like recess arising from the renal pelvis (Fig. 9.6a). In the area of parenchymal thinning glomeruli are very sparse or absent and tubules are

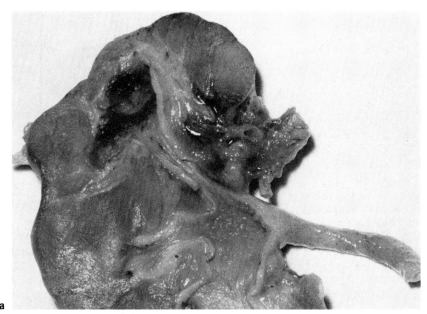

a

Fig. 9.6. The Ask-Upmark kidney in a 10-year-old girl with a history of vesicoureteric reflux, urinary infection, and hypertension: **a** Club-shaped upper pole calyx with thinning of the overlying cortex; **b** tubular loss and glomerular sclerosis with prominent thick walled arteries. (Elastin/van Gieson; 300 ×) Courtesy of the Editor of *Pediatric Radiology*.

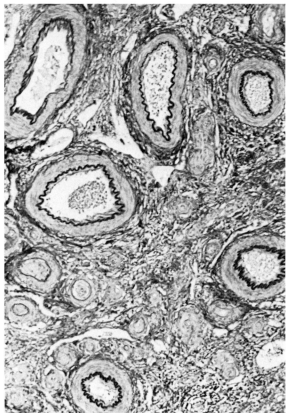

b

varied. Although Royer et al. (1971) consider the segmental areas to be developmental abnormalities, it is difficult to exclude the possibility of acquired disease. Differences in the reported incidence of the condition in different countries (it appears to be much commoner in France than in Great Britain and America) also suggest differences in interpretation. It is of interest that vesicoureteric reflux is a relatively commonly associated abnormality, and an 'overlap' between segmental hypoplasia and so-called reflux nephropathy (see p. 429) is a distinct possibility.

In the reported cases of Ask-Upmark kidney severe arterial hypertension has been the chief clinical abnormality. In unilateral cases nephrectomy occasionally relieves hypertension, but often fails to do so.

2.6.2. Renal Dysplasia

Renal dysplasia is a developmental abnormality of the kidney resulting from anomalous metanephric differentiation (Risdon 1971). The condition is recognized histologically by disorganization of the renal parenchyma, by the presence of abnormally developed, immature nephronic and ductal structures resembling those found during fetal life, and sometimes by cyst formation. These changes may involve the whole kidney, or they may affect the organ only focally or segmentally, so that part of the parenchyma is normal (Risdon 1971). Affected kidneys may be distorted, and if cyst formation is marked they can be larger than expected. A wide variety of macroscopical appearances is thus encountered, and simple hypoplasia and cystic disease

markedly atrophic (Fig. 9.6b). Meshes of thick-walled blood vessels are apparent in the atrophic area, and Ljungqvist and Largergren (1962) describe the vascular arrangement as both cortical and medullary in type, though the medullary portion is greatly reduced. Interpretations of this lesion have of the kidneys may have to be considered in the differential diagnosis.

It is clear that a precise diagnosis of renal dysplasia can only be made on histological grounds, by recognizing the various immature structures that suggest embryonic maldevelopment. The most important of these are *primitive ducts* (Ericsson and Ivemark 1958), which are tubular structures lined with columnar and sometimes ciliated epithelium, surrounded by mantles of cellular mesenchyme in which smooth muscle can sometimes be demonstrated (Fig 9.7a). These are regarded as persistent derivatives of the ureteric bud. Bars of metaplastic cartilage, thought to represent aberrant differentiation of the metanephric blastema (Bigler and Killingworth 1949), are also important markers of renal dysplasia (Fig 9.7b). Other immature nephronic and tubular structures are encountered, including primitive glomeruli with prominent layers of cuboidal cells enveloping the tuft and primitive tubules lined with low cuboidal epithelial cells with darkly basophilic nuclei. Multiple, often fibrous-walled, cysts are present in variable numbers, but these are not confined to renal dysplasia and are a frequent finding in other congenital and some acquired conditions of the kidney (Bernstein 1971; Baxter 1961; Ekström 1955; Elkin and Bernstein 1969). Immature glomeruli and tubules may also occur in acquired renal disease, e.g., infections, ischaemia, or in scars resulting from renal biopsy (Berstein 1968). It follows that the findings of primitive ducts and metaplastic cartilage are the only features peculiar to renal dysplasia, and a histological diagnosis of this condition should be confined to cases in which one or other of these elements is recognized.

The diagnosis of renal dysplasia is helped by the recognition that the renal parenchymal maldevelopment is almost always associated with other congenital abnormalities of the ureter or of the lower urinary tract—ureteric reduplication, ureteric ectopia, and ureterocele or posterior urethral valves (Rubenstein et al. 1961). For this reason, dysplasia is best regarded as an anomaly of the whole urinary tract and not solely of the kidney. Classification of the various types of dyplasia can then be based not just on the presence of extent of any renal parenchymal maldevelopment, but rather on the pattern of the co-existing urinary tract abnormalities. This is important since the clinical outcome, in terms both

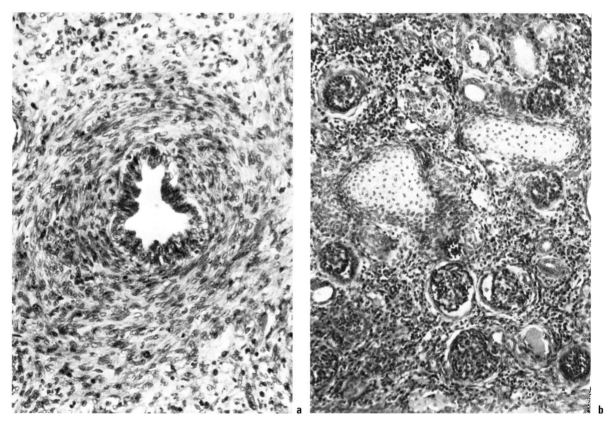

Fig. 9.7. a and **b** Renal dysplasia: **a** Primitive duct lined by columnar epithelium and surrounded by mesenchymal cells. (H and E; 300 ×) **b** Primitive glomeruli and bars of metaplastic cartilage. (H and E; 100 ×) Courtesy of the Editor of the *Journal of Clinical Pathology*.

of likely complications, such as infection and nydronephrosis, and of the probable success of surgical treatment, depends largely on the type of urinary tract abnormality present. It is also true that in a minority of individual examples of complex dysplastic anomalies, such as ectopic ureterocele, definite dysplastic markers in the kidney may be inapparent or masked by acquired disease. Since, however, these cases are indistinguishable in other respects, separate classification of them appears illogical.

The frequent co-existence of renal dysplasia with other urinary tract anomalies has led to the concept that the metanephric maldevelopment results from urinary obstruction or vesicoureteric reflux operating from the early phases of organogenesis (Bialestock 1965). Obstructive lesions developing later in intrauterine life, such as pelviureteric stenosis, are not associated with parenchymal dysplasia. Microdissection studies of grossly cystic dysplastic kidneys (Osathanondh and Potter 1964) reveal diminished branching of the ureteric bud, often with failure of nephron induction and cystic dilatation of the ureteric bud branch.

2.6.2.1. Multicystic, Aplastic, and Small Dysplastic Kidneys. It is best to think of multicystic, aplastic, and small dysplastic kidneys as variants on a continuum. Intermediate forms exist, making too rigid a separation inappropriate. Multicystic and aplastic kidneys constitute the most severe degrees of parenchymal dysplasia, in which the whole kidney is malformed. The multicystic kidney is enlarged, sometimes weighing several hundred grams, and is grossly cystic with an irregular outline (Fig. 9.8). The

largest cysts are usually immediately beneath the capsule, and the renal pelvis and calyces are absent or severely attenuated. Aplastic kidneys are extremely small, functionless, rudimentary organs consisting of a tiny cluster of cysts or a small nubbin of grossly dysplastic renal tissue. In both varieties the draining ureter is atretic for part (usually the upper part) or all of its length, and occasionally it is absent.

Small dysplastic kidneys are misshapen and sometimes contain cysts. Varying amounts of normally differentiated renal parenchyma are present, however, and serve to distinguish this entity. A number of ureteric anomalies may accompany small dysplastic kidneys. These include ureteric narrowing and hypoplasia, hydroureter, often with vesicoureteric reflux, and ureteric ectopia with or without a ureterocele. Rarely, and usually where the degree of parenchymal maldevelopment is minimal, the ureter may be normal.

Renal dysplasia of these types may be unilateral or bilateral. In bilateral multicystic or aplastic kidneys the renal maldevelopment is so gross as to be incompatible with life and the clinical presentation is like that of renal agenesis. Although ureteric atresia has been considered to be universal in multicystic kidneys, it is not uncommon in bilateral disease for the ureters to be patent although hypoplastic. Distinction from polycystic disease is important in such cases, since the genetic implications are quite different. Apart from rare heritable varieties, renal dysplasia is a sporadic phenomenon.

On the whole, unilateral multicystic or aplastic kidneys have a good prognosis. However, Pathak and Williams (1963) have emphasized that unilateral multicystic kidneys are not uncommonly associated with stenosis of the contralateral ureter, either at the

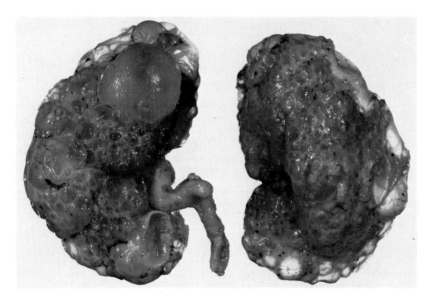

Fig. 9.8 Multicystic dysplastic kidney with atretic ureter.

pelviureteric junction or elsewhere along its length. This may be associated wtih hydronephrosis or infection of the remaining functioning kidney, so that early radiological recognition and surgical treatment of this condition are imperative. A similar association with contralateral ureteric stenosis may occur in unilateral small dysplastic and aplastic kidneys. Unilateral multicystic kidneys presenting as a loin mass in a young infant or neonate may be misdiagnosed as a congenital nephroblastoma. In fact congenital Wilm's tumours are extremely rare, if they occur at all (see p. 650), and with this presentation the multicystic kidney is a far more likely diagnosis.

The prognosis in infants with small dysplastic kidneys depends on the amount of functional renal tissue, the amenability of the associated urinary tract anomalies to surgical correction, and the associated complications, both short-term (infection, obstruction and vesicoureteric reflux) and long-term (arterial hypertension).

With all three varieties of dysplasia there is a greater-than-chance association with major anomalies in other systems. These include ventricular septal defect, preductal aortic coarctation, duodenal, oesophageal, and rectal atresia, the Arnold–Chiari malformation, and meningomyelocele.

2.6.2.2. Renal Dysplasia and Double (Duplex) Kidneys.

Duplex kidney with ectopic ureterocele (Fig. 9.9.) is a complex anomaly in which the dysplastic upper pole of a double kidney is drained by a separate renal pelvis and ureter inserted ectopically at its lower end. Here it forms a cystic swelling, or ureterocele, which bulges into the bladder. The upper pole ureteric orifice is usually beneath the internal sphincter at the bladder neck or in the upper urethra, while the lower-pole ureter is inserted separately in the normal position in the trigone. The upper pole ureter is nearly always obstructed, tortuous, and dilated, and the dysplastic upper pole of the kidney is hydronephrotic. The ureterocele at the insertion of the upper pole ureter is not invariably present.

The lesion can be unilateral or bilateral; in the former instance there is a tendency for the right side to be affected more often than the left. In about 10% of cases the double kidney is bilateral, but in most cases the ureters on the contralateral side join together and have a single, normal insertion. The full ectopic ureterocele is seldom bilateral. Ectopic ureterocele is much commoner in females. Patients with this condition usually present with recurrent urinary tract infections, and sometimes with dribbling incontinence owing either to the ectopic ureter or to cystitis. Occasionally the ureterocele obstructs

both the lower pole and the upper pole ureters. The results of surgery are generally good.

Much less commonly a duplex kidney exhibits dysplasia of the lower rather than of the upper pole. Such kidneys have double ureters, both of which are inserted into the trigone. The lower pole ureter, which is tortuous, dilated, and subject to vesicoureteric reflux, is inserted *above* the upper pole ureter in the trigone (Williams 1962).

2.6.2.3. Renal Dysplasia and Lower Urinary Tract Obstruction.

Congenital lower urinary tract obstruction occurs most commonly in infant boys with posterior urethral valves (Fig. 9.10). Rare causes include urethral stenosis, urethral fibroelastosis (Williams 1968), and Marion's disease (Marion 1940). Obstruction produces bilateral hydronephrosis, hydroureters, and bladder hypertrophy. Renal dysplasia is common in individuals with severe obstruction who present in the neonatal period but is not seen in patients whose obstruction is less complete and who present later. Dysplastic

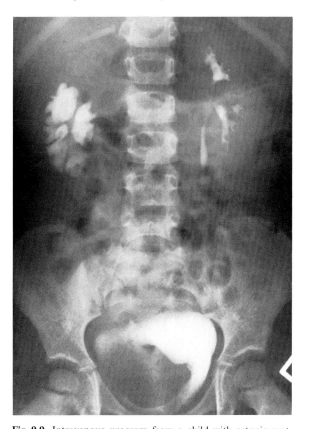

Fig. 9.9. Intravenous urogram from a child with ectopic ureterocele. Note absence of excretion by dysplastic right upper pole, filling defect in bladder owing to ureterocele, and dilatation of right lower pole calyces owing to obstruction of lower pole ureter by ureterocele.
Courtesy of the Editor of *Pediatric Radiology.*

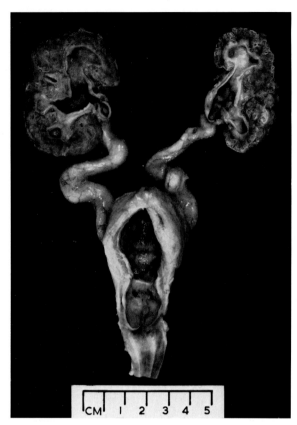

Fig. 9.10. Bilateral hydronephrosis and hydroureters with cysts in the outer renal cortex owing to posterior urethral valves. A staghorn calculus is visible in the renal pelvis on the left side.
Courtesy of the Editor of the *Journal of Clinical Pathology.*

changes and cyst formation are often most prominent in the outer cortex and involve the nephrons that develop last.

In patients with the 'prune belly' syndrome (congenital absence of the anterior abdominal wall musculature with wrinkling of the overlying skin; Williams and Burkholder 1967), similar bilateral hydroureters and bladder hypertrophy may occur, although mechanical lower urinary tract obstruction can seldom be demonstrated. These patients are almost exclusively male; their kidneys commonly exhibit severe renal dysplasia and the testes fail to descend.

2.6.2.4. Familial Forms of Renal Dysplasia. Cystic lesions of the kidneys occur in a number of familial syndromes (see p. 405). The pathology of these lesions often varies in different examples of the same syndrome, and has been inadequately described in reported cases, being labelled rather vaguely as 'polycystic disease' or 'renal dysplasia'. Renal lesions that can be regarded as dysplastic according to the criteria given here do occur in some familial syndromes, and occasionally as an isolated heritable

malformation. In both these situations dysplasia is bilateral, and unlike the much more common sporadic types, is not associated with other malformations of the urinary tract.

The best-described examples of hereditary cystic dysplasia occur in Meckel's syndrome of microcephaly and posterior encephalocele associated with polydactyly, cleft palate and lip and genital anomalies (Opitz and Howe 1969). This syndrome appears to be inherited as an autosomal recessive trait. In the kidneys large fibrous-walled cysts and primitive ducts are the most prominent feature. Metanephric elements (glomeruli and tubules) are extremely sparse and corticomedullary differentiation is absent. Another constant feature is an hepatic lesion closely resembling the hepatic fibrous and bile duct changes (congenital hepatic fibrosis) seen in infantile polycystic kidneys (see p. 406).

Similar renal dysplastic changes sometimes occur in Jeune's asphyxiating thoracic dystrophy and Zellweger's cerebrohepatorenal syndrome.

In the Beckwith–Wiedemann syndrome of macroglossia, omphalocele, endocrine anomalies, and visceromegaly the kidneys are enlarged and lobulated. Dilated collecting ducts and primitive ducts are present in the medullae but the cortex is normally formed, i.e., dysplasia is largely medullary.

Jeune's thoracic dystrophy, Zellweger's syndrome, and Beckwith–Wiedemann syndrome are all inherited as autosomal recessive traits.

3. Cystic Diseases of the Kidney

Cysts in the kidney, particularly when multiple, are often regarded as evidence of anomalous development, but it is now recognized that cystic dilatation is frequently a secondary change, which can occur in any part of a normally differentiated nephron or collecting duct. Renal cysts occur under a wide variety of circumstances and the cause is usually unknown. The concept that cystic change is merely a manifestation of what is vaguely described as polycystic disease is evidently an oversimplification. In fact a number of different varieties of cystic kidney can be distinguished by their clinical presentations and pathological characteristics, and since some types are heritable their accurate diagnosis is important for genetic counselling purposes.

3.1. Simple Renal Cysts

One or more cysts can be found in the kidneys at necropsy in up to 50% of patients over the age of 50 years. Their comparative rarity in younger adults and children strongly supports the concept that they are acquired lesions. The cysts are usually cortical, often solitary, and they vary in size from a few millimetres to several centimetres in diameter. They can be unilocular or, less commonly, multilocular; they have a fibrous wall with a single lining layer of flattened epithelial cells. They appear to develop from local blockage of nephrons as a result of focal scarring. Such cysts are particularly common in arteriosclerotic kidneys.

Multiple simple cysts have been noted to develop in severely scarred (end-stage) kidneys in patients on renal dialysis or those who have had renal transplants for some years but have not had their own kidneys removed (Dunnill et al. 1977).

3.2. Renal Dysplasia

Cystic change is common in renal dysplasia and may be the dominant pathological finding. The multicystic dysplastic kidney is the variety of renal dysplasia most likely to be confused with polycystic disease. Unilateral multicystic dysplasia should present no problems, since true polycystic disease is invariably bilateral. Bilateral multicystic kidneys are recognized histologically by the presence of dysplastic elements (see p. 401).

3.3. Polycistic Disease

At least two distinct varieties of renal polycystic disease are recognized, the so-called adult and infantile varieties.

Adult. Adult polycystic kidneys, whilst by no means common, have probably been encountered by all general pathologists. The label *adult* is attached because the vast majority of cases present in adult life, symptoms most commonly developing during the fourth decade. The clinical picture is of progressive renal failure, usually with hypertension. Without renal transplantation or dialysis patients rarely survive more than 3 years after presentation. The condition is inherited as an autosomal dominant trait, but about 50% of cases result from a new mutation, so that a family history is not always obtained.

Cysts of varying size are present throughout both kidneys, which at the time of diagnosis are usually enlarged (sometimes grossly) and have lost their reniform shape (Fig. 9.11). Cysts may arise in any part of the nephron or in collecting ducts and may distort the pelvicalyceal system. Intravenous urography, ultrasonography, or computerized axial

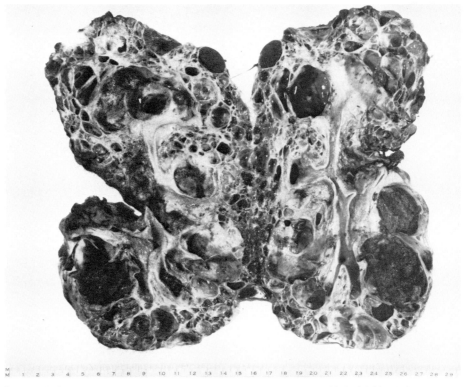

Fig. 9.11. Adult polycystic disease. The kidney weighed 800 g. Note the irregularly sized cysts, some filled with blood clot.

tomography, may allow a diagnosis to be made before the kidneys become palpably enlarged or renal insufficiency develops. Haemorrhage into the cysts may produce loin pain and haematuria, and renal infection may be a complication, particularly terminally.

Cysts may be present in other organs, such as the pancreas and lung, and particularly in the liver, where thin-walled and sometimes multilocular cysts are present in 30% of cases. There is no associated hepatic fibrosis and hepatic function is unimpaired. Berry aneurysms of the cerebral arteries are also common, and rupture of these aneurysms is the cause of death in about 10% of cases.

The pathogenesis of adult polycystic disease is unknown. Those relatively rare cases presenting in early adult life or during childhood usually exhibit less severe degrees of cystic change, and it seems probable that the cysts develop gradually over the years as a result of cystic transformation of initially normally differentiated nephrons and collecting ducts. Only when sufficient parenchyma has become cystic, or has been destroyed by pressure from adjacent cysts, does renal insufficiency develop and the condition become symptomatic. The clear autosomal dominant mode of inheritance has led to the suggestion (Darmady et al. 1970) that cystic transformation might result from the excretion of an unidentified abnormal metabolite produced by a genetically transmitted enzyme defect. Whilst this is an attractive hypothesis it must be admitted that cysts do not develop in renal allographs transplanted into patients with this condition, as might be expected if they were excreting a cystogenic substance.

Infantile. Infantile polycystic disease is inherited as an autosomal recessive trait. Though of more relevance in the paediatric age group, the overall incidence of this form of cystic disease is much less than that of the adult variety. Classically, the condition presents in infants who are stillborn or die in the neonatal period. Both kidneys are grossly enlarged, sometimes to a degree that causes difficulty during delivery. Despite their often huge size the kidneys retain their reniform shape, and fetal lobulation is usually exaggerated. The pelvis, calyces and ureter are normal. The smooth renal surface is studded with innumerable small cysts of uniform size, which on cutting the kidney are seen as radially orientated fusiform or cylindrical dilatations throughout the cortex and medulla (Figs. 9.12 and 9.13a). Microdissection studies (Osathanondh and Potter 1964) suggest that the disease is attributable to dilatation and hyperplasia of the interstitial portions of the branches of the ureteric bud, which form the collecting ducts. These branches retain their ability to induce nephron formation, and the number of nephrons appears to be normal.

Abnormalities of other systems are confined to the liver. In every case the intrahepatic bile ducts are increased in number in every portal tract and exhibit a curious angulated branching and occasional cystic dilatation. This is associated with a varying degree of portal fibrosis and the lesion is referred to as congenital hepatic fibrosis (Fig. 9.13b).

In the classic form of the disease affected infants are usually anuric. This is difficult to explain, since there is no anatomical obstruction, and indeed it is increasingly recognized that a minority of affected infants may survive into childhood with varying

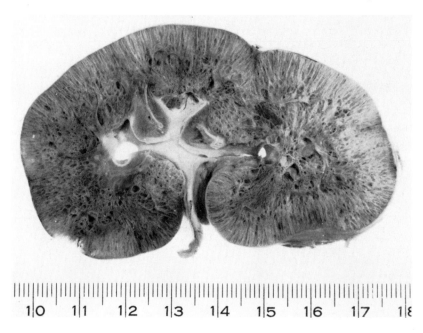

Fig. 9.12. Infantile polycystic disease. Radially aligned, fusiform cysts.

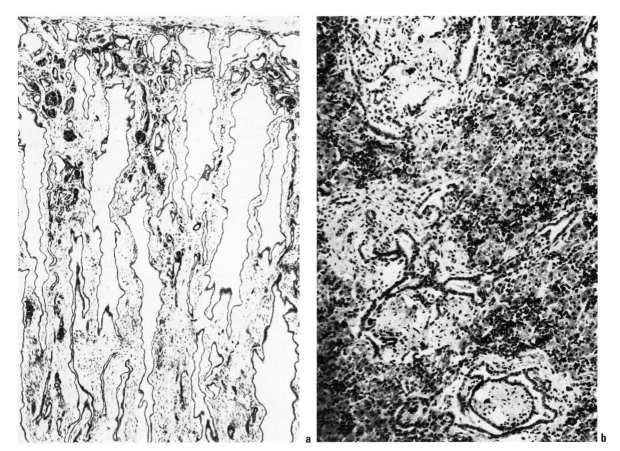

Fig. 9.13. a Infantile polycystic disease. The renal cysts are seen as fusiform dilations of collecting ducts. (H and E; 25 ×) **b** Liver in infantile polycystic disease. Note the angulated branching of bile ducts which appear to run in the plane of the section and the increase in portal fibrous tissue. (H and E; 250 ×)

degrees of renal functional impairment.

The relationship of infantile polycystic kidneys to congenital hepatic fibrosis has not been clarified. All patients with classic infantile polycystic disease have congenital hepatic fibrosis. However, congenital hepatic fibrosis also occurs in association with lesser degrees of renal cystic disease. The individual renal cysts in these cases are identical with those in the classic form, the essential difference being that only a proportion of the parenchyma is involved, the remainder appearing normal. Where the degree of renal cystic change is slight enough to be compatible with long-term survival, hepatic fibrosis may be progressive and eventually give rise to portal hypertension with complications such as bleeding from oesophageal varices. Although in all cases the mode of inheritance appears to be autosomal recessive, Blyth and Ockendon (1971) have shown that within a particular family the relative renal and hepatic involvement appears to breed true, and on this basis they have suggested that a number of different mutant genes may operate.

Congenital hepatic fibrosis is also described as occurring in the absence of renal cystic disease. However, minor degrees of cystic change may be overlooked if the kidneys are not examined minutely. Cysts may apparently be confined to the papillary collecting ducts and may give rise to an appearance identical with that of the so-called medullary sponge kidney on intravenous urography. Such cases, occurring in association with congenital hepatic fibrosis, are described by Reilly and Neuhauser (1960), and the present author has encountered a 60-year-old woman said to have medullary sponge kidneys on radiological assessment, who was found on liver biopsy to have congenital hepatic fibrosis. In this patient biochemical analysis had revealed no hepatic or renal impairment; laparotomy was performed for renal calculi and the liver was found to be small and firm.

In addition, congenital hepatic fibrosis has occasionally been described in association with other varieties of renal cystic disease, notably bilateral multicystic dysplastic kidneys in Meckel's syndrome, juvenile nephronophthisis (Delaney et al. 1978) and Jeune's thoracic dystrophy.

3.4. Medullary Cysts

Cystic changes confined to, or occurring pre-dominantly in, the renal medulla are found in two quite distinct conditions—medullary sponge kidney and medullary cystic disease (or juvenile nephron-ophthisis).

Medullary Sponge Kidney. The medullary sponge kidney is a radiological rather than a patho-logical entity. It is diagnosed at intravenous urog-raphy by the presence of dilated medullary collecting ducts that fill with contrast medium ('ductal ectasia') (Ekström et al. 1959). Flecks of medullary calcifi-cation may also be evident radiologically. Patients with this condition are usually asymptomatic and the diagnosis is ordinarily made in adult life. The radiological findings are commonly incidental to the investigation of other disease, and renal function is unimpaired. Occasionally complicating infection or stone formation bring it to the physician's attention. The condition is usually bilateral, and affected kid-neys are of normal size or slightly enlarged. A family history is not usually obtained (Habib et al. 1965), although it has occasionally been reported (Morris et al. 1965). Associated abnormalities are rare, although hemi-hypertrophy is an occasional finding.

Since the condition is usually discovered radi-ologically, its pathology is not adequately defined. Cystic dilatation is generally described as confined to the medullary collecting ducts, and the renal cortex is normal. However, similar radiological changes may be seen in some cases of infantile polycystic disease (Habib et al. 1965), and the medullary sponge kidney as defined radiologically is evidently an heterogeneous condition.

Medullary Cystic Disease (Juvenile Nephronoph-thisis). Medullary cystic disease and juvenile nephronophthisis were first described as separate entities (Smith and Graham 1945; Fanconi et al. 1951), the former characterized pathologically by the presence of prominent medullary cysts, and the latter as an hereditary nephropathy, apparently with an autosomal recessive mode of inheritance, causing polyuria and renal failure in children. The reali-zation that the two conditions have many clinical and pathological features in common (Strauss and Sommers 1967) and the fact that the two conditions may occur in the same family (Sworn and Eisinger 1972) have led to the idea that they are identical even though their aetiology is quite unknown. The spect-rum of juvenile nephronophthisis and medullary cystic disease is not entirely homogeneous, however, and in particular there is growing evidence of *genetic* heterogeneity. Cases presenting in childhood, when by common usage the condition is called juvenile

nephronophthisis, usually exhibit an autosomal re-cessive inheritance, whilst cases presenting in adult life, when the term usually applied is medullary cystic disease, are either sporadic or inherited as an autosomal dominant trait. A further complication is the occurrence of a third group, in which juvenile nephronophthisis/medullary cystic disease is as-sociated with extrarenal anomalies, predominantly pigmentary degeneration of the retina and cataracts (Schimke 1971; Fairley et al. 1963) or congenital hepatic fibrosis (Boichis et al. 1973; Delaney et al. 1978). These examples show an autosomal recessive inheritance.

The pathological features of juvenile nephronophthisis/medullary cystic disease are fairly constant. Both kidneys are uniformly contracted, and both cortex and medulla are involved (Fig. 9.14). There is widespread periglomerular fibrosis, glomerular sclerosis, tubular atrophy and interstitial fibrosis with focal interstitial chronic inflammation (Fig. 9.15). Typically, tubular and interstitial changes are more prominent than glome-rular alterations, particularly in the early stages of the disease, which are sometimes encountered in biopsy specimens. Thickening and lamination of tubular basement membranes is often marked. Cysts occur in both the cortex and medulla; large and macroscopically obvious medullary cysts are the distinguishing features of cases that have been labelled medullary cystic disease. Microdissection studies (Sherman et al. 1971) show the cysts as diverticula normally limited to the distal convoluted tubules. The medullary cysts are most prominent near the corticomedullary junction, a feature that contrasts with the medullary sponge kidney where cysts occur near the papillary tips.

In cases of juvenile nephronophthisis presenting in childhood the clinical features are characteristic. There is marked growth retardation and the main complaints are usually of polyuria, nocturia, poly-dipsia, and craving for salt. The urine is dilute proteinuria is trivial or absent, and there is no excess of cells in the urine deposit. A normochronic, normocytic anaemia is present and may be dispro-portionate to the degree of renal failure. Salt wasting is a further characteristic feature. In the later stages symptoms due to renal failure develop and renal osteodystrophy is apparent. Without renal transplantation death usually occurs towards the end of the first decade. Juvenile nephronophthisis is now recognized as the second commonest cause of chronic renal failure in childhood (Betts and Forrest-Hay 1973; Lancet 1979). The clinical fea-tures in adult cases are similar. They may develop a salt-wasting syndrome, which is clinically not unlike Addison's disease except that there is no response to mineralocorticoid therapy (Thorn et al. 1944).

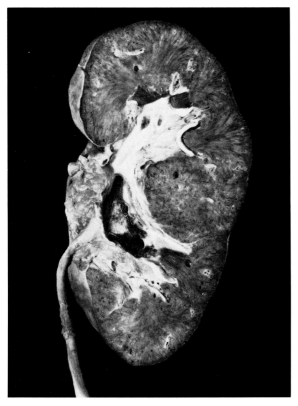

Fig. 9.14. Juvenile nephronophthisis. The kidney, from a 6-year-old girl, weighed 45 g (about half the expected weight). It is diffusely contracted and a few tiny cysts are visible, mainly at the corticomedullary junction. Photographed in UV light.
Courtesy of the Editor of *Pediatric Radiology*.

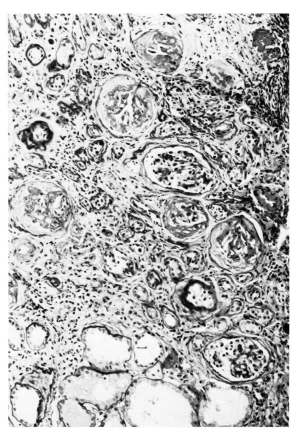

Fig. 9.15. Juvenile nephronophthisis. Note widespread tubular atrophy and loss and glomerulosclerosis. (PAS; 200 ×)
Courtesy of the Editor of *Pediatric Radiology*.

3.5. Multilocular Cyst

Multilocular cyst is a rare cystic malformation of the kidney with the following characteristics (Powell et al. 1951):

i) There is a solitary, well-demarcated, multilocular cystic lesion, usually several centimetres in diameter, which replaces most of the kidney;

ii) The lesion is unilateral;

iii) The cysts are filled with fluid and are discrete, i.e., they communicate neither with each other nor with the collecting system of the kidney;

iv) The cysts are lined with flattened epithelium and the septa between them contain only nondescript mesenchyme and no differentiated renal elements.

Most cases present in childhood, usually as unilateral cystic renal masses. The cases are sporadic, with no evidence of a genetically determined cause. Intravenous urography reveals distortion of the pelvicalyceal system and sometimes evidence of obstruction, caused by the tendency of daughter cysts to prolapse into the renal pelvis and block the pelvicalyceal junction. The distinction from nephro-

blastoma cannot be made clinically, radiologically, or even with certainty on inspection during laparotomy, but only on pathological examination following nephrectomy. Even then, careful microscopic examination of a number of blocks from the lesion is required to exclude the rare multicystic variety of nephroblastoma.

3.6. Renal Cysts and Multiple Malformation Syndromes

Multiple renal cortical cysts developing in glomeruli, convoluted tubules, and collecting ducts are not uncommon in a number of syndromes of multiple malformations, notably the autosomal trisomy D and E syndromes (Warkany et al. 1966) and Zellweger's cerebrohepatorenal syndromes (Poznaski et al. 1970).

The cysts are generally small and widely spaced, and are not usually associated with any functional impairment. Very occasionally the cystic change is associated with histological evidence of dysplasia, i.e., with evidence of metanephric maldifferentiation, but usually such changes are absent. There may be focal tubular and glomerular sclerosis associated with the cysts, so that it is probable that in these cases at least, the cystic change is a secondary phenomenon occurring in normally differentiated nephrons.

The renal lesion seen in Jeune's asphyxiating thoracic dystrophy (a familial abnormality of chest wall development) is rather different (Herdman and Langer 1968). Renal cystic change is often marked, and progressive renal insufficiency is sometimes evident clinically. There is often histological evidence of renal dysplasia, and in addition varying degrees of glomerular tuft hypercellularity and glomerulosclerosis are seen. The liver shows changes in the portal areas of bile-duct proliferation with branching and focal microcystic dilatation very similar to that seen in infantile polycystic disease and Meckel's syndrome. The renal lesions in this condition are a rather confusing mixture of metanephric maldifferentiation and hereditary nephropathy.

In the tuberous sclerosis complex a distinctive and probably hamartomatous cystic lesion is occasionally seen. The cysts are lined with large eosinophilic cells with abundant granular cytoplasm, which resemble somewhat hyperplastic proximal tubular cells. Occasionally these cells form solid nodules, which may show central dissolution to form cysts. This lesion differs from the better-known angiomyolipoma.

4. Renal Diseases Principally Affecting the Glomeruli (Table 9.2)

4.1. Glomerulonephritis

Much clinical and experimental evidence indicates that many forms of inflammatory glomerular disease are immunologically mediated. Although the exact pathogenic mechanisms in man are far from clear, current concepts, derived from clinical and pathological studies and correlation with experimental models in animals, suggest that there are two basic patterns (Unanue and Dixon 1967; Dixon 1968). These are:

1) Fixation of antiglomerular basement membrane antibodies to the glomerular basement membrane (anti-GBM disease);

2) Deposition of immune (antibody–antigen) complexes from the circulation in the glomerulus (soluble-complex disease).

Table 9.2. Classification of glomerular disease

A. *Acquired*
   1. *Primary*
      i) Acute diffuse exudative glomerulonephritis (including post-streptococcal glomerulonephritis)
     ii) Glomerulonephritis with crescents
    iii) Mesangial proliferative glomerulonephritis
    iv) Membranoproliferative glomerulonephritis
     v) Membranous (epimembranous) nephropathy
    vi) Minimal change disease
    vii) Focal glomerulosclerosis
   viii) Focal glomerulonephritis (some types)

   2. *Secondary*
      i) Lupus nephritis
     ii) Glomerulonephritis secondary to other 'autoimmune' systemic diseases (e.g., polyarteritis nodosa, Schönlein–Henoch purpura, etc.)
    iii) Diabetic nephropathy
    iv) Amyloidosis

B. *Congenital*
      i) Hereditary nephropathies (e.g., Alport's syndrome, familial nephrotic syndrome, etc.)

Of these the latter is by far the most frequent in human glomerulonephritis. In both anti-GBM and immune-complex disease glomerular damage is thought to result from activation of the complement system with associated release of enzymes from polymorphonuclear leucocytes and sometimes initiation of blood-clotting mechanisms (Unanue and Dixon 1967).

Dixon (1961) has demonstrated that a crucial factor determining glomerular trapping of immune complexes lies in their size and that it is the soluble complexes found in conditions of antigen excess that are important in initiating this form of glomerulonephritis. Small complexes (with sedimentation rates less than 19S) found in states of marked antigen excess remain in the circulation and are not deposited in the glomeruli. Large, insoluble antigen–antibody aggregates found in conditions of antibody excess are cleared rapidly by the reticuloendothelial system, and glomerular trapping is at most a fleeting phenomenon. Complex size may also be related to antibody affinity (Soothill and Steward 1971). It has been suggested that low-affinity antibody may bind antigen poorly, to produce relatively small, soluble, nonprecipitating complexes of the type associated with immune-complex disease. Germuth and Rodriguez (1972) have produced evidence relating the size of soluble complexes to the pattern of morphological changes in the glomeruli. Smaller soluble complexes tend to penetrate the GBM and are trapped either within the GBM or at the slit pores on the epithelial side of the GBM, whilst larger soluble complexes fail to penetrate the GBM and are deposited in the mesangium or along the subendothelial aspect of the GBM. In the latter instance, proliferation of mesangial cells and mesangial matrix is usually a feature at some stage in the process.

4.1.1. Acute Diffuse Exudative Glomerulonephritis

Classically, acute diffuse exudative glomerulonephritis follows streptococcal infections, and it is assumed to be a soluble-complex nephritis developing during the immune response to the infecting organism. This is a group A, β-haemolytic streptococcus, usually of type 12, 4, or 1. Characteristically there is a latent period of 5–30 days between the infection and the onset of symptoms of nephritis, which are generally haematuria and proteinuria, oliguria, facial oedema, and sometimes hypertension. Acute nephritis of this type is an increasingly rare complication of streptococcal infections, but may still affect children. Cases may be sporadic, or may occur in epidemics following an outbreak of infection. This happens commonly with skin infections by a nephritogenic streptococcus, as in the Red Lake incident in North America (Kleinman 1954; Anthony et al. 1967).

The evidence that the nephritis is immunologically mediated is compelling. The latent period between the infection and the onset of nephritis is compatible with the time required to develop antibodies. The kidney, blood, and urine are sterile, indicating that the renal lesion is not a direct result of infection. Serum complement levels are low during the episode of acute nephritis, implying the involvement of the complement system as a mediator of an immune response. Titres of antistreptolysin 0 are often raised, suggesting that an immune reaction to streptococcal antigens occurs, although this particular antibody has not been implicated in the nephritis. Electron-dense deposits thought to represent the complexes can be seen in the glomeruli during the acute phase in renal biopsy specimens, and immunofluorescence microscopy reveals immunoglobulins (usually IgG), complement, and sometimes fibrin within the glomeruli. Treser et al. (1970) have shown by immunofluorescence that the serum of patients recovering from post-streptococcal glomerulonephritis contains an antibody that binds to the glomeruli in biopsy specimens taken during the acute phase of the disease. This binding could be blocked by absorption of the convalescent serum with the plasma membranes of certain types of group A streptococci, providing strong indirect evidence of the presence within the glomeruli of antigens that either were streptococcal or at least cross reacted with streptococcal antigens.

On light microscopy during the acute phase all the glomerular tufts appear swollen and hypercellular, virtually filling the urinary spaces (Fig. 9.16). There is a proliferation of intracapillary (mainly mesangial) cells, which virtually obliterate the tuft capillary lumina. Infiltration of the glomerular tufts by polymorphonuclear leucocytes is usually a prominent feature. The tubular epithelium is usually well preserved, but there is a variable degree of interstitial oedema and mononuclear cell infiltration.

On electron microscopy, electron-dense deposits (presumed to be complexes) are seen to occur predominantly on the epithelial side of the GBM, and especially large deposits (termed 'humps') may occasionally be seen (Fig. 9.17). Less frequently, deposits on the epithelial side of GBM may be seen, and occasionally a mesangiocapillary type of glomerular lesion has been seen following strepotococcal infection (Turner 1978).

In the great majority of cases (probably 90% of children and some 60% of adults) the disease is not progressive and the glomerular lesion completely resolves or leaves a minimum of glomerular scarring.

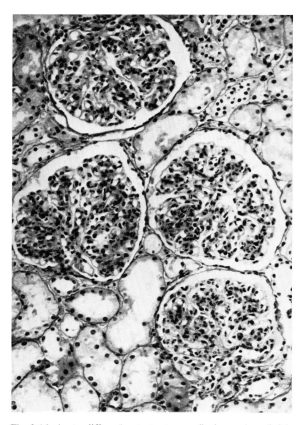

Fig. 9.16. Acute diffuse (post-streptococcal) glomerulonephritis in a 10-year-old boy. Note diffuse glomerular involvement, marked hypercellularity of glomerular tufts and the presence of numerous polymorphs within the tufts. (MSB; 400 ×)

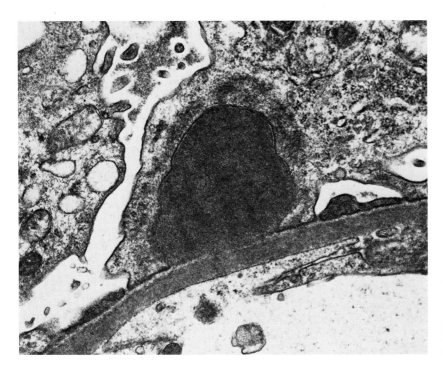

Fig. 9.17. Acute post-streptococcal glomerulonephritis. An electron photomicrograph showing an electron-dense hump on the epithelial side of the glomerular basement membrane and surrounded by epithelial cell cytoplasm. (10 000 ×)

This implies that the circulation and glomerular trapping of soluble complexes is usually short-lived. Certainly deposits can no longer be seen with the electron microscope in biopsies taken more than 6 weeks after the onset of disease from patients who subsequently recover completely. Increased mesangial hypercellularity may persist for some months, however, and may be accompanied clinically by proteinuria.

In a minority of patients glomerular abnormalities persist for more than a year and the disease is said to have entered a 'latent phase' (Jennings and Earle 1961). In an unknown percentage of such patients chronic glomerulonephritis develops (Schacht et al. 1976). Progressive hyalinization and scarring of glomeruli with secondary tubular and interstitial changes develop, and there is a gradual diminution of renal function ending in chronic renal failure. Hypertension may also supervene and the accompanying vascular changes add a component of ischaemic damage to the kidneys.

A very small minority of patients die in the acute phase of the disease from such complications as acute left ventricular failure with pulmonary oedema or cerebral haemorrhage.

With a diminishing incidence of poststreptococcal glomerulonephritis (Meadow 1975) it is becoming clear that by no means all cases of acute diffuse proliferative glomerulonephritis follow streptococcal infections. From these cases it is evident that other antigens, possibly of bacterial or viral origin, may precipitate this type of immune complex disease. A histologically similar form of glomerulonephritis (which sometimes has features of a mesangiocapillary glomerulonephritis) has been seen as a rare complication of infective endocarditis or infected ventriculo-atrial shunts inserted for the relief of hydrocephalus (so-called shunt nephritis). These forms of glomerulonephritis may be mediated by soluble complexes containing microbial antigens derived from bacterial vegetations on the infected valves or from the infected shunt.

4.1.2. Glomerulonephritis with Crescents

The term 'glomerulonephritis with crescents' describes a form of glomerulonephritis in which the predominant histological feature is the proliferation of extracapillary cells between the gomerular tuft and Bowman's capsule. These cells often produce crescentic masses (capsular crescents), which fill and obliterate the urinary space (Fig. 9.18). Proliferation of intracapillary (endothelial and mesangial) cells is usually present but may not be conspicuous if, as is often the case, the crescents are so large that the glomerular tuft becomes compressed. The extracapillary cells forming the crescents are usually regarded as being derived from epithelial cells covering the glomerular tuft and lining Bowman's capsule, although recently it has been suggested that macrophages are an important component of the crescentic masses (Atkins et al. 1976; Holdsworth et al. 1978). The condition is also referred to as rapidly progressive crescentic glomerulonephritis.

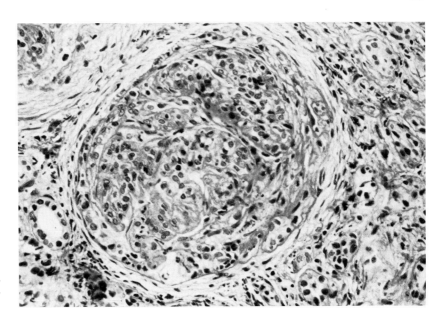

Fig. 9.18. Proliferative glomerulo-nephritis with capsular crescent formation. (MSB; 500 ×)

Occasional crescents affecting a minority of glomeruli are not uncommon in a number of varieties of proliferative glomerulonephritis, but the description glomerulonephritis with crescents is usually reserved for cases in which the majority (80 %–100 %) of the glomeruli show crescents. Fibrin may be demonstrated between the cells forming the crescents, particularly in the early stages, and crescent formation is usually regarded as a reaction to the presence of fibrin in the urinary space. Thus the change is not specific to any particular underlying pathogenic mechanism. The justification for classifying various forms of glomerulonephritis with prominent capsular crescent formation separately is the fact that they generally have a rapid downhill course. Severe renal insufficiency and oliguria or anuria may be present from the onset or develop in the course of a few weeks. Deterioration in renal function is usually irreversible.

Crescentic glomerulonephritis is a very rare sequel of streptococcal infections and may also occur in association with polyarteritis nodosa (see p. 420), systemic lupus erythematosus (see p. 420) or Schönlein–Henoch purpura (see p. 420). Occasionally mesangiocapillary glomerulonephritis (see p. 414) may be accompanied by prominent crescent formation. Often the cause is entirely unknown, although immunofluorescence and electron microscopy indicate an immune complex type of glomerulonephritis. Patients with Goodpasture's syndrome, an association of glomerulonephritis and lung haemorrhage, often exhibit crescentic glomerulonephritis on renal biopsy. Although rare, this syndrome is occasionally seen in childhood. Its particular interest is that it is the only documented

form of human anti-GMB glomerulonephritis. Immunofluorescence microscopy reveals a linear deposition of immunoglobulins (usually IgG) and complement (C_3) along all the glomerular basement membranes. Free anti-GMB antibody can be demonstrated in the sera of patients after bilateral nephrectomy prior to transplantation and in kidney eluates (Lerner et al. 1967).

Thus crescentic glomerulonephritis is by no means a homogeneous entity, but merely a description of a glomerular reaction to a variety of immunological insults, which probably have in common only the deposition of significant amounts of fibrin in the urinary space.

4.1.3. Mesangial Proliferative Glomerulonephritis

The form of diffuse glomerulonephritis in which changes are confined to the centrilobular (mesangial) regions of the glomerular tufts is described as mesangial proliferative glomerulonephritis. There is a varying, although usually mild, degree of mesangial cell proliferation and an increase in the amount of mesangial matrix (Fig 9.19). The capillary loops at the peripheries of the glomerular tufts are widely patent and there is no thickening of the capillary walls.

Classically, this appearance is described in the resolving phase of poststreptococcal glomerulonephritis (Jennings and Earle 1961), and in this situation it has a generally excellent prognosis. In recent years, however, it has become recognized that similar appearances can be seen in biopsies from some patients (often children) with recurrent haematuria or a nephrotic syndrome of insidious

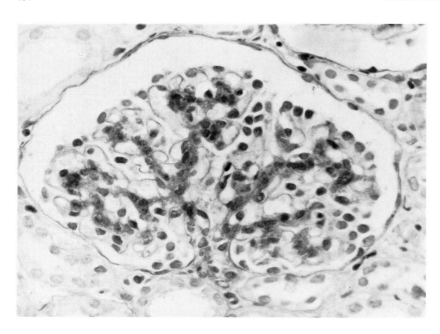

Fig. 9.19. Mesangial proliferative glomerulonephritis. Note widely patent glomerular capillary loops, mild centrilobular hyper cellularity and increase in mesangial matrix. (PAS; 1000 ×)

onset, often accompanied by haematuria (Glasgow et al. 1970; White et al. 1970). In these patients there has been no acute nephritic episode and no firm evidence of a preceding streptococcal infection.

Some children presenting with recurrent haematuria and mesangial proliferative glomerulonephritis have IgA and sometimes IgG and C_3 deposited in the mesangial regions of the glomeruli and fall within the spectrum of Berger's disease (see p. 420). In such patients episodes of haematuria are often precipitated by upper respiratory tract infections, and proteinuria often accompanies the haematuria. Biopsies from children with mesangial proliferative glomerulonephritis associated with the nephrotic syndrome are usually negative on immunofluorescence or show only C_3 deposition, and immune deposits cannot be convincingly demonstrated on electron microscopy. Because of its morphological resemblance to resolving poststreptococcal glomerulonephritis, it has been regarded as a form of immune reaction to a clinically inapparent streptococcal infection. This view is hard to justify, however, in the absence of any real evidence of such an infection. The nephrotic syndrome in these patients is usually resistant to therapy with either steroids or immunosuppressive agents, but in most cases the proteinuria ceases spontaneously over a varying period of months to years. In our ignorance of the pathogenesis and lack of certainty as to whether the histological lesion represents a distinct entity or a particular glomerular response to a variety of insults, it is difficult to give a precise prognosis. All that is known is that in the majority of children with this lesion the prognosis is good and steroid therapy is unlikely to be of benefit.

4.1.4. Membranoproliferative (Mesangiocapillary) Glomerulonephritis

In recent years a form of proliferative glomerulonephritis has been recognized that has morphological similarities to poststreptococcal glomerulonephritis but much more sinister clinical implications. Whilst uncommon, it is an important cause of renal failure in older children and young adults (West et al. 1965).

Light microscopy reveals uniform involvement of all glomeruli, which are enlarged and show prominent lobulation of the glomerular tufts. A variable degree of proliferation of mesangial cells and an increase in mesangial matrix is associated with diffuse thickening of glomerular capillary walls (Fig. 9.20a). Ultrastructurally the capillary wall thickening may be of two main types, and cases are subdivided on this basis (Berger and Galle 1963; Levy et al. 1973).

4.1.4.1. Double-contour Variety. Thickening of the capillary wall is due to the extension of mesangial cell cytoplasm and matrix around the circumference of the capillary loop between the GBM and the lining endothelium. A second layer of basement membrane-like material is seen between the mesangial layer and the endothelium; this can be seen by light microscopy if silver methenamine staining methods are used, producing a 'tramline' or 'double-contour' effect (Fig. 9.20b). Electron-dense deposits are seen both along the endothelial aspect of the GBM and in the mesangium. Immunofluorescence microscopy reveals immunoglobulins (predominantly IgG) and complement (C_3) in a similar

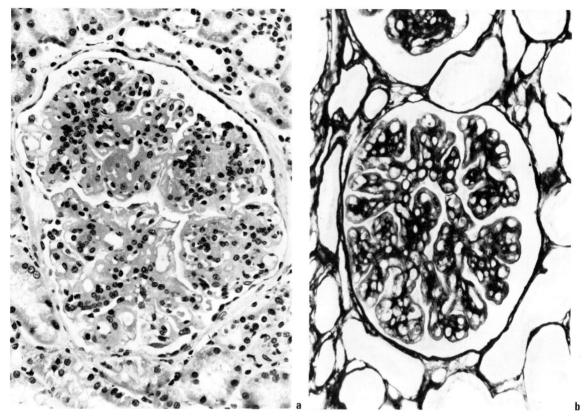

Fig. 9.20. a and **b** Membranoproliferative (mesangiocapillary) glomerulo nephritis. **a** Note the lobulation of the glomerular tuft with marked hyper cellularity and thickening of capillary walls. (H and E; 800 ×) **b** Silver methamine stain to show double contouring of capillary walls. (600 ×).

distribution. This variety of mesangiocapillary glomerulonephritis is occasionally seen in association with infective endocarditis, infected ventriculo-atrial shunts, and plasmodium malarial infection.

4.1.4.2. Linear Dense-deposit Variety. Thickening is due to ribbon-like electron-dense deposits within the basement membrane itself. These deposits extend diffusely along the capillary walls and often involve the basement membrane of Bowman's capsule and the renal tubules. The deposits are particularly well seen on light micro-scopy in plastic-embedded sections stained with toluidine blue, for which they have a high affinity (Fig. 9.21). They are not argyrophilic, and in paraffin sections stained with methenamine silver the paucity of silver staining of the thickened glomerular capillary walls is a useful pointer to this diagnosis. On immunofluorescence microscopy, deposits of C_3 (but not Clq) and absence of immunoglobulin deposition are characteristic findings. With C_3b right granules in the mesangium are associated with weaker linear deposits on the basement membrane.

Mesangiocapillary glomerulonephritis is generally progressive, and the lesion often evolves into a 'lobular' glomerulonephritis in which tuft lobulation is associated with relatively acellular centrilobular hyalinization.

The pathogenesis of this lesion is unknown, but an interesting association is the persistent decrease in the level of serum complement found in particular in cases of linear dense-deposit disease. The association of hypocomplementaemia and the glomerular lesion appears to be indirect. Low complement levels are due partly to decreased synthesis and partly to a serum factor (termed 'C_3 nephritic factor'), which initiates consumption of complement by the alternative pathway (Spitzer et al. 1969).

Mesangiocapillary glomerulonephritis, almost always the linear dense-deposit variety, may also occur in association with partial lipodystrophy (Peters et al. 1973; Peters and Williams 1975). In this condition there is a symmetrical loss of subcutaneous fat from the face and sometimes from the arms, trunk, and hips. The lower extremities, however, show a normal or even increased deposition of fat. Males are affected four times as frequently as females. Patients with partial lipodys-

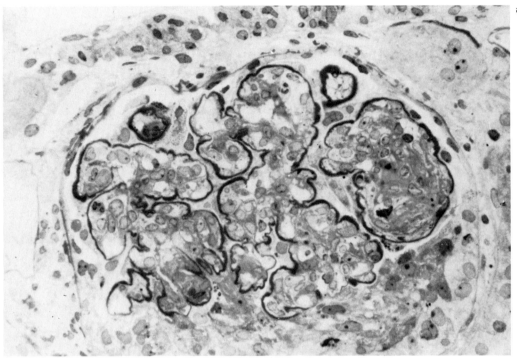

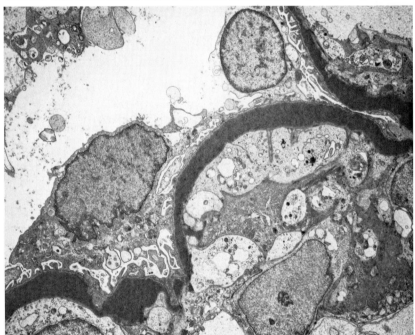

Fig. 9.21. a Membranoproliferative (mesangiocapillary) glomerulo nephritis, 'dense deposit' type. Note the linear deposits in the glomerular basement membrane. (Epon section, toluidine blue; 800 ×) **b** Electron photomicrograph of the same case (10 000 ×)

trophy and mesangiocapillary glomerulonephritis almost invariably exhibit hypocomplementaemia. Occasionally lipodystrophy and hypocomplementaemia occur in the absence of demonstrable renal disease and this has been taken as further evidence that the association between hypocomplementaemia and mesangioglomerulonephritis is indirect.

4.2. Membranous Nephropathy

The glomerular lesion in membranous nephropathy is characterized histologically by a diffuse thickening of the walls of all the glomerular capillaries without significant cellular proliferation (Ehrenreich and Churg 1968). Clinically it is usually associated with the nephrotic syndrome. In Britain and North

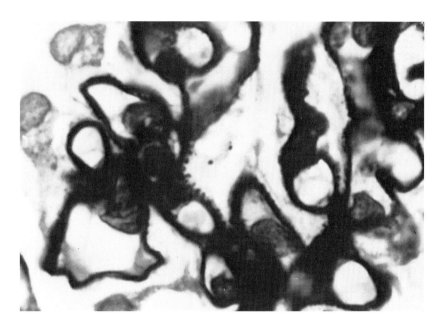

Fig. 9.22. Membranous (epi-membranous) nephropathy. Note the argyrophilic spikes on the epithelial aspect of the basement membrane. (Jones' silver methenamine Stain; 1500 ×)

America it is a relatively uncommon cause of the nephrotic syndrome in children and is certainly much less common in this age group than in adults.

Special staining techniques (trichrome stains and silver methenamine methods) for light microscopy, and electron microscope examination reveal that the glomerular capillary thickening is caused by discrete deposits closely applied to the outer (epithelial) aspect of the GBM. As the lesion progresses, spike-like extensions of the GBM protrude between the deposits like the teeth of a comb (Fig. 9.22). Immunofluorescence microscopy demonstrates the deposits, which contain both IgG and C_3, as a beaded array following the same distribution along the epithelial aspect of the GBM as seen on electron microscopy.

Further progression of the glomerular capillary wall thickening results from the deposition of more basement membrane material around the deposits, which gradually become less distinct and are finally incorporated in the now greatly thickened GBM. Collapse and obliteration of capillary loops by this process leads to gradual hyalinization of whole glomeruli.

In children, membranous nephropathy affects boys more often than girls and may occur at any age including the first year of life. The lesion is less likely to be progressive in children, although about 10% go on to terminal renal failure. Others undergo remission of their nephrotic syndrome but this may be followed by relapse. In some cases complete resolution appears to occur (Habib and Kleinknecht 1975).

4.3. Minimal Change Disease

It has long been recognized (Dunn 1934) that the majority of children (80% or more) and a much smaller percentage of adults who present with the nephrotic syndrome show an absence of glomerular changes on light microscopy, or only trivial ones. In the great majority of such cases immunofluorescence microscopy also fails to demonstrate any glomerular deposition of immunoglobulins, complement, or fibrin. In untreated cases, electron microscopy reveals diffuse fusion and coalescence of epithelial cell foot processes, but this is probably a consequence rather than a cause of the massive proteinuria (Vernier et al. 1960). Renal tubular cells usually show marked 'hyaline droplet' change, again reflecting the massive proteinuria. Lipid deposition is often conspicuous both in tubular cells and in macrophages in the interstitium, a consequence of the derangement of lipid metabolism that occurs in the nephrotic syndrome.

The pathogenesis of minimal change disease is unknown. Suggestions that the increased glomerular permeability for plasma proteins is immunologically mediated are based on indirect evidence, such as changes in the levels of circulating immunoconglutinin and complement (Ngu et al. 1970), but are not supported by immunofluorescence studies.

The peak incidence of minimal change disease associated with the nephrotic syndrome is between 2 and 4 years. Boys are affected about 3 times as often as girls. The severe proteinuria is not generally accompanied by haematuria, which, if present at all, is usually only detected on microscopy of the urine deposit. In affected children proteinuria is nearly always selective, i.e., the urine contains predominantly low molecular weight proteins such as albumin, implying that the defect in the glomerular molecular sieve is partial, and the ability to retain larger macromolecules within the vascular compartment is largely retained (Cameron and White 1965).

Characteristically, children with minimal change disease respond to large doses of steroids or treatment with immunosuppressive drugs such as cyclophosphamide by losing their proteinuria completely. This is most unusual in other types of glomerular disease. A successful response to steroid therapy is accompanied by resolution of the epithelial foot process fusion so that this ultrastructural feature is not seen in renal biopsy specimens taken during remission.

The clinical outcome in children with minimal change disease is generally good. About 20% have only one or two nephrotic episodes before going into permanent remission. In the remainder, although steroid therapy controls the proteinuria, cessation of treatment results in relapse after a shorter or longer period. In about half these patients relapse occurs almost immediately steroids are withdrawn. These steroid-dependent patients pose a difficult clinical problem in view of the large dose of steroid needed to control their proteinuria. More satisfactory remissions can sometimes be obtained with immunosuppressives (Barratt and Soothill 1970) but the long-term effects of such agents, particularly on the gonads, have not yet been established.

4.4. Focal Glomerular Lesions

The glomerular lesions so far described are diffuse, i.e., all the glomeruli are involved in the process. Focal glomerular lesions are those in which only a proportion of glomeruli show recognizable histological lesions, whilst others appear morphologically normal. Although such a distinction has some practical use, the concept of focal glomerular involvement may often be spurious. Examination of serial sections, despite apparently normal glomeruli in these cases, often reveals changes that were not apparent in the initial section at a different level in the glomerulus. In cases of focal glomerulonephritis, immunofluorescence microscopy often shows diffuse immunoglobulin deposition in all glomeruli, even those that appear normal on light microscopy. Focal glomerular scarring may also represent the aftermath of a diffuse glomerular disease in which pathological changes have completely resolved in some glomeruli but have produced scars in others.

Two main varieties of focal glomerular disease are usually described.

4.4.1. Focal Glomerular Sclerosis

Glomerular sclerosis affecting some glomeruli but not others is the hallmark of focal glomerular sclerosis (Churg et al. 1970; Habib and Gubler 1971). The sclerosis may be segmental, i.e., involving part of a glomerular tuft but sparing the remainder, or global, i.e., involving the whole tuft, which is converted to a hyalinized ball. The segmental lesion is characterized by collapse of the capillary loops and an increase in mesangial material or deposition of subendothelial hyaline substance without cellular proliferation (Fig. 9.23). Adhesion of the scarred segment to Bowman's capsule is frequent and material with the staining properties of fibrin may be present, usually in a subendothelial distribution. Immunofluorescence microscopy is frequently negative, but may demonstrate IgM deposition within the segmental lesions.

The tubules associated with the scarred glomeruli, both those with global and those with segmental involvement, are usually atrophic. They show reduction in their cross-sectional diameter, flattening of the lining epithelium, thickening of the tubular basement membrane, and fibrosis in the surrounding interstitium.

In renal biopsy specimens glomerular lesions may be sparse. The presence of areas of tubular atrophy, particularly when the biopsy is from a child, is a useful pointer to the diagnosis. Serial sections of the biopsy will then often reveal glomerular changes not apparent in the initial section.

The pathogenesis of focal glomerulosclerosis is unknown. Clinically, the most common presentation is with the nephrotic syndrome, even in those cases where glomerular scarring is minimal and affects only a small minority of glomeruli. It is clear, therefore, that protein leakage occurs through all glomeruli. Although focal glomerulosclerosis, unlike the minimal change lesion, is often a progressive lesion in which increasing glomerular scarring and secondary tubular and interstitial damage may gradually lead to renal insufficiency, it may be that the two conditions are related. The glomerular scarring that distinguished focal glomerular sclerosis may be an epiphenomenon occurring in a minority of cases of minimal change disease and accounting for the poorer prognosis. However, glomerular scarring may be pronounced even in renal biopsy specimens taken soon after presentation, and the clinical characteristics of the nephrotic syndrome differ from those in minimal change disease (see below). Also, progression from mesangial proliferative glomerulonephritis to focal glomerular sclerosis has been seen in serial biopsy specimens (Habib and Gubler 1973), suggesting a different pathogenesis in these cases at least. It is

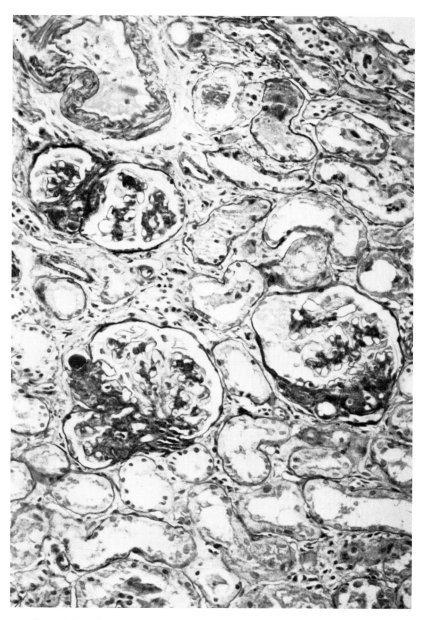

Fig. 9.23. Focal glomerulosclerosis.
Three glomeruli showing segmental
hyalinosis. (PAS; 300 ×)

probable, as in many other glomerulopathies, that the changes in focal glomerular sclerosis merely represent one way in which the glomerulus reacts to injury that is in no way specific.

About 10% of nephrotic children have focal glomerular sclerosis. Unlike minimal change disease, only about 30% respond to steroid or immunosuppressive therapy, and often the response is incomplete, i.e., the proteinuria is lessened but not completely cleared. Protein loss is usually non-selective or may become so in the course of the disease in those who initially show selectivity. Co-existent haematuria is also more common than in minimal change disease. The outcome is variable, but in more than half the cases the disease is progressive. Non-response to steroids and accompanying haematuria are bad prognostic factors (Habib and Gubler 1975).

Diagnosis of focal glomerular sclerosis in renal biopsy specimens, and particularly the distinction from minimal change disease, may be difficult when only a small minority of glomeruli exhibit focal lesions. The distribution of scarred glomeruli, although focal, is not random. Rich (1957) demonstrated that the juxtamedullary glomeruli are the first affected—this region of the kidney may be missed in a renal biopsy specimen. Reference to foci of tubular atrophy as an indicator of glomerular lesions has already been made. Occasional totally sclerosed glomeruli in the *absence* of tubular atrophy are not enough to allow a diagnosis of focal glomerulosclerosis, since this finding may be present in normal children, particularly in the early years of life. Such sclerosed glomeruli probably represent developmental defects where nephrons have failed to establish their proper connection with branches of the ureteric bud.

4.4.2. Focal and Segmental Proliferative Glomerulonephritis

Focal and segmental proliferative glomerulonephritis is an unsatisfactory description, for the reasons already mentioned. In some examples of proliferative glomerulonephritis changes may appear to affect some glomeruli and spare others. Proliferation of both intracapillary (mainly mesangial) and extracapillary cells may occur, often with a segmental distribution, i.e., apparently involving only part of the tuft. Focal scarring and focal fibrinoid necrosis of glomerular tufts may also be seen. Serial sectioning or immunofluorescence microscopy may indicate a more diffuse glomerular involvement despite the apparently focal nature of the lesion. It is probable that the varying *degree* of involvement of individual glomeruli and the presence of different stages in the evolution of the glomerular lesion account for their apparently focal distribution.

This histological picture is seen in a number of different clinical settings. In approximately half the cases of focal and segmental glomerulonephritis in children there is associated systemic disease. The most common is Schönlein–Henoch purpura, others, such as systemic lupus erythematosus, polyarteritis nodosa, and Goodpasture's disease being much less common (see also p. 413). In Schönlein–Henoch purpura, haematuria and proteinuria indicate renal involvement. Occasionally, progressive kidney disease develops, particularly in those cases in which recurrent attacks occur. In the majority, however, the renal lesion resolves completely, although some residual glomerular scarring may be evident. Even in cases that eventually resolve, haematuria and proteinuria may persist for months or even years.

Berger (1969) has shown that many cases of focal glomerulonephritis in children and young adults are associated with mesangial IgA deposition in the glomerular tufts. These cases usually present with recurrent haematuria and often mild proteinuria, but renal function in other respects is generally normal. Haematuria is often precipitated by upper respiratory tract infections, without any latent period. Histologically there is a usually mild focal or diffuse mesangial proliferative glomerulonephritis; immunofluorescence reveals deposits of IgA, C_3 and often IgG in the mesangial regions of the glomerular tufts. Recurrent attacks may occur, but follow-up over a number of years usually (though not invariably) fails to reveal evidence of renal functional deterioration.

4.5. Lupus Nephritis

Systemic lupus erythematosus is a multisystem disorder of apparent 'autoimmune' origin, which may occur during childhood. A number of circulating antibodies may be found, and lupus nephritis, which appears to be a soluble-complex disease caused by glomerular (and sometimes tubular) deposition of deoxyribonucleic acid (DNA)–anti-DNA complexes, is a common and serious manifestation of the disease.

Histologically, a number of glomerular lesions are encountered. There may be swelling and proliferation of intracapillary (mesangial and endothelial) cells, infiltration by leucocytes, foci of tuft necrosis (Fig. 9.24a) and fibrin deposition, and capsular crescent formation. Individual capillary loops may be obstructed with eosinophilic material (so-called hyaline thrombi) and occasionally granular 'haematoxyphil bodies' may be identified. Thickening of tuft capillary walls may be of two main types:

1) Resulting from deposition of material staining as fibrin beneath the endothelial lining to produce the so-called wire loop lesion (Fig. 9.24b); and

2) Membranous transformation, as described in membranous nephropathy (see p. 416).

Destruction of segments of the glomerular tufts results in focal tuft sclerosis with obliteration of capillary lumina and the formation of capsular adhesions. Progressive damage may lead to widespread glomerular scarring with secondary tubular and interstitial changes; this is accompanied clinically by gradual deterioration in renal function leading to renal failure often complicated by hypertension.

Electron microscopy also reveals a varied picture. Electron-dense deposits, presumably immune complexes, may be situated on either side of, or within, the GBM. Structures that some reports have suggested might be viral particles may occasionally be seen within endothelial cells and the GBM. These include tubular formations within the endoplasmic reticulum and organized structures in the basement membranes, composed of a lattice of concentric curves resembling fingerprints. The presence of these structures has been advanced as evidence that viral infection may be involved in the pathogenesis of lupus nephritis, perhaps by interference with the recognition of self antigens.

Immunofluorescence microscopy reveals glomerular and sometimes tubular deposition of IgA, IgG, IgM, C_3 and often fibrinogen. Elution studies have confirmed that anti-DNA antibodies are present in the kidneys.

The pattern of pathological changes shows some correlation with the clinical manifestations and response to treatment in lupus nephritis (see Table 9.3).

4.6. Diabetic Nephropathy

A number of renal diseases, including pyelonephritis (p. 429), necrotizing papillitis, and nephrosclerosis, can complicate diabetes mellitus. The term diabetic nephropathy is usually reserved for a more distinctive glomerular lesion occurring in patients with long-standing diabetes. It is characterized clinically by persistent proteinuria and sometimes by the nephrotic syndrome, and pathologically by nodular or diffuse glomerular lesions, which may occur separately or together in any individual case. The nodular, or Kimmelsteil-Wilson, lesion consists of

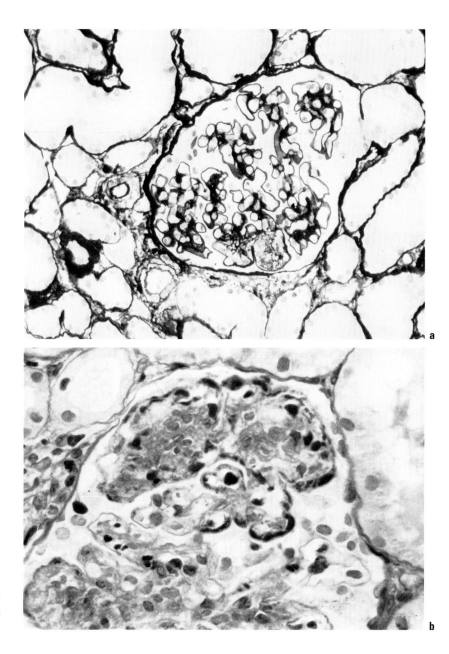

Fig. 9.24. a and **b** Lupus nephritis: **a** Focal glomerular lesion. (Jones' Silver Methanamine Stain; 600 ×) **b** wire loop lesion. (MSB; 1500 ×)

Table 9.3. Pathological changes and clinical manifestations in different forms of renal disease affecting principally the glomeruli

Pathology	Clinical manifestations
Focal glomerulonephritis	Mild proteinuria and haematuria. May remit with steroid therapy. Renal insufficiency rare, but disease can be progressive
Diffuse glomerulonephritis. Varying severity; may be prominent capsular crescents	Severe proteinuria (often with nephrotic syndrome). Haematuria, renal insufficiency, and hypertension common. Disease progressive and rarely responds to treatment
Membranous nephritis. Membranous transformation the principal change. Rare	Nephrotic syndrome, often with haematuria. Renal insufficiency and hypertension less marked. Sometimes responds to therapy; usually progressive

rounded, homogeneous, eosinophilic, hyaline deposits situated in the peripheries of the glomerular tuft lobules in the axial regions. These nodules, which vary in size, often affect more than one lobule in a single tuft. The diffuse lesion consists of widespread mesangial thickening in all glomeruli, accompanied by thickening of tuft capillary walls. In both patterns the hyaline material has ultrastructural characteristics resembling basement membrane material. Characteristically severe arteriolar sclerosis with hyaline thickening of the arteriolar walls accompanies diabetic nephropathy. The pathogenesis of the lesion is unknown, but the deposits have been interpreted as accumulations of fibrin-derived products altered by ageing, which originally seep from the glomerular capillaries as a result of the increased capillary permeability associated with diabetes, or alternatively, as a reflection of abnormal basement membrane synthesis resulting from deranged carbohydrate metabolism.

Although clinical evidence of diabetic nephropathy is rare in children, pathological involvement of the renal glomeruli has been described on a number of occasions in this age group (Urizar et al. 1969; Balodimos et al. 1975; Westberg and Michael 1972). In general the incidence of significant renal involvement increases with duration of the diabetes (White 1956).

4.7. Renal Amyloidosis

Detailed discussion of renal amyloidosis is inappropriate, since the condition is rare in children and differs in no significant way from the adult disease. Occasional cases of secondary amyloidosis with renal involvement occur in this age group but are uncommon with modern treatment of the causative disorders. Familial forms of amyloidosis, such as Mediterranean fever, may develop renal manifestations during childhood (Sohar et al. 1967).

4.8. Hereditary Nephropathy

A number of uncommon or very rare, and usually progressive, forms of renal disease of unknown aetiology are distinguished by their familial incidence. They can be classified to a limited extent by their clinical associations, pathological features, and mode of inheritance, but in most cases information on all these points is sparse and often conflicting. Only the more familiar varieties are dealt with here and the reader is referred to Kissane (1973) for detailed consideration of the topic.

4.8.1. Hereditary Chronic Nephritis

Hereditary chronic nephritis is sometimes referred to as Alport's syndrome after his report (Alport 1927) of progressive renal failure associated with haematuria and deafness in 16 members of a single family. The renal involvement tends to be more severe in males, who develop progressive renal impairment and hypertension during the second and third decades. Affected females have intermittent or persistent haematuria but renal function is otherwise not affected, so that life expectancy is often, though not invariably, normal. Renal function may be impaired during pregnancy. Gross haematuria is usually episodic and can be precipitated by infections. Microscopic haematuria is almost always present between attacks, however, and is the most sensitive indicator of involvement in asymptomatic relatives. Proteinuria is generally slight, but proteinuria of nephrotic proportions has occasionally been described (Knepshield et al. 1965).

The renal disease is accompanied by perceptive deafness in about one-third of reported cases; this usually becomes apparent about the time of puberty. The hearing loss is most marked for high tones (4000–8000 Hz). Ocular abnormalities (keratoconus or cataracts) have been described. It should be emphasized that the majority of cases of Alport's syndrome are not deaf and only a small minority have ocular defects. Where haematuria is the only discernible clinical abnormality, the distinction of hereditary nephritis from other diseases, such as poststreptococcal glomerulonephritis or Berger's nephropathy, may depend on an accurate family history.

The pathological changes in hereditary nephritis are variable and depend to a large extent on the stage of the disease. In young individuals without renal impairment, renal biopsy specimens may be normal or may show minor changes (mild hypercellularity of the glomerular tufts or erythrocytes within the renal tubules). In more advanced cases, or in patients dying from the disease, the pathological features are a mixture of glomerular and interstitial nephritis (Krickstein et al. 1966). The glomeruli show a variety of 'inflammatory' changes with tuft hypercellularity, segmental and global sclerosis, capsular adhesions, and occasional fibroepithelial crescents. Tubular atrophy is generally marked and accompanied by diffuse interstitial fibrosis and irregular chronic inflammation. Foci of foam cells containing cytoplasmic lipid may also be present in the interstitium and are most commonly seen near the corticomedullary junction. Much has been made of this feature, although it is by no means invariably

present and may occur in other types of renal disease, usually those accompanied by the nephrotic syndrome. Recent ultrastructural studies (Hinglais et al. 1972) have shown changes in the glomerular basement membrane, consisting of thickening with distortion of the lamina densa, which is transformed into a network of strands enclosing electron-lucent areas containing tiny granules 500 Å in diameter (Fig. 9.25). These changes have been interpreted as specific for hereditary nephritis, although this has been disputed by some workers (Hill et al. 1974). No evidence of immune complexes has been described either with electron or with immunofluorescence microscopy.

The mode of inheritance in hereditary nephritis is not clear; although it occurs in successive generations transmission is not of the simple autosomal dominant type. Perkoff et al. (1958) suggested partial sex linkage of a dominant gene. Alternative suggestions include autosomal dominant inheritance with varying expression in males and females, or autosomal dominant inheritance with nonrandom segregation of the relevant chromosome with an X chromosome.

4.8.2. Hereditary Multifocal Osteolysis with Nephropathy

Hereditary osteolysis is a rare disorder in which sclerosis, gradual lysis, and collapse affect the carpal and tarsal bones. Osseous involvement commences in early childhood and the disease becomes static by adult life, when deformity may be marked. Inheritance is usually described as autosomal dominant in type, with variable expressivity.

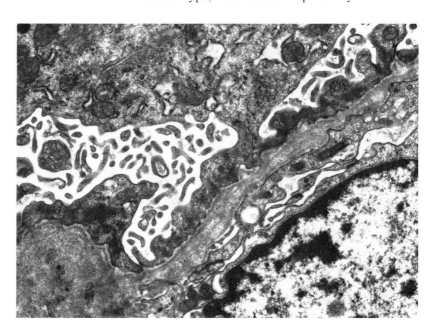

Fig. 9.25. Alport's syndrome. An electron photomicrograph showing foot process fusion, irregular basement membrane thickening and distortion and splitting of the lamina densa. (9000 ×)

Some patients with hereditary osteolysis develop progressive renal disease with hypertension. Most of the few pathological descriptions of the renal lesion have indicated chronic glomerulonephritis. This has usually been reported in adult patients (Marie et al. 1963), but it does also occur in children (Counahan et al. 1975).

4.8.3. Hereditary Onycho-osteodysplasia (Nail–Patella Syndrome)

The nail–patella syndrome is a curious disorder inherited as an autosomal dominant trait with variable expressivity closely allied to that for ABO blood groups and characterized by abnormal development of the finger- and toenails and hyperplasia or absence of the patellae. Malformations of the radii and asymptomatic osseous spurs projecting from the ilium may also be seen. About one-third of the patients affected have evidence of renal disease with proteinuria, sometimes accompanied by haematuria. Renal insufficiency develops very slowly and late in the course of the disease. The morphological changes in the kidney are nonspecific and usually mild, with focal thickening of glomerular capillary walls, irregular glomerular sclerosis, and areas of tubular atrophy.

4.9. Congenital Nephrotic Syndrome

Children with congenital nephrotic syndrome present in the first 6 months of life, unlike those with acquired forms, who only very exceptionally develop symptoms in the first year. In the congenital disease nephrotic manifestations are generally apparent at birth, or in the first few days or weeks. Less commonly, affected infants are apparently normal in the neonatal period and develop symptoms after a few weeks or months. There is a marked familial incidence with an apparently autosomal recessive mode of inheritance, and many of the reported cases are of Finnish extraction. Lack of response to corticosteroid therapy and a fatal outcome are usual in the first 2 years. Affected infants are usually small and often premature, show radiological evidence of abnormal intrauterine calcification of bones, and have large, oedematous placentae, which sometimes weigh more than the infants themselves (Kouvalainen et al. 1962).

Proteinuria can usually be detected on the first post-delivery day. Microscopic haematuria may be also present. The proteinuria may be nonselective or initially selective, becoming nonselective as the disease progresses. This change in selectivity is unusual, and is seen in acquired forms of the nephrotic syndrome only in occasional cases of focal glomerular sclerosis (see p. 418). The proteinuria fails to respond to corticosteroids or immunosuppressives, and the high incidence of intercurrent infection and poor growth rate of these infants are contraindications for steroid treatment.

The pathological changes in the glomeruli are variable. Early in the course of the disease the glomeruli may be normal. Varying degrees of tuft hypercellularity and segmental or global hyalinization are seen later. Cystic dilatation of proximal convoluted tubules may be sufficiently marked to warrant the description 'microcystic disease'. Immunofluorescence microscopy fails to reveal any consistent pattern of immunoglobulin deposition, and ultrastructural examination reveals no evidence of immune complexes.

5. Renal Vascular Disease

5.1. Arterial Hypertension

Essential hypertension is rarely diagnosed in the paediatric age group, and for this reason secondary forms are of greater practical importance than in adults. However, concepts regarding the nature of hypertension are currently changing. The practical importance of a raised arterial blood pressure, apart from its direct effects, lies in the increased risk of complications such as cerebrovascular accidents and ischaemic heart disease. However, hypertension is not a disease in the generally accepted sense. Amongst individuals in a particular population arterial pressure is normally distributed, and although the risk of complications increases as blood pressure rises further beyond the mean, there is is no arbitary level that defines the 'normal' value. Recent work suggests that an individual becomes fixed on a particular blood pressure centile for the population as a whole early in life, perhaps even in infancy (see Berry 1978 for discussion). Genetic factors are undoubtedly important, since pressures tend to be higher in infants one or both of whose parents are hypertensive (Zinner et al. 1971; Beresford and Holland 1975). Since blood pressure tends to increase with age, a child with an arterial pressure significantly above the mean will tend to become hypertensive as an adult, even though his or her pressure in early life may be below that usually associated with an increased risk of complications. The practical implications of these ideas, particularly whether treatment with hypotensive agents is justified in children with persistent arterial pressures significantly above average, have yet to be clarified.

In both essential and secondary forms of hypertension, persistent elevation of the arterial blood pressure may be associated with changes in arterial vessels throughout the body, including those in the kidneys. The nature of these changes depends on the rapidity with which hypertension develops and on the degree of elevation of the arterial pressure. In general, changes in vessels in children with hypertension are not different from those in adults, but complicating factors (atherosclerosis and age-related changes) are absent. Essential hypertension-related renal damage takes many years to develop and is seldom evident in childhood, but in malignant hypertension secondary nephrosclerosis is marked and proliferative changes, even capsular crescent formation and focal necroses, may be apparent in the glomerular tufts. Malignant hypertension may give rise to renal failure, or an increase in intracranial pressure, which can be recognized clinically by the presence of papilloedema.

5.2. Causes of Secondary Hypertension in Children

Glomerulonephritis is the commonest cause of hypertension in children. In acute poststreptococcal glomerulonephritis hypertension is usually transient, and most reports suggest that it results from overload of the extracellular fluid space or an imbalance in the normal humoral regulatory mechanisms. Persistent hypertension may be a feature of any chronic glomerulonephritis, particularly when chronic renal failure develops. Allen et al. (1960) found hypertension in about a quarter of patients with nephritis following Schönlein–Henoch purpura, and it is a prominent feature in about half of all children with the haemolytic uraemic syndrome (p. 427). Hypertension may also occur in children subjected to renal transplantation either immediately following transplantation or during rejection episodes.

The pathology of chronic pyelonephritis and reflux nephropathy is considered in detail on p. 429. Hypertension is sometimes present, particularly in patients with severe bilateral disease. It is rarely present in children without evidence of renal failure, but is occasionally seen in patients without azotaemia and in those with unilateral involvement. The mechanisms involved are disputed (see Heptinstall 1974b), and it is probable that a number of different factors are involved in individual cases.

Segmental renal hypoplasia (the Ask–Upmark kidney) commonly presents with hypertension, which is often severe and may occur with unilateral or bilateral disease. As discussed on p. 399, there is some confusion about the exact nature of this condition. The fact that 'segmental hypoplasia' is not uncommonly associated with vesicoureteric reflux raises the possibility that it is an acquired disease rather than a congenital anomaly, and may be just a form of reflux nephropathy (Johnson and Mix 1976). The separation of cases of segmental hypoplasia may merely represent clinical selection of those cases presenting with hypertension. The associated vesicoureteric reflux may be regarded as insignificant; it may be overlooked if not specifically looked for; or it may indeed have ceased by the time the patient is investigated, since vesicoureteric reflux resolves in a majority of children (see p. 433).

Both renal dysplasia and polycystic disease (see p. 399 and p. 405) may be accompanied by hypertension. As with pyelonephritis, renal dysplasia is seldom complicated by hypertension except where severe bilateral involvement has led to renal failure. Superadded chronic infection is common in these instances. Hydronephrosis may also be accompanied by hypertension and a few cases of unilateral hydronephrosis with ureteric obstruction are on record where complicating hypertension was relieved by surgical removal of the obstruction (Belmen et al. 1968; Palmer et al. 1970).

Children with renal tumours may develop hypertension. Nephroblastoma, according to some reports, is commonly associated with a raised arterial blood pressure (Campbell 1951), and occasionally hypertension can be severe (Mitchell et al. 1970). Renal tumours may cause hypertension by perirenal compression of the kidney, or distortion of the renal arteries causing a renovascular type of hypertension. In addition, some renal tumours, including some examples of nephroblastoma, produce a pressor substance with renin-like activity (Mitchell et al. 1970; Robertson et al. 1967).

Hypertension may follow irradiation of the kidneys, usually following treatment of nephroblastoma or, less commonly, adrenal neuroblastoma.

A number of renovascular lesions can cause hypertension during childhood. Localized changes, including hypoplasia of the aorta or renal artery, or more commonly single or multiple stenoses of the renal arteries affecting one or both sides, may be found. In some cases stenotic lesions of other vessels may be present. Occasionally congenital renal arterial aneurysms may lead to hypertension by thrombosis or compression of branch arteries. Rarely, in children with von Recklinghausen's neurofibromatosis hypertension has been found to complicate coarctation of the aorta, renal artery stenosis, renal arterial aneurysms, or compression of the renal artery by retroperitoneal neurofibromatous tissue.

Arterial hypertension is commonly seen in regions of the body proximal to a coarctation of the aorta. It may also be due to the hormonal effects of functioning adrenal or extra-adrenal chromaffin tumours, congenital hyperplasia of the adrenal cortex, or mineralcorticoid-producing tumours of the adrenal cortex (see p. 580).

Some causes of hypertension in childhood are summarized in Table 9.4.

Table 9.4. Causes of hypertension in childhood

Renal
  Glomerulonephritis (all forms)
  Pyelonephritis and reflux nephropathy
  Ask-Upmark kidney
  Renal dysplasia
  Hydronephrosis
  Polycystic disease
  Renal tumours
  Renal parenchymal damage following irradiation

Vascular
  Coarctation of the aorta
  Renal artery anomalies (stenosis, dysplasia,
    arteritis, aneurysms, neurofibromatosis)

Other
  Adrenal tumours (neuroblastoma, phaeochromocytoma)
  Adrenogenital syndrome
  Cushing's syndrome
  Primary aldosteronism

5.3. Renal Hypoperfusion

Circulatory failure may result in acute renal failure, which may be rapidly reversed without structural damage to the kidney if the underlying circulatory disturbance can be corrected. More prolonged renal hypoperfusion can cause renal injuries that do not recover immediately on restoration of a normal circulation. These lesions include renal tubular necrosis, renal cortical necrosis, renal medullary necrosis, and renal vein thrombosis, and in infants and young children suffering from renal hypoperfusion a combination of these lesions is often present. In such patients the underlying cause of the circulatory failure may be a cardiac abnormality, reduction in blood volume from haemorrhage, reduction of plasma volume from hypoalbuminaemia, loss of extracellular fluid (as in severe burns or sodium depletion), crushing injuries, or severe bacterial infection.

Acute tubular necrosis following hypoperfusion usually affects both the proximal and distal convoluted tubules and the loops of Henle. Tubular necrosis may also follow direct poisoning by heavy metals such as mercury and arsenic, organic solvents such as carbon tetrachloride, and drugs such as sulphonamides and methoxyflurane. Toxic damage of this type is usually confined to the proximal convoluted tubules. With successful clinical management regeneration of the necrotic tubular epithelial cells can be anticipated.

In infancy, and particularly during the first 2 months of life, renal vein thrombosis is likely to complicate renal hypoperfusion. Clinically this is recognized by the development of an enlarged, firm renal mass in a sick infant with oliguria and haematuria. Disseminated intravascular coagulation and thrombocytopenia may also be present. Dehydration following gastrointestinal disturbances is a common underlying cause. Involvement may be unilateral or bilateral, and the thrombus may occlude the main renal vein and all its tributaries, or merely some of the tributaries. Depending on the degree of thrombosis and other factors, part or all of the kidney may undergo venous infarction. Sometimes venous infarction is confined to the renal medulla.

Medullary and cortical necrosis frequently coexist, and aetiological factors giving rise to these lesions in the newborn include severe anaemia, asphyxia, severe haemolytic disease, and disseminated intravascular coagulation. Recently haemorrhagic infarction of the renal medullae and inner adrenal cortex has been described in infants dying from echovirus II infections (Nagington et al. 1978). In older infants and young children, severe gastroenteritis with vomiting and diarrhoea leading to marked dehydration, other severe bacterial infections, postoperative shock, diabetic ketosis, or the haemolytic uraemic syndrome may also cause these lesions. Unilateral or bilateral renal involvement occurs and the kidneys may show patchy or diffuse changes. The deep juxtamedullary cortex and a thin rim of subcapsular cortex are generally spared even in severe bilateral symmetrical cortical necrosis. In the acute phase of the disease the kidneys are swollen and enlarged, but in patients who survive for several weeks the kidneys become shrunken and show marked nodularity because of hypertrophy of the surviving parenchyma. Calcification of the necrotic cortical tissue occurs and may be visible on radiological examination. When there is accompanying medullary necrosis pelvicalyceal deformities are present, giving rise to a radiological picture on intravenous urography that closely resembles that seen in chronic pyelonephritis (Chrispin 1972).

5.4. Renal Infarction

Obstruction of the renal arterial blood supply may produce infarction of the whole kidney or of a segment. Extreme venous engorgement following venous obstruction may also give rise to infarction.

Arterial occlusion is usually the result of thromboembolism, the emboli arising, for example, from vegetations on heart valves or a coarcted aortic segment. Thrombosis of the renal artery is a rare complication of polyarteritis nodosa and other forms of arteritis during childhood.

5.5. Nephropathy in Sickle-cell Anaemia

Diffuse intravascular sickling with agglutination of distorted red cells characteristically occurs in haemolytic crises in patients with sickle-cell anaemia. Patchy ischaemic lesions may then develop in various organs including the kidneys. In patients who survive a number of such crises, widespread renal scarring is not unusual and may result in renal failure. Ischaemic medullary fibrosis is the probable underlying cause of the diminished ability to concentrate the urine, which is an almost invariable feature of sickle-cell anaemia.

5.6. Haemolytic–Uraemic Syndrome

The haemolytic–uraemic syndrome usually affects children, most commonly during the first year of life, and in over 90 % of cases it occurs in patients under 4 years of age. The sexes are equally affected and there is a seasonal variation, the disease being more common in the summer and autumn in the northern hemisphere. An acute infection, usually of the gastrointestinal tract, very commonly precedes the attack by a few days. This is followed by a haemolytic anaemia, jaundice, and thrombocytopenia. A blood film shows deformity and fragmentation of red blood cells, but the direct Coomb's test is negative. Acute renal failure develops and is often accompanied by hypertension and congestive cardiac failure, and sometimes by pulmonary oedema (Piel and Phibbs 1966; Liberman et al. 1969; Brain 1969).

Variable changes occur in the kidney during this acute phase (Lieberman et al. 1969; Courtecuisse et al. 1967). Occasionally there is massive renal cortical necrosis. More commonly the changes are as follows: in the glomeruli swelling and proliferation of endothelial and mesangial cells occur, different glomeruli being affected to varying degrees. Segmental necrosis and focal thickening of tuft capillary walls may be observed, as may occasional capsular crescents. In some tuft capillaries and small arterioles there may be obstruction by eosinophilic granular material with some of the staining properties of fibrin. Ultrastructurally electron-dense material resembling fibrin may be observed in the widened subendothelial space and within the mesangium. Some capillaries may be occluded by a mixture of aggregated platelets, fibrin, and deformed red

cells. Immunofluorescence microscopy reveals fibrinogen along tuft capillary walls, within capillary lumina, and in the mesangium. Immunoglobulins and complement are consistently absent.

The pathological findings in the glomeruli have been interpreted as a reaction to the deposition of fibrin, occurring as a result of intravascular coagulation. Whether or not intravascular coagulation is confined to the renal microvasculature is unclear, although some reports indicate that microthrombi may be seen in other organs if searched for carefully. It is probable that the damage to the microvasculature causes the accompanying haemolytic anaemia by its mechanical effect on the red cells, causing both lysis and the bizarre distorted forms ('burr' cells) seen in the peripheral blood film. The mechanism triggering intravascular coagulation is not known. Suggestions have included viral infection leading to damage to the vascular endothelium and the possibility of a generalized Shwartzmann reaction. In either event, the preceding infection so commonly noted clinically may be relevant.

Evolution of the renal lesion varies and is related to the severity of the initial attack. In a minority of cases, usually those with prolonged anuria during the acute attack, glomerular scarring is severe. Whole glomeruli and segments of glomeruli become solidified and acellular. Associated tubular atrophy and interstitial fibrosis are marked and haemosiderin deposition may be conspicuous, reflecting the considerable haemoglobinuria that may occur during the acute phase. Arterioles and small arteries exhibit marked concentric intimal hyperplasia with severe narrowing or occlusion of their lumina. Clinically hypertension may be severe, and death in uraemia is common. In the majority of cases whose intitial attack is less severe, renal scarring is less pronounced and the outcome is favourable. Such patients tend to be in the younger age group.

5.7. Interstitial Nephritis

A number of disease processes of widely differing aetiologies produce renal parenchymal damage that affects predominantly the tubules and interstitial tissues (and in some cases the blood vessels), rather than the glomeruli. A varying degree of interstitial inflammation is also often present. Since it is impossible to tell on microscopical examination of the kidney alone whether the primary lesion is of tubules, interstitial tissues, or blood vessels, the noncommittal term 'interstitial nephritis' has proved useful to describe these parenchymal changes. The fact that this description is rather vague is valuable, since it emphasizes the need for careful clinicopathological evaluation to seek a possible underlying cause. Not uncommonly, even after thorough investigation the aetiology remains obscure, but gradually more and more factors producing this type of renal damage are becoming recognized.

Renal infection, particularly chronic pyelonephritis, is a significant cause of interstitial nephritis in paediatric practice, and this will be discussed below. In the past, however, it has not been sufficiently appreciated that a number of other types of interstitial nephritis can produce a very similar histological picture to that seen in chronic pyelonephritis. This label has been attached rather indiscriminately to cases where renal infection is either not involved in the pathogenesis or is merely a complication of another underlying renal lesion.

6. Renal Infection

Infection of the urinary tract may be serious, particularly in the neonate, because of the risks both of spread of infection and of septicaemia, but the usual clinical concern is the possibility of involvement of the renal parenchyma (pyelonephritis). It is important to recognize, however, that renal involvement is by no means invariable or even particularly common in urinary tract infections.

Pyelonephritis occurs in both acute and chronic forms and may or may not be associated with obstructive lesions of the urinary tract. In this section the mechanisms whereby urinary infection may spread to the renal parenchyma are discussed and the pathology of acute and chronic pyelonephritis is considered.

6.1. Spread of Infection to the Kidneys

Pyelonephritis usually follows established lower urinary tract infection, and this sequence may be influenced by a number of factors.

Theoretically organisms might gain access to the kidneys by three routes:

1) *Lymphatic spread*; there is little or no clinical or experimental evidence that this mechanism is important.

2) *Haematogenous spread* undoubtedly occurs in some instances. The kidney may be infected in man in the course of septicaemia following staphylococcal infections such as boils, carbuncles, oesteomyelitis, or endocarditis. Haematogenous spread of gram-negative organisms to the kidney sometimes complicates instrumentation or surgical operations on the urethra (Scott 1929; Barrington and Wright 1930).

3) *Direct ascent from the lower urinary tract* is widely accepted as the most frequent route by which infection of the kidneys occurs, although infections of the bladder and urethra are usually confined to the lower urinary tract. The long intramural and submucosal segment of the ureter at the vesicoureteric junction provided an efficient valvular mechanism, which normally prevents the return of the bladder urine and any organisms it might contain into the ureter and upper tract. In some patients, however, congenital or acquired defects of the vesicoureteric junction render it likely to permit reflux or urine during detrusor contraction at micturition. A congenital lack of obliquity of the intramural and submucosal ureter may render the vesicoureteric junction incompetent. This defect can occur as an isolated lesion, which sometimes has a familial incidence (Bredin et al. 1975; Dwoskin 1976; de Vargas et al. 1978), and also in combination with other urinary tract anomalies, such as posterior urethral valves, megacystis–megaureter, ectopic ureter, and ectopic ureterocele. Acquired incompetence of the vesicoureteric junction leading to vesicoureteric reflux can occur in patients with a 'neurogenic' bladder, and even bladder infection itself can produce sufficient mucosal inflammation and oedema to convert the submucosal segment of the ureter into a rigid tube, resulting in reflux.

During micturition intravesical pressure rises, and in patients with incompetence of the vesicoureteric junction the increased pressure is transmitted directly to the renal pelvis. This results in reversal of the normal pressure gradient between the tubular system of the kidney and the renal pelvis. Thus refluxed urine may pass retrogradely into the papillary ducts and renal tubules in the kidney parenchyma. This process of *intrarenal reflux* (Hodson et al. 1976) provides a mechanism whereby any organisms in the bladder urine may be carried directly into the renal substance, where infection can become established. This explains many of the features of pyelonephritic scarring and is dealt with in more detail in the section on chronic pyelonephritis.

When vesicoureteric reflux is gross the ureters become dilated and tortuous. Urine that refluxed into such capacious ureters during micturition returns to the bladder when voiding is complete. This residual urine provides a suitable medium in which organisms can multiply. This predisposes to urinary infection and helps to perpetuate established infection.

6.2. Urinary Tract Obstruction

Obstructive lesions anywhere in the urinary tract are

associated with a 20-fold increase in the incidence of pyelonephritis (Campbell 1951). In infants and children urinary obstruction is most commonly caused by congenital anomalies such as posterior urethral valves, congenital ureteric stenosis, ureterocele, etc., but may result from acquired lesions such as urolithiasis. A neurogenic bladder complicating spina bifida, for example, may produce functional obstruction. The normal bladder is relatively resistant to colonization with micro-organisms. Voiding during micturition empties the bladder efficiently and flushes out any organisms that might be present. In addition, the bladder mucosa has a number of antibacterial protective mechanisms, which help to maintain the sterility of the urine. However, abnormalities such as outflow obstruction leading to a stagnant residual urine provide a medium in which organisms can multiply. It is now recognized that even a healthy urethra often harbours micro-organisms; these may be a source of urinary infection, particularly following trauma during urethral instrumentation such as catheterization. The mechanism whereby organisms gain access to the kidney in urinary obstruction uncomplicated by vesicoureteric reflux is not clear-cut. There is evidence, based on mathematical considerations, that they can ascend within the lumen of of the ureter against the flow of urine (Shapiro 1967), but spread to involve the renal parenchyma is more difficult to explain. Severe pyogenic inflammation of the upper tract occurring with, for example, pyeonephrosis or infective urolithiasis can probably extend into the renal substance directly. It is probable, however, that lower urinary tract infection in the presence of urinary obstruction often involves the kidney via the haematogenous route. Obstruction slows the passage of urine through the kidneys and any organisms filtered from the blood will therefore become established more easily in the renal parenchyma. Transient bacteraemia certainly occurs with lower urinary tract infections, particularly during catheterization.

6.3. Renal Factors

It is an old experimental observation that infection within the kidney tends to localize in areas of pre-existing damage (de Navasquez 1956). Histological evidence of parenchymal infection (the presence of pus cells within tubules) is not infrequently found at necropsy in the diseased kidneys of patients dying with chronic glomerulonephritis, diabetic glomerulosclerosis, or cystic kidneys. Renal infections of this nature are usually a terminal event and are probably the result of haematogenous infection. Pyelonephritis is a common complication of renal dysplasia

and this too has been attributed to an abnormal susceptibility of the malformed kidney to infection (Marshall 1953; Ericsson and Ivemark 1958). However, as previously emphasized, renal dysplasia is almost invariably associated with other urinary tract anomalies, which are either obstructive or accompanied by vesicoureteric reflux. It is probable that these factors are the principal predisposing causes of parenchymal infection in renal dysplasia (Risdon 1971).

6.4. Acute Pyelonephritis

Descriptions of the pathology of acute pyelonephritis usually relate to cases seen at necropsy with severe fulminating infection, associated with urinary obstruction, or staphylococcal septicaemia (the so-called pyaemic kidney). This condition is illustrated in Fig. 9.26.

Grossly the kidney is swollen and small yellow abscesses are usually visible through the capsule. On section the bulging cut surface is discoloured by wedge-shaped areas of cortical congestion and pallor and by yellowish radial streaks. In cases with urinary obstruction the pelvicalyceal system is dilated and the lining mucosa is congested, oedematous, and covered with pus. Sometimes the renal papillae are yellow and necrotic (necrotizing papillitis).

It is important to recognize that this severe and diffuse inflammation may not be typical of the much commoner milder cases of acute upper tract infection seen clinically. It is quite possible that many patients with urinary infections and symptoms of upper tract involvement such as loin pain, may have infection confined to the ureter and renal pelvis (acute pyelitis) without renal parenchymal involvement (Heptinstall 1974a).

6.5. Chronic Pyelonephritis (Reflux Nephropathy)

On gross examination the kidney affected by chronic pyelonephritis is smaller than expected and is coarsely scarred. Renal involvement is usually, but by no means invariably, bilateral. When both kidneys are affected the degree of reduction in renal size is usually unequal, and it is common for one kidney to be appreciably smaller than the other. Characteristically the scarred segments of parenchyma directly overlie a renal calyx that is misshapen and dilated ('clubbed'). The scarred areas tend to be wedge-shaped, the parenchyma in these zones is thinned, and corticomedullary demarcation

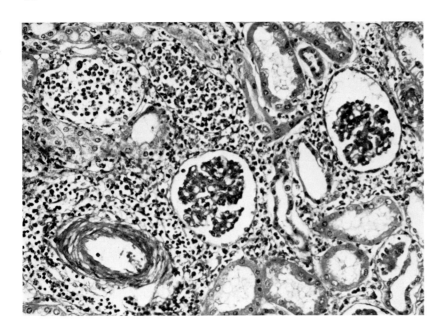

Fig. 9.26. Acute pyelonephritis. Note acute interstitial inflammation and oedema with acute inflammatory tubular destruction. (H and E; 250 ×)

is blurred. In cases with urinary obstruction or severe vesicoureteric reflux the pelvicalyceal system is generally dilated; calyceal clubbing results partly from scarring and contraction of the renal papilla. With long-standing obstruction or reflux, generalized parenchymal atrophy accompanies pelvicalyceal dilatation and the segmental nature of the scarring is much less easy to appreciate. The mucosa lining the renal calyces and pelvis is thickened and its surface is granular.

Microscopically there is considerable interstitial fibrosis and chronic inflammation accompanied by tubular atrophy and loss. There is infiltration by lymphocytes, together with some histiocytes and plasma cells, and well-formed lymphoid follicles are often present (Fig. 9.27a). Sometimes aggregates of atrophic tubules lined with homogeneous eosinophilic material give a 'thyroid-like' appearance. Glomerular damage is variable but is usually less conspicuous than the tubular and interstitial changes. The glomeruli in the scarred zones usually appear crowded together as a result of tubular loss and interstitial fibrosis. Some glomeruli are totally destroyed and converted to rounded acellular scars. Others appear relatively normal or show concentric periglomerular fibrosis. The overall number of glomeruli is frequently diminished, suggesting that some destroyed glomeruli are subsequently absorbed. Vascular changes, particularly fibroelastic intimal thickening of arteries and arterioles, are prominent in the scarred areas even in cases uncomplicated by arterial hypertension. Luminal narrowing of these vessels may be extreme and it is

likely that some of the parenchymal damage is due to, or augmented by, ischaemia. Chronic inflammatory cell infiltration of the subepithelial tissues in the renal calyces, pelvis, and ureter is present (Fig. 9.27b). The intensity of this chronic inflammatory infiltrate varies, but when marked is often accompanied by lymphoid follicle formation.

The pathogenesis of chronic pyelonephritis is far from being completely understood.

In children, urinary obstruction, usually attributable to congenital anomalies, and vesicoureteric reflux are the most important associated conditions. Intrarenal reflux accompanying vesicoureteric reflux provides a convincing mechanism whereby pathogenic organisms present in the urine could gain access to the renal parenchyma and also explains some of the pathological features of the segmental pyelonephric scar (its wedge shape, its often sharp demarcation from surrounding normal parenchyma, and its relation to the renal papilla). These associations are confirmed by clinical, radiological, and experimental observations (Rolleston et al. 1974; Hodson et al. 1975; Ransley and Risdon 1978). Vesicoureteric reflux in children, particularly when severe, shows a significant correlation with segmental scar formation.

Anatomical studies of the renal papillae in both piglets and young children have demonstrated two distinct forms (Ransley and Risdon 1975a, b). One is a simple conical structure resembling the classic description of the renal papilla in anatomical textbooks. Papillary ducts open obliquely into its convex tip in a way that causes them to close when

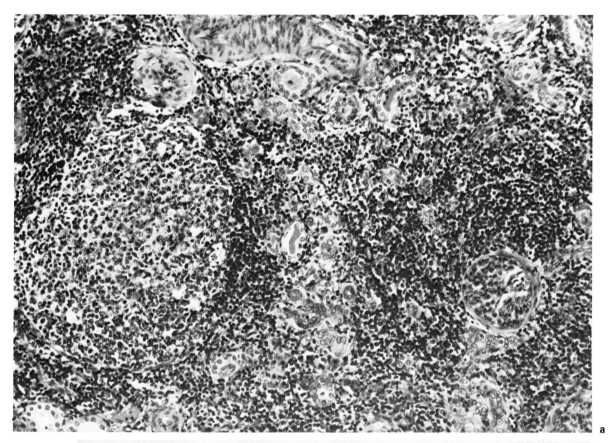

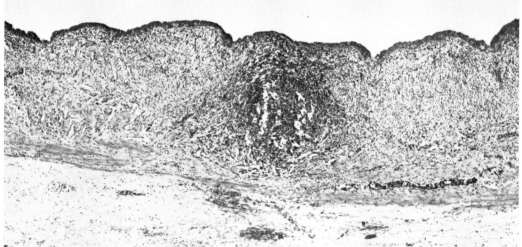

Fig. 9.27. Chronic pyelonephritis. **a** Chronic interstitial inflammation with lymphoid follicle formation. (H and E; 150 ×) **b** Chronic inflammation of the subepithelial connective tissue in the renal pelvis. (H and E; 25 ×)
Courtesy of the Editor of the *Journal of Clinical Pathology*.

the intracalyceal pressure around the tip of the papilla rises (Fig. 9.28a). Thus the papillary duct openings possess a 'check-valve' mechanism, which protects them from intrarenal reflux during an episode of vesicoureteric reflux. These simple nonrefluxing papillae occur principally in the mid-zones of the kidney, where segmental scar formation is relatively uncommon.

The other type of papilla is a compound structure formed by the fusion of a number of papillary units. The calyceal surface is flattened, concave, or deeply indented and the papillary ducts open directly onto this surface (Fig. 9.28b). Thus there is no protective check-valve mechanism, so that such papillae are freely susceptible to intrarenal reflux in the presence of vesicoureteric reflux. Segmental pyelonephritic scarring is most common in the polar regions of the kidney in areas of parenchyma drained by these refluxing papillae.

The suggestion has been made that intrarenal reflux of sterile urine may cause segmental scarring by its hydrodynamic effects alone. This hypothesis has been advanced as an explanation of segmental renal scarring in children who have no clinical evidence of urinary infection (Bailey 1973, 1977). However, experimental studies indicate that intrarenal reflux of infected urine may cause segmental scarring with dramatic speed in the course of only a few days (Ransley and Risdon 1978). Thus the lack of clinical documentation of renal infection is not

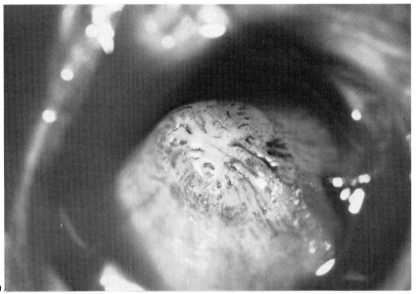

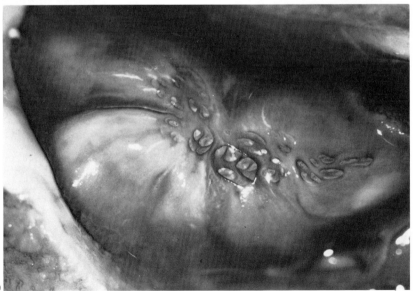

Fig. 9.28. a 'Non-refluxing' papilla (pig). Note the conical shape, domed area cribrosa and slit-like papillary duct orifaces. This type of papilla is not associated with intrarenal reflux. b 'Refluxing' papilla (pig). Note the compound structure with a concave area cribrosa and wide open papillary duct orifices. This type of papilla is associated with intrarenal reflux.
Courtesy of the Editor of the *British Journal of Radiology*.

evidence that it has never occurred. Clinical observations indicate that renal scarring usually occurs
very early in life when for a variety of reasons
urinary infection may be difficult to detect. In fact, in
most children with renal scars the scars are already
present when the child is first seen, and the
development of new scars is relatively rare. Changes
in the radiological appearances can usually be
attributed to growth of the surrounding normal
parenchyma. This strongly supports the concept
advanced by Ransley and Risdon (1978) that
scarring usually occurs in the very young, probably
in infancy in association with episodes of urinary
infection that may not be detected clinically (Lancet
1978).

It is also true that some children do not develop
scars even in the presence of vesicoureteric reflux and
after repeated urinary infections. Anatomical studies of the kidneys from infants and young children
indicate that about one-third (33%) do not possess
any refluxing papillae (Ransley and Risdon 1975b).
Such kidneys would be immune from intrarenal
reflux, and this presumably explains the lack of scars
in such cases.

Renal scars are also relatively frequently detected
in older children who have sterile urine and no
vesicoureteric reflux. Clinical studies on vesicoureteric reflux indicate, however, that in a high proportion of cases reflux ceases spontaneously. Thus
the absence of reflux in an older child does not
necessarily mean that it has never occurred (Ransley
1978).

It is also recognized that progressive renal damage
occurs after a period of years in some patients with
segmental scarring. Various mechanisms have been
postulated, including ischaemic changes following
alterations in renal blood vessels, particularly in
patients who become hypertensive, and secondary
immunological damage. Experimental studies based
on fluorescence microscopy have occasionally demonstrated residual bacterial antigens in pyelo-
nephrotic scars (Cotran 1969) but the evidence link-
ing this with progressive renal destruction is tenuous.
Recently Kincaid-Smith (1979) has reported significant proteinuria in some patients with reflux nephropathy progressing to renal failure. The majority of
such patients exhibit glomerular lesions of focal
sclerosis and hyalinosis (Bhathena et al. 1979).

6.6. Renal Tuberculosis

Tuberculous infection of the kidney is considered
separately from other renal infections. The infection
is invariably blood-borne, usually from a primary
source in the lungs, less commonly in other sites. The
primary source of infection may heal and disappear,
leaving the renal lesion as the dominant site of
tuberculosis (so-called isolated-organ renal involvement).

Renal tuberculosis may (1) be part of a generalized
systemic haematogenous spread (miliary tuberculosis), when numerous small, discrete tubercles are
scattered throughout the renal parenchyma, or (2)
involve massive nodular areas of conglomerate
caseous necrosis affecting both cortex and medulla.
There is often cavitation and sloughing of the renal
pyramids, with considerable calcification and fibrosis and tuberculous ulceration into the pelvicalyceal system. Spread to the mucosa lining the renal
pelvis and ureter may cause stricture formation. The
dilated pelvicalyceal system becomes filled with
caseous material and the renal parenchyma is
reduced to a thin surrounding shell (*tuberculous
pyonephrosis*). Histologically the appearance is that
of a typical tuberculous reaction, and acid-fast
bacilli can usually be demonstrated.

Renal tuberculosis may be unilateral or bilateral
and may involve one or several segments of the
kidney. In all forms of renal involvement there is
usually associated tuberculous cystitis, which is
clinically significant since it is more likely to give rise
to symptoms than is the renal tuberculosis.

7. Urolithiasis

Calculi can form at any level in the urinary tract, and
the incidence at the various sites differs in different
parts of the world. In Great Britain they are
commonest in the pelvicalyceal system.

Stones are composed of crystalloid bound by a
complex mucoprotein matrix, usually arranged in
concentric layers around a nucleus of organic or
crystalloidal material. Common crystalloid constituents are calcium oxalate, calcium phosphate,
triple phosphates, and uric acid, whilst less frequent
components are the amino acids cystine and xanthine. Stones can occur in pure forms, but are much
more commonly mixed.

Phosphate stones are off-white or grey in colour,
smooth, and often crumbly. Large phosphate stones
may fill the pelvicalyceal system to form the so-called
staghorn calculi.

Oxalate stones are much harder and have a spiny
exterior (the so-called mulberry stone). They are
usually dark brown or black owing to blood staining
caused by trauma.

Uric acid stones are moderately hard and yellow-
brown in colour.

Cystine stones are usually multiple and small.

They are smooth and rounded, yellowish in colour, and waxy in consistency.

The mechanisms leading to stone formation are incompletely understood. Urine is a complex mixture of many substances including crystalloids, which are present in concentrations that in ordinary aqueous solution would be supersaturated. It is believed that various colloid constituents of urine help to maintain the crystalloids in solution, and factors that disturb this balance may influence stone formation.

Changes in urine pH are important in this respect. Uric acid and cystine stones form in acid urine, and both these substances are much less soluble at low pH. Phosphate stones form in alkaline solution, and urinary infection with urea-splitting organisms such as *Proteus*, which keep the urinary pH high, are particularly associated with stones of this kind. Dehydration may also be important in stone formation, by increasing the concentrations of crystalloids.

Calculus formation is a recognized complication of various conditions in which there is increased urinary excretion of the various constituent crystalloids.

Hypercalcuria may occur without obvious predisposing cause (idiopathic hypercalcuria) or as a complication of hyperparathyroidism, sarcoidosis, Cushing's syndrome, prolonged immobilization owing to illness, primary renal tubular acidosis, and the milk-alkali syndrome, all of which can occur in childhood. In some patients with these conditions deposits of calcium are also present in the kidneys (nephrocalcinosis).

The condition of *primary hyperoxaluria* is associated with oxalate stone formation and deposits of calcium oxalate in organs throughout the body including the kidneys, but most oxalate stones are not associated with increased urinary oxalate excretion.

Cystine and xanthine stones are rare, and occur almost exclusively in the metabolic disorders cystinuria and xanthinuria, when urinary excretion of these amino acids is high.

Local factors are also probably involved in stone formation. A nucleus of organic or crystalloidal material can usually be found at the centre of a calculus, which presumably acts as a nidus around which aggregates of crystals can form. Tiny blood clots, fibrin, cellular debris, or collections of bacteria have been suggested as possible foreign bodies that could initiate stone formation. Small areas of calcification (*Randall's plaques*) can sometimes be found in the collecting ducts near the apices of the renal pyramids, and these have been suggested as a possible focus for crystal deposition leading to calculus formation. They are, however, fairly common even in individuals who do not form stones, and are often absent when stones are present.

8. Hereditary Abnormalities of Renal Tubular Transport

A number of hereditary disorders of renal tubular transport are described, but the pathological changes produced in the kidney are seldom of great help in making a specific diagnosis. For this reason a brief account only is given in table form (Table 9.5). The classification used is based on that of Kissane (1973).

8.1. Bartter's Syndrome

Bartter's syndrome is a familial disorder of renal potassium excretion, characterized clinically by hypokalaemic, hyperchloraemic alkalosis associated with a normal blood pressure despite elevated blood angiotensin levels and an increased urinary aldosterone excretion. Hyposthenuria is usual and shows no response to vasopressin. Renal biopsy in affected patients revealed marked hyperplasia of the juxtaglomerular apparatus (JGA).

Symptoms may develop shortly after birth but diagnosis is occasionally delayed, sometimes until early adult life. Early symptoms include failure to thrive, polyuria, polydipsia, constipation, muscular weakness, and craving for salt. Growth retardation is common in children, and many are mentally retarded.

The syndrome has been reported in siblings, including twins, but has been described in more than one generation of a kindred. Inheritance is thought to be through a mutant autosomal recessive gene.

The principal morphological abnormality in the kidney is marked hyperplasia and increased granularity of the JGA (Fig. 9.29). The macula densa is usually prominent. The glomeruli exhibit varying degrees of mesangial cell hypercellularity and some increase in the amount of mesangial matrix. Focally, glomeruli with an immature appearance similar to that seen in the fetal kidney may be present. Tubular lesions associated with potassium deficiency are sometimes seen.

The pathogenesis is unknown. The mechanism initially suggested (Bartter et al. 1962) was a primary resistant of peripheral arterioles to the pressor action of angiotensin, leading to inappropriate stimulation of the renin/angiotensin system with hyperplasia of the JGA, promoting increased adrenal production of aldosterone and consequent urinary potassium

Table 9.5. Familial abnormalities of tubular transport

	Disorder	Inheritance	Functional abnormality	Morphological changes in kidneys	Clinical effects
1. Specific disorders of amino-acid transport	(a) Cystinuria	Autosomal recessive	Proximal tubular defect→ increased urinary excretion of cystine, lysine, arginine, and ornithine	–	Cystine calculi in the urinary tract
	(b) Hartnup disease	Autosomal recessive	Proximal tubular defect→ increased urinary excretion of alanine, glutamine, asparagine, nistidine, serine, theonine, phenyl-alanine, tyrosine, and tryptophan	–	Pellagra-like skin rash. Attacks of cerebellar ataxia
	(c) Iminoglycinuria	Autosomal recessive	Proximal tubular defect→ increased urinary excretion of glycine, proline and hydroxyproline	–	Urinary tract calculi
2. Nonspecific disorders of amino-acid transport	(a) Cystinosis (de Toni–Faconi–Lignac–Debré syndrome)				
	(i) Childhood form	Autosomal recessive	Proximal tubular defect→ aminoaciduria, hyper-phosphaturia, acidosis, and hypokalaemia. May be proteinuria	Deposition of cystine crystals in tubules, glomerular epithelial cells, and interstitium (as well as elsewhere in the body). Swan-neck deformity of nephrons on microdissection	Vomiting, fever, polyuria. Vitamin D-resistant rickets. Occasionally pitressin-resistant diabetes insipidus. Renal failure
	(ii) Idiopathic form	autosomal recessive and dominant described	Proximal tubular defect→ glycosuria, aminoaciduria, hypophosphaturia	No cystine deposition	Milder disease than (i). Usually affects adults but may be present in childhood
	(b) Lowe's syndrome	Sex-linked recessive	Proximal tubular defect→ aminoaciduria, hypophosphaturia. Acidosis, proteinuria, and inability to concentrate the urine	Tubular atrophy and glomerulosclerosis	Congenital glaucoma, cataracts, mental retardation, rickets, and renal failure
3. Tubular defects owing to endogen-ous poisons	(a) Galactosaemia	Autosomal recessive	Galactose-1-phosphate uridyl transferase deficiency→galactose retention. Effect on proximal tubules→ aminoaciduria and proteinuria	– –	Cataracts, mental deficiency, and hepatic cirrhosis
	(b) Wilson's disease	Autosomal recessive	Defect of copper metabolism associated with reduced serum caeruloplasmin and deposition of copper. Effect on proximal tubules→ aminoaciduria	– –	Extrapyramidal symptoms, Kayser–Fleischer rings, hepatic cirrhosis

continued next page

Table 9.5. *(continued)*

	Disorder	Inheritance	Functional abnormality	Morphological changes in kidneys	Clinical effects
4. Disorders of other transport mechanisms	(a) Renal glycosuria	Autosomal dominant	Prominent tubular defect→ glycosuria	–	–
	(b) Vitamin D-resistant rickets	Sex-linked dominant	Increased clearance of phosphate owing to reduced reabsorption in the proximal tubules	– –	Rickets refractory to therapy with vitamin D
	(c) Vasopressin-resistant diabetes insipidus	Probably sex-linked dominant with variable expressivity	Distal tubular defect resulting in unresponsiveness to vasopressin	Microdissection indicates diminution in proximal tubule convolutions	Vasopressin-resistant diabetes insipidus
	(d) Primary renal acidosis (i) Infantile form	Autosomal recessive	Distal tubular defect→ inability to acidify urine	Reduction in renal size and nephro-calcinosis in some cases	Vomiting, failure to thrive, de-hydration and hypotonia. Complete recovery following treatment usual. ? Failure in maturation of tubular function
	ii) Late form	Autosomal dominant with increased penetration in females	As in (i) Increased potassium loss in urine may occur	May be cortical scarring and urolithiasis	More serious disorder than (i). May develop periodic paralysis, rickets, and renal stones

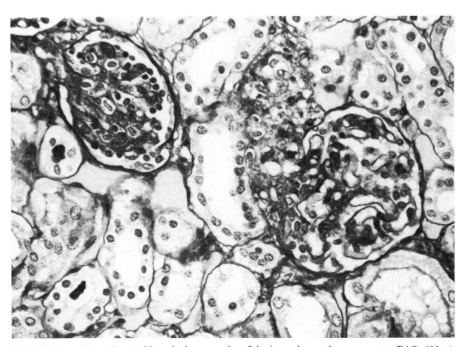

Fig. 9.29. Bartter's syndrome. Note the hypertrophy of the juxtaglomerular apparatus. (PAS; 400 ×)

loss. However, total adrenalectomy fails to correct the potassium wastage. More recently it has been suggested that there is a defect in sodium reabsorption in the proximal tubule (Cannon et al. 1968), so that the macula densa is presented with a urine that is hyperosmolar with respect to sodium, thus stimulating the JGA. The absence of hypertension and the lack of response to exogenous angiotensin have not been satisfactorily explained.

9. Renal Tumours

Malignant nephroblastoma (Wilm's tumour), which is described in Chap. 15, is the commonest solid (i.e., nonleukaemic) malignant tumour outside the central nervous system occurring in the paediatric age group. Other renal tumours and hamartomas are rare and a description of the more important entities is included in this section.

9.1. Benign Tumours and Hamartomas

9.1.1. Congenital Mesoblastic Nephroma

Congenital mesoblastic nephroma, usually recognized clinically in the neonatal period or in early infancy, has only recently been separated from nephroblastoma (Bolande et al. 1967). This distinction is important, since the majority of congenital mesoblastic nephromas reported have behaved as benign neoplasms cured by surgery. The previous confusion of these tumours with Wilm's tumour

probably accounts, at least in part, for the unexpectedly good prognosis in some series of malignant nephroblastomas diagnosed during the first year of life. In addition, the vigorous treatment consisting in surgery followed by radiotherapy and chemotherapy carries an appreciable morbidity and mortality, particularly in very young children, and though necessary for Wilm's tumour it is inappropriate for congenital mesoblastic nephroma (Hilton and Keeling 1973).

Macroscopically the congenital mesoblastic nephroma is a bulky, usually spherical tumour mass up to about 5 cm in diameter, replacing part of the kidney from which it appears fairly well demarcated. The surface is smooth and covered by the expanded renal capsule. The cut surface presents a white, whorled appearance very like that of a myometrial fibroid.

Microscopically, the tumour is composed of interlacing bands of closely packed spindle cells with eosinophilic cytoplasm and round or oval vesicular nuclei. A characteristic finding is the presence of foci of glomeruli and tubules throughout the tumour (Fig. 9.30). These often have a rather immature appearance and appear to represent normal nephronic structures trapped within the expanding tumour. The margin of the neoplasm extends to incorporate parenchymous elements adjacent to it and the tumour is not encapsulated. Within the tumour mass mitotic figures may be frequent, although this is not an indication of malignant transformation. These lesions are generally regarded as hamartomatous developmental anomalies (Kay et al. 1966). The cell of origin is uncertain and ultrastructural studies have identified cells which have been regarded as of smooth muscle origin and as undifferentiated mesenchyme.

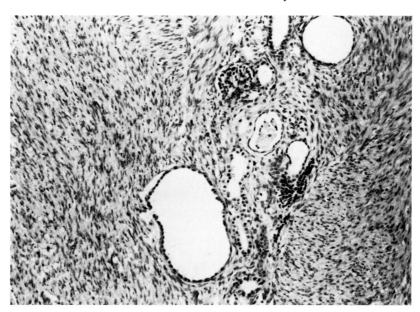

Fig. 9.30. Congenital mesoblastic nephroma. Interlacing sheets of spinde-shaped cells with entrapped glomerular and tubular structures. (H and E; 80×)

9.1.2. Angiomyolipoma

Angiomyolipomas are hamartomatous lesions that can be single or multiple and occur in the renal cortex, usually immediately beneath the renal capsule. They are rounded, sharply circumscribed but unencapsulated swellings often forming nodular projections from the renal surface. They are usually only 2–3 cm in diameter or less, but occasional larger lesions have been described (Moolten 1942).

Microscopically they consist of a disorderly arrangement of smooth muscle cells, abnormal thick-walled blood vessels, and adipose tissue, in varying proportions. A few renal parenchymal elements may be incorporated at the margins of the lesion.

Their importance lies in their frequent association with tuberous sclerosis, particularly when they are multiple, and they are usually regarded as part of the tuberous sclerosis complex. About 80 % of patients with tuberous sclerosis have renal tumours, and about 50 % of patients with renal angiolipomas have other stigmata of tuberous sclerosis.

Another renal cortical hamartoma consisting of nodular collections of cells with abundant eosinophilic cytoplasm resembling enlarged renal tubular epithelial cells is also occasionally encountered in tuberous sclerosis, and very rarely with other phakomatoses. A feature of this lesion is that the centres of the nodules sometimes break down to give a pseudocystic appearance.

9.2. Other Primary Renal Tumours

Renal cortical adenomas similar to those seen in adults occur in children but are extremely rare.

Connective-tissue tumours such as haemangiomas, lipomas, liposarcomas, leiomyomas, osteomas, and chondromas occurring in or adjacent to the kidney have been described in children but are also rare. Benign teratomas have also been described in the kidney (Walker 1897), but need to be distinguished carefully from retroperitoneal teratomas, which merely compress the adjacent kidney.

Although Wilm's tumour is by far the most important malignant renal tumour occurring in children, renal cell carcinomas also occur very occasionally in this age group. In 1961 Scruggs and Ainsworth collected 51 reports of renal cell carcinoma in children. These tumours have the same histological appearances as and behave in a similar fashion to those in adults.

Recently Marsden and Lawler (1978) have described a malignant renal tumour of childhood which, although macroscopically similar to nephroblastoma, can be distinguished by its microscopi-

cal appearance. It consists of pale round, spindle, or stellate cells with round or oval nuclei showing a delicate chromatin pattern. These have a 'packeted' arrangement separated by fibrovascular septa (Fig. 9.31). The densely cellular darkly staining 'blastema' of Wilm's tumour is lacking. Marsden and Lawler describe 15 such tumours occurring in children aged between 18 months and 10½ years. Of the 15 tumours, 13 were in boys. There was a high incidence (9/15 cases) of bone metastases, which are a very rare feature of nephroblastoma.

9.3. Metastic Tumours

The most frequent metastatic involvement of the kidney during childhood occurs in leukaemia. The kidneys are often diffusely enlarged, producing easily palpable bilateral loin masses. Renal function is rarely impaired even with massive involvement, but leukaemic cells may be demonstrated in the urine deposit.

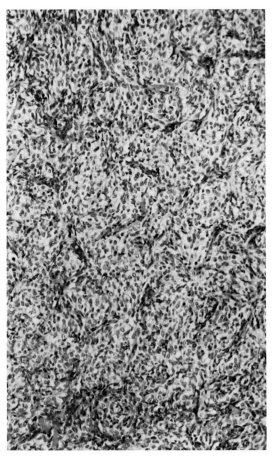

Fig. 9.31. Bone-metastasizing renal tumour. Note the packeted appearance of the tumour cells and the prominent vascular stroma. (H and E; 80 ×)

10. Renal Pelvis, Ureter, Bladder, and Urethra — Embryology

The ureter and renal pelvis develop from the metanephric duct, itself formed as an off-shoot with a cranial course from the lower end of the mesonephric (Wolffian) duct. The ureter is formed by the caudal (unbranched) portion of the metanephric duct, whilst the renal pelvis and calyces are derived by coalescence of the first generations of dichotomous divisions of its cranial portion, which occur when the advancing tip impinges on the metanephric blastema (see p. 395).

Distally, the metanephric duct joins with the terminal portion of the mesonephric duct to form a short common excretory duct that drains into the cloaca. The cloaca is continuous with three endodermal tubes — the hind gut, the allantois, and the blind-ending diverticulum of the tail gut; it is marked externally by a shallow depression covered by the cloacal membrane. At about the 5-mm stage, a septum (the urogenital septum) develops above, in the angle between the allantois and the hind-gut. This septum gradually extends caudally until it reaches and fuses with the cloacal membrane at about the 16-mm stage. The cloaca is thus divided into a smaller dorsal portion (the primitive rectum) and a larger ventral part (the primitive urogenital sinus).

The common excretory ducts from each side join the urogenital sinus, dividing it into an upper portion above the ducts (the vesicourethral canal from which the bladder and upper urethra develop) and a lower portion below the ducts (the definitive urogenital sinus).

The vesicourethral canal is an elongated cylinder, slightly flattened dorsoventrally, which is continuous cranially with the allantois. With the growth of the anterior abdominal wall below the umbilicus, the bladder segment of the vesicourethral canal enlarges and the definitive urogenital sinus becomes flattened from side to side and elongated dorsoventrally.

Probably as a result of dilatation of the common excretory duct and its subsequent absorption into the wall of the vesicourethral canal, the mesonephric and metanephric ducts come to drain separately into the vesicourethral canal. With further development, the ureteric orifices move progressively cranially and laterally in relation to the mesonephric duct openings, which remain close together near the mid-line. In the male the mesonephric duct persists as the epididymis, vas deferens, seminal vesicle, and common ejaculatory duct. In the female the mesonephric duct degenerates, starting at about the 30-mm stage, and apart from the vesitigial epo-

ophoron and Gärtner's ducts, disappears. The triangular zone between the ureteric orifices and the mesonephric duct openings forms the trigone of the bladder. Unlike the rest of the bladder, which is an endodermal structure, the trigone is a mesodermal derivative. The upper part of the bladder is continuous with the allantois, which regresses early and is replaced by a solid fibrous cord (the urachus).

In the female, the primitive urethra, which is derived from the lower part of the vesicourethral canal, forms almost all the definitive urethra. In the male, however, the primitive urethra forms only the upper part of the prostatic urethra. The lower portion of the prostatic urethra and the membranous urethra are derived from the upper (pelvic) portion of the urogenital sinus. The penile urethra is formed by fusion of the urethral folds on each side of the ventral surface of the developing phallus. The groove between these folds (the urethral groove) is formed by a plate of cells (the urethral plate), which extends from the lower (phallic) portion of the urogenital sinus. Fusion of the urethral folds in the mid-line occurs from behind forwards, and posteriorly it is marked externally by the median raphe. This process of fusion extends distally only as far as the circular coronary sulcus, which delineates the glans penis. A cord of ectodermal epithelial cells grows through the glands to reach the distal closed tip of the urethra. This later becomes canalized and its lumen becomes continuous with that of the urethra, thus forming its terminal (glandular) portion and the urethral meatus.

The prostate gland in the male develops at about the 55-mm stage as a series of buds from the primitive urethra and from the adjacent upper portion of the urogenital sinus.

11. Renal Pelvis and Ureter

11.1. Congenital Abnormalities

11.1.1. Duplications

Duplications of the renal pelvis and ureter are common, some degree of pelviureteric duplication being present in about 5% of unselected necropsies. The extent of duplication varies from a mere bifurcation of the extrarenal portion of the renal pelvis draining into a single ureter to complete duplication of the whole system, with separate lower ureteral openings into the bladder. Females are more commonly affected than males. Rare instances of triplication or even quadruplication of the ureters occur. The usual type of duplication is the conjoint ureter (Stephens 1956), in which the upper part of the ureter is divided, the two arms joining to form a single lower ureter that drains normally into the trigone of the bladder. In the great majority of cases the upper system is the smaller, the majority of the renal calyces draining into the lower system. In a small minority of instances (less than 1%), and usually with complete duplications, the ureter is ectopic (see below).

Only 20% of duplications are bilateral. Clinically the condition is usually entirely asymptomatic, but in rare cases obstruction occurs, usually owing to stenosis of the upper system in conjoint ureters. Complicating hydronephrosis or urinary infection may bring the condition to light.

11.1.2. Ureteral Ectopia

An ectopic ureter drains to a site other than the trigone of the bladder. In females an ectopic ureter may open into the urethra, the vagina, or the rectum. In males it may drain into the urethra, the seminal vesicle, or the rectum. In females ureteral ectopia is usually associated with dribbling incontinence of urine. In males, when the ectopic ureter drains into the urethra or seminal vesicle urinary continence is unaffected, since the insertion of the ureter is almost always above the venumontanum and contraction of the urethral sphincter prevents incontinence.

11.1.3. Ureterocele

A ureterocele is a saccular expansion of the lower end of the ureter about its orifice, involving the intramural segment in the bladder wall and the submucosal portion that extends beneath the bladder mucosa immediately above the orifice. Ureteroceles are usually associated with upper tract obstruction and hydronephrosis. Radiologically, the kidney drained by a ureter with a ureterocele may not excrete contrast medium, but the diagnosis can be made by the presence of a globular filling defect in the bladder caused by the ureterocele. Sometimes the ureterocele obstructs the bladder neck and causes bilateral hydronephrosis.

Ureteroceles may occur with a normally sited ureteric orifice, but are more commonly associated with ureteral ectopia and ureteral duplication. The term 'ectopic ureterocele' (Berdon et al. 1968) is usually applied to a complex anomaly, which consists of a duplex kidney with two separate ureters. The ureter draining the lower part of the double kidney is inserted normally in the trigone of the bladder. The ureter draining the upper pole is inserted ectopically and is associated with a ureterocele. The insertion is below and medial to that of the lower pole ureter, usually into the upper urethra.

The ectopic ureter is dilated and tortuous as a result of obstruction, and the upper pole of the kidney, apart from showing changes secondary to obstruction, is very commonly dysplastic (see p. 403). Ectopic ureterocele is much commoner in females. There is often duplication of the contralateral ureter, but this is usually of the conjoint type, and the full ectopic ureterocele is only rarely bilateral. Symptoms are variable. Recurrent urinary infection is the usual presentation but in girls there may be dribbling incontinence; occasionally the ureterocele prolapses into the urethra and may be visible externally. Surgical excision of the ectopic ureter, ureterocele, and upper pole of the kidney usually gives excellent results.

11.2. Vesicoureteric Reflux

The importance of vesicoureteric reflux in the pathogenesis of pyelonephritis and renal scarring is well recognized and has already been discussed (see p. 429). The clinical aspects of this complication, and the other consequences of vesicoureteric reflux in childhood, for example its possible effects on renal growth, have led to considerable controversy regarding appropriate management. These topics are expertly discussed by Ransley (1978).

Vesicoureteric reflux (VUR) does not occur under normal conditions. An abnormality of the vesicoureteric junction producing reflux may be isolated ('primary' reflux) or may occur in association with other abnormalities, such as posterior urethral valves, ureteral duplication, or a neuropathic bladder ('secondary' reflux). There is a tendency for primary VUR to disappear as the affected child grows, a change most marked in children with milder degrees of reflux (assessed by the degree of ureteral dilatation on micturating cystography), 80% of whom eventually stop refluxing spontaneously.

The abnormality of the vesicoureteric junction associated with VUR may often be recognizable on cystoscopy, particularly when the degree of reflux is gross. The ureteric orifice appears as a rounded hole ('golf-hole' orifice) rather than the normal semilunar slit. Direct inspection is not a reliable method of diagnosing or assessing VUR; however, this is usually done radiologically by micturating cystography.

The great majority of children with VUR present as a result of urinary infection. Conversely, about 50% of infants, and about 30% of older children with urinary tract infections, can be shown to have VUR (Shannon 1970). In a proportion of cases, particularly of those considered to have gross reflux judged by the degree of upper tract dilatation on micturating cystography, the kidney may be dysplastic. This has led to the suggestion of a developmental abnormality in cases involving the whole upper tract (Bialestock 1966). It is of interest that some infants with renal dysplasia and VUR also have an abnormal urethra with a smooth, symmetrical narrowing at the level of the external sphincter. The consequent urinary obstruction is freely communicated to the upper tract, which acts like a bladder diverticulum. It can be assumed that this process occurs in utero and probably accounts for the dysplastic renal development (Beck 1971).

Although VUR is relatively uncommon, affecting less than 0.5% of the general population, there is a much higher incidence of between 8% and 26% in families where one member is known to be affected (Bredin et al. 1975; Dwoskin 1976; de Vargas et al. 1977). This suggests that screening for VUR, which is impractical on a population basis, would be of value in affected families.

11.3. Retrocaval Ureter

In the rare anomaly of retrocaval ureter the upper ureter passes behind the inferior vena cava and descends into the pelvis medial to it. The malformation results from the formation of the distal inferior vena cava from the lateral cardinal veins rather than from the posterior cardinal veins, which is the normal pattern. Incomplete obstruction of the ureter results from its retrocaval course.

11.4. Hydronephrosis

The term 'hydronephrosis' describes a dilatation of the renal pelvis and calyces and the secondary effects on the renal parenchyma. The usual cause is a localized narrowing in the ureter, most commonly at the pelviureteric junction. Stenosis may also occur at the vesicoureteric junction and less commonly, elsewhere in the ureter. Such ureteral narrowings may be congenital or acquired defects. Rarer causes of hydronephrosis in infancy and childhood include anomalous inferior polar renal arteries (White and Wyatt 1942) and ureteral valves (Wall and Wachter 1952).

The degree of upper tract dilatation and renal parenchymal atrophy depends partly on the degree of stenosis and partly on the duration of obstruction. Macroscopic changes in the kidney include blunting of the renal papillae and parenchymal thinning. Microscopically there is dilatation of collecting ducts, which run tangentially rather than radially in the medulla, and varying degrees of tubular atrophy and interstitial fibrosis. Atrophy is most marked in the medulla rather than the renal cortex, except in extreme examples, when the whole parenchyma is reduced to a thin rim composed largely of fibrous tissue surrounding the grossly dilated collecting system. Renal infection and stone formation are common complications, particularly in cases of long standing.

12. Bladder

12.1. Congenital Abnormalities

12.1.1. Agenesis

Absence of the bladder is an extremely rare anomaly; it is usually associated with other severe congenital abnormalities and is generally found in stillborn infants. Glenn (1959) described a case of bladder agenesis in a 3–year-old girl and collected less than ten previously reported cases. As in Miller's case (Miller 1948), also a girl, the urethra was blind and the ureters were inserted into the vagina. Lepoutre (1939) reported a male child with absence of the bladder, in whom the ureters were inserted into the rectum.

12.1.2. Urachal Anomalies

During embryonic life the urachus extends from the umbilicus to the dome of the bladder. Persistence of the urachus results in a fistula opening at the umbilicus. Partial persistence results in a urachal diverticulum, which is usually asymptomatic but may be associated with stone formation (Dreyfuss and Fliess 1941).

Occasionally the mid-part of the urachus persists, with obliteration of the two ends to produce a urachal cyst, which may occasionally become infected.

12.1.3. Duplications

A review of bladder duplication has been made by Abrahamson (1961).

Duplications of the bladder may be classified as complete or incomplete. In complete duplication two separate bladders lie side by side in a common adventitial sheath. Each bladder has a separate urethra with a separate external meatus. Duplication of the hind-gut is almost always present, and a rectourethral fistula involving one side is present in over half the reported cases. Other associated rectal and genital anomalies are common.

In incomplete duplication there are two bladders side by side. These are joined at the base and have a single urethra and external meatus.

12.1.4. Septation

When a *complete saggital septum* is present the bladder appears either normal or bilobed from the outside. The complete saggital septum is found on opening the bladder. If a ureter drains into the obstructed side hydronephrosis is present on that side. Sometimes the obstructed half may also obstruct the half draining into the urethra, and bilateral hydronephrosis then results.

If the *saggital septum* is *incomplete* no obstruction occurs, but other anomalies frequently co-exist.

In the presence of an *incomplete frontal septum* the bladder is incompletely divided into anterior and posterior cavities by a septum.

Kohler (1940) described a case of *multiseptate bladder* with complete obstruction of both upper tracts in an infant dying in uraemia.

In the *hourglass bladder* the shape probably reflects a partial persistence of the urachus.

12.2. Extrophy

Bladder extrophy is the commonest manifestation of a series of congenital abnormalities resulting from a failure of mid-line fusion of the mesodermal elements in the anterior abdominal wall below the umbilicus, involving the anterior wall of the bladder and urethra, the genital tubercle, and the pubis. This spectrum of anomalies ranges from minor degrees of epispadias, involving the penis with exposure of the terminal urethra, to a gross abnormality where there is ectopia vesicae and vesico–intestinal fistula and where gross bowel anomalies accompany the bladder lesion.

In bladder extrophy the infraumbilical abdominal wall is shortened and a mid-line defect is present. The size of this varies from a small hole through which the bladder trigone protrudes on straining to an extensive defect through which the entire posterior wall of the bladder protrudes. Some degree of diastasis of the pubis and epispadias are invariably present.

Secondary changes (squamous metaplasia, cystitis cystica, cystitis glandularis) invariably occur in the exposed bladder mucosa, and squamous or adenocarcinoma may develop in patients who survive childhood. Vesicoureteric reflux is common in patients with extrophy of the bladder following surgical reconstruction.

12.3. Diverticula

Bladder diverticula appear as herniations of the bladder mucosa through the detrusor muscle and generally occur at a weak point 1–2 cm behind and lateral to the ureteric orifice. In children they are usually small and single, but larger examples may cause ureteric obstruction. Focal cystitis and stone formation are commoner complications (Forsythe and Smyth 1959).

12.4. Outflow Obstruction (Marion's Disease)

Obstruction of the bladder outflow may have mechanical causes, such as posterior urethral valves, congenital urethral stenosis, and ectopic ureterocele, or may be associated with a neurogenic bladder. When such obvious causes are excluded, many cases remain in which difficulty in voiding, incontinence, and recurrent urinary infection are associated with hypertrophy and trabeculation of the bladder. Vesicoureteric reflux can often be demonstrated radiologically, and progressive dilatation of the bladder and ureters may develop (megacystic–megaureter). Ureteric peristalsis can be demonstrated at first, but with increasing dilatation this may fail and gross hydronephrosis with abundant residual urine results. The underlying cause is obscure. Early reports (Andreassen 1953) suggested deficiencies in the autonomic innervation of the bladder, analogous to Hirschsprung's disease of the intestine, but other authors (Winkelman 1967) describe a normal bladder innervation. Bodian (1957) performed extensive histological studies of the bladder neck and urethra in a number of these patients, and demonstrated elongation of the prostatic urethra with increased amounts of fibroelastic tissue in the submucosa of the bladder neck. Urethral fibroelastosis is accepted as a cause of bladder outflow obstruction in some cases, but it is likely that other lesions are also responsible, and it must be admitted that their pathology has been inadequately studied.

12.5. Tumours

Benign bladder tumours are rare in children. Neurofibromas, usually multiple, may occur as an isolated lesion or as part of generalized neurofibromatosis (von Recklinghausen's disease). Haemangiomas and leiomyomas (Williams and Schistad (1961) also occur.

The most frequent bladder tumour in childhood is the embryonal rhabdomyosarcoma. Macroscopically this consists of a translucent, grape-like, lobulated mass, which partially or almost completely fills the bladder (sarcoma botryoides) and often originates from the region of the trigone. The tumour often extends to involve the urethra and the

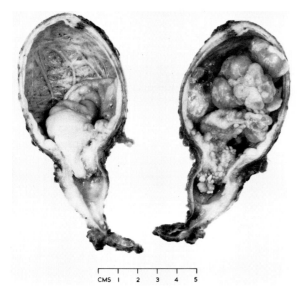

Fig. 9.32. Embryonal rhabdomyosarcoma of the bladder.

lower ureters, which may become obstructed. Embryonal rhabdomyosarcoma of the bladder usually presents in the first few years of life and is commoner in boys. Histologically the tumour is composed of small spindle cells with hyperchromatic nuclei, set in an often abundant myxoid stroma (Fig. 9.32). Cellular pleomorphism is seldom marked and the overlying epithelium is usually intact. These features, particularly in a small biopsy specimen, may give rise to a misleadingly benign appearance. Characteristic strap cells with cross-striated cytoplasm may be found if searched for carefully, and these help to establish the diagnosis. These tumours are aggressive and invade locally. Local excision results in prompt recurrence, but radical surgery may be curative in up to 30% of patients (Williams and Schistad 1964) (see also p. 657).

Epithelial bladder tumours (transitional cell carcinomas) are extremely rare, but have been reported in children (Waller and Roll 1957).

13. Urethra

13.1. Congenital Abnormalities

13.1.1 Atresia

Urethral atresia is a very rare anomaly, usually occurring at the level of the membranous urethra. Drainage of the bladder may be effected via a co-existing rectourethral or urachal fistula. In some cases there is a concomitant prune belly syndrome (congenital absence of the anterior abdominal wall muscles), and rectal agenesis may also co-exist.

13.1.2. Duplication

Complete duplications of the urethra are usually found in association with complete duplication of the bladder or diaphallus. Occasionally, in males, the urethra divides and has one normally situated urethral meatus and a second meatus opening at the perineum.

13.1.3. Valves and Strictures

Congenital urethral stenosis may result from strictures resulting from faulty coaptation of the genital tubercles (in males) or from membranous mucosal diaphragms; in either case they can be single or multiple. Meatal stenosis is the most common variety.

Urethral valves in infant boys are the commonest cause of congenital urethral obstruction. These are usually situated in the posterior urethra, and the three varieties described by Young and McKay (1929) are shown diagrammatically (see Fig. 9.33).

Acquired strictures of the posterior urethra are almost always the result of urethral rupture following fracture of the pelvis.

13.2. Diverticula

Urethral diverticula are rare, and most occur in males.

14. Disorders of Differentiation of the Genital Tract

This account presents a simplified view of anomalies of genital tract differentiation. They are sometimes extremely complex, and for a more extensive review and bibliography the texts of Shapiro (1977) and Warkany (1971) should be consulted.

14.1. Anomalies of Genetic Origin

Alterations in the sex chromosomes may be transmitted by one parent (gonadal dysgenesis) or may occur in the embryo although the initial stages of fertilization were normal (true hermaphroditism).

Gonadal dysgenesis results from nondisjunction of the sex chromosomes during gametogenesis, and may result in Klinefelter's syndrome (XXY) or Turner's syndrome (XO) with ovarian agenesis, or other genetically complex anomalies. True hermaphroditism is associated with failure of disjunc-

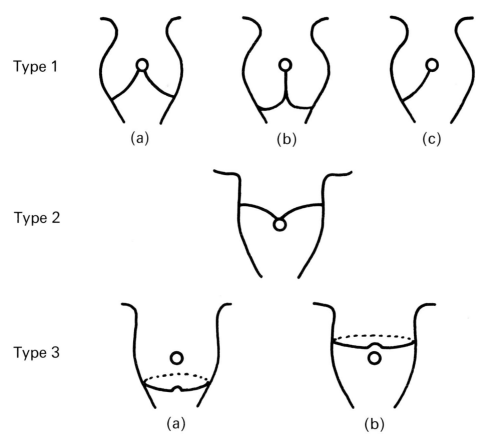

Type 1

(a)   (b)   (c)

Type 2

Type 3

(a)   (b)

Fig. 9.33. Congenital urethral valves. After Young and McKay 1929.

tion of sex chromosomes during the first cleavage mitoses of the egg, leading to XY/XX or XY/XO mosaicism. The relative proportions of the components of the mosaic greatly affect the phenotypic expression of the anomaly.

14.2. Sexual Anomalies of Hormonal Origin

Hormone-conditioned sexual anomalies in individuals with normal genetic constitution. Primary and secondary characteristics may be ambiguous, depending on the degree of exposure to endogenous or exogenous androgen.

14.2.1. Male Pseudohermaphroditism

In a normal XY male pseudohermaphroditism may occur because of deficient androgen production. The abnormalities produced will depend on the stage of development at which the deficiency becomes manifest; in the later stages a small penis, hypo-

spadias, and vulviform appearance of the scrotum may be evident, but severe deficiency in early stages may permit the persistence of a Müllerian system; in this case a vagina and uterus co-exist with normal vasa deferentia. The external genitalia are female and the testes ectopic.

14.2.2. Female Pseudohermaphroditism

Virilization of a femal fetus with normal ovaries and an XX karyotype results in female pseudohermaphroditism. Changes may be caused by androgen production by the fetal adrenal, or by administration of progestagens or anabolic steroids with androgenic effects.

The Müllerian system develops normally, but the Wolffian system, which would normally involute in the female, persists to varying degrees owing to the influence of androgen, which also causes changes in the external genitalia, with clitoral hypertrophy, a tendency to closure of the urogenital sinus, and fusion of the labia majora.

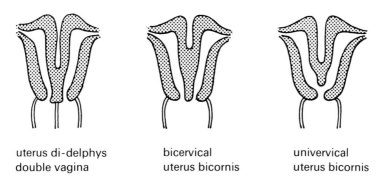

(a) Partial or complete fusion of lower part of Müllerian ducts

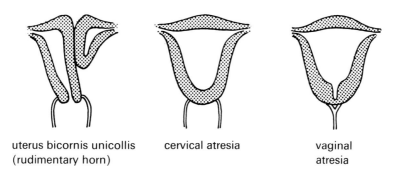

(b) Partial or total atresia of the lower part of one or both Müllerian ducts

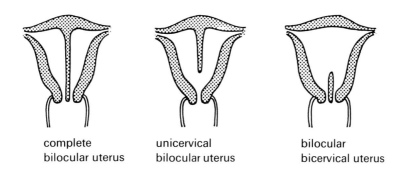

(c) Persistant utero-vaginal septum after fusion of Müllerian ducts

Fig. 9.34. Abnormalities of Müllerian development. After Tuchman-Duplessis and Haegel 1974.

14.3. Malformations of the Uterus and Vagina

In uterine and vaginal malformations the Müllerian system develops as bilaterally symmetrical elements that fuse in their lower parts, giving rise to the upper part of the vagina, the cervix uteri and body of the uterus, and the Fallopian tubes. Various abnormalities of fusion occur, and atresia of all or part of the primordia may also occur (see Fig. 9.34).

14.4. Morphological Abnormalities of the Male Genital Tract

14.4.1. Penis

Absence of the penis is usually associated with complex urogenital malformations (Campbell 1951). Duplication of the penis is extremely rare and is also associated with other anomalies. In the severe forms of anorectal agenesis abnormalities of the genitalia are common (see p. 252).

Failure of fusion of the urogenital groove at around the 11th or 12th week of gestation results in the production of hypospadias, which may be balanic (simple ectopia of the urethral meatus) penile–scrotal (where the urethra opens on the shaft of the penis or scrotum), or perineal. In these severe forms there is an associated abnormality of the scrotal swellings, which coalesce giving rise to a vulviform appearance, and the penis is usually small.

14.4.2. Testes

14.4.2.1. Absence.
Absence of the testis, unilateral or bilateral, may accompany renal agenesis, but is extremely rare as an isolated abnormality. There are less than 100 reports in the literature, most of which were published more than 40 years ago and are not accompanied by chromosome studies. Supernumerary and fused testes are also very rare.

14.4.2.2. Incomplete Descent.
Incomplete descent of the testis is a manifestation of imperfect coordination of the development of the posterior abdominal wall and the various derivatives of the meso- and metanephros. The elongation of the parietes and the active descent of the testis and appendages becomes asynchronous, and although hormonal mechanisms are known to be involved (pituitary gonardotrophins have a significant effect), their precise role is far from clear. The testis normally reaches the orifice of the inguinal canal by the 6th month, descends through it during the 7th, and reaches its definitive intrascrotal position towards the end of the 8th month.

The undescended testis may be in the inguinal canal (80%) or in an intra-abdominal situation (20%). Occasionally a presumed intra-abdominal testis is absent. Nondescent is commoner on the right but can be bilateral. An ipsilateral inguinal hernia is found in most instances.

Histological changes have been described by Farrington (1969). The normal sequence of events in testicular development, with a static phase (0–4 years), a growth phase (4–10 years), and maturation (10 years to puberty) is not well defined in undescended testes, which have fewer germinal cells by the time the age of 6 years is reached, although the tubules may continue to grow normally. Interstitial fibrosis may also occur, with peritubular hyalinization in the older testis.

There are a number of possible complications of cryptorchidism. The inguinal testis is more susceptible to trauma, the intra-abdominal testis to torsion. Fertility may be impaired, and bilaterally cryptorchid males are likely to be sterile if orchiopexy is delayed. Secondary sexual characteristics develop normally. Cryptorchidism is undoubtedly associated with neoplasia, and although estimates vary widely, risks between 15 and 40 times the normal risk are given. There is no evidence to suggest that this risk is modified by ochiopexy, however early this is performed, but earlier diagnosis is practicable with an intrascrotal testis. The subject is discussed in detail by Whitaker (1976).

14.4.2.3. Ectopic Testis.
Ectopic testes do not follow the normal course of testicular descent. The classification of Wattenberg et al. (1949) is generally used. The testis may be:

a) Superficial, inguinal, or interstitial, i.e., lodged superficially in the inguinal region or at the base of the scrotum;

b) Pubopenile, i.e., lodged at the base of the penis;

c) Femoral, i.e., lodged subcutaneously in the superomedial aspect of the thigh;

d) Transverse, i.e., lodged high in the scrotum but lying transversely;

e) Perineal, i.e., posterior to the scrotum in the subcutaneous tissue (Wattenberg et al. 1949).

References

Abrahamson J (1961) Double bladder and related anomalies, clinical and embryologic aspects and a case report. Br J Urol 33: 195

Allen DM, Diamond LK, Howell DA (1960) Anaphylactoid purpura in children (Schönlein–Henoch syndrome): Review with a follow-up of the renal complications. Am J Dis Child 99: 833

Alport AC (1927) Hereditary familial congenital haemorrhagic nephritis. Br Med J i: 504

Andreassen M (1953) Vesical neck obstruction in children. Acta Chir Scand 105: 398

Anthony BF, Kaplan EL, Chapman SS, Oyie PG, Wannamaker LW (1967) Epidemic acute nephritis with reappearance of type-49 streptococcus. Lancet 2: 787

Ask-Upmark E (1929) Über juvenile maligne Nephrosklerose und ihr Verhältnis zu Störungen in der Nierenentwicklung. Acta Pathol Microbiol Scand 6: 383

Atkins RC, Holdsworth SR, Glasgow EF, Matthews EF (1976) The macrophage in human rapidly progressive glomerulonephritis. Lancet 1: 830

Bailey RR (1973) The relationship of vesico-ureteric reflux to urinary tract infection and chronic pyelonephritis—reflux nephropathy. Clin Nephrol 1: 132

Bailey RR (1977) The relationship of vesico-ureteric reflux. (Letter) Arch Dis Child 52: 804

Balodimos MC, Legg MA, Bradley RF (1971) Diabetic glomerulosclerosis in children. Diabetes 20: 622

Barratt TM, Soothill JF (1970) Controlled train of cyclophosphamide in steroid-sensitive relapsing nephrotic syndrome of childhood. Lancet 2: 479

Barrington FJF, Wright HD (1930) Bacteraemia following operations on the urethra. J Pathol Bacteriol 33: 871

Bartter FC, Pronove P, Gill JR Jr, MacCardle RC (1962) Hyperplasia of the juxtaglomerular complex with hyperaldosteronism and hypokalemic alkalosis: A new syndrome. Am J Med 33: 811

Baxter TJ (1961) Morphogenesis of renal cysts. Am J Pathol 38: 721

Beck AD (1971) Effects of intra-uterine obstruction upon the development of the fetal kidney. J Urol 105: 784

Belman AB, Kropp KA, Simon NM (1968) Renal-pressor hypertension secondary to unilateral hydronephrosis. N Engl J Med 278: 1133

Berdon WE, Baker DH, Becker JA, Uson AC (1968) Ectopic ureterocele. Radiol Clin North Am 6: 205

Beresford SAA, Holland WW (1973) Levels of blood pressure in children: a familial study. Proc R Soc Med 66: 1009

Berger J (1969) IgA glomerular deposits in renal disease. Transplant Proc 1: 939

Berger J, Galle P (1963) Deposits denses au sein des membranes basales du rein. Presse Med 49: 2351

Bernstein J (1968) Developmental abnormalities of the renal parenchyma—renal hypoplasia and dysplasia. Pathol Annu 3: 213

Bernstein J (1971) Heritable cystic disorders of the kidney. Pediatr Clin North Am 18: 435

Bernstein J, Meyer R (1964) Some speculations on the nature and significance of developmentally small kidneys (renal hypoplasia). Nephron 1: 137

Bernstein J, Meyer R (1972) Parenchymal maldevelopment of the kidney. In: Kelley V (ed) Brennemann's practice of pediatrics, vol 3, chap 26. Harper & Row, Hagerstown

Berry CL (1978) Hypertension and arterial development: long-term considerations. Br Heart J 40: 709

Betts PR, Forrest-Hay I (1973) Juvenile nephronophthisis. Lancet 2: 475

Bhathena DB, Weiss JH, Holland NH, McMorrow RG, Curtis JJ, Lucas BA, Luke RC (1979) Focal and segmental glomerulo-sclerosis in reflux nephropathy (chronic pyelonephritis). Am J Med 63: 886

Bialestock D (1965) Studies of renal malformations and pyelonephritis in children, with and without associated vesico-ureteral reflux and obstruction. Aust NZ J Surg 35: 120

Bigler JA, Killingworth WP (1949) Cartilage in the kidney. Arch Pathol 47: 487

Blyth H, Ockendon BG (1971) Polycystic disease of the kidneys and liver presenting in childhood. J Med Genet 8: 257

Bodian M (1957) Some observations on the pathology of congenital 'idiopathic bladder-neck obstruction' (Marion's disease). Br J Urol 29: 393

Boichis H, Passwell J, David R, Miller H (1973) Congenital hepatic fibrosis and nephronophthisis. A family study. Q J Med 165: 221

Bolande RP, Brough AJ, Izant RJ (1967) Congenital mesoblastic nephroma of infancy. Pediatrics 40: 272

Brain MC (1969) The haemolytic uraemic syndrome. Semin Hematol 6: 162

Bredin HC, Winchester P, McGovern JH, Degnan M (1975) Family study of vesico-ureteral reflux. J Urol 113: 623

Burk D, Beaudoin AR (1977) Arsenate-induced renal agenesis in rats. Teratology 16: 247

Cameron JS, White RHR (1965) Selectivity of proteinuria in children with the nephrotic syndrome. Lancet 1: 463

Campbell MF (1951) Clinical pediatric urology. Saunders, Philadelphia, p 698

Cannon PJ, Leeming JM, Sommers SC, Winters BW, Laragh JH (1968) Juxtaglomerular cell hyperplasia and secondary aldosteronism (Bartter's syndrome): A re-evaluation of the patholophysiology. Medicine 47: 107

Chrispin AR (1972) Medullary necrosis in infancy. Br Med Bull 18: 233

Churg J, Habib R, White RHR (1970) Pathology of the nephrotic syndrome in children: A report for the International Study of Kidney Disease in Children. Lancet 1: 1299

Coppoletta JM, Wolbach SB (1933) Body length and organ weights of infants and children: Study of body length and normal weights of more important organs of the body between birth and 12 years of age. Am J Pathol 9: 55

Cotran RS (1969) The renal lesion in chronic pyelonephritis: Immunofluorescence and ultrastructural studies. J Infect Dis 120: 109

Counahan R, Simmons MJ, Charlwood GJ (1976) Multifocal osteolysis with nephropathy. Arch Dis Child 51: 717

Courtecuisse V, Habib R, Monnier C (1967) Non-lethal hemolytic and uremic syndromes in children. An electron microscope study of renal biopsies from six cases. Exp Mol Pathol 7: 327

Darmady EM, Offer J, Woodhouse MA (1970) Toxic metabolic defect in polycystic disease of the kidney. Evidence from microscopic studies. Lancet 1: 547

Delaney V, Mullaney J, Bourke E (1978) Juvenile nephron-ophthisis congenital hepatic fibrosis and retinal hypoplasia in twins. Q J Med 186: 281

De Navasquez S (1956) Further studies in experimental pyelo-nephritis produced by various bacteria with special reference to renal scarring as a factor in pathogenesis. J Pathol 71: 27

de Vargas A, Rosenberg A, Barratt TM, Ransley PG, Williams DI, Carter CO (1978) Vesico-ureteric reflux—a family study. J Clin Genet 15: 85

Dixon FJ (1961) Experimental glomerulonephritis. The pathogenesis of a laboratory model resembling the spectrum of human glomerulonephritis. J Exp Med 113: 899

Dixon FJ (1968) The pathogenesis of glomerulonephritis. Am J Med 44: 493

Dreyfuss ML, Fliess M (1941) Patient urachus with stone formation. J Urol 46: 77

Dunn JS (1934) Nephrosis or nephritis? J Pathol Bacteriol 39: 1

Dunnill MS, Millard PR, Oliver D (1977) Acquired cystic disease of the kidneys: A hazard of long-term intermittent maintenance haemodialysis. J Clin Pathol 30: 868

Dwoskin JY (1976) Sibling uropathology. J Urol 115: 726

Ehrenreich T, Churg J (1968) Pathology of membraneous nephropathy. Pathol Annu 3: 145

Ekström T (1955) Renal hypoplasia. A clinical study of 179 cases. Acta Chir Scand [Suppl] 203

Ekström T, Engfeldt B, Lagergren C, Lindvall N (1959) Medullary sponge kidney. Almqvist & Wicksell, Stockholm

Elkin M, Bernstein J (1969) Cystic disease of the kidney. Clin Radiol 20: 65

Ericsson NO, Ivemark BI (1958) Renal dysplasia and urinary tract infection. Acta Chir Scand 115: 58

Ericsson NO, Ivemark BI (1958) Renal dysplasia and pyelon-ephritis in infants and children. 2. Primitive ductules and abnormal glomeruli. Arch Pathol 66: 264

Fairley KF, Leighton PW, Kincaid-Smith P (1963) Familial visual defects associated with polycystic kidney and medullary sponge kidney. Br Med J i: 1060

Fanconi G, Hanhart E, von Albertini A, Euhlinger R, Dohvo E, Prader A (1951) Die familiäre juvenile Nephronopthise. Helv Paediatr Acta 6: 1

Fantel AG, Shepard RH (1975) Potter syndrome: Nonrenal features induced by oligoamnios. Am J Dis Child 129: 1346

Farrington GH (1969) Histologic observations in cryptor-chidism: The congenital germinal-cell deficiency of the undescended testis. J Pediatr Surg 4: 606

Fetterman GH, Habib R (1969) Congenital bilateral olig-onephronic renal hypoplasia with hypertrophy of nephrons (oligomeganephronie): Studies by microdissection. Am J Clin Pathol 52: 199

Forsythe IW, Smyth BT (1959) Diverticulum of the bladder in children: A study of 13 cases. Pediatrics 24: 322

Germuth FG Jr, Rodriguez E (1972) Immunopathology of the renal glomerules: Immune complex deposit and antibasement membrane disease. Little Brown, Boston

Glasgow EF, Moncrieff MW, White RHR (1970) Symptomless

haematuria in childhood. Br Med J ii: 687

Glen JF (1959) Agenesis of the bladder. JAMA 169: 2016

Habib R, Gubler MC (1971) Les lésions glomérulaires focales des syndromes néphrotiques idiopathiques de l'enfant: à propos de 49 observations. Nephron 8: 382

Habib R, Gubler MC (1973) Focal sclerosing glomerulonephritis. In: Kincaid-Smith P, Mathew TH, Becker EL (ed) Glomerulonephritis. Wiley, New York, p 263

Habib R, Gubler MC (1975) Focal glomerulosclerosis, associated with idiopathic nephrotic syndrome. In: Rubin MI, Barratt TM (ed) Pediatric nephrology. Williams & Wilkins, Baltimore, p 499

Habib R, Kleinknecht C (1975) Membranous nephropathy (extramembranous glomerulonephritis). In: Rubin MI, Barratt TM (ed) Pediatric pathology. Williams & Wilkins, Baltimore, p 515

Habib R, Mouzet Massa MT, Coutecuisse V, Royer P (1965) L'ectasie tubulaire précalicielle chez l'enfant. Ann Pediatr 12: 288

Heptinstall RH (1974b) Pyelonephritis: Pathologic features. In: Pathology of the kidney, 2nd edn. Little Brown, Boston, p 878

Heptinstall RH (1974b) Pyelonephritis: Pathologic features. In: Pathology of the kidney, 2nd edn. Little Brown, Boston, p 913

Herdman RC, Langer LO (1968) The thoracic asphyxiant dystrophy and renal disease. Am J Dis Child 116: 192

Hill GS, Jenis EH, Goodloe S Jr (1974) The nonspecificity of the ultrastructural alterations in hereditary nephritis. Lab Invest 31: 516

Hilton C, Keeling JW (1973) Neonatal renal tumours. Br J Urol 46: 157

Hinglais N, Grünfeld J-P, Bois E (1972) Characteristic ultrastructural lesion of the glomerular basement membrane in progressive hereditary nephritis (Alport's syndrome). Lab Invest 27: 473

Hodson CJ, Maling TMJ, McMamamon PJ, Lewis MG (1975) The pathogenesis of reflux nephropathy (chronic atrophic pyelonephritis). Br J Urol Suppl 13

Holdsworth SR, Thomson NM, Glasgow EF, Dowling JP, Atkins RC (1978) Tissue culture of isolated glomeruli in experimental crescentic glomerulonephritis. J Exp Med 147: 98

Jennings RB, Earle DP (1961) Post-streptococcal glomerulonephritis: Histopathologic and clinical studies of the acute, subsiding acute and early chronic latent phases. J Clin Invest 40: 1525

Johnson HL, Mix LW (1976) The Ask–Upmark kidney: a form of ascending pyelonephritis? Br J Urol 48: 393

Kay S, Pratt CB, Salzberg AM (1966) Hamartoma (leiomyomatous type) of the kidney. Cancer 19: 1825

Kincaid-Smith P (1979) Glomerular lesions in atrophic pyelonephritis (PN). In: Hodson CJ, Kincaid-Smith P (eds) Reflux nephropathy. Masson, New York, p 268

Kissane JM (1973) Hereditary disorders of the kidney. II. In: Rosenberg HS, Bolande RP (ed) Perspectives in pediatric pathology, vol 1. Year Book Medical Publishers, Chicago, p 117

Kleinman H (1954) Epidemic acute glomerulonephritis at Red Lake. Minn Med 37: 479

Knepshield JH, Roberts PL, Davies CJ, Moser RH (1968) Hereditary chronic nephritis complicated by nephrotic syndrome. Arch Intern Med 122: 156

Kohler HH (1940) Multiseptate bladder. J Urol 44: 63

Kouvalainen K, Hjelt L, Hallman N (1962) Placenta in congenital nephrotic syndrome. Ann Paediatr Fenn 8: 181

Krickstein HI, Gloor IJ, Blagk K (1966) Renal pathology in hereditary nephritis with nerve deafness and renal foam cells. Arch Pathol Lab Med 82: 506

Lancet (1978) (V.U.R. + I.R.R.) + U.T.I. = C.P.N. (Leading article) Lancet 2: 301

Lancet (1979) Nephronophthisis—just a pretty name? (leading article) Lancet 1: 141

Landing BH, Hughes ML (1962) Analysis of weights of kidneys in children. Lab Invest 11: 452

Lepoutre C (1939/40) Sur un cas d'absence congénital de la vessie (persistance du cloaque). J Urol Med Chir 48: 334

Lerner RA, Glassock RJ, Dixon FJ (1967) The role of antiglomerular basement membrane antibody in the pathogenesis of human glomerulonephritis. J Exp Med 126: 989

Levy M, Loirat C, Haibb R (1973) Idiopathic membranoproliferative glomerulonephritis in children (correlations between light, electron, immunofluorescent microscopic appearances and serum C_3 and C_3 levels). Biomedicine [Express] 19: 447

Lieberman E, Heuser E, Donnell GN, Landing B, Hammond GD (1969) Hemolytic uremic syndrome. Clinical and pathological considerations. N Engl J Med 281: 833

Ljungqvist A, Largergren C (1963) The Ask–Upmark kidney: a congenital renal anomaly studied by micro-angiography and histology. Acta Pathol Microbiol Scand 56: 277

Marie J, Lévêque R, Lyon G, Bêbe M, Watchi J-M (1963) Acroostéolyse essentielle compliquée d'insuffiscance rénale d'évolution fatale. Presse Med 71: 249

Ngu JL, Barratt TM, Soothhill JF (1970) Immunoconglutinin and complement changes in steroid-sensitive relapsing nephrotic syndrome of children. Clin Exp Immunol 6: 109

Opitz JM, Howe JJ (1969) The Meckel syndrome (dysencephalia splanchnocystica, the Gruber syndrome). Birth Defects 5: 167

Osthanondh V, Potter EL (1963a) Development of human kidneys as shown by microdissection. I. Preparation of tissue with reasons for possible misinterpretation of observations. Arch Pathol 76: 271

Osthanondh V, Potter EL (1963b) Development of human kidneys as shown by microdissection II. Renal pelvis, calyces and papillae. Arch Pathol 76: 277

Osthanondh V, Potter EL (1963c) Development of human kidneys as shown by microdissection. III. Formation and interrelationships of collecting tubules and nephrons. Arch Pathol 76: 290

Osthanondh V, Potter EL (1964) Pathologenesis of polycystic kidneys: historical survey; type 1 due to hyperplasia of interstitial portions of collecting tubules; type 2 due to inhibition of ampullary activity; type 3 due to multiple abnormalities of development; type 4 due to urethral obstruction; survey of results of microdissection. Arch Pathol 77: 459

Osathanondh V, Potter EL (1966a) Development of human kidneys as shown by microdissection. IV. Development of tubular portions of nephrons. Arch Pathol 82: 391

Osathanondh V, Potter El (1966b) Development of human kidneys as shown by microdissection. V. Development of vascular glomerulus. Arch Pathol 82: 403

Palmer JM, Zweiman FG, Assay Keen TA (1970) Renal hypertension secondary to hydronephrosis with normal plasma renin activity. N Engl J Med 283: 1032

Pathak IG, Williams DI (1963) Multicystic and cystic dysplastic kidneys. Br J Urol 36: 318

Perkoff GT, Nugent CA Jr, Dolowitz DA, Stephens FE, Carnes WH, Tyler FH (1968) A follow-up study of hereditary chronic nephritis. Arch Intern Med 102: 733

Peters DK, Williams DG (1975) Pathogenic mechanisms in glomerulonephritis. In: Jones NF (ed) Recent advances in renal disease. Churchill Livingston, Edinburgh, p 90

Peters DK, Williams DG, Charlesworth JA, Boulton-Jones JM, Sissons JGP, Evans DJ, Kourilsky O, Morel-Maroger L (1973) Mesangiocapillary nephritis, partial lipodystrophy and hypocomplementaemia. Lancet 2: 535

Piel CF, Phibbs RH (1966) The hemolytic uremic syndrome. Pediatr Clin North Am 13: 295

Marsden HB, Lawler W (1978) Bone metastasising renal tumour of childhood. Br J Cancer 38: 437

Marshall AG (1953) Persistence of foetal structures in pyelo-nephritic kidneys. Br J Surg 41: 38

Meadow SR (1975) Post-streptococcal glomerulonephritis—a rare disease. Arch Dis Child 50: 379

Miller HL (1948) Agenesis of the urinary bladder and urethra. J Urol 59: 1156

Mitchell JD, Baxter TJ, Blair-West JR, McCredie DA (1970) Renin levels in nephroblastoma (Wilm's tumour). Report of a renin-secreting tumour. Arch Dis Child 45: 376

Moolten SE (1942) Hamartial nature of tuberous sclerosis complex and its bearing on the tumour problem: A report of a case with tumour anomaly of the kidney and adenoma sebaceum. Arch Intern Med 69: 589

Morris RC, Yamacuchi H, Pulubinskas AJ, Howenstein J (1965) Medullary sponge kidney. Am J Med 38: 883

Nagington J, Wreghitt TG, Gandy G, Robertson NRC, Berry PJ (1978) Fatal echovirus 11 infections in outbreak in special care baby unit. Lancet 2: 725

Potter El (1946) Facial characteristics of infants with bilateral renal agenesis. Am J Obstet Gynecol 51: 885

Powell T, Schackmann R, Johnson HD (1951) Multilocular cysts of the kidney. Br J Urol 23: 142

Poznanski AK, Nosanchuk JS, Baublis J, Holt JF (1970) The cerebro-hepato-renal syndrome (CHRS) (Zellweger's syndrome). Am J Roentgenol 109: 313

Ransley PG (1978) Vesico-ureteric reflux: continuing surgical dilemma. Urology 12: 246

Ransley PG, Risdon RA (1975a) Renal papillary morphology and intrarenal reflux in the young pig. Urol Res 3: 105

Ransley PG, Risdon RA (1975b) Renal papillary morphology in infants and young children. Urol Res 3: 111

Ransley PG, Risdon RA (1978) Reflux and renal scarring. Br J Urol Suppl 14

Reilly BJ, Neuhauser EBD (1960) Renal tubular ectasia in cystic disease of the kidney and liver. Am J Roentgenol 84: 546

Rich AR (1957) Hitherto undescribed vulnerability of juxtamed-ullary glomeruli in lipoid nephrosis. Bull Johns Hopkins Hosp 100: 173

Richart R, Benirschke K (1960) Penile agenesis: Report of a case, review of the world literature and discussion of pertinent embryology. Arch Pathol 70: 252

Risdon RA (1971) Renal dysplasia I. A clinico-pathological study of 76 cases. II. A necropsy study of 41 cases. J Clin Pathol 24: 57 and 65

Risdon RA (1975) Gross anatomy of the kidney. In: Rubin MI, Barratt TM (ed) Pediatric nephrology. Williams & Wilkins, Baltimore, p 2

Robertson PW, Klidjian A, Harding LK, Walters G, Lee MR, Robb-Smith AHT (1970) Hypertension due to a renin-secreting tumour. Arch Dis Child 45: 476

Rolleston GL, Maling TMJ, Hodson CJ (1974) Intrarenal reflux and the scarred kidney. Arch Dis Child 49: 531

Roosen-Runge EC (1949) Retardation of postnatal development of kidneys in persons with early cerebral lesions. Am J Dis Child 77: 185

Royer P, Habib R, Mathieu H, Courtevuisse V (1962) L'hypoplasie rénale bilatérale congénital avec reduction du nombre et hypertrophie des néphrons chez l'enfant. Ann Pediatr 9: 1330

Royer P, Habib R, Broyer M, Nauaille Y (1971) Segmental hypoplasia of the kidney in children. In: Advances in neph-rology, vol 1. Year Book Medical Publishers, Chicago, p. 145

Rubenstein M, Meyer R, Bernstein J (1961) Congenital abnor-malities of the urinary system. I. A postmortem survey of developmental anomalies and acquired congenital lesions in a childrens' hospital. J Pediatr 58: 356

Schacht RG, Gluck MC, Gallo GR, Baldwin DS (1976) Progression to uremia after remission of acute post-streptococcal glomerulonephritis. N Engl J Med 295: 977

Schimke RN (1971) Hereditary renal-retinal dysplasia. Ann Intern Med 74: 47

Scorer CG (1956) Incidence of incomplete descent of the testicle at birth. Arch Dis Child 31: 198

Scott WW (1929) Blood stream infections in urology: A report of 82 cases. J Urol 21: 527

Scruggs CD, Ainsworth T (1961) Renal cell carcinoma in children: Review of the literature and report of two cases. J Urol 86: 728

Shannon FT (1970) The significance and management of vesico-ureteric reflux in infancy. In: Kincaid-Smith PE, Fairley KF (ed) Renal infection and renal scarring. Mercedes, Melbourne, p 241

Shapiro AH (1967) Pumping and retrograde diffusion in peristaltic waves. In: Glen JF (ed) Proceedings of a Workshop in Ureteral Reflux in Children. National Academy of Sciences–National Research Council, Washington, p 109

Shapiro, LR (1977) Disorders of femal sex differentiation. In: Blaustein A (ed) Pathology of the femal genital tract. Springer, New York Heidelberg Berlin, p. 420

Sherman FE, Studnicki FM, Felterman GH (1971) Renal lesions of familial juvenile nephronophthisis examined by microdissec-tion. Am J Clin Pathol 55: 391

Smith CH, Graham JB (1948) Congenital medullary cysts of the kidney in severe refractory anemia. Am J Dis Child 69: 369

Smith DR (1969) Critique on the concept of vesical neck obstruction in children. JAMA 207: 1686

Sohar E, Gatni J, Pras M, Heller H (1967) Familial mediterranean fever: A survey of 470 cases and review of the literature. Am J Med 43: 227

Soothill JF, Steward MV (1971) The immunopathological significance of the heterogeneity of antibody affinity. Clin Exp Immunol 9: 193

Spitzer RE, Vallota EH, Forristal J, Sudora E, Stitzel A, Davis NC, West CD (1969) Serum C_3 lytic system in patients with glomerulonephritis. Science 164: 436

Stephens FD (1956) Double ureter in the child. Aust NZ J Surg 26: 81

Strauss MB, Sommers SC (1967) Medullary cystic disease and familial juvenile nephronophthisis. N Engl J Med 277: 863

Sworn MJ, Eisinger AJ (1972) Medullary cystic disease and juvenile nephronophthisis in separate members of the same family. Arch Dis Child 47: 278

Thorn G, Koepf GF, Clinton M Jr (1944) Renal failure simulating adrenocortical insufficiency. N Engl J Med 231: 76

Treser G, Semar M, Ty A, Sagel I, Franklin MA, Lange K (1970) Partial characterization of antigenic streptococcal plasma membrane components in acute glomerulonephritis. J Clin Invest 49: 762

Turner DR (1978) Glomerulonephritis. In: Anthony PP, Woolf N (ed) Recent advances in histopathology, vol 10. Churchill Livingstone, Edinburgh, p 245

Unanue ER, Dixon FJ (1967) Experimental glomerulonephritis: Immunological events and pathogenic mechanisms. Adv Immunol 6: 1

Urizar RE, Schwartz A, Top F, Vernier RL (1969) The nephrotic syndrome in children with diabetes mellitus of recent origin. N Engl J Med 281: 173

Vernier RL, Papermaster BW, Olness K, Binet E, Good RA (1960) Morphologic studies of the mechanisms of proteinuria. Am J Dis Child 100: 476

Whitaker RG (1976) Congenital disorders of the testicle. In: Blandy J (ed) Urology. Blackwell Scientific, Oxford, p 1157

White P (1956) Natural course and prognosis of juvenile diabetes. Diabetes 5: 445

White RHR, Glasgow EF, Mills RJ (1970) Clinicopathological study of nephrotic syndrome in childhood. Lancet 2: 1353

White RR, Wyatt GM (1942) Surgical importance of the aberrant renal vessel in infants and children. Am J Surg 58: 48

Williams DI (1962) Reflux in double ureters. Proc R Soc Med 55: 423

Williams DI (1968) Renal dysplasia. In: Williams DI (ed) Paediatric urology. Butterworths, London, p 36

Williams DI, Burkholder GF (1967) The prune belly syndrome. J Urol 98: 244

Williams DI, Schistad G (1961) Lower urinary tract tumours in children. Br J Urol 36: 51

Winkelman J (1967) Coexistent megacolon and megaureter: Report of a case with normal vesical autonomic innervation. Pediatrics 39: 258

Walker EW, (1897) A floating kidney containing three dermoid cysts and several serous cysts: Laparotomy; recovery. Trans Am Surg Assoc 15: 591

Wall B, Wachter HE (1952) Congenital ureteral valve. Its role as a primary obstructive lesion: Classification of the literature and report of an authentic case. J Urol 68: 684

Waller JF, Roll WA (1957) Bladder carcinoma in a teen-age girl. J Urol 78: 764

Warkany J (1971) Congenital malformations. Year Book Medical Publishers, Chicago

Warkany J, Passarge E, Smith LB (1966) Congenital malformations in autosomal trisomy syndromes. Am J Dis Child 112: 502

Wattenberg CA, Rape MG, Beare JB (1949) Perineal testicle. J Urol 62: 858

West CD, McAdams AJ, McConville JM, Davies MC, Holland NH (1965) Hypocomplementemic and normocomplementemic persistent (chronic) glomerulonephritis: Clinical and pathological characteristics. J Pediatr 67: 1089

Westberg NG, Michael AF (1972) Immunohistopathology of diabetic glomerulosclerosis. Diabetes 21: 163

Young HH, McKay RW (1929) Congenital valvular obstruction of the prostatic urethra. Surg Gynecol Obstet 48: 509

Zinner SH, Levy PS, Kass EH (1971) Familial aggregation of blood pressure in childhood. N Engl J Med 284: 401

becomes the fibrocartilage of the intervertebral disc. The semigelatinous nucleus pulposus of the disc contains notochondral remnants.

1.5. The Postnatal Ossification of Bones

A fetus can be assumed to be full-term if there are centres of ossification present for the calcaneus, the talus, and the lower femoral epiphysis. Postnatal ossification centres in the epiphyses show a regularity in sequence and time of appearance, and sets of normal values (standards) have been established for large numbers of carefully repeated radiological examinations in children from socioeconomic backgrounds that ensure well-balanced diets and thus optimal developmental conditions. The chronology of skeletal development as a whole can be assessed by radiological examination of the limbs and general skeletal status is well reflected in the hand and wrist alone. The age rating of a child in skeletal terms is based on the demonstration of the most recently ossified centre. Alterations in the ossification of the hand and wrist are likely to be present in children suffering severe illness or prolonged nutritional defects. Protracted illness during childhood disturbs the sequence of appearance of ossification centres, the delay in ossification being proportional to the duration and intensity of the illness. Endocrine disturbances such as hypothyroidism and hypopituitarism delay the appearance and retard the growth of postnatal ossification centres, while accelerated endochrondral ossification at the epiphyseal plates results in initial acceleration of growth in precocious puberty and is followed by premature epiphyseal fusion, the final height being below average.

A further factor that should be borne in mind when assessing skeletal status is the sex of the subject. Girls are in advance of boys in the time of appearance of ossification centres even at full term, and by 5 years of age they are up to 1 year ahead (Table 10.1). Fusion of many epiphyses occurs 2–3 years earlier in girls than boys (Table 10.2). The data given in Tables 10.1 and 10.2 represent approximate values obtained from several sources. Readers wishing to obtain more precise information or details relating to other bones should refer to the book by Jaffe (1972) or the papers by Francis and Werke (1939), Francis (1940), Fleckes (1942) and Acheson (1957).

Table 10.1. Time of appearance of some ossification centres in children aged up to 10 years

	Girls	Boys
Calcaneus	Birth	Birth
Talus	Birth	Birth
Distal femur	Birth	Birth
Proximal femur	Birth	Birth
Humeral head	Birth to 1 month	Birth to 1 month
Capitate	2–3 months	2–3 months
Hamate	2–3 months	3–4 months
Lat. cuneiform	3–4 months	4–5 months
Femoral head	3–4 months	4–5 months
Distal tibia	3–4 months	4 months
Distal fibula	9 months	12 months
Distal radius	9–10 months	12–13 months
Med. cuneiform	15–16 months	20–24 months
Patella	$2\frac{1}{2}$–3 years	4 years
Greater trochanter	$2\frac{1}{2}$ years	$3\frac{1}{2}$ years
Proximal radius	4 years	5 years
Distal ulna	4–5 years	7 years
Calcaneus, epiph.	5 years	7 years
Olecranon	7–8 years	9–10 years
Talus, epiph.	7–8 years	8–9 years
Lesser trochanter	8–9 years	9–11 years
Tibial tubercle	9–10 years	11–12 years

Table 10.2. Times of fusion of epiphyses of limb bones (years)

	Girls	Boys
Upper humerus	16–17	16–18
Lower humerus	13	15–16
Prox. radius	14	14–16
Distal radius	16–18	17–19
Priximal femur	13–14	14–17
Greater trochanter	14	16
Distal femur	14–17	16–19
Proximal tibia	14–15	16–18
Distal tibia	13–14	15–17
Calcaneus, apophysis	13–14	15–17

2. Abnormal Development

2.1. Teratogenic Agents and Limb Development

A large number of chemical agents have been demonstrated to alter limb development, though their effects are usually not specific just to the limbs. Some teratogens can selectively cause limb defects if administered over a limited period of time in pregnancy. The limb is not equally sensitive at all stages of development, susceptibility beginning at the start of limb bud elongation and ending when the rudimentary skeleton is formed in cartilage. The stages in development of the forelimb precede those of the hind limb by 2–3 days, so that there is a cephalo-caudal sensitivity gradient as well as a proximodistal one. Specific effects of teratogens on the skeleton have been reviewed by Berry (1978).

2.2. Dwarfism

Shortness of stature may be present at birth or may develop during childhood. Dwarfism is classified into certain broad categories.

In achondroplasia, there is a pronounced shortening of the extremities with minimal changes in the trunk. There are several rarer forms of short-limbed (micromelic) dwarfism, and their modes of inheritance are shown in Table 10.3. These disorders, together with even rarer abnormalities, are sometimes collectively termed the osteochondrodystrophies or chondrodysplasias.

Dwarfism may be related to inborn errors of metabolism, most notably in the mucopolysaccharidoses, a group of disorders in which further subtypes are always being defined.

Two other types are the *ateliotic* dwarf, who remains infantile in appearance, and the subject with '*progeria*', whose appearance becomes that of a shrivelled old person even when young. Neither of these shows skeletal disproportion.

Short stature may also be present in certain endocrine disorders (hypopituitarism, hypothyroidism, cretinism, pseudopseudohypoparathyroidism), and renal disease in childhood sometimes results in dwarfism.

Table 10.3. Types of osteochondrodysplasia according to presence or absence of spinal involvement (after Beighton 1978)

Osteochondrodysplasia without significant spinal involvement

Achondroplasia
Hypochondroplasia
Achondrogenesis
Thanatophoric dwarfism
Asphyxiating thoracic dysplasia
Chondroectodermal dysplasia
Multiple epiphyseal dysplasia
Chondrodysplasia punctata
Metaphyseal chondrodysplasia
Mesomelic dwarfism
Rhizomelic dwarfism
Campomelic dwarfism

Osteochondrodysplasia with significant spinal involvement

Pseudoachondroplasia
Spondyloepiphyseal dysplasia
Spondylometaphyseal dysplasia
Schwartz syndrome
Metatropic dwarfism
Kniest syndrome
Diastrophic dwarfism
Dyggue–Melchior–Clausen syndrome
Parastremmatic dwarfism

2.3. Achondroplasia

The commonest of the chondrodysplasias is achondroplasia. It is considered to result from a primary disturbance of endochondral ossification in early fetal life, which has become well established by the time of birth. Severely affected fetuses die towards the end of gestation. Achondroplastics surviving the neonatal period normally grow to adulthood and such milder cases are usually of normal intelligence.

The achondroplastic neonate shows well-marked abnormalities, and those born dead have very severe shortening of the limbs. Pathological examination of achondroplastic neonates reveals long bones as little as half the normal length with considerable enlargement of epiphyses, which may extend up to half the length of the bone. The intervening shaft widens to surround the enlarged epiphysis at either end of the bone (Fig. 10.2). The most notable skull changes occur in the sphenoid and basal part of the occipital bone near the foramen magnum, which may be narrowed. The vertebral bodies are cartilaginous, containing underdeveloped ossification centres. The costochondral junctions are increased in diameter (beading) and shifted towards the axilla because of the shortness of the ribs.

Histologically, deficiency in cartilage cell proliferation is best seen at epiphyseal–diaphyseal junctions of long bones.

There have been few pathological studies of the changes present in achondroplastic children and adults. Biopsy studies in some typical achondroplastics have shown apparently regular and well-organized endochondral ossification (Fig. 10.3), and it has been suggested that the defect is a quantitative decrease in the rate of endochondral ossification. Periosteal ossification is normal and thus relatively increased compared with endochondral bone formation. Periosteal overgrowth results in the cupping at bone ends seen on radiological examination (Rimoin et al. 1976).

In purely descriptive terms, the following features may be present in the achondroplastic. Apart from the actual shortening of the limbs, the ends of the long bones are enlarged and the cortices thickened. There may be coxa vara and genu varum. The position of the fibula relative to the tibia distinguishes the achondroplastic, the head of the fibula reaching to the level of the upper surface of the tibia. The skull is increased in circumference and there is frontal protuberance. Shortness of the base of the skull gives rise to the abnormal 'pug-shaped' nose and there may be prognathism. Lordosis and dorsolumbar kyphosis are often present in the spine. The ribs are abnormally broad, while the most important pelvic abnormality is anteroposterior flattening at the inlet, which gives rise to obstetric problems.

Achondroplasia shows autosomal dominant inheritance. More than 80% of achondroplastics, however, are sporadic cases with normal parents (Scott 1976) and therefore represent new mutations.

2.4. Other Osteochondrodysplasias

Brief accounts of some of the other osteochondrodysplasias are given below.

The osteochondrodysplasias have been divided into two groups by Beighton (1978), and this classification is summarized in Table 10.3. The reader wishing to obtain further clinical, radiological, and genetic details about these disorders is referred to the book by Beighton (1978) and the radiological atlas by Cremin and Beighton (1978).

A summary of the differential diagnosis of short-limbed stillborn and newborn dwarfism is shown in Table 10.4. Some of these disorders are described briefly in the following account and in Table 10.5. Some of the terms used may be a source of confusion. 'Micromelia' is used to mean shortening of all segments of the limbs. 'Rhizomelia' denotes shortening of the proximal segment, while 'mesomelia' and 'acromelia' describe shortening of the middle (i.e., forearm and leg) and distal segments, respectively.

Table 10.4. The differential diagnosis of short-limbed dwarfism at birth

Stillborn (lethal)	Achondrogenesis
	Thanatophoric dwarfism
	Achondroplasia
	Asphyxiating thoracic dysplasia
	Short-rib polydactyly syndromes
	Chondroectodermal dysplasia
	Chondrodysplasia punctata (some)
	Campomelic dwarfism
	Osteogenesis imperfecta
	Hypophosphatasia
Newborn (nonlethal: survival usual)	Achondroplasia
	Mesomelic dwarfism
	Rhizomelic dwarfism
	Spondylepiphyseal dysplasia
	Spondylometaphyseal dysplasia
	Metatropic dwarfism
	Diastrophic dwarfism

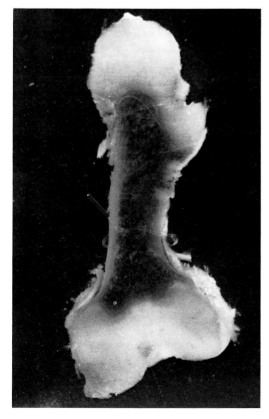

Fig. 10.2. Left femur of a full-term stillborn achondroplastic, showing widened irregular lower metaphysis and widening of the lower epiphysis.

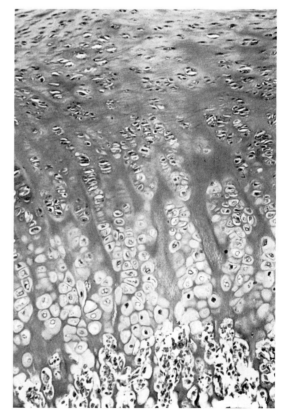

Fig. 10.3. Well-organized endochondral ossification in the lower epiphysis of the femur of a stillborn achondroplastic. (H and E; 400 ×)

Table 10.5. Some conditions resulting in dwarfism

	Type	Features	Inheritance
1. Incompatible with life	Thanatophoric dwarfism	a) Severe micromelia b) Long narrow thorax c) Large cranial vault with depressed base d) Short ribs e) Reduced height of vertebral bodies	Mutation
	Achondrogenesis	a) Severe micromelia b) Ossification defects in various bones, notably vertebral bodies not ossified, wide metaphyses in limbs	Autosomal recessive
	Short-rib polydactyly syndromes	a) Various types b) Features include thoracic narrowing, polydactyly, micromelia, congenital heart disease, anomalies in genito-urinary and gastrointestinal tracts, cleft lip and palate	Autosomal recessive
2. Compatible with life	Achondroplasia	a) Micromelia, dwarfism b) Craniofacial changes c) Small foramen magnum (see text for description)	Autosomal dominant Many sporadic
	Spondylo-epiphyseal dysplasia	a) Dwarfism with short trunk b) Delays in ossification and fragmented epiphyseal ossification centres c) Platyspondyly, talipes equinovarus d) Kyphoscoliosis and thoracic deformity develop in childhood	Autosomal dominant
	Chondroectodermal dysplasia (Ellis–von Creveld syndrome)	a) Micromelia b) Polydactyly with hypoplasia or absence of nails c) Congenital heart disease d) Ectodermal dysplasia e) Normal intelligence (see text for description)	Autosomal recessive
	Asphyxiating thoracic dysplasia	a) Short limbs b) Long narrow thorax, short ribs with costochondral beading c) Head and spine normal d) Polydactyly in some (resemble Ellis–von Creveld) e) Respiratory difficulties, pneumonia, etc., majority die in infancy	Autosomal recessive
	Diastrophic dwarfism (dysplasia)	a) Micromelic dwarfism b) Club foot c) Posterior cleft palate d) Contractures of many joints e) External ear deformity (at 1 or 2 months of age) f) Later develop changes in epiphyses, genu valgum, scoliosis (but spine may be deformed at birth)	Autosomal recessive
	Metatrophic dwarfism (dysplasia)	a) Micromelic dwarfism with trumpet-shaped metaphyses b) Skull and face usually normal c) Kyphoscoliosis with reduced height of vertebral bodies (more marked in childhood) d) Pigeon chest (childhood)	Autosomal recessive (In infancy, differentiate from achondroplasia; in childhood, differentiate from Morquio's disease)

Table 10.5. (Continued)

	Type	Features	Inheritance
2. Compatible with life (*continued*)	Mesomelic dwarfism (dysplasia)	a) Severe micromelia selective to the forearm and leg b) Curved radius, fibular aplasia, genu valgum, club feet, etc., in different types	Autosomal dominant and autosomal recessive types
	Chondrodysplasia punctata	a) Micromelic dwarfism b) Cataract c) Skin manifestations d) Spotty calcification of epiphyses and vertebrae (see text for description)	Autosomal dominant and autosomal recessive types
	Campomelic dysplasia	a) "Bent limbs"—bowing of tubular bones, especially legs b) Calcaneovalgus or equinovarus c) Flat face, low ears, micrognathia, cleft palate d) Platyspondyly, hypoplastic scapulae e) Death from respiratory insufficiency	Sporadic

2.4.1. Histological and Ultrastructural Studies of the Chondrodystrophies

Recent studies are beginning to throw light on the pathology of the chondrodystrophies. The histopathological abnormalities appear to be characteristic in achondrogenesis, diastrophic dwarfism, and thanatophoric dwarfism. In other disorders there is considerable heterogeneity and no clear correlations are yet possible (e.g., spondyloepiphyseal dysplasia). Cartilage is relatively normal in achondroplasia, hypochondroplasia, and multiple epiphyseal dysplasia, so that histological examination is not of much diagnostic value. Ultrastructural studies show differences between some of the chondrosyplasias. The reader is referred to the articles by Rimoin et al. (1976), Sillence et al. (1979) and Hwang et al. (1979) for further details.

2.4.2. Chrondoectodermal Dysplasia (Ellis–von Creveld Syndrome)

Abnormal cartilage development, ectodermal dysplasia, and polydactyly are the main features of the disorder first described by Ellis and von Creveld (1940). Other malformations, including congenital heart disease, may be present. In the newborn, the diagnosis can be made by the presence of short extremities, polydactyly with the extra digit on the ulnar side, and absence or hypoplasia of the nails. Small peg-shaped teeth may be present at birth or appear prematurely. Bronchial defects and hypoplasia of the lungs may contribute to early respiratory death. Babies with severe heart disease die soon after birth. A large series of cases has been described by McKusick et al. (1964).

2.4.3. Chondrodysplasia Punctata (Stippled Epiphyses, Chondodystrophia Calcificans Congenita, Dysplasia Epiphysealis Punctata)

The rare disorder chondrodysplasia punctata is characterized by the presence of multiple punctate foci of calcification in the cartilaginous parts of the neonatal and infant skeleton. The presence of stippled epiphyses is a striking feature on X-ray examination, but it is a radiological sign which is not wholly diagnostic.

Many affected infants are stillborn or die soon after birth. The head and trunk are enlarged, the extremities are short with a proportionally greater reduction in length of proximal parts, and there may be flexion deformities of the hips, knees, and shoulders. Localized skeletal abnormalities include unilateral micromelia, club foot, and dislocation of the hip. Cataracts may be a feature and skin manifestations, namely dyskeratosis, seborrhoeic dermatosis, hyperkeratosis, or icthyosis, may occur.

Irregular focal calcification (stippling) is seen both in the epiphyses of the femur, tibia, humerus, and iliac crest and in the posterior ends of the ribs and vertebral bodies on radiological examination. Pathological examination has been performed in a number of cases. Endochondral bone formation is markedly abnormal. The chondrocytes are not organized into columns and there is diminished mineralization of matrix associated with decreased vascularization of the cartilage. Resting cartilage contains areas of mucoid degeneration, with calcification and fragmentation (Rimoin et al. 1975).

Similar changes have been described in warfarin embryopathy (see p. 80).

2.4.4. Multiple Epiphyseal Dysplasia

Multiple epiphyseal dysplasia is a relatively rare disorder of skeletal development, which is inherited as a dominant trait. Characteristically, there are abnormalities in the growth of ossification centres with resultant shortness of stature. Growth abnormalities become apparent during the second or third years of life rather than at birth, and include knock knees, bow legs, short stubby digits, and minor wedge or biconcave deformities of the vertebral bodies.

Ossification centres are delayed in appearance and irregular in outline, appearing fragmented when present. The fragments eventually coalesce to form a single centre with an irregular outline. Alterations in structure are likely to be detectable in the hip, ankle, and shoulder joints on X-ray examination. Little is known of the detailed pathological features in the human since the condition is not lethal. Prematurely developing osteoarthrosis is a frequent complication. The study by Rasmussen (1975) of multiple epiphyseal dysplasia in the dog is of some interest, since it was possible to follow the development of pathological changes. Initially, there was an accumulation of abnormal cartilage matrix in relation to chondrocytes. This was followed by liquefaction and cyst formation, and later by focal calcification.

2.4.5. Metaphyseal Dysostosis (Metaphyseal Chondrodysplasia)

A disturbance of the metaphyses of long bones occurs in the group of conditions known collectively as metaphyseal dysostosis, which are very rare. The affected persons are of small stature and have coxa vara and genu vara. The changes may be mild, or severe and deforming. In young children cupping of the metaphyses of long bones and expansion of the anterior ends of the ribs reflect the presence of large amounts of calcifying and ossifying cartilage. The chief problem is in differential diagnosis from rickets, where similar expansions of the ends of bones occurs.

The epiphyses, skull, and trunk are essentially normal. Several types of metaphyseal chondrodysplasia that have associated abnormalities, have been described, e.g., cartilage-hair hypoplasia, malabsorption and neutropenia, thymolymphopenia,

asymptomatic hypercalcaemia. The reader is referred to specialist accounts for further details.

Histological examination shows disorganization of the growth plate and extension of cartilage into the metaplysis. Larger than normal chondrocytes are arranged in clusters instead of columns, and the intervening matrix has a fibrillar appearance. There is irregularity of vascular invasion resulting in irregular spicules of calcified cartilage and bone (see Rimoin et al. 1975).

2.5. Cleidocranial Dysostosis

Cleidocranial dysostosis is inherited as an autosomal dominant, but occasional sporadic cases occur. Although the principal abnormalities occur in the clavicles and calvarium, anomalies in bones formed in cartilage have been noted, including deficient ossification or even absence of parts of the pubic bones, hip-joint deformities, spina bifida occulta, and abnormalities in dentition.

The clavicles are incompletely formed in typical cases. They are composed of fragments, which articulate normally with the sternum but have non-articulating lateral ends. They are either freely mobile or joined by fibrous bands to the choranoid process, acromion, first rib, or glenoid cavity. In some cases, the clavicles may consist of lateral and medial ends separated by a wide gap containing fibrous tissue. They may be completely absent.

The defective calvarium has wide fontanelles and greatly separated sutures. These are gradually closed in later life by irregular islands of bone but a large frontal defect often persists. The calvarium comprises a mosaic of small bones representing unfused ossification centres. There are large frontal bosses and the skull is flattened laterally.

2.6. Neurospinal Dysraphism

The various forms of neurospinal dysraphism involve defects in the closure of the neural tube and its surroundings to different degrees. The primary fault occurs in the neural tube and not in the related mesoderm. The severest deformity is total myeloschisis, in which all the vertebral arches are deficient and the whole spinal cord is laid open to the exterior. The number of vertebrae is often reduced and there may be a lordosis in the cervical region. In some cases even the vertebral bodies themselves may be divided.

In localized myeloschisis or myelocele, one or more vertebral arches are defective and other local spinal anomalies may co-exist.

2.7. Congenital Dislocation of the Hip

Typical congenital dislocation of the hip does not exist at birth, and almost all examples of the disorder are the result of hip-joint anomalies that predispose to dislocation (see Hass 1951).

True congenital dislocation of the hip, with bilateral displacement, is rarer and is often known as atypical congenital dislocation of the hip. In this form, the hip-joint socket is diminished in size and flattened by the accumulation of cartilaginous connective tissue. The femoral neck is shortened. Other abnormalities that may be associated include torticollis, spina bifida, agenesis of the sacrum, knee contractures, fibular and femoral hypoplasia, and club foot.

The common form of congenital dislocation of the hip occurs more frequently in some families than in the general population (see p. 75). In the predisposed neonate, the cartilaginous portions of the joint are almost intact but there is hypoplasia of the osseous nuclei, especially those of the acetabulum. The obliquity of the acetabular roof is increased, the socket is flattened, and anteversion of the femoral head is increased in the stage before luxation. Ossification of the femoral head is retarded, the centre appearing later on the affected side.

In subluxation, the femoral head may still remain in contact with the original articular surface but protrudes from the acetabulum. The flattened acetabular roof becomes elongated and has a depression at the site where the femoral head rests. The femoral head is flattened and at a later stage moves over the rim of the acetabulum, losing contact with the original socket. Displacement is always upwards but may in addition be anterior, posterior, or lateral. A secondary socket is formed opposite the dislocated femoral head, which is itself reduced in size. The direction of the femoral neck may be altered, resulting in coxa vara or coxa valga deformities. Newly formed fibrocartilage formed in the fat pad around the ligamentum teres fuses with the hyaline cartilage of the original socket, which is flattened. Further information on the growth of the acetabulum in the normal child and the changes in congenital hip dysplasia is available in the recent publications of Ponseti (1978a, b).

2.8. Club Foot (Talipes Equinovarus)

Any foot deformity involving the talus is called 'talipes'. Club foot (talipes equinovarus) is one of the most frequent skeletal malformations present at birth. About 20 % of affected neonates are not viable owing to associated malformations, especially neurospinal dysraphism. Club foot is a composite deformity in which the sole is turned medially so that the lateral margin of the foot touches the ground (varus) and the toes are held lower than the heel (equinus). The talus and calcaneus show the most marked changes. The talus is thickened, with its body turned forward and its elongated neck deflected inward and downward. The calcaneus is in a position of plantar flexion and the heel elevated.

2.9. Congenital Talipes Calcaneovalgus

In congenital talipes calcaneovalgus the foot is dorsiflexed and everted. The dorsum readily touches the anterolateral surface of the leg and plantar flexion ceases at mid-position. It may be mistakenly diagnosed where there is congenital vertical talus, especially in very young babies. Vertical talus is distinguishable because there is subtalar rigidity and the heel is in equinus.

3. Skeletal Abnormalities Developed Later in Childhood or Adolescence

3.1. Juvenile Kyphosis (Preadolescent and Adolescent Kyphosis)

Juvenile kyphosis is not an uncommon condition, and it affects males and females equally. The abnormality is usually first recognized between 13 and 17 years of age, and is either asymptomatic or causes backache. On examination, there is lower thoracic or thoracolumbar kyphosis often associated with scoliosis. The main radiological and pathological features may be a mild increase in the normal thoracic curvature of the spine, with anterior narrowing of the intervertebral spaces. In more advanced cases the vertebral bodies show marked anterior narrowing in the affected region and disc protrusions cause indentations of the vertebral bodies so that the margin between disc and bone is irregular or there are Schmorl's nodes.

The cartilaginous growth plates of the vertebral bodies on either side of the affected intervertebral disc are subjected to undue pressure by the discs, causing changes in endochondral bone formation in the vertebral bodies, which may undergo extensive destruction. Changes in the disc result in a tendency to narrowing of the intervertebral space, but since the bodies are held posteriorly by the apophyseal joints only the anterior parts of the vertebral bodies move closer together. Inhibition of growth resulting from pressure on the anterior parts of the vertebral body results in the progressive development of a wedge-shaped vertebra. Areas of prolapsed disc in the vertebral bodies are eventually surrounded by osseous tissue and vascular fibrous tissue extends into the disc, so that an immobile fibrous union between adjacent vertebral bodies results.

3.2. Osteochondritis Dissecans

'Osteochondritis dissecans' is the term used to describe a condition in which a small piece of articular cartilage with related subchondral bone becomes detached and is found free in the joint space as an osteochondral body. It affects mainly males aged between 15 and 20 years and has a familial tendency.

The knee is affected in 90 % of cases, usually on the lateral surface of the medial femoral condyle. The elbow, hip, ankle, and shoulder may occasionally be involved. Radiological examination may show irregularity of the bone at the joint surface, a well-delineated lesion that is partly attached, or a completely free body, usually lying in the anterior compartment when the knee joint is affected.

In early cases there are cracks and fissures in the involved cartilage on macroscopical examination. An osteochondral body loosely attached to cartilage or lying free in the joint space is elliptical. The surface cartilage of the body is normal or increased in thickness and the related subchondral bone is necrotic (Fig. 10.4).

3.3. Perthes' Disease

Perthes' disease is a condition in which there is partial or complete aseptic necrosis of the ossification centre of the femoral head. Males are affected four times more often than females, 90 % of cases are unilateral, and the usual age of presentation is 5–9 years. Alterations in the femoral head are associated with certain changes in the femoral neck and acetabulum almost from the time of onset; and although the changes regress with appropriate treatment, the morphology of all three components may not be normal by the end of the growth period.

Necrosis of the capital ossification centre probably takes place over a short period of time. The contour of the femoral head remains unaltered for a while, after which there is collapse of areas of bone, with amorphous debris present in the intertrabecular spaces. The cartilaginous part of the femoral head remains completely viable since it receives its nutrition from the synovial fluid. With revascularization of the epiphysis (by vessels from the femoral neck, bone marrow, and ligamentum teres), there is appositional new bone formation on the necrotic trabeculae. The femoral head may be flattened and the neck shorter and broader than normal when remodelling is completed (Fig. 10.5).

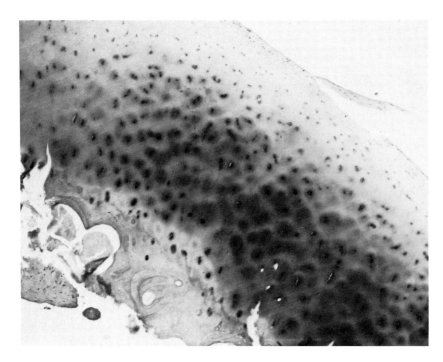

Fig. 10.4. Loose body from the knee of a 20-year-old male with osteochondritis dissecans, showing normal viable hyaline cartilage and necrotic subchondral bone. (H and E; 150×)

Deformity of the femoral head and acetabulum predispose to the development of secondary osteoarthrosis, a common sequel of Perthes' disease.

3.4. Slipped Capital Femoral Epiphysis

Gradual slipping of the femoral head off the neck occurs a little more commonly in males and presents at age 10–16 years in boys, a year or so earlier in girls. Many of the patients are taller and heavier than is normal for their age. The slipping of epiphyses may be unilateral or bilateral, though it is rarely synchronously bilateral. Subsequent involvement of the opposite side is more likely with unilateral disease.

The epiphysis itself is not altered in an uncomplicated case. The epiphyseal cartilage plate shows fragmentation, reduplication, and folding, with occasional islands of cartilage being displaced into the epiphysis. Slipping of the epiphysis thus follows disruption of the epiphyseal cartilage plate (Suto 1935; Ponseti and McClintock 1956). Increased vascularity with fibrous tissue and new bone formation are seen in the region of the plate. Reunion (synostosis) eventually occurs with the femoral head and neck malaligned. Complications include ischaemic necrosis of the slipped capital epiphysis and, more rarely, necrosis of the femoral and acetabular articular cartilages, which presumably results from altered synovial fluid formation. Secondary osteoarthrosis may develop.

4. Osteogenesis Imperfecta (Fragilitas Ossium)

The relatively uncommon disease of osteogenesis imperfecta is inherited as an autosomal dominant and is variable in severity and time of onset. It is often somewhat artifically subdivided into prenatal (osteogenesis imperfecta fetalis) and postnatal (osteogenesis imperfecta tarda) types.

In the severe fetal type, multiple fractures take place in utero or at birth. The infant is small and underweight, with shortened deformed limbs and ribs showing fractures at various stages of healing (Fig. 10.6). Fractures first appear in infancy and childhood in the less severe form and the patient becomes short in stature because of skeletal deformities, which comprise mainly malaligned fractures of the lower limb and abnormal curvatures of the vertebral column. The fractures are provoked by minimal physical force.

Blue sclerae are present in both types and are seen in practically all surviving postnatal cases. Severe bone disease may be associated with white sclerae (Ibsen 1967; King and Bobechko 1971). Deafness may result from otosclerosis in late childhood and adolescence.

The basic defect found on pathological examination is one of ossification, disordered osteoblastic activity resulting in the laying down of poorly

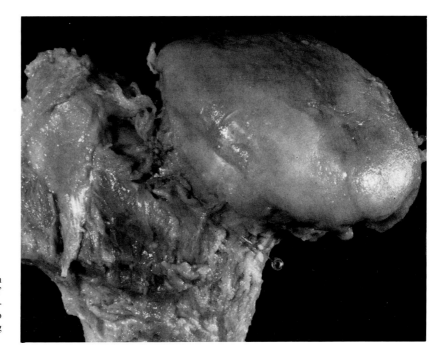

Fig. 10.5. Femoral head from an adult male with a history of Perthes' disease in childhood, showing typical flattening of the femoral head to a mushroom shape and shortening of the femoral neck.

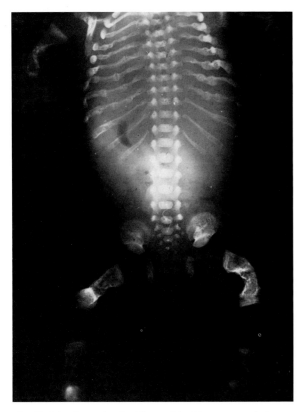

Fig. 10.6. Radiograph of stillborn girl with osteogenesis imperfecta showing fractured left femur, right humerus, and multiple healed fractures of the ribs.

organized collagen in deficient amounts. In the fetal form, the skull comprises either a thin shell of individual bones separated by wide sutures and large fontanelles or only a fibrous membrane containing small islands of bone. The easily cut long bones show a thinned cortex and sparse trabecular bone. The epiphyseal–metaphyseal junctions are sharply delineated in the normal way but bone is meagre on microscopical examination.

Little pathological information is available on the changes present in the less severe postnatal form of the disorder. Those post-mortem and amputation specimens examined show failure of proper organization of the cortical bone into haversian systems.

Biochemical investigations have shown differences in collagen synthesis in the skin of patients with osteogenesis imperfecta (Bauze et al. 1975; Penttinen et al. 1975) but no pronounced changes in the collagen of bone (Eastoe et al. 1973). The rate of biosynthesis of collagen is increased in the skin of patients with osteogenesis imperfecta according to Kovac et al. (1974). Dickson et al. (1975) found evidence of an abnormality of noncollagenous bone matrix proteins.

5. Osteopetrosis (Albers–Schönberg Disease; Marble Bone Disease)

Increased density of bone on radiographic examination is the characteristic feature of osteopetrosis, which often becomes apparent during infancy and has occasionally been diagnosed in utero. It may not present until late childhood, or even adult life in milder cases. The condition is sometimes subdivided into a severe infantile form (osteopetrosis fetalis) and a less severe type (osteopetrosis tarda).

In the severe neonatal form there may be hydrocephalus, anaemia, hepatosplenomegaly, lymphadenopathy, blindness, fractures, and growth retardation. Fracture, usually of a long bone, is often the first manifestation. Anaemia is related to displacement of bone marrow by dense bone, and when it is severe, extremedullary haematopoiesis is responsible for the hepatomegaly and superficial lymphadenopathy. Cranial nerve injury occurs and most often this takes the form of optic nerve atrophy owing to narrowing of the optic foramen, though any nerve can be similarly involved.

Bony encroachment of the sella turcica upon the pituitary may result in hypopituitarism, which in turn explains the short stature and sexual underdevelopment of some patients with osteopetrosis. The increased density and thickening of bones, together with the features of bony encroachment in the skull, are all visible on X-rays. Radiological examination of the spine shows increased density with horizontal more radiolucent bands in the mid-zone of the vertebral bodies. The radiodensity of the long bones may be so increased that the medullary cavity cannot be distinguished.

Examination of bones from severe cases forms the basis of knowledge of the pathological processes. The cut surfaces of the long bones may show complete merging of the cortices, with dense bone in the interior replacing all myeloid tissue (Fig. 10.7). The cortex may be thickened externally by appositional periosteal bone. The vertebrae show similar changes and there is beading at the costochondral junctions. Postnatal ossification centres are retarded in development and made up of compact bone. Microscopic examination of areas of endochondral ossification show abnormally wide zones of proliferating cartilage. Areas of calcified cartilage are present in the intramedullary region and confluent masses of non-lamellar bone in relation to this show sparse cellular (osteoblastic and osteoclastic) activity.

Attention has been paid to the osteoclasts in osteopetrosis at the light and electron microscopic

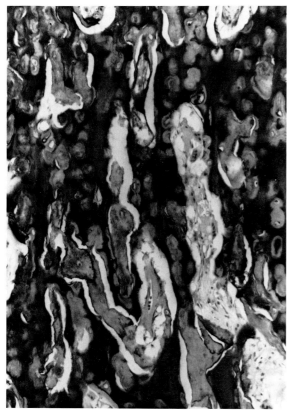

Fig. 10.7. Dense bone in the interior of the shaft of the femur in the severe infantile form of osteopetrosis, showing replacement of the myeloid tissue. (von Kossa; 400 ×)

levels (Bonucci et al. 1975; Shapiro et al. 1980). Although numbers of these cells are present, they lack ruffled borders, suggesting that they are functionally defective (Shapiro et al. 1980). There are lethal forms of osteopetrosis in rodents (Milhaud and Labat 1978; Loutit and Nisbet 1979) and in these animals the basic defect appears to be a failure of endosteal bone resorption. Injection of bone marrow cells from normal littermates into osteopetrotic rats (Milhaud et al. 1975) and mice (Walker 1975) has proved an effective way of restoring resorptive activity. Bone marrow transplantation has been applied recently with some success to the treatment of the lethal form of osteopetrosis in human infants (Ballet et al. 1977; Coccia et al. 1980).

6. Inborn Errors of Metabolism

The errors of metabolism affecting lipid and mucopolysaccharide will be dealt with in this section.

Other disorders that may have effects on the skeletal system include alkaptonuria, in which pigmentation of cartilages, disc calcification, and premature development of arthritis occur. These changes are not a particular feature of the disease in childhood, though patients are of short stature in adult life because of the effects of the disease process on development.

6.1. The Mucopolysaccharidoses (p. 621)

Classification of the mucopolysaccharidoses is becoming more complicated and the number of deficiencies recognized increases as biochemical investigations are carried out. The mucopolysaccharidoses comprise a group in which there is excessive intracellular storage of mucopolysaccharide (glycosaminoglycan). The biochemical basis of this group of disorders is considered briefly below, followed by descriptions of individual disease entities.

6.1.1. Biochemical Abnormalities in the Mucopolysaccharidoses

All the classified mucopolysaccharidoses, with the exception of Morquio's syndrome, involve a disturbance in the lysosomal catabolism of dermatan sulphate and heparan sulphate, either singly or together. Both are polymers made up of alternating sulphated hexosamine (glucosamine or galactosomine) and uronic acid (glucuronic or L-iduronic acid), and the major pathways for their degradation involve lysosomal glycosidases and sulphatases acting sequentially. A distinct enzyme is required to remove each chemical group and several enzymes are needed to degrade each chain. If any one enzyme is missing the degradative sequence is interrupted, and breakdown by hyaluronidase to large fragments of the chains is the only method of catabolism available. Storage of these large fragments in cells is responsible for the pathological changes. The lysosomal defects and the primarily affected metabolites are summarized in Table 10.6, which also gives some clinical features of the disorders and their modes of inheritance. Further details of the biochemical disorders present in the mucopolysaccharidoses are available in the articles by Neufeld (1974) and Neufeld et al. (1975).

Table 10.6. The mucopolysaccharidoses: Features, inheritance, and biochemical defects

Disorder	Features	Inheritance	Enzyme defect	Metabolite affected

Hurler's syndrome	Dwarfism
	Mental retardation
	Hepatosplenomegaly
	Corneal opacities
	Altered facies
	Skeletal changes, including
	  bowed limbs and kyphosis
	  (see text)
		Autosomal
		recessive
			α-L-Iduronidase	Dermatan
				sulphate
				
				Heparan
				sulphate

Hunter's syndrome	Dwarfism
	Mental retardation
	Hepatosplenomegaly
	Altered facies
	Cardiac abnormalities,
	  deafness
	Corneal changes *not* present
	  (see text)
	(Slower course than Hurler's)
		Sex-linked
		recessive
			Iduronate
			sulphatase
				Dermatan
				sulphate
				
				Heparan
				sulphate

Sanfilippo's syndrome	Severe mental deficiency Deafness Altered facies Few skeletal changes	Autosomal recessive	Heparan N-sulphatase or N-acetyl-α-glucosaminidase (2 subtypes)	Heparan sulphate
Scheie's syndrome	Normal stature Normal intelligence Corneal opacities Hepatosplenomegaly Claw hands, hypertrichosis Variable skeletal changes	Autosomal recessive	α-L-Iduronidase	Dermatan sulphate Heparan sulphate

Maroteaux–Lamy	No mental retardation
	Growth retardation
	Altered facies
	Lumbar kyphosis, short
	  limbs
	Corneal and auditory
	  involvement variable
		Autosomal
		recessive
			N-Acetylgalactosamine
			sulphatase
				Dermatan
				sulphate

Morquio's
syndrome
	Dwarfism
	Kyphoscoliosis, flat
	  vertebrae
	No limb shortening
	Hip deformity
	Mental retardation not
	  usually present
		Autosomal
		recessive
			N-Acetylhexosaminase
			6-SO_4-sulphatase
				Keratan
				sulphate

6.1.2. Hurler's Syndrome (Gargoylism)

Features of Hurler's syndrome become manifest in the early years of life, though affected individuals are considered normal for some months after birth. The clinical features comprise skeletal abnormalities, corneal opacities, hepatosplenomegaly, and progressive mental retardation. The face becomes altered in appearance, with wide-set eyes, depressed nose, bulging cheeks, large mouth, and thick lips. Subsequently bowing deformities of the limbs, shortness of the neck, dorsolumbar kyphosis, stubbiness of the fingers, and limitation of joint movement develop. Retardation of growth, the spinal changes, and the bowing of the lower limbs all contribute to dwarfism.

Radiological features include generalized rarefaction of tubular bones with widening of their metaphyseal ends, delay in the appearance of epiphyseal ossification centres, and later cortical thinning with rounded or tapered ends to long bones. The kyphosis is the result of failure of ossification of the anterior half of at least one vertebral body (usually D_{12} or L_1), which gives rise to a conspicuous 'beak-like' appearance on X-ray examination. Sagittal section of the lumbar vertebral bodies reveals oval and irregular outlines and the presence of cartilage, not bone, in the upper anterior part of each of the beaked dorsolumbar vertebrae. The skull is thickened, sutures close prematurely, and there are osteophyte-like protrusions on the floor of the middle and posterior fossae, with narrowing of the foramen magnum. The ends of tubular bones show widened irregular epiphyseal plates and discoloured gelatinous articular cartilage, which is abnormally thick in places.

Histologically, marked disturbances of endochondral ossification are present, with loss of height in the cartilage proliferation zone at the ends of long bones and reduction in the amount of cartilage bordering epiphyseal ossification centres. Osseous tissue is present next to the epiphyseal plate and the cartilage of the epiphyseal ossification centres, there being no intermediate stages of capillary ingrowth and cartilage calcification. Collections of glycosaminoglycan-containing macrophages fill the bone-marrow spaces and similar collections in periosteal connective tissue cells may produce cortical defects. Chondrocytes are larger than normal and have a granular cytoplasm, which on electron microscopy is found to represent lysosomal vacuoles containing apparently undegraded proteoglycan (Rimoin et al. 1975). The cells seen in Sanfilippo's and Morquio's syndromes show similar changes.

6.1.3. Hunter's Syndrome

Onset of symptoms is delayed in Hunter's syndrome, but abnormal behaviour, feeding problems, and mental retardation are usually manifest by age 3 years. The features include growth retardation, coarse facial features, enlargement of the head, hepatosplenomegaly, stiffness and contractures of the joints, cardiac abnormalities, and deafness. Corneal changes are not present.

6.1.4. Sanfilippo's Syndrome

Skeletal and visceral lesions are less marked in Sanfilippo's syndrome, which is characterized by severe mental retardation, deafness, altered facies, clumsy gait, contractures, and respiratory and feeding difficulties.

6.1.5. Maroteaux–Lamy Syndrome (Polydystrophic Dwarfism)

Lack of growth between the ages of 2 and 3 years and the development of facial features of Hurler's syndrome are present in the Maroteaux–Lamy syndrome. Indeed, the lumbar kyphosis, with a wedge-shaped deformity of the dorsolumbar vertebrae (D_{12} and L_1) seen on radiology, is similar to that present in Hurler's syndrome. The limbs and the trunk are short and there is platyspondyly. Corneal and auditory involvement are variable.

6.1.6. Morquio's Syndrome

The most marked abnormalities in Morquio's syndrome occur in the vertebral column, in which there is kyphoscoliosis, most marked in the dorsolumbar region. It is this change that is mostly responsible for the shortness of stature of the patients, though knock knees, dislocation of the hip, and the holding of the hips in semi-flexion all contribute, as does general growth retardation. The hands reach down to mid-thigh level, so that patients resemble rachitic rather than micromelic dwarfs.

Platyspondyly is a marked feature of the vertebral column and is more pronounced in the dorsal region. The flattened vertebral bodies are increased in diameter anteroposteriorly and transversely and have irregular upper and lower borders, which slope towards each other anteriorly. Centres of ossification are delayed in appearance and development. They may resemble multiple epiphyseal dysplasia on radiological examination.

6.2. Gaucher's Disease (p. 623)

Gaucher's disease is characterized by the presence of cerebroside-laden histiocytes in the lymphoreticular system and bone marrow. The enzyme deficiency is one of β-glucosidase and the accumulated metabolite is glucosylceramide. The clinical course of the disease varies, but it is not usually manifest until childhood.

In the skeletal system, accumulation of Gaucher's cells in the bone marrow (Fig. 10.8) may show necrosis and accompanying fibrosis. Thinning of the bone cortex in relation to the collections of Gaucher's cells may be present. The diploic spaces of the skull and medullary cavity of long bones may be replaced, and vertebral bodies so severely involved as to become collapsed. Necrosis of Gaucher's cells in the femoral head with accompanying partial collapse and deformity may simulate Perthes' disease.

6.3. Niemann–Pick Disease (p. 630)

Abnormal accumulation of phospholipid (sphingomyelin) occurs in histiocytes in the lymphoreticular system. Little information is available on the

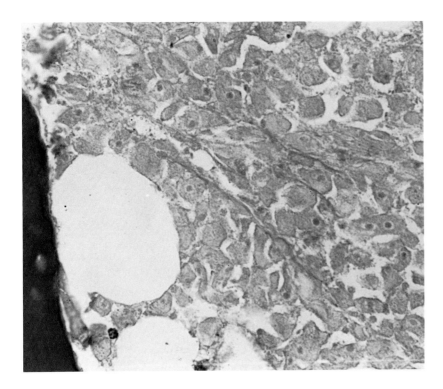

Fig. 10.8. Replacement of the bone marrow by Gaucher cells, with necrosis of adjacent bone. (Azan; 1000 ×)

pathological appearances of the bones in this condition. Accumulation of lipid-laden cells in the bone marrow causes this to show yellow-coloured areas, and thinning of cortical and trabecular bone is seen. The appearance of secondary ossification centres is delayed but this is related to general poor health (see p. 552) rather than to specific bone effects. Collapse of the femoral head has not been described and localized areas of bone marrow infiltration are not seen, in distinction from Gaucher's disease.

6.4. Hypophosphatasia

In hypophosphatasia, a group of inborn errors of metabolism that have an autosomal recessive mode of inheritance, there is a deficiency in alkaline phosphatase in both the blood and the tissues. These conditions are fatal in infancy when severe, but milder cases survive into adult life. The current state of knowledge concerning the biochemical abnormalities is discussed by Gorodischer et al. (1976).

Extensive skeletal involvement is present at birth in the affected neonate, which has a globular head, soft calvarium, shortening and bowing of the limbs, and costochondral beading. Externally, clinical features may suggest a diagnosis of achondroplasia, but radiological examination shows poorly mineralized, underdeveloped bones, sometimes with fractures and deformities in long bones. Widening of

epiphyseal growth plates with a disorderly arrangement of cells and failure of mineralization of cartilage matrix are present on pathological examination. Nephrocalcinosis is related to the hypercalcaemia present.

When the underlying defect is less severe, skeletal changes are not evident until some time after birth. In older infants and young children there may be only slight widening of epiphyseal cartilage plates (Fig. 10.9). The cortices of the long bones are thinner and more porotic than normal, and the epiphyses more radiolucent. Histological examination has shown changes similar to those occurring in rickets.

7. Metabolic Disorders Related to Bones

7.1. Rickets

Rickets is a disorder affecting endochondral ossification in growing long bones and membranous ossification in some bones. Its pathogenesis varies and includes renal and intestinal causes. Nutritional rickets principally affects infants and young children (6 months to 3 years) who may have insufficient exposure to sunlight, or pigmented skin in areas of moderate sunshine, concomitant low vitamin D intake, and dietary calcium and phosphorus deficiency all favouring the development of the disease.

Widening of calvarial sutures and the anterior fontanelles may be the only manifestations at 3 or 4 months of age. Progressive development of deformities occurs, so that by the age of 2 years many of the features described in Table 10.7 may be present.

Table 10.7. Clinicopathological features of rickets

Craniotabes, parietal bossing, depressed anterior fontanelle, which may remain open until age 3 or 4 years
Pigeon-breasted appearance
Rickety rosary at costochondral junctions
Enlargement of ends of long bones (especially at wrists, ankles, elbows, knees)
Bow legs or knock knees
Pelvic changes giving rise to serious problems in childbirth

The long bones show enlargement of epiphyseal–metaphyseal junctions, which on histological examination show a zone of disorganized and intermingled bone and cartilage. The changes consist in:

a) Deficient calcification of the proliferating cartilage;

b) Disordered vascular penetration of cartilage with impaired chondrocyte proliferation;

c) Abnormal amounts of cartilage accumulation;

d) Deposition of osteoid in the metaphysis by osteoblasts.
Increased osteoid formation in the calvarium of an infant with rickets is shown in Fig. 10.10. Increased curvature of the shaft of long bones results from the effects of weight-bearing, there is tilting of epiphyses with misdirection of growth, and greenstick fractures are found. Bow legs (genu varum) and knock knees (genu valgum) are the most typical deformities.

Enlargement of the costochondral junction (rickety rosary) has the same pathological basis as the widening at epiphyseal–metaphyseal junctions seen in long bones. These changes at the costochondral junction initiate anterior protrusion of the sternum to give a pigeon-breast deformity.

7.2. Disorders Giving Rise to Rickets

Apart from nutritional deficiency, rickets may result from any one of a series of disease processes. Briefly, malabsorption from whatever cause may result in sufficient lack of vitamin D absorption to cause bone disease. Gluten-sensitive enteropathy and cystic fibrosis of the pancreas (fibrocystic disease) are two important conditions in this respect. Disordered renal function, including Fanconi's syndrome, may

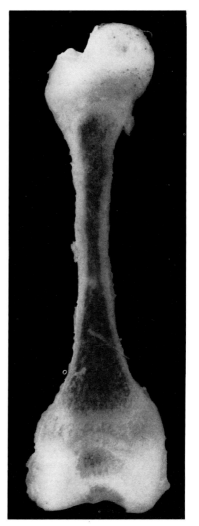

Fig. 10.9. Femur from a young child with hypophosphatasia, showing widening of the lower epiphysis.

result in rickets, while renal failure occurring in children may cause dwarfism, rickets, or the bone changes related to hyperparathyroidism, the latter more frequently in older children. A rare cause of rickets in infants and young children is congenital biliary atresia.

8. Endocrine Disorders and the Skeleton (see also Chapter 13)

8.1. Primary Hyperparathyroidism

Primary hyperparathyroidism is extremely rare in children, and a detailed description of the related

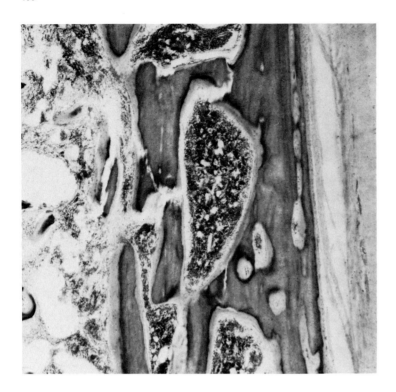

Fig. 10.10. Frontal bone of a 5-month-old boy with rickets, showing wide osteoid seams on the bone of the outer table. (von Kossa; 150 ×)

bone changes, known rather unsatisfactorily as 'osteitis fibrosa cystica' need not be given here. Reference should be made to any of the standard texts on pathology for details.

The bone lesions of hyperparathyroidism may be focal, simulating an osteoclastoma radiologically and histologically, or diffuse. The pathological process characteristically shows proliferation of spindle-cell masses, with fibrosis on bone surfaces and increased numbers of osteoclastic giant cells. Osteoblastic activity is unimpaired, so that evidence of bone regeneration may also be seen.

8.2. Secondary Hyperparathyroidism

The skeletal changes of hyperparathyroidism secondary to chronic renal disease may be conspicuous in children, and hyperparathyroidism in a child of less than 10 years is much more likely to be secondary than primary.

The changes are usually relatively mild and comprise increased resorptive activity on trabecular surfaces with fibrosis. Biochemical evidence (hypercalcaemia, hypophosphataemia, raised serum alkaline phosphatase) and radiological changes of hyperparathyroidism may be entirely lacking in patients with histological changes present on bone biopsy. In cases with protracted renal insufficiency, bone changes may be indistinguishable from those of primary hyperparathyroidism. Bone growth will

usually be stunted in these patients and there may be co-existing changes of rickets.

8.3. Hyperpituitary Gigantism

Hyperpituitarism due to an eosinophil adenoma of the adenohypophysis results in gigantism in young patients, as growth hormone has a direct stimulatory effect at the epiphyseal cartilage plates. Growth hormone-producing tumours are rare in childhood, and little is known of the detailed histopathology of the condition.

8.4. Hypopituitary Dwarfism

Hypopituitary dwarfs have normal skeletal proportions and grow at a normal rate during the first years of life. The primary causes are intracranial lesions damaging either the adenohypophysis or the hypothalamohypophyseal system and are outlined in Table 10.8.

There is delay in the appearance of postnatal ossification centres and arrest or retardation of ossification at the epiphyseal plates, which persist beyond the ages at which they would normally disappear. Since epiphyseal growth is retarded, the bone age of the child is less than the chronological age. The ossification centres are not abnormal in form, in contrast to hypothyroid dwarfism.

Table 10.8. Primary causes of hypopituitarism

Craniopharyngioma
Gliomas of the optic chiasm
Hand–Schüller–Christian disease
Pituitary chromophobe adenoma
Basal meningitis, fracture or haemorrhage
Maldevelopment of the pituitary or pituitary fossa

8.5. Hyperthyroidism

Accelerated bone growth may occur in hyper-thyroidism in childhood and adolescence. Osteoporosis may develop where hyperthyroidism is long-standing.

8.6. Hypothyroid Dwarfism

Babies with cretinism show evidence of stunted physical development and mental retardation from the very first months of life. The effects of hypo-thyroidism on the skeleton of a child are similar to those of hypopituitarism, namely, delayed appearance and retarded growth of postnatal ossification centres, retarded growth at epiphyseal cartilage plates, and persistence of these plates and calvarial sutures beyond the age at which they would normally disappear. The skull develops a brachycephalic appearance because growth retardation is more severe at the base than the vault. Postnatal ossification centres show areas of cystic degeneration of the epiphyseal cartilage, and differentiation from 'stippled epiphyses. and Perthes' disease may be difficult. Collins (1966) believed it possible that some cases of stippled epiphyses described as dysplasia epiphysealis punctata represented cases of unrecognized hypothyroidism.

8.7. Cushing's Syndrome

Osteoporosis is one of the features of Cushing's syndrome, the spine and other cancellous bone being prominently affected. Decreased osteoblastic activity with no increase in osteoclastic resorption is the basis of the abnormality. Detailed pathological changes need not be described here and are available in standard textbooks of pathology. There are no other special features to the osteoporosis occurring in Cushing's syndrome or induced by steroid treatment in childhood.

8.8. Eunuchism and Gonadal Dysgenesis

Males castrated in childhood grow tall, with a slender gracile skeletal structure. Excess growth tends to be greatest in the femur. The pelvis develops a female configuration. Epiphyseal cartilage plates persist longer than in normal development, and, in contrast to hypopituitarism and hypothyroidism, are functionally active.

Patients with gonadal dysgenesis tend to be of short stature, with radiological changes resembling dysplasia epiphysealis multiplex. Features said to be helpful in the diagnosis include hyperplasia of the first cervical vertebra, tibia vara, wrist changes, and shortening of the fourth metacarpal bone. There may be no skeletal abnormalities in some cases of gonadal dysgenesis in girls.

8.9. Adrenogenital Syndrome

Adrenal virilization associated with precocious puberty in young children is usually seen in boys. If the underlying tumour is not malignant, accelerated initial growth is followed by premature closure of epiphyseal cartilage plates, so that the patient eventually fails to reach average height.

8.10. Diabetes Mellitus

Children with diabetes mellitus of recent onset may have postnatal ossification centres present slightly ahead of the normal chronological age and be of above-average height. Postnatal ossification centres are less well developed in long-standing childhood diabetics. Growth-arrest (Harris's) lines are often present in the metaphyses of long bones.

9. Skeletal Changes in Haematological Disorders

Bone changes occur in sickle-cell anaemia, thalassaemia and haemophilia. Each is dealt with briefly below.

9.1. Sickle-cell Anaemia

The pathological features of sickle-cell anaemia may be considered under three main headings:

a) Erythroid hyperplasia of the bone marrow, resulting in local bone resorption, widening of the trabecular bone area, and thinning of the related cortical bone;

b) Blockage of small blood vessels by masses of sickle cells, giving rise to infarction in the territory supplied. Such ischaemic bone necrosis may occur in any bone and at any site. The shaft or articular ends of long bones are frequent sites of necrosis, especially the femoral head (Chung and Ralston 1969). This may resemble that seen in Perthes' disease on X-ray. Fibrous tissue replaces necrotic bone marrow and there is new bone formation;

c) Osteomyelitis, usually involving bone in which there has been infarction. The organism is frequently of the Salmonella group and the route of infection is via the blood.

The X-ray changes reflect marrow encroachment on bone, with increased radiolucency in the mandible, widening of the diploic region of the calvarium, and rarefaction of the vertebral bodies with cup-shaped outlines to their upper and lower surfaces, owing to expansion of the discs into the thinned bone.

9.2. Thalassaemia

Thalassaemia results from abnormal synthesis of either the α- or the β-chains of haemoglobin. The severity of the disease is related to whether the patient is homozygous (thalassaemia major) or heterozygous (thalassaemia minor).

Thalassaemia major is seen mainly in infants and young children who have progressive anaemia with evidence of haemolysis and hepatosplenomegaly. There may be changes in the facial bones to give a mongoloid appearance. The affected child often dies in early life. Severe cases of long duration show retarded skeletal maturation and growth.

Pathological examination of the thickened skull shows deep red hyperplastic bone marrow with thinning of the outer table. The amount of bone marrow is also increased at many other sites, including ribs, vertebrae, femora, and iliac bones. The vertebrae are porotic and show concave cup-shaped superior and inferior surfaces with thinned cortical shells like those seen in sickle-cell disease. Histological examination shows bone atrophy with hyperplastic bone marrow containing islands of foam cells and iron-laden macrophages.

The pathological changes are reflected in the radiological appearances as rarefaction of bones. The skull of the child with thalassaemia major shows thickening of the calvarium with a 'hair-on-end' appearance, comprising radially arranged striations and a poorly defined outer table.

9.3. Haemophilia

Haemorrhages may occur at any site of trauma in haemophilia, and in the skeletal system the main results are arthropathy and the relatively uncommon haemophilic pseudotumour.

The overall incidence of arthropathy in haemophilia is high. First evidence of joint involvement is unusual before age 2 years, but the incidence increases with increasing age and arthropathy is notable by 8–14 years. The knee is most commonly affected, followed by the elbow, ankle, hip, shoulder, and wrist. Initially there are simple haemarthroses, but after several episodes in a given joint, chronic haemophilic arthritis develops. The pathological findings depend on the severity and chronicity of the haemorrhages. The thickened synovial membrane is discoloured brown when repeated haemorrhages have occurred, and there is marked proliferative reactive inflammation with formation of numerous vascular pigment-stained synovial villi. Haemosiderin pigment is concentrated in the superficial layers of the synovium. The articular surface is also discoloured and may have defects filled with pigmented fibrous tissue, areas of cartilage loss down to subchondral bone, and eburnation, changes that indicate progression to osteoarthrosis.

Haemophilic pseudotumour is a haematoma that appears radiologically as a large radiolucent area expanding the affected bone. It is important because it can be mistaken for a true bone neoplasm. The local bone cortex may undergo resorption due to pressure from the haematoma, which also causes periosteal elevation. There may be an accompanying pathological fracture.

9.4. Christmas Disease

The clinical and pathological features of Christmas disease in bones and joints are essentially the same as those of haemophilia.

10. Chronic Polyarthritis

Juvenile chronic polyarthritis (juvenile rheumatoid arthritis in the United States) is a condition that presents, by definition, before the age of 16 years. There is arthritis (manifest as any two of pain, swelling, or limitation of movement) present for a minimum period of 3 months, and other diseases causing arthritis must have been excluded (see Table 10.9).

Classification within this definition is into three main subgroups according to the type of presentation, namely with

a) Systemic illness
b) Polyarthritis

Table 10.9. Conditions to be excluded in diagnosis of chronic arthritis

A.	*Infections* 1) Bacterial arthritis (including tuberculosis) 2) Viral and fungal arthritides	D.	*Haematological disorders* 1) Haemophilia 2) Sickle-cell disease
B.	*Other connective tissue disorders* 1) Systemic lupus erythematosus 2) Polymyositis and dermatomyositis 3) Sjögren's syndrome 4) Vasculitides (Henoch–Schönlein purpura, serum sickness, mucocutaneous lymph node syndrome, infantile polyarteritis) 5) Progressive systemic sclerosis 6) Mixed connective-tissue disorder 7) Polyarteritis nodosa 8) Arthritis in ulcerative colitis, regional enteritis, psoriasis, Reiter's and Behcet's syndromes 9) Rheumatic fever	E.	*Other bone and joint conditions* 1) Gout and pyrophosphate arthropathy 2) Osteochondritis 3) Slipped femoral capital epiphysis 4) Trauma: battered child syndrome, fractures, soft-tissue injuries 5) Chondromalacia patellae 6) Villonodular tenosynovitis 7) Bone tumours (osteoid osteoma, osteosarcoma, etc.)
C.	*Neoplastic disease* 1) Leukaemia 2) Lymphoma 3) Neuroblastoma		

c) Pauciarticular disease (four or fewer joints affected).

The age of onset, sex incidence, and subsequent natural history of these differ, as outlined below. The eponym Still's disease is often used interchangeably with juvenile chronic arthritis, rather than in its original and more specific sense of polyarthropathy, splenomegaly, and leukopenia.

Detailed recent information on this group of disorders may be obtained in the published proceedings of a symposium in the American Rheumatism Association (1977). A briefer account is that by Schaller (1977).

10.1. Systemic-onset Chronic Arthritis

Systemic-onset chronic arthritis is the main subgroup of childhood chronic arthritis and has the features originally described by Still. Systemic involvement consists of fever, skin rashes, lymphadenopathy, hepatosplenomegaly, and pericarditis. Lymphadenopathy is a much more prominent feature of juvenile chronic polyarthritis than of classic adult rheumatoid arthritis.

The patients are seronegative, and two-thirds are aged under 5 years at onset. Boys are affected more frequently than girls. The joints especially involved are those of the wrist and ankle, often with small joints of the toes. Hip-joint involvement and tenosynovitis of some of the flexor tendons of the hand also often occur. The cervical spine is affected fairly frequently. The earlier the onset of the disease, the more likely are erosive joint changes and alterations in growth to develop.

10.2. Polyarticular Chronic Arthritis

The subgroup of polyarticular chronic arthritis is similar to adult rheumatoid arthritis. Girls are affected more often than boys, and although the onset may be as early as 5 years of age most patients are aged 10 years or more. The presence of IgM rheumatoid factor is usually noted soon after onset and about one-fifth of cases have rheumatoid nodules at the elbow. The polyarthritis is symmetrical and involves distal limb joints (hands, feet, wrists, ankles, knees) more than proximal. Persistent activity in joints with erosive changes and joint destruction within a year of onset is common.

10.3. Pauciarticular Chronic Arthritis

Pauciarticular arthritis usually occurs in young children (age 1–5 years) and affects girls more frequently than boys. Chronic iridocyclitis, a common feature in these patients, may lead to blindness or severe visual impairment. Tests for rheumatoid factor are negative, but 80% of cases have antinuclear antibody at the time of diagnosis.

The ankles, knees, and elbows are the joints chiefly involved and the hips are rarely affected. Sacroiliitis does not develop (see Section 10.4). Those patients developing chronic iridocyclitis have a high incidence of a newly described HLA histocompatibility group, at present known as HLA-D TMLO.

10.4. Juvenile Ankylosing Spondylitis

Pauciarticular arthritis in older children may be ankylosing spondylitis. Boys are affected about five times more often than girls and the age of onset is usually 8–12 years. The lower limb joints (hips, knees, ankles) are most commonly affected, and approximately half of all cases subsequently develop sacroiliitis. Atlantaxial subluxation may occur in the late teens or early twenties. Acute iridocyclitis is seen in about 20% of cases. A quarter of these patients have a family history of ankylosing spondylitis, and 90% are of the HLA B27 histocompatibility group. Children with this disorder satisfy the criteria for a childhood chronic arthritis early in its course, and only subsequently do the features of ankylosing spondylitis become apparent (Fig. 10.11).

10.5. Pathological Appearances in Juvenile Chronic Arthritis

On macroscopical examination, the joints in juvenile chronic arthritis resemble those of rheumatoid arthritis, with pannus formation in established cases. The articular cartilage of childhood and juvenile joints is thicker than that of adults and this may have some protective effect, i.e., the joints are destroyed

more slowly and the stage of reversibility of the changes is prolonged. The histological features of the synovitis are indistinguishable from those of adult rheumatoid arthritis (Fig. 10.11). Marginal erosions, eburnation, and the development of secondary osteoarthrosis are features in the late stage, but osteophyte formation is much less pronounced than in adults. Fibrous ankylosis is fairly common where there is hip- and knee-joint involvement.

Growth arrest may occur, with premature ossification of epiphyses and changes at the epiphyseal cartilage plates. The resultant 'rheumatic dwarfism' must be distinguished from the arrest of growth brought about by long-term corticosteroid treatment.

Nodules over bony pressure points and in tendons show the classic features of rheumatoid nodules in seropositive cases, with central necrosis and pallisaded surrounding histocytes. Seronegative cases have nodules that appear more like those found in rheumatic fever, with proliferating fibroblasts and irregular areas of fibrinous exudate.

There are often early indications of cervical spinal involvement, especially in the seronegative juvenile chronic arthritis group. The apophyseal joints are primarily affected and undergo ankylosis, especially at the second and third cervical vertebrae. Subsequent loss of movement and lack of growth of the vertebrae, with later fusion of vertebral bodies may occur. Atlanto-occipital subluxation is rare in comparison with cervical subluxation in adult rheumatoid arthritis.

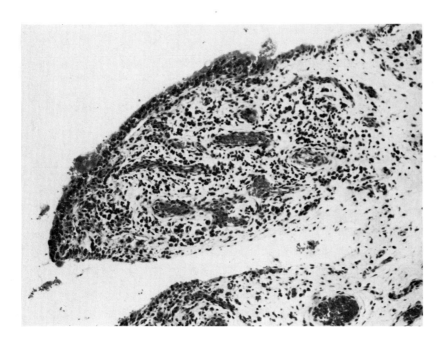

Fig. 10.11. Synovium from the knee of an 8-year-old boy presenting with monarticular arthritis, showing non-specific chronic inflammatory cell infiltrate, synovial lining cell hyperplasia and surface fibrin deposition. This patient subsequently developed features of ankylosing spondylitis and was HLA B27–positive. This case was kindly provided by Dr A. I. D. Prentice.

11. Infections of Bones and Joints

11.1. Bacterial Infections

Only special features of bone and joint infections as they occur in childhood will be described in this section. Reference should be made to standard textbooks of pathology for detailed accounts.

11.1.1. Septic Arthritis

Septic arthritis normally involves a single joint, most frequently the knee, followed by the hip, elbow, and ankle. Small joints are only rarely affected. The incidence of infection with different organisms varies with age. *Haemophilus influenzae* accounts for the vast majority of cases aged 2 years and under. *Staphylococcus aureus* is also an important organism, though it is less often involved in the very young, most such infections occurring with increasing frequency from 3 years onwards, so that older children and adolescents are most often affected. A long list of other organisms could be included, and a few are summarized in Table 10.10, the data for which have been taken from Fink et al. (1977).

Table 10.10. Organisms causing septic arthritis in childhood, (after Fink et al. 1977)

Organism	Percentage of cases affected	Notes
H. influenzae	19	95% of cases age <2 years
Staph. aureus	18	69% of cases aged 2–10 years
Streptococci	9	Approx. 30% in each of the age ranges <2, 2–5 and 6–10 years
N. gonorrhoea	5	Unusual under 2 years
Staph. epidermidis	2	80% of cases aged 0–5 years
N. meningitidis	2	80% of cases aged 0–5 years
Enterobacter spp.	2	
Salmonella spp.	1	
Others	9	
Organism unknown	33	

Septic arthritis is one of the most common complications of osteomyelitis and is much more frequent in this form in infants and young children than in adults. Since the ends of long bones are the sites of predilection for osteomyelitis, nearby joints are likely to be affected by the direct spread of organisms. Joints are otherwise involved by direct synovial infection with bloodborne organisms.

Establishment of infection in a joint leads to acute inflammation of the synovial membrane with abundant polymorphs in the synovial fluid and destruction of the articular cartilage. Abscesses may develop, depending on the responsible organism. Necrotic fragments of cartilage become sequestrated in the joint space and immobilization by fibrous adhesions and bony ankylosis may occur.

11.1.2. Osteomyelitis

Pyogenic osteomyelitis is due to *Staph. aureus* infection in the large majority of cases. Infection is usually bloodborne rather than direct from compound fractures or infected wounds. The haematogenously spread organisms lodge in the juxtaepiphyseal and metaphyseal regions of the bones.

Staphylococcal osteomyelitis is most frequent in the age range 3–15 years, though it is not rare in babies and infants. Osteomyelitis due to *Strep. pyogenes* occurs more often in babies and young children than older patients, and *H. influenzae* and *Strep. pneumoniae* infections, although less common, also occur in this age group. Children with sickle-cell anaemia are especially likely to get *Salmonella* osteomyelitis. The results recorded in a series by Fink et al. (1977) are summarized in Table 10.11.

Table 10.11. Organisms causing osteomyelitis in childhood (after Fink et al. 1977)

Organism	Percentage of cases affected	Notes
Staph. aureus	59	All ages, but nearly 70% aged 2–10 years
Streptococci	9	70% of cases less than 5 years old
Staph. epidermidis	4	70% of cases less than 2 years old
H. influenzae	3	80% of cases less than 2 years old
Pseudomonas aeruginosa	2	
Others	8	Includes *salmonella* spp., which account for 1% of cases
Organism unknown	15	

Almost any bone may become infected, but the common sites are in the lower limb (75% in the femur or tibia at their proximal or distal ends). The lumbar region is the most frequent site of haematogenous infection of the vertebral column.

When organisms lodge in the bone marrow of the metaphysis abscess formation occurs, with death and fragmentation of trabecular bone. Extension of suppuration into haversian systems causes death of large areas of cortical bone, pieces of which become separated from living bone as sequestra, while increased osteoblastic activity of surviving living bone surrounds the necrotic bone with new bone (involucrum).

The complications of osteomyelitis include septicaemia, pathological fracture, sinus formation, and the development of septic arthritis in children.

Osteomyelitis may accompany middle ear infection, sinus infection or severe dental sepsis.

11.1.3. Brodie Abscess

A chronic bone abscess (Brodie abscess) is a sharply delineated infective focus occurring predominantly in those who have not yet completed skeletal growth. It is usually solitary, and a common site is the distal end of the tibia, though other bones, including the radius and femur, may be affected. The abscess contains fluid of variable consistency and appearance and has a wall lined with inflammatory granulation tissue surrounded by a connective tissue layer and sclerotic bone.

11.1.4. Tuberculosis

Skeletal tuberculosis in children occurs mostly in the age range 3–15 years, and is rare in the first year of life. Haematogenous dissemination to bones and joints occurs in children who have a primary lesion in the lung.

The main sites of involvement are the vertebral column, the hip, and the knee. Detailed descriptions of the pathology of the disease in children will not be given here, since the histological changes are the same as in the adult. Long bones tend to be involved at the epiphyseal ends near the articular surface, while the diaphysis is the site of infection in short bones. Spinal infection starts in the vertebral bodies and spreads from the marrow cavities through the bone to extend beneath the longitudinal ligaments to the margins of the intervertebral discs. Tuberculosis almost never starts in the discs, although this is theoretically possible because the discs still have blood vessels in children.

Collapse of vertebral bodies and discs gives rise to severe spinal deformities, and extension into the related soft tissues may give rise to a paravertebral abscess.

Radiologically tuberculous involvement of the hip may be mistaken for Perthes' disease, and syphilitic arthritis (Clutton's joints) of the knee may resemble tuberculosis in children. Tuberculosis in the shaft of a long bone is often indistinguishable from pyogenic osteomyelitis.

Tuberculous involvement of synovial tissues occurs by two mechanisms, namely haematogenous and local spread, the latter from tuberculous osteomyelitis in the end of the neighbouring bone. The pathological appearances of tuberculous arthritis are variable, depending on the severity of involvement. The synovial fluid may vary from thin yellow fluid to thick purulent material. The synovial membrane may be only moderately thickened, with an inflamed injected appearance, or grossly thickened, with abundant surface fibrin. Histological examination shows typical tuberculoid granulomas, though the amount of caseation is variable. Cartilage destruction by tuberculous inflammatory tissue occurs and if it is present in a subchondral position there is undermining of the cartilage, which may become separated.

11.2. Syphilis

Congenital syphilis has become rare in developed countries but still occurs commonly in parts of Africa. The pathological features in the skeleton of the fetus, newborn, and young infant are osteochondritis, osteomyelitis of the diaphysis, and periostitis.

Osteochondritis involves all sites of endochondral ossification, which show widening of the provisional calcification zone. Where there is severe involvement, syphilitic inflammatory tissue may cause separation of the metaphysis from the epiphysis, and such epiphyseal separation occurs mostly in long bones of neonates and infants up to 3 months of age. Diaphyseal osteomyelitis arises independently or by extension of subchondral inflammation present in the late stages of osteochondritis. Foci of osteomyelitis with microscopic areas of bone necrosis result. In ossifying periostitis bone deposits are present along the shafts of long bones and the surfaces of flat bones such as the ilium.

In patients with syphilitic infection that has been mild, unrecognized, or inadequately treated during infancy, late manifestations of congenital syphilis occur, usually from 4 years of age onwards. The bone lesions are of two main types, namely gummatous and nongummatous osteomyelitis and periostitis. A number of time-honoured descriptions exist for the changes, such as saddle-nose deformity and sabre tibia. Detailed descriptions of the changes can be found in the standard texts on pathology of bone.

11.3. Viral Infections

A small percentage of children surviving smallpox have been reported to have had osteomyelitis, and foci of bone-marrow necrosis have been noted in the long bones at autopsy in patients dying with the disease. Shortening of long bones in adults who suffered from smallpox during childhood has been ascribed to changes in the epiphyses and epiphyseal–metaphyseal junctions. Bone involvement following smallpox vaccination is excessively rare (Jaffe 1972).

Rubella is well known to cause abnormalities in the developing fetus. As well as the congenital rubella syndrome, skeletal changes are evident radiologically in the metaphyseal region of long bones, where linear and ovoid areas of radiolucency appear. There is thickening of osteoid trabeculae, which are poorly mineralized (Singer et al. 1967). They disappear within a few months of birth.

Joint symptoms in viral infections are infrequent, usually acute, and self-limiting. True arthritis is unusual, arthralgia being the main manifestation. Children develop arthralgia with rubella infection or after vaccination, though less frequently than adults. Symptoms develop at about the time of appearance of circulating antibodies. Involvement is usually nonarticular and symptoms last for 1–2 weeks. Histology of the synovial membrane is nonspecific.

A serum sickness-like illness that includes polyarthralgia, and less often polyarthritis, occurs in some adults during the incubation period of type B viral hepatitis. This has also recently been recognized in children. The synovial membrane shows nonspecific vascular changes with a sparse inflammation reaction.

Certain arboviruses commonly cause arthritis in Africa and Australia, but not in the Western Hemisphere. Children are affected less frequently and less severely than adults. The viruses are mosquito-borne and comprise Chikungunya and O'nyong nyong in Africa and Ross River (epidemic polyarthritis) in Australia.

Rare cases of arthritis have been reported in children with mumps and chickenpox. The reader is referred to the recent review of viral arthritis in children by Phillips (1977) for further details and references to these conditions.

12. Tumours and Tumour-like Conditions

Many tumours other than those described here may occasionally affect children, but the majority of neoplasms seen in childhood fall into the categories described.

12.1. Chrondroblastoma

Chondroblastoma is a rare tumour, affecting males more often than females and usually occurring in the epiphyseal part of a bone. The femur, humerus, and tibia are the most common sites. The age range is 10–20 years. Radiologically there is a radiolucent defect in the epiphyseal region, which may extend into the metaphysis and be surrounded by a narrow margin of sclerosis. Macroscopically, this well-demarcated lesion has a gritty blue-grey or grey-brown surface. Microscopy shows it to be composed of chondroblasts, which are polygonal, round, or spindle-shaped, with oval nuclei (Fig. 10.12). Some chondroid matrix and giant cells are also present. Spotty calcification is a helpful feature in the differential diagnosis (Spjut et al. 1970).

12.2. Chondromyxoid Fibroma

Chondromyxoid fibroma is a localized benign tumour characterized by lobulated areas of spindle-shaped or stellate cells and abundant myxoid or

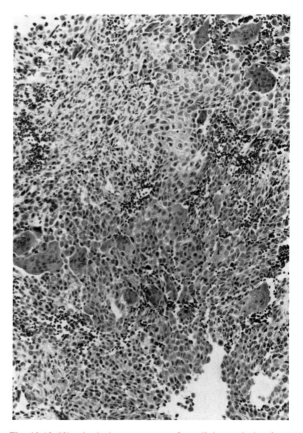

Fig. 10.12. Histological appearances of a radiolucent lesion from the region of the lower femoral epiphysis of a 15-year-old girl, showing polygonal and spindle-shaped chondroblasts, with intermingled giant cells. Chondroblastoma. (H and E; 400 ×)

chondroid intercellular matrix. These areas are separated by more cellular tissue with abundant spindle-shaped cells and variable numbers of giant cells.

Chondromyxoid fibroma occurs in the 10- to 30-year age group and the sexes are more or less equally affected. The metaphyseal region of a long bone, especially in the lower limb, is a common site (Spjut et al. 1970). It is a well-circumscribed, lobulated solid grey-white to tan mass that expands and erodes the cortex of the bone.

Confusion with chondrosarcoma may occur when large pleomorphic tumour cells are present (Jaffe and Lichtenstein 1948).

Recurrence may occur after curettage, but cases with malignant change have been questioned as not being true examples (Dahlin 1967). Sarcomatous change, if it occurs, is a pathological rarity (Dahlin 1978).

12.3. Osteochondroma (Osteocartilaginous Exostosis)

Osteochondromas are cartilage-capped bony projections. They are fairly common and occur most frequently in childhood; their growth usually ceases at the time of skeletal maturation. Osteochondromas are located on the external surface of the metaphyseal portions of long bones, commonly at the lower end of the femur, upper tibia, and upper humerus (Fig. 10.13) (Dahlin 1978). They may be solitary or multiple, multiple tumours occurring in the condition known as multiple osteocartilaginous exostosis (diaphyseal aclasis; hereditary deforming dyschondroplasia; hereditary multiple exostoses).

Patients with this particular disorder may have bowing and shortening of the extremities and pelvic or pectoral girdle asymmetry (Spjut et al. 1970).

Malignant change is rare in solitary osteochondroma and occurs more frequently in cases with multiple exostoses (Jaffe 1958; Dahlin 1978). Cartilaginous exostoses have been described in children (usually less than 3 years of age) following radiotherapy for neuroblastoma, Wilm's tumour, and eosinophilic granuloma. They occur within or near the field of radiation treatment (Murphy and Blount 1962; Cole and Darte 1963).

12.4. Osteoid Osteoma

Osteoid osteoma is a benign osteoblastic tumour, which is clearly demarcated, less than 1 cm in diameter (Byers 1968) and surrounded by new bone formation. Males are affected two or three times more often than females. The great majority of cases occur between the ages 5 and 24 years (Byers 1968), and the diaphyses of long bones in the lower limb (tibia, femur) are most often involved. The lesions are generally painful.

A friable red-grey discrete 'nidus' surrounded by sclerotic new bone is seen on macroscopic examination, and gives the radiologically classic appearance of a small central radiolucent or dense area with a dense periphery. Histologically the nidus is composed of cellular, highly vascular tissue containing islands of closely associated osteoid trabeculae having irregular borders and surrounded by osteoblasts. Some calcification may be present and there is no evidence of cartilage formation. Well-organized newly formed trabeculae make up the surrounding

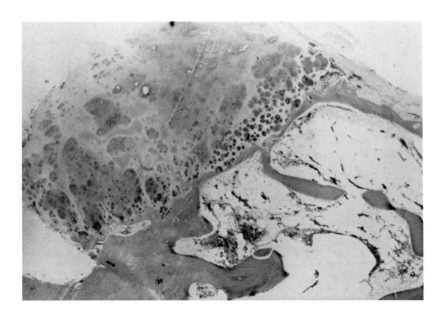

Fig. 10.13. Osteochondroma from the upper end of the humerus of a 15-year-old boy. (H and E; 100 ×)

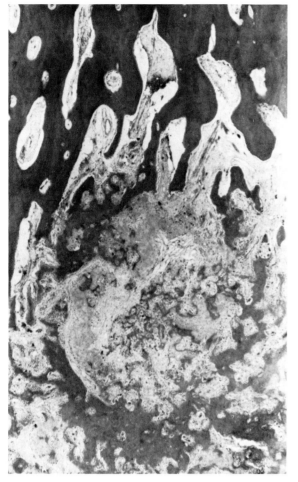

Fig. 10.14. Painful lesion from the mid-shaft region of the tibia of a 20-year-old male, showing central nidus of an osteoid osteoma with surrounding sclerotic bone. (H and E; 100 ×)

sclerotic bone (Spjut et al. 1970; Schajowicz et al. 1972) (Figs. 10.14 and 10.15).

12.5. Osteoblastoma

Osteoblastoma is related to osteoid osteoma and there are no specific histological criteria for their separation. The chief differences are the site, clinical presentation, radiological appearance, and changes in the surrounding bone. Reactive new bone is usually absent in relation to osteoblastomas.

The vertebrae, ilium, ribs, and bones of the hand and foot are most commonly affected by osteoblastoma and the patients are usually aged 10–35 years (Jaffe 1958; Lichtenstein 1965; Spjut et al. 1970). Some pain may be present but this is not as marked a feature as in osteoid osteoma. The radiological appearances lack specificity and may be mistaken for those of osteosarcoma, aneurysmal bone cyst, chondrosarcoma, or osteoid osteoma (Pochachevsky et al. 1960).

The lesions are usually over 1 cm in diameter, well circumscribed, and have a dark purple, red-grey or brown gritty cut surface. On histological examination the highly vascular osteoblastic stroma shows formation of osteoid and primitive bone, so that the tumour closely resembles osteoid osteoma (Jaffe 1958; Spjut et al. 1970).

12.6. Osteosarcoma (Osteogenic Sarcoma)

Osteosarcoma is a malignant tumour showing evidence of osteoid or bone formation by the tumour

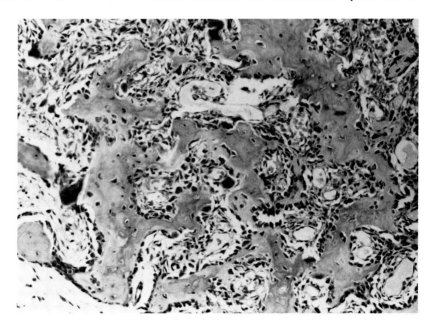

Fig. 10.15. High-power view of the nidus of an osteoid osteoma, showing vascular fibrous tissue containing irregular trabeculae of osteoid surrounded by osteoblasts. (H and E; 400 ×)

cells. Most cases occur between the ages 10 and 20 years and boys are affected more often than girls. Any bone can be affected but the metaphyseal ends of long bones (lower femur, upper tibia, upper femur, upper humerus) are the most frequently involved, especially in young patients (see Table 10.12). The most common symptoms are pain and local swelling.

Radiological appearances usually include evidence of bone destruction, new bone formation in relation to cortical destruction, and subperiosteal new bone formation. These X-ray appearances are often thought to be specific, but a large minority of cases have none of the characteristic features, and occasional cases have the appearances of a benign lesion.

Macroscopically, the tumour arises centrally and has usually penetrated the cortex and invaded soft tissues by presentation. The naked-eye appearances vary with the amount of cartilaginous, fibrous, or osseous tissue in the tumour. Some are highly vascular. The histological features are also variable, depending on the amount of tumour bone production, the pleomorphism of the tumour cells, and the extent to which fibrous, myxoid, and cartilaginous elements are present (Spjut et al. 1970; Schajowicz et al. 1972). Classically, a malignant stroma of spindle-shaped and oval cells with variable numbers of mitoses and some multinucleate cells contains malignant osteoid or bone. The bone consists of islands of these osseous tissues surrounded by pleomorphic osteoblasts. Some tumours may contain vascular areas with numerous thin-walled vessels. Telangiectatic osteogenic sarcoma, having cystic spaces lined with anaplastic spindle cells, has a poorer prognosis according to Matsuno et al. (1976).

Histochemical studies have demonstrated the presence of alkaline phosphatase in tumour cells (Jeffree and Price 1965), and if available, this method may help in the identification of osteosarcoma.

Osteosarcoma metastasizes almost exclusively by the haematogenous route and 90% of cases die with secondary deposits in the lung. Metastases sometimes occur in other organs, other bones, and lymph nodes.

12.7. Ewing's Sarcoma

Ewing's sarcoma, an uncommon primary malignant bone tumour, arises in almost any bone, although the mid-shaft or metaphysis of the femur, humerus, and tibia, the ilium, and the ribs are the usual sites. Children and adolescents are most often affected, two-thirds of cases presenting before the age of 20 years (Dahlin et al. 1961; Spjut et al. 1970). The radiological appearances are nonspecific (see, e.g., Vohra 1967) and may be mistaken for those of osteosarcoma, chondrosarcoma, malignant lymphoma, osteomyelitis, or eosinophilic granuloma of bone.

Macroscopically, the tumour is situated in the medullary cavity, and is soft and grey-white in

Table 10.12. Site of involvement with osteosarcoma in five large series (percentage of cases)

	Hayles et al. (1960)[a]	Lindbom et al. (1961)	Weinfeld and Dudley (1962)	McKenna et al. (1966)	Dahlin and Coventry (1967)
Skull			1	<1	2
Jaw	2		7	5	
Vertebra	1		3		3
Sternum		3			
Clavicle	1	3		<1	<1
Ribs	1	2		2	2
Scapula		3		1	2
Humerus	10	13	11	13	11
Radius					1
Ulna		3	2	<1	<1
Wrist and hand			3		<1
Pelvis	4	5	5	3	9
Femur	58	39	45	52	46
Tibia	22	26	17	18	19
Fibula	1		4	3	6
Ankle and foot	1	2	1	1	1
Total number of cases	129	96	94	258	600

[a]Specifically children (aged <16 years).

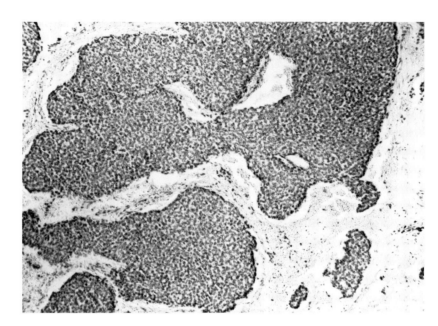

Fig. 10.16. Replacement of the bone marrow by sheets of small round cells in Ewing's sarcoma. (H and E; 80×)

colour, with haemorrhagic areas sometimes present. On histological examination the tumour is found to be made up of small round cells (Figs. 10.16 and 10.17), which are larger than lymphocytes and present in sheets, cords and nests, characteristically separated by fibrous septa. It is richly vascular and may show the presence of a rosette pattern due to the collection of tumour cells around vascular spaces. The chief problems in the histological differential diagnosis are metastatic neuroblastoma, poorly differentiated lymphoma, and metastatic carcinoma, notably oat-cell carcinoma, though this usually occurs in a much older age group (Spjut et al. 1970).

Careful attention to the clinical details, especially the possible presence of an adrenal mass, is required in the differential diagnosis of neuroblastoma and Ewing's sarcoma. The determination of levels of catecholamine metabolites is a useful discriminant (Gitlow et al. 1970) and should be recommended to clinicians. The formation of rosettes in neuroblastoma is often quoted as a feature (e.g., Spjut et al. 1970). While this may be true of primary neuroblastoma, metastatic tumour is not likely to show this appearance (Jaffe 1958). The presence of glycogen granules in the cells of Ewing's sarcoma has been demonstrated by Schajowicz (1959) by light microscopy, and confirmed in an ultrastructural study by Friedman and Gold (1968). The demonstration of glycogen granules by electron microscopy is of limited value according to Llombart-Roche et al. (1978). Reticulum-cell sarcoma of bone contains no glycogen (Schajowicz 1959) and there are PAS-positive granules present in neuroblastomas (Spjut

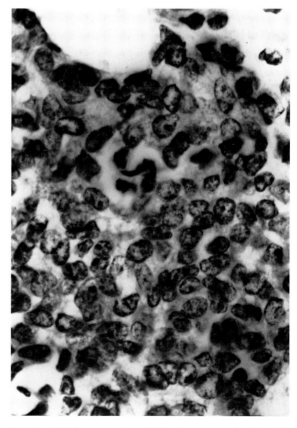

Fig. 10.17. High-power view of Ewing's sarcoma, showing cells with indistinct cytoplasmic outlines and well-defined nuclear membranes. (H and E; 1500×)

et al. 1970). The paper by Llombart-Roche et al. (1978) describes the ultrastructural features of Ewing's sarcoma and discusses the differentiation from reticulum-cell sarcoma and other round-cell sarcomas. Differentiation of Ewing's sarcoma from lymphoblastic lymphoma may be difficult. Lennert (1978) states that Ewing's sarcoma and metastatic neuroblastoma show cells tightly packed together, whereas the cells of lymphoblastic lymphoma of convoluted-cell type (see Chap. 12) are isolated from one another. Lymphoblastic lymphoma of Burkitt type may also sometimes be present in bone marrow. Convoluted-cell lymphoblastic lymphoma shows the presence of a diastase-resistant PAS-positive reaction in a single clumped pattern in the cytoplasm of tumour cells. The cells of Burkitt-type lymphoblastic lymphoma are not PAS-positive (Lennert 1978).

More than a quarter of patients with Ewing's sarcoma have metastases at the time of presentation. Common sites are other bones (especially the skull), the lungs, lymph nodes, and other viscera.

Rarely the tumour may present as an extraskeletal lesion.

12.8. Reticulum-cell Sarcoma (Primary Malignant Lymphoma)

Malignant lymphoma primarily involving bone is a rare occurrence in childhood, especially under 10 years of age. The classification of malignant lymphomas is in general a subject of debate in pathology, and nowhere is this more so than in the case of poorly differentiated lymphoreticular malignancies. The term reticulum-cell sarcoma is usually considered synonymous with poorly differentiated lymphoma.

Reticulum-cell sarcoma of bone presents as a focally destructive lesion on X-ray examination and on naked eye examination is a homogeneous grey or reddish-grey with areas of necrosis. The histological appearances are varied. The round pleomorphic tumour cells have nuclei with prominent nucleoli, and are mixed to a variable degree with other cells, including lymphocytes and occasional multinucleate giant cells in some tumours. The appearances in some cases are similar to those in poorly differentiated malignant lymphomas, while in others derivation from the histiocyte line is suggested. Differentiation of reticulum-cell sarcoma of bone from Ewing's sarcoma is partly aided by special stains. Stains for glycogen are usually positive and reticulin is sparse in the latter; whereas reticulin staining, though variable, is often increased in reticulum-cell sarcoma of bone. For further details of the lymphoreticular neoplasms see Chap. 12.

12.9. Leukaemia

Most children with acute leukaemia have radiographic bone changes. Leukaemic infiltration results in a rounded osteolytic lesion seen in X-rays and failure of normal bone formation with radiolucent lines near the epiphyses. There may be large areas of bone necrosis (Thomas et al. 1961).

12.10. Tumour-like Conditions

12.10.1. Histiocytic Disorders

The histiocytic disorders are nonneoplastic conditions characterized by the abnormal proliferation of the monocyte–macrophage (histiocyte) series. The histiocytic disorders have been recently reviewed by Cline and Golde (1973). They include Letterer–Siwe disease, Hand–Schüller–Christian disease, and eosinophilic granuloma, and are sometimes collectively known as 'histiocytosis X'. Although they may be related pathologically, they are quite distinct in clinical manifestations (p. 554).

The unifying aspect of this group of disorders is the presence of histiocytes with no cytological features of malignancy, intermingled with variable numbers of eosinophils, giant cells, neutrophils, foamy macrophages, and areas of fibrosis. The histiocytes contain intracytoplasmic granules of a characteristic appearance and similar to those seen in Langerhans cells of the skin (Basset et al. 1972). The ultrastructural appearances have recently been described by Corrin and Basset (1979) and the enzyme histochemistry of the cells by Elema and Poppema (1979).

12.10.1.1. Letterer–Siwe Disease. Most cases of Letterer–Siwe disease present in infancy or early childhood (up to the age of 2 years), and occasional congenital cases have been described. Most affected infants die within weeks or months of the onset; a few survive for 1 or 2 years. The clinical features are those of a febrile illness with a skin rash, hepatosplenomegaly, lymphadenopathy, a bleeding diathesis with purpura, and 'tumours' of bones. These last are destructive lesions present especially in the calvarium, mandible, and basisphenoid regions of the skull.

The basic pathological finding is one of generalized increases in non-lipid-containing macrophages in the many affected organs, either as nodules or diffusely. Small numbers of lymphocytes, plasma cells, and eosinophils are intermingled with the histiocytes. The histiocytes may contain phagocytosed material including red cells or haemosiderin. Long-standing lesions may have fibrous scarring and foamy histiocytes resembling those seen in Hand–Schüller–Christian disease.

12.10.1.2. Hand–Schüller–Christian Disease.

Hand–Schüller–Christian disease is a rare histiocytic disorder of childhood, the great majority of cases occurring in the age group 4–10 years. In its classic form it comprises the triad of diabetes insipidus, exophthalmos, and defects in bone, notably of the skull, but it is rare for all these features to be present in a single case. Radiologically, the common sites of the osteolytic lesions are the calvarium, petrous and mastoid bones, mandible, and maxilla.

The histological features differ from those of Letterer–Siwe disease although there is some similarity. The lesions consist of focal accumulations of histiocytes (Fig. 10.18), many with a foamy cytoplasm, and collagenous fibrous tissue. Some lymphocytes, plasma cells, neutrophils, and eosinophils may be present.

12.10.1.3. Eosinophilic Granuloma.

Eosinophilic granuloma of bone generally presents before the age of 10 years, usually as a single focus, but multifocal changes are not rare. Almost any bone can be affected, and common sites are the calvarium, mandible, ribs, femur, humerus, pelvis, and vertebrae (Table 10.13). The lesion nearly always occurs in the shaft when present in a long bone. Epiphyseal involvement is very rare (Ochsner 1966). Vertebral involvement may lead to collapse of vertebral bodies into a wedge-shape. Multifocal disease suggests an overlap with Hand–Schüller–Christian disease. The lesions are osteolytic on radiological examination and may be round and confined to the bone (e.g., in a

Table 10.13. Common sites of eosinophilic granuloma

Frontal and parietal bones
Mandible
Humerus
Ribs
Proximal metaphysis of femur

long bone). There may be radiographic confusion with osteomyelitis and Ewing's sarcoma (Spjut et al. 1970).

The findings on histological examination are variable and depend on the age of the lesion, the presence of repair reactions, and whether there has been pathological fracture. In a typical case there are sheets of large histiocytes with which eosinophils and multinucleate giant cells are mixed (Fig. 10.19). The histiocytes have large single or double nuclei and many contain phagocytosed red or white cells. Variable numbers of neutrophils, lymphocytes, and plasma cells may be present. When there are few eosinophils and the histiocytes predominate, appearances may resemble those of Hodgkin's disease.

12.11. Fibrous and Cystic Defects

12.11.1. Metaphyseal Fibrous Defect (Nonossifying Fibroma)

Metaphyseal fibrous defect is a nonneoplastic lesion occurring in the metaphyseal region of long bones of growing children and adolescents, the lower end of the femur or either end of the tibia being commonly affected. There may be pain or pathological fracture at presentation, but the lesions are often entirely

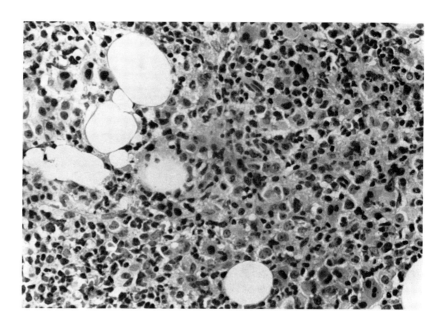

Fig. 10.18. Osteolytic lesion from the ilium comprising mainly histiocytes with small numbers of lymphocytes, neutrophils, and eosinophils. Hand–Schuller–Christian disease (histiocytosis X). (H and E; 1000 ×)

asymptomatic. Selby (1961) found such fibrous cortical defects in 27% of apparently normal children.

Metaphyseal fibrous defects take the form of well-localized osteolytic areas in the cortex or marrow space, containing fibrous tissue with a whorled appearance, multinucleate giant cells (Fig. 10.20), foamy macrophages, and haemosiderin pigment. The giant cells are widely scattered or may be present in small nests. The lesion has sometimes been confused with giant-cell tumour of bone (Spjut et al. 1970). The interlacing and whorled pattern of the stroma is a helpful feature in this differential diagnosis.

Fibrous cortical defect is a small asymptomatic lesion confined to the cortex of the bone in the region of the metaphysis. Nonossifying fibroma is considered by Jaffe (1958) to represent a more advanced form of this lesion, which is no longer confined to the cortex.

12.11.2. Fibrous Dysplasia

Fibrous dysplasia is a benign, relatively uncommon abnormality of unknown aetiology made up of fibrous tissue with a characteristic whorled pattern, which contains trabeculae of immature woven nonlamellar bone (Fig. 10.21). These islands of bone

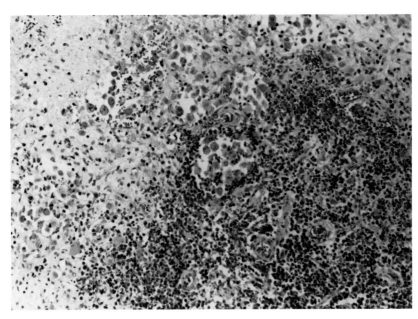

Fig. 10.19. Osteolytic lesion from the frontal bone of an 18-year-old male presenting with a palpable mass. There are numerous large histiocytes intermingled with eosinophils, some lymphocytes, and neutrophils. Eosinophilic granuloma (histiocytosis X). (H and E; 400 ×)

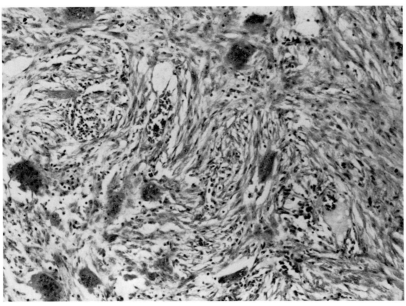

Fig. 10.20. Metaphyseal fibrous defect from the lower end of the radius of a 12-year-old girl, showing whorled pattern of fibrous tissue and giant cells. (H and E; 400 ×)

usually lack osteoblasts at the surface. Presentation is in childhood or adolescence; the condition can be monostotic or polyostotic, and is one of the commonest benign lesions of the ribs. The femur, tibia, and facial skeleton are also often affected. Dysplastic lesions at the base of the skull or in the jaw are sometimes classified as ossifying fibromas, osteoid fibromas, or fibro-osteomas. They are regarded as variants of fibrous dysplasia by Dahlin (1978). Radiological examination reveals a characteristic 'ground-glass' appearance.

Polyostotic lesions, which are predominantly unilateral, when combined with cutaneous pigmentation and, in girls, precocious puberty, form the complex known as Albright's syndrome (Albright et al. 1938; Harris et al. 1962). Osteogenic sarcoma developed in one of the cases of Harris and colleagues. The present author has seen one similar case.

12.11.3. Solitary Bone Cyst (Simple or Unicameral Bone Cyst)

Solitary bone cysts are benign and occur in children and adolescents, affecting boys three times more frequently than girls (Bosecker et al. 1968). They consist of a fluid-filled cavity most frequently situated in the metaphysis at the upper end of the humerus or femur, abutting the epiphyseal plate in many cases. Distal long bones are also sometimes affected. Fractures are present in approximately two-thirds of cases where the long bones are involved. Radiological examination is essential in the diagnosis of solitary bone cyst (Lodwick 1958).

The cyst is lined with loose vascular connective tissue, which forms a membrane of variable thickness and may contain giant cells, osteoid and bone trabeculae. Most of these cysts contain some granulation tissue and show evidence of previous haemorrhage, fibrin, calcified material, and cholesterol clefts (Spjut et al. 1970; Schajowicz et al. 1972).

12.11.4. Aneurysmal Bone Cyst

Aneurysmal bone cyst usually presents in patients under 30 years of age and involves the metaphyseal region of long bones and the vertebral column, but involvement of almost all bones has been described. The distribution of lesions in one large series is shown in Table 10.14. It is an eccentrically placed osteolytic lesion consisting of blood-filled spaces of variable size outlined by fibrous septa containing osteoid, bone trabeculae, or osteoclastic cells in granulation tissue. Differentiation from a giant-cell tumour of bone may be difficult or impossible, especially where curettings are submitted for a histological opinion. As with other bone tumours, the examination of adequate biopsy material and careful review of clinical and radiological features are essential for a correct diagnosis (see Spjut et al. 1970; Reed and Rothenberg 1964; Dahlin 1978).

Table 10.14. Distribution of aneurysmal bone cyst in 193 cases (Dabska and Buraczewski 1969)

Lower limb	53%
Vertebrae	27%
Upper limb	18%
Thorax	9%
Pelvis	7%
Skull and mandible	3%

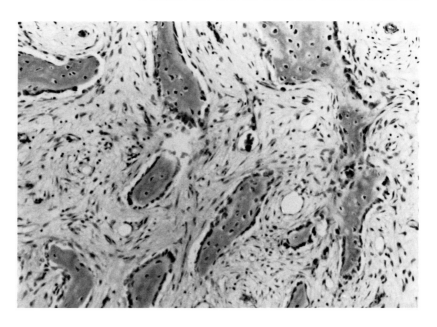

Fig. 10.21. Slowly growing lesion from the mandible of a 7-year-old male showing the presence of immature osseous trabeculae in fibrous tissue. The trabeculae show the presence of appositional osteoblasts. Fibro-osseous dysplasia (ossifying fibroma). (H and E; 400×)

References

Acheson RM (1957) The Oxford method of assessing skeletal maturity. Clin Orthop 10: 19

Albright F, Scoville B, Sulkowitch HW (1938) Syndrome characterized by osteitis fibrosa disseminata, areas of pigmentation and a gonadal dysfunction. Further observations including the report of two more cases. Endocrinology 22: 411

American Rheumatism Association (1977) [Proceedings of a symposium devoted to pediatric rheumatology.] Arthritis Rheum 20/2: [Suppl]

Ballet JP, Griscelli C, Coutris G, Milhaud G, Maroteaux P (1977) Bone marrow transplantation in osteopetrosis. Lancet 2: 1137

Basset F, Escaig J, Le Crom M (1972) A cytoplasmic membranous complex in histiocytosis X. Cancer 29: 1380

Bauze RJ, Smith R, Francis MJO (1975) A new look at osteogenesis imperfecta. J Bone Joint Surg [Br] 57: 2

Beighton P (1978) Inherited disorders of the skeleton. Churchill Livingstone, Edinburgh London New York (Genetics in medicine and surgery series)

Berry CL (1978) Drugs and the developing skeleton. Invest Cell Pathol 1: 129

Bonucci E, Sartori E, Spina M (1975) Osteopetrosis fetalis. Report on a case, with special reference to the ultrastructure. Virchows Arch [Pathol Anat] 368: 109

Boseker EH, Bickel WH, Dahlin DC (1968) A clinico-pathologic study of simple unicameral bone cysts. Surg Gynecol Obstet 127: 550

Byers PD (1968) Solitary benign osteoblastic lesions of bone. Osteoid osteoma and benign osteoblastoma. Cancer 22: 43

Chung SMK, Ralston EL (1969) Necrosis of the femoral head associated with sickle cell anaemia and its genetic variants. J Bone Joint Surg [Am] 51: 33

Cline MJ, Golde DW (1973) A review and re-evaluation of the histiocytic disorders. Am J Med 55: 49

Coccia PF, Krivit W, Cervenka, J, Clawson C, Kersey JH, Kim TH, Nesbit ME, Ramsay NKC, Warkentin PI, Teitelbaum SL, Kahn AJ, Brown DM (1980) Successful bone-marrow transplantation for infantile malignant osteopetrosis. N Engl J Med 302: 701

Cole ARC, Darte JMM (1963) Osteochondromata following irradiation in children. Pediatrics 32: 285

Collins DH (1966) Pathology of bone. Butterworths, London

Corrin B, Basset F (1979) A review of histiocytosis X with particular reference to eosinophilic granuloma of the lung. Invest Cell Pathol 2: 137

Cremin BJ, Beighton P (1978) Bone dysplasias of infancy. A radiological atlas. Springer, Berlin Heidelberg New York

Dabska M, Buraczewski J (1969) Aneurysmal bone cyst. Pathology, clinical course and radiologic appearances. Cancer 23: 371

Dahlin DC (1967) Chondromyxoid fibroma. In: Bone tumours, 2 edn. Thomas, Springfield Ill

Dahlin DC (1978) Bone tumours, 3rd edn. Thomas, Springfield Ill

Dahlin DC, Coventry MB (1967) Osteogenic sarcoma. A study of six hundred cases. J Bone Joint Surg [Am] 49: 101

Dahlin DC, Coventry MB, Scanlon PW (1961) Ewing's sarcoma. A critical analysis of 165 cases. J Bone Joint Surg [Am] 43: 185

Dickson IR, Millar EA, Veis A (1975) Evidence for abnormality of bone matrix proteins in osteogenesis imperfecta. Lancet 2: 586

Eastoe JE, Martens P, Thomas NR (1973) The amino-acid composition of human hard tissue collagens in osteogenesis imperfecta and dentigenesis imperfecta. Calcif Tissue Res 12: 91

Elema JD, Poppema S (1978) Infantile histiocytosis X (Letterer–

Siwe disease). Investigation with enzyme histochemical and sheep erythrocyte rosetting techniques. Cancer 42: 555

Ellis RWB, Van Creveld S (1940) A syndrome characterised by ectodermal dysplasia, polydactyly, chondroplasia and congenital morbus cardis. Arch Dis Child 15: 65

Fink CW, Dick VQ, Howard J, Nelson JD (1977) Infection of bone and joints in children. Arthritis Rheum 20 [Suppl 2]: 578

Flecker H (1942) The time of appearance and fusion of ossification centres as observed by roentgenographic methods. Am J Roentgenol 47: 97

Francis CC (1940) The appearance of centres of ossification from 6 to 15 years. Am J Phys Anthropol 27: 127

Francis CC, Werle PP (1939) The appearance of centres of ossification from birth to 5 years. Am J Phys Anthropol 24: 273

Friedman B, Gold H (1968) Ultrastructure of Ewing's sarcoma of bone. Cancer 22: 307

Gitlow SE, Bertani LM, Rausen A, Gribetz O, Dziedzig SW (1970) Diagnosis of neuroblastoma by qualitative and quantitative determination of catecholamine metabolites in urine. Cancer 25: 1377

Gorodischer R, Davidson RG, Mosovich LL, Yaffe SJ (1976) Hypophosphatasia: a developmental anomaly of alkaline phosphase? Pediatr Res 10: 650

Harris WH, Dudley GR, Barry RJ (1962) The natural history of fibrous dysplasia. An orthopedic, pathological and roentgeographic study. J Bone Joint Surg [Am] 44: 207

Hass J (1951) Congenital dislocation of the hip. Thomas, Springfield Ill

Hayles AB, Dahlin DC, Coventry MB (1960) Osteogenic sarcoma in children. JAMA 174: 1174

Hwang WS, Tock EPC, Tan KL, Tan LKA (1979) The pathology of cartilage in chondrodysplasias. J Pathol 127: 11

Ibsen KH (1967) Distinct varieties of osteogenesis imperfecta. Clin Orthop 50: 279

Jaffe HL (1958) Tumors and tumorous conditions of the bones and joints. Lea and Febiger, Philadelphia

Jaffe HL (1972) Metabolic, degenerative and inflammatory diseases of bones and joints. Lea and Febiger, Philadelphia

Jaffe HL, Lichtenstein L (1948) Chondromyxoid fibroma of bone. A distinctive benign tumor likely to be mistaken especially for chondrosarcoma. Arch Pathol 45: 541

Jeffree GM, Price CHG (1965) Bone tumours and their enzymes. A study of the phosphatases, non-specific esterases and beta-glucuronidase of osteogenic and cartilaginous tumours, fibroblastic and giant cell lesions. J Bone Joint Surg [Br] 47: 120

King JD, Bobechko WP (1971) Osteogenesis imperfecta. An orthopaedic description and surgical review. J Bone Joint Surg [Br] 53: 72

Kovac MH, Wolf JW, Thompson RC, Schwartz ER (1974) The biosynthetic rate and hydroxylysine content of collagen in osteogenesis imperfecta. J Bone Joint Surg [Am] 56: 859

Lennert K (1978) Malignant lymphomas. Springer, Berlin Heidelberg New York

Lichtenstein L (1965) Bone tumors. 3rd edn. Mosby, St. Louis

Lindbom A, Söderberg G, Spjut HT (1961) Osteogenic sarcoma. A review of 96 cases. Acta Radiol 56: 1

Llombart-Bosch A, Blache R, Pedro-Olaya A (1978) Ultrastructural study of 28 cases of Ewing's sarcoma. Cancer 41: 1362

Lodwick GS (1958) Juvenile unicameral bone cyst. A roentgen reappraisal. Am J Roentgenol 80: 495

Loutit JF, Nesbit NW (1979) Resorption of bone. Lancet 2: 26

Matsuno T, Unni KK, McLeod RA, Dahlin DC (1976) Telangiectatic osteogenic sarcoma. Cancer 38: 2538

McKenna RJ, Schwinn CP, Soong KY, Higinbotham NL (1966) Sarcomata of the osteogenic series (osteosarcoma, fibrosarcoma, chondrosarcoma, parosteal osteogenic sarcoma, and sarcomata arising in abnormal bone). An analysis of 552 cases. J Bone Joint Surg [Am] 48: 1

McKusick VA, Egeland JA, Eldridge R, Krusen DE (1964)

Dwarfism in the Amish. The Ellis–van Creveld syndrome. Bull Johns Hopkins Hosp 115: 306

Milhaud G, Labat M-L (1978) Thymus and osteopetrosis. Clin Orthop 135: 260

Milhaud G, Labat M-L, Graf B, Juster M, Balmain N, Moutier R, Toyama K (1975) Démonstration cinétique, radiographique et histologique de la guérison de l'ostéopétrose congénitale du rat. CR Acad Sci (Paris) [D] 280: 2485

Murphy FD, Blount WP (1962) Cartilaginous exostoses following irradiation. J Bone Joint Surg [Am] 44: 662

Neufeld EF (1974) The biochemical basis for mucopolysaccharidoses and mucolipidoses. Prog Med Genet 10: 81

Neufeld EF, Lim TW, Shapiro LJ (1975) Inherited disorders of lysosomal metabolism. Annu Rev Biochem 44: 357

Ochsner SF (1966) Eosinophilic granuloma of bone; experience with 20 cases. Am J Roentgenol 97: 719

Penttinen RP, Lichtenstein JR, Martin GR, McKusick VA (1975) Abnormal collagen metabolism in cultured cells in osteogenesis imperfecta. Proc Natl Acad Sci USA 72: 586

Phillips PE (1977) Viral arthritis in children. Arthritis Rheum 20 [Suppl 2]: 584

Pochaczesky R, Yen YM, Sherman RS (1960) The roentgen appearance of benign osteoblastoma. Radiology 75: 429

Ponseti IV (1978a) Growth and development of the acetabulum in the normal child. J Bone Joint Surg [Am] 60: 575

Ponseti IV (1978b) Morphology of the acetabulum in congenital dislocation of the hip. J Bone Joint Surg [Am] 60: 586

Ponseti IV, McClintock R (1956) The pathology of slipping of the upper femoral epiphysis. J Bone Joint Surg [Am] 38: 71

Rasmussen PG (1975) Multiple epiphyseal dysplasia. II. Morphological and histochemical investigation of cartilage matrix, particularly in the pre-calcification state. Acta Pathol Microbiol Scand [A] 83: 493

Reed RJ, Rothenberg M (1964) Lesions of bone that may be confused with aneurysmal bone cyst. Clin Orthop 35: 150

Rimoin DL, Silberberg R, Hollister PW (1976) Chondro-osseous pathology in the chondrodystrophies. Clin Orthop 114: 137

Schajowicz F (1959) Ewing's sarcoma and reticulum cell sarcoma of bone with special reference to the histochemical demonstration of glycogen as an aid to differential diagnosis. J Bone Joint Surg [Am] 41: 349

Schajowicz F, Ackerman LV, Sissons HA (1972) Histological typing of bone tumours. International histological classification of tumours, no. 6. World Health Organization, Geneva

Schaller JG (1977) Arthritis of childhood onset. Clin Rheum Dis 3: 333

Scott CI (1976) Achondroplastic and hypochondroplastic dwarfism. Clin Orthop 114: 18

Selby S (1961) Metaphyseal defects in the tubular bones of growing children. J Bone Joint Surg [Am] 43: 395

Shapiro F, Glimcher MJ, Holtrop ME, Tashjian AH, Brickley-Parsons D, Kenzora JE (1980) Human osteopetrosis. J Bone Joint Surg [Am] 62: 284

Sillence DO, Horton WA, Rimoin DL (1979) Morphologic studies in the skeletal dysplasias. Am J Pathol 96: 813

Singer DB, Rudolph AJ, Rosenberg HS, Rawls WE, Boniuk M (1967) Pathology of the congenital rubella syndrome. J Pediatr 71: 665

Spjut HJ, Dorfman HD, Fechner RE, Ackerman LV (1970) Tumours of bone and cartilage. Armed Forces Institute of Pathology, Washington DC (Atlas of tumour pathology, 2nd ser, fasc 5)

Sutro CJ (1935) Slipping of the capital epiphysis of the femur in adolescence. Arch Surg 31: 345

Thomas LB, Forkner CE, Frei E, Besse BE, Stabenau JR (1961) The skeletal lesions of acute leukaemia. Cancer 14: 608

Vohra VG (1967) Roentgen manifestations of Ewing's sarcoma. A study of 156 cases. Cancer 20: 727

Walker DG (1975) Bone resorption in osteopetrotic mice by transplants of normal bone marrow and spleen cells. Science 190: 784

Weinfeld MS, Dudley HR (1962) Osteogenic sarcoma. A follow up study of the ninety-four cases observed at the Massachusetts General Hospital from 1920–1960. J Bone Joint Surg [Am] 44: 269

Chapter 11

Muscle and Peripheral Nerve

Michael Swash

The development of new techniques for the histological study of muscle and peripheral nerve has led to fresh concepts of the pathogenesis and classification of these disorders, and to a more rational and hopeful approach to both diagnosis and treatment. Naturally, new problems and controversies have also arisen.

In this chapter a general account of the pathological reactions of muscle and nerve will be given, together with brief descriptions of the characteristic features of those disorders that occur in infancy and childhood. Much of the chapter will relate to biopsy material but some attention will also be given to autopsy findings.

1. Muscle Biopsy Techniques

Fixation in formol–saline, with subsequent paraffin embedding, is now little used in diagnostic work. The availability of unfixed, frozen material allows the use of enzyme histochemical and immunohistochemical techniques. With these methods, subcellular organelles can be studied by light microscopy, and different fibre types can be identified. In addition, the classic histological stains, adapted for frozen material, can still be used. Many of the newer techniques produce permanent results so that slides can be stored for future study. The blocks of frozen tissue can themselves be stored indefinitely in liquid nitrogen.

Techniques for snap-freezing muscle are well described in other texts (see Dubowitz and Brooke 1973). To avoid artefacts it is important to take particular care to prepare small cylindrical blocks of tissue (3 x 2 mm) from the fresh biopsy specimen. The muscle should be kept moist in buffered saline or Ringer's solution to avoid any drying-artefact before freezing. It is preferable to freeze the tissue, attached to a small disc of cork by a blob of Tissue-Tek, in isopentane cooled to near its freezing point in a thermos of liquid nitrogen. When cutting sections in the cryostat sudden changes in temperature, such as would be caused by a warm cryostat knife or warm slides, must be avoided to prevent the development of ice-crystal artefact. This can sometimes be cleared from a block by allowing it to thaw at room temperature and then refreezing, although this manoeuvre usually results in the loss of some enzyme activity. A series of up to 12 transverse sections, each 5–8 μm thick, should be cut. Longitudinal sections, which are difficult to produce because of imperfect orientation of muscle fibres in most blocks, are also useful. In each case, small pieces of fresh tissue should be fixed in glutaraldehyde so that, if necessary, sections can be prepared for electron microscopy.

1.1. Histological Methods

The haematoxylin and eosin method provides general information about the biopsy (Fig. 11.1). The elastin–van Gieson stain is sometimes useful, particularly in assessing connective tissue changes. The modified Gomori trichrome stain has become popular, since it allows delineation of nuclei, fibrous tissue, myofibrillar material (bluish), and intermyofibrillar substance (red). Trichrome stains may also differentiate two muscle fibre types, the red and pale fibres of older workers, but this is not always very obvious.

A variety of enzyme-histochemical reactions are available for histological work, and in most laboratories a routine series is used. This series should provide a clear differentiation of fibre type and should yield a variety of organelle-specific reaction products so that mitochondria, sarcoplasmic lipid droplets, myofibrils, cell membranes, and sarcoplasmic glycogen, and perhaps also ribonucleic acid and acid phosphatase, can be identified by light microscopy. The nicotine adenine dinucleotide tetrazolium reductase (NADH) technique is particularly useful, as it produces a permanent preparation with good contrast (Fig. 11.2), which allows fibre type differentiation to be recognized approximately. The reaction product is localized in mitochondria and, nonspecifically, in the tubular system of the intermyofibrillar sarcoplasm. Succinic dehydrogenase (SDH) is located only in mitochondria but the reaction product is often less easily visualized.

Fibre typing is conventionally performed in myofibrillar adenosine triphosphatase (ATPase) preparations (see Dubowitz and Brooke 1973). This reaction produces different results depending on the pH of the pre-incubation (Figs. 11.3 and 11.4). Pre-incubations are carried out at pH 9.4, 4.5, and 4.3. In good preparations there should be a pattern reversal between the pH 9.4 and pH 4.3 pre-incubations, fibres which are dark in the former (type 2 fibres) being pale in the latter (Figs. 11.3 and 11.4). In the intermediate (pH 4.5) pre-incubation some type 2 fibres show an intermediate reaction-product density (type 2 B fibres). Myophosphorylase, located at the cross-bridges of the active component of the myofilament, can also be demonstrated, but this method does not produce permanent results.

Neutral lipid droplets are most satisfactorily demonstrated by the oil red O method; a counterstain of Ehrlich's haematoxylin enables basophilic fibres and sarcolemmal nuclei to be recognized. A number of other stains can be used for neutral lipid, e.g., Sudan black, but they are generally less satisfactory. Glycogen granules and cell membranes, together with other myofibrillar membranous structures, can be demonstrated by the periodic acid-Schiff (PAS) method. Predigestion with diastase allows proof of the presence of glycogen in the untreated sections. The sections should be fixed on the slides with alcohol for the most uniform results. Acid phosphatase, localized in lysosomes, can be demonstrated in abnormal fibres, particularly in those undergoing autolysis. A summary of the enzyme-histochemical reactions in fibres of different histochemical types is given in Table 11.1.

Comparison of this histochemical classification of fibre types with physiologically based classifications of muscle fibres has led to controversy (see Brooke and Kaiser 1970). Type 1 fibres probably correspond to slow-contracting, oxidative fibres, type 2 B to fast-contracting, glycolytic fibres, and type 2 A to fast-contracting, oxidative/glycolytic fibres (Peter et al. 1972).

In addition to these routine histological and histochemical methods, the use of frozen tissue enables immunohistochemical techniques to be employed for demonstration of immunoglobulins and complement in blood vessels (Whitaker and Engel 1972). Acetylcholine receptor protein in motor end-plates or in the cell membrane of denervated muscle fibres can also be demonstrated in frozen sections. The method (Ringel et al. 1976) utilizes a sandwich technique, based on the demonstration of antibody to an irreversible acetylcholine receptor blocking agent, α-bungarotoxin, by immunoperoxidase. There are several well-tried methods for the demonstration of cholinesterase at the synaptic folds of motor end-plates, one of which is combined with silver to show the nerve terminals themselves (Pestronk and Drachman 1978). In fresh unfrozen muscle, motor end-plates and the terminal innervation can readily be demonstrated by supravital methylene blue staining (Coërs and Woolf 1953) (Fig. 11.5).

Electron microscopy is useful in some instances to examine the ultrastructure of cellular abnormalities detected by light microscopy, for example, to study paracrystalline inclusions in mitochrondria in ragged-red fibres, or to study tubular aggregates. It is not generally useful in routine diagnosis, although

Table 11.1. Summary of the enzyme-histochemical reactions in fibres of different histochemical types

	Type 1	Type 2A	Type 2B
ATPase pH 9.4	Pale	Dark	Dark
ATPase pH 4.5	Dark	Pale	Dark
ATPase pH 4.3	Dark	Pale	Pale
NADH	Dark	Intermediate	Intermediate
Glycogen	Pale	Dark	Intermediate
Myophosphorylase	Pale	Dark	Dark
Neutral lipid	Plentiful	Sparse	Sparse

Fig. 11.1. In this transverse section the close interdigitation of ▷ normal muscle fibres is clearly seen. The muscle fibre nuclei are almost all subsarcolemmal. The muscle fibres are arranged in fascicles. Normal muscle. (H and E; 140 ×)

Fig. 11.2. A mosaic arrangement of fibres of various staining ▷ intensity is seen in this serial section. Type 1 fibres are darkly-stained, type 2 fibres are relatively pale. Type 2A fibres tend to be darker than type 2B fibres. The intermyofibrillar substance has a finely granular appearance. Arteriolar walls also stain positively. (NADH tetrazolium reductase; 140 ×)

Fig. 11.3. In this reaction type 1 fibres are pale and type 2 fibres are ▷ dark. Serial section. (ATPase pH 9.4; 140 ×)

Fig. 11.4. The mosaic pattern has reversed: type 1 fibres are dark ▷ and type 2 fibres are very pale. Serial section. (ATPase pH 4.3; 140 ×)

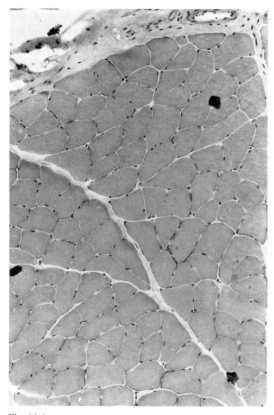

Fig. 11.1.

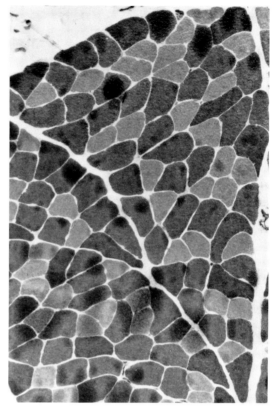

Fig. 11.3.

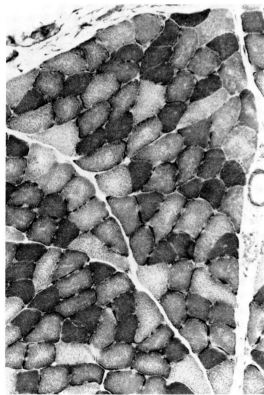

Fig. 11.2.

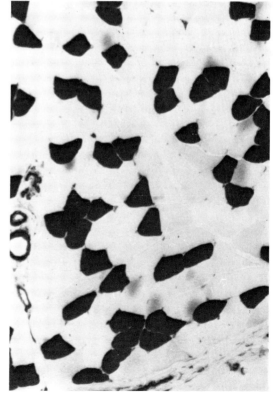

Fig. 11.4.

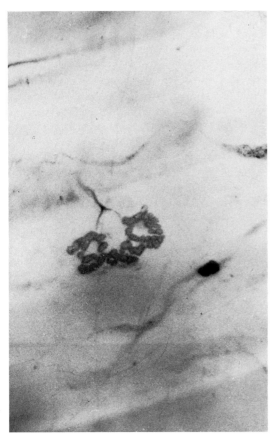

Fig. 11.5. The terminal axon branch innervates the ending, which consists of an arborization of subterminal expansions forming the neural part of the motor end-plate. Normal motor end-plate. (Supravital methylene blue; 140 ×)

semi-thin sections of plastic-embedded muscle stained with toluidine blue or paraphenylenediamine provide a useful adjunct to light microscopy of frozen sections. The striations, mitochondria, triads of the sarcotubular system, and intermyofibrillar granular sarcoplasm are shown in longitudinal section in Fig. 11.6.

2. Histological Features of Neuromuscular Disease

2.1. Statistical Methods

The changes found in the distribution and size of type 1 and type 2 fibres can be described by simple statistical methods. These descriptions give important information about selective involvement of fibre types (see Engel 1970).

2.2. Fibre-type Predominance

The proportions of fibres of each histochemical type vary in different muscles (Brooke and Engel 1969a, b; Johnson et al. 1973). For example, extensor hallucis longus normally contains a majority of type 1 fibres. However, in the three muscles commonly biopsied in clinical practice, quadriceps, biceps brachii, and deltoid, type 2 fibres are found in greater numbers than type 1 fibres. A change in the proportion of either fibre type is termed fibre type predominance; type 1 fibre predominance is present when more than 55 % of fibres in one of these three muscles are type 1 fibres, and type 2 predominance when more than 80 % of fibres are type 2 fibres (see Dubowitz and Brooke 1973).

2.3. Fibre Diameter

Atrophy and hypertrophy are difficult to assess subjectively, and it is useful to calculate the means of the lesser diameter of at least 100 fibres, including fibres of both fibre type, to compare these with normal values (Polgar et al. 1972; Dubowitz and Brooke 1973). Since muscle fibres in children are smaller than those of adults, and their diameters vary at different ages, these measurements are less important in paediatric practice, but selective atrophy of type 1 or type 2 fibres may occur in certain diseases and this may be important in diagnosis (Brooke and Engel 1969b).

Selective atrophy of type 2 fibres is common; it is a feature of disuse atrophy of any cause and can therefore occur in patients immobilized in bed for orthopaedic procedures, in cachexia, in cortispinal tract lesions, in myasthenia gravis, or in arthropathies of any cause. It may also occur in collagen–vascular diseases (Engel 1965) and in steroid myopathy and osteomalacia. Atrophy of type 1 fibres is less common. It is a particular feature of myotonic dystrophy (Engel and Brooke 1966), but also occurs in myotubular myopathy, nemaline myopathy, and congenital fibre type disporportion (see below). In collagen–vascular disease, such as dermatomyositis of childhood (Banker and Victor 1966), selective atrophy of fibres of both histochemical types may occur at the periphery of the fascicles: this phenomenon is known as perifascicular atrophy. This is probably due to capillary shutdown from arteriolar or capillary involvement, leading to ischaemia of the periphery of the fascicle and so to atrophy or even necrosis of these fibres (Carpenter et al. 1976).

2.4. Central Nucleation

Centrally placed nuclei are found in less than 3 % of fibres in normal muscle biopsies. Central nucleation occurs in hypertrophied fibres as a feature associated with fibre splitting (Fig. 11.7) and in regenerating fibres (Fig. 11.8), and is especially prominent in centronuclear myopathy and myotonic dystrophy.

2.5. Fibre-type Grouping

Muscle fibres are normally arranged in a random mosaic distribution of fibre types within fascicles (James 1971). Most fibres supplied by a single motor axon are widely dispersed within the muscle (Edstrom and Kugelberg 1968).

The finding of groups of fibres of similar histochemical type is evidence that reinnervation of denervated fibres has occurred, probably by collateral sprouting from nearby motor axons (Fig. 11.9). This is therefore evidence of effective functional compensation, indicating a neurogenic disorder of some chronicity. By convention, fibre-type grouping is said to occur when two or more fibres of the same histochemical type are enclosed, at all points on their circumference, by other fibres of the same histochemical type. This usually means that there are at least ten fibres in the group, but this clearly depends on fibre size. When fibre-type predominance exceeds about 80 % enclosed fibres will become frequent (Johnson et al. 1973), without this necessarily implying that fibre-type grouping is present. Fibre-type predominance is itself a factor that should lead to the suspicion of a neurogenic disorder.

Groups of small pointed fibres indicate that irreversible denervation has occurred. When this is due to a chronic disorder, in which there has been opportunity for collateral reinnervation of isolated denervated fibres, the group of denervated fibres may be very large, even occupying whole fascicles. Clusters of three to six small angular narrow fibres—disseminated neurogenic atrophy—typically occur

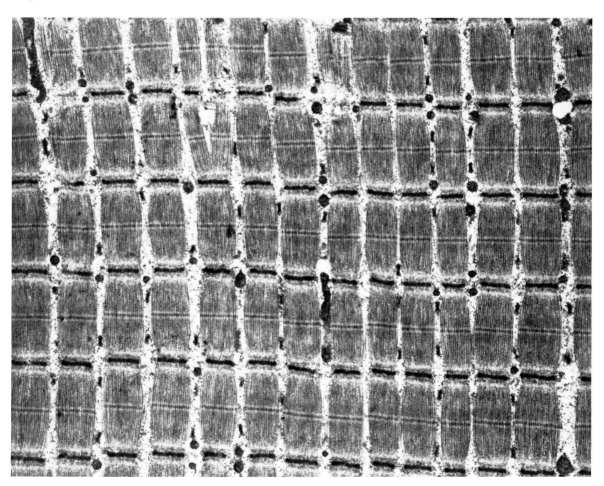

Fig. 11.6. Normal contracted muscle, longitudinal section. Mitochondria (*M*) and triads of the sarcotubular system (*T*) are located near the Z line (*Z*). (EM: 22 500 ×)

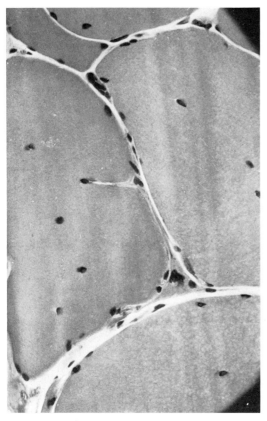

Fig. 11.7. Central nucleation and fibre splitting in a chronic neurogenic disorder. (H and E; 360 ×)

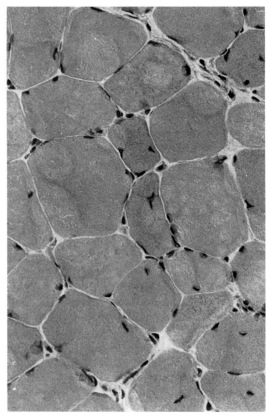

Fig. 11.8. Central nucleation in regenerating muscle fibres in acute polymyositis. The two fibres in the centre of the field are slightly basophilic. The slight variation in staining intensity in the other fibres are 'architectural changes', which are commonly found in polymyositis. (H and E; 360 ×)

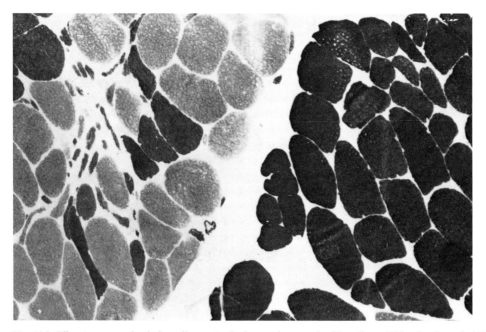

Fig. 11.9. Fibre-type grouping in juvenile-onset spinal muscular atrophy (Kugelberg–Welander disease). (ATPase pH 9.4; 140 ×)

in more rapidly progressive, or poorly compensated, neurogenic disorders when collateral reinnervation has failed (Fig. 11.10).

2.6. Degenerative Changes

2.6.1. Necrotic Fibres

Necrotic fibres are a common feature of the myopathies, but they are also found in biopsies from patients with chronic neurogenic disorders (Cazzato 1970; Schwartz et al. 1976). They appear pale and hyaline. Later they lose their eosinophilic character, become pale and patchily stained, and begin to undergo phagocytosis (Fig. 11.11). Sometimes an endomysial cellular reaction occurs around them, composed of endothelial capillary nuclei and sarcolemmal nuclei. Necrotic fibres usually contain prominent acid phosphatase-positive material. If the blood supply to a region of fibre necrosis is impaired the endomysial tubes and basal lamina scaffold may remain intact, producing an appearance of rings of empty endomysial tubes, i.e., subendomysial necrosis. This is seen particularly in polymyositis (Schmalbruch 1976) and in other acute necrotizing myopathies usually found in adults (Urich and Wilkinson 1970). Large rounded hyaline fibres are particularly characteristic of Duchenne muscular dystrophy.

2.6.2. Granular Fibres

Granular fibres (Brooke 1966) appear coarsely granular in haematoxylin and eosin preparations. The granular material is faintly basophilic and is usually distributed in the sarcoplasm; it is particularly prominent at the periphery of the affected fibres. This material stains red in the Gomori trichrome preparation, is dark in NADH and SDH preparations, and does not stain in ATPase preparations (Fig. 11.12). Affected fibres are almost always type 1 fibres. In addition, this material is usually faintly basophilic and is often associated with droplets of neutral lipid. These fibres, usually known as

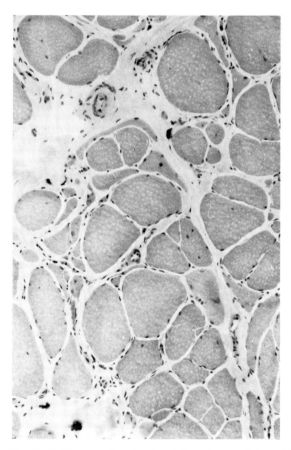

Fig. 11.10. Clusters of small pointed fibres, in association with larger rounded fibres. Interstitial fibrosis has occurred. Spinal muscular atrophy. (H and E; 140 ×)

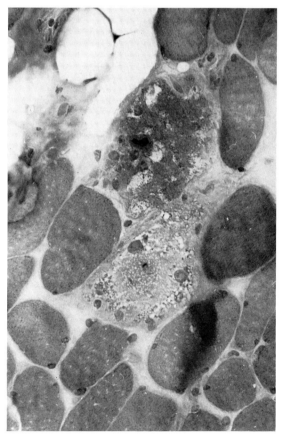

Fig. 11.11. Two necrotic fibres undergoing phagocytosis. (Modified Gomori trichrome; 560 ×)

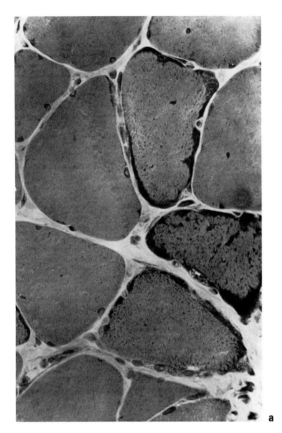

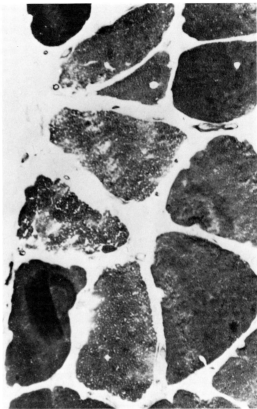

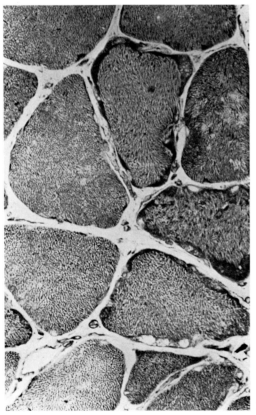

Fig. 11.12. a–c Ragged-red fibres, transverse section. (560 ×) **a** Gomori trichrome three fibres appear granular and show an irregular darkly staining (red) rim; **b** NADH The pattern of intermyofibrillar reaction is disturbed in the ragged-red fibres. The rims of these fibres stain darkly, but not uniformly; **c** ATPase pH 4.3 The abnormal material does not stain.

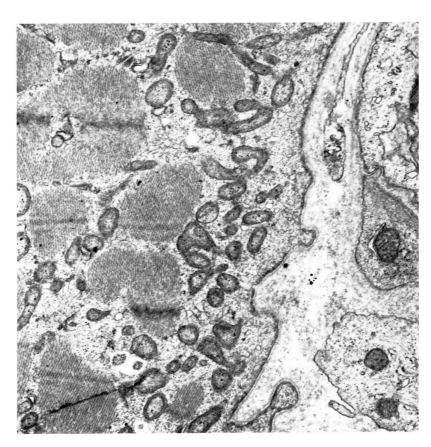

Fig. 11.13. Peripherally located aggregates of mitochondria. These show abnormal cristae, and contain osmiophilic dense bodies. Deltoid biopsy from patient with progressive external ophthalmoplegia. (EM; 15 000 ×)

ragged-red fibres (Fig. 11.12), are found as an isolated phenomenon in patients with progressive ophthalmoplegia (Engel 1971) associated with a mild proximal myopathy, but they have also been reported in a variety of other disorders (Swash et al. 1978a), including a number of rare cases of myopathies associated with defective mitochondrial oxidation (Morgan-Hughes et al. 1978). Electron microscopy reveals that the granular appearance results from an accumulation of mitochrondria (Fig. 11.13), which may show morphological abnormalities and which often contain osmiophilic bodies and paracrystalline material (Fig. 11.14).

2.6.3. Tubular Aggregates

Tubular aggregates appear similar to ragged-red fibres although they do not usually produce a generally granular appearance, the abnormal red material being limited to a peripheral segment of affected fibres. Further, they are found in type 2 B fibres, and although the abnormal zones are darkly stained in oxidative enzyme reaction they are negative in SDH preparations. Electron microscopy demonstrates the characteristic stacked tubules

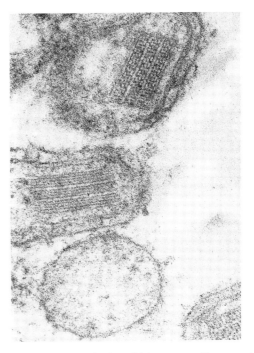

Fig. 11.14. Intramitochrondrial paracrystalline material. (EM; 90 000 ×)

(Fig. 11.15). Although in itself a highly characteristic finding, this change is not specific for any particular disorder (Dubowitz and Brooke 1973). Nevertheless, some patients with this abnormality have been reported as having myopathy with tubular aggregates.

2.6.4. Fibre Splitting

Fibre splitting is found particularly in chronic disorders. It is a feature of chronic neurogenic muscle disease, such as intermediate spinal muscular atrophy, when it particularly affects the hypertrophied type 1 fibres. Splitting usually begins from the periphery of affected fibres, the line of separation running into the centre of the fibre toward a centrally placed nucleus (Fig. 11.16). The cleft is usually basophilic and the nuclei associated with it may be vesicular (Schwartz et al. 1976). Sometimes a fibre is split into multiple fragments, some of which can become separated from the 'parent' fibre, resulting in denervation of the separated segment (Swash and Schwartz 1977). Splitting of this type is probably due to mechanical stress associated with functional overload of weakened muscles (Hall-Craggs 1972; Schwartz et al. 1976). Similar splitting occurs in Duchenne-type dystrophy (Bell and Conen 1968), limb-girdle myopathies, and polymyositis (Swash et al. 1978b). It may be important in functional compensation in these disorders (Swash and Schwartz 1977), and in chronic neurogenic disorders it can lead to an appearance of combined fibre necrosis and regeneration, with variability in fibre size and central nucleation (Fig. 11.17), called secondary 'myopathic' change (Drachman et al. 1967; Schwartz et al. 1976). Fibre splitting is a normal phenomenon near musculotendinous insertions (Bell and Conen 1968). It must not be confused with subendomyosial regeneration (Fig. 11.18) occurring after fibre necrosis (see Schmalbruch 1976; Swash et al. 1978a).

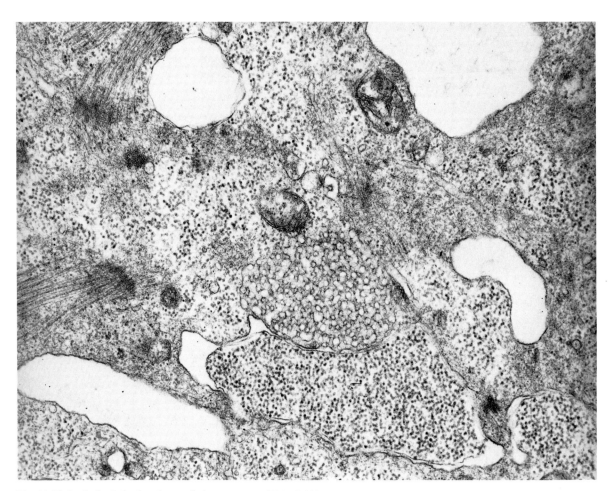

Fig. 11.15. Stacked tubules forming a tubular aggregate. (EM; 60 000 ×)

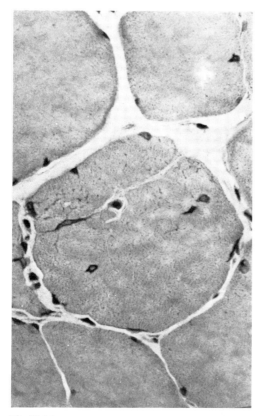

Fig. 11.16.

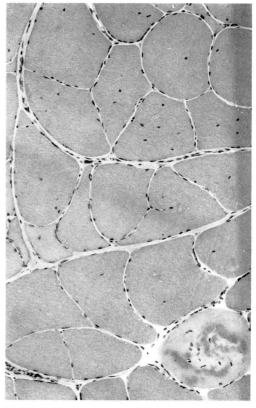

Fig. 11.17.

Fig. 11.16. Fibre splitting and its relation to a central nucleus. The cleft of incomplete splitting is basophilic. (H and E; 560 ×)

Fig. 11.17. Fibre splitting in hypertrophied fibres, with prominent central nucleation. There are several narrow atrophic fibres, which are probably denervated. A large fibre is necrotic. These are the features of secondary myopathic change in a chronic neurogenic disorder: Kugelberg–Welander disease. (H and E; 140 ×)

Fig. 11.18. Subendomysial regeneration. Individual endomysial tubes contain immature regenerating fibres. These muscle fibres stain irregularly. (H and E; 560 ×)

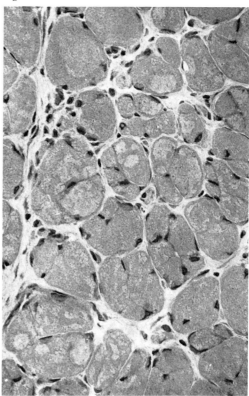

Fig. 11.18.

2.6.5. Target Fibres

Target fibres (Engel 1961) are best seen in ATPase and NADH preparations (Fig. 12.19). These fibres contain a central unstained zone, surrounded by a densely stained intermediate zone, and a third, relatively normal outer zone. Most affected fibres are type 1 fibres. Target fibres are usually associated with denervation, especially that associated with neuropathies, but they have been produced experimentally by tenotomy (Engel et al. 1966).

2.6.6. Central Cores

It is often difficult to distinguish central cores from target fibres. The core consists of a central zone of myofibrillar disruption, nonreactive in NADH preparations, which extends the length of the fibre. A distinction has been drawn between fibres with structured (ATPase-positive) and unstructured (ATPase-negative) cores (Neville and Brooke 1971), but it is doubtful whether this is useful in practice. The latter are sometimes called core-targetoid fibres, a term that illustrates the difficulties.

2.6.7. Moth-eaten Fibres

Moth-eaten fibres (Brooke and Engel 1966) are fibres in which the normally regular intermyofibrillar network seen in the oxidative enzyme reactions is disturbed. Type 1 fibres are preferentially affected. The abnormality often consists of a whorled appearance, and areas of nonreactivity to NADH are often present near these whorls (Fig. 11.20). This change is not specific for any single disorder, but is particularly associated with inflammatory myopathies.

2.6.8. Rod Bodies

The Gomori preparation gives the best visualization of rod bodies. They consist of small, red, rod-like bodies, scattered in the sarcoplasm of affected fibres (Fig. 11.21). These rods are faintly visible as basophilic structures in haematoxylin and eosin stains, and are derived from Z-band material (Fig. 11.22). They were first described in a familial, nonprogressive myopathy with hypotonia by Shy et al. (1963)

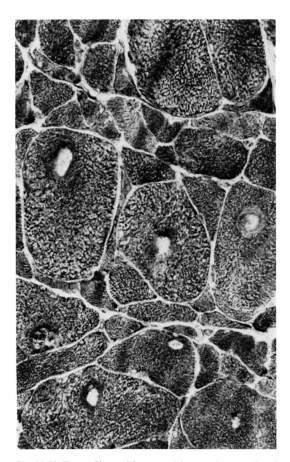

Fig. 11.19. Target fibres with grouped denervation atrophy after a peripheral nerve injury. (NADH; 560 ×)

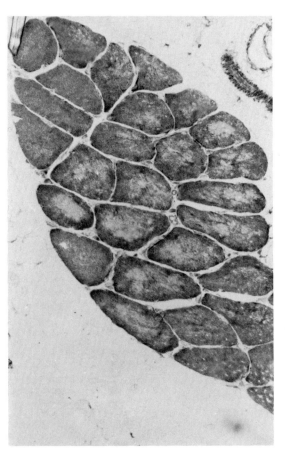

Fig. 11.20. Moth-eaten fibres in dermatomyositis. (NADH; 140 ×)

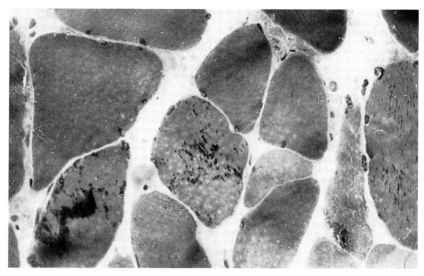

Fig. 11.21. Rod bodies. There is abnormal variability in fibre size with interstitial fibrosis. (Gomori trichrome; 560 ×)

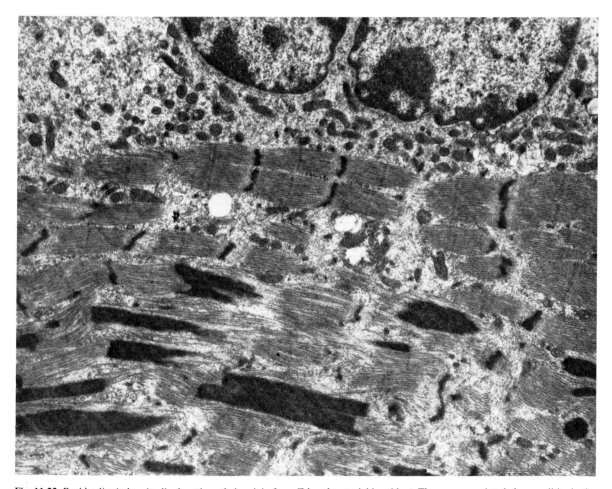

Fig. 11.22. Rod bodies in longitudinal section; their origin from Z-band material is evident. There are associated abnormalities in the organization of the structure of myofibrils. (EM; 22 500)

and were termed nemaline myopathy by these authors. However, they have also been reported in adult limb-girdle myopathies, polymyositis (Sato et al. 1971), and a variety of other disorders.

2.6.9. Cytoplasmic Bodies

Cytoplasmic bodies, consisting of small eosinophilic, PAS-positive zones within otherwise normal muscle fibres, have been particularly associated with collagen vascular disease, such as dermatomyositis (Fig. 11.23), but when present in small numbers their significance is doubtful.

2.6.10. Ring Fibres

Although formerly associated with myotonic dystrophy, ring fibres (Fig. 11.24) can occur in many other chronic disorders. Nevertheless they are most frequently encountered in myotonic dystrophy and are then often associated with *sarcoplasmic masses*. Ring fibres (*Ringbinden*) consist of fibres in which a displaced myofibrillar strand has taken up a spiral position around the periphery of the fibre. Sarcoplasmic masses consist of peripheral zones of sarcoplasm, devoid of myofibrils and of other cell organelles (Klinkerfuss 1967).

2.7. Regenerative Changes

Regeneration occurs after necrosis or injury in most tissues of the body, and muscle fibres, which are particularly susceptible to injury in everyday life, have considerable regenerative potential. After fibre necrosis, which may be limited to a segment of the muscle fibre, regeneration can occur either in continuity with the undamaged portions of the fibre (continuous repair) or from myoblast formation in the necrotic segment itself (discontinuous repair). Regeneration thus begins at a stage when phagocytosis of necrotic material is still incomplete, while mononucleated cells are abundant in the interstitium around the necrotic fibre.

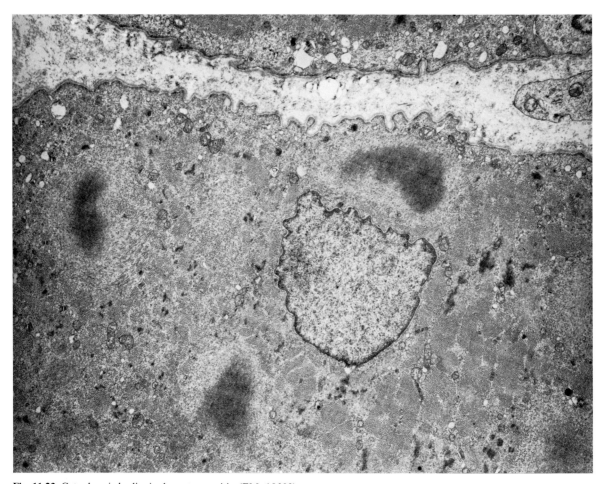

Fig. 11.23. Cytoplasmic bodies in dermatomyositis. (EM; 15 000)

Regenerating fibres are usually smaller than neighbouring normal fibres (Fig. 11.18). Their sarcoplasm is basophilic and contains neutral lipid droplets. The nuclei are centrally located, large, and vesicular and contain prominent nucleoli. Cytoplasmic RNA can be demonstrated with special stains.

In discontinuous regeneration, repair proceeds from mononucleated myoblasts (Sloper and Pegrum 1969), which are probably themselves derived from activation of satellite cells (Reznik and Engel 1970), and these myoblasts form long basophilic multinucleated ribbon-like cells, which later fuse, forming a new fibre (Reznik 1973). Satellite cells are found in normal muscle fibres as a nucleus, surrounded by sparse granular sarcoplasm containing abundant free fibrosomes, Golgi apparatus, endoplasmic reticulum, and mitochondria, but devoid of myofilaments. The satellite cell is limited by plasma membrane, and is situated beneath the basement membrane of the muscle fibre. The numbers of such cells in muscle are increased after injury (Reznick 1973) and after denervation (Ontell 1974). Reznik (1973) has recently reviewed the ultrastructural sequence of changes found in these cells, giving rise to myoblast formation during regeneration after cold-induced injury.

Webb (1977) has recently drawn attention to the importance of programmed cell death of myotubes during embryonic myogenesis. The stimulus for cell death is unknown, but a similar phenomenon probably occurs during differentiation of myoblasts in regenerative repair, since several developing myotubes are found in the early stages of repair before fusion occurs and the single myofibre is reconstituted. It is possible that the achievement of functional reinnervation, which can only occur when the fibre is reconstituted across the necrotic segment, is important in this process.

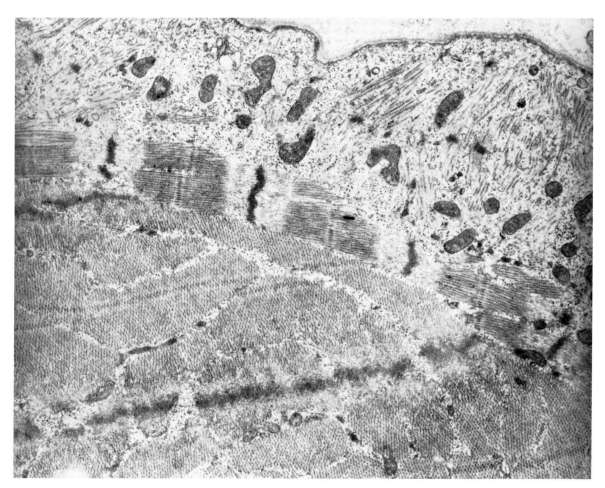

Fig. 11.24. Myotonic dystrophy. Ring fibres consist of a displaced myofibril, or group of myofibrils, situated at the periphery of a fibre. There are peripheral sarcoplasmic masses containing myofibrillar debris. (EM; 30 000 ×)

2.8. Other Features

2.8.1. Motor End-plates

Motor end-plates (Fig. 11.5) are seen occasionally in random biopsies, but can be studied more easily in motor point biopsies. Their morphology has been reviewed by Gauthier (1976).

2.8.2. Blood Vessels

Blood vessels, including arterioles, veins, and capillaries, are found in all muscle biopsies. Abnormalities in blood vessels are uncommon, except in polymyositis and polyarteritis, when necrosis of the arteriolar wall, hyaline change, thrombosis, and, most frequently, infiltration by small round cells and plasma cells may occur. The capillaries have been little studied, although it has been suggested that the perifascicular atrophy found in inflammatory myopathies may be due to capillary necrosis or shut-down (Carpenter et al. 1976), and tubular inclusions have been reported in these endothelial cells in childhood dermatomyositis. In childhood dermatomyositis Whitaker and Engel (1972) found depositions of immune complexes in the walls of capillaries and arterioles, but this observation has not been confirmed.

2.8.3. Connective Tissue

The connective tissue in the endomysium is increased in any chronic neuromuscular disease, but marked fibrosis is an especially typical feature of Duchenne-type muscular dystrophy.

Small *nerve fascicles* are often found in muscle biopsies, and it is occasionally possible to recognize abnormalities such as demyelination, or congenital absence of myelination (Karch and Urich 1975), and the axonal change of 'dying-back' neuropathies. Methylene blue impregnations performed by the supravital method (Cöers and Woolf 1956) are valuable in the assessment of such disorders, but they are time-consuming and are rarely performed in routine laboratory practice (Harriman 1961).

2.8.4. Muscle Spindles

Muscle spindles (Fig. 11.25) are found fairly frequently in muscle biopsies. Normal muscle spindles consist of a capsule of perineurial cells, fibrocytes, and collagen enclosing a periaxial space containing several small intrafusal muscle fibres, the nuclear bag and nuclear chain fibres, a bundle of small nerve fibres, and a few capillaries. There are normally at least two bag fibres (Fig. 11.25) and three to ten chain fibres. These fibres receive a complex motor and sensory innervation (Swash and Fox 1972). They undergo characteristic changes, consisting in fragmentation of intrafusal muscle fibres (Fig. 11.26) in myotonic dystrophy (Swash and Fox 1975a, b), and abnormalities also occur (Swash and Fox 1976) in Duchenne-type muscular dystrophy (Fig. 11.27) and in motor and sensory denervation (Fig. 11.28) (Swash and Fox 1974).

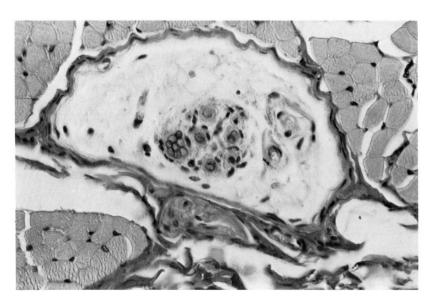

Fig. 11.25. Normal muscle spindle. The spindle consists of a capsule enclosing a mucopolysaccharide-filled periaxial space and a cluster of intrafusal muscle fibres. In this transverse section the nuclear bag and nuclear chain fibres can be recognized. In children, as in this illustration, extrafusal muscle fibres are not much larger than the intrafusal muscle fibres. (van Gieson, 560 ×)

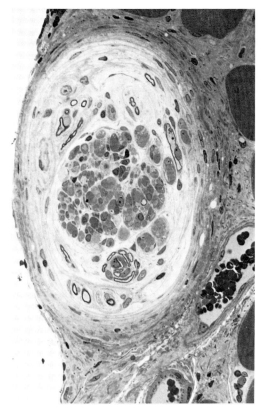

Fig. 11.26.

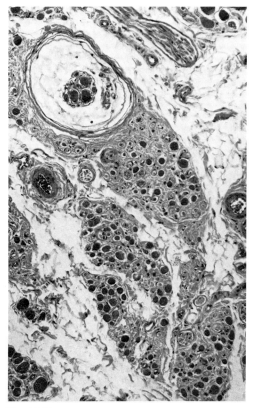

Fig. 11.27.

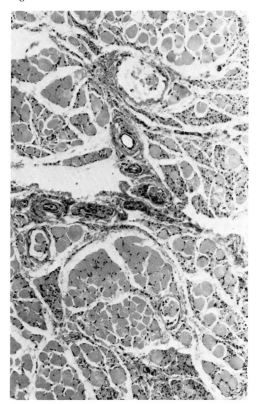

Fig. 11.26. The intrafusal muscle fibres are fragmented and the pattern of innervation is abnormal in this case of myotonic dystrophy. (Toluidine blue, semi-thin section; 560 ×)

Fig. 11.27. Duchenne-type muscular dystrophy: autopsy specimen. There is dense fibrosis with fat replacement. Remaining muscle fibres are rounded. The muscle spindle shows fibrosis of the intrafusal muscle fibre bundle with dilatation of the periaxial space and capsular thickening. (van Gieson; 140 ×)

Fig. 11.28. Werdnig–Hoffmann disease: autopsy specimen. The spindle to the *right* shows dilatation of the periaxial space. There is a slight increase in the number of intrafusal muscle fibres and these are smaller than normal. Atrophy of extrafusal muscle fibres has resulted in crowding and prominence of the spindle capsules. (van Gieson; 140 ×)

Fig. 11.28.

3. Classification of Neuromuscular Disorders

The classification of neuromuscular disorders introduced by the World Federation of Neurology (Gardner-Medwin and Walton 1974) is comprehensive, but it is cumbersome to use because it takes no account of the extreme rarity of many of the disorders included in it. Neuromuscular diseases are broadly classified into myopathic and neurogenic disorders. Although there has been controversy in recent years about the role of neurogenic factors in the pathogenesis of the muscular dystrophies (McComas 1977), this is largely of theoretical interest. There are clearly recognizable differences in the histological changes found in disorders ordinarily classified as myopathies and those found in the neurogenic disorders (Table 11.2).

4. Myopathic Disorders

4.1. Muscular Dystrophies

The term muscular dystrophy refers to a group of genetically determined diseases characterized by progressive degenerative changes in muscle fibres without primary abnormality in the lower motor neuron. They are classified (Table 11.3) according to their clinical, morphological, and genetic characteristics.

Table 11.2. Changes found in myopathic and in neurogenic disorders

Myopathic	Neurogenic
1. Prominent degenerative and regenerative changes in individual fibres	1. Fibre-type grouping
2. Increased variability in fibre size	2. Fibre-type atrophy
3. Fibrosis may be prominent	3. Clusters of small pointed fibres, often dark in NADH and nonspecific esterase preparations
4. Architectural changes prominent	4. Type 1 fibre hypertrophy
5. Various specific morphological abnormalities	5. Only rare degenerative changes
6. Type 2 fibre atrophy	6. Rare architectural changes
7. Perifascicular atrophy	7. Little fibrosis
8. Blood vessels abnormal in inflammatory myopathies	8. Blood vessels normal
9. Fibre-type grouping uncommon	9. Target fibres or core fibres

Table 11.3. Classification of neuromuscular disorders in childhood

A. *Myopathic disorders*

  1. *Muscular dystrophies*
  (i)   Duchenne-type muscular dystrophy
  (ii) Becker muscular dystrophy
  (iii) Limb-girdle muscular dystrophy
  (iv) Facio–scapulo–humeral muscular dystrophy
  (v)   Congenital muscular dystrophy
  (vi) Muscular dystrophy with external ophthalmoplegia

  2. *Benign congenital myopathies*
  (i)   Central-core and multicore disease
  (ii) Nemaline myopathy
  (iii) Myotubular myopathy
  (iv) Congenital fibre-type disproportion
  (v)   Mitochondrial myopathies
  (vi) Other myopathies

  3. *Myotonic syndromes*
  (i)   Myotonic dystrophy (Steinert's disease)
  (ii) Myotonic congenita (Thomsen's disease)
  (iii) Paramyotonia congenita (Eulenburg's disease)
  (iv) Other myotonic syndromes

  4. *Metabolic and endocrine myopathies*
  (a) Metabolic myopathies:
       (i)   Glycogenoses
       (ii) Abnormalities of lipid metabolism
       (iii) Periodic paralysis
       (iv) Myopathies with myoglobinuria
       (v)   Malignant hyperpyrexia
  (b) Endocrine myopathies
       (i)   Thyroid disorders
       (ii) Parathyroid disorders and osteomalacia
       (iii) Pituitary and adrenal disorders

  5. *Myasthenia gravis*

  6. *Inflammatory myopathies*
  (i)   Dermatomyositis and polymyositis
  (ii) Infective myositis

  7. *Floppy infant syndrome*

  8. *Arthrogryposis multiplex*

B. *Neurogenic disorders*

  1. *Spinal muscular atrophies*
  (i)   Severe (infantile) spinal muscular atrophy (Werdnig–Hoffman disease)
  (ii) Intermediate spinal muscular atrophy
  (iii) Mild spinal muscular atrophy (Kugelberg–Welander disease)
  (iv) Motor neurone disease

  2. *Heredo-familial sensorimotor peripheral neuropathies*
  (i)   Type 1 (peroneal muscular atrophy)
  (ii) Type 2 (Neuronal type of peroneal muscular atrophy)
  (iii) Type 3 (hypertrophic neuropathy of Dejerine and Sottas)
  (iv) Type 4 (hypertrophic neuropathy with phytanic acid storage—Refsum's disease)
  (v)   Type 5 (neuropathy with spastic paraplegia)
  (vi) Scapuloperoneal syndrome
  (ii) (Other types see Table 11.5)

  3. *Acquired Neuropathies*
  (see Table 11.6)

4.1.1. Duchenne-type Muscular Dystrophy

Duchenne-type muscular dystrophy is a progressive myopathy inherited in a sex-linked recessive pattern, so that it is carried by females and expressed only in males. It presents in infancy with delay in the achievement of motor developmental milestones, especially walking, and is often characterized by hypertrophy and hardness of the calf and shoulder muscles on palpation. Weakness is principally proximal at first, but as the disease progresses, weakness becomes generalized, although distal muscles are always relatively spared and the external ocular muscles are apparently never affected. Scoliosis, dysphagia, and cardiomyopathy develop and there is often a degree of mental retardation. Boys affected by the condition never learn to run, and death occurs before the 18th year in almost all cases. The blood creatine phosphokinase level is greatly raised, often to values several hundred times the normal range, and this abnormality is present before the disease is recognizable clinically. Female carriers of the gene for Duchenne dystrophy usually also show slightly raised levels of creatine phosphokinase in their blood, both at rest and after exercise

(Dreyfus et al. 1960), and this may be useful for detection of the carrier state during genetic counselling.

Muscle biopsies show the typical features of myopathy, but these abnormalities vary in severity according to the stage of the disease and the muscle biopsied. In the early stages there is abnormal variation in fibre size, with prominent focal areas of small, basophilic regenerating fibres. The muscle fibres usually appear unusually rounded. Even at this stage of the disease there may be increased interfascicular and endomysial fibrous tissue. Rounded, large, dark-staining fibres (hyaline fibres), which are markedly eosinophilic and stain red in trichrome preparations, are a prominent feature (Fig. 11.29). Scattered necrotic fibres undergoing phagocytosis and small clusters of regenerating fibres are also present (Fig. 11.30). Fibre splitting may be prominent at this early stage of the disease. As the disorder progresses fibrosis becomes more evident. In severely affected muscles the fascicular pattern of the muscle is destroyed, and the remaining muscle fibres become arranged in irregular bundles surrounded by adipose and fibrous tissue

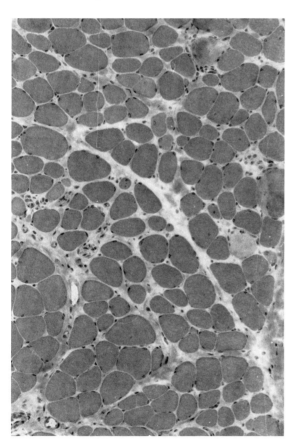

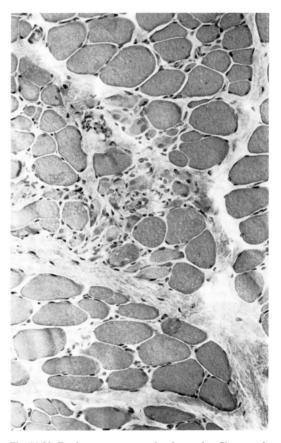

Fig. 11.29. Duchenne-type muscular dystrophy. The muscle fibres are unusually rounded. There is abnormal variability in fibre size. (Gomori trichrome; 140 ×)

Fig. 11.30. Duchenne-type muscular dystrophy. Clusters of small regenerating fibres are a characteristic feature. Several larger, rounded fibres have undergone hyaline change. (H and E; 140 ×)

(Fig. 11.27). Nerve fascicles are relatively spared, but muscle spindles are involved, and are eventually destroyed (Swash and Fox 1976). In the early stages it is not uncommon for regenerating clumps of fibres to form small groups of fibres of similar histochemical type, but fibre-type grouping is not a feature of the disease (Schwartz et al. 1977). Biopsies usually show type 1 fibres to be predominant (Fig. 11.31), and the normally clear differentiation of type 1 and type 2 fibres in the ATPase reaction at pH 9.4 is impaired, so that many fibres appear to be of intermediate histochemical type in this preparation.

Electron microscopy shows degenerative and regenerative changes, which are not specific. However, it has recently been suggested on the basis of electron microscopic studies that plasma membranes of necrotic (Milhorat et al. 1966) and of apparently normal muscle fibres in Duchenne dystrophy are defective, allowing abnormal permeability and thus leading to swelling and focal necrosis of fibres (Mokri and Engel 1975). This abnormality might also explain the presence of focal 'hypercontraction bands' in muscle fibres in this disorder, an abnormality that seems to underlie the formation of the darkly staining hyaline fibres. Studies in which the freeze-fracture technique was used to visualize the details of membrane ultrastructure have shown a reduction in the numbers of intramembrane particles in the two faces of the fractured membrane from dystrophic muscle fibres, and extensive areas in which only a few particles were seen. In particular, the number of 'square-array' pits in the membrane was reduced. It has been suggested that this abnormality, which may be distributed more widely than in muscle alone, may be the primary defect in Duchenne muscular dystrophy (Schotland 1977).

At autopsy most of the proximal muscles are found to be replaced by fat and fibrous tissue. The peripheral nerves and spinal cord are normal and there is a normal number of anterior horn cells, evidence that the electrophysiological finding of reduced numbers of functioning motor units in Duchenne muscular dystrophy is due to the abnormality in the muscle, rather than a primary neurogenic phenomenon. However, in the brain abnormal patterns of gyral development, pachygyria, and microscopic heterotopias have been observed, and the weights of brains from boys with Duchenne dystrophy are less than those of normal brains (Rosman and Kakulas 1966).

The carrier state can be detected by muscle biopsy in many instances. In addition to elevation of the serum creatine phosphokinase level, there may be slight myopathic changes consisting of increased variability in fibre size, excess central nucleation and, more rarely, of focal necrosis, and regeneration of single fibres. These findings have been taken as evidence supporting the hypothesis that expression of the gene for Duchenne dystrophy in females depends on variations in the degree of inactivation of paternal or maternal X chromosomal material (Pearce et al. 1966).

4.1.2. Becker-type Muscular Dystrophy Becker-type muscular dystrophy disorder is similar to Duchenne dystrophy but of lesser severity, so that survival into adult life with preservation of the ability to walk, is a criterion for diagnosis. Like Duchenne dystrophy, it is inherited as an X-linked recessive disorder. It has been associated with deutan colour blindness and the Xg blood group, suggesting that it is genetically distinct from Duchenne muscular dystrophy (Becker 1962; Emery et al. 1969). Muscle biopsy generally reveals similar features to those of Duchenne dystrophy, but the abnormalities may be less severe, and there are sometimes large numbers of small fibres, some of which appear pointed and resemble denervated fibres (Bradley et al. 1978).

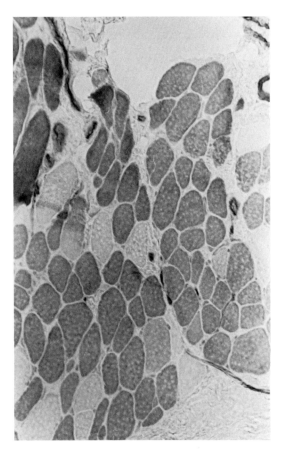

Fig. 11.31. Duchenne-type muscular dystrophy. The rounded fibres are well shown. There is quite prominent type 1 fibre predominance. (ATPase, pH 4.3; 140 ×)

4.1.3. Limb-girdle Muscular Dystrophy Muscular dystrophy in a limb-girdle distribution, with proximal weakness affecting the legs more than the arms, is difficult to distinguish from Becker dystrophy. However, limb-girdle dystrophy is inherited in an autosomal recessive pattern. The disease may progress rapidly or slowly, and it is probable that this pattern of muscular weakness does not represent a specific disease entity, but rather results from a number of different biochemical disorders. In the past, juvenile-onset spinal muscular atrophy (Section 3.2.1.) was often misclassified as limb-girdle dystrophy, but modern enzyme-histochemical methods have eliminated this problem. The creatine phosphokinase is usually slightly or moderately elevated in limb-girdle dystrophy.

Muscle biopsy shows fibres of varying size, with increased central nucleation, a few scattered necrotic or regenerating fibres, and striking hypertrophy of some fibres. Fibre-type grouping is absent. Oxidative enzyme preparations show fibres, particularly larger fibres, with a whorled appearance, indicating an abnormal distribution of lipid and mitochondria and therefore an abnormal pattern of myofibrils. PAS preparations show a similar abnormality. Electron microscopy shows no specific abnormality.

4.1.4. Facio–Scapulo–Humeral Muscular Dystrophy. The shoulder girdle and facial muscles are principally affected in facio–scapulo–humeral muscular dystrophy. The syndrome probably results from a number of different causes, including muscular dystrophy, myasthenia gravis, various congenital myopathies (especially myotubular myopathy), nemaline myopathy, central-core disease, and mitochrondrial myopathies (van Wijngaarden and Bethlem 1971), polymyositis, and chronic denervating disorders. Cases resulting from idiopathic dystrophy are a minority in this list of causes, and in these cases changes found in biopsies of affected muscles are often surprisingly slight. Scapuloperoneal myopathy forms a rare sub-group of this disorder in which weakness principally affects periscapular and peroneal muscles; the extensor digitorum brevis muscles are strikingly spared. This latter disorder also has a neurogenic form (see Kaeser 1965).

4.1.5. Congenital Muscular Dystrophy The syndrome of congenital muscular dystrophy presents from birth with hypotonia and generalized weakness. Contractures develop. There may be associated mental retardation. In some cases improvement occurs with increasing age. The muscle biopsy shows striking myopathic changes with marked endomysial fibrosis and accumulations of adipose tissue.

The muscle fibres are often strikingly small. This syndrome is one of the causes of arthrogryposis multiplex (Section 3.1.6.4.).

4.1.6. Muscular Dystrophy with Involvement of External Ocular Muscles Cases of progressive external ophthalmoplegia with ptosis (Kiloh and Nevin 1951), oculopharyngeal myopathy, often associated with some skeletal muscular weakness (Victor et al. 1962; Barbeau 1966), and external ophthalmoplegia with limb-girdle weakness, sometimes associated with cerebellar ataxia, retinitis pigmentosa, heart block, and an elevated cerebrospinal fluid protein (Kearns and Sayre 1958) and other features (Drachman 1975; Berenberg et al. 1977) form a distinct group of syndromes.

It is striking that external ophthalmoplegia does not occur in other myopathies or dystrophies, although it is also a feature of myasthenia gravis.

In these syndromes with external ophthalmoplegia, biopsy of a proximal upper limb muscle may reveal a characteristic abnormality, consisting of lightly vacuolated fibres, rimmed with red material in the Gomori stain—ragged red fibres (Fig. 12.12). This abnormality predominantly affects type 1 fibres. Other myopathic features, including slightly increased variability in fibre size, increased central nucleation, and increased endomysial fibrous tissue, may be seen. Ultrastructural studies reveal mitochondrial abnormalities similar to those found in other 'mitochondrial myopathies' (p. 508).

4.2. Congenital Myopathies

Congenital myopathic disorders present at birth or in early infancy as the floppy infant syndrome, or later in childhood as proximal or generalized muscular weakness. In some cases, principally those with mitochondrial abnormalities, external ocular muscles are involved. In most instances these disorders are nonprogressive, or only very slowly progressive, and the creatine phosphokinase level is often normal.

4.2.1. Central-core Disease Shy and Magee (1956) defined central-core disease as a nonprogressive congenital myopathy beginning shortly after birth, but more recently cases have been described that are apparently of later onset (Bethlem et al. 1966) and some that have been associated with congenital dislocation of the hip (Armstrong et al. 1971). Hypotonia is a prominent feature, and weakness is not severe. The disorder is usually dominantly inherited. The muscle biopsy shows type 1 fibre predominance or, sometimes, poorly differentiated fibres with a core of tissue devoid of enzyme reactivity in oxidative enzyme preparations. Electron microscopy shows that these cores contain few mitochondria and little sarcoplasmic reticulum; various myofibrillar abnormalities, including streaming of the Z-line, occur in this region (Seitelberger et al. 1961). The cores have a predilection for type 1 fibres (Dubowitz and Roy 1970) and must be distinguished from target fibres, an abnormality found in denervated muscle. Cores may be 'structured', retaining their myofibrillar pattern and thus being demonstrable in ATPase preparations, or unstructured, losing their myofibrillar and intermyofibrillar structure (Neville and Brooke 1973).

In multicore (minicore) disease, a similar but sporadic or autosomal recessive disorder, muscle biopsy shows multiple areas of focal decrease in mitochondrial oxidative enzyme activity, usually associated with focal degenerative changes in myofibrils. These areas, unlike the cores of classic central-core disease, do not extend throughout the length of affected fibres but are relatively sharply circumscribed (Currie et al. 1974). Central nucleation is usually prominent.

4.2.2. Nemaline Myopathy (Rod-body Myopathy)

Shy and Magee (1956) and Gonatas et al. (1966) described rod-like structures in the muscle biopsies of several infants that had been floppy since birth and showed weakness of the arms more than of the legs. Other workers (Hopkins et al. 1966) have recognized that this disorder was the same as had previously been termed Krabbe's universal muscular atrophy. The disease is probably inherited as an autosomal dominant characteristic. Respiratory difficulties are common in infancy. The severity of the disorder varies widely from case to case, and the nosological position of nemaline myopathy is made particularly controversial by reports of the occurrence of similar nemaline bodies in a variety of other disorders, including denervation, psychosis, myotonic dystrophy, polymyositis, and Adie's syndrome, and after experimental tenotomy (see Dubowitz and Brooke 1973; Swash and Fox 1976). Late-onset cases also occur (Engel and Resnick 1966).

In some cases of nemaline myopathy the biopsy has been normal, apart from the presence of the rods, but in many instances there is increased variability in fibre size (the rod bodies being more prominent in the smaller fibres) and increased central nucleation. In oxidative enzyme preparations whorled fibres are sometimes seen. The rod bodies are difficult to recognize in haematoxylin and eosin preparations, but in Gomori stains (Figs. 11.21 and 11.22) they appear as short, bright red masses and are usually predominantly subsarcolemmal in location. Aggregates of rods appear as negatively stained areas in ATPase preparations.

Either or both fibre types may be affected. Electron microscopy reveals that the rods are derived from Z-band material (Figs. 11.14 and 11.27), and Shafiq et al. (1967) have suggested that they are derived from tropomyosin, a protein devoid of tryptophan. Rod bodies have been reported to co-exist with central cores (Afifi et al. 1965), and there may thus be similarities between these two apparently dissimilar disorders.

4.2.3. Myotubular Myopathy

Myotubular myopathy (Spiro et al. 1966), also known as centronuclear myopathy (Sher et al. 1967), is a rare disorder characterized by hypotonia with delayed motor developmental milestones in infancy, followed by a slowly progressive myopathy involving facial and sometimes external ocular musculature. Adult-onset examples have also been reported (Bethlem et al. 1968). These have usually affected females, and in one family there was an association with diabetes mellitus (Swash et al. 1970). Central nucleation is found in nearly all the fibres in the biopsy. In the central regions of affected fibres oxidative enzyme activity is absent or abnormally intense, and myofibrillar ATPase is absent in these regions. In some cases type 1 fibre hypertrophy has been described (Bethlem et al. 1969).

4.2.4. Congenital Fibre-type Disproportion

The characteristic feature of congenital fibre-type disproportion is only evident on muscle biopsy (Brooke 1973). Clinically, affected infants have been floppy or even very weak from birth, but after 2 years of age there is usually some improvement. The disorder is associated with congenital dislocation of the hip, low body weight and short stature, kyphoscoliosis, a high-arched palate, and foot deformities. The biopsy shows small type 1 fibres and normal or enlarged type 2 fibres. No other abnormality is present (Fardeau et al. 1975). The differential diagnosis must include severe infantile spinal muscular atrophy, which has a much poorer prognosis, congenital myotonic dystrophy, and myotubular myopathy with type 1 fibre hypotrophy. The pattern of inheritance is variable.

4.2.5. Mitochondrial Myopathies

In mitochondrial myopathies a characteristic morphological abnormality is present in mitochondria, resulting in the occurrence of *ragged-red fibres* (Section 2.6.2). On electron microscopy these fibres are found to show an abnormal myofibrillar pattern; their mitochondria show abnormalities consisting of an increase in number, reduplication of their double limiting membranes, and the presence of round, osmiophilic dense bodies and of intermembranous paracrystalline bodies (Fig. 11.28). These abnormalities occur in a number of clinically different neuromuscular disorders, including ocular myopathies, Kearns–Sayre syndrome, limb-girdle myopathies with defects of mitochondrial oxidation (Morgan-Hughes et al. 1978), uncoupled oxidative phosphorylation leading to weight loss, hypothyroidism, facio–scapulo–humeral weakness, carnitine deficiency, and polymyositis. However, ragged-red fibres are most commonly found in biopsies of limb muscles from patients with progressive external ophthalmoplegia. Ragged-red fibre change is virtually restricted to type 1 fibres in all these conditions. The red material consists not only of aggregated mitochondria but also of lipid droplets, which are particularly conspicuous in carnitine deficiency. More than 1 % of type 1 fibres should be affected by ragged-red fibre change before the abnormality is regarded as significant.

Swash et al. (1978b) have suggested that ragged-red fibre change can occur as one aspect of regeneration of fibres. This would account for their occurrence in muscle biopsies in conditions other than the myopathies associated with progressive external ophthalmoplegia.

4.2.6. Other Congenital Myopathies In a number of reports, individual patients or families have been described in whom myopathies beginning in infancy have been associated with muscle fibre abnormalities that are, as yet, unclassified. These include myopathies with subsarcolemmal 'fingerprint' inclusions (Engel et al. 1972), myopathies with abnormal sarcotubular systems, zebra-body myopathy (Lake and Wilson 1975), and myopathies with cytoplasmic bodies or tubular aggregates. Dubowitz (1978) has proposed the term 'minimal change myopathy' to described cases such as these, in which the muscle biopsy shows only minimal myopathic abnormalities without more specific features.

4.3. Myotonic Syndromes

The group of myotonic syndromes involves patients in whom myotonia, a state of delayed relaxation or of sustained contraction of muscle fibres, occurs alone or in association with myopathic muscular weakness. Myotonia, although recognizable clinically, must be differentiated by electromyographic criteria from other forms of persistent contraction of muscle fibres. It is probably due to an abnormality in ionic conductance in the muscle fibre membrane (Barchi 1975).

4.3.1. Myotonic Dystrophy In myotonic dystrophy, myotonia is typically associated with muscular weakness and wasting, frontal baldness, testicular atrophy, ptosis, dysphagia, and cataract.

Cardiomyopathy and diabetes mellitus and some degree of mental retardation are common. The disease usually begins in adult life or in adolescence, and the weakness is most evident in facial, sternomastoid, neck extensor, and distal limb muscles. The tendon reflexes are usually absent. In childhood the disease can also present with these features, but in the congenital form of myotonic dystrophy the clinical manifestations are somewhat different. There is hypotonia and failure to thrive, with respiratory difficulties in the perinatal period. Facial weakness is very prominent but myotonia is usually absent. If the infant survives cardiomyopathy and mental retardation become evident. This form of the disease is particularly common in children of *mothers* with the disease (Harper 1975). Myotonic dystrophy is inherited as a Mendelian dominant characteristic.

In both adult- and congenital-onset cases the creatine phosphokinase is usually normal. Abnormalities in IgG and IgM concentration and metabolism have been reported (Wochner et al. 1966; Bundey et al. 1970). In the adult type of the disease muscle biopsies show marked changes. There is increased variability in fibre size with type 1 fibre atrophy, and some degenerative changes in single fibres, consisting both in fibre necrosis and in patchy myofibrillar degeneration, often with the formation of peripherally placed masses of granular sarcoplasm free of myofibrils (Fig. 12.24) (Klinkerfuss 1967). Fibrosis is a feature only in very wasted muscles. There may be a number of other abnormalities, including fibres with a moth-eaten appearance in the NADH preparation, and a variety of inclusions are seen in ultrastructural studies. Rod bodies have also been reported in myotonic dystrophy. A striking feature is central migration and proliferation of muscle fibre nuclei, resulting in the occurrence of long chains of centrally placed vesicular nuclei in longitudinal sections. Displaced myofibrils, forming *Ringbinden* (Fig. 12.24), are also common in this disease.

The muscle spindles show a characteristic abnormality consisting of fragmentation of intrafusal muscle fibres (Fig. 11.26), which is more marked in their polar than their equatorial regions, with proliferation of the motor and sensory innervation (Swash and Fox 1972, 1975a, b). The muscle spindle abnormality is not uniformly distributed, some spindles being more severely affected than others.

Small pointed fibres that are strongly positive for NADH and for nonspecific esterase and contain pyknotic nuclei are commonly found in myotonic dystrophy, suggesting that denervation occurs in the disease. The innervation of the extrafusal muscle fibres in myotonic dystrophy is abnormal. Motor end-plates show proliferative changes, with extensive subterminal axonal branching and expansion of the end-plate zone, but there is some doubt as to whether these abnormalities are primary or secondary to the dystrophic changes in the muscle fibres themselves (Allen et al. 1969).

In the less common congenital form of myotonic dystrophy the muscle biopsy shows similar abnormalities, but the main feature is the presence of small round fibres with central nuclei and atrophy of type 1 fibres.

4.3.2. Myotonia Congenita Thomsen's disease, otherwise known as myotonia congenita, consists of myotonia, beginning in childhood and aggravated by cold, fatigue, or sudden voluntary muscular contraction. This type of myotonia, which can be disabling and painful, is associated with marked muscular hypertrophy, but weakness is uncommon. The disease may be inherited as a recessive or dominant trait, and the recessive form is more likely to be accompanied by muscular weakness, although this is rarely severe. Muscle biopsies do not show myopathic changes, but absence of type 2B fibres has been reported (Crews et al. 1976).

4.3.3. Paramyotonia Congenita Eulenberg's disease consists of myotonia induced or aggravated by cold. There is some controversy as to whether this syndrome is a distinct disorder, since reports of patients with paramyotonia congenita have shown overlapping features with Thomsen's myotonia congenita and with hyperkalaemic periodic paralysis (see Dubowitz 1978).

4.3.4. Others Myotonia is a minor feature in some patients with periodic paralysis, in whom it is particularly evident in the upper eyelids. Myotonia is also a feature of the Schwartz–Jampel syndrome, consisting of myotonic lid-lag, muscle weakness, dwarfism, and a characteristic facies.

4.4. Metabolic Myopathies

Metabolic myopathies are a group of myopathies of varying severity, associated with biochemical defects. In some a fixed or progressive myopathy develops, but in others there are recurrent episodes of muscular weakness, often associated with transient myoglobinuria and muscular pain.

4.4.1. Glycogenoses The glycogen storage diseases are all uncommon, and muscular involvement does not occur in all of them. Myopathy is prominent, among other manifestations, in acid maltase deficiency (type 2 glycogenosis), in amylo 1–6 glucosidase deficiency (type 3 glycogenosis), in myophosphorylase deficiency (type 5 glycogenosis:

McArdle's disease) and in phosphofructokinase deficiency (type 7 glycogenosis), but only in the last two are muscular symptoms the only manifestation.

In the infantile, autosomal recessive variety of acid maltase deficiency, proximal weakness, often associated with enlargement of the heart, liver, and tongue, develops. Death usually occurs from cardiorespiratory failure before the age of 1 year. A milder form of the disease, leading to death in the second decade, resembles Duchenne dystrophy in its clinical manifestations. An adult-onset form has also been reported (Engel et al. 1973).

In acid maltase deficiency the creatine phosphokinase is slightly raised and muscle biopsy shows a marked vacuolar myopathy. The normal histological pattern of the muscle is destroyed by glycogen-containing PAS-positive vacuoles. These vacuoles are also strongly reactive for acid phosphatase (A.G. Engel 1970a). The autophagic nature of the vacuoles is confirmed by electron microscopy, which reveals glycogen granules packed free in the sarcoplasm, in whorled, membrane-bound glycogen bodies, and in autophagic vacuoles (A.G. Engel 1970a).

Type 3 glycogenosis involves liver and muscle. Although muscular involvement is relatively slight the muscle biopsy shows a prominent vacuolar myopathy (Fig. 11.32). The vacuoles contain glycogen, but unlike those found in type 2 glycogenosis, these vacuoles are not lysosomal in origin and are negative in stains for acid phosphatase (Illingworth et al. 1956; Brunberg et al. 1971).

In myophosphorylase (McArdle 1951; Schmid and Mahler 1959) and phosphofructokinase deficiency (Tarui et al. 1965), easy fatiguability is followed, in late childhood or adolescence, by severe muscular cramps with weakness on exertion. Transient myoglobinuria may occur in these episodes. Later mild permanent proximal weakness may develop. Although an autosomal recessive pattern of inheritance is usual, McArdle's syndrome is commoner in boys than girls. The blood creatine phosphokinase levels are raised after exertion in both syndromes, and during ischaemic exercise the venous lactate fails to rise (Mellick et al. 1962). The muscle biopsy shows only minor histological changes. There are some small PAS-positive subsarcolemmal vacuoles and PAS staining shows an excess of sarcoplasmic glycogen. Necrotic or small fibres occur and internal nucleation is common. Histochemical stains for phosphorylase demonstrate no reaction in McArdle's disease and a similar absence of phosphofructokinase has been demonstrated in type 7 glycogenosis (Tarui et al. 1965). Ultrastructurally, glycogen deposition is prominent both in intermyofibrillar sarcoplasm and in the subsarcolemmal vacuoles.

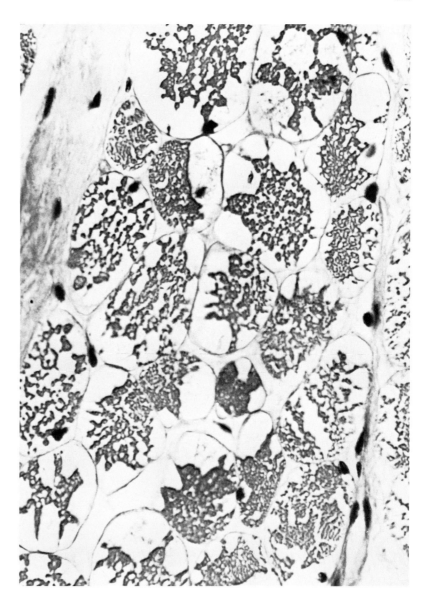

Fig. 11.32. Glycogen storage disease, type 3 rectus abdominis muscle. The vacuoles are filled with glycogen, which is invisible with this stain. (H and E; 950 ×)

4.4.2. Abnormalities of Lipid Metabolism Myopathies caused by abnormal lipid metabolism are characterized by the accumulation of neutral lipid in muscle fibres and by a variety of degenerative changes, including ragged-red fibres, in individual fibres. Carnitine deficiency and carnitine palmityl transferase deficiency are the best-documented examples. These two disorders are also classified as mitochondrial myopathies, because they are due to defects of mitochondrial metabolism and are accompanied by characteristic morphological changes in mitochondria in affected fibres (Section 2.5.). Weakness and myoglobinuria, with muscular pain, occur after exercise. In carnitine deficiency plasma, muscle and hepatic carnitine levels are low and there is sometimes hypoglycaemia. There is gross wasting and cachexia. In carnitine palmityl transferase deficiency cachexia is not a feature. Fasting can induce attacks of weakness and myoglobinuria, together with a rise in blood triglycerides. The muscle biopsy in carnitine palmityl transferase deficiency is usually normal, but in carnitine deficiency there is a severe, destructive myopathy with prominent lipid-containing acid phosphatase-positive vacuoles (see Karpati et al. 1975; Bank et al. 1975). Diagnosis of these disorders rests on demonstration of the primary biochemical disorder by quantitative biochemical studies, although it may be possible to suggest the likely defect from the clinical, biochemical, and histological features.

4.4.3. Other Causes of Myoglobinuria Myoglobinuria can occur whenever there is acute necrosis of muscle, as in polymyositis, acute toxic myopathies, etc. (see Table 11.4.).

Table 11.4. Classification of myoglobinuric myopathies

Metabolic	(e.g., Glycogenoses, lipid storage myopathies, malignant hyperpyrexia)
Toxic	(e.g., Carbon monoxide poisoning, alcohol, drugs)
Traumatic	
Ischaemic	(Anterior tibial compartment syndrome)
Postinfection	
Idiopathic rhabdo-myolysis	

4.5. Periodic Paralyses

Periodic paralyses are inherited as autosomal dominant traits and are characterized by attacks of flaccid paralysis of varying severity associated with a low, normal, or high serum potassium during the attacks. The term adynamia episodica hereditaria has been used to describe the normokalaemic variety (Gamstorp 1956), and in some patients attacks of weakness have been observed with normal and with raised serum potassium levels. The clinical features of these three forms of periodic paralysis overlap. In hypokalaemic periodic paralysis weakness often begins during sleep although, as in hyperkalaemic periodic paralysis, a period of rest after vigorous exercise may also induce attacks. Weakness may be provoked in the hypokalaemic variety by a heavy carbohydrate meal, cold, anxiety, or a glucose load. Insulin will also induce an attack. The attacks of weakness are usually more severe and more prolonged in hypokalaemic paralysis than in the other forms of periodic paralysis, but death in an attack is uncommon. The disease usually begins in infancy or childhood, and after several attacks of severe weakness it may become apparent that there is some fixed or even progressive proximal weakness. This is often asymmetrical. Myoglobinuria is obvious only in severe attacks. In Oriental races a form of hypokalaemic paralysis may be a presenting feature of thyrotoxicosis (Cheah et al. 1975).

Biopsies taken between attacks of weakness may show little or no abnormality, but in attacks there are often large vacuoles in muscle fibres (Fig. 11.33). In severe attacks some fibres become necrotic and the typical sequence of necrosis, ingestion by macrophages, and basophilic regeneration, usually subsarcolemmal, then occurs. Although the vacuoles appear empty in haematoxylin and eosin stains they usually contain traces of PAS-positive material. However, electron microscopy reveals that the vacuoles are membrane-bound (Fig. 11.34) and continuous with the sarcoplasmic reticulum and T-tube system (Howes et al. 1966; A.G. Engel 1970b). Other, nonspecific, tubular abnormalities have also been described (Bradley 1969). Weller and McArdle (1971) demonstrated calcium salts (hydroxyapatite) in the vacuoles and in the muscle fibres themselves in biopsies from patients with long-standing periodic paralysis. The fixed myopathy found in some patients with these syndromes is associated with typical but nonspecific histological features of a myopathy, including variability in fibre size, central nucleation, single-fibre necrosis and regeneration, and increased endomysial fibrous tissue (Fig. 11.33). However, even in these cases there is sometimes vacuolation of fibres, and this can be an important clue in diagnosis.

4.5.1. Other Forms of Hypokalaemic Paralysis Severe hypokalaemia of any cause can induce muscular weakness with typical vacuolar changes in

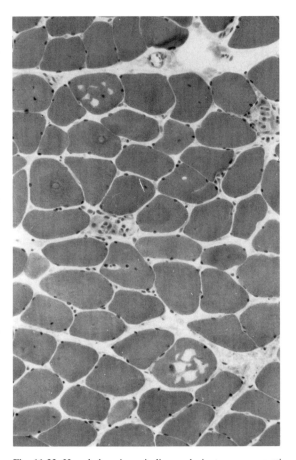

Fig. 11.33. Hypokalaemic periodic paralysis, transverse section. Several fibres contain large vacuoles: two others have undergone necrosis with phagocytosis. These are the features of long-standing periodic paralysis, with a recent acute attack. (H and E; 140 ×)

the muscle biopsy. For example, hypokalaemia resulting from diuretic therapy, renal disease, or liquorice ingestion may occasionally be sufficiently severe to induce weakness.

4.5.2. Malignant Hyperpyrexia In malignant hyperpyrexia a mild or even subclinical myopathy, dominantly inherited, is associated with a tendency for fatal hyperpyrexia to develop during general anaesthesia. The hyperpyrexia seems to result from heat produced by intense and generalized muscular rigidity with tachycardia, tachypnoea, cyanosis, and severe metabolic acidosis. Extensive muscular necrosis follows, with myoglobinuria, a very high serum creatine phosphokinase, and sometimes renal failure. Recovery is usually complete in patients who survive the hyperpyrexia, hyperkalaemia, and acid-osis. The underlying metabolic disorder is ill-defined, but it has been suggested that certain anaesthetic drugs release sarcoplasmic and sarco-tubular calcium ions, causing muscular contraction. Susceptibility can sometimes be recognized by provocation tests on muscle tissue obtained by biopsy in an in vitro test (Moulds and Denborough 1972; Ellis et al. 1973).

Muscle biopsies taken after an attack of hyperpyrexia show extensive muscle fibre necrosis, followed by regeneration. Biopsies taken from susceptible subjects who are otherwise not affected show minor abnormalities consisting of slightly increased variability in fibre size with increased central nucleation. The serum creatine phosphokinase may be slightly raised in these patients (Isaacs and Barlow 1970).

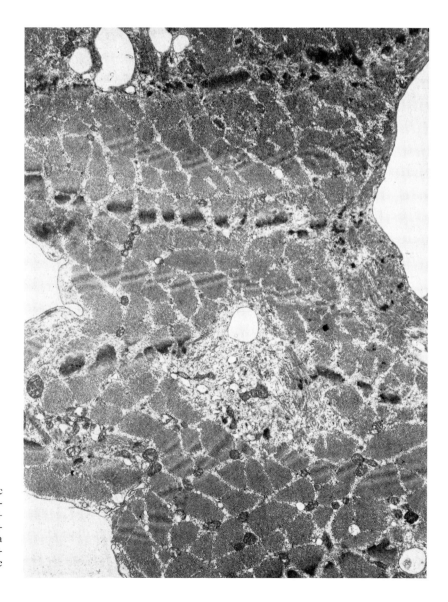

Fig. 11.34. Hypokalaemic periodic paralysis. The vacuoles are continuous with tubules of the sarcoplasmic reticulum and T-tube system, and are therefore bound by a single layered membrane. Myofibrils near these vacuoles have become disrupted. (EM; 1500 ×)

4.6. Endocrine Myopathies

Muscular weakness may complicate thyrotoxicosis, hypothyroidism, hyperparathyroidism, osteomalacia, acromegaly, and both Cushing's disease and steroid therapy. In these disorders, myopathy is rarely severe, and histological changes may be very slight. Atrophy of type 2 fibres occurs, especially in steroid myopathy and in osteomalacia, and in acromegaly there may also be hypertrophy of type 1 fibres.

4.6.1. Myasthenia Gravis Myasthenia gravis is characterized by fluctuating weakness, particularly affecting cranial muscles but consisting principally in abnormal fatiguability after sustained activity, with improvement after rest. The disease is commonest in young adults, affecting women 3 times more frequently than men, but several childhood forms exist: (a) Juvenile myasthenia, a disorder similar to the adult disease; (b) Congenital (or infantile) myasthenia; (c) Transient neonatal myasthenia in infants born to myasthenic mothers.

Juvenile myasthenia gravis is an uncommon condition. Although a quarter of all patients with myasthenia gravis present before the age of 20 years, less than 5% present before the age of 10 years (Bundey 1972). Myasthenia beginning before the age of 2 years is usually termed congenital myasthenia. Although the clinical features of congenital and juvenile myasthenia may be similar, patients with— congenital myasthenia tend to have a benign, non-progressive course (Namba et al. 1971) and ocular manifestations may be prominent (Whiteley et al. 1976). The term infantile myasthenia is better reserved for cases of *severe* myasthenia beginning before the age of 2 years (Whiteley et al. 1976), since this disorder may present with bulbar and respiratory problems (Conomy et al. 1975). In both congenital and infantile myasthenia siblings are also commonly affected, an uncommon feature in adult or juvenile myasthenia (Bundey 1972), but the association of myasthenia with HLA–B1, HLA–B8 and HLA–DW3 haplotypes found in about 70% of patients with juvenile or adult myasthenia (Behan et al. 1973; Pirskanen 1976) is not found in the congenital form (Whiteley et al. 1976). Neonatal myasthenia is a transient disorder. About 15% of infants born to myasthenic mothers are floppy and weak, requiring anticholinesterase therapy during the first month after birth (Osserman 1958; Stern et al. 1964). Finally, myasthenia is occasionally associated with thyrotoxicosis and with polymyositis.

In juvenile myasthenia lymphoid hyperplasia and an increase in the number and size of germinal centres occurs in the thymus in about two-thirds of patients, but thymoma in infants and children is very rare (Namba et al. 1978). In congenital and infantile myasthenia the thymus is usually normal. Muscle biopsies in myasthenia of any type reveal little abnormality in most cases. Lymphorrhages, usually related to blood vessels, are common (Russell 1953), but are not specific for myasthenia, having been reported in neurogenic disorders and in polymyositis (Dubowitz and Brooke 1973). Engel and McFarlin (1966) found atrophy of type 2 fibres in about half their patients, and lymphorrhages in only a quarter. Dubowitz and Brooke (1973) noted that type 2 fibre atrophy was often irregularly distributed within the biopsy, suggesting that it was not necessarily a nonspecific phenomenon. Scattered small pointed fibres, or even fibre-type grouping have also been reported, which suggests that denervation and reinnervation occur during the course of the disease (Fenichel and Shy 1963; Brownell et al. 1972). Denervation has usually been attributed to myasthenic damage to motor end-plates, but it has been shown that treatment with anticholesterase drugs itself causes morphological and functional changes in motor end-plates (Schwartz et al. 1977).

Cöers and Desmedt (1959) described characteristic abnormalities in the motor innervation in myasthenia gravis (Fig. 11.35), consisting of elongated motor endings without evidence of axonal sprouting (dysplastic pattern) and increased collateral ramification of motor axons (dystrophic pattern) with the formation of multiple end-plates (Cöers and Telerman-Toppet 1976). Cöers (1975) has suggested that the dystrophic pattern is a feature of older patients and the dysplastic pattern of younger patients. In patients with a dystrophic pattern the terminal innervation ratio may be increased (Cöers and Telerman-Toppet 1976), an observation suggesting that denervation has occurred. Schwartz et al. 1977) considered that this might be due to the effect of prolonged anticholinesterase therapy, rather than to the myasthenia itself. Ultrastructural studies of motor end-plates in myasthenia have shown that the possynaptic region is smaller than normal, with loss (simplification) of the postsynaptic folds. The mean nerve terminal area is also smaller in myasthenic end-plates, but the numbers of synaptic vesicles are normal (Santa et al. 1972).

The area of postsynaptic membrane capable of binding α-bungarotoxin, a snake venom with specific affinity for acetylcholine receptors at motor end-plates, is reduced (Engel et al. 1977), as is the total amount of α-bungarotoxin bound at an end-plate (Fambrough et al. 1973). In myasthenia gravis this loss of functioning acetylcholine receptors is due to an interaction between the receptor protein itself and a circulating acetylcholine-receptor antibody found within the immunoglobulin G fraction of the serum proteins. Such antibodies to extracted human acetylcholine receptor protein can be demonstrated in 90% of patients with myasthenia gravis (Lindstrom et al. 1976). This antibody does not occupy the acetylcholine-binding site of the receptor moiety; rather its effect is to cause loss of acetylcholine receptor protein from the postsynaptic membrane (Lindstrom and Lambert 1978). Receptor degradation is thus accelerated in this condition (Drachman et al. 1978). The site of synthesis of acetylcholine-receptor antibody in myasthenia gravis, and the role of the thymus or thymus-dependent lymphocytes in this humoral disorder, are uncertain. Vincent et al. (1978) demonstrated that cells from one of four thymus glands and three of five thymic lymphocyte preparations synthesized the acetylcholine-receptor antibody.

Passive transfer of immunoglobulin G from myasthenic patients to the mouse (Toyka et al. 1975) causes myasthenic weakness in the recipient mouse, and neonatal myasthenia, recently shown to be associated with gradually declining levels of acetylcholine receptor antibody in the serum of affected infants (Keesey et al. 1977), may result from a similar passive transfer mechanism. However, the severity of myasthenic weakness in juvenile myasthenia does not correlate readily with levels of circulating acetylcholine receptor antibody. Further, in congenital myasthenia acetylcholine-receptor antibody may not be demonstrable and this disorder is probably due to one or more of several different congenital defects of the postsynaptic membrane. These newer concepts of myasthenia gravis have led to rationalization of the role of anticholinesterase drugs, of immuno-suppressant therapy, and of thymectomy in the management of the disease.

4.6.2. Inflammatory Myopathies Walton and Adams (1958) classified the inflammatory myopathies into four subgroups: (a) Polymyositis, beginning in childhood (before the age of 16 years) or in adult life, and acute, subacute, or chronic in course; (b) polymyositis, with some skin changes, or with associated features of other connective-tissue disorders, e.g., polyarthropathy; (c) Severe connective-tissue disease with slight muscular involvement; (d) Polymyositis or dermatomyositis associated with malignant disease.

This classification is based on Walton's and Adams' predominant experience of polymyositis in adults (see Bohan and Peter 1975).
Dermatomyositis of childhood is a distinct but uncommon disorder, presenting with muscular weakness, skin lesions, and systemic symptoms. Muscular weakness is usually proximal, sometimes very severe, and usually also involves facial muscles. The skin lesion, as in adult poly-

myositis/dermatomyositis, may be florid or quite inconspicuous. It is more prominent in exposed skin. There is usually muscular pain and tenderness, with fever and weight loss, and hepatosplenomegaly, fleeting polyarthropathy, cardiac involvement, and calcification of the muscle and skin (Cook et al. 1963); ulceration of skin and gastrointestinal tract also occurs in some cases (Banker and Victor 1966). The creatine phosphokinase and the ESR are usually, but not always, both raised and in patients with widespread muscular damage the creatine phosphokinase may be raised to as much as several hundred times the normal value.

The muscle biopsy shows increased variability in fibre size with atrophy of both fibre types. Fibre hypertrophy is uncommon, but in chronic cases there may be some hypertrophy of type 1 fibres. In these patients fibre splitting may occur (Swash et al. 1978a). Scattered small angular fibres that are intensely reactive for NADH are usually present, indicating the presence of denervation, which results

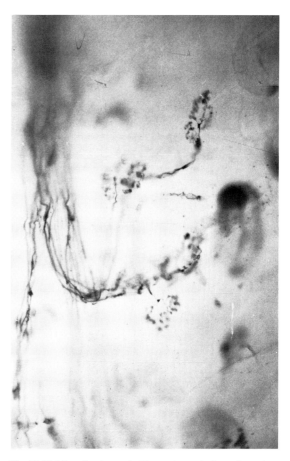

Fig. 11.35. Myasthenia gravis. The motor end-plates show sprouting and elongation. (Supravital methylene blue impregnation; 350×)

either from damage to the peripheral nerves, as in polyarteritis nodosa or, in most cases, from infarction of small nerve twigs in the muscles themselves. Fibre-type grouping is seen in some biopsies, but the numbers of fibres within these groups are small compared with the numbers in biopsies from neurogenic disorders. Necrotic, and basophilic regenerating fibres are common, especially if patients with a subacute course, and central nucleation is frequent. In patients with an acute onset there may be patchy but widespread subendomysial necrosis of fibres, often in a fascicular distribution (Fig. 11.36), suggesting a vascular causation (Banker and Victor 1966; Swash et al. 1978a). Architectural changes in individual fibres are common, particularly in those at the periphery of a fascicle (Fig. 11.37). These changes include loss of ATPase reaction in the centre of a fibre, patchy loss, and accentuation of the NADH and PAS reactions, causing a pronounced moth-eaten appearance or even a 'ghost' fibre that is unreactive in all enzyme preparations (Fig. 11.36). Cytoplasmic bodies and ring fibres also occur.

Inflammatory changes, often predominantly perivascular, occur in about 75% of biopsies in polymyositis (Dubowitz and Brooke 1973). Fibrosis occurs as the disease progresses.

Banker has emphasized the vascular origin of the childhood forms of dermatomyositis (Banker and Victor 1966), suggesting that the muscular and systemic features of the disorder are due to a vasculitis affecting arterioles, small veins, and capillaries in affected muscles and other organs. The finding of extensive perifascicular atrophy and architectural changes supports this concept. Whitaker and Engel (1973) found deposits of immunoglobulin and complement in small blood vessels, particularly in veins, in childhood dermatomyositis, but this observation has not been confirmed and cell-mediated mechanisms have recently gained more support in hypotheses on the pathogenesis of the disorder (Dawkins and Mastaglia 1973). Nonetheless, the finding that muscle capillary endothelial cells contain undulating tubular cytoplasmic inclusions, and evidence that these cells are thicker

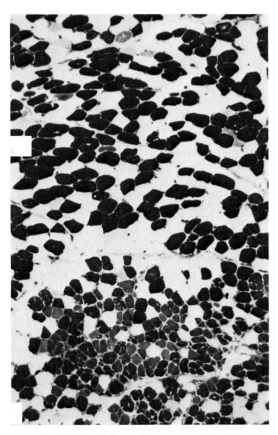

Fig. 11.36. Childhood form of dermatomyositis. Subendomysial necrosis and regeneration is limited by the fascicular planes of the muscle, suggesting a vascular causation. Many of the regenerating fibres are intermediate in histochemical type. (ATPase pH 4.3; 140 ×)

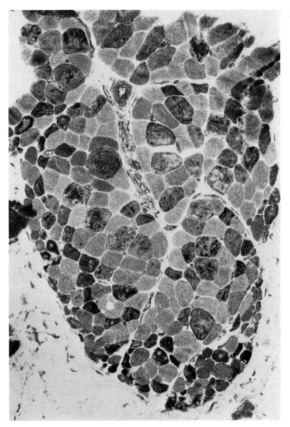

Fig. 11.37. Childhood form of dermatomyositis. Perifascicular atrophy with prominent architectural change, whorled and moth-eaten fibres. (NADH; 140 ×)

than normal and are often surrounded by reduplicated basal lamina (Jerusalem et al. 1974; Banker 1975), have led Carpenter et al. (1976) to suggest that capillary necrosis is the primary lesion in the childhood form of dermatomyositis, leading to the characteristic perifascicular distribution of the changes in muscle fibres in the disease. Undulating tubules and evidence of capillary necrosis have not been reported as characteristic features of the adult form of polymyositis, but capillary damage does occur in adult-onset polymyositis and in polymyositis associated with connective tissue disorders, such as rheumatoid arthritis (Carpenter et al. 1976).

Although a viral aetiology has been suggested, only a few cases associated with high antibody titres, especially for Coxsackie B virus (Chou and Gutmann 1970) and myxovirus (Chou 1968) have been reported. It is possible, however, that the disease may be triggered as an allergic response to a preceding viral infection, since muscular symptoms commonly follow banal 'influenzal' symptoms (see Schwartz et al. 1978).

4.6.3. Floppy Infant Syndrome The floppy infant syndrome is a syndrome of weakness and hypotonia in infancy, due to any of a number of congenital or acquired myopathies, neurogenic disorders, or brain diseases of infancy. It is not a disease entity. This syndrome may also be caused by disorders of elastic tissue, such as Ehlers–Danlos disease.

4.6.4. Arthrogryposis Multiplex Similarly, arthrogryposis is a syndrome of varying causation. The term refers to a complex clinical deformity, usually due to a progressive disorder, consisting of muscular wasting and joint and skeletal deformities. The child is usually unable to stand or walk. The onset is in infancy. This syndrome may occur in a number of progressive, congenital myopathies, in spinal muscular atrophy, or in chronic, infantile polyneuropathies.

5. Neurogenic Disorders

Neurogenic disorders are due to diseases of the motor unit which is composed of the lower motor neurone (anterior horn cell, motor nerve fibre, motor end-plates), and of the individual muscle fibres innervated by these structures. These disorders can be grouped into those due to disease of the anterior horn cells themselves, the *spinal muscular atrophies*, and those in which the motor nerve fibres are primarily affected, the *motor neuropathies*. In the latter group of diseases there can be damage to axons or to Schwann cells, and in many there is associated

involvement of sensory nerve fibres in some cases. These peripheral neuropathies are discussed in Section 3.3.

5.1. Spinal Muscular Atrophies

The spinal muscular atrophies, which affect only the lower motor neurone, are probably the commonest of the neuromuscular disorders of childhood. Subclassification of these cases into severe infantile, intermediate, and mild types is at best arbitrary, since the age of onset of all three groups overlaps and classification can only be finally determined by the outcome (Fried and Emery 1971). However, there are pathological differences between them.

The *severe infantile form* (Werdnig–Hoffman disease) has a well-defined genetic basis, being inherited as an autosomal recessive trait, but sporadic cases also occur. Severe generalized weakness with hypotonia becomes evident during the first few days of life, or may even be noticed by the mother before birth since fetal movements become progressively weakened in some cases. Bulbar palsy develops and death usually occurs before the age of 1 year, although survival to about 3 years occurs in a somewhat milder form of the disorder. In a rare variant of spinal muscular atrophy the bulbar nuclei may be selectively involved, causing a progressive bulbar paralysis (Fazio–Londé syndrome).

In *intermediate spinal muscular atrophy* disability is less marked, but the child is usually unable to walk or stand unaided. Weakness is symmetrical and is accompanied by marked wasting of affected muscles. Proximal muscles are almost always predominantly affected. Fasciculation is not a usual feature, but the tendon reflexes are usually absent. The disorder usually begins between 3 and 15 months of age. It is only slowly progressive and survival into adolescence is common; some patients may improve a little. Cardiac muscle is not involved. Both autosomal recessive and dominant forms occur.

Mild spinal muscular atrophy (Kugelberg–Welander disease) begins in adolescence or in early adult life. The course is only very slowly progressive, and the ability to stand and walk is retained. Weakness is predominantly proximal and the presentation may be similar to that of muscular dystrophy. Occasionally, a neurogenic disorder, due either to a sensorimotor neuropathy or to a form of spinal muscular atrophy presents in a scapuloperoneal distribution. In this disorder the scapular weakness and the characteristic sparing of the extensor digitorum brevis muscles excludes Charcot–Marie–Tooth syndrome. Scapuloperoneal weakness can also be myopathic in origin.

Motor neurone disease (amyotrophic lateral sclerosis) is very rare in childhood.

Muscle biopsies in spinal muscular atrophy show similar features in the severe and intermediate varieties. There is atrophy of both type 1 and type 2 fibres and atrophic fibres are usually arranged in large groups, even affecting whole fascicles (Figs. 11.7 and 11.37). Some fascicles contain smaller groups of hypertrophied fibres of uniform histochemical type. In Werdnig–Hoffman disease atrophic fibres can retain their mosaic pattern of histochemical type, suggesting that denervation has occurred without compensatory reinnervation. Interpretation of atrophy of this type is very difficult without fibre-type grouping or hypertrophy in a biopsy. It has been suggested that these sheets of small rounded, atrophic and poorly differentiated fibres are persistent fetal or immature fibres that have never reached their motor innervation, the disorder having begun in utero. Because atrophy can be very severe, the muscle spindles, which show changes due to denervation only in more chronic disorders (Swash and Fox 1974), may be unusually conspicuous in severe spinal muscular atrophy.

Degenerative changes in single muscle fibres are not a primary feature of this disease, but in chronic, milder forms, especially in Kugelberg–Welander syndrome, such changes are common. These consist of increased interstitial fibrosis, degenerative and regenerative changes in single muscle fibres, fibre hypertrophy, especially affecting type 1 fibres, fibre splitting, increased central nucleation, and fibres with cores, whorls, or a moth-eaten myofibrillar pattern in NADH preparations (Schwartz et al. 1976). In haematoxylin- and eosin-stained sections these secondary myopathic changes may be so prominent (Fig. 11.17) that an erroneous diagnosis of primary myopathy may be suggested unless ATPase preparations show fibre-type grouping.

Clusters of narrow pointed fibres are relatively uncommon in spinal muscular atrophies, although this is a characteristic feature of other acquired forms of denervation. In mild spinal muscular atrophy supravital methylene blue stains will reveal terminal axonal branching and sprouting, illustrating the effectiveness of the collateral reinnervation associated with fibre type grouping. In the central nervous system anterior horn cells are lost and remaining anterior horn cells and somatic motor neurones in the bulbar nuclei show degenerative changes, consisting of chromatolysis, pyknosis, neuronophagia, and gliosis.

6. Diseases of Peripheral Nerve

6.1. Anatomy

Peripheral nerves consist of bundles of myelinated and unmyelinated axons, arranged in fascicles surrounded by connective tissue, collagen, and perineurial cells (Fig. 11.38). The endoneurial space contains small blood vessels. The peripheral nerves tend to be associated with arteries and veins, forming neurovascular bundles. Even small nerve branches situated in muscles show this relationship. Almost all peripheral nerves contain both motor and sensory fibres. During development there is a close interdependence between motor and sensory nerves, growing out from anterior horn cells of the spinal cord and from posterior root ganglia respectively, in the 4th to 6th weeks of intrauterine life. Mesodermal/neural interactions are also important; if the limb nerves are damaged experimentally or fail to grow during this time the appropriate mesodermal somites do not develop properly, leading to congenital anomalies of the limbs.

The *epineurial sheath,* consisting of an outer layer of connective tissue, binds the nerve fascicles together. Each nerve fascicle is surrounded by concentric layers of flattened cells separated by collagen. Each thin cellular layer is surrounded by a layer of basement membrane, and tight junctional complexes and pinocytotic vesicles are prominent features of these cells. These *perineurial* cells form a permeability barrier between the endoneurial space and blood and other extracellular tissue compartments. In the nerve roots the perineurial layer is continuous with the arachnoid cellular layer that surrounds the central nervous system. The cerebrospinal fluid and the endoneurial space are thus potentially in continuity. The *endoneurial space* contains nerve fibres, Schwann cells and blood vessels. Thin cellular septa, fibroblasts and longitudinally orientated collagen fibrils (Fig. 11.39), together with bundles of randomly orientated collagen fibrils, fibroblasts, and acid mucopolysaccharide ground substance, called Renaut bodies, are also found in the endoneurial space. The function of

Fig. 11.39. Normal sural nerve, transverse section. There is a ▷ large, thickly myelinated nerve fibre. The internal and external mesaxon of its Schwann cell, and the dot-like neurofilaments and peripherally situated neurotubules, mitochondria, and lipid droplets of its axon can be seen. Collagen filaments and part of a fibroblast separate this nerve fibre from an adjacent fibre sectioned through a node of Ranvier. Note the dense axonal membrane. Unmyelinated nerve fibres surrounded by thin layers of Schwannian cytoplasm occupy the remainder of the field. (EM; 22 500 ×)

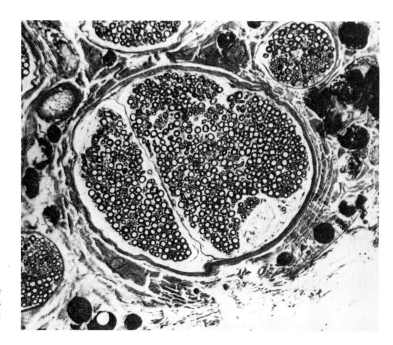

Fig. 11.38. Normal median nerve, TS. The normal distribution of myelinated nerve fibres in fascicles in the nerve can be seen. Osmium method for myelin.

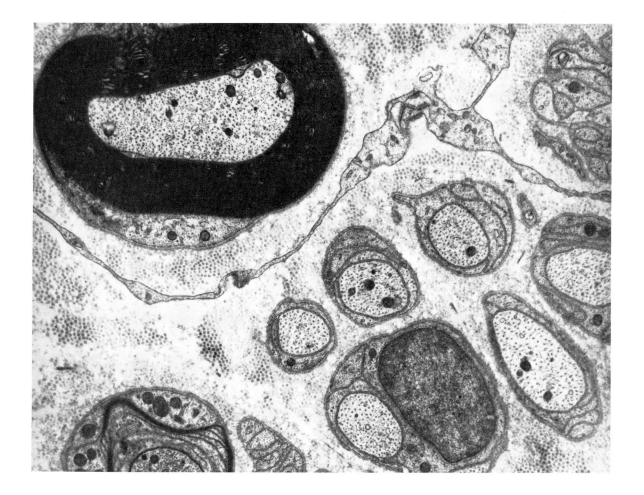

Renaut bodies is obscure (Asbury 1973).

The proportions, diameters, and numbers of myelinated and unmyelinated nerve fibres vary in different peripheral nerves, but normal values are available for several human nerves, including the sural nerve, which is the one most commonly biopsied (Ochoa and Mair 1969; Dyck 1975). In this nerve unmyelinated fibres ($30000/mm^3$) are four times more numerous than myelinated fibres ($8000/mm^3$). Unmyelinated fibres in this nerve range from 0.5 to 0.3 μm in diameter and myelinated fibres range from 2.0 to 17.0 μm in diameter, with bimodal peaks of diameter at 5.0 μm and 13.0 μm. There are slight variations from these figures for very young children and elderly subjects.

Myelinated nerve fibres can be demonstrated in sectioned material or in teased preparations of single nerve fibres. Myelin is formed by layers of Schwannian membranes wrapped concentrically around the axon. The numbers of Schwann cells associated with individual nerve fibres are determined in fetal life;

during development these cells elongate to take account of increasing axonal length. The gap between individual Schwann cells, called the node of Ranvier, is specialized to allow electrolyte exchange during the process of saltatory conduction of the nervous impulse. The thickness of the myelin sheath is related to axonal diameter.

Axons of myelinated nerve fibres can be shown up for light microscopy by silver impregnation. With electron microscopy they are seen as lucent cytoplasm containing dot-like neurofilaments and more peripherally located neurotubules, surrounded by a layer of plasma membrane (Fig. 11.40). Mitochondria and smooth endoplasmic reticulum can usually be recognized (Figs. 11.39 and 11.40). The Schwann cells are closely invested by a layer of basement membrane, which enables them to be distinguished from fibroblasts in sectioned material; several axons can be myelinated by a single Schwann cell. The ultrastructure of Schwann cells, with their nodes of Ranvier and Schmidt–Lanterman incisures, is com-

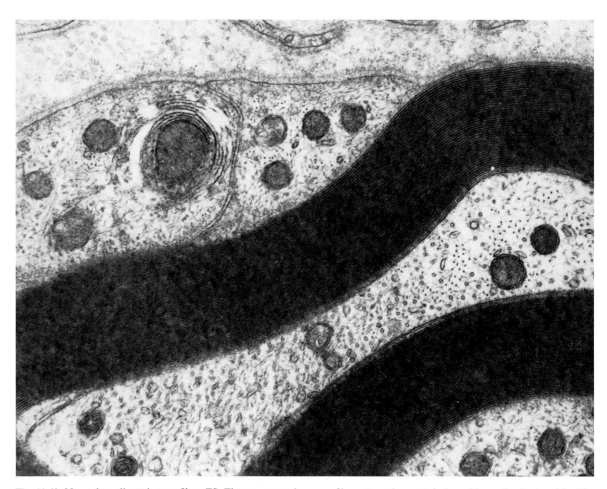

Fig. 11.40. Normal myelinated nerve fibre, TS. The axon contains neurofilaments and neurotubules, with small mitochondria. The myelin lamellae and the Schwann cell covering surrounded by a layer of basement membrane can be clearly seen. ($60000 \times$)

plex (Fig. 11.41). Detailed descriptions of the structure of myelinated nerve fibres are available elsewhere (Landon and Hall 1976).

Unmyelinated nerve fibres (Fig. 12.39) are also associated with Schwann cells, but myelin lamellae are not present (see Ochoa 1976). Typically, Schwann cells are associated with groups of unmyelinated axons (Fig. 11.42). Motor end-plates and sensory receptors in skin and muscle, including muscle spindles (Swash and Fox 1972a, b) have also been studied in peripheral neuropathies, but they are not routinely evaluated.

6.2. Peripheral Nerve Biopsy

The sural nerve is usually selected for biopsy. This nerve is distally located, and thus likely to show abnormalities in patients with peripheral neuropathy. It is superficially located near the ankle and thus easily approached surgically, and it is purely sensory, supplying a small area of skin on the dorsolateral surface of the foot near the ankle. Occasionally, in very severe chronic neuropathies, it may be justifiable to biopsy other nerves, such as the median nerve. The superficial branch of the radial nerve, near the dorsal surface of the base of the thumb may also be selected for biopsy. During biopsy it is important not to squeeze or apply tension to the nerve, because this leads to artefactual folding, tearing, and even disruption of myelin lamellae. Even cutting the nerve with scissors may result in significant artefact. A short length of nerve is removed, and this can be prepared for light and electron microscopy after fixation in glutaraldehyde and embedding in epoxy resin. Toluidine blue staining of semi-thin sections is particularly useful. It is helpful to soak a small piece of the nerve biopsy in isopentane–liquid nitrogen so that histochemical stains for amyloid, and sometimes for complement and immunoglobulins, can be employed. A full discussion of the biopsy technique has been given by Stevens et al. (1975).

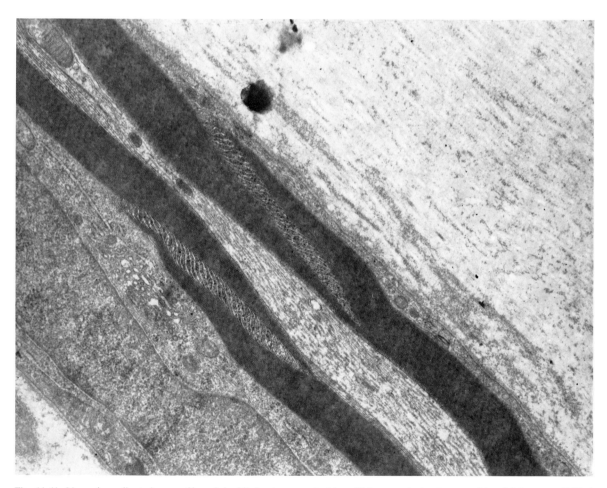

Fig. 11.41. Normal myelinated nerve fibre. Schmidt–Lantermann incision. This normal structure consists of Schwann cell-filled separations of the myelin lamellae.

6.3. Pathological Reactions of Nerve Fibres

The pathological reactions of peripheral nerve fibres are grouped broadly into axonal and demyelinating neuropathies. In the former the axon is damaged and in the latter the Schwann cell is affected. Degeneration of an axon may lead to Wallerian changes in its Schwann cell covering.

6.3.1. Axonal Degeneration Axonal degeneration is the consequence of failure of the metabolic machinery of the neurone itself, resulting in impaired transport of metabolites and proteins along the axon to the periphery. If the neuronal cell body dies axonal degeneration occurs along the length of the axon, with resultant *Wallerian changes* (Figs. 11.43 and 11.44). Such a process will be selective, affecting only certain populations of neurons and their axons.

6.3.2. Distal Axonal Degeneration Distal axonal degeneration (dying-back neuropathy) occurs when metabolism of the distal parts of certain axons fails (Cavanagh 1964). It is thought that this usually results from impaired metabolism of the perikaryon of the nerve cell itself, but local abnormalities in distal axonal metabolism could also produce the change. Myelin breakdown, often segmental in character, occurs in the region of the axonal degeneration, which takes the form of irregularities in axonal size and shape (Fig. 11.45) and of degeneration of axoplasmic constituents and of the axonal terminations themselves, e.g., sensory receptors and motor end-plates (Fig. 11.43). Recovery from this process is possible if the metabolic abnormality can be corrected, e.g., by replacement of vitamin deficiency or cessation of exposure to

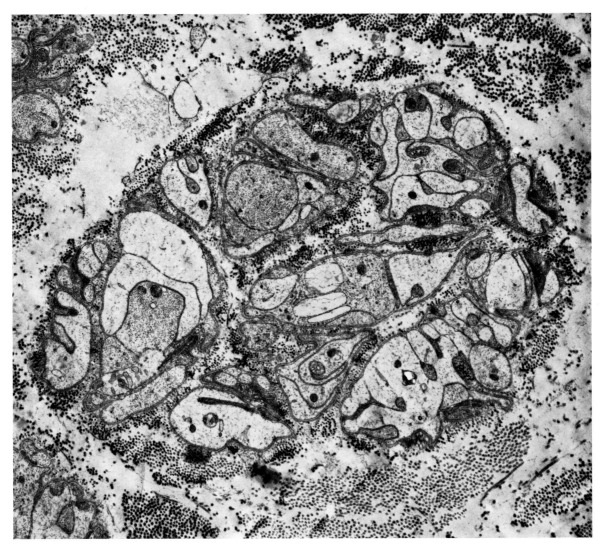

Fig. 11.42. Normal unmyelinated axon, TS. There is a profusion of unmyelinated axons and Schwann cell cytoplasm. (22 500 ×)

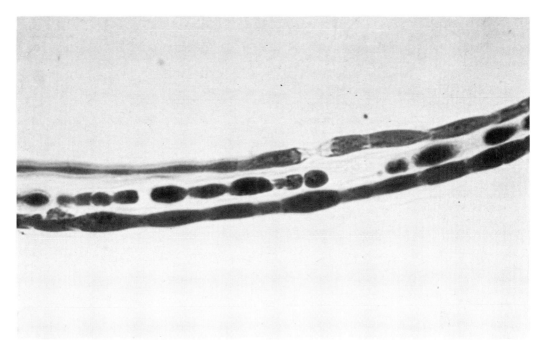

Fig. 11.43. Teased osmicated nerve fibres. One fibre has undergone Wallerian degeneration, with myelin ovoid formation. (160 ×)

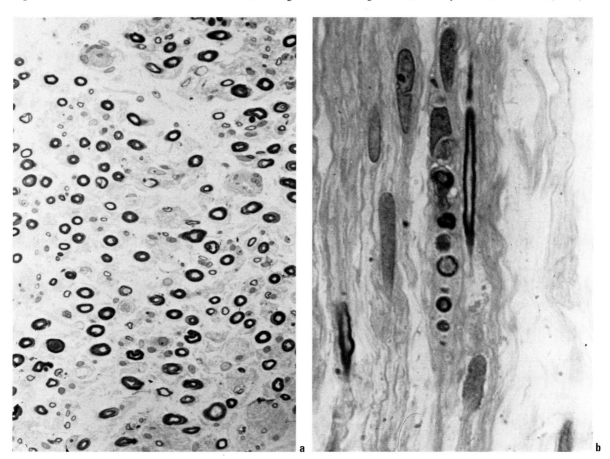

Fig. 11.44. a Axonal neuropathy, transverse section. There is a reduction in the number of myelinated axons. (Toluidine blue; 500 ×) **b** Wallerian degeneration secondary to axonal degeneration, longitudinal section. (Toluidine blue; 1800 ×)

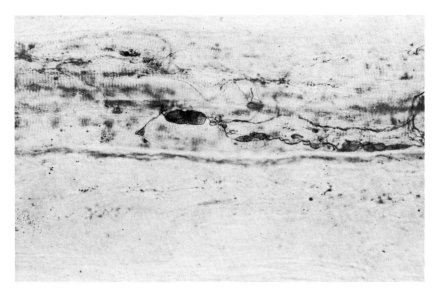

Fig. 11.45. Axonal degeneration, longitudinal section. In this muscle spindle, in a patient with tabes dorsalis, a sensory ending shows degenerative changes, with the terminal axonal swelling and constriction typical of a dying-back process. (Barker and Ip teased preparation; 950 ×)

neurotoxic drugs or industrial chemicals. Distal axonal atrophy also occurs in inherited neuropathies.

The cell body proximal to a sectioned axon undergoes *chromatolysis*, a reversible change that is probably part of a regenerative response. The cell body becomes rounded and enlarged, the nucleus and nucleolus enlarge, and the nucleus becomes displaced towards the side of the cell away from the axon hillock. The Golgi apparatus moves away from the nucleus towards the cell periphery and slightly cytoplasmic agyrophilia develops. The light microscopic changes correspond to the ribosomal dispersion, proliferation of endoplasmic reticulum, and increase in the numbers of mitochondria and neurofilaments seen in electron microscopic studies of chromatolysis.

6.3.3. Segmental Demyelination Segmental demyelination occurs in neuropathies, including those caused by diphtheria toxin or lead poisoning, in which the Schwann cells are selectively damaged. Myelin breakdown occurs and may be restricted to individual Schwann cells so that degeneration is limited by the nodes of Ranvier. This abnormality is particularly easily recognized in teased, osmicated preparations but it can usually also be discerned in longitudinal sections of plastic-embedded material (Fig. 11.46). During the process of remyelination, shortened, 'intercalated' nodes are formed, a characteristic finding indicating that segmental demyelination and remyelination 'onion bulbs' (Fig. 11.47) are formed. This term refers to the presence of circumferential leaflets of Schwann cell processes surrounding an axonal core. The outer leaflets are interspersed with collagen fibrils and

fibroblasts. This proliferation of interstitial elements may result in palpable enlargement of affected nerves (hypertrophic neuropathy).

Compression of a nerve that is sufficient to produce segmental demyelination at the site of injury usually produces Wallerian degeneration in some fibres. There is controversy concerning the role of increased pressure within nerves, e.g., in amyloidosis, ischaemic swelling, or the inflammatory polyneuropathies, as a factor leading to axonal or Schwann cell injury.

6.4. Heredofamilial Sensorimotor Neuropathies

These disorders have been classified by Dyck and Lambert (1968a, b) according to clinical, genetic, and electrophysiological criteria. Because of their variety no classification is entirely satisfactory, and in all of them there is progressive distal weakness and wasting, beginning in early childhood. Pes cavus or curling of the toes (hammer toes) may be the first abnormality noticed. Sensory impairment is usually present in the feet before the hands and may be slight. Distal tendon reflexes are lost. The type 1 disorder is associated with hypertrophied peripheral nerves, and nerve conduction velocities are usually less than half normal. The CSF protein is raised. This disorder is similar to type 2 hereditary sensorimotor neuropathy, but in the latter symptoms usually begin later, the peripheral nerves are *not* enlarged, distal atrophy is not so marked (although weakness may be more severe), and nerve conduction velocities are usually normal, indicating that axonal degeneration is the primary abnormality. The onset of the type 2 disorder may be delayed into

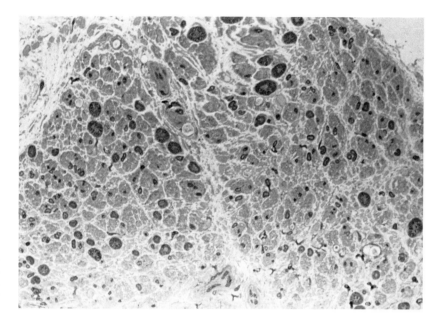

Fig. 11.46. Segmental de-myelination, TS. There is a marked absence of myelin rings, although the axons can still be seen. (Tolu-idine blue; 400 ×)

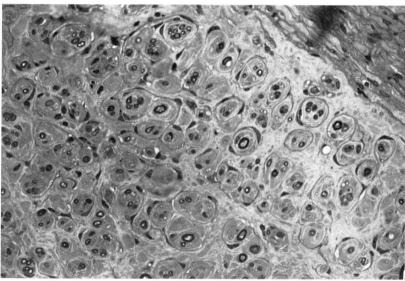

Fig. 11.47. 'Onion-bulbs' in burnt-out leprosy, semi-thin section. Single axon or small clusters of axons are surrounded by rings of hypertrophied Schwann cells and fibrous tissue (Toluidine blue; 350 ×)

adult life. Both type 1 and type 2 hereditary sensori-motor neuropathies have an autosomal dominant inheritance.

Dejerine–Sottas disease (type 3) is inherited as an autosomal recessive trait. Motor milestones are delayed, but the ability to walk is retained into adult life. There is mild distal sensory loss, and ataxia may be a feature. The peripheral nerves are enlarged and the nerve conduction velocity is slowed, indicating segmental demyelination, a suggestion confirmed by pathological studies. The onset of this rare disorder is in infancy.

In Refsum's disease (type 4) a hypertrophic sensorimotor neuropathy, usually beginning in-sidiously in childhood or adolescence, is associated with ataxia and other cerebellar signs, night blind-ness, retinitis pigmentosa, neural deafness, cardiomyopathy, cataracts, pupillary abnormalities, dry scaly skin, and epiphyseal abnormalities. The neuropathy may undergo sudden periods of deterioration and the CSF protein is raised (Refsum 1946). The disease is associated with inability to metabolize dietary phytanic acid, resulting in stor-age of this material in affected tissues (Steinberg et al. 1966) and in high blood levels of phytanic acid. Hereditary spastic paraplegia (type 5) is sometimes associated with a mild sensorimotor neuropathy. The scapuloperoneal syndrome, consisting of proximal weakness in the upper limbs and distal weakness in the legs, with a predominantly scapular and peroneal distribution, respectively, is a hetero-geneous syndrome due either to a primary myopathy (Thomas et al. 1972) or to a neurogenic disorder resembling spinal muscular atrophy (Kaeser 1965). Davidenkow (1939) described a group of cases with neurogenic scapuloperoneal atrophy and distal sensory loss (Schwartz and Swash 1975).

Muscle biopsies in these disorders show the typical features of neurogenic disorders. In the type 2 disorder, thought to be neuronal in origin, these changes are pronounced (Haase and Shy (1960) with fibre-type atrophy and fibre-type grouping affecting both type 1 and type 2 fibres. Clusters of small, narrow, angulated fibres, darkly stained in the NADH preparations are common, and there may be compensatory fibre hypertrophy with mild second-ary 'myopathic' change in the more chronic cases (Schwartz et al. 1976). Terminal axonal sprouting can be demonstrated in methylene blue preparations (Cöers and Woolfe 1953) but degenerative and end-plate changes, including axonal expansions and fusion of end-plate expansions into ill-formed masses, also occur (Harriman 1976). By contrast, in types 1, 2, 3, and 4 hereditary sensorimotor neuropathy, neurogenic atrophy is less prominent in muscle biopsies. In these disorders the neuropathy results from an abnormality in the Schwann cells, leading to a demyelinating neuropathy with relative preservation of the axis cylinders themselves.

Nerve biopsies in these hypertrophic neuropathies show enlargement of the diameter of the nerve fascicle, which contains excess collagen fibrils. The perineurium is thickened, due to extra layers of perineurial cell cytoplasm and fibrosis. There is only a slight loss of nerve fibres. Large axons may be unmyelinated or surrounded by only thin myelin rings, an appearance suggesting that remyelination is occurring. Further, clusters of axons, or single axons, become enveloped in multiple rings of Schwannian cytoplasm—the onion bulbs seen on light microscopy (Fig. 11.47). Sometimes Schwann cell cytoplasm envelops a few collagen fibrils, for-ming 'collagen pockets'. Teased fibre preparations confirm that segmental demyelination is present in these cases (Gutretcht and Dyck 1966). In Refsum's disease (type 4) small sudanophilic droplets have been found in the endoneurial spaces, Schwann cells, meninges, and glia, and there is loss of Purkinje cells.

In all the axonal neuropathies or neuronal dis-orders in the classification of Dyck and Lambert (1968a, b), an axonal reaction occurs in anterior horn cells and there is degeneration in the posterior columns secondary to the peripheral lesions. Nerve biopsy in the neuronal type of peroneal muscular atrophy (type 2) shows loss of larger axons, with relative preservation of smaller myelinated axons and of unmyelinated fibres. Wallerian change occurs

and this can readily be recognized by light micros-copy (Figs. 11.45 and 11.44). Cardiomyopathy may be a feature of all these disorders. The myocardium shows focal scarring and fibrosis similar to that found in Friedreich's ataxia.

6.5. Other Inherited Neuropathies

A number of very rare neuropathies due to met-abolic disorders, in addition to Refsum's disease, may present in infancy and childhood (Table 11.5). Detailed reviews of the pathology of these disorders are available elsewhere.

Table 11.5. Very rare neuropathies due to metabolic disorders

Infantile polyneuropathy with defective myelination
Metachromatic leukodystrophy (sulphatidosis)
Krabbe's disease (globoid-cell leukodystrophy)
Fabry's disease (angiokeratoma corporis diffusum)
Refsum's disease
Tangier disease (α-lipoprotein deficiency)
Bassen–Kornzweig's disease (β-lipoprotein deficiency)
Acute intermittent porphyria
Chediak–Higashi syndrome
Late infantile and juvenile amaurotic idiocy
Cockayne's syndrome
Congenital insensitivity to pain

6.5.1.   Infantile Polyneuropathy Infantile poly-neuropathy with defective myelination (Karch and Urich 1975) is a disorder that was first reported by Lyon (1969), in which hypotonia is noted from early infancy, with absent tendon jerks, distal wasting, and delayed motor milestones. Death may occur in infancy. Biopsies of sural nerve reveal preservation of axons, but absence of myelin sheaths. There is mild endoneurial fibrosis. Electron microscopy in one case revealed concentric whorls or reduplicated basal laminae, with scanty Schwann cell processes resembling onion bulbs. Similar findings have been described in an autopsied case (Karch and Urich 1975). The relation of this disorder to hypertrophic neuropathy beginning in infancy is uncertain (Dyck 1966; Joosten et al. 1974). These disorders form part of the spectrum of diseases responsible for the floppy infant syndrome.

6.5.2.   Metachomatic   Leucodystrophy Meta-chromatic leucodystrophy (sulphatidosis) occurs in two forms: arylsulphatase A deficiency and multiple sulphatase deficiency (mucosulphatidosis). In both these variants motor signs are prominent, but epilepsy and mental retardation are also features, as in other leucodystrophies. The onset is usually at about 2 or 3 years of age, but juvenile- and adult-onset forms have also been described. In the central nervous system there is demyelination, loss of oligodendroglia, and accumulation of metachromatic sulphatide lipid granules within neurones. In the peripheral nervous system metachromatic granules are found in Schwann cells and endoneurial macrophages. Large-diameter myelinated fibres are usually lost, with very extensive segmental demyelination. Ultrastructurally, the sulphatide deposits consist of groups of rounded inclusions about 1 μm in diameter, often situated near a myelinated nerve fibre. Metachromatic lipid can also be found in desquamated renal tubular cells in the urine. Diagnosis can thus be established by examination of the urine, or by sural nerve biopsy. The underlying biochemical defect can be confirmed in cultures of skin fibroblasts (Kamensky et al. 1973).

Segmental demyelination is also a feature of the peripheral nerve abnormality (Bischoff 1975) found in *Krabbe's globoid cell leucodystrophy* (cerebroside sulphotransferase deficiency). The Schwann cell cytoplasm contains crystalline deposits and increased acid phosphatase activity (Dunn et al. 1969), and posterior root ganglia may show degenerative changes (Sourander and Olsson 1968).

In *Fabry's disease* (*angiokeratoma corporis diffusum*) sural nerve biopsy may show reduction of myelinated nerve fibres with lamellated glycolipid (ceramide trihexoside) deposits in the perineurium (Kocen and Thomas 1970). However, the diagnosis is more easily made by skin biopsy.

Two inherited lipoprotein disorders are associated with neuropathy. *Tangier disease*, due to absence of high-density α-lipoproteins in the blood with low blood cholesterol levels, presents in childhood with tonsillar enlargement due to accumulation of cholesterol ester producing an orange-flecked tonsillar surface. The viscera may also be enlarged, and a progressive sensorimotor neuropathy with moderately slowed nerve conduction velocities develops. Histologically this neuropathy is characterized by loss of myelinated and unmyelinated nerve fibres without segmental demyelination but with accumulations of cholesterol esters in the Schwann cells (Kocen et al. 1973). In a *β-lipoproteinaemia* (Bassen–Kornzweig disease) a variety of other clinical manifestations occur besides peripheral neuropathy, including acanthocytosis, retinitis pigmentosa, progressive posterior column degeneration, loss of anterior horn cells, mental retardation, steatorrhoea, and hypocholesterolaemia (Mars et al. 1969). The peripheral neuropathy in this disorder probably results partly from axonal damage and partly from segmental demyelination.

Late infantile and juvenile variants of amaurotic idiocy, including Bassen–Bielschowsky syndrome, some cases of Niemann–Pick disease, and Spielmeyer–Vogt syndrome may be diagnosed by a combination of biochemical and ultrastructural studies or sural nerve biopsies. Diagnosis is usually made more easily by biochemical examination of blood and other tissues. Pompe's disease can also be recognized in sural nerve biopsies by glocogen deposition in both cytoplasm and lysosomes in macrophages, fibroblasts and Schwann cells (Goebel et al. 1977).

In acute intermittent porphyria and in porphyria variegata, acute spontaneous or drug-induced attacks of mainly motor neuropathy are a characteristic manifestation. The disease usually presents in adolescence. Porphobilinogen and δ-aminolaevulinic acid are excreted in the urine in attacks. The lower limbs are particularly affected and wasting can be very severe. The ankle jerks are sometimes unexpectedly preserved (Ridley 1969). Recovery is often slow and incomplete (Hierons 1957). This neuropathy is a typical example of a selective axonal neuropathy. The distal portions of large motor fibres are predominantly affected, especially in proximal muscles (Cavanagh and Mellick 1965), suggesting that the neuropathy is attributable to a dying-back process (Cavanagh 1964), although the largest motor fibres are unexpectedly spared in most cases of this disease. Wallerian degeneration is a prominent feature and there is central chromatolysis in anterior horn cells of the spinal cord. The biochemical disorder has been reviewed by Sweeney et al. (1970) and by Ridley (1975).

In *Chediak–Higashi syndrome*, a disorder characterized by partial albinism, hepatosplenomegaly, and peroxidase-positive granules in polymorphonuclear leucocytes (see p. 549), cranial and peripheral neuropathy can be associated with spinocerebellar degeneration and mental retardation. Intracytoplasmic inclusions are found in neurones and axons and perivascular infiltrates are sometimes found, in both the central and the peripheral nervous systems (Sheramata et al. 1971). *Cockayne's* syndrome of mental and physical retardation, with dwarfism, deafness, retinitis pigmentosa, and other defects may be complicated by peripheral neuropathy (Moosa and Dubowitz (1970).

Congenital indifference to pain, a disorder in which normal pain sensation is absent, may be due to a hereditary sensory neuropathy, but the nosological position of this syndrome is dubious. It has also been reported in patients with familial dysautonomia (*Riley–Day syndrome*) and in the *Lesch–Nyhan syndrome.*

The familial amyloid neuropathies have been reported only in adults.

6.6. Acquired Neuropathies

There are many acquired neuropathies, and these are itemized in Table 11.6.

Table 11.6. Acquired neuropathies

Traumatic neuropathies
Entrapment and compressive neuropathies
Toxic neuropathies (e.g., drug-induced neuropathies, lead poisoning
Inflammatory polyradiculoneuropathy (Guillain-Barré syndrome)
Viral infections (Herpes zoster, poliomyelitis)
Leprosy
Neuropathies associated with arteritis
Metabolic neuropathies (diabetes, uraemia, vitamin deficiencies)

6.6.1. Traumatic Neuropathies These commonly occur after penetrating trauma but they may also be caused by excessive stretching during injury. Several grades of severity of nerve injury have been described, on the basis of the varying degree of recovery expected (Sunderland 1968).

1) The nerve may be severed, when there is axonal discontinuity resulting in Wallerian degeneration in the distal stump and denervation atrophy of muscles supplied by the nerve. Regeneration occurs by axonal sprouting from the proximal end of the severed nerve (Fig. 11.45); the effectiveness of this regeneration depends on the presence of empty perineurial tubes and on the absence of a fibrous barrier (scar formation). Without surgical apposition of the cut ends, or insertion of an autogenous graft, the prognosis for functional recovery is poor (Tallis et al. 1978);

2) If the nerve is stretched or crushed, resulting in axonal severance, but continuity of the perineurial tissues, or even of Schwann tubes is maintained, more effective regeneration is possible. Axon regeneration occurs at a rate of about 1–2 mm growth per day (Young 1942);

3) Transient failure of function may occur after acute compressive injury without anatomical disruption of tissue. Recovery usually occurs within about 3 weeks. The neurological disorder is probably due to the disruption of myelin lamellae (Ochoa et al. 1971).

Traumatic lesions occur most commonly in superficially placed nerves, e.g., the ulnar nerve at the olecranon groove on the medial side of the elbow and the common peroneal nerve at the head of the fibula. The radial nerve can be damaged by supracondylar fractures of the humerus or by injury in the spiral groove, and the median nerve is susceptible during arterial or venous puncture in the antecubital fossa. The sciatic nerve is occasionally injured by injection into the buttock. Trauma, especially in road accidents, can cause stretch injury, or even rupture of anterior or posterior nerve roots. The posterior roots are more commonly affected and the lower cervical roots are most vulnerable, usually during sudden torsional injuries to the neck.

6.6.2. Entrapment and Compressive Neuropathies
In many respects the pathogenesis of entrapment and compressive neuropathies is similar to that described above. The classic example, the carpal tunnel syndrome, is scarcely ever found in childhood, except occasionally in children with rheumatoid arthritis or mucopolysaccharidosis, in which the transverse carpal ligaments sometimes become thickened. Entrapment can also occur at the intervertebral foramina, by protruded disc material after injury. In these neuropathies there is compression with intussusception of myelin lamellae in the paranodal regions, leading to paranodal demyelination and conduction block (Ochoa et al. 1971). The underlying lesion, therefore, is segmental demyelination, but in severe examples axonal degeneration occurs. Repeated stretching probably plays a role in the pathogenesis of the lesion (McLellan and Swash 1976).

6.6.3. Toxic and Drug-induced Neuropathies
Neuropathies occur after exposure to a variety of compounds, including organic solvents, drugs, heavy metals, and bacterial toxins. Most drugs and many organic and nonorganic substances used in solvents and in industry cause an axonal degeneration of the dying-back type discussed by Cavanagh (1964). The morphological changes are those most obvious in intramuscular nerve fibres and motor end-plates, and in sensory receptors in skin and muscle. Segmental demyelination occurs after exposure to diphtheria toxin and in lead poisoning. The earliest changes occur in the paranodal regions. Full discussions of these neuropathies and of the substances that cause them are available elsewhere, (Dyck et al. 1975; Argov and Mastaglia 1979; Schaumberg and Spencer 1979).

6.7. Inflammatory Polyradiculoneuropathy

Inflammatory polyradiculoneuropathy, or the Guillain–Barré syndrome, is an acute disorder characterized by weakness, paraesthesiae, muscle tenderness, absent tendon reflexes, and a raised cerebrospinal fluid protein level, with a normal cell count (Guillain et al. 1916). The disease is often preceded by an ill-defined febrile illness, and relapsing and chronic varieties, some with central manifestations, are also recognized (Arnason 1975;

Swash 1978). Cranial nerves, especially the facial nerves, are often affected, and there may be autonomic involvement. A similar, subacute type of polyneuritis occurs after specific virus infections, such as mumps, measles, vaccinia, Herpes zoster, and infectious mononucleosis, and after rabies vaccination (see Urich 1976; Swash 1978). Pathologically, the characteristic feature of the acute disorder is segmental demyelination, which affects nerves throughout their length, even involving nerve roots, accompanied by perivascular lymphocytic infiltration. The latter is particularly prominent near demyelinated nerve. Macrophages and plasma cells also infiltrate affected nerve fascicles. Axonal degeneration occurs in some of these areas, resulting in denervation atrophy in some muscles. In most cases recovery is rapid, disrupted myelin being rapidly reconstituted, but in severe cases recovery is delayed. Electron microscopic studies have shown that macrophages penetrate basement membranes of affected nerve fibres and displace Schwann cell cytoplasm from the myelin sheath, leading to separation of axons from their myelin envelopes (Prineas 1972). In relapsing and chronic cases nerve hypertrophy, with typical Schwannian onion bulbs surrounding demyelinated and remyelinated axons and a sparser inflammatory cell infiltrate, is found. This histological appearance is similar to that found in experimental allergic neuritis, an experimental demyelinating neuropathy induced by treatment with peripheral nerve protein (Thomas et al. 1969).

Autonomic neuropathy sometimes complicates Guillain–Barré syndrome, perhaps accounting for sudden death, which occurs in a small proportion of patients. A few cases of subacute autonomic neuropathy occurring without motor or sensory abnormalities, but similar in other respects to subacute Guillain–Barré syndrome, have been reported in childhood (Thomashevksy et al. 1972).

6.8. Virus Infections

Two viruses, poliomyelitis and Herpes zoster, can invade the peripheral nervous system, although others, especially Herpes simplex virus and rabies virus, may enter the nervous system by passing along endo- or perineurial tissues from distal sites of entry. Herpes zoster is uncommon in childhood, although it does occur in children with debilitating disorders and during chemotherapy for malignant disease. The poliomyelitis virus causes a form of leptomeningitis with perivascular lymphocytic cuffing in the spinal cord and brain stem and phagocytosis of infected, dead anterior horn cells. Axonal degeneration and neurogenic muscular atrophy follow.

6.9. Leprosy

Leprosy is widespread in tropical and subtropical zones, and cases occur in temperate climates among immigrant populations. The disease is acquired only after prolonged contact in overcrowded conditions. Many people appear not to be susceptible to the disease, perhaps because of previous exposure to *Mycobacterium tuberculosis*. The factors leading to susceptibility are complex and largely determine the course and clinical type of the disease in individual patients. Nutritional and immunological factors are particularly important, but children are generally more susceptible than adults. Infection can occur through the skin or upper respiratory tract. Clinical manifestations of leprosy vary (Cochrane and Davey 1964; Sabin and Swift 1975), and several different types of the disease are recognized. Figure 11.48 shows the various possible outcomes of exposure to *M. leprae*.

6.9.1. Indeterminate Indeterminate leprosy is an early lesion most commonly found in children. There is an indolent, hypopigmented skin lesion, which may be anaesthetic. Biopsy of this lesion shows a few inflammatory cells neear neurovascular bundles, and *M. leprae* may be present in small cutaneous nerves.

6.9.2. Lepromatous In lepromatous leprosy there is little immunological check to bacterial proliferation, and the skin and peripheral nervous system are extensively involved, particularly in cooler body areas such as the nose, exposed areas of the limbs, the cheeks, and the pinna. Skin lesions are often difficult to see, even when very extensive. Large numbers of bacilli can be seen in acid-fast stains of skin biopsies. The bacilli are usually located within histiocytes, which may be distended by masses of bacilli. Nasal or skin scrapings usually reveal abundant bacilli in acid-fast stains.

The peripheral nerve trunks are grossly enlarged by fusiform rather than nodular swellings, and small cutaneous nerves are usually similarly palpably

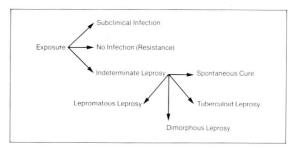

Fig. 11.48. Possible consequences of exposure to *M. leprae*.

enlarged. Affected nerves are often tender. Histologically these nerves are oedematous, with relative preservation of their fascicular architecture. The perineurium is infiltrated by foamy histiocytes, and bacilli, oriented longitudinally to the nerve trunk, are prominent. Teased preparations of single nerve fibres show demyelinated or thinly myelinated axons, with short intercalcated segments, consistent with segmental demyelination.

6.9.3. *Tuberculoid* In tuberculoid leprosy the cutaneous nerves are enlarged by firm nodules, often in association with a nearby skin lesion. The affected nerves show extensive destructive changes with loss of the fascicular pattern, prominent axonal changes, and epithelioid and giant cell granulomas. Onion bulb formation may be prominent (Fig. 11.47). Only sparse bacilli are found in the nerves, and almost none in the skin in tuberculoid leprosy.

6.9.4. *Other Forms* Dimorphous leprosy represents an intermediate disorder between the lepromatous and tuberculoid forms. Clinically, dimorphous leprosy is unstable, and reversion to either of the major forms may occur. Histologically there are features of both forms, depending on the immunological state of the patient.

6.10. Diabetic Neuropathy

Neuropathy has been recognized as a complication of diabetes mellitus for more than 100 years. It is common only in adult diabetic patients, however, and its incidence increases with increasing age. The incidence in childhood is probably about 2%, but a higher incidence has been recorded (Lawrence and Locke 1963). Symmetrical, predominantly sensory, and mononeuropathic types occur. The last group includes isolated cranial nerve palsies and diabetic amyotrophy. Only the symmetrical sensory neuropathy is recorded in paediatric practice. Autonomic neuropathy may complicate this disorder. Pathologically, features of both axonal neuropathy and segmental demyelination are present (Greenbaum et al. 1964; Thomas and Lascelles 1966). These degenerative changes are most marked peripherally, but the spinal roots, particularly the posterior roots, may be involved (Olsson et al. 1968) and loss of posterior root ganglion cells and anterior horn cells has also been observed (Greenbaum et al. 1964).

6.11. Lead Poisoning

In children lead poisoning causes anaemia, convulsions, and encephalopathy far more commonly than neuropathy. When it occurs in childhood lead neuropathy usually presents as foot drop, unlike the more familiar wrist drop of adults. The neuropathy, which remits when blood lead levels fall with treatment, is due to segmental demyelination.

6.12. Others

Neuropathies associated with arteritis and with various acquired metabolic disorders, such as uraemia, hepatic disease, etc., are rare in childhood and will not be discussed here. They have been reviewed by Dyck et al. (1975).

References

Afifi AK, Smith JW, Zellweger H (1965) Congenital nonprogressive myopathy: Central core and nemaline myopathy in one family. Neurology (Minneap) 15: 371

Allen DE, Johnson AG, Woolf AL (1969) The intramuscular nerve endings in dystrophia myotonica: A biopsy study by vital staining and electron microscopy. J Anat 105: 1

Argov Z, Mastaglia FL (1979) Drug-induced peripheral neuropathies. Br Med J i: 663

Armstrong RM, Königsberger R, Mellinger J, Lovelace RE (1971) Central core disease with congenital hip dislocation: A study of two families. Neurology (Minneap) 21: 369

Arnason BGW (1975) Inflammatory polyradiculoneuritis. In: Dyck PJ, Thomas PK, Lambert EH (eds) Peripheral neuropathy, vol 2. Saunders, London Philadelphia, p 1110

Asbury AK (1973) Renaut bodies: A forgotten endoneurial structure. J Neuropathol Exp Neurol 32: 334

Bank WJ, DiMauro S, Bonilla E, Capcizzi DM, Rowland LP (1975) A disorder of lipid metabolism and myoglobinuria. N Engl J Med 292: 443

Banker BQ (1975) Dermatomyositis of childhood: Ultrastructural alterations of muscle and intramuscular blood vessels. J Neuropathol Exp Neurol 34: 46

Banker BQ, Victor M (1966) Dermatomyositis (systemic angiopathy) of childhood. Medicine (Baltimore) 45: 261

Barbeau A (1966) The syndrome of hereditary late-onset ptosis and dysphagia in French Canada. In: Kuhn E (ed) Symposium über progressive Muskeldystrophie. Springer, Berlin, p 102

Barchi RL (1975) Myotonia: An evaluation of the chloride hypothesis. Arch Neurol 32: 175

Becker PE (1962) Two new families of benign sex-linked recessive muscular dystrophy. Rev Can Biol 21: 551

Behan PO, Simpson JA, Dick (1973) Immune response genes in myasthenia gravis. Lancet 2: 1033

Bell CD, Conen PE (1968) Histopathological changes in Duchenne muscular dystrophy. J Neurol Sci 7: 529

Berenberg RA, Pollock JM, DiMauro S, Schotland DL, Bonilla E, Eastwood A, Hays A, Vicale CT, Behrens M, Chutarian A, Rowland LP (1977) Lumping or splitting? Ophthalmoplegia plus or Kearns–Sayre syndrome. Ann Neurol 1: 37

Bethlem J, van Gool J, Hülsmann WC, Meijer AEFH (1966) Familial non-progressive myopathy with muscle cramps after exercise: A new disease associated with cores in the muscle fibres. Brain 89: 569

Bethlem J, Meijer AEFH, Schellens JPM, Uvran JJ (1968) Centronuclear myopathy. Eur Neurol 1: 325

Bethlem J, van Wijngaarden GK, Meijer AEFH, Hülsmann WC (1969) Neuromuscular disease with type 1 fibre atrophy, central nuclei and myotube-like structures. Neurology (Minneap) 19: 705

Bischoff A (1975) Neuropathy in leucodystrophies. In: Dyck PJ, Lambert EH, Thomas PK (eds) Peripheral neuropathy. Saunders, London Philadelphia, p 891

Bohan A, Peter JB (1975) Polymyositis and dermatomyositis. N Engl J Med 292: 344 and 403

Bradley WG (1969) Ultrastructural changes in adynamia episodica hereditaria and normokalaemic periodic paralysis. Brain 92: 379

Bradley WG, Jones MZ, Mussini J-M, Fawcett PRW (1978) Becker-type muscular dystrophy. Muscle Nerve 1: 111

Brooke MH (1966) The histological reaction of muscle to disease. In: Buskey EJ, Cassens R, Trautman J (eds) The physiology and biochemistry of muscle as a food. University of Wisconsin Press, Madison, p 151

Brooke MH, Kaiser KK (1970) Muscle fibre types: How many and what kind? Arch Neurol 23: 369

Brooke MH (1973) A neuromuscular disease characterised by fibre type disproportion. In: Kakulas PA (ed) Clinical studies in myology. Excerpta Medica, Amsterdam, p 147 (ICS no. 295)

Brooke MH, Engel WK (1966) The histologic diagnosis of neuromuscular diseases: A review of 79 biopsies. Arch Phys Med Rehabil 47: 99

Brooke MH, Engel WK (1969a) The histographic analysis of human muscle biopsies with regard to fibre types. 1. Adult male and female. Neurology (Minneap) 19: 221

Brooke MH, Engel WK (1969b) The histographic analysis of human muscle biopsies with regard to fibre types, 4 children's biopsies. Neurology (Minneap) 19: 591

Brownell B, Oppenheimer DR, Spalding JMK (1972) Neurogenic muscle atrophy in myasthenia gravis. J Neurol Neurosurg Psychiatry 34: 311

Brunberg JA, McCormick WF, Schochet SS Jr (1971) Type 3 glycogenosis: An adult with diffuse weakness and muscle wasting. Arch Neurol 25: 171

Bundey S (1972) Genetic study of infantile and juvenile myasthenia gravis. J Neurol Neurosurg Psychiatry 35: 41

Bundey S, Carter CO, Soothill JF (1970) Early recognition of heterozygotes for the gene of dystrophia myotonica. J Neurol Neurosurg Psychiatry 33: 279

Carpenter S, Karpati G, Rothman S, Watters G (1976) The childhood type of dermatomyositis. Neurology (Minneap) 26: 952

Cavanagh JB (1964) The significance of the 'dying back' process in experimental and human neurological disease. Int Rev Exp Pathol 7: 219

Cavanagh JB, Mellick RS (1965) On the nature of the peripheral nerve lesions associated with acute intermittent perphyria. J Neurol Neurosurg Psychiatry 28: 320

Cazzato G (1970) Myopathic changes in denervated muscle: A study of biopsy material in various neuromuscular diseases. In: Walton JN, Canal N, Scarlato G (eds) Muscle disease. Excerpta Medica, Amsterdam, p 392 (ICS no. 199)

Cheah JS, Tock EPC, Tan Sp (1975) The light and electron microscopic changes in the skeletal muscles during paralysis in thyrotoxic periodic paralysis. Am J Med Sci 269: 365

Chou SM (1968) Myxovirus-like structures and accompanying nuclear changes in chronic polymyositis. Arch Pathol 86: 649

Chou SM, Gutmann L (1970) Picornavirus-like crystals in subacute polymyositis. Neurol (Minneap) 20: 205

Cochrane RG, Davey TF (eds) (1964) Leprosy in theory and practice, 2nd edn. Wright, Bristol

Cöers C (1975) Motor innervation of myasthenic muscles related to age. Lancet 2:55

Cöers C, Desmedt JE (1959) Mise en évidence d'une malformation caracteristique de la jonction neuromusculaire dans la myasthenie. Acta Neurol Belg 59: 539

Cöers C, Telerman-Toppet N (1976) Morphological and histological changes of motor units in myasthenia. Ann NY Acad Sci 274: 6

Cöers C, Woolf AL (1953) The innervation of muscle. Blackwell, Oxford

Cook CD, Rosen FS, Banker BQ (1963) Dermatomyositis and focal scleroderma. Pediatr Clin North Am 10: 979

Conomy JP, Levinsohn M, Fanaroff A (1975) Familial infantile myasthenia gravis: A cause of sudden death in young children. J Pediatr 87: 428

Crews J, Kaiser KK, Brooke MH (1976) Muscle pathology of myotonia congenita. J Neurol Sci 28: 449

Currie S, Naronha M, Harriman DGF (1974) 'Minicore' disease (Abstract). Third International Congress on Muscle Disease. Excerpta Medica, Amsterdam, p 12 (ICS no. 334)

Davidenkow S (1939) Scapulo-peroneal amyotrophy. Arch Neurol 41: 694

Dawkins RL, Mastaglia FL (1973) Cell-mediated cytotoxity muscle in polymyositis. N Engl J Med 288: 434

Drachman DA (1968) Ophthalmoplegia plus: The neurodegenerative disorders associated with progressive external ophthalmoplegia. Arch Neurol 18: 654

Drachman DB, Angus CW, Adams RN, Michelson JD, Hoffman GJ (1978) Myasthenic antibodies cross-link acetylcholine receptors to accelerate degradation. N Engl J Med 298: 1116

Drachman DB, Murphy SR, Nigam MP, Hills JR (1967) 'Myopathic' changes in chronically denervated muscle. Arch Neurol 16: 14

Dreyfus JS, Shapiro G Demos J (1960) Etude de la creatinekinase serique chez les myopathies et leur familles. Revue Française d'Etudes Cliniques et Biologiques 5: 384

Dubowitz V (1978) Muscle disorders in childhood. In: Major problems in clinical pediatrics, vol XVI. Saunders, London

Dubowitz V, Brooke MH (1973) Muscle biopsy: A modern approach. Saunders, London

Dubowitz V, Roy S (1970) Central core disease of muscle: Clinical histochemical and electron microscopal studies of an affected mother and child. Brain 93: 133

Dunn HG, Lake BD, Dolman CL, Wilson J (1969) The neuropathy of Krabbe's infantile cerebral sclerosis (globoid cell leucodystrophy). Brain 92: 329

Dyck PJ (1966) Histologic measurements and fine structure of biopsied sural nerve: Normal and in peroneal muscular atrophy, hypertrophic neuropathy and congenital sensory neuropathy. Mayo Clin Proc 41: 742

Dyck PJ (1975) Pathologic alterations of the peripheral nervous system of man. In: Dyck PJ, Thomas PK, Lambert EH (eds) Peripheral neuropathy. Saunders, London Philadelphia p 296

Dyck PJ, Lambert EH (1968a) Lower motor and primary sensory neuron diseases with peroneal muscular atrophy. I. Neurologic, genetic and electrophysiologic findings in hereditary polyneuropathies. Arch Neurol 18: 603

Dyck PJ, Lambert EH (1968b) Lower motor and primary sensory neuron diseases with peroneal muscular atrophy. II. Neurologic, genetic and electrophysiologic findings in various neuronal degenerations. Arch Neurol 18: 619

Dyck PJ, Lambert EH, Thomas PK (1975) Peripheral neuropathy (2 vols). Saunders, London Philadelphia

Edstrom L, Kugelberg E (1968) Histochemical composition, distribution of fibres and fatiguability of single motor units. Anterior tibial muscle of the rat. J Neurol Neurosurg Psychiatry 31: 424

Ellis FR, Kearney NP, Harriman DGF (1973) Histopathological and neuropharmacological aspects of malignant hyperpyrexia. Proc R Soc Med 66: 60

Emery AEH, Smith CAB, Sanger R (1969) The linkage reactions of the loci for benign (Becker type) X-borne muscular dystrophy, colour blindness and the Xg blood groups. Ann

Hum Genet 32: 261

Engel AG (1970a) Acid maltase deficiency in adults: Studies in four cases of syndrome which may mimic muscular dystrophy or other myopathies. Brain 93: 599

Engel AG (1970b) Evolution and content of vacuoles in primary hypokalaemic periodic paralysis. Mayo Clin Proc 45: 774

Engel AG, Angelini C, Gomez MR (1972) Finger-print body myopathy. Mayo Clin Proc 47: 377

Engel AG, Gomez MR, Seybold ME, Lambert EH (1973) The spectrum and diagnosis of acid maltase deficiency. Neurology (Minneap) 23: 95

Engel AG, Lindstrom JM, Lambert EH, Lennon VA (1977) Ultrastructural localization of the acetylcholine receptor in myasthenia gravis and its experimental autoimmune model. Neurology (Minneap) 27: 307

Engel AG, Mokri B, Jerusalem F, Sakakibara H, Paulson OB (1977) Ultrastructural clues in Duchenne dystrophy. In: Rowland CP (ed) Pathogenesis of human muscular dystrophies. Excerpta Medica, Amsterdam, p 310 (ICS no 404)

Engel WK (1961) Muscle target fibres, a newly recognised sign of denervation. Nature 191:389

Engel WK (1965) Muscle biopsy. Clin Orthop 39: 80

Engel WK (1970) Selective and non-selective susceptibility of muscle fibre types: A new approach to human neuromuscular disease. Arch Neurol 22: 97

Engel WK (1971) 'Ragged-red fibres' in opthalmoplegia syndromes and their differential diagnosis. In: Abstract. Second International Congress on Muscle Diseases. Excerpta Medica, Amsterdam, p 28 (ICS no. 237)

Engel WK, Brooke MH (1966) Histochemistry of the myotonic disorders. In: Kuhn E (ed) Progressive Muskeldystrophie, Myotonie, Myästhenia. Springer, Berlin Heidelberg New York, p. 203

Engel WK, McFarlin De (1966) Discussion. Ann NY Acad Sci 135: 68

Engel WK, Resnick JS (1966) Late-onset rod myopathy: A newly recognised, acquired and progressive disease. Neurology (Minneap) 16: 308

Engel WK, Brooke MH, Nelson PG (1966) Histochemical studies of denervated or tenotomized cat muscle, illustrating difficulties in relating experimental animal conditions to human neuromuscular diseases. Ann NY Acad Sci 138: 160

Famborough D, Drachman DB, Satyamart S (1973) Neuromuscular junction in myasthenia gravis: Decreased acetylcholine receptors. Science 182: 293

Fardeau M, Harpey J-P, Caille B (1975) Disproportion congénitales des différentes types de fibre musculaire avec petitesse relative des fibres de type 1: Documents morphologiques concernant les biopsies musculaires prélevées chez trois membres d'une même famille. Rev Neurol (Paris) 131: 745

Fenichel GM, Shy GM (1963) Muscle biopsy experience in myasthenia gravis. Arch Neurol 9: 237

Fried K, Emery AEH (1971) Spinal muscular atrophy Type II: A separate genetic and clinical entity from type 1 (Werdnig-Hoffman disease) and type III (Kugelberg-Welander disease). Clin Genet 2: 203

Gamstorp I (1956) Adynamia episodica hereditaria. Acta Paediatr 108: 1

Gardner Medwin D, Walton JN (1974) Clinical examination of voluntary muscles In: Walton JN (ed) Disorders of voluntary muscle, 3rd edn. Churchill Livingstone, London, p 546

Gauthier GF (1976) The motor end-plate: Structure. In: Landen DN (ed) The peripheral nerve. Chapman & Hall, London, p 464

Goebel HH, Lenard HG, Kohlschütter A, Pilz H (1977) The ultrastructure of the sural nerve in Pompe's disease. Ann Neurol 2: 111

Gonatas NK, Shy GM, Godfrey EH (1966) Nemaline myopathy: The origin of nemaline structures. N Engl J Med 274: 535

Greenbaum D, Richardson PC, Salmon MV, Urich H (1964) Pathological observations in six cases of diabetic neuropathy. Brain 87: 201

Guillain G, Barré JA, Strohl A (1916) Sur un syndrome de radiculo-névrite avec hyperalbuminose du liquide céphalorachidien sans un réaction cellulaire. Remarques sur les caractères cliniques et graphiques des reflexes tendineux. Bulletin Societé Medicale des Hôpitaux de Paris 10: 146

Gutretcht JA, Dyck PJ (1966) Segmental demyelinization in peroneal muscular atrophy nerve fibres teased from sural nerve biopsy specimens. Mayo Clin Proc 41: 775

Haase GR, Shy GM (1960) Pathological changes in muscle biopsies from patients with peroneal muscular atrophy. Brain 83: 631

Hall-Craggs ECB (1972) The liquificance of longitudinal fibre division in skeletal muscle. J Neurol Sci 15: 27

Harper PS (1975) Congenital myotonic dystrophy in Britain, 1. Clinical aspects. 2. Genetic aspects. Arch Dis Child 50: 505 514

Harriman DGF (1961) Histology of the motor end plate (motor point muscle biopsy). In: Licht S (ed) Electrodiagnosis and electromyography, 2nd edn. Licht, New Haven, p 134

Harriman DGF (1976) Diseases of muscle. In: Blackwood W, Corsellis JAN (eds) Greenfield's neuropathology. Arnold, London, p 849

Hierons R (1957) Changes in the nervous system in acute perphyria. Brain 80: 176

Hopkins IJ, Lindsey JR, Ford FR (1966) Nemaline myopathy: A long-term clinicopathologic study of affected mother and daughter. Brain 89: 299

Howes EL Jr, Price HM, Blumberg JM (1966) Hypokalaemic periodic paralysis: Electron microscopic changes in the sarcoplasm. Neurology (Minneap) 16: 242

Illingworth B, Cori GT, Cori CF (1956) Amylo 1,6 glucosidase in muscle tissue in generalized glycogen storage disease. J Biol Chem 218: 123

Isaacs H, Barlow MB (1970) Malignant hyperpyrexia during anaesthesia: Possible association with subclinical myopathy. Br Med J i: 295

James NT (1971) The distribution of muscle fibre types in fasciculi and their analysis. J Anat 110: 335

Jerusalem F, Rakuska M, Engel AG, MacDonald PD (1974) Morphometric analysis of skeletal muscle capillary ultrastructure in inflammatory myopathies. J Neurol Sci 23: 391

Johnson MA, Polgar J, Weightman D, Appleton D (1973) Data on the distribution of fibre types in thirty six human muscles: An autopsy study. J Neurol Sci 18: 111

Joosten E, Gabreëls F, Bagreëls-Festen A, Vrensen G, Karten J, Notermans S (1974) Electron microscopic heterogeneity of onion-bulb neuropathies of the Déjerine–Sottas type. Two patients in one family with the variant described by Lyon. Acta Neuropathol (Berl) 27: 105

Kaeser HE (1965) Scapuloperoneal muscular dystrophy. Brain 88: 407

Kamensky E, Philippart M, Cancilla P, Frommes SP (1973) Cultured skin fibroblasts in storage disorders: An analysis of ultrastructural features. Am J Pathol 73: 59

Karch S, Urich H (1975) Infantile polyneuropathy with defective myelination: An autopsy study. Dev Med Child Neurol 17: 504

Karpati G, Carpenter S, Engel AG, Watters G, Allen J, Rothman S, Klassen G, Mamer OA (1975) The syndrome of systemic carnitine deficiency. Neurology (Minneap) 25: 16

Kearns TP, Sayre GP (1958) Retinitis pigmentosa, external ophthalmoplegia and complete heart block. Arch Ophthalmol 60: 280

Keesey J, Lindstrom J, Cokely H, Herrmann C Jr (1977) Antiacetylcholine receptor antibody in neonatal myasthenia gravis. N Engl J Med 296: 55

Kiloh LG, Nevin S (1951) Progressive dystrophy of the external ocular muscles (ocular myopathy). Brain 24: 115

Klinkerfuss GH (1967) An electron microscopic study of myotonic dystrophy. Arch Neurol 16: 181

Kocen RS, Thomas PK (1970) Peripheral nerve involvement in Fabry's disease. Arch Neurol 22: 81

Kocen RS, King RHM, Thomas PK, Haas LF (1973) Nerve biopsy findings in two cases of Tangier disease. Acta Neuropathol (Berl) 26: 317

Lake BD, Wilson J (1975) Zebra body myopathy: Clinical, histochemical and ultrastructural studies. J Neurol Sci 24: 437

Landon DB, Hall SM (1976) The myelinated nerve fibre. In Landon DN (ed) The peripheral nerve. Chapman & Hall, London, p 1

Lawrence DG, Locke S (1963) Neuropathy in children with diabetes mellitus. Br Med J ii: 784

Lindstrom JM, Lambert E (1978) Content of acetylcholine receptor and antibodies bound to receptor in myasthenia gravis, experimental autoimmune myasthenia gravis and Eaton-Lambert syndrome. Neurology (Minneap) 28: 130

Lindstrom JM, Seybold ME, Lennon VA, Whittingham S, Duane DD (1976) Antibody to acetylcholine receptor in myasthenia gravis: Prevalence, clinical correlates and diagnostic value. Neurology (Minneap) 26: 1054

Lyon G (1969) Ultrastructure of a nerve biopsy from a case of early infantile chronic neuropathy. Acta Neuropathol (Berl) 13: 131

Mars H, Lewis LA, Robertson AL, Butkus A, Williams GH (1969) Familial hypo β lipoproteinaemia. Am J Med 46: 886

McArdle B (1951) Myopathy due to a defect in muscle glycogen breakdown. Clin Sci Mol Med 10: 13

McComas AT (1977) Neuromuscular function and disorders. Butterworths, London

McLellan DL, Swash M (1976) Longitudinal sliding of the median nerve during movement. J Neurol Neurosurg Psychiatry 38: 506

Morgan-Hughes JA, Daviniza P, Kahn SN, Landon DN, Sherratt RM, Land SM, Clark JB (1978) A mitochondrial myopathy characterized by a deficiency in reducible cytochromes. Brain 100: 617

Moulds RFW, Denborough MA (1972) Procaine in malignant hyperpyrexia. Br Med J iv: 526

Mellick RS, Mahler RF, Hughes BP (1962) McArdle's syndrome: Phospharylase deficient myopathy. Lancet 1: 1045

Milhorat AT, Shafiq SA, Goldstone L (1966) Changes in muscle structure in dystrophic patients, carriers and siblings seen by electron microscopy: Correlation with levels of serum creatine phospholeinase Ann NY Acad Sci 138: 246

Mokri B, Engel AG (1975) Duchenne dystrophy—electron microscopic findings pointing to a basic or early abnormality in the plasma membrane of the muscle fibre. Neurology (Minneap) 25: 1111

Moosa A, Dubowitz V (1970) Peripheral neuropathy in Cockayne's syndrome. Arch Dis Child 45: 674

Namba T, Brunner NG, Brown SB, Mugurama M, Grob D (1971) Familial myasthenia gravis. Arch Neurol 25: 49

Namba T, Brunner NG, Grob D (1978) Myasthenia gravis in patients with thymoma with particular reference to onset after thymectomy. Medicine (Baltimore) 57: 411

Neville HE, Brooke MH (1971) Central core fibres: Structured and unstructured (Abstract). Excerpta Medica, Amsterdam, p 31 (ICS no. 237)

Neville HE, Brooke MH (1973) Central core fibres: Structured and unstructured. In: Kakulas BA (ed) Basic research in myology, part I. Excerpta Medica, Amsterdam, p 497 (ICS no. 294)

Ochoa J (1976) The unmyelinated nerve fibre. In: Landon DN (ed) The peripheral nerve. Chapman & Hall, London, p. 106

Ochoa J, Mair WG (1969) The normal sural nerve in man. 1. Ultrastructure and numbers of fibres and cells. Acta Neuropathol (Berl) 13: 197

Ochoa J, Danta G, Fowler TJ, Gilliatt RW (1971) Nature of the nerve lesion caused by a pneumatic tourniquet. Nature 233: 265

Olsson Y, Säve-Soderbergh J, Sourander P, Angerwall L (1968) A patho-anatomical study of the central and peripheral nervous system in diabetics of early onset and long duration. Pathol Eur 3: 62

Ontell M (1974) Muscle satellite cells: A validated technique for light microscopic identification and a quantitative study of changes in their population following denervation. Anat Rec 178: 211

Osserman KE (1958) Myasthenia gravis. Grune & Stratton, New York

Pearce GW, Pearce JMS, Walton JN (1966) The Duchenne type muscular dystrophy: Histopathological studies of the carrier state. Brain 89: 109

Pestronk D, Drachman DB (1978) A new method for demonstrating sprouting at neuromuscular terminals. Muscle Nerve 1: 40

Peter JB, Barnard VR, Edgerton VR, Gillespie CA, Stempel KE (1972) Metabolic profiles of three fibre types of skeletal muscles in guinea pigs and rabbits. Biochemistry 11: 2627

Polgar J, Johnson MA, Weightman D, Appleton D (1972) Data on fibre size in thirty-six human muscles. J Neurol Sci 19: 307

Pirskanen R (1976) Genetic association between myasthenia gravis and the H-LA system. J Neurol Neurosurg Psychiatry 39: 23

Prineas JW (1972) Acute idiopathic polyneuritis: An electron microscopic study. Invest 26: 133

Refsum S (1946) Heredopathia atactica polyneuritiformis: A familial syndrome not hitherto described. Acta Psychiatr Scand [Suppl] 38 1: 303

Reznik N (1973) Current concepts of skeletal muscle regeneration. In: Pearson CM (ed) The striated muscle. Williams & Wilkins, Baltimore, p 185

Reznik M, Engel WK (1970) Ultrastructural and histochemical correlations of experimental muscle regeneration. J Neurol Sci 11: 167

Ridley A (1969) The neuropathy of acute intermittent porphyria. Q J Med 38: 307

Ridley A (1975) Porphyric neuropathy. In: Dyck PJ, Lambert EG, Thomas PK (eds) Peripheral neuropathy, vol 2. Saunders, London Philadelphia, p 942

Ringel SP, Bender AN, Engel WK (1976) Extrajunctional acetylcholine receptors: Alterations in human and experimental neuromuscular diseases. Arch Neurol 33: 751

Rosman NP, Kakulas BA (1966) Mental deficiency associated with muscular dystrophy: A neuropathological study. Brain 89: 769

Russell DS (1953) Histological changes in the striped muscles in myasthenia gravis. J Pathol Bacteriol 65: 279

Sabin TD, Swift TR (1975) Leprosy In: Dyck PJ, Thomas PK, Lambert EH (eds) Peripheral neuropathy, vol 2. Saunders, London Philadelphia, p 1166

Santa T, Engel AG, Lambert EH (1972) Histometric study of neuromuscular junction. 1 myasthenia gravis. Neurology (Minneap) 22: 71

Sato T, Walker DL, Peters HA, Reese HH, Chou SM (1971) Chronic polymyositis and myxovirus-like inclusions: Electron microscopic and viral studies. Arch Neurol 24: 409

Schaumberg HH, Spencer PS (1979) Toxic neuropathies. Neurology (Minneap) 29: 429

Schmalbruch H (1976) Muscle fibre splitting and regeneration in diseased human muscle. Neuropathol Appl Neurobiol 2: 3

Schmid R, Mahler R (1959) Chronic progressive myopathy with myoglobinuria: demonstration of a glycogenolytic defect in the muscle. J Clin Invest 38: 2044

Schotland DL (1977) Duchenne dystrophy—a freeze fracture study. In: Rowland LP (ed) Pathogenesis of human muscular dystrophies. Excerpta Medica, Amsterdam, p 562 (ICS no 404)

Schwartz MS, Swash M (1975) Scapulo-peroneal atrophy with

sensory involvement: Davidenkow's syndrome. J Neurol Neurosurg Psychiatry 38: 1063

Schwartz MS, Sargeant M, Swash M (1976) Longitudinal fibre splitting in neurogenic muscular disorders: Its relation to the pathogenesis of 'myopathic' change. Brain 99: 617

Schwartz MS, Moosa A, Dubowitz V (1977a) Correlation of single fibre EMG and muscle histochemistry using an open biopsy recording technique. J Neurol Sci 31: 309

Schwartz MS, Sargeant MK, Swash M (1977b) Neostigmine-induced end-plate proliferation in the rat. Neurology (Minneap) 27: 289

Schwartz MS, Swash M, Gross M (1978) Benign post-infection polymyositis. Br Med J ii: 1256

Seitelberger F, Wanko T, Gavin MA (1961) The muscle fibre in central core disease: histochemical and electron microscopic observations. Acta Neuropathol (Berl) 1: 223

Shafiq SA, Dubowitz V, Peterson HdeC, Milhorat AT (1967) Nemaline myopathy: Report of a fatal case, with histochemical and electron microscopic studies. Brain 90: 817

Sher JH, Rimalovski AB, Athanassiades TJ, Aronson SM (1967) Familial centronuclear myopathy: A clinical and pathological study. Neurology (Minneap) 17: 727

Sheramata W, Kott S, Cyr DP (1971) The Chediak–Higashi–Steinbrinck syndrome. Arch Neurol 25: 289

Shy GM, Magee KR (1956) A new congenital non-progressive myopathy. Brain 79: 610

Shy GM, Engel WK, Somers JE, Wanko T (1963) Nemaline myopathy: A new congenital myopathy. Brain 86: 793

Sloper JC, Pegrum GD (1967) Regeneration of crushed mammalian skeletal muscle and effects of steroids. J Pathol 93: 47

Sourander P, Olsson Y (1968) Peripheral neuropathy in globoid cell leucodystrophy (Morbus Krabbe). Acta Neuropathol (Berl) 11: 69

Spiro AJ, Shy GM, Gonatas NK (1966) Myotubular myopathy. Arch Neurol 14: 1

Stern GM, Hall JM, Robinson DC (1964) Neonatal myasthenia gravis. Br Med J 2: 284

Steinberg D, Mize C, Avigan J, Falls HM, Eldjarn L, Try K, Stokke O, Refsum S (1966) On the metabolic error in Refsum's disease. Trans Am Neurol Assoc 91: 168

Stevens JC, Lofgren EP, Dyck PJ (1975) Biopsy of peripheral nerves. In: Dyck PJ, Thomas PK, Lambert EH (eds) Peripheral neuropathy. Saunders, London Philadelphia, p 410

Sunderland S (1978) Nerves and nerve injuries. Churchill Livingstone, Edinburgh

Swash M (1979) Guillain-Barré syndrome: Clinical aspects. J R Soc Med 12: 670

Swash M, Fox KP (1972) Muscle spindle innervation in man. J Anat 112: 61

Swash M, Fox KP (1974) The pathology of the muscle spindle: Effect of denervation. J Neurol Sci 22: 1

Swash M, Fox KP (1975a) Abnormal intrafusal muscle fibres in myotonic dystrophy: A study using serial sections. J Neurol Neurosurg Psychiatry 38: 91

Swash M, Fox KP (1975b) The fine structure of the spindle abnormality in myotonic dystrophy. Neuropathol Appl Neurobiol 1: 171

Swash M, Fox KP (1976) The pathology of the muscle spindle in Duchenne muscular dystrophy. J Neurol Sci 29: 17

Swash M, Schwartz MS (1977) Implications of longitudinal fibre splitting in myopathic and neurogenic disorders. J Neurol Neurosurg Psychiatry 40: 1152

Swash M, van den Noort S, Craig JW (1970) Myopathy associated with diabetes mellitus in two sisters. Neurology (Minneap) 20: 694

Swash M, Sargeant MK, Schwartz MS (1978a) Pathogenesis of longitudinal splitting of muscle fibres in neurogenic disorders and polymyositis. Neuropathol Appl Neurobiol 4: 99

Swash M, Schwartz MS, Sargeant MK (1978b) The significance of ragged-red fibres in neuromuscular disease. J Neurol Sci 36: 347

Sweeney VP, Pathak MA, Asbury AK (1970) Acute intermittent porphyria: Increased ALA synthetase activity during an acute attack. Brain 83: 369

Tallis R, Staniforth P, Fisher TR (1978) Neurophysiological studies of autogenous sural nerve grafts J Neurol Neurosurg Psychiatry 41: 677

Tarui S, Oluno G, Ikura Y, Tanaka T, Suda M, Nishikawa M (1965) Phosphofructokinase deficiency in skeletal muscle: a new type of glycogenosis. Biochem Biophys Res Commun 19: 517

Thomas KP, Calne DB, Elliott CF (1972) X-linked scapulo-peroneal syndrome. J Neurol Neurosurg Psychiatry 35: 208

Thomas PK, Lascelles RG (1966) The pathology of diabetic neuropathy. Q J Med 35: 489

Thomas PK, Lascelles RG, Hallpike JF, Hewer RC (1969) Recurrent and chronic relapsing Guillain–Barré polyneuritis. Brain 92: 589

Van Wijngaarden GK, Bethlem J (1971) The facioscapulohumeral syndrome. In: Kakulas BA (ed) Second International Congress on Muscle Diseases. Excerpta Medica, Amsterdam, p 54 (ICS no. 237)

Victor M, Hayes R, Adams RD (1962) Oculopharyngeal muscular dystrophy. A familial disease of late life characterized by dysphagia and progressive ptosis of the eyelids N Engl J Med 267: 1267

Vincent A, Scadding GK, Thomas HC, Newsom Davis J (1978) In-vitro synthesis of anti-acetylcholine receptor antibody to thymic lymphocytes in myasthenia gravis. Lancet 1: 305

Walton JN, Adams RD (1958) Polymyositis. Williams & Wilkins, Baltimore

Webb JN (1977) Cell death in developing skeletal muscle: Histiochemistry and ultrastructure. J Pathol 123: 175

Weller RO, McArdle B (1971) Calcification within muscle fibres in the periodic paralyses. Brain 94: 263

Whitaker JN, Engel WK (1972) Vascular deposits of immunoglobulins and complement in idiopathic inflammatory myopathy. N Engl J Med 286: 333

Whitaker JN, Engel WK (1973) Mechanisms of muscle injury in idiopathic inflammatory myopathy. N Engl J Med 288: 434 and 289: 107

Whiteley AM, Schwartz MS, Sachs JA, Swash M (1976) Congenital myasthenia gravis: Clinical and HLa studies in two brothers. J Neurol Neurosurg Psychiatry 39: 1145

Wochner RD, Dres G, Strober W, Waldmann TA (1966) Accelerated breakdown of IgG in myotonic dystrophy: A hereditary error of immunoglobulin catabolism. J Clin Invest 45: 321

Young JZ (1942) Functional repair of nervous tissue. Physiol Rev 22: 318

Chapter 12

Spleen, Lymph Nodes and Immunoreactive Tissues

Colin L. Berry and Peter A. Revell

The varied functions of spleen, lymph nodes, and thymus result in their being involved in a widely disparate group of disease processes. A number of these, e.g., metabolic disease, are dealt with elsewhere in the volume, and this chapter is concerned with certain specific abnormalities, including the pathology of immune deficiency states and of lymphomas.

1. Embryogenesis and Development

The brief account of the embryology of the thymus given here is based on the studies of Hammar (1911, 1921) and Kingsbury (1915), together with an examination of human fetal thymuses obtained from Dr. H.E.M. Kay.

The primordial thymus develops from the third and probably fourth endodermal pouches during the 6th week of development approximately 7–10 days after the appearances of these structures (10- to 12-mm stage). The pouches are simple epithelial cell masses with, initially, a cleft-like lumen. The narrower caudal portion of the third pouch arising from the pharynx forms the corresponding half of the thymus, which at this stage is connected to the pharynx by the ductus pharyngobrachialis III. This later becomes solid, and then breaks (12 mm). Remnants of this duct may become parathyroid or thyroid 'rests' or form epithelial cysts.

The walls of the pouch thicken and obliterate the lumen, and the cell mass moves caudally and medially. The parathyroid precursor generally separates from the thymic rudiment at around the 20-mm stage. The thymic precursor thickens caudally and this part is included in the developing thoracic cavity, where it fuses with the similar component of the other side. This fusion is limited to the connective tissue component. With differential growth of the neck and relative descent of the heart and great vessels the thymus is drawn down into the thorax. The cervical portion becomes elongated and thinned, and extends into the neck in a very variable manner.

At 35–37 mm (approx. 56 days) the dense epithelial mass is surrounded by a mesenchymal condensation, and a lobulated structure develops following vascular invasion of the gland. At around the 40-mm stage the thymic medulla and cortex can be differentiated. Further development of the epithelial component occurs when large cells with eosinophilic cytoplasm appear, collect in small aggregates and become granular and more eosinophilic, and form Hassall's corpuscles. Personal observations suggest that this may occur at around 9–10 weeks after conception, a little earlier than generally suggested. Lymphocytes appear in the gland at the 30- to 35-mm stage (7–8 weeks) (Gilmour 1941) and are derived from immigrant stem cells of a haematopoietic origin.

Ultrastructural studies of the 10- to 38-mm embryonic thymus have been performed by Pinkel (1968), who described the gland as an epithelial network enclosing lymphocytes and segregating them into groups. A haemo–thymic vascular barrier was described, preventing penetration of antigen into the gland, backed up by a highly phagocytic zone of epithelial cells. Evidence for lymphocyte digestion was found in Hassall's corpuscles, supporting the suggestion of Siegler (1964) that this was an important function of these structures. Essentially similar ulstrastructural findings were described by Goldstein et al. (1968), but lymphocytes were seen in passage across the walls of thymic blood vessels in their study.

In Fig. 12.1 the appearances of the gland in early and late pregnancy are shown.

1.1. Embryology of Lymph Nodes and Spleen

The spleen first appears as a mesenchymal condensation in embryos of approximately 10 mm, in the dorsal mesogastrium. It is supplied by a branch of the coeliac artery to the greater curve of the stomach, which will become the adult splenic artery. At around 30 mm (8–9 weeks) a series of anastomosing trabeculae become visible, in the spaces of which haematopoiesis develops by the 90-mm stage. It is during this stage that splenic sinusoids are formed. Follicular structures are seen by the end of the second trimester (Fig. 12.2).

Accessory masses of splenic tissue often become detached from the main body to form accessory spleens or splenunculi, which are commonly seen at autopsy in childhood.

Lymph nodes can be identified in the neck at the 25-mm stage. During early development erythropoiesis occurs in nodes, but this ceases early in intrauterine life. By 50 mm, when nodes are found in large numbers, the proliferating cells in their stroma are almost entirely lymphoid (Fig. 12.3). Rates of cell division in the fetus are low (Metcalf and Brumby 1966).

1.2. Histological Change in the Thymus with Age

Hammar (1926) and Boyd (1932) have discussed in some detail the changes occurring in the thymus gland with age. The latter author has also included in her description a quantitative assessment of the numbers of Hassall's corpuscles and their size distribution from prenatal life to the ninth decade.

In general the initial appearance of closely packed lobules of thymic tissue changes at puberty owing to enlargement of interlobar septa. At about 15–17

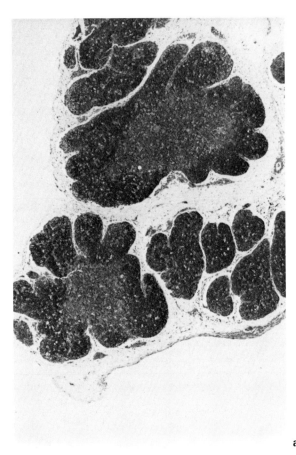 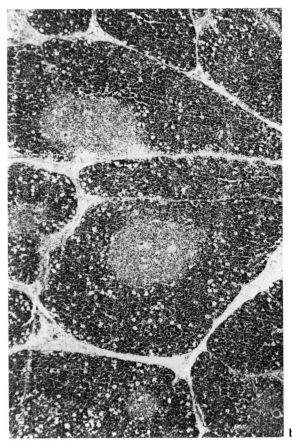

a   b

Fig. 12.1. a and **b** Thymic appearances in early (**a**) and late gestation. Initially the lymphocytic component is small and the gland appears to be predominantly epithelial. **a** Thymus at 12 weeks. (H and E; 40 ×) **b** Thymus at 26 weeks. (H and E; 160 ×)

years of age the thymus reaches its maximum weight, and progressive decrease in size then ensues, with more rapid loss of cortex than medulla. Fat appears in the interlobular septae and eventually the gland remains as a series of epithelial strands separated by fat. A thin rim of cortical lymphocytes is seen. Goldstein and Mackay (1967) have confirmed Boyd's finding that Hassall's corpuscles decrease in number with increasing age—from 12/mm² of medulla at birth to 2/mm² at 70 years of age.

1.3. Development and Function of Immunoreactive Tissues

Some knowledge of the developmental changes of the immunoreactive tissues is essential to a proper understanding of immune deficiency states. The system and its functions are phylogenetically ancient.

In many primitive animals, e.g., the arthropods and protostomes (annelid worms and molluscs) there are specialized phagocytic cells, which engulf injected or foreign particles and fragments of damaged tissue. Specialized lymphocytes first occur in the early vertebrates; both the agnathia and the lampreys and hagfishes have lymphocytes and can reject allografts. Recent work suggests that a self-recognition system, although not very effective, may exist in all animals. It seems likely, in view of the importance of complex cell-surface characteristics in a number of processes in development, that a sensitive recognition system developed in association with this type of change, which explains the widespread presence of such systems.

The combination of functions expressed in an immune system capable of recognizing and rejecting allografts, maintaining a memory for previously experienced antigens, and producing specifically reactive families of immunoglobulins is confined to the vertebrates. How is the system formed?

The immunodeficiency states provide a clear example of how animal studies and the careful examination of congenital defects in structure and function in man have led to a better understanding of how a system works. What follows is a synthesis

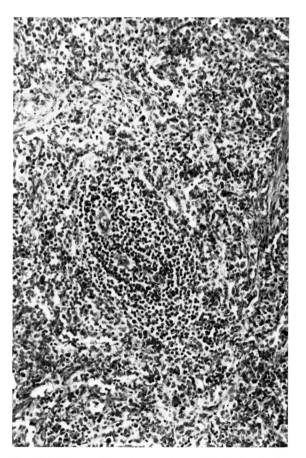

Fig. 12.2. Spleen at 24 weeks, showing early follicular development. (H and E; 240 ×)

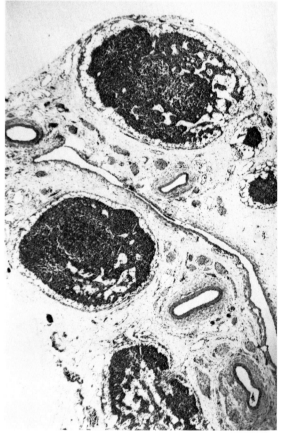

Fig. 12.3. Lymph nodes with well-defined lymphocytic populations but a wide subcapsular sinus (26 weeks). (H and E; 40 ×)

of views on the development of the cellular components of the immunoreactive tissues.

Multipotent haematopoietic stem cells are first found in the vessels of the embryonic yolk sac. These cells give rise to subpopulations of stem cells, some of which persist throughout life but which in early stages of development migrate to different organs. There they are induced by local tissue to migrate further, forming specialized cell colonies of stable cells capable of clonal proliferation. We may concern ourselves initially with two main routes of differentiation, to T or B lymphocytes (Fig. 12.4).

1.3.1. T Cells

Cells from the yolk sac, fetal marrow, and liver migrate to the thymus, where they proliferate and differentiate. The cells are altered in a way that causes them to express a number of markers of T cell activity, differing subpopulations being concerned with cytotoxic reactions and suppressor and helper aspects of the immune reaction.

Around 75% of circulating lymphocytes are T cells, assessed by their capacity to form rosettes with sheep erythrocytes. Absolute numbers are 1620–4320/mm³ at 1 week of age, and 590–3090/mm³ at 18 months (Fleisher et al. 1975). This population may be subdivided by means of antisera into two principle groups, in one of the cells which proliferate in mixed lymphocyte cultures, produce lymphocyte mitogenic factor, and act as 'helper' and 'killer' cells, and a second which proliferates in response to soluble antigens but does not perform the other functions described. Both populations proliferate in response to phytohaemagglutinin.

Tests of T cells function performed clinically include

1) *Delayed skin tests*: to agents such as mumps virus, PPD, *Candida*, etc., or keyhole limpet haemocyanin if confirmation of absent response is required;

2) *Capacity of lymphocytes to proliferate*: in response to such stimuli as phytohaemagglutinin (nonspecific) or to previously experienced antigens

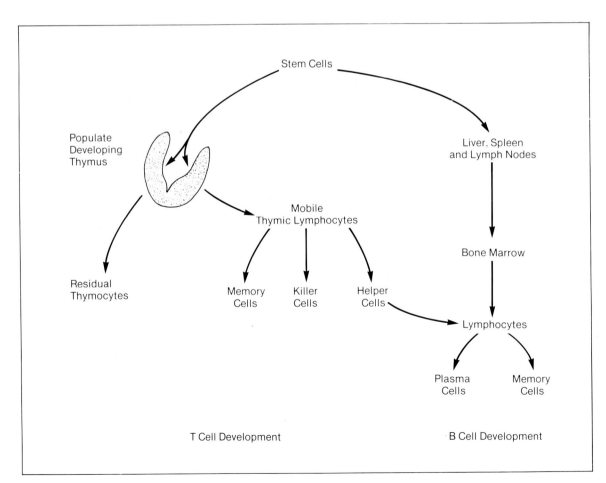

Fig. 12.4. Differentiation of stem cells into T cells and B cells.

(tetanus, PPD, *Candida*, etc.). Stimulation by a one-way mixed leucocyte reaction can also be measured;

3) *Tests of helper, killer and suppressor functions*: These are usually performed in a way that permits the assessment of the effects of adding cells to a standardized in vitro antibody-producing cell culture (see Waldmann and Broder 1978 for review).

1.3.2. B Cells

So-called pre-B cells (large rapidly dividing cells that synthesize small amounts of monomeric IgM) are found in the fetal liver. They do not have the stable surface immunoglobulin receptors that characterize B lymphocytes. These cells migrate to bone marrow, where they divide. They do not yet possess other characteristics of mature B cells (Fc receptors for IgG, receptors for C_3) and this may protect them from involvement with antigen, complexes, and activated C_3, permitting them to generate great clonal diversity. Later some cells become modified, from the production of IgM to the production of IgG, A, or E, although the antibody specificity within any clone remains identical. This stage is reached early in the second trimester.

None of the stages described thus far involves T cells. When B cells with all these receptors are stimulated by antigen and helper T cells; they give rise to *memory* B cells and plasma cells.

The testing system usually used for B cell function involves the polyclonal response of cells in vitro to pokeweed mitogen (PWM) (see Cooper et al. 1978 for review). PWM is capable of inducing B cell lymphocytes to proliferate and to mature into antibody producing cells of all classes but it is necessary for helper T cells to be present for this response to occur. These helper cells may facilitate the linkage of antigen and B cell.

are exposed to rubella virus (Banatvala et al. 1971). Complement components are the next to appear, at around 15 weeks (C3) and 18 weeks (C4) (Adinolfi 1972). By 20 weeks all components of complement are present.

It used to be argued that the absence of plasma cells in fetal tissues supported the contention that immunoglobulins were not produced in the fetus, despite observations at the turn of the century that plasma cells were seen in congenital syphilis and more recently that they may be found in toxoplasmosis. These difficulties are resolved by modern techniques of demonstrating specific proteins by immunofluorescence or enzyme reactions, when immunoglobulin-producing cells of non-plasma-cell morphology are demonstrated. The relative paucity of plasma cells during gestation is largely related to lack of stimulus. The timing of antibody production and the sequence in which the various classes appear are apparently under genetic control, and from Silverstein's work (see Silverstein 1972) this control appears to be finely tuned. In man, following intrauterine infections IgM and IgG antibodies may be found in the serum of newborns, for example, in *Toxoplasma gondii*, cytomegalic inclusion disease, and herpes simplex infection. Antibodies to *Listeria monocytogenes* and gram-negative organisms have been found in apparently normal neonates (Cohen and Norins 1968) and the blood group anti-A and anti-B agglutinins of nonmaternal origin have been detected in cord sera (Perchalski et al. 1968).

IgG and IgM antibodies are produced in very low concentrations in neonates, and the synthesis of IgD commences after birth. There is some evidence to suggest that IgE may be produced in utero (See Adinolfi 1974). Holland and Holland (1966), using what would now be regarded as relatively insensitive techniques, demonstrated antibody production in the 2-month-old child of an aglobulinaemic mother.

2. Fetal Immunoreactivity

There is a considerable body of evidence documenting the immunological competence of the human fetus and its capacity to react to infection. The morphological appearance of the tissues described above is followed by the appearance of lymphocytes in the blood at around the 10th week at a level of approximately 1000 cells/mm³. At 12 weeks lysozyme (muramidase), a basic protein with a molecular weight of around 15 000 and with pronounced bacteriolytic properties, is produced. Interferon is also found if cells from fetuses older than 18 weeks

3. Immune-deficiency States

Infection may be defined as the entry of self-replicating antigens into the tissues of the host, producing significant injury to the tissues. The establishment of an infection by a virus, fungus, or bacterium is dependent on the virulence of the agent concerned, its number, mode of entry, and the resistance of the host. Establishment of bacteria in tissues implies a breach of the first line of defence—the integrity of mucous membranes or skin with the associated activity of lysozyme, secretory IgA, etc. The bacteria in the tissues are then exposed to a variety of humoral agents with growth-inhibitory or opsonizing effects. Phagocytosis may occur, by granulocytes or mononuclear cells, and intracellular destruction follows, although a number of infective agents may continue to proliferate intracellularly following phagocytosis. The process of intracellular digestion presents antigenic material to responsive cells and the efferent limb of the immune response (specific antibody production, establishment of delayed hypersensitivity, etc.) is activated.

Immune-deficiency states may be considered to affect primarily the 'phagocytosis/digestion/antigen recognition' or *afferent* limb of the immune response, or the *efferent* limb, as defined above. However, it will be seen later that such diseases are complex, both in their causation and in the effects of the particular defect considered. The distinction between afferent and efferent limb defects or between cellular or humoral immunity is often not sharply defined, and alterations in one component may indirectly affect another.

3.1. T cell-deficiency States

Patients with T cell-deficient conditions present with clinical manifestations that include severe or overwhelming infection with ordinarily nonpathogenic bacteria (BCG) or fungi, or with agents that do not normally give rise to serious illness (zoster, varicella, herpes simplex, cytomegalovirus). There may be acute or chronic graft-versus-host disease in those transfused with viable allogenic lymphocytes. Subtle T cell-deficient states may be manifest in localized mucosal infections, immunoglobulin deficiency, or autoimmunity.

In general, clinical syndromes occur in a way that suggests that all stages of the development of the immunoreactive system may be faulty, with specific effects.

We describe here a number of histopathological entities before making a clinicopathological synthesis. We would emphasize that accurate delineation of these syndromes requires sophisticated laboratory investigation in life, but that in previously unsuspected or uninvestigated causes useful data can be obtained from autopsy and histological examination.

3.2. Reticular Dysgenesis

Reticular dysgenesis was first described by de Vaal and Seynhaeve (1959) in twins, and few other reports have since been made. The thymus is absent, there is lymphopenia, agranulocytosis, and agammaglobulinaemia. Little or no development of peripheral lymphoid tissue is seen, and in a personal case a roll preparation of the entire mesentery revealed no lymph nodes after examination by step sectioning at 100 µm intervals.

The disease is thought to be due to deficiencies of the haematopoietic stem-cell precursor, giving rise to the lymphocytic and granulocytic population. Red cells and platelets are present (see also Gitlin et al. 1964b).

3.3. Thymic Agenesis (Di George Syndrome)

In 1965 Di George, in the discussion of a paper, described four cases of thymic agenesis associated with absence of the parathyroid glands. The immunological function of one of these infants was studied and normal immunoglobulin levels were found. Plasma cells were present in lymph node biopsies but there was no demonstrable capacity to develop delayed hypersensitivity reactions. 'Runting' was a feature of the clinical syndrome.

In the great majority of reported cases of the syndrome abnormalities of the aortic arch and heart have been present in association with thymic and parathyroid agenesis. Dische (1968) has reported an instance of associated tracheo-oesophageal fistula and oesophageal atresia. There is one familial report (Steele et al. 1972) and the disease can occur in either sex.

The expression of the defect of the third and fourth arches is clearly variable: some patients have small thymic masses present, and in only 7 of the 19 patients reported by Lischner and Huff (1975) was the thymus completely absent. The fragments present are usually histologically completely normal. Parathyroid glands can be found in cases with completely absent thymic tissue.

There is a reduction in the thymic-dependent area of the peripheral lymph nodes in most cases, although Huber et al. (1967) have described tonsils, spleen, gut, and lymph nodes as all having a normal structure and lymphoid population.

In five personal cases of thymic agenesis the presenting symptoms have been those of congenital heart disease in two, death occurring within 7 days of birth. One further child presented aged 10 days with congenital heart disease and hypocalcaemic tetany, and another at 6 weeks with hypocalcaemic tetany. The heart lesions present in these cases were truncus arteriosus with right-sided aortic arch (2), transposition of the great arteries, and ventricular septal defect with gross preductal aortic arch hypoplasia and persistent ductus arteriosus.

Aortic branching was anomalous in three cases. In one further case, from which a thoracic pluck was examined, absence of the thymus was confirmed by serial sectioning (at 20 μm intervals) of the superior mediastinum, and a small nodule of parathyroid tissue was found. Tests with a functional basis had shown severe defects in T cell activity (failure of sensitization with dinitrochlorobenzene and prolonged survival of allogenic skin grafts). Humoral immune functions are usually well preserved. In general, the results of such tests in these cases suggest that the defect in the Di George syndrome is not at the level of the stem cell giving rise to the T cell population, but is a defect in the thymus anlage, which prevents the proper processing of stem cells to T cells (Waldmann and Broder 1978).

3.4. Thymic Dysplasia and Combined Immune-deficiency Syndromes

The term 'thymic dysplasia' is used to describe an abnormality of thymic epithelial development resulting in gross reduction in number or complete absence of Hassall's corpuscles from the medulla of the gland. This change is accompanied by severe lymphocyte depletion.

When this criterion is used to select cases, a number of immune-deficiency syndromes may be found when clinical records are examined (Berry 1968; Berry and Thompson 1968). In general these have the features of the 'combined immunity-deficiency syndrome' ('Swiss-type' hypo-γ-globulinaemia; Glanzmann and Riniker 1950), but cases of the type described by Nézelof et al. (1964), with defective cellular immunity and normal circulating immunoglobulins, are also seen. The

Wiskott–Aldrich syndrome (see below and Aldrich et al. 1954) is also associated with thymic dysplasia.

3.5. Pathological Findings

3.5.1. Thymus

The thymus gland is small, weighing less than 2 g in most cases, although weights up to 12 g have been recorded. The abnormal gland tends to be found largely above the innominate vein. Histologically a fetal pattern is preserved, with a simple lobular architecture with conspicuous connective tissue. Corticomedullary demarcation is not marked (Fig. 12.5). The lobules are composed of a mass of mesenchymal and endothelial cells, with fewer epithelial cells and only occasional lymphocytes, although in some instances variable numbers of these cells are seen. Hassall's corpuscles are absent or grossly reduced in numbers (Fig. 12.6). Reticulin stains confirm the 'alveolar' pattern seen at the periphery of the lobules of some glands.

The changes are distinct from those seen in the thymus after involution, in which cortical lymphocyte loss may be extreme, with collapse of the periphery of the gland. Medullary lymphocytes persist and the medulla has a crowded appearance with many Hassall's corpuscles, which may be cystic (Fig. 12.7).

3.5.2. Lymph Nodes

The lymph nodes may be absent, with no trace of such structures despite extensive search by serial section (Berry 1970).

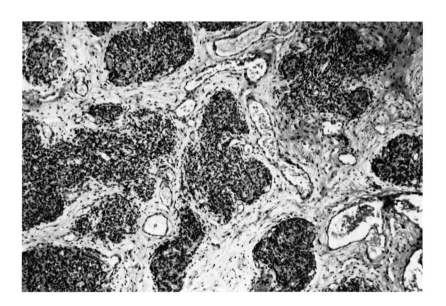

Fig. 12.5. Lobular pattern of thymus, without corticomedullary demarcation. (H and E; 40 ×)

In cases in which nodes are present they may be represented as open-work lattices of supporting tissue, with few sinusoidal histocytes and virtually no lymphocyte population, or as simple masses of ill-organized vessels and connective tissue only recognizable by the distinct subcapsular sinus (Fig. 12.8). Occasionally follicular collections of lymphocytes are seen, and plasma cells may be present. Varied appearances may be seen in different nodes in the same case, but follicular structures, if present, are found in most nodes. Haemophago-cytosis is not uncommon.

3.5.3. Spleen

In 26 personal autopsy cases the spleen has been present and within the normal weight range for the age. Few lymphocytes may be present in the pulp, but small perivascular lymphocyte cuffs are usually seen about penicillar arteries, although grossly diminished in size compared with age-matched controls (Fig. 12.9).

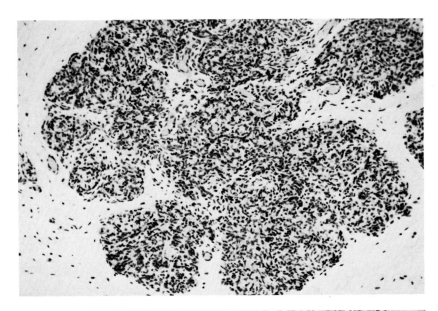

Fig. 12.6. A lobule with no evident development of Hassall's corpuscles. (H and E; 240 ×)

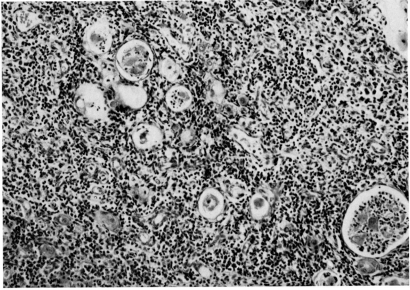

Fig. 12.7. Cystic Hassall's corpuscles with peristence of medullary lymphocytes. The collapsed cortex (*top right*) is lymphocyte-depleted. (H and E; 240 ×)

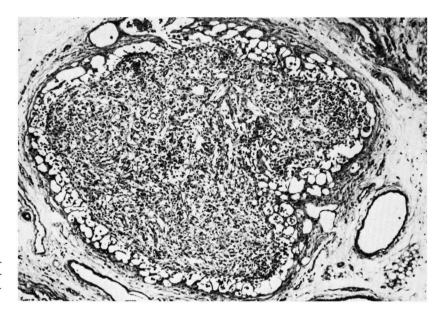

Fig. 12.8. A small lymph node without follicular differentiation or significant lymphocyte population. (H and E; 40 ×)

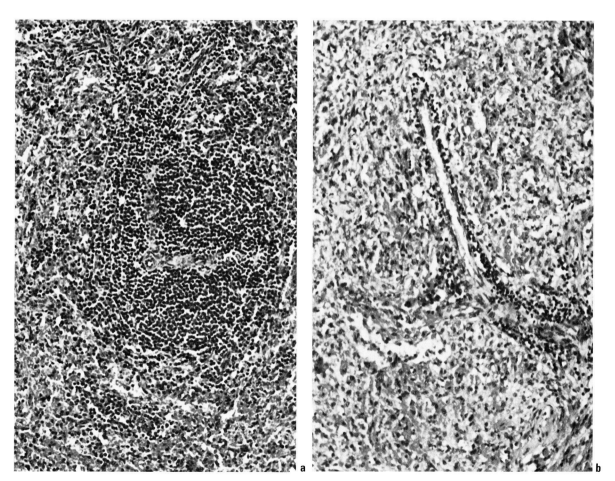

Fig. 12.9. a Control spleen. Normal lymphocytes around artery in 4-month-old child. (H and E; 120 ×) **b** Combined immunity-deficiency syndrome with small lymphocyte population around penicillary vessel. (H and E; 140 ×)

3.5.4. Gut-associated Lymphoid Tissue

The tonsils, appendix and Peyer's patches and lymphoid follicles of the gut are here considered as an entity. In personally studied autopsy cases absence of lymphoid tissue in the tonsillar fossa has invariably been associated with absence of Peyer's patches and appendiceal lymphoid tissue (Fig. 12.10).

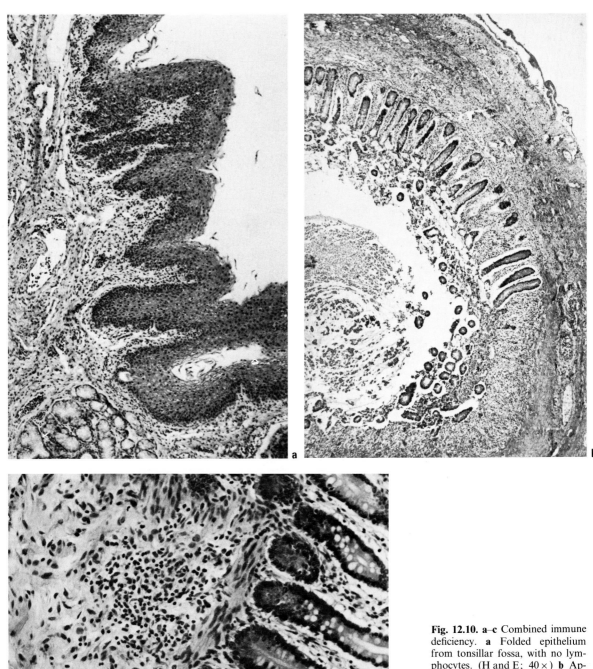

Fig. 12.10. a–c Combined immune deficiency. **a** Folded epithelium from tonsillar fossa, with no lymphocytes. (H and E; 40×) **b** Appendix, with no follicular development. (H and E; 20×) **c** Small lymphoid collection in colon. This is not so large as to interrupt the continuity of the muscularis mucosa, here or in subsequent sections. (H and E; 140×)

The changes found in this group of syndromes are apparently related to an arrest of thymic development at around the 30-mm stage (Blackburn and Gordon 1967) or earlier (Berry 1970), with subsequent changes in the other lymphoid tissues.

Reconstitution therapy has been attempted by grafting of fetal thymus and stem cell transfusion. Graft-versus-host disease may develop in these immunologically incompetent hosts (Robertson et al. 1971) (Fig. 12.11), and this may apparently occur as a result of materno–fetal transfusion during pregnancy (Kadowaki et al. 1965).

It must be emphasized that this morphological grouping of cases cuts across clinical syndromes, and is intended to be useful in histopathological diagnosis of the unsuspected case. Nowhere is the value of keeping infant viscera available until after histopathological examination of selected blocks more clearly seen than in these syndromes, in which accurate diagnosis may have important consequences for genetic counselling. Blocks of the tonsillar bed and appendix are seldom taken for 'routine' histology.

More recent reviews of the pathology of combined immune-deficiency syndromes (Heymer et al. 1977) suggest a specificity of association of particular syndromes with morphological findings that in our view is difficult to support.

3.6. Antibody-deficiency Syndromes

In X-linked infantile agammaglobulinaemia, first described by Bruton (1952), the symptomatology is that of recurrent bacterial infection with pathogenic organisms (pneumococci, streptococci, staphylococci and *H. influenzae*). These infections, involving the middle ear, lungs, skin, or gut usually occur from 3 months of age. Immunoglobulin is present in very small amounts and blood-group isoagglutinins may be absent. Antibodies are not formed in response to immunization with conventional antigens (e.g., tetanus toxoid). For a useful review see Rosen and Janeway (1966).

3.6.1. Pathological Findings

Lymphoid tissue is greatly reduced in amount and lymph nodes are difficult to find. The tonsils and adenoids are virtually absent. The thymus is of normal size and form.

Histopathologically there is an absence of reactive two-component follicles in lymphoid tissue. Plasma cells are rarely found in this site. In some cases small follicular structures may be seen and plasma cells discovered; this is presumably the structural expression of the low but detectable immunoglobulin levels present. Lymphoid tissue is found in reduced amounts in the Peyer's patches and appendix. The thymus shows lymphocyte depletion, but the epithelial component is well represented and Hassall's corpuscles are present in normal numbers.

The sequelae of the disease include abscess formation and bronchiectasis, the lesions of which show no specific features, apart from the paucity of plasma cells in the inflammatory exudate.

Various different forms of agammaglobulinaemia have been defined, following the application of specific tests for lymphocyte functions. The defect in the X-linked form described above is known to be

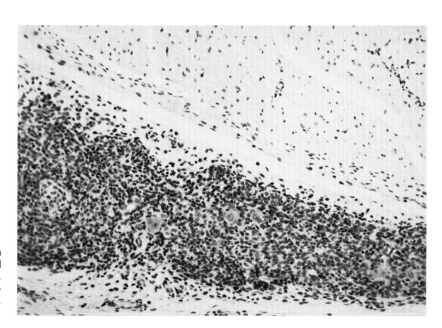

Fig. 12.11. Grafted fetal thymus in rectus sheath in case of combined immunity deficiency syndrome. Note presence of Hassall's corpuscles in normal fetal gland. (H and E; 130 ×)

due to a regulatory gene effect that affects pre-B cell differentiation. These boys have few B cells, but pre-B cells are present in normal numbers (Pearl et al. 1978) in patients with late-onset hypogammaglobulinaemia, and about one-third have low numbers of circulating B lymphocytes. Patients have been described who produce no antibody with kappa chains or who show an imbalance between kappa and lambda light chain ratios.

Selective deficiency of immunoglobulin production also exists. Isolated reduction in the levels of IgM in the serum was reported by Hobbs et al. (1967), and is particularly associated with meningitis. Isolated IgA deficiency is present in about 1:1000 adults, but not all of these individuals are symptomatic.

3.7. Neutropenia

Repeated staphylococcal infection, mainly of the skin, and oral ulceration of uncertain aetiology, may occur in so-called benign or cylic neutropenia, where episodes of neutropenia lasting 7–10 days occur at 3–6 week intervals. Histopathological findings resemble those seen in areas of infection following drug-induced neutropenia and are characterized by absence of cellular response in the infected areas, with a marked tendency to necrosis and ulceration. A more severe form of the disease has been described by MacGillivray et al. (1964).

Neutropenia associated with exocrine atrophy of the pancreas may be associated with increased susceptibility to infection (Burke et al. 1967).

3.8. Chronic Granulomatous Disease

Granulomatous disease was first described by Landing and Shirkey (1957). Although it appears as one disease phenotypically, there are two distinct modes of inheritance, X-linked recessive, which is the more common (Windhorst et al. 1968), and autosomal recessive (De Chatelet et al. 1976).

The fundamental defect is failure of the phagocyte to increase its respiratory activity, which is necessary in the destruction of certain phagocytosed bacteria. Cell motility, phagocytosis and granule enzyme content and degranulation are essentially normal (see review by Babior 1978). Staphylococci and the enterobacteriacae are not killed once engulfed, but pneumococci and streptococci are; this difference depends on the fact that the latter organisms themselves produce H_2O_2. This is used by the neutrophil to kill them, whilst staphylococci and enterobacteriacae are 'protected' by their own catalases.

Other immune functions in these individuals are normal; immunoglobulin levels are often high, presumably as a result of chronic infection.

The effect of the persistence of an indestructible agent in phagocytic cells is to induce a granulomatous response in the host. This essential abnormality produces the lesions seen in the disease.

In the skin, discrete tuberculoid granulomas with giant cells are often seen at the site of inflammation (Fig. 12.12) but granulation tissue indistinguishable from that seen around any chronic inflammatory sinus may be seen, with plasma cells present in normal numbers. Regional lymph nodes show reactive changes and the brown pigmented histiocytes described by some authors may be present. In our experience of 18 cases, these cells are by no means invariably found, but the pigment is found to be sudanophilic and weakly acid-fast (Fig. 12.13). PAS reactivity is variable. Central necrosis may develop in granulomas in lymph nodes; degenerate polymorphonuclear cells are often seen in the centre of such areas. The spleen is invariably large (Fig. 12.14) and in autopsy material areas of necrosis surrounded by a granulomatous inflammatory reaction may be seen. The liver shows a variety of changes; discrete focal intraparenchymal granulomas (Fig. 12.15), granulomatous inflammation in the portal tracts, portal fibrosis, and areas of necrosis and repair may all be seen at different stages. A similar range of appearances may be seen in the kidney (Fig. 12.16).

In the lungs the effects of the disease are often masked by superimposed bronchiectatic changes or abscess formation. Granulomatous masses with central necrosis occur and occasional isolated granulomas may be present, but histological material from mildly affected individuals or those in the early stages has not been studied. Symchych et al. (1968) have commented on the frequency with which pigmented histiocytes may be found in the lamina propria of the gut; this is true in our material and in that of Corson et al. (1965). Involvement of bone is not infrequent and destructive osteomyelitis may ensue (Fig. 12.17).

The organisms involved in these lesions are often 'nonpathogenic'; from personal cases *Aspergillus nidulans* has been isolated from the vertebral bodies, *Serrata marsecens* from the lung, and *Staphylococcus albus* from the renal parenchyma.

3.9. Other Granulocyte Defects

A clinical picture closely resembling that of chronic granulomatous disease may occur in glucose-6-phosphate dehydrogenase deficiency (see Babior 1978). These patients have similar defects of phagocyte function but the disease usually presents after the first 5 years of life. In myeloperoxidase deficiency and glutathione deficiency there is no enhancement of susceptibility to infection, but glutathione per-oxidase deficiency is associated with the phenotype of chronic granulomatous disease (see Matsuda et al. 1976).

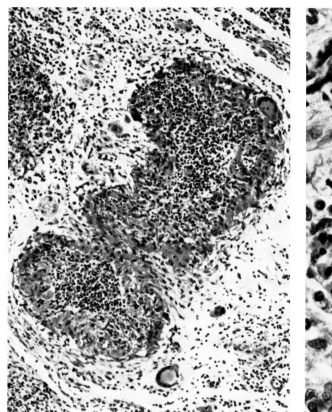

Fig. 12.12. Granuloma in skin from case of chronic granulomatous disease. *Staph. albus* cultured. (H and E; 120 ×)

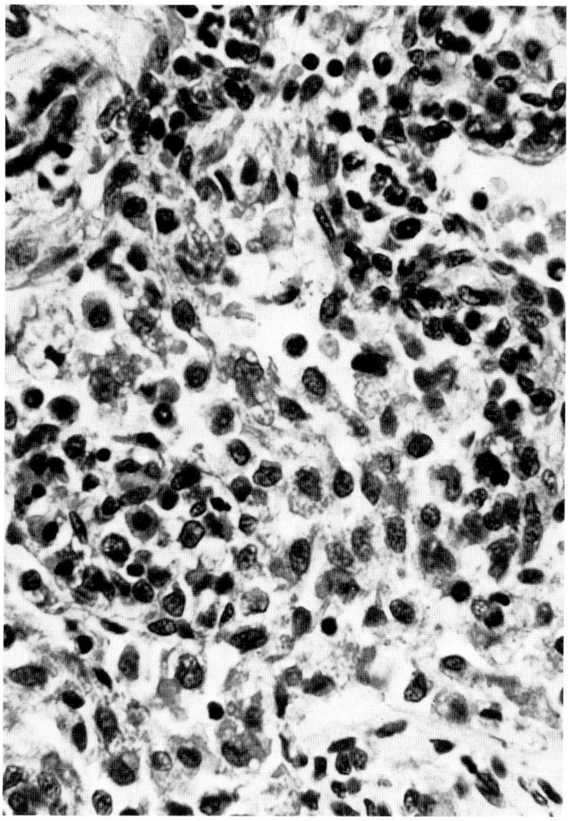

Fig. 12.13. Pigment-containing histiocytes in lymph node. (H and E; 240 ×)

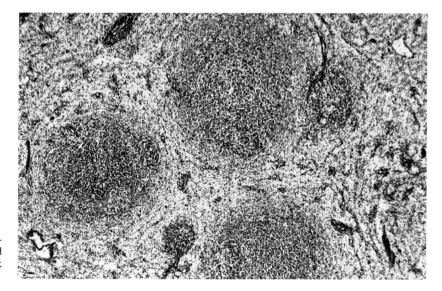

Fig. 12.14. Spleen in chronic granulomatous disease, showing marked sinusoidal hyperplasia. (H and E; 80 ×)

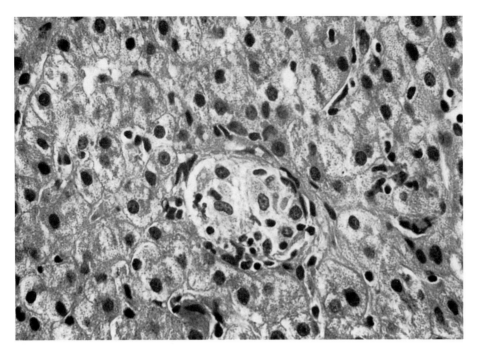

Fig. 12.15. Granuloma in liver parenchyma. (H and E; 240 ×)

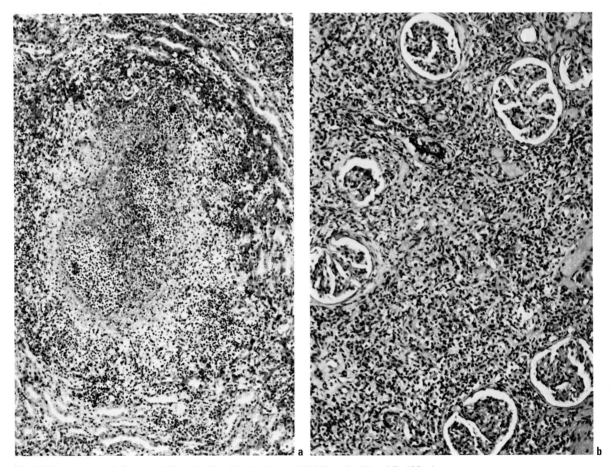

Fig. 12.16. a Intrarenal abscesses. (H and E; 80 ×) **b** Renal interstitial fibrosis. (H and E; 120 ×)

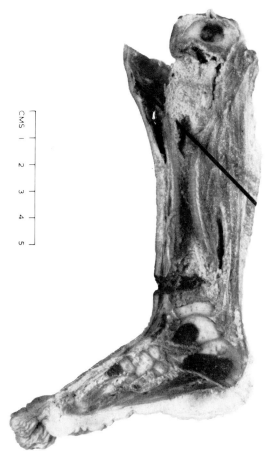

Fig. 12.17. Osteomyelitis with sinus formation and massive bony necrosis in chronic granulomatous disease.

3.10. Ataxia Telangiectasia

There are many distinctive features of ataxia telangiectasia. It is inherited as an autosomal recessive characteristic with multisystem effects including cerebellar ataxia, oculocutaneous telangiectasia, recurrent pulmonary infections, and a variable immunodeficiency state. There may also be café-au-lait spots, vitiligo, and grey hair. Carbohydrate metabolism may be abnormal (for a review see McFarlin et al. 1972). The lung infection occurs intermittently but may be progressively destructive, producing pulmonary crippling. A further long-term risk is the development of neoplasia, mainly lymphomatous but including gastric carcinoma, CNS malignancy, and ovarian tumours (dysgerminoma).

Detailed immunological studies show normal IgG levels, low IgA and E, and abnormal IgM (low molecular weight). The low levels of IgA and E are due to decreased synthesis (Strober et al. 1968). Immune response to test antigens is poor. Cellular immunity is variable, only $15\%–20\%$ of patients responding to common skin test antigens, and there is delayed rejection of skin grafts.

Histopathologically the changes in the lymphoid tissues are those described under thymic dysplasia. Additional lesions include cerebellar atrophy, demyelination of the posterior columns, and anterior horn cell loss. The pathology of the cutaneous lesions (e.g., café-au-lait spots) has no special features. Recently patients with the disease have been shown to have a defect in the repair of DNA and to be extremely sensitive to irradiation. Chromosome breaks are common. These changes may explain why large cells with bizarre nuclei are seen in many organs in this condition. α-Fetoprotein levels are high in most cases (Waldmann and McIntire 1972), and this is considered to be an indicator of a widespread failure of gene regulation. Recently Cox et al. (1978) have suggested that the radiosensitivity of cultured skin fibroblasts be used as a diagnostic test in this condition.

3.11. Chediak–Higashi Syndrome

A rare familial disorder, Chediak–Higashi syndrome involves partial oculocutaneous albinism (blue eyes, decreased retinal pigmentation associated with photophobia) and severe recurrent infections. Hepatosplenomegaly is common, and the disease causes death in infancy or childhood from infection or neoplasia, the oldest reported survivor being 18 years of age (Kritzler et al. 1964). A history of consanguinity is common, and an autosomal recessive mode of inheritance has been proposed.

Pathologically the classic feature of the disease is the presence of massive intracellular inclusions of lysosomal origin. These are 2–4 µm in diameter, and myeloperoxidase- and lysozyme-positive; they occur in leucocytes, renal tubular epithelial cells, gastric mucosa, pancreas, thyroid, melanocytes, and glial cells. The coincidence of enzyme reactivity attributable to more than one type of intracellular inclusion suggests an origin from fused azurophilic and specific granules (Rausch et al. 1978).

Defects of leucocyte function have been described, affecting both their chemotactic response and their bactericidal abilities. The massive inclusions are slow to fuse with phagocytic vacuoles, and this presumably underlies the failure of intracellular bacterial killing.

3.12. Wiscott–Aldrich Syndrome

Wiscott–Aldrich syndrome is inherited as a sex-linked recessive disorder, and is characterized by thrombocytopenic purpura, eczematoid dermatitis, and recurrent infections. The platelets of affected individuals are small and show a failure to aggregate when exposed to ADP, collagen, or epinephrine. Recently Shapiro et al. (1978) have devised a test whereby the carrier state can be detected by assessment of the response of platelets to metabolic stimuli.

Affected individuals may die of infection, haemorrhages or tumours (Table 12.1). The only effective therapeutic measure appears to be bone marrow transplantation (Parkman et al. 1978). Immunoglobulins are present in most cases, but the response to bacterial capsular antigens is poor. Histopathologically there is a varied picture, many cases having relatively normal, although lymphocyte-depleted, thymus and lymph nodes while others are affected by changes resembling those described for thymic dysplasia. The skin lesions are those of a typical eczematous dermatitis.

3.13. Immunodeficiency States Caused by Protein Loss or Acquired Cellular Defects

Protein-losing enteropathy from any cause is often associated with immunoglobulin deficiency. In intestinal lymphangiectasia, injected labelled immunoglobulin has a short half-life owing to excretion via the gut. These patients may have absolute lymphopenia with loss of T cells and failure of cellular immune functions (Strober et al. 1967).

Protein loss in the nephrotic syndrome may lower circulating immunoglobulin levels. Cytotoxic drug therapy may have similar effects, and certainly affects lymphocyte populations.

3.14. Enzyme Defects and Immunodeficiency States

There have been a number of descriptions of specific enzyme defects associated with immune-deficient states. Absence of adenosine deaminase gives rise to the severe combined immune-deficiency syndrome (probably accounting for half of all cases of the non-X-linked form); purine nucleoside phyrophosporylase to a cellular immune deficiency syndrome; absence of transcobalamine II to agammaglobulinaemia; and diminished activity of nucleotidase to hypogamma-globulinaemia. The absence of these various enzymes may lead to damage to stem cells or B cells by accumulation of metabolites, or as in the case of transcolalamine II, to failure of transport of vitamin B_{12} into rapidly growing cells. The subject is extensively reviewed by Hirschhorn and Martin (1978).

3.15. Tumours and Immunodeficiency States

Enhanced tumour susceptibility occurs in a number of syndromes of immune deficiency. The reasons for this are discussed in detail elsewhere (Berry, to be published), and Table 12.1 summarizes reported findings.

Table 12.1. Immune-deficiency syndromes and tumours

Disease	Tumours reported
Ataxia telangiectasia	Leukaemia; lymphomas; carcinoma of stomach, skin, parotid Glioma; medulloblastoma; dysgerminoma
Wiskott–Aldrich syndrome	Leukaemia; lymphomas; astrocytoma; leiomyosarcoma
Congenital agammaglobulinaemia (Bruton type)	Leukaemia; lymphomas
Combined immunity-deficiency syndromes	Leukaemia; lymphoma; carcinoma of stomach, breast, bladder, buccal cavity
Isolated IgA deficiency	Carcinoma of colon, lung, stomach, breast, oesophagus, skin Gliomas
Isolated IgM deficiency	Lymphomas; neuroblastoma

3.16. Infectious Mononucleosis and Duncan's Disease

Infectious mononucleosis has no specific features in childhood, closely resembling the more usual adolescent disease. Death is rare, and is usually attributable to neurological involvement or to rupture of the spleen (Penman 1971). However, in certain sibships an anomalous response to the Epstein–Barr virus (EBV) may result in other changes, which were first described in a family called Duncan (see Purtilo et al. 1977 for review).

In glandular fever EBV infects B lymphocytes. The clinical disease is the manifestation of a 'war between lymphocytes', with T cells attacking and destroying B cells. In Duncan's disease, an abnormality inherited as an X-linked recessive, this war may result in complete destruction of B cells, producing agammaglobulinaemia. Alternatively, malignant transformation of B cells may occur, with the development of a proliferative state such as

Burkitt's lymphoma, plasmacytoma or immuno-blastic sarcoma. This change is presumably due to failure of T cells to control the EBV-containing B cells.

4. Other Diseases of the Thymus

4.1. Neoplasms

Thymic tumours, which are rare in all age groups, are relatively much commoner in adults than in children. In the assessment of previous reports the designation 'malignant thymoma', often the only pathological description, is unhelpful; however, of the three cases aged 15 years or less in the series of 55 cases reported by Friedman (1967), two were benign teratomas and one a malignant teratocarcinoma. In the series of Berg et al. (1968) and Watson et al. (1968), in a total of 59 cases there were three malignant thymomas in individuals less than 15 years of age; these were apparently lymphoepithelial in type. Further confusion with the term 'lymphosarcoma' occurs, owing to the frequent involvement of the thymus in leukaemia. Examination of the tissues of so-called primary lymphosarcomas of the thymus often reveals evidence of leukaemia, and in a series of 49 autopsy cases of lymphoblastic leukaemia examined by one of us, 43 cases showed evidence of infiltration of the thymus. Of 18 thymic tumours in individuals aged 15 years or less seen by the present authors, seven were teratomas (patients' ages 3, 4, 8, and 9 months and 1½, 8 and 14 years). None of these was malignant, and it is generally true that malignancy in this group of teratomas is manifest in the second decade. Nine cases of benign thymoma or thymic hyperplasia were seen; none of these were associated with myasthenia.

One lymphoepithelial thymoma was removed from a boy of 7 years, who was active and well 6 years after resection. A further example, removed when the patient was 4 years old proved rapidly fatal. Lynch (1975) has described a lymphoepithelial tumour associated with myasthenia in a 12-year-old (see p. 514) for an account of myasthenia in childhood).

Cases of thymic tumour with acquired immunoglobulin deficiency (Rubin et al. 1964) have not been recorded in children, and among 94 reported cases of thymic tumour and hypoplasia of the bone marrow, only one was in a child (aged 5 years) (Talerman and Amigo 1968).

4.2. Thymolipoma

Although described as a distinct condition, it seems likely that thymolipoma is a lipoma occurring in the anterior mediastinum. These lesions are rare in infancy, but may be massive in size.

4.3. Germinal Follicles

The appearance of germinal follicles in the thymus has been reported in a number of conditions associated with autoimmunity. In infancy and childhood germinal follicles (two cellular component-reactive follicles) are undoubtedly commoner than in adults (Henry 1968), but criteria of what constitutes a follicle and methods of study, e.g. section frequency, have varied widely, accounting for the enormous range of normal described as 1% (Okabe 1966) or 50% (Middleton 1967).

4.4. Cysts

Dyer (1967) has suggested that a number of anterior mediastinal cysts are of thymic origin. If the term is confined to cysts having their origin in the thymus or its analogue, however, they are apparently rare, and are generally regarded as remnants of the ductus phangiobrachialis. They are often lined with a ciliated or columnar epithelium (Fig. 12.18), but other varieties may be seen. For further discussion see Bieger and McAdams (1966) and Indeglia et al. (1967).

4.5. Respiratory Obstruction

Sealy et al. (1965) described seven patients in whom the thymus apparently compressed the trachea at the thoracic inlet and caused respiratory obstruction.

It seems from their description that some of these cases may be instances of cartilaginous abnormality of the trachea, which was described as 'slit-like' and collapsing in some instances. It is also possible that the compression had affected the viability of the tracheal wall, as has occurred in one case of thymic hyperplasia seen personally.

5. Anatomical Abnormalities of the Spleen

Abnormalities of number and position of spleens are common. Splenunculi are often found in neonatal autopsies (in 10%–15%), and in view of an apparently lower incidence in adult life many presumably involute. There is evidence that they may hypertrophy following splenectomy in adult life, e.g., in myelofibrosis and uncommonly in congenital spherocytic anaemia. Congenital polysplenia, a term used to describe the presence of many splenunculi rather than a single spleen, is associated with malrotation of the gut, congenital anomalies of the

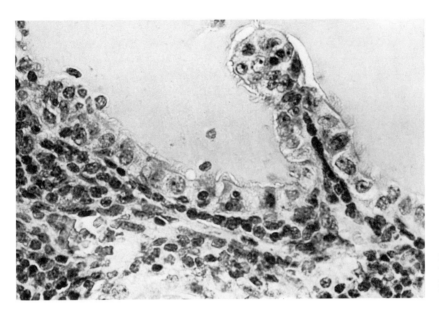

Fig. 12.18. Ciliated epithelium in a thymic cyst 6 cm in diameter, removed surgically from a 5-year-old boy. (H and E; 240 ×)

heart, and the presence of two lobes in each lung.

Absence of the spleen is also invariably associated with other congenital abnormalities, notably of the cardiovascular system (see p. 139), and with various forms of malposition of the viscera.

6. Effects of Splenectomy

Splenectomy may be necessary following trauma, or may be indicated in conditions as diverse as congenital spherocytic anaemia, thrombocytopenic purpura, Gaucher's disease, and thalassaemia. There has been considerable discussion, over a period of 30 years, of the risks attending splenectomy in the young (see Eraklis and Filler 1972). In general it is agreed that septicaemia is commoner in splenectomized patients and that the commonly associated organisms are *Streptococcus pneumoniae* and other encapsulated bacteria (*H. influenzae, N. meningitidis*), and less commonly *E. coli*. Classically an overwhelming infection occurs within 2–3 years of the operation and is associated with a mortality of up to 80%. Although it has been suggested that post-traumatic splenectomy is less likely to be associated with later infection, a recent study by Singer (1973) suggests that this is not so. Because of this a conservative approach to the traumatized spleen is now adopted in some centres (Aronzon et al. 1977).

A more recent problem is infection in young patients splenectomized during staging laparotomy for Hodgkin's disease or other lymphoma. A recent report (Chilcote et al. 1976) documented 20 episodes of meningitis and septicaemia in 18 of 200 children after splenectomy during staging. The pneumococci, streptococci, *H. influenzae* and meningococci were the organisms involved in the 75% of cases in which a diagnosis was made (in 25% the causative organism was not identified).

Sepsis may also occur in congenital asplenia (Kevy et al. 1968).

7. Cysts

Splenic cysts are rare, but McNamara and his colleagues (1968) reported five cases, all in females. They presented between 9 and 15 years of age, with progressive abdominal swelling. Splenectomy revealed pseudocysts (fibrous cavities around areas of presumed necrosis) or epidermoid cysts.

The differential diagnosis includes hydatid disease, lymphangioma and haemangioma (see also Qureshi et al. 1964).

8. Storage Disorders

The diagnosis of storage disorders is described in detail elsewhere. Splenomegaly is a feature of a number of storage disorders, which will be briefly considered here.

8.1. Gaucher's Disease

Gaucher's disease is a disease in which glucocerebrosides accumulate in the histiocytes of the entire reticuloendothelial system. The commonest form is characterized by hepatosplenomegaly, lymphadenopathy, and bone marrow involvement, causing bone pain and various haematological complications including thrombocytopenia, haemolytic anaemia, and neutropenia. The severity of these complications determines the clinical course; the disease is compatible with long life. Macroscopically tissues involved by Gaucher's disease show an irregular pattern of yellowish-white deposits. These may be confluent in the liver, and the bone marrow appears yellowish-white. Gaucher cells are seen in vast numbers in affected tissues; they are typically massive (up to 120 μm), with granular cytoplasm showing a striated or folded pattern. Figures 12.19 and 12.20 show cells from a 9-year-old boy with the disease who died following a tonsillectomy after

haemorrhage associated with thrombocytopenia. The cells are sudanophilic and stain positively with PAS. Electron microscopy shows large inclusions with a single limiting membrane.

Neuropathic Gaucher's disease presents in the first year of life, with failure of neurological development followed by marked regression. Massive hepatosplenomegaly develops and the disease is rapidly fatal. There is no direct cerebral involvement by cerebroside storage, changes in the brain are degenerative and nonspecific.

The two forms of the disease appear to be genetically distinct. The nonneuropathic form only is commoner in Jews.

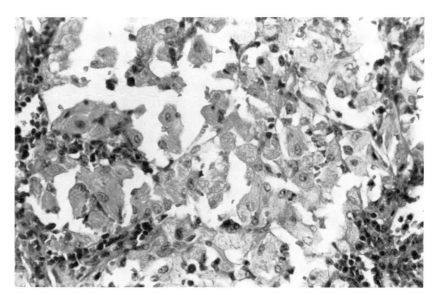

Fig. 12.19. Gaucher cells in spleen, granular cytoplasm. (H and E; 240 ×)

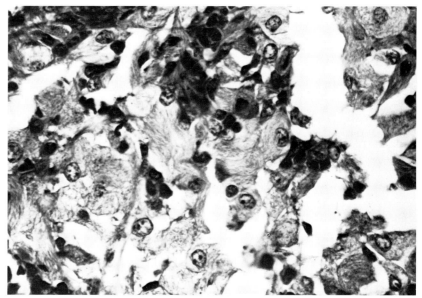

Fig. 12.20. 'Folded' cytoplasmic appearance in Gaucher cells. (Azan stain; 240 ×)

8.2. Niemann–Pick Disease

Niemann–Pick disease also occurs in two forms, and involves sphingomyelin accumulation within the reticuloendothelial system and neurones. In the year of life and include progressive mental and motor retardation, progressive cachexia, and death usually by 2–3 years of age. Massive hepatosplenomegaly occurs, and lymph nodes may enlarge sufficiently to be palpable. In rare cases, neurological involvement is absent and the disease presents later and has a chronic course. An autosomal recessive mode of inheritance seems likely; the infantile form is commoner in Jews.

Macroscopically the brain appears firm and shrunken, while the liver and spleen are hard and uniformly yellowish-white. Reticuloendothelial cell involvement is manifest in the presence of foamy cells up to 80 μm in diameter with a cytoplasm containing multiple small vacuoles, which are sudanophilic and PAS-positive, and in frozen sections fluoresce under ultraviolet light. Electron microscopy shows multilamellate inclusions and some amorphous deposits (see p. 631). Similar cytoplasmic deposits are found in neurones and in the dura.

8.3. Wolman's Disease

Wolman's disease, often diagnosed clinically by the presence of calcification in the adrenals in a child with hepatosplenomegaly and malabsorption, is characterized by the storage of cholesterol esters. Foamy macrophages can be seen in the marrow, spleen, liver, lymph nodes, and lamina propria of the intestine. The central nervous system is not involved (see also p. 619).

9. Histiocytosis X

There have been many disputes and much discussion on whether it is appropriate to consider the disease syndromes generally considered under this heading as part of one disease. The syndromes include Letterer–Siwe disease (disseminated nonlipid histiocytosis). Hand–Schüller–Christian disease, and eosinophilic granuloma of bone. From the pathological viewpoint a unifying concept is attractive, since not only are there histological similarities between the three groups but there is also evidence, from cases with intermediate features, of some structural unity. Lichtenstein also pointed out the virtue of the brevity of the term 'histiocytosis X', compared with the eponyms.

The review of Sims (1977) described 43 cases of histiocytosis X presenting in children under 12 years of age over a 29-year period. Approximately one-third had died, low age at presentation and soft-tissue involvement being associated with a poor prognosis. Of the survivors, about half had residual disability, including diabetes insipidus, pancytopenia, and abnormal lung function tests. Defects of immune function were not found in survivors. Ten of the 29 survivors developed diabetes insipidus, two only temporarily. Histologically, bone lesions often resembled typical eosinophil granuloma (see below) but a 'granulomatous' reaction with varying numbers of histiocytes, eosinophils, plasma cells, lymphocytes, and polymorphs often led to the diagnosis 'compatible with histiocytosis X'. Sims' review emphasizes the heterogeneous nature of this disease, and although pathological findings of typical entities are described below, mixed patterns are commonplace (see also Avery et al. 1957; Newton and Homoudi 1973).

9.1. Aetiology

Pentalaminar cytoplasmic inclusions (Shamoto 1970) have been seen in the cytoplasm of histiocytes from cases of all three types of histiocytosis X, but are probably a non-specific finding (Basset et al. 1972). Surface receptors of IgG and receptors for immune complexes (C_3) are present on the histiocytes of the lesions (Nézelof et al. 1977), confirming that the neoplastic cells are of mononuclear phagocyte origin. Atypical response to infection, graft-versus-host disease, and metabolic abnormalities have all been suggested as the predisposing factor for generation of the granulomatous proliferation that characterizes histiocytosis X, but there is no real evidence to support any hypothesis.

9.2. Letterer–Siwe Disease

Letterer–Siwe disease presents in infancy with generalized symptoms including fever, irritability, and anorexia. Lymphadenopathy and hepatosplenomegaly develop, together with a curious scaly papular dermatitis affecting the scalp and trunk, which may be haemorrhagic (Figs. 12.21 and 12.22). At autopsy, liver, spleen, and lymph nodes are enlarged and firm and their cut surfaces appear irregularly speckled with greyish dots. Histologically the structure of the organs is disturbed by a proliferation of well-defined histiocytes with ample cytoplasm and typical reniform nuclei and neucleoli. Cellular atypia is uncommon, but cells with two or three nuclei are not. These cells are associated with lymphocytes, other mononuclears and some eosinophils in the cellular infiltrate (Fig. 12.23). A similar cellular infiltration may affect the lung in a very diffuse distribution.

9.3. Hand–Schüller–Christian Disease

Hand–Schüller–Christian disease is typically characterized by multiple lytic lesions in bone and the syndrome of dwarfism, diabetes insipidus, and exophthalmos, a collection of symptoms and signs that is uncommonly seen. Systemic involvement is common and may present as hepatosplenomegaly, lymphadenopathy, or honeycomb lung; pancytopenia develops when marrow involvement is severe.

Microscopically the typical lesion is composed of a granulomatous cellular mass, with many histiocytes and eosinophils. Multinucleate forms are common and lipid accumulates in these cells and in histiocytes. This cellular infiltrate may be found microscopically in many organs, including the skin. Involvement of the ear is common and in our experience a common presentation is of a nonresolving middle ear infection and an excoriated external auditory meatus, associated with X-ray appearances showing temporal bone destruction (see also p. 481).

9.4. Eosinophil Granuloma

Eosinophil granulomas typically occur as solitary lesions in bones, usually flat bones, although the authors have seen examples in the thyroid and lung. The skull, the ribs, or the vertebrae are commonly involved, and lesions are occasionally multiple. X-ray appearances suggest a circumscribed lesion, although a distinct margin may not always be evident. Pathologically the lesions are pinkish-grey

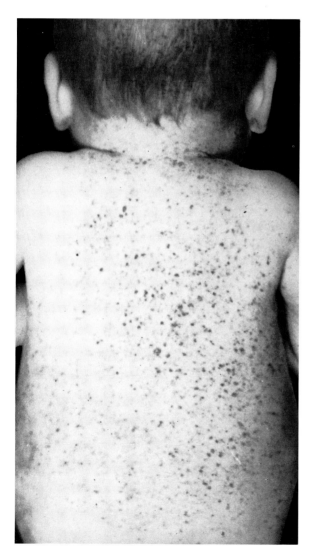

Fig. 12.21. Rash in typical distribution of Letterer–Siwe disease. Notice abdominal swelling owing to hepatosplenomegaly.

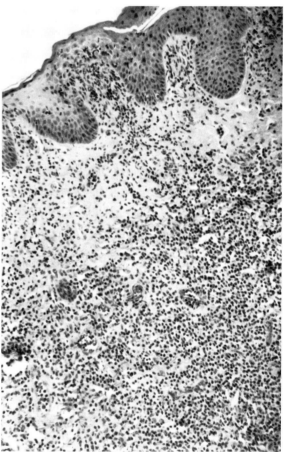

Fig. 12.22. Skin biopsy. The infiltrate is seen in the upper dermis. (H and E; 120 ×)

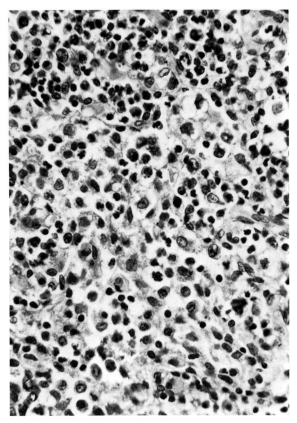

Fig. 12.23. Pleomorphic infiltrate including histiocytes, lymphocytes, occasional polymorphs and eosinophils. Lymph node. (H and E; 180 ×)

or grey, variable in texture, and occasionally gritty due to reactive new bone formation or healing of a fracture. Masses of histiocytes with variable numbers of eosinophils are seen microscopically; giant cells are common. Foam cells and cells containing haemosiderin pigment may also be present (see also p. 480).

10. Leukaemia

Although leukaemia is the commonest neoplastic disease of infancy and childhood, detailed consideration of this group of disease is not appropriate here, being dealt with in specialist texts (see Willoughby 1977).

Acute lymphoblastic leukaemia (ALL) is the commonest form of the disease in childhood, and is itself a mixture of cases of T cell ALL, B cell ALL, common ALL and null-ALL, T cell lesions having the worst prognosis. A large mediastinal mass visible on X-ray is an ominous prognostic sign in all forms. Customarily undifferentiated stem cell leukaemia is included in this group in most series. Acute myeloblastic and monocytic leukaemias are less common

but still more frequently found than chronic myeloid leukaemia (CML), which accounts for less than 2% of all cases.

CML is seen in two forms, a juvenile, rapidly progressive type, with infection, skin lesions, white cell counts of less than 100 000 mm³, and absence of the Philadelphia chromosome as features, and a more typical adult form with gradual onset, higher white cell counts, and the presence of the Philadelphia chromosome.

There is an increased incidence of both forms of acute leukaemia in children with Down's syndrome. The ratio of ALL to AML is the same as in other children (Rosner et al. 1972). The view often expressed that AML is more frequently seen in these children is probably due to the facility with which they mount leukaemoid reactions.

Histopathological findings are similar in many types of leukaemia. In autopsied cases there may be evidence of local (often necrotizing) infections, including stomatitis, and haemorrhage. Moderate hepatosplenomegaly is usual, and lymph node enlargement may be found. The bone marrow is fleshy and pink and may closely resemble the homogeneous, usually darker red, splenic pulp. The liver is uniformly enlarged but the cut surface may appear normal. Diffuse renal involvement is also common, with often massive enlargement of the kidneys. Focal deposits are sometimes found. Gonadal involvement is common, and the gonads seem to be an important site from which recurrences may begin, as is the central nervous system. Leukaemic masses may be seen in the retina with the ophthalmoscope; meningeal and perivascular intracerebral cuffing with leukaemic cells are all commonly found. Changes in an untreated case of ALL in a case of Down's syndrome are seen in Figs. 12.24–12.27.

Therapy produces important modifications of the histopathological findings. Leukaemic cells may almost disappear, the marrow may become hypoplastic, and drug-associated changes may be seen in a number of tissues (Fig. 12.28).

11. Malignant Lymphomas

Lymphomas are now divided into a large number of different categories and according to several different classifications. The classification of lymphomas is a problem for most pathologists. A battery of investigative methods is available for their differentiation, including immunological, cytochemical, histochemical, and ultrastructural studies. The reader is referred to the book by Lennert (1978) for more detailed descriptions. The most important points are outlined below.

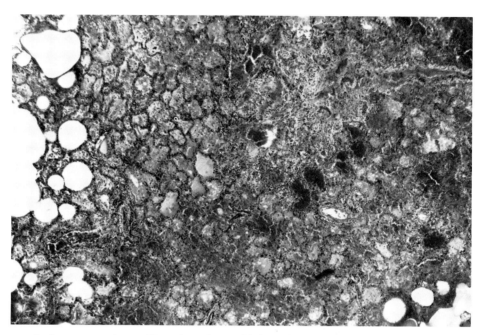

Fig. 12.24. Necrotizing pneumonia, from untreated case of Down's syndrome with ALL. (H and E; 60 ×)

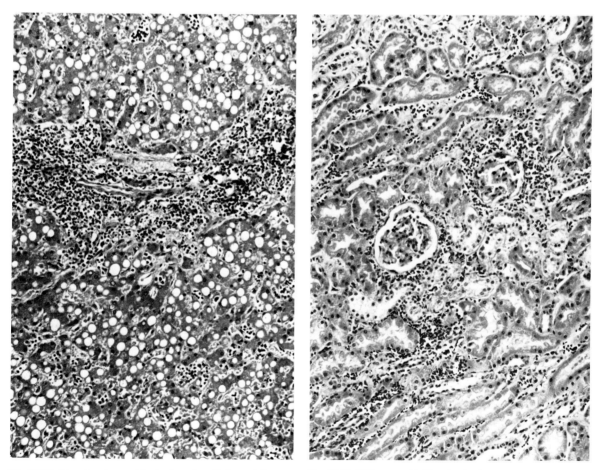

Fig. 12.25. Liver involvement by leukaemic cells in portal tracts (same case as in Fig. 12.24). (H and E; 120 ×)

Fig. 12.26. Diffuse renal infiltration in the same case as illustrated in Figs. 12.24 and 12.25. (H and E; 120 ×)

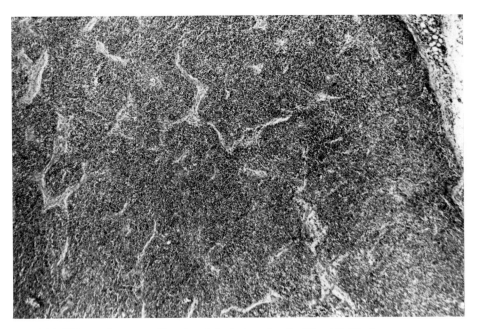

Fig. 12.27. Diffuse replacement of lymph node by leukaemic cells. (H and E; 60 ×)

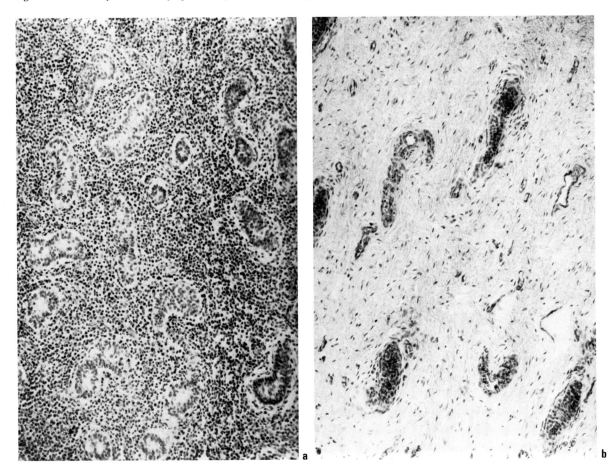

Fig. 12.28. a Testis showing marked interstitial infiltration by leukaemic cells. (H and E; 120 ×) **b** Testis after combination chemotherapy. The gonads had been diffusely enlarged before treatment. Interstitial fibrosis replaces the cellular infiltrate. (H and E; 120 ×)

11.1. Classification

The classification of non-Hodgkin malignant lymphomas is currently in a state of flux. It is not proposed to give details of each classification that has been suggested over recent years. The reader is referred to individual authors (e.g., Rappaport 1966; Lukes and Collins 1974; Dorfman 1974; Bennett et al. 1974; Lennert et al. 1975a and b).

The Kiel classification (as presented by Gerard-Merchant et al. [1974] and modified by Lennert [1978]) will be used in the descriptions below. The main categories of lymphoma in this classification are shown in Table 12.2. Many of these types of lymphoma are either not seen in childhood or are excessively rare. The majority of childhood lymphomas are of high-grade malignancy. Lennert (1978) describes the low-grade tumours that very occasionally occur in childhood.

Modern ideas about the classification of lymphomas centre around the concept of the 'follicle centre cells'. Camera lucida studies were used by Lukes and Collins (see for example, Lukes and Collins 1975) to differentiate the types of cell present in lymphomas on the basis of their similarity to the cells present in normal germinal centres. These follicle centre cells (FCC) are divided into cleaved and noncleaved types. The former are small to medium-sized, having a notch or indentation in the nucleus, and are referred to as centrocytes by Lennert (see Lennert 1978). The noncleaved cells are medium or large in size and have round or oval nuclei with several prominent nucleoli, which are usually close to the nuclear membrane. They are called centroblasts by Lennert. The reader wishing to familiarize himself with this concept should refer to Lukes and Collins (1975) or the first section of the book by Lennert (1978).

11.2. Investigation

Biopsied lymph nodes should ideally be received in the laboratory in the fresh state to enable imprint preparations, histochemistry and other methods to be used. Some of the applicable techniques with discriminatory functions are listed below with the tissues and preparations on which their use is appropriate.

PAS reaction with diastase	Sections and imprints Diastase-sentitive (juvenile rhabdomyosarcoma, Ewing's sarcoma, lymphoblastic lymphoma [rarely]) Diastase-insensitive (immunoglobulin-producing cells, mast cells)
Chloracetate esterase	Sections and imprints (myeloid and monocytic leukaemia, mast cells)

Table 12.2. Classification systems for malignant lymphomas

Kiel classification of ML (Lennert 1978)		Rappaport (1966)[a]		Lukes and Collins (1975)
Low-grade malignancy				
ML lymphocytic		ML lymphocytic, WD, D		Small lymphocyte
ML lymphoplasmacytic/lymphoplasmacytoid		ML lymphocytic, with plasmacytoid features		Plasmacytoid lymphocyte
ML plasmacytic				
ML centrocytic		ML WD and PD, N or D		FCC, cleaved
ML centroblastic-centrocytic:	Follicular	ML lymphocytic, WD		
	Follicular and diffuse	ML lymphocytic, PD	N or D	FCC large and small, cleaved and noncleaved, follicular or diffuse
	Diffuse	ML lymphocytic/histiocytic		
		ML histiocytic		
High-grade malignancy				
ML centroblastic		ML histiocytic ML undifferentiated	N or D	
ML lymphoblastic		ML undifferentiated, D ML lymphocytic, PD, D		
ML immunoblastic		ML histiocytic, D		

[a]WD, well differentiated; PD poorly differentiated; N, nodules; D, diffuse.

Acid phosphatase | Imprints Tartrate-sensitive (monocytes, lymphoblastic lymphoma, convoluted cell type)

α-Naphthylacetate esterase | Imprints (monocytic leukaemia, true histiocytic malignancy)

Immunological methods of examination to differentiate T and B cells are well described (e.g., Raff 1970; Bianco et al. 1970; Jondal et al 1972; Coombs et al. 1970).

The markers for B cells include:
a) Surface immunoglobulin (immunofluorescence or immunoperoxidase methods)
b) Cytoplasmic immunoglobulin, in secretory B cells (immunofluorescence)
c) Complement receptor, demonstrated by EAC (erythrocyte-antibody-complement) rosette formation
d) IgG-Fc receptor (antibody opsonic adherence), which is also present on activated T cells and is demonstrated by a rosette-forming reaction
e) Formation of rosettes with mouse red cells.

Spontaneous rosette formation by human lymphocytes with sheep red cells is a marker for T cells.

11.3. Lymphoblastic ML

Lymphoblastic MLs comprise a group in which the malignant cells are small to medium-sized blast cells having round nuclei and some basophilic cytoplasm.

They are subdivided as follows:
1) ML lymphoblastic, Burkitt type
2) ML lymphoblastic, convoluted cell type
3) ML lymphoblastic, unclassified.

All three subtypes occur frequently in childhood.

11.4. Lymphoblastic ML, Burkitt-type (Burkitt's lymphoma)

The occurrence of ML characterized by tumours of the jaw or orbit or by enlargement of abdominal lymph nodes was first described in African children by Burkitt (1958/59). Morphological studies of this lymphoma were performed by O'Connor (1961) and Wright (1963). Similar tumours were soon found in many different parts of the world, for example, an American variant described by Dorfman (1965). A World Health Organization booklet gives a histo-pathological definition of Burkitt's lymphoma and contains excellent colour photographs (Berard et al. 1969).

A virus of the herpes group (Epstein–Barr Virus, EBV) was identified in cell cultures of Burkitt's lymphoma cells (Epstein et al. 1964) and a number of EBV-specific antigens have now been demonstrated (e.g., Klein 1975). The EBV can be demonstrated in practically all cases of Burkitt's lymphoma (97% according to Klein 1975), whereas only a small percentage of cases of morphologically similar cases from other parts of the world contain EBV. It thus seems likely that although the histological appearances of this type of lymphoblastic lymphoma are similar, the aetiology may be different in different parts of the world. It is for this reason that the tumour is classified as ML lymphoblastic, Burkitt-type, rather than Burkitt's lymphoma, the latter title being strictly applicable only to EBV-associated cases.

Clinical features. Boys are affected two or three times more frequently than girls (Burkitt 1970a; Levine et al. 1975; Lennert 1978). The age distribution shows a peak at 4–7 years in Africa according to Burkitt (1970a), and involvement over the age of 14 years is rare. The available data for American and European series show a similar predominance of cases in the first decade, but Burkitt-type lymphoblastic lymphoma also occurs in adult life in these parts of the world (Levine et al. 1975; Banks et al. 1975; Lennert 1978).

Tumours of the jaw are present in over half the African cases, while abdominal masses (25%) and ovarian tumours (30% of girls) are also frequent (Wright 1970; Burkitt 1970b). Lymph node involvement was found at autopsy in 69% of affected children (Wright 1970). Co-existent lymphoblastic leukaemia (see below) in African Burkitt's lymphoma is rare. Peripheral lymph node involvement is rare at the outset in African cases (Wright 1970; Burkitt 1970). Lymphoblastic lymphoma of Burkitt type occurring in Continental Europe involved mainly cervical, then abdominal lymph nodes according to Lennert (1978), whereas abdominal involvement was a prominent feature in the series described by Banks et al. (1975) in the United States.

Histological features. Burkitt's lymphoma is lymphoblastic in type, being made up of medium-sized lymphoid cells with uniform nuclei showing a coarse chromatin pattern and several prominent nucleoli. Mitoses are frequent. Almost invariably there are macrophages with abundant clear cytoplasm, containing cellular debris or intact tumour cells scattered throughout the tumour (Fig. 12.29). These give rise to the typical 'starry-sky' appearance on low-power microscopy (Fig. 12.30).

The appearance of ML lymphoblastic, Burkitt-type in imprint preparations and in histochemical

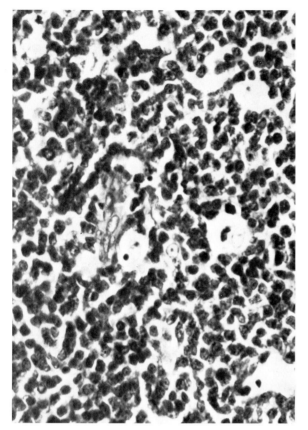

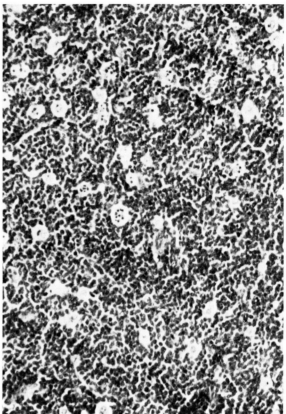

Fig. 12.29. Malignant lymphoma lymphoblastic, Burkitt type. Section of cervical lymph node showing macrophages with clear cytoplasm containing cellular debris. The surrounding lympho-blastic tumour cells show uniform nuclei with nucleoli that are mostly centrally placed. (H and E; 1000 ×)

Fig. 12.30. Malignant lymphoma lymphoblastic Burkitt type. Low-power view showing starry-sky appearance; the mac-rophages contain cellular debris. Cervical lymph node. (H and E; 400 ×)

and electron microscopical studies are well described in the WHO booklet (Berard et al. 1969) and by Lennert (1978). Briefly, the tumour cells contain sudanophilic granules and there are large amounts of neutral fat in the starry-sky macrophages. Alkaline phosphatase and nonspecific esterase are absent from the tumour cells but present in the macrophages.

Although bone marrow involvement is usually considered to occur late, Brunning et al. (1977) have recently described eleven cases who had bone marrow replacement at the onset of their disease. All had a rapid clinical course despite chemotherapy. None was frankly leukaemic.

Differential diagnosis. While a large number of undifferentiated malignant neoplasms may oc-casionally cause problems, the chief difficulties arise with respect to acute lymphoblastic leukaemia, acute myeloblastic leukaemia, and undifferentiated malig-nant lymphomas. The different features of these neoplasms are discussed in the WHO publication (Berard et al. 1969).

11.5. Lymphoblastic ML, Convoluted-cell Type

An ill-defined group of mediastinal sarcomas with associated leukaemia in children was frequently described in the past as Sternberg sarcoma, follow-ing an original description by Sternberg (1908).

More recently a definite entity has become recognized by Lukes and Lennert and their col-leagues (Barcos and Lukes 1975; Lennert et al. 1975b). This lymphoblastic ML of convoluted-cell type is relatively rare.

Clinical features. The presence of a large media-stinal mass (in over 80 % of patients) is the main clinical feature of this type of lymphoma (Lennert 1978). Males are affected about twice as often as females and the peak incidence is between 10 and 15 years of age (Barcos and Lukes 1975; Lennert 1978). There may in addition be peripheral lymph node involvement and a leukaemic blood picture. Bone marrow infiltration usually occurs only late in the course of the disease.

Histological features. The mediastinal mass and replaced lymph nodes comprise a diffuse infiltrate of small to medium-sized lymphoid cells having round or oval nuclei, small nucleoli, and a thin rim of basophilic cytoplasm. Intermingled with these cells are others, which are large and have large nuclei and prominent nucleoli. The diagnostic convoluted cell of this tumour is present only in small numbers. It is larger than most of the other cells and has irregularly shaped nuclei, which may have knob-like projections or appear gyrate in outline (Fig. 12.31). Linear subdivisions across the nucleus give a 'chicken-foot' appearance, as described by Lukes and Collins (1975). Mitoses are frequent.

Imprint preparations show a predominance of small cells, but marked variation of cell size and the presence of large cells with convoluted nuclei.

One of the chief diagnostic features of this type of malignant lymphoma is found on histochemical examination of imprints and frozen sections. Strong focal tartrate-sensitive acid phosphatase activity is present in the paranuclear region of the smaller

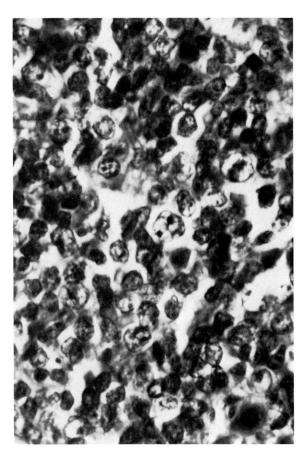

Fig. 12.31. Malignant lymphoma lymphoblastic, convoluted-cell type. Section showing the presence of two larger cells with lobes or gyrate nuclei. Cervical lymph node from 20-year-old male who also had a large mediastinal mass. (H and E; 1750 ×)

tumour cells and can be demonstrated by electron microscopy to be localized in the Golgi apparatus (Catovsky et al. 1975). The large convoluted cells do not show the presence of acid phosphatase reaction product. The tumour cells are also positive by acid nonspecific esterase and β-glucuronidase staining methods, but are negative by other enzyme histochemical methods.

The frequency of thymic involvement, the presence of acid phosphatase activity in tumour cells resembling that of thymocytes, and the formation of sheep red cell rosettes by the tumour cell are all strong evidence that this is a T cell ML (see Catovsky 1975; Ritter et al. 1975).

11.6. Lymphoblastic ML, Unclassified

Lymphoblastic lymphomas that cannot be diagnosed with certainty as belonging to one of the above two groups may be designated as 'unclassified'. It may be in some cases that they are unclassifiable, while insufficient material may be available in others. As with the other two types of lymphoblastic lymphoma, most cases occur in childhood and adolescence. Males are affected about twice as frequently as females.

Clinical features. The main clinical presentation is of lymph node enlargement. This may be accompanied by leukaemia.

Histological features. The lymph nodes are replaced by medium-sized lymphoid cells with several prominent nucleoli in nuclei having a fine chromatin pattern (Fig. 12.32). Mitoses are frequent. Special studies fail to show acid phosphatase, nonspecific esterase, peroxidase, or chloroacetate esterase. The PAS reaction is negative in paraffin sections, but may show granular positivity in imprints.

The problems of differentiation from other childhood tumours and from other types of lymphoma need to be considered, e.g., metastatic neuroblastoma, juvenile rhabdomyosarcoma, and Ewing's sarcoma.

11.7. Centroblastic ML

A diffuse malignant lymphoma in which there is a large proportion of centroblasts (noncleaved FCC) present is recognized by Lukes and Collins (1975) and by the German group (Lennert et al. 1975b). Lennert subdivides centroblastic lymphomas into primary and secondary types, depending on whether there has been previous evidence of a centroblastic/centrocytic ML (follicular lymphoma) in the same patient. According to him, primary centroblastic lymphoma occurs at all ages, including childhood, and may have a nodular or diffuse pattern. The present author has some difficulty separating a diffuse lymphoblastic lymphoma (undifferentiated) from a diffuse centroblastic lymphoma. Lennert (1978) states that centroblastic/centrocytic lymphoma does not occur below the age of 20 years. There are several references in the literature to follicular (or nodular) lymphoma in childhood (e.g., Symmers 1948; Jones et al. 1973; Pinkel et al. 1975; Wollner et al. 1975; Murphy et al. 1975). Follicular lymphoma in childhood is certainly very rare, and when this diagnosis is contemplated the possibility that the lymph node is showing florid reactive hyperplasia should be seriously considered.

11.8. Immunoblastic ML

Lymphomas comprised of large undifferentiated cells were formerly classified as reticulum-cell sarcoma or histiocytic malignant lymphoma. Some of these tumours have now been shown to have B- or T-cell characteristics, either by immunological or by enzyme cytochemical methods. There undoubtedly does exist a group of tumours that show no such markers, and these may be either so poorly differentiated as to not possess particular markers, or be derived from nonlymphocyte precursors.

Immunoblastic malignant lymphoma (immunoblastic sarcoma) does occur in childhood and adolescence, although this is rare (Jones et al. 1973; Murphy et al. 1975; Lennert 1978). Males are affected up to three times more often than females. The histological appearances in the replaced lymph node or other organ comprise diffuse sheets of large cells having oval or round nuclei with one or more prominent nucleoli. The cytological features, including the prominence of nucleoli, are apparent in imprint preparations. The chief problems in differentiation are from other undifferentiated childhood neoplasms, Hodgkin's disease, and true histiocytic malignancies.

11.9. True Histiocytic Malignancy

Some difficulties arise over the use of the term 'histiocytic' in relation to lymphoreticular neoplasms. Rappaport (1966) distinguished lymphocytic, mixed lymphocytic–histiocytic, and undifferentiated lymphomas. Most of these types would not be classified as containing histiocytes in the more recent views of Lukes and Collins (1975) and the Kiel classification (Gerard-Marchant et al. 1974; Lennert 1978) (see Table 12.2).

However, there is undoubtedly a group of disorders in which there is neoplastic proliferation of true histiocytes. They have been reviewed recently by Cline and Golde (1973). Included are such processes as histiocytic medullary reticulosis (Robb-Smith 1938; Scott and Robb-Smith 1939; Marshall 1956), which is part of the malignant histiocytosis group of the American literature (e.g., Rappaport 1966; Huhn and Meister 1978). Although these are mostly disorders of adults, Lennert (1978) describes a condition confined almost exclusively to children as *sarcoma of histiocytic reticulum cells*, which apparently falls within the broad category of malignant histiocytosis. According to Lennert, there is complete replacement of the lymph node by medium-sized to large cells having abundant cytoplasm, round or oval nuclei, and central neucleoli (Fig. 12.33). Variable numbers of binucleate and multinucleate giant cells are present. Mitoses are frequent. Smaller macrophages are interspersed with these tumour cells. Erythrophagocytosis and leucophagocytosis may be present and are best recognized in imprint preparations (Fig. 12.34). Nonspecific esterase is demonstrable in the tumour cells.

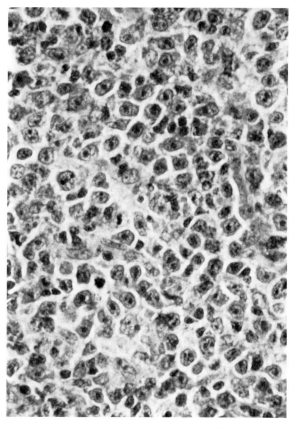

Fig. 12.32. Malignant lymphoma lymphoblastic, unclassified. Section showing medium-sized tumour cells having one or two prominent nucleoli. Cervical lymph node. (Giemsa; 1000 ×)

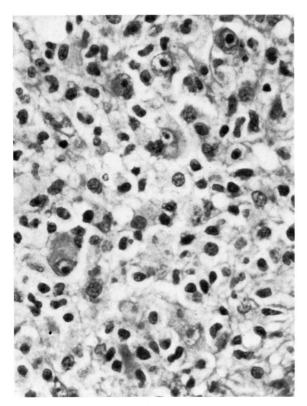

Fig. 12.33. Malignant histiocytosis. Section of lymph node showing tumour cells with abundant cytoplasm and prominent nucleoli. Interspersed are smaller macrophages. (H and E; 1000 ×)

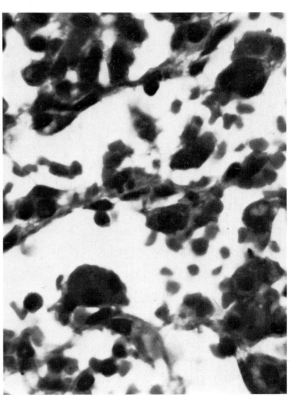

Fig. 12.35. Familial erythrophagocytic lymphohistiocytosis. Section of cervical lymph node of a 10-week-old infant, showing infiltration of the sinuses by histiocytic tumour cells, some of which are binucleate. Note erythrophagocytosis by cells (*bottom left*). Post-mortem revealed histiocytic infiltration of liver, lymph nodes, bone marrow, and spleen. (H and E; 1400 ×)

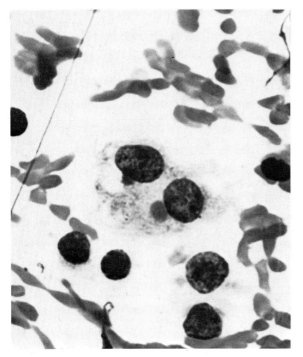

Fig. 12.34. Malignant histiocytosis. Imprint preparation, showing erythrophagocytosis in a binucleate tumour cell. (Leishman; 3000 ×)

11.10. Familial Erythrophagocytic Lymphohistiocytosis

The unusual syndrome of familial erythrophagocytic lymphohistiosis has been described in over 20 families and has recently been reviewed by Perry et al. (1976). Briefly, the age of onset is from 2 weeks to 7 years, and the diseases mostly affect infants. Neither sex predominates and an autosomal recessive inheritance has been suggested. The clinical onset is nonspecific with failure to thrive, pallor, anorexia, and diarrhoea as common features. All affected children have had pyrexia and hepatosplenomegaly at or about the time of onset. Anaemia and progressively deepening jaundice occur, together with bleeding into the skin, gastrointestinal tract, and brain. Patients have usually died with bleeding, sepsis, or development of a lymphocytic meningitis. The pathological features are a diffuse histiocytic infiltration of the liver, spleen, lymph nodes (Fig. 12.35), bone marrow, lungs, gastrointestinal tract, genitourinary tract, and central nervous system. Erythrophagocytosis is often a marked feature, and there are usually lymphocytes intermingled with the histiocytic infiltrate. The disorder has some resemblance to histiocytic medullary reticulosis, but this affects mainly adults and is not familial (apart from one report of an affected father and son by Boake et al. 1965). The histiocytes in familial erythrophagocytic lymphohistiocytosis do not show the marked cellular atypia seen in most cases of malignant histiocytosis (histiocytic medullary reticulosis). Recent investigations have shown the presence of a primary immunological deficiency in patients with familial erythrophagocytic lymphohistiocytosis (Barth et al. 1972; Ladisch et al. 1978).

11.11. Hodgkin's Disease

Hodgkin's disease occurs in childhood, although it is not common. The age range varies from 2½ or 3 years to 15 years in various published series (e.g., Pitcock et al. 1954; Kelly 1965; Franssilla et al. 1967; Jenkin et al. 1967; Keller et al. 1968; Norris et al. 1975; Kolygin 1976). Appearances suggesting Hodgkin's disease in an infant should give rise to the suspicion

of Letterer–Siwe disease. Males are affected one-and-a-half times to twice as often as females in most series, although MacMahon (1966) found 85% of cases in children under age 10 years were males on reviewing over 100 cases in the literature.

Hodgkin's disease is classified according to the Rye Classification (Lukes et al. 1968) into lymphocyte predominant, nodular sclerosis, mixed-cellularity and lymphocyte-depleted types (Figs. 12.36 and 12.37). Details need not be given here and are available in the published proceedings of an American symposium (Lukes and Butler 1966; Rappaport 1966), the book by Kaplan (1972), and standard textbooks of adult histopathology. They are briefly summarized in Table 12.3.

The incidence of these particular histological types in childhood varies in different series. The results of two recent studies are summarized in Table 12.4. Lymphocyte-depleted disease has a low incidence or does not occur in most series (Franssilla et al. 1967; Keller et al. 1968; Aghai et al. 1975; Norris et al. 1975), but is reported by Kolygin (1976). Keller and his colleagues (1968) found mixed cellularity to be most common in the first decade. Nodular sclerosis and lymphocyte predominance were about equal in frequency. In the second decade, they found nodular sclerosis to be much more

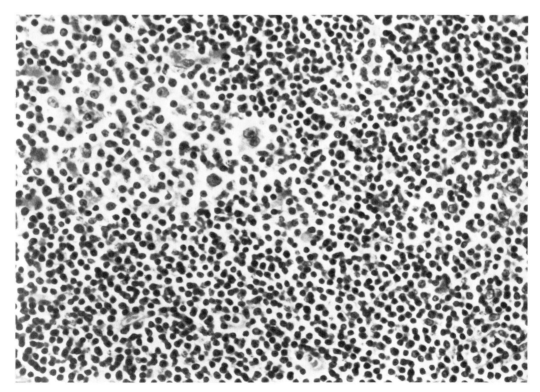

Fig. 12.36. Lymphocyte-predominant Hodgkin's disease. Section of cervical lymph node showing the presence of occasional Hodgkin's cells and a binucleate Reed–Sternberg cell. (H and E; 400 ×)

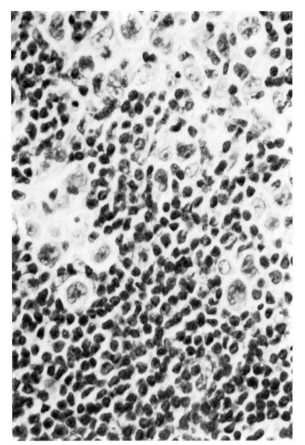

Table 12.4. Incidence of different histological types of Hodgkin's disease in childhood, expressed as percentages

	Total no. of cases	Type of Hodgkin's disease			
		LP	NS	MC	D
Norris et al. (1975)	116	19	58	21	33
Kolygin (1978)	45	29	13	38	20

common, then mixed cellularity, which was in turn more frequent than lymphocyte predominance. Hodgkin's disease was found to be more frequent in the second decade by Franssilla et al. (1967), and the nodular sclerosis group predominated.

Childhood Hodgkin's disease most often presents as lymphadenopathy, which is usually cervical or supraclavicular. Mediastinal involvement is sometimes found in addition (e.g., Kelly 1965; Jenkin et al. 1967). Kelly reported generalized disease to be present in 33 % of cases at presentation, while Jenkin and colleagues found 28 % of their cases had clinical stage III or IV disease.

Fig. 12.37. Hodgkin's disease in the spleen of a 14-year-old girl with a nodular sclerosing pattern in her lymph nodes, showing the presence of Reed–Sternberg and multinucleate tumour cells. (H and E; 600 ×)

Table 12.3. Rye classification of Hodgkin's disease

1.	*Lymphocyte predominance:* (LP)	a)	Lymphocyte (or histiocyte) dominant
		b)	Reed–Sternberg cells seldom numerous
		c)	Eosinophils, neutrophils, plasma cells, sparse or absent
		d)	Little or no fibrosis
2.	*Nodular sclerosis:* (NS)	a)	Collagenous bands separating nodules of lymphoid tissue
		b)	Reed–Sternberg and other large 'Hodgkin's' cells fairly frequent. NB: Lacunar cells formerly said to be specific, occur in other types
		c)	Lymphocytic or mixed infiltrate (lymphocytes, neutrophils, eosinophils, histiocytes)
		d)	May have necrosis
3.	*Mixed-cellularity:* (MC)	a)	Highly cellular with mixed infiltrate of lymphocytes, histiocytes, neutrophils, eosinophils, plasma cells and fibroblasts
		b)	Reed–Sternberg cells and other large malignant cells readily detectable
		c)	Varying degrees of fibrosis but *no collagen*
		d)	May have focal necrosis
4.	*Lymphocyte depletion:* (LD)	a)	Reticular or diffuse fibrosis type
		b)	Numerous Reed–Sternberg and large pleomorphic cells (may be more difficult to discover in fibrosing type)
		c)	Commonly, areas of necrosis

References

Adinolfi M (1972) Ontogeny of components of complement (C'_4 and C'_3) in human fetal and new born sera. Dev Med Child Neurol 12: 306

Adinolfi M (1974) Development of lymphoid tissues and immunity. In: Davis JA, Dobbing J (eds) Scientific foundations of paediatrics. Heinemann, London, p 333

Aghai E, Brenner H, Ramot B (1975) Childhood Hodgkin's disease in Israel. Cancer 36: 2138

Aldrich RA, Steinberg AG, Campbell DC (1954) Pedigree demonstrating a sex-linked recessive condition characterized by draining ears, eczematoid dermatitis and blood diarrhoea. Pediatrics 13: 133

Aronzon DZ, Arnold WS, Arnold HE, Jerrald MB, Schneider TM (1977) Non-operative management of splenic trauma in children: A report of 6 consecutive cases. Pediatrics 60: 482

Avery ME, McAgee JG, Guild HG (1957) The course and prognosis of reticuloendotheliosis (eosinophilic granuloma, Schüller–Christian disease and Letterer–Siwe disease) a study of forty cases. Am J Med 22: 636

Babior B (1978) Oxygen-dependent microbial killing by phagocytes. N Engl J Med 298: 721

Banatavala JE, Potter JE, Best JM (1971) Interferon response to Sendai and Rubella viruses in human foetal cultures, leucocytes and placenta cultures. J Gen Virol 13: 193

Banks PM, Arsenau JC, Gralnick HR, Canellos GP, DeVita VT, Berard CW (1975) American Burkitt's lymphoma: A clinicopathologic study of 30 cases. Am J Med 58: 322

Barcos MP, Lukes RJ (1975) Malignant lymphoma of convoluted lymphocytes: A new entity of possible T-cell type. In: Skinks LF, Godden JO (eds) Conflicts in childhood cancer. An evaluation of current management, vol 4. Liss, New York, p 147

Barth RF, Vergara GG, Khurana SK, Lowman JT, Beckwith JB (1972) Rapidly fatal familial histiocytosis associated with eosinophilia and primary immunological deficiency. Lancet 2: 503

Basset F, Escaig J, Le Crom M (1972) A cytoplasmic membranous complex in histiocytosis X. Cancer 29: 1380

Bennett MH, Farrer-Brown G, Henry K, Jelliffe AM (1974) Classification of non-Hodgkin's lymphomas. (Letter to the Editor). Lancet 2: 405

Berard C, O'Connor GT, Thomas LB, Thorloni H (1969) Histopathological definition of Burkitt's tumour (18 signatories). Bull WHO 40: 601

Berg NP, Rosengren B, Seeman T (1968) Treatment of tumours of the thymus. Scand J Thorac Cardiovasc Surg 2: 65

Berry CL (1968) Clinico-pathological study of thymic dysplasia. Arch Dis Child 43: 579

Berry CL (1970) Histopathological findings in the combined immunity deficiency syndrome. J Clin Pathol 23: 193

Berry CL (to be published) The formation and behaviour of tumours in childhood. In: Davis JA, Dobbing J (eds) Scientific foundations of paediatrics. Heinemann, London

Berry CL, Thompson EN (1968) Clinico-pathological study of thymic dysplasia. Arch Dis Child 43: 579

Bianco C, Patrick R, Nussenzweig V (1970) A population of lymphocytes bearing a membrane receptor for antigen-antibody-complement complexes. J Exp Med 132: 702

Bieger RG, McAdams AJ (1966) Thymic cysts. Arch Pathol 82: 535

Blackburn WR, Gordon DS (1967) The thymic remnant in thymic alymphoplasia. Arch Pathol 84: 363

Boake WC, Card WH, Kimney JF (1965) Histiocytic medullary reticulosis concurrence in father and son. Arch Intern Med 116: 245

Boyd E (1932) The weight of the thymus gland in health and in disease. Am J Dis Child 43: 1162

Brouet JC, Valensi F, Daniel MT, Flandrin G, Preud'homme JL, Seligmann M (1976) Immunological classification of acute lymphoblastic leukaemias: Evaluation of its clinical significance in a hundred patients. Br J Haematol 33: 319

Brunning RD, McKenna RW, Bloomfield CD, Coccia P, Gajl-Peczalska KJ (1977) Bone marrow involvement in Burkitt's lymphoma. Cancer 40: 1771

Bruton OC (1952) Agammaglobulinemia. Pediatrics 9: 722

Burke V, Colebatch JH, Anderson CM, Simons MJ (1967) Association of pancreatic insufficiency and chronic neutropenia in childhood. Arch Dis Child 42: 147

Burkitt DP (1958/59) A sarcoma involving the jaws in African children. Br J Surg 46: 218

Burkitt DP (1970a) General features and facial tumours. In: Burkitt DP, Wright DH (eds) Burkitt's lymphoma. Livingstone, Edinburgh, London, p 6

Burkitt DP (1970b) Lesions outside the jaws. In: Burkitt DP, Wright DH (eds) Burkitt's lymphoma. Livingstone, Edinburgh, London, p 16

Carson MH, Chadwick CA, Brubaker RS, Cleland RS, Landing BH (1965) Thirteen boys with progressive septic granulomatosis. Pediatrics 35: 405

Catovsky D (1975) T cell origin of acid-phosphatase-positive lymphoblasts. Lancet 2: 327

Catovsky D, Frisch B, van Noorden S (1975) B, T and 'null' cell leukaemias. Electron cytochemistry and surface morphology. Blood Cells 1: 115

Chilcote RR, Baehner RL, Hammond D and the Investigators and Special Studies Committee of the Children's Cancer Study Group (1976) Septicemia and meningitis in children splenectomised for Hodgkin's disease. N Engl J Med 295: 798

Cline MH, Golde DW (1973) A review and re-evaluation of the histocytic disorders. Am J Med 55: 49

Cohen IR, Norins LC (1968) Antibodies of IgG, IgM and IgA classes in newborn and adult sera reactive with gram bacteria. J Clin Invest 47: 1053

Coombs RRA, Gurner BW, Wilson AB, Holm G, Lindgren B (1970) Rosette-formation between human lymphocytes and sheep red cells not involving immunoglobulin receptors. Int Arch Allergy Appl Immunol 39: 658

Cooper MD, Chase HP, Lowman JT, Krivit W, Good RA (1968) Immunologic defects in patients with Wiskott–Aldrich syndrome. Birth Defects 4: 378

Cooper MD, Lawton AR, Preud'homme JL, Seligman M (1978) Primary antibody deficiencies. Springer/Berlin Heidelberg New York (Seminars in Immunopathology vol 1, p 265)

Cox R, Hosking GP, Wilson J (1978) Ataxia telangiectasia. Arch Dis Child 53: 386

De Chatelet LR, Shirley PS, McPhail LC (1976) Normal leukocyte glutathione peroxidase activity in patients with chronic granulomatous disease. J Pediatr 89: 598

de Vaal OM, Seynhaeve V (1959) Reticular dysgenesis. Lancet 2: 1123

Di George AM (1968) Congenital absence of the thymus and its immunologic consequences: Concurrence with congenital hypoparathyroidism. Birth Defects 4: 116

Dische MR (1968) Lymphoid tissue and associated malformations in thymic agenesis. Arch Pathol 86: 312

Dorfman RF (1965) Childhood lymphosarcoma in St. Louis, Missouri, clinically and histologically resembling Burkitt's tumour. Cancer 18: 418

Dorfman RF (1974) Classification of non-Hodgkin's lymphoma (Letter to the Editor). Lancet 1: 1295

Dyer NH (1967) Cystic thymomas and thymic cysts. Thorax 22: 408

Epstein MA, Achong BG, Barr YM (1964) Virus particles in cultured lymphoblasts from Burkitt's lymphoma. Lancet 1: 702

Eraklis AJ, Filler RM (1972) Splenectomy in childhood. J Pediatr Surg 7: 382

Fleisher TA, Luckasen JR, Salad A, Gebrts RC, Kersey JH (1975) T and B lymphocytic sub-populations in children. Pediatrics 55: 162

Fransilla KO, Kalima TV, Voutilainen A (1967) Histologic classification of Hodgkin's disease. Cancer 20: 1594

Friedman NB (1967) Tumours of the thymus. J Thorac Cardiovasc Surg 53: 163

Gerard-Marchant R, Hamlin I, Lennert K, Rilke F, Stansfield AG, van Unnink JAM (1974) Classification of non-Hodgkin's lymphomas (Letter to the Editor). Lancet 2: 406

Gilmour JR (1941) Normal haemopoiesis in intra-uterine life. J Pathol Bacteriol 52: 25

Gitlin D, Vawter G, Craig JM (1964) Thymic alymphoplasia and congenital aleukocytosis. Pediatrics 33: 184

Glanzmann E, Riniker P (1950) Essentielle Lymphocytophthise. Ein neues Krankheitsbild aus der Säuglingspathologie. Pediatr Res 175: 1

Goldstein G, Abbot A, Mackay IR (1968) An electron microscopic study of the human thymus: Normal appearances and findings in myasthenia gravis and systemic lupus erythematosus. J Pathol Bacteriol 95: 211

Goldstein G, Mackay IR (1967) The thymus in systemic lupus erythematosus. A quantitative histopathological analysis and comparison with stress involution. Br Med J ii: 475

Hammer JA (1911) Zür gröberen Morphologie und Morphogenie der Mesenchenthymus. Anatomische Hefte 43: 201

Hammar JA (1921) The new views as to the morphology of the thymus gland and their bearing on the problem of the function of the thymus. Endocrinology 5: 543

Hammar JA (1926) Die Menschenthymus in Gesundheit und Krankheit I. Das normale Organ. Z Mikrosk Anat Forsch 6: 107

Helwig H (1976) Zur BCG-Impfstoffaffäre. Paediatrische Praxis 16: 485

Henry K (1968) The thymus in rheumatic heart disease. Clin Exp Immunol 3: 509

Heymer B, Niethammer D, Spanel R, Galle J, Kleihauer E, Haferkamp O (1977) Pathomorphology of humoral, cellular and combined primary immunodeficiencies. Virchows Arch [Pathol Anat] 374: 87

Hirschhorn R, Martin DW (1978) Enzyme defects in immunodeficiency diseases. Springer, Berlin Heidelberg New York (Seminars in Immunopathology, vol 1, p 299)

Hobbs JR, Milner RDG, Watt PJ (1967) Gamma-M-deficiency predisposing to meningococcal septicaemia. Br Med J iv: 583

Holland NH, Holland P (1966) Immunological maturation in an infant of an agamma-globulinaemic mother. Lancet 2: 1152

Huber J, Cholnoky P, Zoethout HE (1967) Congenital aplasia of the parathyroid glands and thymus. Arch Dis Child 42: 190

Huhn D, Meister P (1978) Malignant histiocytosis. Cancer 42: 1341

Indeglia RA, Shea MA, Grage TB (1967) Congenital cysts of the thymus gland. Arch Surg 94: 149

Jenkin RDT, Peters MV, Darte JMM (1967) Hodgkin's disease in children. Am J Roentgenol 100: 222

Jondal M, Holm G, Wigzell H (1972) Surface markers on human T and B lymphocytes. I. A large population of lymphocytes forming non-immune rosettes with sheep red blood cells. J Exp Med 136: 207

Jones SE, Fuks Z, Bull M, Kadin ME, Dorfman RF, Kaplan HS, Rosenberg SA, Kim H (1973) Non-Hodgkin's lymphomas. IV. Clinicopathologic correlation in 405 cases. Cancer 31: 806

Kadowaki JI, Zuelzer WW, Brough AJ, Thompson RI, Woolley PV, Gruber D (1965) XX/XY lymphoid chimaerism in congenital immunological deficiency syndrome with thymic alymphoplasia. Lancet 2: 1152

Kaplan HS (1972) Hodgkin's disease. Harvard University Press, Cambridge

Keller AR, Kaplan HS, Lukes RJ, Rappaport H (1968) Correlation of histopathology with other prognostic indicators in Hodgkin's disease. Cancer 22: 487

Kelly F (1965) Hodgkin's disease in children. Am J Roentgenol 95: 48

Kevy SV, Tefft M, Vawter GF (1968) Hereditary splenic hyperplasia. Pediatrics 42: 752

Kingsbury BF (1915) The development of the human pharynx. I. The pharyngeal derivatives. Am J Anat 18: 329

Klein G (1975) The Epstein-Barr virus and neoplasia. N Engl J Med 293: 1353

Kolygin BA (1976) Combination chemotherapy of Hodgkin's disease in children. Cancer 38: 1494

Kritzler RA, Terner JY, Lindenbaum J, Magidson J, Williams R, Preisig R, Phillips GB (1964) Chediak–Higashi syndrome. Cytologic and serum lipid observations in a case and family. Am J Med 36: 583

Ladisch S, Poplack DG, Holiman B, Blaese RM (1978) Immunodeficiency in familial erythrophagocytic lymphodistiocytosis. Lancet 1: 581

Landing BH, Shirkey HS (1957) A syndrome of recurrent infection and infiltration of viscera by pigmented lipid histiocytes. Pediatrics 20: 431

Lennert K (1978) Malignant lymphomas. Springer, Berlin Heidelberg New York

Lennert K, Mohri N, Stein H, Kaiserling E (1975a) The histopathology of malignant lymphoma. Br J Haematol 31 [Suppl]: 193

Lennert K, Stein H, Kaiserling E (1975b) Cytological and functional criteria for the classification of malignant lymphomata. Br J Cancer 31: Suppl 29

Levine PH, Cho BR, Connelly RR, Berard CW, O'Coner GT, Dorfman RF, Easton JM, DeVita VT (1975) The American Burkitt lymphoma Registry: A progress report. Ann Intern Med 83: 31

Lischner HW, Huff DS (1975) T cell deficiency in Di George syndrome. In: Bergsama D, Good RA, Finstad J, Paul NW (eds) Immuno-deficiency in man and animals. Sinaver, Sunderland p 16

Lukes RJ, Butler JJ (1966) The pathology and nomenclature of Hodgkin's disease. Cancer Res 26: 1063

Lukes RJ, Collins RD (1974) Immunologic characterization of human malignancy lymphomas. Cancer 34: 1488

Lukes RJ, Collins RD (1975) New approaches to the classification of lymphomata. Br J Cancer 31 [Suppl II]: 1

Lukes RJ, Craver LF, Hall TC, Rappaport H, Rubin T (1966) Report of the nomenclature committee. Symposium: Obstacles to the control of Hodgkin's disease. Cancer Res 26: 1311

Lynch RG (1975) Thymus and immune deficiency. In: Kissane JM (ed) Pathology of infancy and childhood. Mosby, St. Louis, p 913

MacGillivray JB, Dacie JV, Henry JRK, Sacker LS (1964) Congenital neutropenia: A report of five cases. Acta Paediatr Scand 53: 188

MacMahon B (1966) Epidemiology of Hodgkin's disease. Cancer Res 26: 1189

Marshall AHE (1956) Histiocytic medullary reticulosis. J Pathol Bacteriol 71: 61

Matsuda I, Oka Y, Taniguchi N (1976) Leukocyte glutathione peroxidase deficiency in a male patient with chronic granulomatous disease. J Pediatr 88: 581

McFarlin DE, Strober W, Waldman TA (1972) Ataxia telangiectasia. Medicine (Baltimore) 51: 281

McNamara JJ, Murphy LJ, Griscom NT, Tefft M (1968) Splenic cysts in children. Surgery 64: 487

Metcalf D, Brumby M (1966) The role of the thymus in the ontogeny of the immune system. J Cell Physiol 67: 149

Middleton G (1967) The incidence of follicular structures in the human thymus at autopsy. Aust J Exp Biol Med Sci 45: 189

Murphy SB, Frizzera G, Evans AE (1975) A study of childhood non-Hodgkin's lymphoma. Cancer 36: 2121

Newton WA Jr, Homoudi AB (1973) Histiocytosis: A histologic classification with clinical correlation. In: Rosenberg HS, Bolande RP (eds) Perspectives in pediatric pathology, vol 1. Year Book Medical Publishers, Chicago, p 251

Nezelof C, Jammet ML, Lortholary P, Labrune B, Lamy M (1964) L'Hypoplasie héréditaire du thymus. Sa place et sa responsabilité dans une observation d'aplasie lymphocytaire normoplasmocytaire et normoglobulinémique du nourisson. Arch Fr Pediatr 25: 897

Nezelof C, Diebold Nicole, Rousseau-Merck, François Marie (1977) Ig surface receptors and erythrophagocytic activity of histiocytosis X cells in vitro. J Pathol 122: 105

Norris DG, Burgert EO, Cooper HA, Harrison EG (1975) Hodgkin's disease in childhood. Cancer 36: 2109

O'Connor GT (1961) Malignant lymphoma in African children. II. A pathological entity. Cancer 14: 270

Okabe H (1966) Thymic lymph follicles. A histopathological study of 1,356 autopsy cases. Acta Pathol Jpn 16: 109

Parkman R, Rappaport J, Geha R, Belli J, Cussaday R, Levey R, Nathan DG, Rosen FS (1978) Complete correction of the Wiskott-Aldrich syndrome by allogenic bone marrow transplantation. N Engl J Med 298: 921

Pearl ER, Voglar LB, Oakas AJ, Crist WM, Lawton AR, Cooper MD (1978) B lymphocyte precursors in human bone marrow. An analysis of normal individuals and patients with antibody deficiency states. J Immunol 120: 1169

Perchalski JE, Clem LW, Small PA (1968) 75 Gamma M immunoglobulins in human cord serum. Am J Med Sci 256: 107

Penman HG (1971) Fatal infectious mononucleosis: A critical review. J Clin Pathol 23: 765

Perry MC, Harrison EG, Burgert EO, Gilchrist GS (1976) Familial erythrophagocytic lymphohistiocytosis. Cancer 38: 209

Pinkel D (1968) Ultrastructure of human fetal thymus. Am J Dis Child 115: 222

Pinkel D, Johnson W, Aur RJA (1975) Non-Hodgkin's lymphoma in children. Br J Cancer 31 [Suppl II]: 298

Pitcock JA, Bauer WC, McGaron MH (1959) Hodgkin's disease in children. Cancer 12: 1043

Purtilo DT, De Florio D, Hutt ML, Bhawan J, Yang JPS, Otho R, Edwards W (1977) Variable phenotypic expression of an X-linked recessive lymphoproliferative syndrome. N Engl J Med 297: 1077

Qureshi MA, Hafner DC, Dorchak JR (1964) Non-parasitic cysts of the spleen. Arch Surg 89: 570

Raff MC (1970) Two distinct populations of peripheral lymphocytes in mice distinguishable by immunofluorescence. Immunology 19: 637

Rappaport H (1966a) Discussion on: The pathology and nomenclature of Hodgkin's disease. Cancer Res 26: 1082

Rappaport H (1966b) Tumours of the haematopoietic system. Atlas of tumour pathology, Sect 3, Fasc 8. Armed Forces Institute of Pathology, Washington DC

Rausch PG, Pryswansky KB, Spitznagel JK (1978) Immunocytochemical identification of azurophilic and specific granule markers in the giant granules of the Chediak-Higashi neutrophils. N Engl J Med 298: 693

Ritter J, Gaedicke G, Winkler R, Beckmann H, Landbeck G (1975) Possible T cell origin of lymphoblasts in acid phosphatase-positive acute lymphatic leukaemia. Lancet 2: 75

Robb-Smith AHT (1938) Reticulosis and reticulosarcoma. A histological classification. J Pathol Bacteriol 47: 457

Robertson NRC, Berry CL, Macaulay JC, Southhill JF (1971) Partial immunodeficiency and graft-versus-host disease. Arch Dis Child 46: 571

Rosen FS, Janeway CA (1966) The gamma globulins: III: The antibody deficiency syndromes. N Engl J Med 275: 769

Rosner P, Lee SL and Acute Leukaemia Group B (1972) Down's syndrome and acute leukaemia: Myeloblastic or lymphoblastic? Report of 43 cases and review of the literature. Am J Med 53: 203

Rubin M, Strauss B, Allen L (1964) Clinical disorders associated with thymic tumours. Arch Intern Med 114: 389

Scott RB, Robb-Smith AHT (1939) Histiocytic medullary reticulosis. Lancet 2: 194

Sealy WC, Weaver WL, Young WG (1965) Severe airway obstruction in infancy due to the thymus gland. Ann Thorac Surg 1: 389

Sell S (1968) Immunological deficiency disease. Arch Pathol 86: 95

Shamoto M (1970) Langerhans cell granules in Letterer-Siwe disease: An electron microscopic study. Cancer 26: 1102

Shapiro RS, Perry GS, Krivit W, Gerrard JM, White JG, Kersey JH (1978) Wiskott-Aldrich syndrome: Detection of carrier state by metabolic stress of platelets. Lancet 1: 121

Siegler R (1964) The morphology of thymuses and their relation to leukaemia. In: Good RA, Gabrielsen AE (eds) The thymus in immunobiology. Harper & Row, New York, p 623

Silverstein AM (1972) Immunological maturation in the fetus: Modulation of the pathogenesis of congenital infectious disease. In: Ontogeny of acquired immunity. Associated Scientific Publications, Amsterdam, p 17 (Ciba Foundation Symposium)

Sims DG (1977) Histiocytosis X. Follow up of 43 cases. Arch Dis Child 52: 433

Singer DB (1973) Post-splenectomy sepsis. In: Rosenberg HS, Bolande RP (eds) Perspectives in pediatric pathology. Year Book Medical Publishers, Chicago, p 285

Steele RW, Limas C, Thurman GB, Schulein M, Bauer H, Bellanti JA (1972) Familial thymic aplasia. Attempted reconstitution with fetal thymus in a millipore diffusion chamber. N Engl J Med 87: 787

Sternberg C (1908) Über Leukosarkomatose. (Cited by Lennert 1978.) Wien Klin Wochenschr 21: 475

Strober W, Wochner AD, Carbone PP, Waldmann TA (1967) Intestinal lymphangiectasia: A protein losing enteropathy with hypogammaglobulinemia, lymphocytopenia and impaired homograft rejection. J Clin Invest 46: 1643

Strober W, Wochner AD, Barlow MH, McFarlin DE, Waldmann TA (1968) Immunoglobulin metabolism in ataxia telangiectasia. J Clin Invest 47: 1905

Symchych PS, Wanstrup J, Anderson V (1968) Chronic granulomatous disease of childhood. Acta Pathol Microbiol Scand 74: 179

Symmers D (1948) Lymphoid diseases. Arch Pathol 45: 73

Talerman A, Amigo A (1968) Thymoma with aplastic anaemia in a five year old child. Cancer 22: 445

Waldmann TA, Broder S (1978) T Cell disorders in primary immunodeficiency diseases. Springer, Berlin Heidelberg New York (Seminars in Immunopathology, vol 1, p 239)

Waldmann TA, McIntire KR (1972) Serum alpha-fetoprotein levels in patients with ataxia telangiectasia. Lancet 2: 1112

Watson RR, Weisel W, O'Connor TM (1968) Thymic neoplasms. Arch Surg 97: 230

Willoughby MN (1977) Leukaemia and related disorders. In: Willoughby MN (ed) Paediatric haematology. Churchill Livingstone, Edinburgh London New York p 372

Windhorst DB, Page AR, Holmes B (1968) The pattern of genetic transmission of the leukocyte defect in fatal granulomatous disease of childhood. J Clin Invest 47: 1026

Wollner N, Burchenall JH, Leiberman PH, Exelby P, D'Angio G, Murphy ML (1975) Non-Hodgkin's lymphoma in children. A comparative study of two modalities of therapy. Cancer 37: 123

Wright DH (1963) Cytology and histochemistry of the Burkitt lymphoma. Br J Cancer 17: 50

Wright DH (1970) Gross distribution and haematology. In: Burkitt DP, Wright DH (eds) Burkitt's lymphoma. Livingstone, Edinburgh London, p 64

Chapter 13

Endocrine Pathology in Paediatrics

Christopher L. Brown

1. Adrenal Cortex

1.1. Development

The cortical tissue of the adrenals arises in the posterior coelomic mesoderm close to the genital ridge and can be identified at the 10-mm stage (6th week). At birth their combined weights average 6.5 g, with the bulk of this relatively large mass comprising a specific fetal cortical zone. This is composed of masses of large eosinophil cells that show ultrastructural characteristics similar to those of the adult adrenal cortex. The definitive cortex forms a sharply contrasting narrow zone of small cortical-type cells beneath the gland capsule. Degenerative involution of the fetal cortex starts at or shortly before birth and is virtually complete within the first few months of postnatal life, though remnants may occasionally be found up to the end of the first year. The definitive cortex shows conspicuous evidence of growth by the 4th day after birth and the zona glomerulosa and zona faciculata are defined by the 6th week. As a result of involution of the fetal zone the combined weights decrease from birth to an average of 3.5 g at 3 months, after which they increase steadily in size in relation to body weight to reach 6 g at about 12 years of age. The normal development of both the fetal and the definitive cortex is to a large extent dependent on normal hypothalmic and pituitary function since the fetal zone is found to be markedly reduced and the definitive cortex less conspicuously so in cases of anencephaly (Fig. 13.1). Similar failure of development of the rat adrenal can be induced experimentally by destruction of the hypothalamus. The fetal

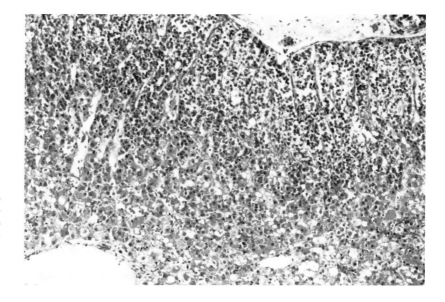

Fig. 13.1. Adrenal from an anencephalic stillborn female. The combined weight of the two glands was 0.2 g. The fetal cortical zone seen in the *lower half* of the picture is greatly reduced, appearing similar in thickness to the definitive cortex. (H and E; 120 ×)

zone is observed to be of increased size in babies born to mothers with diabetes mellitus and in cases of postmaturity.

During intrauterine development the cells of the definitive cortex appear undifferentiated in the electron microscope, whilst those of the fetal zone are large and are active in steroid synthesis. The factors involved in the maintenance and control of the fetal cortex remain uncertain. There is a close functional link between the placenta and the adrenals, the latter producing oestrogen and androgen precursors by removal of a two-carbon side chain from placental progesterone, a step requiring 17-hydroxylase and desmolase, which the placenta lacks.

1.2. Developmental Abnormalities

Absence of one adrenal gland is rare. Failure of both glands to develop probably only occurs in examples of congenital monsters (Benirschke et al. 1956). Occasionally one or both glands are misplaced and are then usually found still related to the urogenital tract. An adrenal has been discovered, well formed, within the skull (Wiener and Dallgaard 1959). Such misplaced glands are usually well organized into the various zones and the medulla is found separately, near the upper renal pole. Ectopic islands of cortical tissue are commonly found adjacent to the main gland, in the retroperitoneal tissues, in the capsule of the liver and kidneys, and in the vicinity of the testes and ovaries. Such islands may become enlarged and prominent in conditions of diffuse hyperplasia of the adrenal cortex, and have been responsible for relapse

in some cases of Cushing's disease treated by adrenalectomy.

Congenital hypoplasia is rare but may affect several members in a single family. Two major types are recognized (Kerenyi 1961). In the first the adrenals are small and similar in detail to those seen in anencephaly (vide infra). Accompanying abnormalities involving aplasia or hypoplasia of the pituitary and maldevelopment involving the hypothalamus are usually found. In occasional cases of adrenal hypoplasia of anencephalic type the hypothalmus and pituitary appear to be normal and the small adrenals might reflect their unresponsiveness to trophic hormone. In the second type, with primary congenital adrenocortical hypoplasia, the adrenal cortex is disorganized and consists of clusters of large pleomorphic cells that may reach 100 μm in diameter. Their cytoplasm is eosinophilic and vacuolated and their nuclei are hyperchromatic, some being very large, and often show 'inclusions' of invaginated cytoplasm (Fig. 13.2; Oppenheimer 1970; Borit and Kosek 1969). This 'cytomegaly' is accompanied by electron microscopical appearances that suggest cellular activity (Oppenheimer 1970; Borit and Kosek 1969). The pituitary and hypothalamus appear normal. The condition is inherited as an X-linked recessive trait (Weiss and Mellinger 1970). In both types the adrenal medulla is uninvolved, though in some of the cytomegalic cases it may be formed into several islands.

Evidence of adrenal insufficiency is earlier and more severe in the anencephalic type. With better recognition of neonatal 'salt-losing' syndromes and the possibility of successful treatment, occasional cases of congenital adrenal insufficiency are being

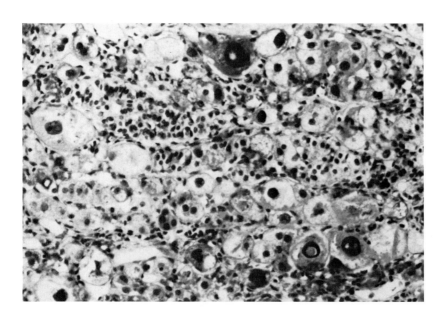

Fig. 13.2. Cytomegaly involving a high proportion of the cells of the fetal adrenal cortex. The enlargement involves both nucleus and cytoplasm, and large infoldings of the nuclear membrane are common, resulting in apparent nuclear inclusions. (H and E; 240×)

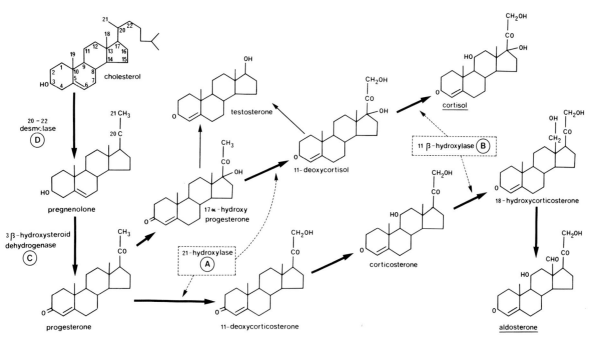

Fig. 13.3. Schematic representation of the major pathways for the synthesis of cortisol and aldosterone. The points at which enzyme defects are most commonly involved in the syndromes of congenital adrenal hyperplasia are indicated (A, B, C, and D).

recorded in whom associated gonadatrophin deficiency has become apparent (Kelly et al. 1977; Marek 1977; Black et al. 1977). Adrenal cytomegaly is not limited to cases of idiopathic hypoplasia. Similar changes are seen in occasional cells of the fetal zone in normal infants and have been observed in the adrenals in 1 % of infants stillborn or dying in the neonatal period (Kohler 1963). In the Beckwith–Wiedemann syndrome there is extensive cytomegaly in the fetal zone (Beckwith 1969; Wiedemann 1964), and in some cases of autoimmune Addison's disease the surviving cortical cells may appear similar.

In anencephaly adrenal development has been noted to be normal up to the 20th gestational week. The fetal zone then involutes prematurely and the definitive cortex remains smaller than normal, so that at birth the combined weight of the two glands is commonly about 1 g, with the definitive cortex contributing the greater part of the mass. Similar changes were found in the adrenals of five of 25 infants with hydrocephalus (Benirschke et al. 1956).

1.3. Congenital Hyperplasia

Lack of specific enzymes involved in the synthesis of steroid hormones (Fig. 13.3) underlies a group of abnormalities inherited as autosomal recessive diseases in which impaired cortisol production is accompanied by enormous adrenal cortical hyperplasia (Fig. 13.4) and formation of large quantities

of alternative steroid hormones and their precursors. The resulting clinical picture depends on the severity of the particular enzyme defect, which is consistent in any one pedigree, and its position in the chain of reactions leading to the synthesis of the various hormones. The incidence of these disorders varies

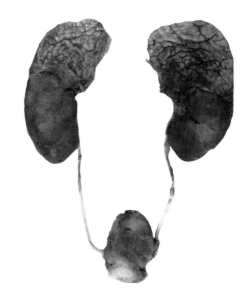

Fig. 13.4. Congenital adrenal hyperplasia. Male aged 14 weeks. Post-mortem specimen showing bilateral extreme diffuse adrenal cortical hyperplasia with characteristic wrinkling of the cortical layers.

greatly in different communities, and for the commonest types has been estimated as 1 in 67 000 births in Maryland (Childs et al. 1956), whereas in an Alaskan Eskimo tribe the incidence is about 1 in 500 (Hirschfield and Fleshman 1969).

1) *21-Hydroxylase deficiency* accounts for about 90 % of cases and occurs as a severe salt-losing form and a less severe virilizing form. In the latter form the increased stimulation of the adrenals results in adequate cortisol output but only at the cost of greatly increased production of the precursor 17α-hydroxyprogesterone, which is converted to testosterone and the excretory product pregnanetriol. There is evidence that the disturbed steroid synthesis is established as early as week 9 of gestation (Kelley et al. 1952), and the consequence of the increased levels of testosterone is virilization of the fetus, resulting in female pseudohermaphrodites and macrogenitosomia praecox in males. Whilst the effects on a female fetus are clinically obvious it appears that a proportion of the less severely affected male infants go unrecognized. If untreated the hormonal imbalance produces somatic changes. Linear growth is accelerated and muscular development increased. Skeletal maturation is even more advanced, however, so that early fusion of the epiphyses results in a reduced final height. Growth of pubic hair may occur as early as 2 years of age, followed by the appearance of axillary, facial, and body hair in masculine distribution. Gonadal maturation may be inhibited, the small testes contrasting with the penile development in boys whilst in girls breast development and menstruation fail to occur.

The salt-losing form is a little less common than the pure virilizing form, accounting for about one-third of all cases. The more severe defect is accompanied by deficient aldosterone production, but the precise mechanism involved in this further defect is still not understood. The impaired renal salt conservation manifests clinically about the 8th to 10th postnatal day in most cases but may sometimes be delayed until towards the end of the 2nd month. The manifestations resemble acute Addisonian crisis with vomiting, diarrhoea, dehydration, and circulatory insufficiency. Without steroid therapy deterioration is rapid and death may occur.

2) *11β-Hydroxylase deficiency* is the second commonest cause of congenital adrenal hyperplasia, but even so accounts for only about 5 % of cases. There is an increase in 11-deoxy precursors of cortisol, the most important of which is 11-deoxycorticosterone, its strong mineralocorticoid effects resulting in hypertension. There is also excess production of androgens and consequent virilization.

3) *3β-Hydroxysteroid dehydrogenase deficiency* affects a very early step in steroid hormone synthesis, affecting cortisol and aldosterone production and allowing formation of only weak androgenic steroids. There is a severe salt-losing syndrome in most cases without virilization, and many cases die despite full replacement therapy.

In all these three forms of the disease the gross and histological changes in the adrenals are similar. The high levels of pituitary ACTH result in hyperplasia of compact cells, which expand the zona reticularis, with only occasional lipid-containing cells forming the small peripheral zona fasciculata. Large bizarre cortical cells can occur and reflect the high level of cell function. The zona glomerulosa is variously described as increased or decreased in size. The medulla is normal. The weight of each gland averages 15 g, as against the normal weight in children of 1.5–3 g. When untreated they are brown in colour; their size continues to increase and they may exceed 30 g in weight. Multiple nodules may develop.

4) *Congenital lipid hyperplasia* is a very rare fourth type of congenital hyperplasia, which produces different appearances in the adrenals. There is a deficiency of 20–22 desmolase, so that conversion of cholesterol to pregnenolone cannot proceed, with consequent impairment of the formation of all steroid hormones including those formed in the gonads. Each gland may exceed 3 g in weight; the enlarged cortex is pale, disorganized and nodular, composed mostly of large lipid filled cells; and there may be deposits of cholesterol. Since virilizing hormones cannot be synthesized the genital tract in affected male fetuses develops towards the female type (Siebenmann 1957).

1.4. Wolman's disease

Wolman's disease is a primary familial xanthomatosis in which the adrenals, amongst other organs, are involved and appear enlarged with calcification in the inner cortex (Wolman et al. 1961). There is no substantial evidence of functional deficiency (Marshall et al. 1969). (See also p. 619.)

1.5. Acquired Adrenocortical Insufficiency

Haemorrhage into the adrenals is seen commonly in newborn infants and is related to prematurity, birth trauma and asphyxia. From their findings in postmortems de Sa and Nicholls (1972) observed an incidence of 1.7 per 1000 in perinatal deaths. Minor lesions do not cause adrenal insufficiency but

Christopher L. Brown
575

massive haemorrhage may result in acute adreno-cortical insufficiency. Calcification is a common secondary change in these lesions. Focal cortical necroses with or without haemorrhage may be found complicating bacterial and viral infections. Haemorrhage into the adrenals sometimes occurs in cases of leukaemia and other bleeding disorders and into metastatic tumour deposits.

1.6. Waterhouse–Friderichsen Syndrome

The term 'Waterhouse–Friderichsen syndrome' should be reserved for those cases that conform to the classic clinical and pathological picture of this well-defined condition. The illness is abrupt in onset, with rapid appearance of shock and cyanosis, usually with an accompanying petechial rash (Fig. 13.5). Often despite prompt treatment death occurs within 6–24 h. Most cases occur in previously healthy children and young adults as a complication of a septicaemia, usually involving *Neisseria meningitidis*. Cases have been described with infection by *Haemophylus influenzae* or pneumococci, and in association with varicella. At post-mortem both adrenals are found to be greatly expanded by haemorrhage into the central cortex (see Fig. 13.6).

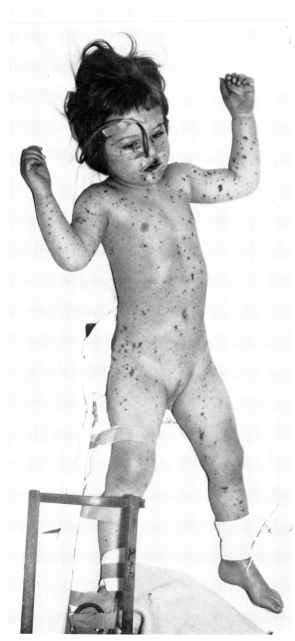

Fig. 13.5. Female aged 3 years. Haemorrhagic rash accompanying meningococcal septicaemia.

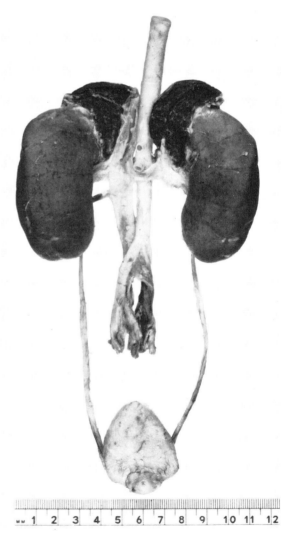

Fig. 13.6. Post-mortem specimen from a girl aged 2 years who died of meningococcal septicaemia with bilateral adrenal haemorrhages (Waterhouse–Friderichsen syndrome).

The exact causal mechanism of the haemorrhage remains uncertain. Experimentally the lesion can be induced in heparinized animals, suggesting that thrombosis of the vascular sinuses and disseminated intravascular coagulation are not primary events. It may be a direct effect of bacterial toxins acting on the stimulated highly vascular gland (Levin and Cluff 1965). Although the syndrome was originally thought to be the result of acute adrenocortical failure this has not been substantiated. Occasional clinically typical cases have been described in which the adrenals have been normal at post-mortem (Hardman 1968), and in cases that recover adrenal function is usually found to be normal.

1.7. Cystic Change in the Definitive Cortex

The appearance of multiple small cysts in the definitive cortex has repeatedly been observed at post-mortem in some stillborn fetuses and cases of perinatal death, and has usually been regarded as part of normal development. The studies of Oppenheimer (1969), however, suggest that prematurity and fetal infection are important predisposing factors and that the changes are the result of focal cortical cell degeneration as a consequence of intrauterine stress.

1.8. Addison's Disease

Chronic adrenal insufficiency in childhood is uncommon. In infants it can result from congenital hypoplasia and in some cases follows haemorrhage and calcification in the adrenals. Most other cases are seen in later childhood and adolescence, sometimes from infection by the tubercle bacillus or *Histoplasma capsulatum*, but more often from acquired atrophy. This is usually the result of autoimmune adrenalitis, as originally suggested by Anderson et al. (1957). Not only are circulating antibodies to adrenal cortical cells frequently present, but in some cases there are manifestations of autoimmune disease involving other endocrine organs, when the total condition is referred to as autoimmune polyendocrinopathy. A history of involvement of other family members with varying combinations of endocrine disturbances is usually found in these cases and in addition tissues outside the defined endocrine glands may be involved, most notably with resulting pernicious anaemia, areas of cutaneous vitiligo, and sometimes loss of all hair. In cases presenting with these other autoimmune diseases circulating antibodies to adrenal cortex may be present without clinical or laboratory evidence of deficient adrenal function (Blizzard et al. 1962).

In the cases resulting from tuberculous infection the adrenals are almost totally destroyed and enlarged, consisting of central necrotic material and a peripheral inflammatory zone. The infective process does not usually extend beyond the adrenal capsule. There may be extensive calcification in old lesions. In the autoimmune cases the glands are very small and may be misshapen. In some instances no adrenal tissue can be found. Microscopically there are islands of large eosinophilic compact-type cells surrounded by the collapsed vascular reticulin framework of the original cortex but no fibrosis. There may be a moderate lymphoid infiltration with some involvement of the medulla, which is otherwise normal.

1.9. Cushing's Syndrome

Cushing's syndrome is rare in children and more often results from a functioning adrenal adenoma or carcinoma than from pituitary-driven adrenocortical hyperplasia. More than three-quarters of cases occur in females. Clinical manifestations vary largely according to the underlying cause. In most cases there is some degree of virilization, and if this is marked there is usually associated carcinoma. When androgenic steroid effects are dominant accelerated muscular and skeletal development are prominent, which is in contrast to the findings in cases where cortisol effects dominate. In these more usual cases of Cushing's syndrome obesity with the classic truncal, shoulder, and face distribution, impairment of linear growth, and osteopoenia are the major effects and are regularly associated with acne, hirsutism, and a flushed face to produce a highly typical clinical picture (Fig. 13.7). Glucose intolerance is nearly always demonstrable and there may be symptomatic diabetes. A diastolic blood pressure above 90 mmHg is found in the majority of cases. Adolescent girls usually have amenorrhoea. 'Pure' Cushing's syndrome, in which the virilizing effects are not seen, is usually due to an adenoma or primary adrenocortical nodular dysplasia (vide infra). Occasional tumours, usually carcinomas, are oestrogen-producing and give rise to feminization and abnormal uterine bleeding in young girls, whilst in adolescent boys there may be testicular atrophy and gynaecomastia. Most cases show some acne and growth of sex hair. Aldosterone-producing tumours are particularly rare, and nonfunctioning carcinomas are also uncommon.

Adrenal cortical tumours associated with Cushing's syndrome occur in all age groups. Adenomas are rounded, encapsulated, firm, and pale or brownish with patches of yellow lipid. They vary in size, usually weighing less than 50 g and rarely exceeding 100 g. Their cells are recognizable as adrenal cortical and are arranged in columns and solid nests separated by a delicate vascular network. The cytoplasm is eosinophilic, like that of the cells of the normal adrenal reticularis, and may contain obvious lipofuscin in pigmented tumours. The nuclei are large, whilst pleomorphic and bizarre forms are common. These strikingly abnormal nucleated cells may be grouped in well-defined areas in the tumour. Clusters of small and large clear cells correspond to the visible lipid-rich patches. Occasional mitoses may be found. There is atrophy of the cortex of both adrenal glands and the brown zona reticularis is barely visible on the cut surface.

An adrenal cortical carcinoma is the commonest cause of Cushing's syndrome in childhood, being recorded in up to three-quarters of cases, though a lower proportion may be more appropriate (Neville and Symington 1972). The history in these cases is usually shorter and features of virilization are more prominent. The tumours (Fig. 13.8a) are soft and lobulated, with a pale or brownish cut surface. Most weigh more than 100 g, occasional cases reaching a very large size. Evidence of malignancy may be obvious from the finding of metastases in local lymph nodes and vascular invasion, but on purely histological grounds their recognition is uncertain more often than not. Apart from the larger size, other findings suggesting malignancy are the presence of areas of necrosis, marked disproportionate nuclear enlargement, the presence of monster cells, often with multiple nuclei, and numerous mitoses. It is well for the pathologist to bear in mind that metastasizing tumours that appear histologically innocent have been described and that benign endocrine tumours may show marked nuclear pleomorphism and mitotic activity. All large adrenal cortical tumours should be regarded with suspicion. In carcinomas the cells are mostly of the compact type with few and scattered lipid-containing cells (Fig. 13.8b).

Occasional cases of pure Cushing's syndrome are described, usually in girls, with onset in later childhood and into early adulthood, in which both adrenals contain numerous pigmented nodules up to 3 mm in diameter throughout a shrunken yellow cortex. The combined weights of the glands have varied from well below to somewhat above normal.

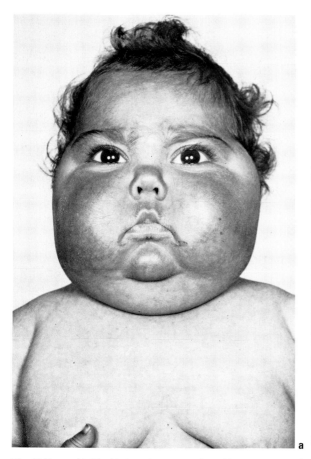 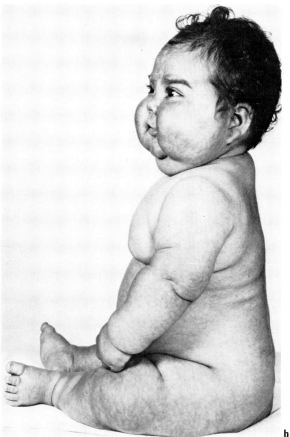

Fig. 13.7. a and **b** Florid clinical features of Cushing's syndrome due to an adrenal carcinoma in a male infant aged 14 months.

a

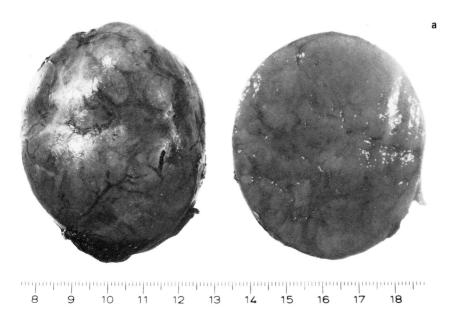

```
||||||||||||||||||||||||||||||||||||||||||||||||||||||||||||||||||||||||||||||||||||||||||||||||||||||||||||
   8    9    10    11    12    13    14    15    16    17    18
```

b

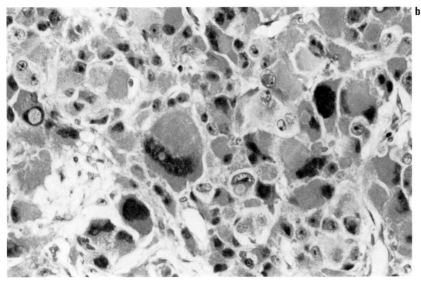

Fig. 13.8. a External and cut surfaces of an adrenal tumour weighing 84 g, removed from an 11-year-old girl with mixed Cushing's syndrome. The cut surface is solid and evenly tan coloured with no visible lipid-rich areas. **b** An area of bizarre compact-type adrenal cortical cells from the same tumour. Such cytological changes are not an indication of malignancy. (H and E; 300 ×)

The nodules consist of large, pigmented, compact cells with small nuclei, and are sharply demarcated from the rest of the cortex but are not encapsulated. The residual cortex is described as atrophic and composed of clear cells, and in some cases it shows a focal lymphocytic infiltrate. The zoning of the cortex is preserved and the medulla is normal. The condition was identified and described as primary adrenocortical nodular dysplasia by Meador et al. (1967), and was further described by Ruder et al. (1974). Corticotrophin is undetectable and the abnormality appears to be a primary disturbance of the adrenal cortex. It must be distinguished from nodularity in bilateral diffuse adrenal cortical hyperplasia.

Pituitary-driven bilateral adrenocortical hyperplasia accounts for about 35% of childhood Cushing's syndrome, mostly in adolescents and only very rarely before the age of 8 years (Neville and Symington 1972). These authors found the weights of the adrenal glands usually fell within the normal adult range (4.0–6.0 g each). In all cases, however, there is clear histological evidence of hyperplasia (Fig. 13.9). Compact cells of zona reticularis type occupy from one-third to a half the thickness of the cortex, forming a well-defined regular inner band. The zona glomerulosa is conspicuous, with frequent short columns of cells projecting down into the outer zona fasciculata. Microscopical nodules composed of clear cells are found related to the central vein and at the periphery of the cortex. In occasional cases multiple nodules ranging from a few millimetres to 2 cm in diameter may be visible throughout the cortex. The glands in such cases may be much heavier and of markedly unequal size. Histologically the intervening cortex shows diffuse hyperplasia, with the zona reticularis occupying about half the cortical thickness. The nodules usually consist of small compact cells with prominent nuclei.

Almost all cases of Cushing's syndrome in which bilateral adrenal cortical hyperplasia is present are the result of excessive pituitary ACTH secretion (true Cushing's disease), which characteristically is found at a constant concentration in the blood throughout the 24 h rather than at a clearly abnormal elevated level on any single estimation. Recent experience gained from the treatment of cases of Cushing's disease by pituitary microsurgical techniques show that a pituitary adenoma, often very small, is found in almost every case. The removal of the adenoma is accompanied by cure of the disease and eventual return of normal hypothalamic–pituitary–adrenal function without loss of other pituitary functions (Salassa et al. 1978; Tyrrell et al. 1978). This is the only form of treatment that regularly achieves complete cure, and constitutes strong evidence that the primary abnormality is a pituitary tumour in most, or possibly all cases, rather than a functional hypothalamic disturbance. Radiological evidence of a pituitary tumour prior to treatment is found in a minority of cases, but following treatment by adrenal ablation Hopwood and Kenny (1977) found increasing pigmentation in 18 and enlargement of the pituitary fossa in 8 (Nelson's syndrome) of 31 children treated for Cushing's disease from 1 to 5.5 years previously. This is a much higher incidence of this complication than is recorded in adults similarly treated. Very good results can be obtained from the treatment of childhood Cushing's disease with pituitary irradiation, without risk of occurrence of Nelson's syndrome (Jennings et al. 1977).

The adenomas found in the pituitary in cases of Cushing's syndrome are mostly basophil or chromophobe, and sometimes mixed. Rarely an acidophil tumour is found. In Nelson's syndrome the tumour enlarges progressively and tends to infiltrate surrounding structures. This is sometimes regarded as evidence of malignant change, but although pulmonary metastases have been described the tumours do not usually appear less well-differentiated histologically. The corticotrophs in the pituitary gland show Crooke's hyaline change in all cases of active Cushing's syndrome from whatever cause. The cells of a basophil adenoma when present do not show the change.

The rarest form of Cushing's syndrome in children

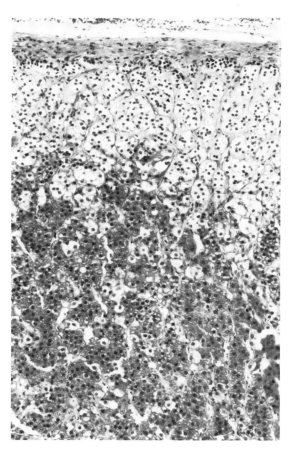

Fig. 13.9. Diffuse adrenal cortical hyperplasia in Cushing's disease. The darkly staining compact cells of the zona reticularis (*left*) have expanded to fill the inner three-quarters of the thickened cortex. The zona glomerulosa forms a distinct narrow band of small clear cells beneath the capsule. The combined weight of the two adrenals was 16.1 g. They were removed from a male aged 15 years who had probably been suffering from Cushing's disease for the preceding 6 years. At the time of treatment clinical features were obvious and severe osteoporosis had resulted in loss of height. (H and E; 120 ×)

is seen when bilateral adrenal cortical hyperplasia results from ACTH secretion by a nonpituitary tumour. Eleven cases of tumours in children with evidence of ectopic ACTH production are recorded in the review by Omenn (1971). Tumours of neuroblast origin form the largest group and almost all of the remainder are accounted for by tumours of the thymus, pancreatic islets, and anaplastic carcinoma of the lung. Medullary carcinoma of the thyroid has also been noted in this context (Williams et al. 1968).

1.10. Virilizing Tumours

Virilizing adrenal cortical tumours without features of Cushing's syndrome are relatively more common in children than in adults, and practically all the examples described in males have been in children. More than three-quarters of cases occur in females, and carcinomas account for a similarly large majority. The contralateral adrenal is atrophic in less than 30% of cases, an indication that most of these tumours produce insignificant amounts of cortisol. The anabolic effects of the androgens prevent the growth inhibition and muscle wasting caused by cortisol when present in excess, so that clinically there is precocious growth and muscular development in addition to virilization. Virilizing tumours usually consist exclusively of compact-type cells with eosinophilic granular cytoplasm. Distinction between benign and malignant tumours on histological grounds is often difficult, as has already been discussed (see p. 577). Virilization in a male child is also seen in late-onset congenital adrenal cortical hyperplasia, interstitial tumours of the testis, true precocious puberty, and gonadotrophin-secreting tumours. An androgen-secreting ovarian stromal tumour is a rare cause in females.

1.11. Feminizing Tumours

Feminizing adrenal cortical tumours are very rare in children, and though such tumours are in general mostly carcinomas a relatively high proportion in children are adenomas (Gabrilove et al. 1965). Their gross and microscopical features are not specifically different from those of other functioning adrenal tumours. In a girl distinction from true precocious puberty and from an oestrogen-producing ovarian tumour must be made.

1.12. Nonfunctioning Tumours and Hypoglycaemia

Adrenal cortical carcinomas that show no evidence of hormone production are very rare in children. Occasional large tumours have been associated with episodes of spontaneous hypoglycaemia. In the case involving a girl of 16 recorded by Scholz et al. (1967) immunoreactive insulin was undetectable in the blood during hypoglycaemia, and insulin-like activity could not be detected. The relationship of hypoglycaemia and adrenal carcinoma is complicated since in some cases the tumour has been a part of the Beckwith–Wiedemann syndrome, in which pancreatic islet hyperplasia occurs (Weinstein et al. 1970).

1.13. Aldosteronism

Aldosteronism is rare in children. Males are affected more often, and symptoms are typically severe and can usually be traced to infancy (New and Petwoon 1966). The commonest change in the adrenals is cortical hyperplasia, often with multiple cortical nodules composed of large clear cells of zona fasciculata type. Grim et al. (1967) discuss nine cases under the age of 18 years, including one case of their own. Seven of the cases were in males, the youngest aged 9 years. In six cases the adrenals were described as hyperplastic, and they were nodular in three. In the remaining three the adrenals were thought to be normal. Three reported cases of Conn's adenoma in children aged from 3 to 15 years are quoted by New and Petwoon (1966).

2. Adrenal Medulla and Paraganglia

The adrenal medulla and the extra-adrenal chromaffin tissue differentiate from stem cells (sympathicogonia) of neural crest ectodermal origin. Sympathicogonia migrate laterally in the dorsal wall of the coelom to reach the area of the adrenal mesenchyme by the 6th gestational week. Clusters of these migrant cells penetrate to a central position in the adrenal mesenchyme through the succeeding week, with additional small numbers of cells continuing to arrive through most of the period of gestation. Differentiation of the adrenal medullary sympathicogonia to form chromaffin cells is slow and mostly occurs in early postnatal life, normally being complete by the end of the third year. Groups of primitive cells, sometimes forming rosettes, may be found related to the adrenal vein in neonatal infants. Large collections are not uncommon and have been regarded as localized neuroblastomas (see discussion on p. 643). Sympathicogonia outside the adrenal differentiate into the paraganglial chromaffin tissue. This matures quickly and is most prominent during intrauterine and early postnatal life, principally in relation to the abdominal aorta. The largest of these masses develops at the end of the second gestational month and forms the para-aortic organ of Zuckerkandle, a paired body found at the level of the origin of the inferior mesenteric artery. The extra-adrenal chromaffin tissue involutes as the adrenal medulla develops and is no longer visible by the time of puberty.

Nonchromaffin paraganglial tissue forming autonomic structures related to vessels, nerves and other tissues is widely distributed. Well-defined para-ganglia include the carotid bodies, glomus jugulare, and aortic (arch) body. The principal cells of these structures have been shown to contain electron-dense granules 100–200 μm in diameter, similar to those found in adrenal phaeochromocytes, and some show formalin-induced cytoplasmic fluorescence, indicating the presence of catecholamine. These features are strong evidence in support of the view that the cells of these structures originate from the neural crest. This has been directly confirmed in the case of the carotid body in the chick (Le Dourain et al. 1972).

The systems of chromaffin and nonchromaffin tissues are clinically important because of the tumours that may develop, often as a part of genetically determined syndromes that also involve hyperplasia in the affected structures.

Conventionally the simple neoplasms are neuro-blastoma and its maturing derivatives, phaeo-chromocytoma and paraganglioma. On the basis of the unifying concept of the neurocristopathies this list can be extended to include carcinoid tumours, medullary carcinoma of the thyroid, at least some tumours of pancreatic islet cells, and anterior pituitary and melanotic progonoma of the jaw. Many of these are described in detail elsewhere.

2.1. Phaeochromocytoma

Phaeochromocytomas are rare tumours that occur sporadically and in familial clusters consistent with an autosomal dominant mode of inheritance (Carman and Brashear 1960). Most are found in the adrenal, but they may occur wherever chromaffin tissue is located. Most extra-adrenal tumours are found in the abdomen along the sympathetic chain, whilst occasional cases have been recorded in the neck, mediastinum, and urinary bladder. There is a preponderance in males and in the right adrenal. In children the incidence of bilateral adrenal tumours is higher than the 10% recorded in adults (Hume 1960), at least in part as a consequence of the relatively high proportion of genetically determined cases seen at this age. They are only very rarely malignant. Clinical manifestations are the result of the release from the tumour of large amounts of catecholamines into the blood. Adrenal phaeochromocytomas usually produce both adrenaline and noradrenaline, whereas in extra-adrenal tumours noradrenaline alone is the principal product. In children hypertension is usually sustained rather than paroxysmal, and when severe may produce retinopathy. Noradrenaline-induced cardiomyopathy can occur, producing hypotensive heart failure. Glucose intolerance may produce sympto-matic diabetes mellitus, and weight loss with glocysuria may lead to diagnostic confusion. A large number of cases in children have been reviewed by Stackpole et al. (1963).

The tumours are usually well circumscribed and rounded, and they vary greatly in size, from only a few grams to a kilogram. Figure 13.10 shows an adrenal phaeochromocytoma. The cut surface is grey-brown with haemorrhagic areas, and in parts is often cystic. Fixation of fresh tissue in a chromate–bichromate mixture produces a brown reaction product with the contained catecholamines, and is important in confirmation of the diagnosis. Micro-scopically there is some resemblance to the normal adrenal medulla, with groups of large cells with basophilic granular cytoplasm surrounded by a delicate vascular network. In bichromate-fixed tissue the cytoplasm of many of the tumour cells is coloured brown and 'lakes' of brown pigment are commonly concentrated in the connective tissue around larger vessels. Tumour nuclei are mostly uniform, but scattered large and sometimes bizarre hyperchromatic forms are very typically present. Mitoses are usually difficult to find. Histological recognition of the rare malignant tumour is not possible (Fig. 13.11), and in interpretation of multiple masses of phaeochromocytoma as evidence of malignancy the commoner occurrence of multiple independent tumours must be borne in mind. Good evidence of malignancy is the finding of multiple deposits in unusual sites for chromaffin tissue. Ultrastructural studies show numerous cytoplasmic electron-dense granules 130–270 μm in size that represent the site of catecholamine storage and correspond to the granules seen on light microscopy. In addition, the electron microscope demonstrates two cell populations, light and dark, but this is apparently unrelated to any functional difference.

The diagnosis of phaeochromocytoma depends on the demonstration of excessive levels of circulating catecholamines in the blood and abnormal amounts of their metabolites in 24 h urine specimens. Ectopic hormone production has been described, including ACTH, erythropoeitin, prostaglandins, and possibly a parathormone-like substance.

Study of the ultrastructure of neuroblastomas, nonchromaffin paragangliomas, and melanotic progonomas shows electron-dense neurosecretory granules in greater or lesser numbers. Catecholamine production occurs in a large proportion of neuroblastomas with resulting hypertension in up to 10% of cases. Paragangliomas are generally regarded as nonfunctioning, but occasional cases have been associated with hypertension and increased urinary catecholamine excretion (Weichert 1970). One patient with a melanotic progonoma has been

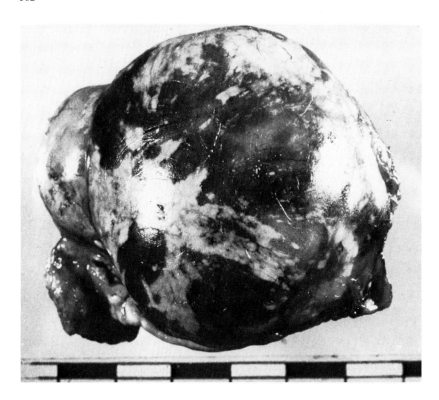

Fig. 13.10. Adrenal phaeochromocytoma weighing 60 g and forming
a soft lobulated deep red tumour.
The pale areas on the surface represent adrenal cortex, whilst the bulk
of the adrenal gland projects from
the lower left surface of the tumour.

reported, in whom elevated catecholamine excretion was recorded. The characteristics of carcinoid tumours relating to their embryological origins have been set out by Williams and Sandler (1963), and their varied endocrine potential is recorded by Weichert (1970).

3. Pancreatic Islets

The pancreatic islets are shown to differentiate from cells of pancreatic duct ectoderm (Pictet et al. 1976) rather than from migratory cells of the neural crest (Pearse et al. 1973). Cell nests are seen budding from the small ducts in the 3rd month of gestation. The connection with the duct system is subsequently lost. Insulin and glucagon can be demonstrated within the islet cells by the 20th gestational week. Islet tissue forms 1%–2% of the pancreatic mass.

3.1. Hypoglycaemic Disorders

Hypoglycaemia occurring in infants and young children is most commonly a consequence of fasting in an otherwise normal individual (ketotic hypo-glycaemia; Chaussain 1973). Liability to hypo-glycaemia is particularly great in premature and small-for-gestational age neonatal infants. Less common causes include hepatic enzyme defects, growth hormone and glucorticoid deficiency, and inappropriate insulin secretion. Most cases of persistent inappropriate insulin secretion occur before the age of 2, and delay in recognition and treatment carries a high risk of permanent neuro-logical and mental damage. The disorder has been attributed to dysfunction of the β cells without consistent demonstrable histological abnormality (Pagliara et al. 1973) and to agenesis of the glucagon-producing islet A cells (Yakovac et al. 1971) in addition to islet hyperplasia, abnormal β cell proliferation, and β cell tumour (Fischer et al. 1974; Misugi et al. 1970).

3.2. Nesidioblastosis

In nesidioblastosis there is continued uncontrolled proliferation of pancreatic ductular endocrine cells, which replace the normal islets of Langerhans and infiltrate amongst the acinar tissue. Apparent budding off of endocrine cells from ductular epi-thelium is seen. Immunohistochemical study has shown near-normal proportions of the different islet-cell types (Heitz et al. 1977). Nesidioblastosis has been observed in a proportion of cases of sudden infant death (Fig. 13.12; Polak and Wigglesworth 1976; Cox et al. 1976) and in cases of hypoglycaemia

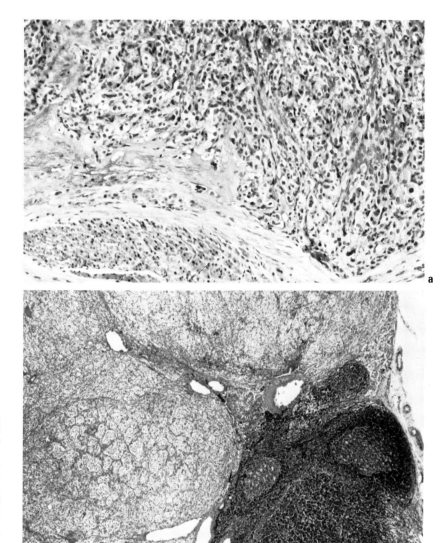

Fig. 13.11. a and **b** Malignant phaeochromocytoma arising in the bladder (**a**) and infiltrating the muscle wall. (H and E; 120 ×)

There are not histological criteria by which malignancy can be recognized in a phaeochromocytoma but in this case a metastasis was present in a local lymph node (**b**; H and E; 30 ×)

Case 1 of Higgins PM, Tresidder GC (1966) *BMJ* ii: 274.

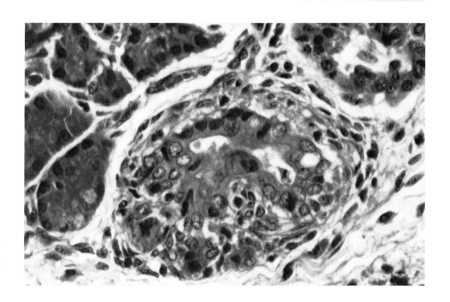

Fig. 13.12. Proliferation of islet cells in a small duct in an infant dying in the postnatal period with nesidioblastosis. (H and E; 480 ×)

that have been clinically recognized. In most of the cases described the proliferation of endocrine cells affects the pancreas diffusely, but on occasion only localized areas may be involved, the remaining pancreatic tissue being histologically normal or containing some enlarged islets (Davidson et al. 1974; Gang 1978).

Hyperplasia of the islets of Langerhans is seen as a temporary change in the pancreas of a proportion of infants of diabetic mothers. It is one of the features seen in the Beckwith syndrome and in some cases of erythroblastosis fetalis.

3.3. Diabetes Mellitus

Diabetes mellitus is the commonest endocrine disease in childhood, affecting males and females with equal frequency. The prevalence in school-age children is similar in England, Sweden, and the United States at about 1.3 per 1000 with a linear increase in incidence from age 5 years to age 16 years (Holmgren et al. 1974; Calnan and Peckham 1977; Kyllo and Huttall 1978). Most cases are of the insulin-deficiency type with acute onset of their disease, though only a minority present with established diabetic ketoacidosis. The major metabolic disturbances are well controlled with insulin but the later complications that affect small and large vessels and are responsible for retinopathy, nephropathy, and large artery occlusion remain.

Factors relating to the occurrence of insulin-deficiency diabetes have become more clearly defined in recent years with investigations of genetic make-up, immune responsiveness, and virus infections currently providing insight into the hereditary and environmental factors concerned in its aetiology. The major genetic susceptibility is determined by a gene in the HLA regions of the chromosome 6 pair associated with HLA8 and W15 antigens at the B locus and DW3 and DW4 antigens at the D locus. Autoimmune organ-specific diseases show an association with the presence of the HLA8 antigen and an association has increasingly been detected between insulin-deficiency diabetes and various autoimmune diseases, including Graves' disease, Hashimoto's thyroiditis, pernicious anaemia, Addison's disease, and myasthenia gravis (Nabarro et al. 1979). Antibodies that react with pancreatic islet cells are present at the onset of the disease in the serum of a high proportion of cases (Irvine et al. 1977; Lernmark et al. 1978; MacLaren et al. 1975), and abnormalities in the T lymphocytes have been demonstrated (Huang and MacLaren 1976). Pure inheritance and altered immunity are not sufficient in themselves to account for the development of the disease, however, since the concordance

rate among pairs of identical twins with one of each pair having insulin-deficiency diabetes is only 50%. Whether virus infections are the necessary environmental triggering agent remains open to speculation, but epidemiological observations suggest that diabetes follows Coxsackie virus B4 infections by weeks, mumps infections by months to a few years, and intrauterine exposure to rubella virus by up to 20 years (Gamble et al. 1969; Sultz et al. 1975; Menser et al. 1978). In the acute fatal case described by Yoon et al. (1979) a variant of Coxsackie virus B4 isolated from the pancreas was shown to survive in cell culture and to infect suitable mice with accompanying β cell damage and hyperglycaemia.

In a small proportion of diabetic children the disease has a different aetiology, usually of obesity-related glucose intolerance, in which case there may be a strong family history of maturity-onset diabetes. A number of rare genetic syndromes account for the remaining occasional cases (Rimoin 1971). In ataxia telangiectasia there is a decrease in the affinity of the insulin receptor probably caused by binding of circulating inhibitors (Bar et al. 1978), whilst in Turner's syndrome there is a reduction in the number of insulin receptors unrelated to obesity (Neufeld et al. 1978).

3.3.1. Changes in the Pancreas

In his study of the pancreas in patients with juvenile diabetes mellitus, Gepts (1965) found abnormalities in the majority of cases both when the disease was clinically of recent onset (less than 6 months) and in those dying after more than 2 years of disease. The weight of the pancreas was found to be normal in the acute group but variably lower than normal in a considerable proportion of chronic cases. Weight deficit, when present, showed no relationship to the severity, duration, or age at onset of the disease. Similar observations were made by Doniach and Morgan (1973), who suggest in explanation cessation of normal pancreatic growth from the time of onset of the disease rather than destruction of exocrine tissue.

The most consistent abnormality is seen histologically to involve the islets of Langerhans (Fig. 13.13). Practically all cases show a reduction, usually marked, in the total number of islets and the number of β cells, and depletion of their cytoplasmic granules in aldehyde-fuschin stained sections that is more marked in cases with long-standing disease. Other changes seen include insular fibrosis, shrinkage of the islet cells, and occurrence of β cells with swollen vacuolated cytoplasm described as hydropic transformation, an appearance resulting from degranulation and accumulation of glycogen.

A proportion of the insular cells in some cases contain large irregular nuclei and hyperchromatic nuclei. Gepts (1965) observed an inflammatory infiltrate within and/or around some islets in nearly 70% of his patients with diabetes of recent onset (insulitis). The infiltrating cells were lymphocytes, macrophages, and a few polymorphs, but included no plasma cells. None of the cases studied by Doniach and Morgan (1973) showed an inflammatory infiltrate.

3.3.2. Changes in Extrapancreatic Structures

Clinical effects resulting from the changes that take place in the small blood vessels and muscular arteries in diabetes generally become evident only after many years and are therefore rarely seen before the age of 18. Since vascular complications are by far the commonest single cause of major illness and eventual death amongst diabetics there is great concern to understand the mechanisms behind their development and so allow the introduction of logical steps to prevent their development from an early stage in the disease. A central theme common to much contemporary investigation is the suggestion that an abnormally elevated concentration of glucose may of itself lead to the vascular and tissue changes. The tissues principally involved in the late complications of diabetes (blood vessels, nerves, eyes) do not require insulin for glucose uptake. It is possible therefore that the accumulation of by-products from the metabolism of the excessive amounts of glucose by the sorbitol pathway leads to damage in these tissues (Gabbay 1975). The nonenzymatic glycosylation of an increased proportion of long-lived proteins that occurs with an increase in glucose concentration can impair their function. Haemoglobin is markedly affected in this way, with an adverse effect on its affinity for oxygen (Koenig et al. 1976).

Thickening of the basement membrane of small blood vessels is typical in young diabetics. The capillaries are most severely affected and have been found to be abnormal in the glomerulus, retina, muscle, subcutaneous tissue, and skin. Thickening of nonvascular basement membrane has also been found in Bowman's capsule, renal tubules, seminiferous tubules, breast, ciliary process of the eye, and sweat glands of the skin. Basement membrane change occurs early and has been observed in biopsies taken at the time of presentation and in asymptomatic children with impaired glucose tolerance.

The evolution of the various complications in a large number of juvenile diabetics has been recorded by Knowles et al. (1965) and by the Public Health Service, National Institutes of Health of the US Department of Health, Education, and Welfare (1977). Retinopathy and glomerulosclerosis begin to appear after about 10 years of disease and are therefore not seen before the mid- to late teens. Knowles et al. recorded retinopathy in as many as 70% of their patients who had had 20 years of disease, and glomerulosclerosis in 30%. About 50% of juvenile diabetic patients eventually die of renal disease. Neuropathy is not usually clinically evident before about 10 years of disease but abnormal electromyographic patterns can be detected much earlier (Eeg-Olofsson and Petersen 1966). The NIH statistics indicate that cataracts are present in at least 5% of diabetic patients under 19 years of age. Accounts of the histological changes in these late diabetic complications are recorded by Bloodworth (1968) and Williams and Porte (1974).

3.4. Tumours of the Pancreatic Islets

Islet-cell tumours of the pancreas are rare in children. Amongst the recorded cases insulin-secreting tumours are commonest and have been found at all ages, including in a newborn child (Salinas et al. 1968). Children are also recorded in small numbers amongst cases of gastrin-secreting tumours. Both benign and malignant tumours occur, and they have similar pathological and behavioural characteristics to the much commoner adult examples. With better availability of specific antibodies for immunocytochemical use, practice now has moved towards classification of islet-cell tumours according to their secretory product as well as by traditional morphological and staining characteristics (Jones and Dawson 1977; Nieuwenhuijzen Kruseman et al. 1978; Larsson 1978). A proportion of cases of islet-cell tumour show a familial incidence, and many are coincident with abnormalities in other endocrine tissues. This should be considered particularly when more than a single tumour is found in the pancreas and when islets of abnormal appearance are found in the surrounding gland (see p. 587).

4. Multiple Endocrine Neoplasia Syndrome

The syndromes of multiple endocrine neoplasia are familial disorders in which hyperplasia or tumours involve more than one endocrine gland. The pathogenesis of the syndromes is unknown, but they are apparently disorders principally affecting structures

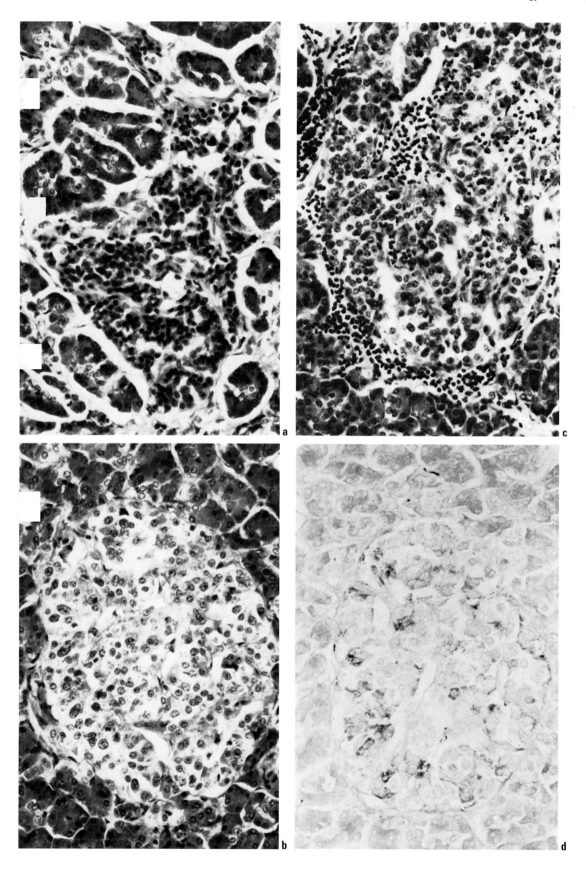

of neuroectodermal origin and are inherited as an autosomal dominant trait. Their clinical manifestations reflect the local effects and the effects of secretory activity of the particular tumours involved, this usually being the production of the hormone normal for the cell of origin, though sometimes there is ectopic hormone secretion. Evidence of multiple organ involvement may be present at the outset, but in some cases disease of a single organ may be the only apparent abnormality and in others there may be several years' delay in the appearance of disease in the different organs. Although these are uncommon diseases expression of the abnormality is the rule, so that the identification of a case may bring to light a large number of cases amongst relatives. In some instances, however, no further cases are found amongst the family members of a patient with an apparently typical multiple endocrine syndrome and some of these are undoubtedly examples of mutation.

4.1. Type 1 (Wermer's Syndrome)

The anterior pituitary, parathyroids, and pancreatic islets are the structures most commonly involved in type 1 (Wermer 1974). Adenoma of the pituitary, usually single, is recorded in about half the studied cases. This may be of acidophil, basophil, chromophobe or mixed-cell type, and may interfere with the normal function of the pituitary or produce gigantism and acromegaly or Cushing's disease as a consequence of secretory activity. The parathyroids and pancreas are found to be abnormal in the great majority of cases. Nodular chief-cell hyperplasia involving all four parathyroids is usual, though adenomas have been described. The pancreatic islets (Fig. 13.14) show hyperplasia that may be diffuse, multiple adenomas, and carcinomas. All these changes may be found in the same gland. The tumours may be several centimetres in diameter or may be microscopical, in which case distinction from

a large hyperplastic islet can be difficult. They may be found outside the pancreas in the wall of the duodenum and stomach. The histological and ultrastructural appearance of the tumour is similar to that seen in sporadic cases, except that a pronounced ribbon pattern is strongly suggestive of genetic disease (Wermer 1974). The distinction between some of the benign and malignant tumours can be problematic. The most frequent clinical manifestations of islet-cell tumour are the Zollinger–Ellison syndrome and hypoglycaemia. Immunohistochemical studies have also identified tumours that contain glucagon and pancreatic polypeptide.

Benign and malignant tumours in other organs have been recorded in some families with sufficient frequency to allow their inclusion as a part of the syndrome. Most notable amongst these are carcinoid tumours and adrenal cortical abnormalities. Carcinoids have been described in bronchi, gut, pancreas, and thymus. Micronodular and diffuse hyperplasia and adenomas of the adrenal cortex are common and may be accompanied by hyperaldosteronism or Cushing's syndrome. Diffuse adrenocortical hyperplasia with Cushing's disease of pituitary origin also occurs. Cases that have developed lipomas of the subcutaneous tissues and viscera and with adenomas and carcinomas of the large bowel are also described.

The commonest clinical manifestations in childhood and adolescence are hypoglycaemic attacks, diarrhoea, and peptic ulceration from pancreatic tumours, and amenorrhoea associated with a pituitary adenoma. Hypercalcaemia is very frequently found but symptomatic hyperparathyroidism is unusual at this age.

4.2. Type 2

The specific association in families of medullary carcinoma of the thyroid with phaeochromocytoma was first recognized by Williams (1965), and the rare further association with mucosal neuromas was described by Williams and Pollock (1966). The parathyroids may also be abnormal, usually showing primary nodular chief-cell hyperplasia. Parathyroid abnormality is sometimes found in cases of sporadic medullary carcinoma of the thyroid but in these cases is not accompanied by elevated levels of serum calcium (Melvin et al. 1972). The simultaneous occurrence of medullary carcinoma of the thyroid, phaeochromocytomas usually in both adrenals, and parathyroid abnormality has been designated multiple endocrine neoplasia type 2 (Steiner et al. 1968). Multiple, and usually bilateral, medullary carcinomas and phaeochromocytomas occur simultaneously in most cases, though in a

Fig. 13.13. a–d Histological changes in islets of Langerhans in insulin-dependent diabetes mellitus of recent onset. **a** Ill-defined islet of irregular outline composed of shrunken cells with small uniform darkly staining nuclei. (H and E; 300 ×) **b** Conspicuous islet, smooth in outline, composed of large cells forming cords separated by prominent capillaries. The nuclei have a well-defined chromatin pattern. There are several unusually large nuclei and small haematoxyphil bodies can be seen in the cytoplasm of many of the cells. (H and E; 300 ×) **c** An infiltrate of inflammatory cells (insulitis), principally lymphocytes with a few polymorphs, may occasionally be seen within and adjacent to some islets. (H and E; 300 ×) **d** Marked decrease in number and intensity of staining of beta cells. (Aldehyde fuchsin; 300 ×)

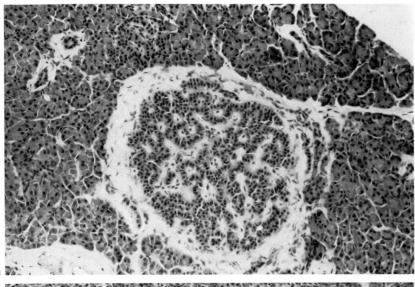

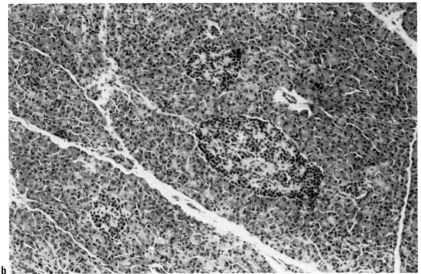

Fig. 13.14. a and b Sections from a partial pancreatectomy specimen from a boy aged 10 years with MEN type I. Episodes of hypoglycaemia had occurred during the previous year. Several small discrete islet cell tumours were visible to the naked eye in the resected pancreas. In addition there were several microscopical islet cell tumours (a; H and E; 150×), and unusually large but otherwise apparently normal islets. (b; H and E; 120×)

small proportion the thyroid or adrenal lesion alone may occur. The adrenal involvement may be very asymmetrical but if one gland is clinically involved the other will almost certainly be found to be abnormal on microscopical examination, and should also be removed. Hypercalcaemia is found in less than 50% of cases and the incidence of parathyroid abnormality is not certain. Keiser et al. (1973), however, found parathyroid hyperplasia or adenoma in most of their 45 patients.

The cases in which mucosal neuromas occur together with medullary carcinoma and phaeochromocytoma have been variously designated multiple endocrine neoplasia type 2b and type 3. This constellation of abnormalities is inherited separately from the other familial medullary carcinoma cases, and is the rarest form seen. The neuromas are most prominent on the eyelids, lips, and margin of the tongue, and are accompanied by diffuse enlargement of the lips and sometimes prognathism, producing a characteristic facial appearance (Schimke et al. 1968; Gorlin et al. 1968). Slit-lamp examination reveals abnormal corneal nerves. Ganglioneuromatosis (Fig. 14.15) throughout the gastrointestinal tract is often found, sometimes with accompanying diverticulosis and megacolon. The hereditary nature of this subtype is seen in only a minority of cases, so that most would appear to be the result of mutation.

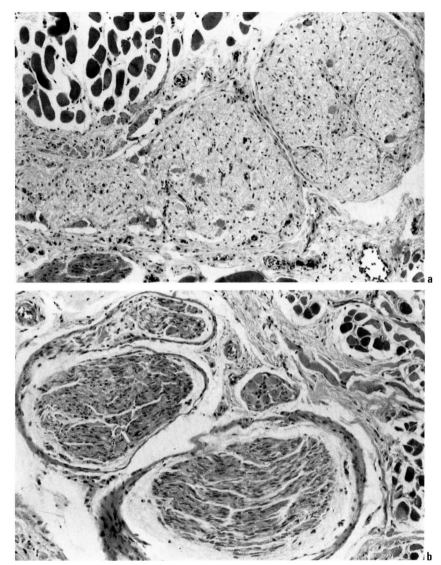

Fig. 13.15. a Ganglioneuromatosis involving the myenteric plexus of the upper oesophagus in a patient with the complete form of familial medullary carcinoma syndrome. (H and E; 120 ×) **b** Similar neuromas in the tongue produced irregular small projections on the surface. (H and E; 120 ×)

A further factor contributing to the rarity of this group is the much earlier presentation than in other forms of medullary carcinoma syndromes. Many patients with this condition die of their thyroid carcinoma whilst still young (Khairi et al. 1975; Norton et al. 1979).

5. Parathyroid Glands

The parathyroids appear as solid cellular proliferations of the third and fourth pharyngeal pouch epithelium, and can be identified by the 7th gestational week. The solid epithelial masses quickly separate from their pharyngeal pouch, those derived from the fourth arch remaining closely related to the lateral lobes of the thyroid whilst those from the third arch associate with the migrating thymus and come to lie close to the inferior poles of the thyroid. The cells that make up the parathyroids of infants and children are similar to those of adult glands except that oxyphil cells are not found much before 5 years of age and thereafter occur as occasional single cells until after the age of 10 years, when small clusters begin to appear. Fat is not found incorporated in the infant parathyroid, appearing during early childhood as isolated fat cells and increasing in amount with age, eventually forming small areas of fatty tissue.

Production and release of parathormone are modulated directly by the blood level of ionized calcium. There is little storage of hormone in the normal gland. The present understanding of the synthesis, structure and actions of parathormone are fully discussed by Habener and Potts (1978) and Martin et al. (1979).

Various aspects of parathyroid development, histology, and anomalies are dealt with in the several publications by Gilmour and associates (1937, 1938, 1939, 1941) (see Table 13.1).

Table 13.1. Parathyroid weights[a]

	Mean combined weight of parathyroid glands (mg)	
	Male	*Female*
Birth to 3 months	6.2	8.8
3 months to 1 year	25.4	15.6
1 year to 5 years	34.9	22.3
6 years to 10 years	49.7	63.3
11 years to 20 years	91.9	95.7

[a]From Gilmour JR, Martin WJ (1937) The weight of the parathyroid glands. *J Pathol Bacteriol* 44: 431.

5.1. Developmental Abnormalities

One and sometimes more of the parathyroid glands are found in an ectopic site in about 10% of individuals. The inferior pair of glands is most commonly involved and is usually found in association with the superior poles of the thymus in the upper mediastinum. It is common to find a small amount of thymic tissue adjacent to the normally situated inferior parathyroids. Occasionally a parathyroid is found embedded within the thyroid, and cases of parathyroid adenoma located posterior to the oesophagus have been described.

Apparent failure of development involving a parathyroid appears to be an uncommon event. Gilmour (1938) found only three parathyroids in 6% of his post-mortem series and was of the opinion that in most of these cases his dissection had failed to locate a gland. Supernumerary concentrations of parathyroid tissue are common, having been detected in 3 of 14 fetuses (Gilmour 1941) and may be found in an ectopic location. Hypoplasia or agenesis involving all parathyroids is associated with the DiGeorge syndrome and also occurs as an accompaniment of congenital malformation in some cases, most conspicuously in those with anomalies involving the head and neck (p. 540).

Cysts involving the parathyroids are usually found in adults as a secondary change in an adenoma. Developmental cysts are rare and most are probably derived from a pharyngeal pouch remnant, with the parathyroid being involved by association. Microscopical cysts or vesicles are a normal histological feature.

5.2. Hypoparathyroidism and Hypocalcaemia

Rapid development of hypocalcaemia involves tetany and convulsions. In more prolonged hypocalcaemia tetany is latent rather than overt and complaints of weakness and pins and needles in the extremities are typical. Chronic hypocalcaemia results in changes in epidermal structures manifesting as scaly, coarse skin with patchy hyperpigmentation. There is a liability to chronic cutaneous and mucosal candiasis. The hair is brittle and there is a tendency for a patchy loss to occur. The nails show deformity with horizontal ridging and become heaped-up when affected by chronic fungous infection. Prolonged hypocalcaemia is likely to be accompanied by soft-tissue calcification, particularly involving the basal ganglia of the brain, the retina, and subcutaneous tissue. The eyes may also be affected by cataracts. Developing teeth are deformed as a result of irregular hypoplasia of the enamel, producing transverse ridging and a predisposition to caries. Tooth eruption is delayed and radiographs show lack of calcification in the tooth root and in some cases a thickening of the lamina densa of the adjacent jaw bone.

The different causes of hypocalcaemia fall broadly into those resulting in hypocalcaemia manifesting in infancy and a second group of causes relevant to hypocalcaemia of later onset. Tetany in the neonatal period can be a complication of prematurity and may follow abnormal labour and pregnancy, where it may result from parathyroid injury. A large phosphate load caused by feeding with an unmodified cows' milk formula can result in a sufficient depression of the calcium concentration to produce tetany, typically about the end of the 1st week of life (Tsang et al. 1973). Hypocalcaemia is likely to complicate conditions primarily producing low blood levels of magnesium. This type has proved more difficult to correct, probably because of the permissive role of magnesium in allowing parathormone to exert its effects (Anast et al. 1972; Suh et al. 1973). A number of instances of neonatal tetany have been described, with onset usually between the 2nd and 20th postnatal days, where the mother has been shown to have primary hyperparathyroidism (Johnstone et al. 1972). On occasion several offspring have been affected (Hutchin and Kessner 1964). A rare sex-linked recessive form of hypoparathyroidism affects males in the first week or early months of life (Peden 1960).

Hypoparathyroidism occurring in later childhood is seen most commonly between 5 and 15 years of age though symptoms may be manifest in infancy. It is usually described as 'idiopathic', but its frequent association with Addison's disease, hypothyroidism, pernicious anaemia, steatorrhoea and diabetes mellitus is well documented, suggesting an autoimmune disorder. Many of the cases have a family history of hypoparathyroidism with or without disturbance involving other endocrine glands (Gorodischer et al. 1970). Circulating antibodies to parathyroid were found in 38% of the patients with idiopathic hypoparathyroidism studied by Blizzard et al. (1966) and in 26% of their patients with Addison's disease without evidence of hypoparathyroidism. Six percent of their controls also had detectable antibodies. In these autoimmune cases, *Candida albicans* infection of the nails and mouth is particularly common and can spread to become generalized. The infection usually antedates the clinical development of hypoparathyroidism and is not affected by restoring the serum calcium concentration to normal. In cases where hypoparathyroidism and autoimmune disorders involving other endocrines are associated it is usual for the parathyroid disturbance to be the first to develop. Addison's disease is the commonest associated disorder. The pathological changes in the parathyroids in these cases have not been widely studied. In some cases no parathyroid tissue could be found. Almost total replacement by fat and also fibrosis with lymphocytic infiltration have been described (Drake et al. 1939; Chu Hsien-Yi et al. 1964).

5.3. Pseudohypoparathyroidism

The syndrome of unresponsiveness of target organs to parathormone and associated characteristic somatic features, particularly short metacarpals and metatarsals, diminished height and rounded face was first described by Albright et al. (1942). The disorder appears to be transmitted as an autosomal recessive trait. The hypocalcaemia is the result of failure of 1-hydroxylation of 25-hydroxy vitamin D in the renal tubules through failure of activation of renal cyclic AMP by parathormone (Drezner et al. 1976). The defect in bone growth results from dyschondroplasia with early fusion of epiphyses and is regarded as an independent genetic trait. Evidence of hyperparathyroid bone disease is found in some cases only, so that the unresponsiveness to para-

thormone usually also involves the skeleton. It might be expected that the parathyroid glands would be hyperplastic. In those few cases in which the parathyroids have been examined histological evidence of hyperplasia has been described in some whilst in others they have been regarded as normal. Raised blood levels of parathormone have been found with normal suppression on restoring the blood calcium to normal (Chase et al. 1969). Cases in which there is evidence of disturbance involving other endocrine glands have been described. These include abnormal thyrotropin and prolactin secretion and decreased responsiveness of the thyroid to thyrotropin (Zisman et al. 1969; Marx et al. 1971; Werder et al. 1975; Carlson et al. 1977). The formation of bone in subcutaneous tissue is commonly present and is probably not directly related to the functional hypoparathyroidism.

Occasional cases involving alternative abnormalities in the synthesis and actions of parathormone have been described and have become entangled incidentally in some of the most confusing nomenclature (summarized by Williams 1978). The distinctive clinical features in pseudohypoparathyroidism and idiopathic hypoparathyroidism are summarized and contrasted by Bronsky et al. (1958).

5.4. Hyperparathyroidism

A sustained increase in secretion of parathormone may be primary or, alternatively, be a response to a depressed level of plasma calcium. Such responsive hyperparathyroidism may eventually lead to the development of parathyroid tumours and autonomous production of excessive amounts of parathormone with resulting hypercalcaemia (tertiary hyperparathyroidism).

5.4.1. Primary Hyperparathyroidism

5.4.1.1. Infantile Hyperparathyroidism with Parathyroid Hyperplasia. A few examples of diffuse, nonnodular, chief-cell hyperplasia involving all or several of the parathyroids have been recorded in infants, with evidence of inheritance as an autosomal recessive characteristic in some cases (Hillman et al. 1964; Bradford et al. 1973; Fretheim and Gardborg 1965). Children with this disorder present with hypotonia, dehydration, feeding difficulties, and respiratory distress resulting from impaired development and fractures of the rib cage. There is pronounced osteitis fibrosa and radiological evidence of generalized lack of skeletal mineralization with subperiosteal resorption.

5.4.1.2. Primary Nodular Hyperplasia. Some cases of primary nodular hyperplasia occur in childhood, mostly in older children and adolescents, though neonatal cases have been recorded (Spiegel et al. 1977). Many are genetically determined and inherited as autosomal dominant disorders. In these cases the parathyroid disorder (Fig. 13.16) may be part of the two syndromes of multiple endocrine neoplasia (MEN 1 and MEN 2), whilst in other cases it is inherited without other endocrine anomalies. Typically, all the parathyroid glands are enlarged and reddish-brown in colour. There may be a marked difference in size amongst the glands in an individual case, one or more of which may be of normal weight. The normal-sized glands may not be obviously abnormal microscopically. Histologically the enlarged glands contain multiple nodules composed of chief cells arranged in a variety and mixture of patterns—solid, trabecular, and follicular. Occasional nodules may consist predominantly of oxyphil cells. If one nodule dominates the resulting appearance is difficult to distinguish from an adenoma. It has been suggested that the presence of intracellular fat serves to distinguish normal from hyperplastic parathyroid glands (Roth and Gallagher 1976). The intrafollicular material has the characteristics of amyloid in a proportion of cases of primary hyperplasia (Leedham and Pollock 1970).

5.4.2. Secondary Hyperplasia

Some degree of parathyroid hyperplasia occurs in any condition in which the ionized calcium concentration tends to be decreased. Formerly the commonest cause was rickets from dietary vitamin D deficiency, a problem that has re-emerged among the Asian immigrant population in Britain. Disease with accompanying malabsorption and severe hep-atic disease have a similar effect. Probably the commonest cause is chronic renal disease, in which phosphate retention is accompanied by a compensatory lowering of calcium levels. This metabolic disturbance is in part the result of an impaired renal excretory capacity but also reflects reduced hydroxylation of 25-hydroxy vitamin D to form the active 1-25-dihydroxy vitamin D, which normally takes place in the renal tubular epithelium. The normal phosphaturic response to parathormone is mediated through the action of the activated vitamin D. A few cases of intrauterine hyperparathyroidism secondary to maternal hypoparathyroidism have been described (Bronsky et al. 1968; Landing and Kamoshita 1970; Gorodischer et al. 1970).

In secondary hyperplasia the parathyroid glands are modestly enlarged and are paler than normal. Microscopically they are uniformly hypercellular, being composed of normal chief cells. Where the stimulus to hyperplasia has been severe and prolonged one or more of the parathyroids may develop one or several nodules and will then appear similar to the parathyroids from cases of primary nodular hyperplasia. The clinical history and chemical changes are important in the interpretation of such cases. In chronic renal disease the size of the parathyroids is generally considered to increase in proportion to the duration of the renal failure. More recently, however, in children maintained on long-term haemodialysis parathyroid size has been observed to be related to the amount of calcium loss during dialysis and was independent of bone disease which correlated with duration of renal disease (Gruskin et al. 1976). Autonomous hyperparathyroidism supervening on responsive hyperplasia (tertiary hyperparathyroidism) appears to be rare in childhood.

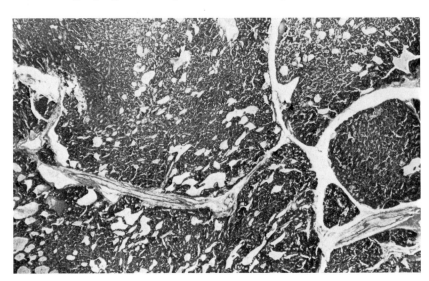

Fig. 13.16. Nodular chief-cell parathyroid hyperplasia in a woman with MEN type 1 manifest in hypercalacaemia, secondary amenorrhoea and an enlarged pituitary fossa. (H and E; 20 ×)

5.5. Other Causes of Hypercalcaemia

5.5.1. Tumours

Hypercalcaemia has been recorded with many kinds of tumour, either as a result of extensive bony metastasis or through the action of parathormone or parathormone-like substances produced by the tumour. Other bone-mobilizing substances may cause hypercalcaemia, particularly prostaglandin (PGE$_2$), which has osteoclastic activity. Tumours that have been associated with parathormone production in children include some bone tumours, neuroblastoma, rhabdomyosarcoma and a number of cases of leukaemia and lymphosarcoma (Joyaraman and David 1977; Ramsay et al. 1979; Myers 1960; Stapleton et al. 1976; Hutchinson et al. 1978).

5.5.2. Iatrogenic Causes

Both vitamins D and A in excess cause hypercalcaemia and, in vitamin faddism, are likely to be taken together. Thiazide diuretics possibly act through potentiation of the calcaemic effect of parathyroid hormone.

Idiopathic hypercalcaemia of infancy with 'elfin facies', mental retardation and supravalvular aortic stenosis appears to be part of the spectrum of Williams' syndrome, in which there is evidence for hypersensitivity to vitamin D. Involvement of more than one member in a family has been observed. Excessive parenteral and dietary intake of vitamin D in infancy has been considered the cause of some cases of supravalvular aortic stenosis and the infantile hypercalcaemia syndrome. Immobilization of an adolescent in the treatment of such problems as fractures and extensive burns can result in a rise in blood calcium level within 4 or 5 days. The rise reaches a peak by the end of 1 week and although in most cases the changes are slight, levels as high as 4.5 mmol per litre have occurred.

Benign familial hypercalcaemia is a rare disorder that is apparently inherited as an autosomal dominant trait. The hypercalcaemia is of modest degree and has no apparent ill effects. The underlying disorder is obscure.

Hypercalcaemia is observed in a small proportion of cases of thyrotoxicosis, probably as a direct effect of thyroid hormone excess on bone resorption (Rude et al. 1976). In Addison's disease hypercalcaemia may occur.

5.6. Effects of Hypercalcaemia

Hypercalcaemia produces clinical manifestations that include muscular weakness with a combination of irritability, listlessness, and lethargy. Examination shows hypotonia and hyperextensible joints, and in young infants there is retardation of all forms of motor development. The bowel is atonic with resulting constipation. Metabolic effects include polyuria as a direct effect of excess calcium or renal tubular water handling. In older children, thirst will tend to compensate for the polyuria unless prevented by nausea, whilst dehydration is likely to occur in infants and in part may be due to feeding difficulties. Nocturnal enuresis may be the first complaint. A rise in blood urea results from the defective renal tubular function and dehydration. Bradycardia and shortening of the Q–T interval on the ECG may be seen.

Metastatic calcification may occur and can involve the conjunctiva and superficial cornea, joint ligaments, cartilage, blood vessels, lungs, and gastric mucosa. In children the kidneys are more often affected by interstitial calcification than stone formation and their involvement results in impairment of function.

6. Pituitary

6.1. Development

The pituitary develops from two separate ectodermal layers. The *infundibular process* forms from an evagination of the floor of the diencephalon and comes to comprise the *median eminence* at the base of the hypothalamus, a connecting neural stalk or *infundibular stem* and the posterior lobe of the pituitary or *pars nervosa*. Rathke's pouch is a dorsal evagination of the primitive stomatodeum. The developing sphenoid bone pinches off the neck of the evagination, leaving a vesicle. The cells of the anterior wall of the vesicle proliferate to form the *adenohypophysis* comprising the *pars distalis* and the *pars tuberalis*. The posterior wall forms the *pars intermedia*, which is vestigial in man, giving rise to the posterior lobe basophils and a group of colloid-filled cysts. The cavity of Rathke's pouch collapses, leaving the hypophyseal cleft, a colloid-filled space between the pars distalis and pars intermedia. Growth hormone has been demonstrated as early as the 9th week of development. A residuum of the neck of Rathke's pouch sometimes persists in the sphenoid bone and is regularly present in the form of clusters of small pituitary type cells, sometimes including nests of squamous cells in the dorsal pharyngeal wall, and known as the pharyngeal pituitary. It is unlikely that these structures serve any pituitary function.

The blood supply to the pituitary is complex with the superior hypophysial arteries, one from each internal carotid, supplying the median eminence and upper pituitary stalk by way of numerous special vascular structures, the gomitoli. The capillaries drain into portal sinuses that run down the surface of the stalk to supply the capillary sinuses that ramify between the cells of the anterior lobe. The final venous drainage is into local dural venous sinuses. The posterior lobe and the lower infundibular stem receive blood from a pair of inferior hypophysial arteries. The effect of this vascular arrangement is to allow releasing and inhibiting hormones produced in cells of the hypothalamic nuclei and conveyed to their axon terminals in the median eminence, to be transferred in the portal blood to target cells in the anterior pituitary. Axons from neurones of the supraoptic and paraventricular nuclei of the hypothalamus pass into the posterior pituitary where their neurosecretions, antidiuretic hormone and oxytocin, are stored prior to release into the blood stream.

6.2. Developmental Abnormalities

Developmental abnormalities of the pituitary are rare and range from harmless separation of the two component parts ('dystopia of the neurohypophysis'; Lennox and Russell 1951) to ectopia (Weber et al. 1977), hypoplasia, and aplasia, usually in association with abnormalities of the brain and skull with clinically obvious external defects (Fig. 13.17; Sadeghi-Nejad et al. 1974; Lundberg and Gemzell 1966). In anencephaly the anterior pituitary is present but small, and being deprived of normal hypothalmic connections is assumed not to function. The constituent cells show electron microscopical evidence of differentiation into the various anterior pituitary cell types. The failure of full development of the fetal zone of the adrenal cortex in this condition is ascribed to lack of pituitary stimulus. There is, however, no notable defect in the development of the thyroid. In holoprosencephaly and septo-optic dysplasia there is failure of pituitary hormone production that often involves growth hormone alone, though sometimes several or all of the anterior and posterior pituitary hormones may be deficient.

Failure of normal growth in childhood is found to be related to growth hormone deficiency in 3%–12% of cases. In about a half of these cases the defect is the result of a local pituitary lesion and there is then usually additional evidence of deficiency of other pituitary hormones or disturbance to local structures. Pituitary hypoplasia is a rare cause, most cases being related to tumours of the pituitary and adjacent structures or other locally destructive lesions such as eosinophil granuloma, tuberculous infection, and autoimmune destruction. Ischaemic necrosis following head injury and birth trauma is rare. In the remaining half no pituitary cause is found and these cases are classed as idiopathic. They are mostly sporadic, but in some instances there is a family history with autosomal recessive inheritance. The growth hormone deficiency may be complete or partial and is usually the sole deficiency in the familial group, whereas in about half the remaining idiopathic cases there is associated deficiency of other pituitary hormones. Thus sexual development may also be impaired and thyroid and adrenal function can be deficient. There are very few post-

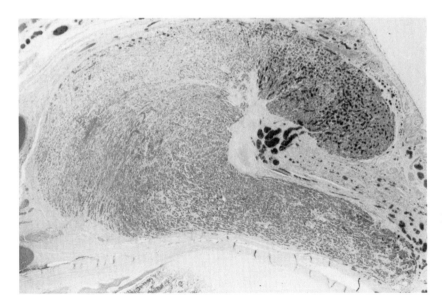

Fig. 13.17. A well-organized mass of anterior pituitary tissue from an anencephalic monster. The base of the skull lies below the gland nodule without forming a fossa. There is a covering of disorganised vascular glial tissue. (H and E; 20 ×)

mortem studies available on the pituitary and hypothalamus in idiopathic cases. The whole pituitary gland tends to be small in dwarfism from any cause, with little evidence of selective depletion in somatotrophs (Russfield and Reiner 1957), though this has been described (Hewer 1944). Evidence thus favours an abnormality involving the hypothalamic nuclei, a suggestion supported by the observation that injection of thyrotropin-releasing hormone (TRH) provokes normal release of TSH in cases with associated thyrotrophin deficiency. Rare cases have been described in which there is evidence of production of an abnormal growth hormone or failure of induction of peripheral somatomedin generation.

There are several lesions that arise from persisting developmental structures that may destroy the pituitary or interfere with its function and compress surrounding structures. Craniopharyngioma is the commonest tumorous lesion. Most are suprasellar in location, with more than half presenting in childhood and adolescence and rare cases being recorded in the newborn (Iyer 1952; Gass 1956; Tabaddor et al. 1974) (p. 198). In instances where part of the tumour occupies the sella turcica greater damage is caused to the pituitary, with resulting hypopituitarism and hypopituitary dwarfism. Suprasellar and dumb-bell cysts are considered to originate from nests of squamous cells commonly found near the junction of the stalk with the pars distalis in adults (Erdheim 1904) and in the newborn (Goldberg and Eshenbaugh 1960). Intrasellar cysts are believed to develop from the hypophyseal cleft that represents the remnant of the cavity of Rathke's pouch. Remnants of the compressed pituitary are found in the outer part of the wall of intrasellar cysts and there is usually at least a partial lining of cuboidal ciliated epithelium. The cyst contents are either fluid or inspissated and discoloured from old haemorrhage. Rare tumours include teratomas of typical and 'atypical pinealoma' types and dermoid and epidermoid cysts that must be distinguished from teratomas in the case of the former whilst the latter should probably be included with the craniopharyngiomas (Russell and Rubinstein 1977a).

6.3. Inflammatory Lesions

Acute hypophysitis can occur as part of a septicaemia or pyaemia and as an extension of infection of the leptomeninges and local air sinuses. The pituitary may be involved diffusely or the inflammation may be localized, most commonly affecting the anterior lobe. Chronic infective disease of the meninges may affect the pituitary either by direct extension of the infection leading to de-

struction or as a result of inflammatory damage to the pituitary stalk. Causes include tuberculosis, coccidiomycosis, and histoplasmosis.

Autoimmune hypophysitis is typically a disease that affects middle-aged and elderly women, but occasionally cases occur in childhood. The process usually involves the anterior lobe only and in most cases giant-cell granulomas are a conspicuous feature, with diffuse lymphocytic and plasma cell infiltration in the intervening pituitary tissue. In some cases there is a diffuse lymphocytic infiltrate with a small proportion of plasma cells but no granulomas.

In Hand–Schüller–Christian disease there is usually evidence of disturbance of neurohypophyseal function. The accumulation of cholesterol-containing macrophages in the sphenoid bone and dura and in the basal leptomeninges, pituitary stalk and its posterior lobe produces erosion of the bone and a yellowish-grey thickening of the soft structures.

Both the anterior and posterior lobes of the pituitary are involved in Hunter–Hurler disease. The cytoplasm of the constituent cells, particularly of the acidophils, become distended by the accumulation of mucopolysaccharide (Schochet et al. 1974) but it is unusual for there to be any evidence of functional disturbance.

In cases of fatal head injury subcapsular haemorrhage and necrosis of both pituitary lobes is a common finding and is often independent of rupture of the stalk. Injury to the hypothalamus may also occur. Similar, though perhaps less severe, lesions in those surviving injury occur, but evidence of anterior pituitary dysfunction is only occasionally documented (Paxson and Brown 1976; Winternitz and Dzur 1976; Landon et al. 1978; Fleischer et al. 1978; Miller et al. 1980). The recognition of pituitary disturbance as separate from hypothalamic damage is problematic. In cases where rupture of the pituitary stalk has occurred diabetes insipidus develops either immediately or after a latent period. If the rupture occurs below the median eminence there may be recovery of hormone production.

6.4. Adenomas of the Adenohypophysis

Pituitary adenomas are rare before adult life. Traditionally they are classified according to their staining characteristics in histological preparations into chromophobe, acidophil, and basophil. In contrast to the high proportion of apparently nonfunctioning chromophobe tumours amongst adult pituitary adenomas, this type is practically unknown in childhood and adolescence (Russell and Rubinstein 1977b). Growth hormone-producing tumours and corticotrophin-producing tumours are recorded occasionally and are associated with acromegalic gigantism and Cushing's disease, respectively. Sometimes the tumour cells contain few secretory granules and can then appear chromophobe. In a proportion of cases an acidophil adenoma is present as part of the hereditary syndrome of multiple endocrine neoplasia type 1 and nodular chief-cell hyperplasia of the parathyroids and tumours of the pancreatic islets may be simultaneously present or may develop subsequently. The histological and ultrastructural characteristics of childhood pituitary adenomas are similar to the findings in equivalent adult cases, which are described by Doniach (1977). In a large proportion of cases of childhood Cushing's disease treated by adrenalectomy there is subsequent enlargement of the pituitary tumour, sometimes with infiltration of the surrounding bone (Hopwood and Kenny 1977), but truly malignant change is extremely rare (Russell and Rubinstein 1977b).

6.5. Pituitary Changes Reflecting Disease in Target Organs

Impaired function in the various endocrine glands is accompanied by changes in the anterior pituitary consequent to the perturbation of hormone levels or the effects of altered metabolic activity on the pituitary.

In hypothyroidism the pituitary enlarges owing to increased size and numbers of thyrotrophs. These can be found in groups within the median wedge and close to the capsule in the anterior and anterolateral areas and are identified in PAS-stained sections from the presence of PAS-positive droplets and the small number of granules in their cytoplasm (Fig. 13.18). In long-standing untreated hypothyroidism granulated acidophils become less numerous.

Cushing's syndrome is accompanied by characteristic changes in the corticotroph basophils as described by Crooke (1935; Fig. 13.19a). There is enlargement of the nucleus and cytoplasm which loses its granules, acquiring a hyaline, slightly refractile appearance. Degranulation occurs first in the cytoplasm adjacent to the nucleus and in a band in the mid-zone of the cell body and is accompanied by the appearance of large clear vacuoles. Eventually the cells are totally degranulated. Electron microscopy shows that the hyaline cytoplasm contains a feltwork of fine filaments (Porcile and Racadot 1966; Fig. 13.19b). Crooke cell change occurs in response to persistently elevated levels of glucocorticoids whether spontaneous or the result of steroid medication. The cells of basophil adenomas in cases of Cushing's disease do not show Crooke cell change but the corticotrophs in the surrounding pituitary do. In untreated Addison's disease the number of partially degranulated basophils is increased and acidophils are reduced in number (Crooke and Russell 1935). Pregnancy and lactation is accompanied by increase in pituitary weight owing to proliferation of prolactin acidophil cells.

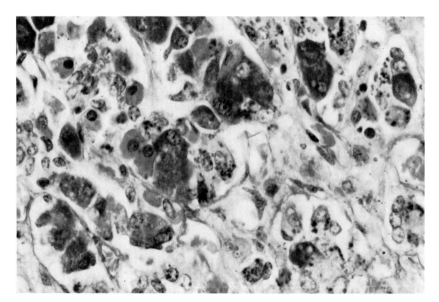

Fig. 13.18. Pituitary from a patient with myxoedema. Several cells with large dark cytoplasmic PAS-positive droplets stand out amongst the large uniformly dark mucoid basophils and lighter acidophils. (PAS, Orange G; 480 ×)

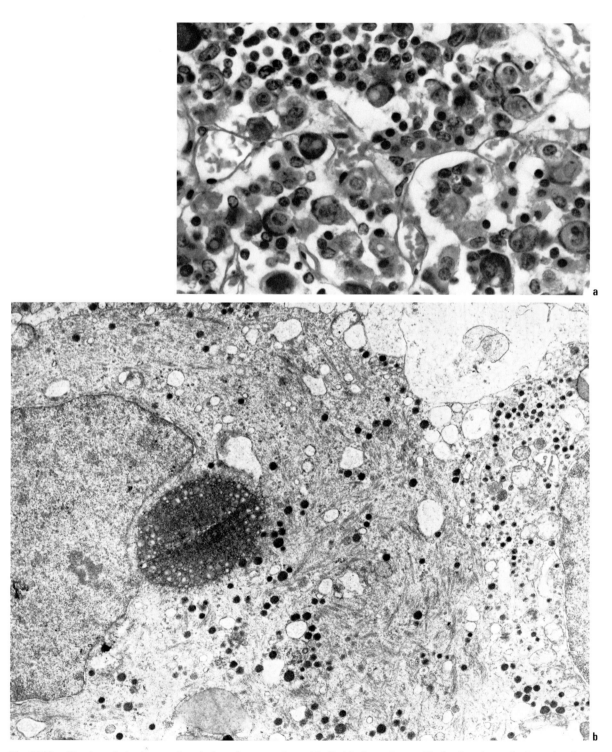

Fig. 13.19. a Crooke cells in the anterior pituitary from a patient with Cushing's syndrome. The hyaline change in the perinuclear cytoplasm and appearance of variable-sized vacuoles is well seen in several of the basophil cells. (PAS, Orange G; 480 ×) **b** Electron photomicrograph of an anterior pituitary basophil cell showing Crooke cell change. The cytoplasm contains arrays of fibrils and the secretory granules are reduced in number. (14 000 ×)

7. Thyroid

7.1. Development

Most, if not the whole of the human thyroid develops from evagination, proliferation, and caudal migration of cells in the mid-line of the ventral fore-gut epithelium, commencing at the end of the 1st month of gestation. A solid, bilobed mass is formed that is attached by a hollow stalk, the thyroglossal duct, to the pharyngeal floor. At the same time a lateral thyroid mass, the ultimobranchial body, forms from the fourth pharyngeal pouch on each side and fuses with the main median mass. The contribution of the lateral thyroid masses to the developing thyroid remains controversial; they commonly show degenerative changes at an early stage and in cases of ectopic sublingual thyroid it is unusual for isotope studies to show any cervical uptake of iodine, so that their capacity to form follicular epithelium appears to be insignificant. Studies in animals have shown that the thyroid C cells, or parafollicular cells, which produce calcitonin are of neural crest origin and migrate to the thyroid via the ultimobranchial bodies (Pearse et al. 1972). It is likely that human thyroid C cells have a similar origin and that the small nests of squamoid and columnar cells commonly found in the lateral thyroid lobes represent remnants of the ultimobranchial body. Further development of the definitive thyroid is by proliferation of its cells in the form of solid cords and later as tubular structures. At about 72 days of gestation an intracytoplasmic vacuole lined by microvilli forms and is followed by the appearance of desmosomes between cell groups, which then extrude their vacuoles to produce an extracellular follicle. Colloid production and the ability to concentrate and bind iodide is established by the 80th gestational day, as has been demonstrated by occasional cases of accidental fetal thyroidectomy resulting from administration of I[131] to the mother for therapeutic purposes occurring only when the isotope has been given after the 70th gestational day (Fisher et al. 1963). These early stages in the development of the thyroid are independent of thyrotrophin, but once colloid and thyroid hormone synthesis is established the activity of the thyroid comes under pituitary control. From the 80-mm stage the thyroid weight is established at about 0.046 % of the body weight, a proportion that persists into adult life.

7.2. Ectopic Thyroid Tissue

Small, and sometimes large, amounts of thyroid tissue are occasionally found outside the normal anatomical site. In most cases the ectopic tissue has been found in the course of the thyroglossal duct as a result of failure of migration early in development. Substantial masses are found most commonly in relation to the posterior part of the tongue (lingual thyroid) and are usually easily visible. Rarely an additional mass separates from the main gland and is found below a lower pole or in the anterior mediastinium with a separate blood supply. It is not very rare to find striated muscle or adipose tissue incorporated in the periphery of a thyroid lobe, and collections of a few thyroid follicles have been demonstrated in cervical lymph nodes in up to 3 % of individuals (Meyer and Steinberg 1969). These might represent developmental 'tangles' or, in the case of the lymph node foci, benign tissue emboli rather than developmental misplacement.

The importance of misplaced thyroid tissue is firstly, that it might be misinterpreted as well-differentiated carcinoma, especially in the case of inclusions within lymph nodes and secondly, a large ectopic mass might represent the total thyroid tissue. This is commonly the case with a lingual thyroid, so that hypothyroidism is a likly consequence of its excision. Most patients with a lingual thyroid present with a swelling in the throat or mouth and many are found to have myxoedema. Both problems are easily corrected with oral thyroxine. Carcinoma has been described and appears to be commoner in lingual thyroids than in normally placed glands (Smithers 1970). It is likely that at least some of the reported cases represent mistaken diagnosis in the presence of a marked hyperplasia accompanying defective thyroid hormone production. Dyshormonogenesis is probably the most frequently associated abnormality, accounting for the observed high incidence of hypothyroidism, goitre and development of tumours.

Development of a cyst from remnants of the thyroglossal duct is common and can present in childhood (Brerton and Symonds 1978) or adult life, and even in old age. They occur in the mid-line between the thyroid and the floor of the mouth, and are often intimately related to the hyoid bone, the mid-portion of which should be resected together with the cyst to ensure comple removal. Excised cysts are found to have a lining of respiratory or squamous epithelium or a mixture of both. They have a thick fibrous capsule, which usually includes a variable amount of lymphoid tissue. Apart from size and the disfigurement these cysts may produce they have a tendency to become infected. Occasionally a papillary carcinoma develops in the course of the thyroglossal duct. Such tumours appear to involve no worse a prognosis than their thyroidal counterpart (Page et al. 1974; Saharia 1975).

7.3. Goitre

7.3.1. Sporadic

Sporadic or euthyroid simple goitre is not seen in young children but does occur after the age of 6 years, most usually in pubertal and adolescent females. There may be an initial phase of diffuse thyroid enlargement prior to the development of a multinodular goitre similar in morphology to its adult counterpart. Routine tests of thyroid function yield normal results.

Areas of endemic goitre where iodine prophylaxis has not been introduced show a high prevalence of goitre in children of both sexes, with cases occurring at birth and in infancy in the most severely affected districts. It is in these severely goitrous districts that endemic cretinism is found. The level of iodine deficiency alone appears to be only a partial explanation of the incidence of thyroid disease, and severe iodine deficiency has been described without the occurrence of goitre or cretinism (Roche 1959). Even in the most severely goitrous areas there is always a proportion of the population that is spared, although the same water supply and diet is shared. The scale of the problem of endemic goitre in world terms is well documented in the detailed survey by Kelly and Snedden (1960). The gross and histological appearances of the thyroid vary according to the severity and duration of the iodine deficiency and also between different goitrous areas. In some endemic cretins the thyroid appears to atrophy during intrauterine development, leaving only a small fibrotic remnant. The more usual endemic goitre shows an initial phase of parenchymal hyperplasia in response to an elevated blood level of TSH. Later the commonly illustrated and often very large colloid goitre that eventually becomes multinodular supervenes.

7.3.2. Dyshormonogenetic

Dyshormonogenetic goitre comprises a group of uncommon conditions in which there is an inborn defect of thyroid hormone synthesis. The subject has been comprehensively reviewed by Stanbury (1978). The capacity of the thyroid to produce hormone is diminished and results in an increased output of thyrotrophine (TSH) from the pituitary, with consequent thyroid hyperplasia. In cases where the block to hormone synthesis is severe goitre and hypothyroidism are present in infancy. In many

instances, however, the disorder is less severe, so that with increased TSH drive the hyperplastic gland maintains sufficient hormone production. The increased demand for thyroid hormone during growth and at puberty often appears to be the time at which a previously compensated defect is revealed by the development of a goitre.

An intrathyroidal metabolic block has been demonstrated to occur at least five steps in hormone synthesis.
1) Failure of iodide trapping
2) Failure of organic binding of intrathyroidal iodide owing to peroxidase deficiency
3) Failure of iodotyrosine coupling
4) Dehalogenase deficiency leading to failure of deiodination of iodotyrosine residues
5) Defect in thyroglobulin synthesis and production of abnormal iodoproteins.

Defects in organification of iodide caused by deficiency in the peroxidase system is by far the commonest of these generally rare inherited disorders and is the defect found in Pendred's syndrome, in which there is an associated perceptive deafness. The disturbance of thyroid function amongst cases of Pendred's syndrome is usually less severe than the apparently similar defect in peroxidase in other cases, so that overt hypothyroidism is uncommon and the size of the goitre is generally modest.

The many cases of Pendred's syndrome that have been described indicate an autosomal recessive mode of inheritance (Nilsson et al. 1964). There appears to be close linkage between the genes determining the thyroidal defect and the deafness, since only very rarely have cases showing the thyroidal disorder alone been described amongst these families. The peroxidase defect may be of variable severity in non-Pendred families so that although a goitre is invariably present not all cases are hypothyroid. The tendency for the hypothyroid cases to be concentrated mainly within certain families suggests genetic heterogeneity in this disorder. An autosomal recessive mode of inheritance also appears to be operating in the other types of dyshormonogenetic goitre and clearly is so in the extensively studied large family of tinkers described by Hutchison and McGirr (1956) and shown to have a defect in deiodinase resulting in goitre, hypothyroidism and, in the majority of their cases, mental retardation.

The identification of the type of defect depends on laboratory investigation. In those with an organification defect iodide is rapidly concentrated in the thyroid but is largely discharged by the subsequent administration of perchlorate, which blocks the iodide-trapping mechanism. In cases with a deiodinase defect the other tissues show the same defect so that a dose of labelled mono- and

di-iodotyrosine injected intravenously can be recovered unchanged in the urine. The rare cases in
which the iodide trap is defective are unable to
concentrate iodide tracer or pertechnetate in their
thyroid. The salivary gland tissues and gastric
mucosa are similarly affected and the consequent
inability to concentrate iodide into their saliva is
demonstrable by cannulation of a salivary gland
duct and administration of labelled iodide. In cases
involving the production of abnormal iodoproteins,
these may be insoluble in butanol and can be
separated by electrophoresis.

The pathological changes in the thyroid are
similar in most of the different types of defect and are
characteristic. The hyperplastic gland can reach an
enormous size, and weights of several hundred
grammes are not uncommon, whilst occasional cases
with a gland weighing in excess of 2 kg have been
recorded. The excised thyroid (see Fig. 13.20) is firm
and fleshy with little visible colloid. Nodules are
almost invariably present and in large specimens
account for the greater part of the mass. Microscopically there is intense parenchymal hyperplasia with
small, usually empty, follicles lined by columnar
epithelium. Pleormorphic nuclei in the thyroid
epithelium are usually prominent, including occasional irregular hyperchromatic giant forms. The
nodules (Fig. 13.21a) vary in size and morphology:
most are cellular, comprising solid and empty
follicles with only a little vascular stroma. Sometimes the stroma is prominent and oedematous and

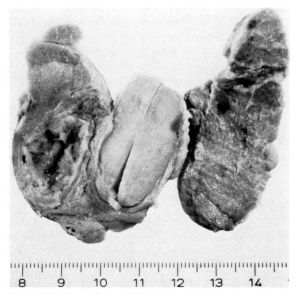

Fig. 13.20. Coronal cut through a dyshormonogenetic goitre
weighing 63 g removed from a 17-year-old clinically euthryoid
female. The cut surface of the thyroid is paler and more fleshy
than normal. An adenoma expands the isthmus and a second
partly cystic adenoma occupies the lower pole on the left. In
addition several small nodules are visible scattered in the parenchyma.

degenerative changes can occur, whilst the epithelial
component can form a wide variety of patterns
including papillary structures and large colloid-filled
follicles (Fig. 13.21b), and may show extreme
nuclear pleomorphism. Individual nodules are
usually surrounded by a well-defined fibrous compression zone but their margin may be ill defined and
the nodular tissue may appear to encroach on the
adjacent parenchyma and even to invade the walls of
blood vessels. The pleomorphism and aggressive
appearances can lead to a diagnosis of carcinoma
but caution is needed in assessment and treatment,
since truly malignant behaviour with metastases is
rare (McGirr et al. 1959; Crooks et al. 1963). In cases
in which an abnormal iodoprotein is found the
pathological changes may be somewhat different
(Kennedy 1969), with a tendency for the goitre to be
much larger with a multicystic appearance to the cut
surface. The colloid in the large cystic follicles
appears pale, fragmented, and filamentous on
microscopic examination. Multiple nodules are
also usually present.

7.4. Cretinism and Hypothyroidism

The term 'cretinism' is liable to some variation in its
use, some authors applying it to all cases of
congenital hypothyroidism, others only to those
where there are associated irreversible mental and
neurological sequelae. Congenital hypothyroidism
is usually divided into cases associated with severe
endemic iodine deficiency and the nonendemic or
sporadic form. This latter group includes a variety of
entities and can be subdivided into goitrous cases
resulting from dyshormonogenesis with a normally
placed or ectopic thyroid and nongoitrous cases
resulting from thyroidal hypoplasia or agenesis. The
reasons for thyroidal hypoplasia and agenesis are
not understood but several specific associations have
been observed, including a high incidence of first-
cousin marriages amongst the parents, a high
incidence of both thyroid antibodies in the mothers'
serum and of hyperthyroidism and hypothyroidism
amongst relatives, and associations with Down's
syndrome and Turner's syndrome. Endemic cretins
may be evident at birth and are found in areas with
extreme iodine deficiency and a high incidence of
goitre, and may account for as much as 8% of the
population (Choufoer et al. 1965; Fiero-Benitez et
al. 1965), and though usually goitrous some cases
occur with a small or impalpable thyroid attributable to associated hypoplasia or agenesis. Sporadic
cretins usually appear normal at birth and tend to be
large, and in those whose cretinism results from
dyshormonogenesis a goitre may be obvious. Reliable early diagnosis is possible by routine assay of

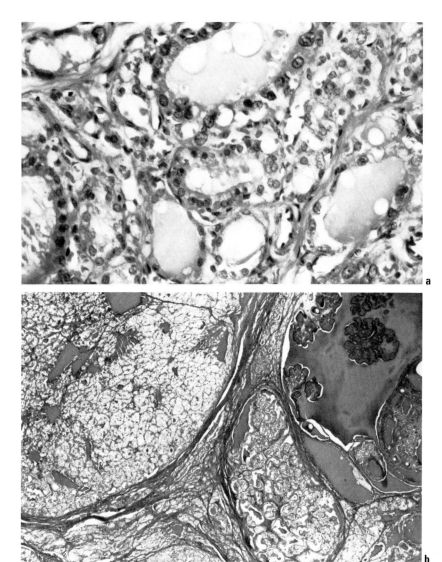

Fig. 13.21. a and **b.** Dyshormono-genetic goitre. **a** There are several nodules with varied histological patterns in the field of view. The parenchyma is diffusely hyper-plastic (*bottom left*). (H and E; 20 ×) **b** Detail from the diffusely hyperplastic parenchyma. The follicles appear empty or contain pale-staining vacuolated colloid. The epithelial cells are cuboid or columnar and in several the nucleus is large and hyperchromatic. (H and E; 300 ×)

serum TSH levels in the neonatal period (Dussault et al. 1975; Hulse et al. 1980). The earliest clinical manifestations of hypothyroidism are undue persistence of physiological jaundice, feeding difficulties and constipation with failure to thrive, an umbilical hernia, and respiratory problems. Later, thickening, dryness and pallor of the skin, poor hair growth, and relative enlargement of the tongue develop, and with time the failure of closure of the fontanelles and retardation of linear growth and mental and motor functions become obvious. The slowing of central nervous development is the most serious effect of fetal and infantile thyroid deficiency, since unlike the other somatic effects, the delay in growth and maturation of the cerebral cortex and cerebellum is irreparable and results in mental defect and motor disturbances in which ataxia, strabismus, severe spasticity, and mild hypotonia are recorded (Hag-

berg and Westphal 1970; Smith et al. 1957; Koenig 1968; Mäenpää 1972). Skeletal abnormalities in infantile and childhood hypothyroidism are constant findings, the appearance of the ossification centres is delayed, and the absence or small size and fragmentation of the distal femoral epiphysis in a full-term infant is good supporting evidence for hypothyroidism (Dorff 1934; Anderson 1973), having otherwise only been described in babies of diabetic mothers (Pedersen and Osler 1958).

Hypothyroidism developing later in childhood is assumed to be caused by autoimmune thyroid destruction in most cases and affects the sexes with equal frequency (Winter et al. 1966). After the age of 3 years intelligence is not usually irreversibly affected but slowing of cerebral activity is a common finding, as are the effects on growth and bone maturation.

7.5. Autoimmune Thyroid Disease

Both Graves' disease and chronic lymphocytic thyroiditis are recorded at all ages. Some 5% of all Graves' disease patients are under 16 years old (Saxena et al. 1964), and more than 40% of childhood nontoxic goitre is attributed to chronic lymphocytic thyroiditis (Saxena and Crawford 1962; Nilsson and Doniach 1964). Girls form the great majority of cases of both disorders. Circulating thyroid antibodies are present, as in the adult disease, and their demonstration is important in diagnosis. A family history of autoimmune thyroid disease is often obtained, and laboratory evidence of thyroid disorder in a parent is very common. The frequent coincidence of autoimmune thyroid disorders in cases with a chromosomal abnormality, notably Down's syndrome (Hollingsworth et al. 1974) and Turner's syndrome (Doniach et al. 1968), is recognized.

The changes seen in the thyroid in childhood Graves' disease are similar to those that occur in adults. There is symmetrical smooth, modest, enlargement as a result of diffuse hyperplasia of the parenchyma, with an accompanying depletion of colloid, markedly increased vascularity, and a focal lymphocytic infiltrate of variable amount in most cases. The systemic manifestations are usually of insidious onset, a rapid pulse rate and accelerated growth rate are often the only changes observed, but enquiry usually draws attention to some falling-off of school performance and an increased appetite. Protuberant exophthalmos from orbital infiltration is rare in children, and sexual maturation is undisturbed in most.

In chronic lymphocytic thyroiditis the gland is enlarged by 2–5 times, usually symmetrically and with a granular firm consistency and easily palpable outline. The development of a goitre is often the only indication of a thyroid abnormality. Clinical or laboratory evidence of hypothyroidism is found in about one-third of the cases (Saxena and Crawford 1962), and in these the goitre tends to be smaller than in euthyroid cases. The more severely hypothyroid patients show diminished growth and may be myxoedematous (Nilsson and Doniach 1964). Only limited studies of the histological changes in the thyroid are available (Clayton and Johnson 1960; Leboeuf and Bongiovanni 1964). There is an extensive interfollicular infiltrate of lymphocytes and formation of lymphoid follicles with germinal centres. The thyroid epithelium is hyperplastic, the follicles small, and the colloid scanty and inspissated. Fibrosis and oxyphil metaplasia are not usually seen except in long-standing cases.

Other inflammatory disorders affecting the thyroid are rare in children. Rare cases of acute bac-terial infection have most often been attributed to β-haemolytic streptococci. De Quervain's subacute giant-cell or granulomatous thyroiditis sometimes occurs in adolescent girls, when it produces the usual symptoms of sore throat and fever followed by painful enlargement of the thyroid, sometimes only one lobe being involved. Symptoms in mild cases resolve in a few days, whilst in others they may last for several months. There is a patchy inflammatory involvement of the thyroid with oedema and an infiltrate of lymphocytes that may sometimes extend through the thyroid capsule. Giant cells and granulomas form at the site of destroyed thyroid follicles and here eventual healing is by fibrosis. There is no permanent disturbance of thyroid function.

7.6. Tumours

Both benign and malignant tumours of the thyroid are less common in children than in adults. This lowered incidence is greater in the case of benign follicular adenomas and colloid nodules, so that the proportion of solitary thyroid nodules presenting in childhood that are found to be carcinomas is comparatively greater and is probably in excess of 20%. Little is known of naturally occurring factors predisposing to the development of thyroid tumours but in the hyperplastic dyshormonogenetic gland adenomas, usually multiple, appear sooner or later. Adenomas are also more common in goitrous districts, and follicular and anaplastic carcinomas may be commoner amongst adults in these areas (Wegelin 1928; Cuello et al. 1969). Papillary carcinoma has a much higher incidence in some countries, notably Japan and Iceland, and it is possible that the high level of dietary iodine may be in part responsible (Williams et al. 1977). Some cases of medullary carcinoma have a familial incidence, with inheritance as a Mendelian autosomal dominant character. There are no data relating to whether chronic lymphocytic thyroiditis has any part to play in the rare cases of childhood thyroid lymphoma. Induction of thyroid tumours in children by irradiation (Winship and Rosvoll 1961; Saenger et al. 1960; Hempelmann et al. 1967) has occurred inadvertently on a wide scale as a consequence of the use of X-rays to shrink the thymus in infants in an attempt to prevent status thymolymphaticus and croup. This was practiced particularly in the United States from about 1925 to 1955, and the thyroid was inevitably included in the treatment field in these small newborn infants. The use of X-rays as a depilatory agent in the management of tinea capitis and for the treatment of inflammatory and other cutaneous lesions has also contributed cases. Both benign and malignant tumours develop with an increased frequency after a period averaging about 9 years, with the risk persisting throughout life. The accident in 1954 in which radioactive fallout from a hydrogen bomb detonated on Bikini affected islanders on nearby Rongelap was followed by the development by 1969 of one carcinoma and small multinodular goitres in 16 of 19 exposed children (Conard et al. 1970). Thyroidal irradiation was principally from radioiodine with a calculated dose to the gland of up to 1400 rads.

Individual thyroid tumours in children are similar pathologically to their adult counterparts, and are classified accordingly (Table 13.2).

Table 13.2. Histological classification of thyroid tumours[a]

1. *Epithelial tumours*
   A. Benign
      Follicular adenoma

   B. Malignant
      Papillary carcinoma
      Follicular carcinoma
      Anaplastic carcinoma
      Medullary carcinoma

2. *Nonepithelial tumours*
   Lymphoma
   Teratoma

[a]Based on the International Histological Classification of Tumours no. 11, World Health Organization.

7.6.1. Adenomas

Adenomas are typically solitary lesions, are encapsulated, and may be subdivided according to whether they are formed from large or small colloid-containing follicles or solid epithelial cords, though no useful purpose is surved by this. Adenomas are usually solitary and mitoses may be easily identified in the more cellular examples. Several sections should be examined to exclude invasion of the capsule and its contained vascular sinuses. This may not be an obvious feature in some of the low-grade follicular carcinomas. Figure 13.22 shows an atypical adenoma.

7.6.2. Carcinoma

The distribution of the different types of carcinoma is a little different when compared with adults. There is an even greater preponderance of papillary tumours, whilst anaplastic carcinomas are uncommon.

7.6.2.1. Papillary. Typically, papillary carcinomas are unencapsulated tumours (Fig. 13.23a), often showing marked central fibrosis and contraction. They are often multifocal. In many cases the primary tumour is less than 2 cm in diameter, and it can be minute. A mixture of neoplastic follicles and papillary structures is usually found (Fig. 13.23b),

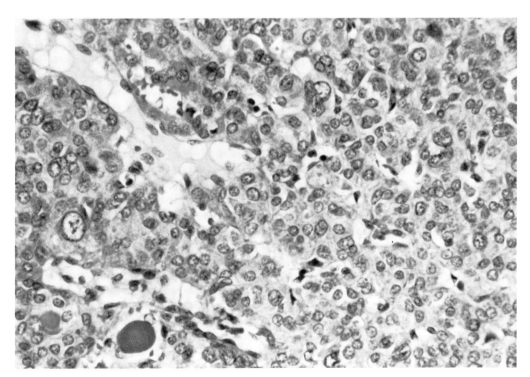

Fig. 13.22. Atypical adenoma. The solid cellular pattern and nuclear pleomorphism are not indications of malignancy. (H and E; 400×)

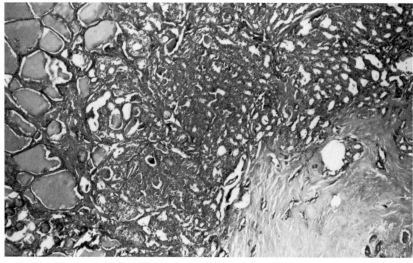

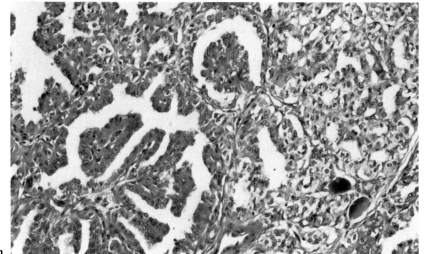

Fig. 13.23. a Papillary carcinoma forming an unencapsulated tumour infiltrating between adjacent thyroid follicles. The centre of the tumour is sclerotic. There are several psammoma bodies at the periphery of the tumour. (H and E; 30×) b A mixture of papillary structures and neoplastic follicles that is typical of papillary carcinoma as a group. The proportions of the two elements vary and cases apparently composed exclusively of one or other can occur. (H and E; 120×)

with a tendency, in children, for a greater proportion of the tumours to have a predominantly papillary pattern, sometimes with numerous psammoma bodies. Cervical lymph node metastases are present in nearly 90% of cases and may be bilateral in up to 25% of cases (Hayles et al. 1963; Harness et al. 1971). Bulky masses are often formed. The prognosis in young people is very good, possibly best in those cases presenting with local lymph node metastases (Woolner et al. 1961). It does not appear to be influenced greatly by any particular current form of treatment (Winship and Rosvoll 1961). Cases in which complete surgical removal of tumour is possible show the best survival figures, but radical surgery may carry high risks of unnecessary damage to recurrent laryngeal nerves and the parathyroids (Richardson et al. 1974). Recorded cases include some that have been observed over several decades, with known metastatic deposits that have shown no evidence of progression.

7.6.2.2. Follicular. Follicular carcinomas are encapsulated tumours that do not form papillary structures. To the naked eye they usually appear solid and fleshy; they are usually more than 2 cm in diameter and as a group they are larger than the papillary carcinomas but similar in size to the adenomas. The majority cannot be distinguished from the more cellular adenomas on the basis of their gross appearance. Invasion of the tumour capsule with penetration of capsular vascular sinuses and, in the more aggressive tumours, invasion of the surrounding thyroid by pushing rounded tumour masses, are the diagnostic features (Fig. 13.24). The invasion of local blood vessels explains the tendency for metastases to involve the lungs and bones. Secondary deposits in cervical lymph nodes are rare. An important source of erroneously diagnosed cases is the inclusion of the often very cellular and sometimes pleomorphic but benign tumours that develop in dyshormonogenetic goitres (see p. 600).

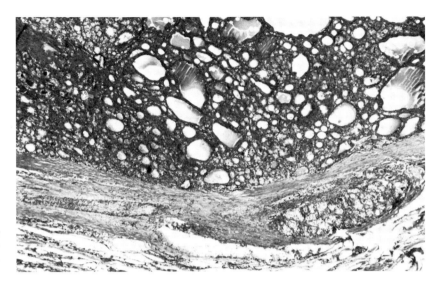

Fig. 13.24. Encapsulated follicular carcinoma identified by tumour invasion into a capsular blood vessel. (H and E; 30×)

Another cause of occasional over-diagnosis is the 'atypical' adenoma with its solid structure, mitoses and, in some cases, markedly pleomorphic nuclei. Microscopical evidence of invasion through the tumour capsule and into blood vessels is conspicuous in the more aggressive cases with a correspondingly greater risk of distant metastases and a worse prognosis. The greater proportion of these tumours are, however, indolent in their behaviour and are recognized by less penetrating invasion of their capsule and involvement only of vascular sinuses within the capsule. Evidence of such invasion in some of these cases requires the examination of many tissue blocks taken to include the capsule, and it is recommended that eight to twelve such blocks should be taken if possible.

7.6.2.3. Medullary. Arising from the parafollicular, or C cells, medullary carcinomas have a distinctive morphology and differ in all respects from the papillary and follicular carcinomas that originate from the follicular epithelium. They probably account for between 5% and 10% of thyroid carcinomas, but an accurate figure is difficult to calculate since recorded personal series are small and liable to distortion if a large pedigree of the inherited variety is included. The genetically determined cases follow an autosomal dominant mode of transmission and can be divided into three subgroups (Williams 1975), one in which thyroid medullary carcinoma alone occurs, a second where medullary carcinoma and phaeochromocytoma are linked, and least commonly, cases with medullary carcinoma, phaeochromocytoma, and multiple mucosal neuromas. In any particular family the subtype to which they belong is maintained from one generation to the next, with the reservation that in those linked with phaeochromocytoma, which is the commonest

form, not all cases will necessarily manifest both the thyroid and adrenal tumours. Sometimes the genetic link can be traced in only two generations. This is particularly so in the cases with neuromatous malformations and suggests a small but definite contribution by mutation. In the familial cases the average age at presentation is lower than in sporadic cases, with the result that relatively more will be seen in children. Another characteristic of the familial type is that in most cases the tumours are multifocal and bilateral, apparently arising in hyperplastic C cell nests.

In about half those cases presenting clinically, local cervical lymph nodes contain metastases. The primary tumour in the thyroid is commonly 2–5 cm in diameter, sharply defined, solid, and often of creamy-yellow colour and gritty when cut. Microscopically the tumour cells are polygonal (Fig. 13.25a) or fusiform and arranged in solid nests and sheets that engulf residual nonneoplastic thyroid follicles. They are broken up by a variable amount of collagenous stroma. Amyloid is usually demonstrable both within the cell masses and in the tumour connective tissue, although on occasions the amount present may be very small. Calcification in amyloid and collagen occurs commonly and can give a characteristic pattern of speckled shadowing on a soft-tissue radiograph. Less common histological patterns occur (Williams et al. 1966), and if amyloid is difficult to demonstrate electron microscopy with demonstration of electron-dense membrane-bound secretory granules can be a help in correct identification. The prognosis in individual cases is difficult to predict. The likelihood of tumour dissemination has been correlated with the presence of cervical lymph node metastases (Woolner et al. 1968) and with evidence of more rapid growth assessed by the finding of mitoses and areas of necrosis, features that are more commonly seen with a pronounced spindle-celled pattern (Fig. 13.25b; Williams et al. 1966). Rapidly fatal cases are uncommon, and even with inoperable or recurrent local disease or distant metastases prolonged survival is more usual.

Calcitonin, the natural product of the C cells, is consistently produced in large quantities by medullary carcinomas. Measurement of levels in the peripheral blood before and after provoked release by alcohol or pentagastrin is a useful test for residual tumour following treatment and for screening of vulnerable members of a family in the genetically determined variants. In some cases additional substances are produced, including ACTH, serotonin, prostaglandin, and histaminase. In as many as a quarter of cases a humoral agent that causes severe watery diarrhoea is produced.

7.6.3. Teratoma of the Neck

Teratomas of the neck are rare tumours; they are usually present at birth, occur equally in the two sexes, are associated with hydramnios in 18% of recorded cases, and occasionally cause obstruction during labour. In the younger age group most are benign, only one case of a malignant teratoma having been recorded in infancy. Distinction between teratomas arising within the thyroid (Fig. 13.26) and those arising in extrathyroidal cervical tissues can be difficult (Silberman and Mendelson 1960).

8. Hormonal Effects of Gonadal Tumours

8.1. Testicular

Except for seminoma a substantial proportion of other germ-cell tumours of the testis occur before adulthood, particularly teratomas, in which extra-embryonic components (yolk sac and trophob-

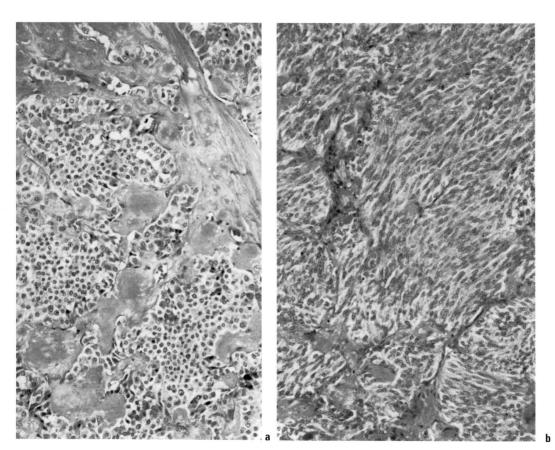

Fig. 13.25. a Medullary carcinoma of polygonal cell type. The tumour cells have granular eosinophilic cytoplasm and are arranged in solid nests separated by fibrous tissue and nodular deposits of amyloid. (H and E; 120 ×) **b** Medullary carcinoma composed of plump spindle cells. Small nodular masses of amyloid are present. (H and E; 120 ×)

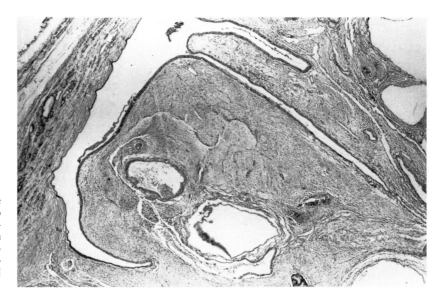

Fig. 13.26. Teratoma within the thyroid removed from a male negro child. The tumour is composed entirely of mature structures of which neuroglia is a prominent solid component. Thyroid follicles are present at the surface of the tumour. (H and E; 20 ×)

last), are prominent histologically. Many of the rare stromal tumours of the testis are seen in childhood. The pathological features and some aspects relating to aetiology and incidence are recorded by Mostofi (1973), and a series of testicular tumours occurring in childhood is recorded by Bormel and Mays (1961).

8.2. Germ Cell Origin

Gynaecomastia occurs in about 30 % of all cases of germ cell tumour (Paulsen 1974), particularly among patients with tumours that include histologically recognizable trophoblast and measurable levels of chorionic gonadotrophin in their blood and urine. Young children form a prominent group of cases, mostly as a result of the occurrence of tumours that consist predominantly of yolk sac or embronal carcinoma at this early age (Giebnink and Ruymann 1974). Pure chorion carcinoma and seminoma have virtually never been recorded before puberty.

8.3. Testicular Stromal Cell Origin

Tumours of interstitial cell (Leydig cell) origin (Fig. 13.27) are rare. In a review of the literature Gabrilove et al. (1975) quote 23 of 94 recorded cases being in children under 15 years of age. In prepubertal cases the tumour is regularly accompanied by virilization and on occasion gynaecomastia develops in addition. Gabrilove et al. (1975) suggest that gynaecomastia may result from disturbance of the normal ratio of concentration of oestrogen to androgen. Gynaecomastia has also been recorded

following administration of methyltestosterone to male eunuchs (McCallagh and Rossmiller 1941). Leydig cell tumours with purely feminizing effects are seen only in adults. Nodules of ectopic hyperplastic adrenal cortical tissue found in relation to the testis in a male infant with congenital adrenal hyperplasia must be distinguished from Leydig cell tumour.

Sertoli cell tumours are usually benign and are most uncommon. Mostofi et al. (1959) found 23 cases recorded in the AFIP (Armed Forces Institute of Pathology) files, ten being under 20 years of age. Weitzner and Gropp (1974) found 22 childhood cases recorded in the literature and added one of their own. Sixteen of these cases were less than 1 year old and in two cases there were tumours in both testes. A testicular swelling was the commonest clinical abnormality. Gynaecomastia or sexual precocity occurred in only a few cases. Examination of the pituitary from an adult dying with a malignant Sertoli cell tumour that had been accompanied by gynaecomastia showed changes interpreted as an indication of hyperplasia of the gonadotrophs (Mostofi et al. 1959).

8.4. Ovarian

Granulosa theca cell tumours of the ovary are uncommon, with approximately 5 % occurring before pubertal age (Lyon et al. 1963) and occasionally even in infancy (Marshall 1965). In most childhood cases the tumours are composed predominantly of granulosa cells. Nonfunctioning and androgen-secreting tumours occur, but the great

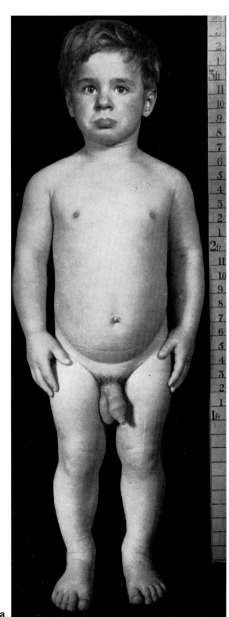

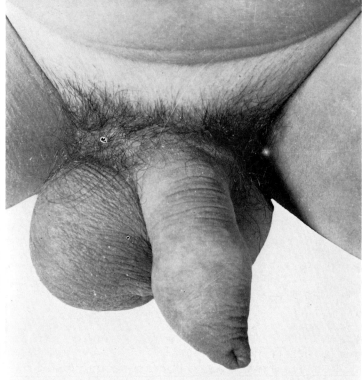

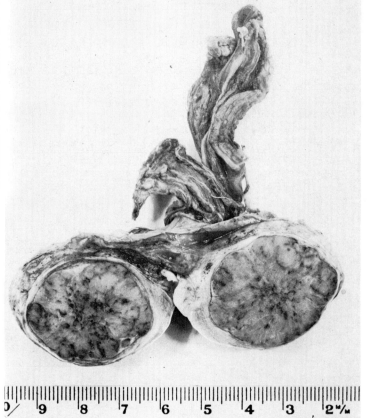

Fig. 13.27. a–c Interstitial cell tumour of the testis in a male aged 2 years 4 months, producing unilateral testicular enlargement, penile development and growth of pubic hair (**a** and **b**). Bisected orchidectomy specimen (**c**) shows the solid sharply circumscribed tumour within the testicular body.

Christopher L. Brown

609

majority produce oestrogens, with resultant development of the breasts and genitalia. The appearance of axillary and pubic hair usually follows, but not invariably. The uterus enlarges and endometrial proliferation may be accompanied by irregular bleeding. The contralateral ovary remains infantile.

Other ovarian stromal tumours are even more of a rarity in children. Hilus (Leydig) cell tumours are recorded by Boivin and Richart (1965), and have been reported in association with gonadal dysgenesis (Warren et al. 1964). Sertoli–Leydig cell tumours (androblastomas), though typically occurring in young women, are rare before menarche (Norris and Jensen 1972). Familial occurrence associated with thyroid adenoma has been recorded in adolescents (Jensen et al. 1974). Both tumours usually produce androgens, resulting in pure virilization before puberty and defeminization in postpubertal girls before overtly virilizing effects.

A substantial proportion of germ-cell tumours of the ovary occur in the first two decades. Forty-four percent of the dysgerminomas in Asadourian's and Taylor's (1969) series were in patients less than 20 years of age. Figure 13.28 shows a dysgerminoma removed from a child. Immature teratoma and embryonal carcinoma are both found predominantly in children and adolescents (Abell et al. 1965). Increased levels of chorionic gonadotrophin in urine and serum suggest that the tumour includes a trophoblastic component and may be accompanied by precocious isosexual development in children, and by menstrual irregularity, amenorrhoea, and breast enlargement in postpubertal cases. Occasionally dysgerminoma and gonadoblastoma are associated with virilization (Usizima 1956; Scully 1953).

Details of the clinical and pathological features of ovarian neoplasms occurring in childhood and adolescence are described by Abell (1977).

9. Ectopic Hormone Syndromes Associated with Tumours

Extensive data have accumulated relating to the production of hormones by tumours of nonendocrine tissues and inappropriate hormones by tumours of endocrine origin in adults (Rees and Ratcliffe 1974; Anderson 1973; Ellison and Neville 1973). Additionally there are examples of hormone-like effects of tumours that it has not been possible to relate to the appropriate hormone (e.g., insulin-like effects). Tumours occurring in children of similar type to those seen in adults have on occasion been reported to produce the same ectopic hormone effects, and additionally there are examples of hormone production by tumours that are more typical of childhood. Many of the reported cases are reviewed by Omenn (1971).

Production of ACTH is well documented. Most childhood cases involve tumours now generally regarded as of endocrine cell origin, such as oat cell carcinoma of lung, carcinoid of the thymus, islet cell tumours, and medullary carcinoma of the thyroid. Of the tumours of childhood those of neuroblast origin are prominent and include phaeochromocytoma.

Hypercalcaemia with hypophosphataemia from parathormone production has been recorded with hepatoblastoma and testicular carcinoma amongst the cases reviewed by Omenn (1971), and in bone sarcoma, neuroblastoma, rhabdomyosarcoma, and a number of cases of lymphosarcoma and leukaemia (Joyaraman and David 1977; Ramsay et al. 1979; Myers 1960; Stapleton et al. 1976; Hutchinson et al. 1978).

Isosexual precocity resulting from gonadotrophin production is recorded in nine males with hepatoblastoma in the review by Omenn (1971). Excluding

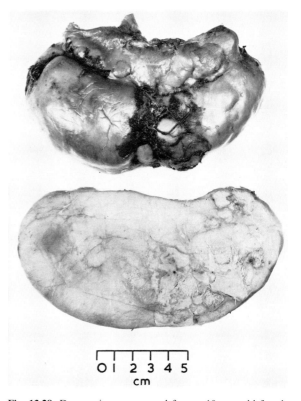

Fig. 13.28. Dysgerminoma removed from a 10-year-old female and apparently restricted to the ovary, though there are some vascular adhesions between the tumour surface and adjacent tissues.

germ cell tumours this appears to be the only tumour to produce truly ectopic gonadotrophin. The gonadotrophin is similar in action to pituitary luteinizing hormone (Root et al. 1968; McArthur 1969), a conclusion supported by both the absence of stimulation of the cells of the seminiferous tubules noted in testicular biopsies and the apparent exclusive occurrence of the syndrome in males. The gonadotrophin in the case studied by Braunstein et al. (1972) was similar to chorionic gonadotrophin and distinct from human pituitary luteinizing hormone. The pituitary from the case studied by Behrle et al. (1963) showed a reduced number of acidophils and chromophobes, with increased numbers of basophils and amphophils. Similar pituitary changes were observed in an adult dying with a malignant Sertoli cell tumour of the testis (Mostofi et al. 1959).

Nine childhood cases of hypoglycaemia associated with large nonpancreatic abdominal tumours are collected in the review by Omenn (1971). Four of the tumours were of connective tissue and included amongst the remainder were two cases of lymphoma, a large adrenal cortical carcinoma, a Wilm's tumour, and a neuroblastoma. The problem of elucidating the cause of the hypoglycaemia associated with tumours of this type, in which low levels of circulating immunoreactive insulin during the hypoglycaemic episode are the usual finding, is discussed by Skrabauek and Powell (1978).

The four tumour-related ectopic hormone and hormone-like conditions so far discussed account for the majority of such syndromes occurring in childhood. Chronic diarrhoea in patients with medullary carcinoma of the thyroid and ganglioneuroma (Green et al. 1959) is mediated by tumour products in much the same way as in the case of some pancreatic islet cell tumours. In many of the latter cases the gut hormone has been identified and many are not truly ectopic. Similarly, hyperthyroidism provoked by placental thyrotopin in cases of trophoblastic tumour (Cohen and Utiger 1970) is not strictly the result of production of hormone foreign to the tumour concerned.

References

Abell MR (1977) Ovarian neoplasms of childhood and adolescence. In: Blaustein A (ed) Pathology of the female genital tract. Springer-Verlag, New York Heidelberg Berlin, p 586

Abell MR, Johnson VJ, Holyz F (1965) Ovarian neoplasms in childhood and adolescence. I. Tumours of germ cell origin. Am J Obstet Gynecol 92: 1059

Albright F, Burnett CH, Smith PH, Parson W (1942) Pseudohypoparathyroidism: An example of 'Seabright-Bantom syndrome': Report of three cases. Endocrinology 30: 922

Anast CS, Mohs JM, Kaplan SL, Burns TW (1972) Evidence for parathyroid failure in magnesium deficiency. Science 177: 606

Anderson G (1973) Paramalignant syndromes. In: Baron DM, Compston MH, Dawson AM (eds) Recent advances in medicine. Churchill Livingston, Edinburgh, p 1

Anderson JR, Goudie RB, Gray KG, Timbury GC (1957) Autoantibodies in Addison's disease. Lancet 1: 1123

Asadourian LA, Taylor HB (1969) Dysgerminoma. An analysis of 105 cases. Obstet Gynecol 33: 370

Bar RS, Lewis WR, Rechler MM, Harrison LC, Siebert C, Podskalany J, Roth J, Muggeo M (1978) Extreme insulin resistance in ataxia telangiectasia: Defect in affinity of insulin receptors. N Engl J Med 298: 1164

Beckwith JB (1969) Magroglossia, omphalocele, adrenal cytomegaly, gigantism, and hyperplastic visceromegaly. Birth Defects 5: 188

Behrle FC, Mantz FA, Olson RL, Trombold JC (1963) Virilization accompanying hepatoblastoma. Pediatrics 32: 265

Benirschke K (1956) Adrenals in anecephaly and hydrocephaly. Obstet Gynecol 8: 412

Benirschke K, Bloch E, Hertig AT (1956) Concerning the function of the fetal zone of the human adrenal gland. Endocrinology 58: 598

Black S, Brook CGD, Cox PJH (1977) Congenital adrenal hypoplasia and gonadotrophin deficiency. Br Med J ii: 996

Blizzard RM, Kyle M, Chandler RW, Hung W (1962) Adrenal antibodies in Addison's disease. Lancet 2: 901

Blizzard RM, Chee D, Davis W (1966) The incidence of parathyroid and other antibodies in the sera of patients with idiopathic hypoparathyroidism. Clin Exp Immunol 1: 119

Bloodworth JMB Jr (1968) Diabetes mellitus: Extra-pancreatic pathology. In: Bloodworth JMB Jr (ed) Endocrine pathology. Williams & Wilkins, Baltimore p 330

Boivin Y, Richart RM (1965) Hilus cell tumours of the ovary. A review with a report of three new cases. Cancer 18: 231

Borit A, Kosek J (1969) Cytomegaly of the adrenal cortex, electron microscopy in Beckwith's syndrome. Arch Pathol 88: 58

Bormel P, Mays HB (1961) Testicular tumours of infancy and childhood. J Urol 86: 119

Bradford WD, Wilson JW, Gaode JT (1973) Primary neonatal hyperparathyroidism—An unusual cause of failure to thrive. Am J Clin Pathol 59: 267

Braunstein GD, Bridson WE, Glass A, Hull EW, McIntire KR (1972) In vivo and in vitro production of human chorionic gonadotropin and alpha-fetoprotein by a virilizing hepatoblastoma. J Clin Endocrinol Metab 35: 857

Brerton RJ, Symonds E (1978) Thyroglossal cysts in children. Br J Surg 65: 507

Bronsky D, Kushner DS, Dubin A, Shapper I (1958) Idiopathic hypoparathyroidism and pseudohypoparathyroidism: Case reports and review of the literature. Medicine 37: 317

Bronsky D, Kramko RT, Moncada R, Rosenthal IM (1968) Intrauterine hyperparathyroidism secondary to maternal hypoparathyroidism. Pediatrics 42: 606

Calnan M, Peckham CS (1977) Incidence of insulin dependent diabetes in the first 16 years of life. Lancet 1: 589

Carlson HE, Brickman AS, Bottazzo GF (1977) Prolactin deficiency in pseudohypoparathyroidism. N Engl J Med 296: 140

Carman CT, Brashear RE (1960) Phaeochromocytoma as an inherited abnormality. N Engl J Med 263: 419

Chase LR, Melson GL, Aurbach GD (1969) Pseudohypoparathyroidism: Defective excretion of 3',5'-AMP in response to parathyroid hormone. J Clin Invest 48: 1832

Chaussain JL (1973) Glycemic response to 24 hour fast in normal children and children with ketotic hypoglycemia. J Pediatr 82: 438

Childs B, Grumbach MM, Van Wyk JJ (1956) Virilizing adrenal hyperplasia: A genetic and hormonal study. J Clin Invest 35: 213

Choufoer JC, Van Rhijn M, Querido A (1965) Endemic goitre in Western Guinea. II. Clinical picture, incidence and pathogenesis of endemic cretinism. J Clin Endocrinol Metab 25: 385

Chu H-Y, Chang C, Yin W (1964) Idiopathic hypoparathyroidism. Report of 14 cases with one autopsy record. Chin Med J [Engl] 83: 723

Clayton GW, Johnson CM (1960) Struma lymphomatosa in children: report of 12 cases. J Pediatr 57: 410

Cohen JD, Utiger RD (1970) Metastatic choriocarcinoma associated with hyperthyroidism. J Clin Endocrinol Metab 30: 423

Conard RA, Dobyn BM, Sutton WW (1970) Thyroid neoplasm as a late effect of exposure to radioactive iodine in fallout. JAMA 214: 316

Cox JM, Guelpa G, Terrapon M (1976) Islet-cell hyperplasia and sudden infant death. Lancet 2: 739

Craig JM, Schiff LH, Boone JE (1955) Chronic moniliasis associated Addison's disease. Am J Dis Child 89: 669

Crooke AC (1935) A change in the basophil cells of the pituitary gland common to conditions which exhibit the syndrome attributed to basophil adenoma. J Pathol Bacteriol 41: 339

Crooke AC, Russell DS (1935) The pituitary gland in Addison's disease. J Pathol Bacteriol 40: 255

Crooks J, Greig WR, Branwood AW (1963) Dyshormonogenesis and carcinoma of the thyroid gland. Scott Med J 8: 303

Cuello C, Correa P, Eisenberg H (1969) Geographic pathology of thyroid carcinoma. Cancer 23: 230

Davidson DC, Blackwood MJ, Fox EG (1974) Neonatal hypoglycaemia with congenital malformation of pancreatic islets. Arch Dis Child 49: 151

de Sa DJ, Nicholls S (1972) Haemorrhagic necrosis of the adrenal glands in perinatal infants. J Pathol 106: 133

Doniach D, Roitt IM, Polani PE (1968) Thyroid antibodies and sex-chromosome anomalies. Proc R Soc Med 61: 278

Doniach I (1977) Histopathology of the anterior pituitary. Clin Endocrinol Metabol 6: 21

Doniach I, Morgan AG (1973) Islets of Langerhans in juvenile diabetes mellitus. Clin Endocrinol 2: 233

Dorff GB (1934) Sporadic cretinism in one of twins. Report of cases with roentgen demonstration of osseous changes that occurred in utero. Am J Dis Child 48: 1316

Drake TG, Albright F, Bauer W, Castleman B (1939) Chronic idiopathic hypoparathyroidism: Report of six cases with autopsy findings in one. Ann Intern Med 12: 1751

Drezner MK, Neelon FA, Haussler M, McPherson HT, Lebovitz HE (1976) 1,25-dihydroxycholecalciferol deficiency: The probable cause of hypocalcaemia and metabolic bone disease in pseudohypoparathyroidism. J Clin Endocrinol Metab 42: 621

Dussault JH, Coulombe P, Laberge C, Letarte J, Guyda H, Khoury K (1975) Preliminary report on a mass screening program for neonatal hypothyroidism. J Pediatr 86: 670

Eeg-Olofsson O, Petersen I (1966) Childhood diabetes neuropathy. A clinical and neurophysiological study. Acta Paediatr Scand 55: 163

Ellison ML, Neville AM (1973) Neoplasia and ectopic hormone production. In: Raven RW (ed) Modern trends in oncology. Butterworth, London, p 163

Erdheim J (1904) Über Hypophysenganggeschwülste und Hirncholesteatome. SB Akad Wiss Wien [3] 113: 537

Fiero-Benitez R, Alban R, Cordova J, Eguiguren L, Franco R, Moreano M, Malo L, Paltan JD, Paredes M, Rivadeneira I, Sanchez-Jaramillo P, Weilbrauer P (1965) Endemic goitre and endemic cretinism in the Equatorial Andes. VIth Pan American Congress of Endocrinology. Excerpta Medica, Internat. Congress Series No 99, Abstract No. 36

Fischer GW, Vazquez AM, Buist NRM, Campbell JR, McCarty E, Egan ET (1974) Neonatal islet cell adenoma: Case report and literature review. Pediatrics 53: 753

Fisher WD, Voorhess ML, Gardner LI (1963) Congenital hypothyroidism in infant following maternal I^{131} therapy. J Pediatr 62: 132

Fleischer AS, Rudman DR, Payne NS, Tyndall GT (1978) Hypothalamic hypothyroidism and hypogonadism in prolonged traumatic coma. J Neurosurg 49: 650

Fretheim B, Gardborg O (1965) Primary hyperparathyroidism in an infant. Acta Chir Scand 129: 557

Gabbay KH (1975) Hyperglycemia, polyol metabolism, and complications of diabetes mellitus. Annu Rev Med 26: 521

Gabrilove JL, Nicolis GL, MiHy HA, Shoval AR (1975) Feminizing interstitial cell tumor of the testis: Personal observations and a review of the literature. Cancer 35: 1184

Gabrilove JL, Sharma DC, Wotiz HH, Dorfman R (1965) Feminizing adrenocortical tumours in the male: A review of 52 cases. Medicine (Baltimore) 44: 37

Gamble DR, Kinsley ML, FitzGerald MG, Bolton R, Taylor KW (1969) Viral antibodies in diabetes mellitus. Br Med J iii: 627

Gang DL (1978) In: Case records of the Massachusetts General Hospital. Case 30. N Engl J Med 299: 241

Gass HH (1956) Large calcified craniopharyngioma and bilateral subdural haematoma present at birth. J Neurosurg 13: 514

Gepts W (1965) Pathologic anatomy of the pancreas in juvenile diabetes mellitus. Diabetes 14: 619

Giebnink GS, Ruymann FB (1974) Testicular tumours in childhood. Am J Dis Child 127: 433

Gilmour JR (1937) The embryology of the parathyroid glands, the thymus and certain associated rudiments. J Pathol 45: 507

Gilmour JR (1938) The gross anatomy of the parathyroid glands. J Pathol 46: 133

Gilmour JR (1939) The normal histology of the parathyroid glands. J Pathol 48: 187

Gilmour JR (1941) Some developmental abnormalities of the thymus and parathyroids. J Pathol Bacteriol 52: 213

Goldberg GM, Eshbaugh DE (1960) Squamous cell nests of the pituitary gland as related to the origin of craniopharyngiomas. A study of their presence in the newborn in infants up to age four. Arch Pathol 70: 293

Gorlin RJ, Sedano HO, Vickers RA (1968) Multiple mucosal neuromas, phaeochromocytoma and medullary carcinoma of the thyroid—a syndrome. Cancer 22: 293

Gorodischer R, Aceto T Jr, Terplan K (1970) Congenital familial hypoparathyroidism: Management of an infant, genetics, pathogenesis of hypoparathyroidism and fetal under-mineralisation. Am J Dis Child 119: 74

Green M, Cooke RE, Lattanzi W (1959) Occurrence of chronic diarrhoea in three patients with ganglioneuroma. Pediatrics 23: 951

Grim CE, McBryde AC, Glenn JF, Gunnells JC (1967) Childhood primary aldosteronism with bilateral adrenocortical hyperplasia: plasma renin activity as an aid to diagnosis. J Pediatr 71: 377

Gruskin AB, Root AW, Duckett GE, Balnarte HJ (1976) Parathyroid function in uremic children during periods of renal insufficiency, haemodialysis and transplantation. J Pediatr 89: 755

Guin GH, Gilbert EE, Jones B (1969) Incidental neuroblastoma in infants. Am J Clin Pathol 51: 126

Habener JF, Potts JT Jr (1968) Biosynthesis of parathyroid hormone. N Engl J Med 299: 635

Hagberg B, Westphal O (1970) Ataxic syndrome in congenital hypothyroidism. Acta Paediatr Scand 59: 323

Hardman JM (1968) Fatal meningococcal infections: The changing pathologic picture in the 60's. Milit Med 133: 951

Harness JK, Thompson HW, Nishiyama RH (1971) Childhood thyroid carcinoma. Arch Surg 102: 278

Hayles AB, Johnson LM, Beahrs OH, Woolner LB (1963) Carcinoma of the thyroid in children. Am J Surg 106: 735

Heitz PU, Klöppel G, Häcki WH, Polak JM, Pearse AGE (1977) Nesidioblastosis: The pathologic basis of persistent hyper-insulinemic hypoglycemia in infants. Diabetes 26: 632

Hempelmann LH, Pifer JW, Burke GJ, Ames WR (1967) Neoplasms in persons treated with X-rays in infancy for thymic enlargement. A report of the third follow-up survey. J Natl Cancer Inst 38: 317

Hewer TF (1944) Ateleiotic dwarfism with normal sexual function: A result of hypopituitarism. J Endocrinol 3: 397

Hillman DA, Scriver CR, Pedvis S, Schragovitch I (1964) Neonatal familial primary hyperparathyroidism. N Engl J Med 270: 483

Hirschfield AJ, Fleshman JK (1969) An unusually high incidence of salt-loosing congenital adrenal hyperplasia in the Alaskan Eskimo. J Pediatr 75: 492

Hollingsworth DR, McKeau HE, Roeckel I (1974) Goitre, immunological observations and thyroid function tests in Down syndrome. Am J Dis Child 127: 524

Holmgren G, Samuelson G, Hermansson B (1974) The prevalence of diabetes mellitus: A study of children and their relatives in a northern Swedish county. Clin Genet 5: 465

Hopwood NJ, Kenny FM (1977) Incidence of Nelson's syndrome after adrenalectomy for Cushing's disease in children. Am J Dis Child 131: 1353

Huang SW, MacLaren NK (1976) Insulin dependent diabetes: A disease of autoaggression. Science 192: 64

Hulse JA, Grant DB, Clayton BE, Lilly P, Jackson D, Spracklan A, Edwards RWH, Nurse D (1980) Population screening for congenital hypothyroidism. Br Med J i: 675

Hume DM (1960) Phaeochromocytoma in the adult and in the child. Am J Surg 99: 458

Hutchin P, Kessner DM (1964) Diagnostic lead to hyperparathyroidism in the mother. Ann Intern Med 61: 1109

Hutchison JH, McGirr EM (1956) Sporadic non-endemic goitrous cretinism: Hereditary transmission. Lancet 1: 1035

Hutchinson RJ, Shapiro SA, Raney RB (1978) Elevated parathyroid hormone levels in association with rhabdomyosarcoma. J Pediatr 92: 780

Irvine WJ, McCallum CJ, Gray RS, Campbell CJ, Duncan LJP, Farquher JW, Vaughan H, Morris PJ (1977) Pancreatic islet-cell antibodies in diabetes mellitus correlated with the duration and type of diabetes, coexistent autoimmune disease and HLA type. Diabetes 26: 138

Iyer CGS (1952) Case report of an adamantinoma present at birth. J Neurosurg 9: 221

Jennings AS, Liddle GW, Orth DM (1977) Results of treating childhood Cushing's disease with pituitary irradiation. N Engl J Med 287: 957

Jensen RD, Norris HJ, Fraumeni JF Jr (1974) Familial arrhenoblastoma and thyroid adenoma. Cancer 33: 218

Johnstone REH, Kreindler T, Johnstone RE (1972) Hyperparathyroidism during pregnancy. Obstet Gynecol 40: 580

Jones RA, Dawson IMP (1977) Morphology and staining patterns of endocrine cell tumours in the gut, pancreas and bronchus and their possible significance. Histopathology 1: 137

Joyaraman J, David R (1977) Hypercalcemia as a presenting manifestation of leukaemia: Evidence of excessive PTH secretion. J Pediatr 90: 609

Keiser HR, Beaven MS, Doppman J, Wells S, Buja LM (1973) Sipple's syndrome: Medullary thyroid carcinoma, phaeochromocytoma and parathyroid disease. Ann Intern Med 78: 561

Kelley VC, Ely RS, Raile RB (1952) Metabolic studies in patients with congenital adrenal hyperplasia. Effects of cortisone therapy. J Clin Endocrinol Metab 12: 1140

Kelly FC, Snedden WW (1960) Prevalence and geographical distribution of endemic goiter. In: Endemic goiter. WHO Monogr Ser 44: 27

Kelly WF, Joplin GF, Pearson GW (1977) Gonadotrophin deficiency and adrenocortical insufficiency in children: A new syndrome. Br Med J 2: 98

Kennedy JS (1969) The pathology of dyshormonogenetic goitre. J Pathol 99: 251

Kerenyi N (1961) Congenital adrenal hypoplasia. Report of a case with extreme adrenal hypoplasia and neurohypophyseal aplasia, drawing attention to certain aspects of etiology and classification. Arch Pathol 71: 336

Khairi MR, Dexter RM, Burzynski MJ, Johnston CC (1975) Mucosal neuroma, phaeochromocytoma and medullary carcinoma: Multiple endocrine neoplasia type 3. Medicine (Baltimore) 54: 89

Koenig MP (1968) Die Kongenital hypothyreose und der endemische Kretinismus. Springer-Verlag, Berlin, Heidelberg, New York

Koenig RJ, Peterson CM, Jones RL, Saudek C, Lehrman M, Cerami A (1976) Correlation of glucose regulation and haemoglobin ALC in diabetes mellitus. N Engl J Med 295: 417

Kohler HG (1963) Karyomegaly of the fetal adrenal cortex. J Clin Pathol 16: 383

Knowles HC Jr, Guest GM, Lampe J, Kessler M, Skillman TG (1965) The course of juvenile diabetes treated with unmeasured diet. Diabetes 14: 239

Kyllo DF, Nuttall FQ (1978) Prevalence of diabetes mellitus in school-age children in Minnesota. Diabetes 27: 57

Landing BH, Kamoshita S (1970) Congenital hyperparathyroidism secondary to maternal hypoparathyroidism J Pediatr 77: 842

Landon H, Adin I, Spitz IM (1978) Pituitary insufficiency following head injury. Isr J Med Sci 14: 785

Larsson L-I (1978) Endocrine pancreatic tumours. Hum Pathol 9: 401

Leboeuf G, Bongiovanni AM (1964) Thyroiditis in childhood. Adv Pediatr 13: 183

Le Dourain N, Le Lievre C, Containe J (1972) Recherches expérimentales sur l'origine embryologique du corps carotidien chez les oiseaux. CR Acad Sci [D] (Paris) 275: 583

Leedham PW, Pollock DJ (1970) Intrafollicular amyloid in primary hyperparathyroidism. J Clin Pathol 23: 811

Lennox B, Russell DS (1951) Dystopia of the neurohypophysis: Two cases. J Pathol 63: 485

Lernmark A, Freedman ZR, Hofmann C, Rubenstein AH, Steiner DF, Jackson RL, Winter RJ, Traisman HS (1978) Islet-cell-surface antibody in juvenile diabetes mellitus. N Engl J Med 299: 375

Levin J, Cluff LE (1965) Endotoxemia and adrenal haemorrhage A mechanism for the Waterhouse-Friederichsen syndrome. J Exp Med 121: 247

Lundberg PO, Gemzell C (1966) Dysplasia of sella turcica. Acta Endocrinol (Kbh) 52: 478

Lyon FA, Sinykin MB, McKelvey JL (1963) Granulosa-cell tumours of the ovary, review of 23 cases. Obstet Gynecol 21: 67

MacLaren NK, Huang SW, Fogh J (1975) Antibody to cultured human insulinoma cells in insulin-dependent diabetes. Lancet 1: 997

Mäenpää J (1972) Congenital hypothyroidism; aetiological and clinical aspects. Arch Dis Child 47: 914

Marek J (1977) Gonadotrophin deficiency and adrenocortical insufficiency in children. Br Med J ii: 828

Marshall JR (1965) Ovarian enlargement in the first year of life: Review of 45 cases. Ann Surg 161: 372

Marshall WC, Ockenden BG, Fosbrook AS, Cummings JN (1969) Wolman's disease. A rare lipoidosis with adrenal calcification. Arch Dis Child 44: 331

Martin KJ, Kruska KA, Freitag JJ, Klahr S, Slatopolsky E (1979) The peripheral metabolism of parathyroid hormone. N Engl J

Med 301: 1092

Marx SJ, Hershaman JM, Aurbach GD (1971) Thyroid dysfunction in pseudohypoparathyroidism. J Clin Endocrinol Metab 33: 822

Meador CK, Bowdoin B, Owen WC, Farmer TA (1967) Primary adrenocortical nodular dysplasia: A rare cause of Cushing's disease. J Clin Endocrinol Metab 27: 1255

Melvin KEW, Tashjian AH Jr, Miller HH (1972) Studies in familial (medullary) thyroid carcinoma. Recent Prog Horm Res 28: 399

Menser MA, Forrest JM, Bransby RD (1978) Rubella infection and diabetes mellitus. Lancet 1: 57

Meyer JS, Steinberg LS (1969) Microscopically benign thyroid follicles in cervical lymph nodes. Cancer 24: 302

Miller WL, Kaplan SL, Grumbach MM (1980) Child abuse as a cause of post-traumatic hypopituitarism. N Engl J Med 302: 724

Misugi K, Misugi N, Sotas J, Smith B (1970) The pancreatic islets of infants with severe hypoglycemia. Arch Pathol 89: 208

Mostofi FK (1973) Testicular tumours. Epidemiologic, etiologic and pathologic features. Cancer 32: 1186

Mostofi FK, Theiss EA, Ashley DJB (1959) Tumours of specialized gonadal stroma in human male patients. Cancer 12: 944

McArthur JW (1969) Discussion. Recent Prog Horm Res 25: 306

McCallagh EP, Rossmiller HR (1941) Methyltestosterone; 1. Androgenic effects and production of gynecomastia and oligospermia. J Clin Endocrinol Metab 1: 496

McGirr EM, Clement WE, Currie AR, Kennedy JS (1959) Impaired dehalogenase activity as a cause of goitre with malignant change. Scott Med J 4: 232

Myers WPL (1960) Hypercalcemia in neoplastic disease. Arch Surg 80: 308

Nabarro JD, Mustaffa BE, Morris DV, Walport MJ, Kuntz AB (1979) Insulin deficient diabetes: Contrasts with other endocrine deficiencies. Diabetologia 16: 5

Neufeld ND, Lippe BM, Sperling M, Kaplan SA (1978) Insulin resistance with reduction in monocyte insulin binding in gonadal dysgenesis. Clin Res 26: 190A

Neville AM, Symington T (1972) Bilateral adrenocrotical hyperplasia in children with Cushing's syndrome. J Pathol 107: 95

New MI, Petwoon RE (1966) Disorders of aldosterone secretion in childhood. Pediatr Clin North Am 13: 43

Nienwenhuijzen Kruseman AC, Knijnenburg G, Burtel de la Riviere G, Bosman FT (1978) Morphology and immunohistochemically-defined endocrine function of pancreatic islet cell tumours. Histopathology 2: 389

Nilsson LR, Doniach D (1964) Autoimmune thyroiditis in children and adolescents: 1. Clinical studies. Acta Pediatr Scand 53: 255

Nilsson LR, Bogfors M, Gamstorp I, Holst H-E, Liden G (1964) Non-endemic goitre and deafness. Acta Paediatr Scand 53: 255

Norris HJ, Jensen RD (1972) Relative frequency of ovarian neoplasms in children and adolescents. Cancer 30: 713

Norton JA, Frooke LC, Farrell RE, Wells SA (1979) Multiple endocrine neoplasia Type IIb. The most aggressive form of medullary thyroid carcinoma. Surg Clin North Am 59(1): 109

Omenn GS (1971) Ectopic hormone syndromes associated with tumours in childhood. Pediatrics 47: 613

Oppenheimer EH (1969) Cyst formation in the outer adrenal cortex; Studies in the human fetus and newborn. Arch Pathol 87: 653

Oppenheimer EH (1970) Adrenal cytomegaly: Studies by light and electron microscopy. Arch Pathol 90: 57

Page CP, Kemmerer WT, Haff RC, Mazzaferri EL (1974) Thyroid carcinomas arising in thyroglossal ducts. Ann Surg 180: 799

Pagliara AS, Karl IE, Haymond M, Kipnis DM (1973) Hypoglycemia in infancy and childhood. I. J Pediatr 82: 365

Pagliara AS, Karl IE, Haymond M, Kipnis DM (1973) Hypoglycemia in infancy and childhood. II. J Pediatr 82: 558

Paulsen CA (1974) The testis. In: Williams RH (ed) Textbook of endocrinology, 5th edn. Saunders, Philadelphia London Toronto, p 362

Paxson CL Jr, Brown DR (1976) Post-traumatic anterior hypopituitarism. Pediatrics 57: 893

Pearse AGE, Polak JM, van Nooreden S (1972) The neural crest origin of the C cells and their comparative cytochemistry and ultrastructure in the ultimobranchial gland. In: Talmage RV, Munson PL (eds) Calcium, parathyroid hormone and calcitonins. Excerpta Medica, Amsterdam, p 29

Pearse AGE, Polak JM, Heath CM (1973) Development, differentiation and derivation of the endocrine polypeptide cells of the mouse pancreas. (Immunofluorescence, cytochemical and ultrastructural studies). Diabetalogia 9: 120

Peden VH (1960) True idiopathic hypoparathyroidism as a sex-linked recessive trait. Am J Hum Genet 12: 323

Pedersen J, Osler M (1958) Development of ossification centres in infants of diabetic mothers. Acta Endocrinol (Kbh) 29: 467

Pictet RL, Rall LB, Phelps P, Rutter WJ (1976) The neural crest and the origin of the insulin producing and other gastrointestinal hormone producing cells. Science 191: 191

Polak JM, Wigglesworth JS (1976) Islet-cell hyperplasia and sudden infant death. Lancet 2: 570

Porcile E, Racadot J (1966) Ultrastructure des cellules de Crooke observées dans l'hypophyse humaine au cours de la maladie de Cushing. C R Acad Sci [D] (Paris) 263: 948

Ramsay NKC, Brown DM, Nesbit ME, Coccia PF, Krivit W, Krutzik S (1979) Autonomous production of parathyroid hormone by lymphoblastic leukaemia cells in culture. J Pediatr 94: 623

Rees LH, Ratcliffe JG (1974) Ectopic hormone production by non-endocrine tumours. Clin Endocrinol (Oxf) 3: 263

Richardson JE, Beaugie JM, Doniach I, Brown CL (1974) Thyroid cancer in young patients in Great Britain. Br J Surg 61: 85

Rimoin DL (1971) Inheritance of diabetes mellitus. Med Clin North Am 55: 807

Roche M (1959) Elevated thyroidal I^{131} uptake in the absence of goitre in isolated Venezuelan Indians. J Clin Endocrinol Metab 19: 1440

Root AW, Bongiovanni AM, Eberlein WR (1968) A testicular interstial cell-stimulating gonadotrophin in a child with hepatoblastoma and sexual precocity. J Clin Endocrinol Metab 28: 1317

Roth SI, Gallagher MJ (1976) The rapid identification of 'normal' parathyroid glands by the presence of intracellular fat. Am J Pathol 84: 521

Rude RK, Oldham SB, Singer FR, Nicoloff JT (1976) Treatment of thyrotoxic hypercalcaemia with propranolol. N Engl J Med 294: 431

Ruder HJ, Loriaux DL, Lipsett MB (1974) Severe osteopenia in young adults associated with Cushing's syndrome due to micronodular adrenal disease. J Clin Endocrinol Metab 39: 1138

Russell DS, Rubinstein LJ (1977a) Pathology of tumours of the nervous system, 4th edn. Arnold, London, p 38

Russell DS, Rubinstein LJ (1977b) Pathology of tumours of the nervous system, 4th edn. Arnold, London, p 312

Russfield AB, Reiner L (1957) The hypophysis in human growth failure: Report of three dwarfs. Lab Invest 6: 334

Sedeghi-Nejad A, Seniar B (1974) Familial syndrome of isolated aplasia of the anterior pituitary. J Pediatr 84: 79

Saenger EL, Silverman FN, Sterling TD, Turner ME (1960) Neoplasia following therapeutic irradiation for benign conditions in childhood. Radiology 74: 889

Saharia PC (1975) Carcinoma arising in thyroglossal duct remnant: Case reports and review of the literature. Br J Surg 62: 689

Salassa RM, Laws ER Jr, Carpenter PC, Northcutt RC (1978) Trans-sphenoidal removal of pituitary microadenoma in Cushing's disease. Mayo Clin Proc 53: 24

Salinas ED Jr, Mangurten HH, Roberts SS, Simon WH, Cornblath M (1968) Functioning islet cell adenoma in the newborn. Pediatrics 41: 646

Saxena KM, Crawford JD (1962) Juvenile lymphocytic thyroiditis. Pediatrics 30: 917

Saxena KM, Crawford JD, Talbot NB (1964) Childhood thyrotoxicosis: A long-term perspective. Br Med J ii: 1153

Schimke RN, Hartmann WH, Prout TE, Rimoin DL (1968) Syndrome of bilateral pheochromocytoma, medullary thyroid carcinoma and multiple neuromas. N Engl J Med 279: 1

Schochet SS, McCormick WF, Halmi NS (1974) Pituitary gland in patients with Hurler's syndrome. Arch Pathol 97: 96

Scholz DA, Horton ES, Lebowitz HE, Ferris DO (1967) Spontaneous hypoglycaemia associated with an adrenocortical carcinoma. J Clin Endocrinol Metab 27: 991

Scully RE (1953) Gonadoblastoma. A gonadal tumor related to the dysgerminoma (seminoma) and capable of sex hormone production. Cancer 6: 455

Siebenmann RE (1957) Die kongenitale Lipoidhyperplasie der Nebennierenrinde bei Nebennierenrindeninsuffizienz. Schweiz Z Pathol 20: 77

Silberman R, Mendelson IR (1960) Teratomas of the neck: Report of 2 cases and review of the literature. Arch Dis Child 35: 159

Skrabauek P, Powell D (1978) Ectopic insulin and Occam's razor: Reappraisal of the riddle of tumour hypoglycaemia. Clin Endocrinol (Oxf) 9: 141

Smith DW, Blizzard RM, Wilkins L (1957) The mental prognosis in hypothyroidism of infancy and childhood: Review of 128 cases. Pediatrics 19: 1011

Smithers DW (1970) Tumours of the thyroid gland. In: Monographs on neoplastic disease. Livingstone, Edinburgh, p 155

Spiegel AM, Harrison HE, Marx SJ, Brown EM, Aurbach GD (1977) Neonatal primary hyperparathyroidism with autosomal dominant inheritance. J Pediatr 90: 269

Stackpole RH, Melicow M, Uson AC (1963) Pheochromocytoma in children. Report of 9 cases and review of the first 100 published cases with follow-up studies. J Pediatr 63: 315

Stanbury JB (1978) Familial goitre. In: Stanbury JB, Wyngaarden JB, Fredrickson DS (eds) The metabolic basis of inherited disease, 4th edn. McGraw-Hill, New York, p 206

Stapleton FB, Lukert BP, Linshaw MP (1976) Treatment of hypercalcaemia associated with osseous metastases. J Pediatr 89: 1029

Steiner AC, Goodman AD, Powers SR (1968) Study of a kindred with pheochromocytoma, medullary thyroid carcinoma, hyperparathyroidism and Cushing's disease: Multiple endocrine neoplasia, type 2. Medicine (Baltimore) 47: 371

Suh SM, Tashjian AH Jr, Matsuo M, Parkinson DK, Fraser D (1973) Pathogenesis of hypocalcaemia in primary hypomagnesaemia: Normal end-organ responsiveness to parathormone. Impaired parathyroid gland function. J Clin Invest 52: 153

Sultz HA, Hart BA, Zielezny M, Schlesinger ER (1975) Is mumps virus an etiologic factor in juvenile diabetes mellitus? J Pediatr 86: 654

Tabaddor K, Shulman K, Dal Canto MC (1974) Neonatal craniopharyngioma. Am J Dis Child 128: 381

Tsang RC, Light IJ, Sutherland JM, Kleinman LI (1973) Possible pathogenetic factors in neonatal hypocalcemia of prematurity. J Pediatr 82: 423

Tyrrell JB, Brooks RM, Fitzgerald PA, Cofoid PB, Forsham PH,

Wilson PB (1978) Cushing's disease: Selective transsphenoidal resection of pituitary microadenomas. N Engl J Med 198: 753

Usizima H (1956) Ovarian dysgerminoma associated with masculinization. Report of a case. Cancer 9: 736

Warren JC, Erkman B, Cheatum S (1964) Hilus-cell adenoma in a dysgenetic gonad with XX/XO mosaicism. Lancet 1: 141

Weber FT, Donnelly WH, Bejar RL (1977) Hypopituitarism following extirpation of a pharyngeal pituitary. Am J Dis Child 131: 525

Wegelin C (1928) Malignant disease of the thyroid gland and its relations to goitre in man and animals. Cancer Treat Rev 3: 297

Weichert RF (1970) III. The neural ectodermal origin of peptidesecreting endocrine glands. Am J Med 49: 232

Weinstein RL, Kliman B, Neeman J, Cohen RB (1970) Deficient 17-hydroxylation in a corticosterone producing adrenal tumour from an infant with hemihypertrophy and visceromegaly. J Clin Endocrinol Metab 30: 456

Weiss L, Mellinger RC (1970) Congenital adrenal hypoplasia an X-linked disease. J Med Genet 7: 27

Weitzner S, Gropp A (1974) Sertoli cell tumor of testis in childhood. Am J Dis Child 128: 541

Werder EA, Illig R, Bernasconi S, Kind H, Prader A, Fischer JA, Fanconi A (1975) Excessive thyrotropin response to thyrotropin-releasing hormone in pseudohypoparathyroidism. Pediatr Res 9: 12

Wermer P (1974) Multiple endocrine adenomatosis; Multiple hormone-producing tumours, a familial syndrome. Clin Gastroenterol 3: 671

Wiedemann HR (1964) Complex malformatif familial avec hernie ombilicale et macroglossie—un 'syndrome nouveau'? J Genet Hum 13: 223

Wiener MF, Dallgaard SA (1959) Intracranial adrenal gland. A case report. Arch Pathol 67: 228

Williams ED (1965) A review of 17 cases of carcinoma of the thyroid and phaeochromocytoma. J Clin Pathol 18: 288

Williams ED (1975) Medullary carcinoma of the thyroid. In: Harrison CV, Weinbred K (eds) Recent advances in pathology, vol 9. Churchill Livingstone, Edinburgh, p 156

Williams ED (1978) The parathyroid glands. In: Symmers W St C (ed) Systemic pathology, vol 4. Churchill Livingstone, Edinburgh London New York, p 2045

Williams ED, Pollock DJ (1966) Multiple mucosal neuromata with endocrine tumours: A syndrome allied to von Recklinghausen's disease. J Pathol Bacteriol 91: 71

Williams ED, Sandler M (1963) The classification of carcinoid tumours. Lancet 1: 238

Williams ED, Brown CL, Doniach I (1966) Pathological and clinical findings in a series of 67 cases of medullary carcinoma of the thyroid. J Clin Pathol 19: 103

Williams ED, Morales AM, Horn R (1968) Thyroid carcinoma and Cushing's syndrome. J Clin Pathol 21: 129

Williams ED, Doniach I, Bjarnason O, Michie W (1977) Thyroid cancer in an iodide rich area. Cancer 39: 215

Williams RH, Porte D Jr (1974) The pancreas. In: Williams RH (ed) Textbook of endocrinology, 5th edn. Saunders, Philadelphia London Toronto, p 566

Winship T, Rosvoll RV (1961) A study of thyroid cancer in children. Am J Surg 102: 747

Winter J, Eberlein WR, Bongiovanni AM (1966) The relationship of juvenile hypothyroidism to chronic lymphocytic thyroiditis. J Pediatr 69: 709

Winternitz WW, Dzur JA (1976) Pituitary failure secondary to head trauma: Case report. J Neurosurg 44: 504

Wolman M, Sterk VV, Gatt SL, Frenkel M (1961) Primary familial zanthomatosis with involvement and calcification of the adrenals. Report of two more cases in siblings of a previously described infant. Pediatrics 28: 742

Woolner LB, Beahrs OH, Black BM, McConahey WM, Keating FR Jr (1961) Classification and prognosis of thyroid carcinoma: A study of 885 observed cases in a thirty year period. Am J Surg 102: 354

Woolner LB, Beahrs OH, Black BM, McConahey WM, Keating FR Jr (1968) Thyroid carcinoma: General considerations and follow-up data on 1181 cases. In: Young S, Inman DR (eds) Thyroid neoplasia. Academic Press, London p 51

Yakovac WC, Baker L, Hummeler K (1971) Beta cell nesidioblas-tosis in idiopathic hypoglycemia of infancy. J Pediatr 79: 226

Yoon JW, Austin M, Onodera T, Notkins AL (1979) Isolation of a virus from the pancreas of a child with diabetic ketoacidosis. N Engl J Med 300: 1173

Zisman E, Lotz M, Jenkins ME, Bartter FC (1969) Studies in pseudohypoparathyroidism: Two cases with a probable selective deficiency of thyrotropin. Am J Med 46: 464

Chapter 14

Metabolic Disorders: General Considerations

Brian D. Lake

The study of metabolic disorders in children has provided significant insight into normal physiological pathways. Following these studies, methods of diagnosis have altered over the years, with the result that diagnostic histopathological examinations are less frequently performed. Education of the biochemist by the histopathologist, and vice versa, has led to the development of diagnostic techniques dependent on the study of urinary excretion products, enzyme assay of white blood cells, or microscopy of blood or bone marrow. In some disorders biopsies are still necessary, but these now make up a minor proportion of cases.

This chapter is devoted to conditions in which microscopy (light and/or electron) can provide a specific diagnosis or permit assignment of a metabolic defect to a particular group. Conditions that show nonspecific changes on microscopy and require biochemical analysis (e.g., maple syrup urine disease, phenylketonuria, etc.) are beyond the scope of this chapter and are well covered in the standard texts (Stanbury et al. 1978).

The simplest possible approach to the problem will often lead to a diagnosis in the shortest time with least discomfort to the patient and minimal involvement of the laboratory. As in all branches of medicine, there is no substitute for a well-informed clinical appraisal, and it is most important to establish a dialogue between the paediatrician and pathologist to ensure adequate investigation. Any surgeon to be involved should also be aware of the reasons for the biopsy and, more importantly, of what should and should not be done to it.

It must be remembered that metabolic disorders affect only a very small proportion of children; thus each disorder is rare and few paediatricians will be familiar with the whole range. It may be better to refer the patient to a specialist centre rather than to attempt a diagnosis with limited experience and expertise. However, some tests which can confirm or exclude the presence of metabolic disease can be performed in most laboratories.

Occasionally a biopsy will arrive in the laboratory without prior warning or consultation, even in the best-regulated centres. Under these circumstances, provided the specimen has arrived fresh and without undue delay, part should be fixed in formalin for routine histopathology, part should be frozen by the most rapid means available for histochemistry and biochemistry, and part should be fixed for electron microscopy. The two best methods for freezing tissue are (1) freezing in isopentane cooled to $-160°C$ in liquid nitrogen; and (2) freezing in hexane cooled to $-79°C$ in an acetone/solid carbon dioxide bath. An adequate, but less desirable method is freezing directly in liquid nitrogen. If these methods are not practicable, freezing on solid carbon dioxide, or in the last resort by placing in a deep freeze, will preserve the tissue for biochemical analysis but may leave it in a state unsuitable for sectioning. Whichever freezing technique is used, the frozen tissue should be carefully wrapped in aluminium cooking foil or parafilm to prevent drying, and stored in a precooled small bottle at $-20°C$ or below. It is a useful principle to 'fix some, freeze some, and take some for electron microscopy' from most biopsies, whether or not they are from patients suspected of having a metabolic disorder.

The sections below set out the principal tests that can be performed in the majority of hospital laboratories. The number of special stains required is not large. Considerable information can be derived from:

a) A periodic acid–Schiff (PAS) reaction to detect glycogen and compounds containing 1:2 glycol groups (e.g., oligosaccharides, gangliosides)

b) Sudan black for lipids. Some indication of the

presence of neutral fat or complex lipids can be inferred from the colour of the stained section

c) A reaction to show acid phosphatase activity. A change in the intensity of the reaction, or of its distribution within the cell, indicates altered cellular function.

Other methods will be necessary from time to time, but these three and a haematoxylin and eosin preparation will allow the general nature of the disorder to be appreciated. Figure 14.1 shows a rectal suction biopsy stained to reveal acid phosphatase activity.

The enzyme defects and substances stored in various types of lysosomal storage disease are shown in Table 14.1.

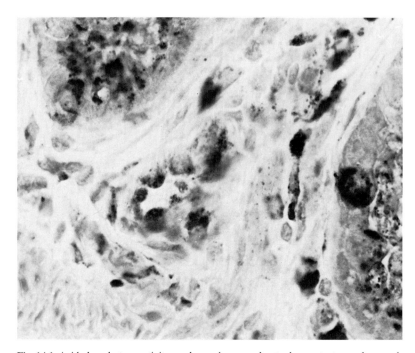

Fig. 14.1. Acid phosphatase activity can be used as a marker to demonstrate an abnormal reaction in an otherwise normal-looking cell. The endothelial cells normally show no acid phosphatase activity, but in this figure their involvement is clearly shown in a suction rectal biopsy from a patient with Niemall–Pick disease. Similar involvement may be demonstrated in Batten's disease and GMI-gangliosidosis. (1000 ×)

Table 14.1. Lysosomal storage disease: Stored substance and enzyme defect

Disorder	Enzyme defect	Stored substance
Pompe (GSD II)	Acid maltase (α-1:4 glucosidase)	Glycogen
Niemann–Pick (A and B)	Sphingomyelinase	Sphingomyelin (and cholesterol)
Gaucher (all forms)	Glucocerebrosidase (β-glucosidase)	Glucocerebroside
Wolman	Acid esterase	Cholesteryl esters and triglycerides
Fabry	α-Galactosidase	Ceramide trihexoside
Cystinosis	Unknown	Cystine
Tay–Sachs	Hexosaminidase A	GM2-Ganglioside
Sandhoff	Hexosaminidases A and B	GM2-Ganglioside
Generalized gangliosidosis	β-Galactosidase	GM1-Ganglioside
Batten's	Unknown	Retinoyl complexes
Ophthalmoplegic lipidosis	Unknown	Unknown
Farber	Ceramidase	Ceramides
Mannosidosis	α-Mannosidase	Oligosaccharides with terminal α-mannose
Cherry-red spot—myoclonus syndrome	Sialidase (2 types)	Oligosaccharides with sialic residues, and gangliosides
Metachromatic leucodystrophy	Arylsulphatase A	Cerebroside sulphate
Krabbe's leucodystrophy	Galactocerebosidase	Galactocerebroside

1. Blood-film Examination

1.1. General

The examination of blood films by light microscopy can help either in making a specific diagnosis or in suggesting a particular direction for further investigation. In many instances a confident diagnosis can be made and confirmed by a specific enzyme assay. In this way valuable time and expensive reagents—some of which have to be prepared and radiolabelled in the laboratory—can be saved. In contrast with this is the blunderbus approach, where the patient is investigated for every condition for which there is an enzyme assay on leucocytes. More often than not, no inborn error is detected under these circumstances. Screening by light microscopy can avoid many of these tests.

Some clues to the type of metabolic disorder can be derived from simple blood films stained with the May–Grunwald–Giemsa sequence (or Wright's, Leishmann or whatever routine haematological stain is preferred). Vacuolation, particularly in lymphocytes, is found in the conditions shown in Table 14.2. The change may be marked, with numerous well-defined large vacuoles in many cells, or minor, with small vacuoles in few cells. Occasionally all lymphocytes contain vacuoles. It should be noted that the vacuolation induced in monocytes by an anticoagulant is coarse, irregular, and without well-defined margins to the vacuoles. Even with prolonged immersion in anticoagulant, similar induced vacuolation is not apparent in neutrophils or lymphocytes.

Table 14.2. Conditions in which vacuolated lymphocytes are found

GMI-Gangliosidosis type 1
Niemann–Pick type A
Pompe's disease
Juvenile Batten's disease
Mannosidosis
I-cell disease
Wolman's disease
Mucopolysaccharidosis (sometimes in some forms)
Aspartylglucosaminuria
One form of ophthalmoplegic lipidosis
Fucosidosis
Cherry red spot—myoclonus syndrome
Mucolipidosis I and II
Salla disease

1.2. Pompe's Disease

In Pompe's disease, the infantile glycogen storage disease type II (see Section 5), each lymphocyte contains one or more small discrete vacuoles in which glycogen can be demonstrated. The demonstration of glycogen is best accomplished by the PAS reaction after a thin protective film of celloidin has been applied to the slide by dipping it in dilute (0.25%) celloidin in ethanol, shaking, and air-drying. A nuclear counterstain is added to define the cell type. Although B lymphocytes contain glycogen deposits, these deposits are usually all round the periphery of the cell; they do not show vacuolation and their proportion of the lymphocyte population is small. The glycogen deposits in Pompe's disease coincide with acid phosphatase activity, showing the lysosomal connection with the storage material.

The milder forms of this disorder, affecting juveniles and adults, also show glycogen deposits within lymphocyte vacuoles, but fewer lymphocytes appear to be affected. Confirmation of the diagnosis is by assay of acid maltase (α-1:4-glucosidase) activity in leucocytes or cultured fibroblasts. Prenatal diagnosis is possible; acid maltase is assayed in cultured amniotic fluid cells. The glycogen content of affected cells is high and the deposits are in discrete membrane-bound vacuoles 1–2 μm in diameter. Similar discrete deposits can be seen in uncultured amniotic fluid cells from affected pregnancies. However, prenatal diagnosis of an affected fetus should not be made by light microscopy. In normal amniotic fluid, glycogen-containing cells are prominent and could cause some confusion, which might lead to a wrong diagnosis. As with all metabolic disorders, first-hand experience of affected cases is necessary before the diagnosis can be made reliably.

1.3. Niemann–Pick Disease

The lymphocytic vacuoles in Niemann–Pick disease type A are also small and discrete, but they do not affect every lymphocyte. The deposited sphingomyelin is difficult to demonstrate since the staining reactions for small amounts are not sufficiently intense. The diagnosis can be confirmed by assay of sphingomyelinase activity in leucocytes or cultured fibroblasts, by examination of bone marrow (see Section 2.3), or by suction rectal biopsy (see Section 4.6). Lymphocytes in Niemann–Pick disease type B (juvenile/adult without neurological involvement) show no significant vacuolation.

1.4. Wolman's Disease

Wolman's disease and cholesteryl ester storage disease show lymphocytic vacuoles similar to those in Pompe's disease and type A Niemann–Pick disease. In this instance the vacuoles contain neutral fat (triglyceride and cholesteryl esters), which is readily stained with Oil Red O or Scharlach R. Deficiency of acid esterase activity can be reliably shown by a histochemical method in which 1-naphthyl acetate is used as substrate (Lake 1971). Large foam cells similar to those in marrow are rarely found in blood films, but have occasionally been seen in the acute infantile form.

1.5. Ophthalmoplegic Lipidosis

Small discrete vacuoles also occur in one form of ophthalmoplegic lipidosis (see Section 2.5), affecting a small but significant proportion of lymphocytes (Hagberg et al. 1978).

1.6. G_{MI}-Gangliosidosis

Numerous larger, but still well-defined, vacuoles occur in the majority of lymphocytes in infantile G_{MI}-gangliosidosis (type 1), but in the late infantile form (type 2) no vacuolation is seen. No storage substance can be shown within the vacuoles, which indicates that whatever is there is probably extremely soluble or that the appropriate staining reaction has yet to be found. The deficiency of β-galactosidase activity in neutrophils and lymphocytes from patients with types 1 and 2 disease can be shown histochemically by means of a substituted indoxyl substrate (Lake 1974).

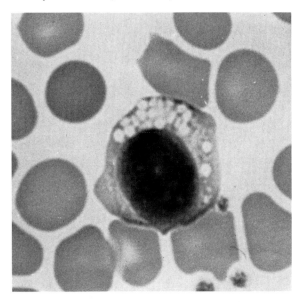

Fig. 14.2. Mannosidosis. Vacuolated lymphocyte in the blood film. Coarse vacuolation similar to this also occurs in G_{MI}-gangliosidosis and juvenile Batten's disease. (May–Grünwald–Giemsa; 2800 ×)

1.7. Mannosidosis

Similar coarse vacuolation, but affecting a smaller percentage of lymphocytes, is found in mannosidosis. In this instance the condition clinically resembles one of the mucopolysaccharidoses, but coarse lymphocytic vacuolation is not a feature of that group of conditions. Whenever the proportion of lymphocytes containing vacuoles is low, these lymphocytes do not occur with significant frequency in the main part of the film used for differential counting of blood cells. Thus a haematology department may well not report gross vacuolation unless they are aware that the affected cells tend to be found in the tail of the film and in the thicker regions. In mannosidosis (Fig. 14.2) the stored substances are water-soluble oligosaccharides, which can be demonstrated by the PAS method for glycogen (Section 1.2) in the affected lymphocytes in the thicker regions of the blood film. Even though the vacuoles are prominent in the tail of the film the stored substance cannot be demonstrated, probably because in this thinly spread region the cells have ruptured and their contents are thus freely soluble. Occasional lymphocytes with numerous small vacuoles occupying almost all the cytoplasm may also be present.

1.8. Batten's Disease

In Batten's disease, the most common group of neurodegenerative disorders seen in children, the type of lymphocyte abnormality varies with the subgroup of the disease. The juvenile type of Batten's disease (also known as Speilmeyer–Vogt or Sjögren disease), shows prominent coarse vacuoles in about 10%–30% of lymphocytes, particularly in the tail of the blood film. The contents of these vacuoles are unknown, and all stains fail to demonstrate anything within them. Electron microscopy shows mainly membrane-bound vacuoles, but in occasional vacuoles an impression of fingerprint bodies can be obtained after prolonged searching. The relatively large number of vacuolated cells with scarcity of fingerprint inclusions makes electron microscopy of lymphocytes in juvenile Batten's disease an unattractive means of diagnosis, and a rectal biopsy is the investigation of choice for confirmation of this condition. In contrast, late-infantile Batten's disease (or Bielschowsky–Jansky disease) is readily identifiable by the presence of curvilinear bodies in many lymphocytes at electron microscopy. No light microscopic abnormality is noted, and in particular no vacuoles are seen. Similarly, in the infantile form (or Santavuori or Hagberg type) no vacuoles are present but electron microscopy of the lymphocytes shows membrane-bound granular osmiophilic deposits (GROD) measuring 0.5–1 µm in diameter, with one or two of these present in about 50% of lymphocytes.

1.9. The Mucopolysaccharidoses (p. 463)

Occasional vacuolation is seen in the lymphocytes from patients with mucopolysaccharidosis, and in some of the vacuoles small densely staining inclusions may be present. The cells correspond to those initially described by Gasser (1950) in a patient with presumed Hurler's disease (MPS 1 H), and can be present in any of the mucopolysaccharidoses (Fig. 14.3). Lymphocytic vacuolation is also found in the mucolipidoses but in this group of disorders there is no mucopolysaccharide deposition and the metachromasia characteristic of the mucopolysaccharidoses is absent.

Table 14.3. Mucopolysaccharidosis: Metachromatic inclusions in lymphocytes

Percentages of lymphocytes containing metachromatic inclusions	Significance
20% or more	Sanfilippo (MPS III) is first choice. Some patients with Hunter (MPS II) may also have high counts
5%–20%	Hurler (MPS 1H) or Hunter (MPS II)
Less than 5%	Hurler–Sheie (MPS 1 H/S) or Scheie (MPS 1 S)

The degree of metachromasia is helpful in predicting the type of mucopolysaccharidosis, and following the staining procedure described by Muir et al. (1963) 100 lymphocytes are examined under an oil-immersion objective and the percentage of those with metachromatic inclusions is recorded. Table 14.3 is a general guide to the conclusions that can be drawn from the percentage of lymphocytes with metachromatic inclusions.

Patients with Morquio's syndrome (MPS IV) (Table 14.4) show no metachromasia, but basophilic inclusions of doubtful significance and specificity are sometimes present in neutrophils (Hansen 1972).

Although lymphocyte metachromasia is present in patients with Maroteaux–Lamy syndrome (MPS VI) the much more striking and specific Alder granulation is the better diagnostic pointer. All neutrophils show what appears to be marked toxic granulation in the routine Giemsa stains and it is almost impossible to differentiate this specific granulation from toxic granulation without special stains. Alder granulation (Fig. 14.4) is not metachromatic with the standard toluidine blue method (neither are toxic granules), but in the more sensitive toluidine blue staining method of Haust and Landing (1961) Alder granulation is basophilic while toxic granulation remains unstained. It is interesting to note that the first description of the Maroteaux–Lamy syndrome must be ascribed to Alder (1939), who in his presentation clearly described two patients with the mild form of Maroteaux–Lamy syndrome (MPS VI B), each of

Table 14.4. The mucopolysaccharidoses

Type[a]		Enzyme defect	Urinary GAG
IH IS IH/S	Hurler Scheie Hurler/Scheie	α-L-Iduronidase	Dermatan sulphate Heparan sulphate
II	Hunter	Sulphoiduronate sulphatase	Dermatan sulphate Heparan sulphate

III A
    B
    C
	Sanfilippo
	Sanfilippo
	Sanfilippo
		Heparan sulphate-N-sulphatase
		N-acetyl-α-D-glucosaminidase
		Acetyl CoA: α-glucosaminide
		   N-acetyltransferase
			Heparan sulphate

IV	Morquio	Chondroitin sulphate—
		   N-acetylhexosamine—
		   sulphate 6-sulphatase
			Keratan sulphate

VI	Maroteaux-Lamy	Chondroitin sulphate-N-
		   acetylgalactosamine sulphate-4
		   sulphatase
			Dermatan sulphate

VII		β-Glucuronidase	Dermatan sulphate

[a] *Type V* is vacant since the Scheie Syndrome (originally type V) was transferred to type I on recognition of its enzyme defect.

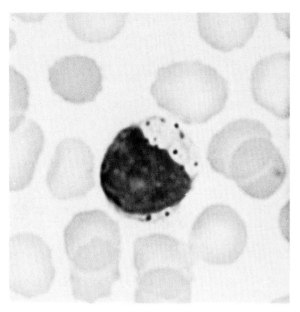

Fig. 14.3. Gasser cell in blood film. Mucopolysaccharidosis. These cells can occur in most mucopolysaccharidoses, but are not specific for any particular type. (May–Grünwald–Giemsa; 2800 ×)

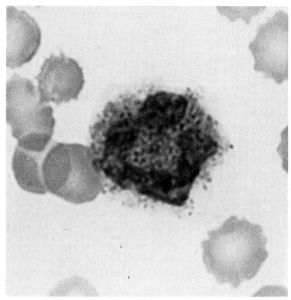

Fig. 14.4. Alder granulation in neutrophil in a blood film from a patient with Maroteaux–Lamy syndrome (MPS VI). (2800 ×)

whom had the neutrophil granules. Similar granulation is reported in cases of mucosulphatidosis (Rampini et al. 1970) and of β-glucuronidase deficiency (Pfeiffer et al. 1977).

Reilly's article (1941) created some confusion since he did not clearly state whether his granules were present in bone marrow cells or leucocytes. Since there are marked differences between bone marrow and blood cells it is not surprising that Reilly granules have not always been seen in mucopolysaccharidosis and consequently have been regarded with some suspicion.

1.10. Other Conditions

Lymphocytic vacuolation occurs in a number of other, much rarer, conditions. Aspartylglucosaminuria, which was first described in England (Jenner and Pollitt 1967) and later found to be relatively common in Finland (Haltia et al. 1975), shows very marked, coarse vacuolation similar to that seen in juvenile Batten's disease, type 1 G_{MI}-gangliosidosis, and Salla disease (Aula et al. 1979).

Some patients with fucosidosis and some with the cherry red spot–myoclonus syndrome, also known as sialidosis (Rapin et al. 1978), show a small number of vacuolated lymphocytes which may be missed without extensive searching.

1.11. Neutrophil Vacuolation

Neutrophil abnormalities are rare in metabolic disorders. In some cases where carnitine deficiency has been established, and in some cases where it is suspected but not proven, lipid deposits can be found in vacuolated neutrophils. This phenomenon, which should not be confused with the less conspicuous neutrophil vacuolation sometimes seen in acute infections, was described by Jordans (1953) in two brothers, who in retrospect may have had carnitine deficiency. However, not all patients with carnitine deficiency have neutrophil vacuolation.

2. Bone-marrow Examination

2.1. General

The judicious use of bone-marrow sampling can be of great help in deciding whether a patient with hepatosplenomegaly has a storage disease or whether the hepatosplenomegaly is caused by malignancy, infection, or some other process. Most histopathologists are unused to looking at marrow films and prefer their samples fixed, embedded, and sectioned. If this practice is followed it will not be possible to draw any conclusions about storage disorders. For the diagnosis of this group of conditions, several films should be made from the aspirate, either directly from the needle or after sequestrene treatment. They should be made by a person experienced in making high-quality films, as opposed to the smear so often offered. A standard haematological stain will show storage cells, which are usually quite numerous, although on rare occasions only a few may be found in an otherwise adequate sample. There is no need to fix the other films, and as long as they remain dry their cytochemical reactions will be preserved for many weeks and can if necessary be sent by post for further study.

It is important that purely histochemical methods are used, so that appropriate conclusions can be made. For example, the Sudan black method commonly used by haematologists does not demonstrate fat but peroxidatic activity. The methods that give the most useful information are Sudan Black for lipids, PAS for carbohydrates and an acid phosphatase reaction for lysosomal activity. Normal bone marrow cells do not show much acid phosphatase activity after short incubation (30 min in a Gomori medium), and the strong activity of histiocytes or macrophages is easily visible under a lower-power objective. Other staining methods may occasionally be necessary.

2.2. Gaucher's Disease (p. 552)

Two main types of storage cell occur in bone marrow, and to the inexperienced eye they can cause problems of identification. The Gaucher cell is large, is sometimes multinucleate, and has a cytoplasm which stains a bluish grey with Giemsa or similar stains (Figs. 14.5 and 14.6). In addition, the cytoplasm is often described as having the appearance of crumpled tissue paper. Many of the cells have this rather stripey look, in complete contrast with the foamy vacuolated appearances of the storage cells in Niemann–Pick disease and most other lipid storage diseases. Gaucher cells stain only weakly with Sudan Black, and moderately with PAS, these two reactions being in keeping with the staining properties of glucocerebroside. Gaucher cells, like all storage cells and histiocytes with activated lysosomal systems, show strong acid phosphatase activity with β-glycerophosphate as substrate. The deficiency of the glucocerebrosidase as a β-glucosidase cannot be shown by histochemical methods.

The number of Gaucher cells is variable, but in general terms the infantile cases show numerous positive cells in a marrow aspirate, while the juvenile and adult forms tend to have fewer Gaucher cells. Cells that are reputedly similar to those in Gaucher's disease have been reported in chronic myeloid leukaemia and thalassemia. In G_{MI}-gangliosidosis type 2 (late infantile) Gaucher-like cells are present, but the cytoplasm is less fibrillar, more closely packed, and stains slightly more intensely blue than that of Gaucher cells in a Giemsa preparation. In these cases the deficiency of β-galactosidase activity can be detected in the marrow sample or in blood films (see Section 1.6).

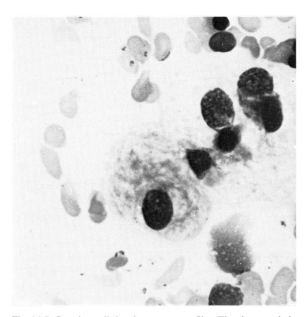

Fig. 14.5. Gaucher cells in a bone-marrow film. The characteristic stripey appearance is not always easily seen. (May–Grünwald–Giemsa; 1000 ×)

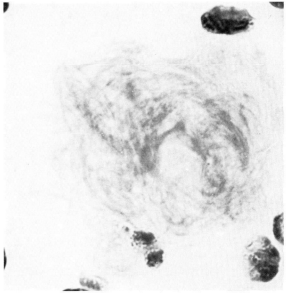

Fig. 14.6. A Gaucher cell in a bone-marrow film. The fibrillar stripey nature of the cytoplasm is clearly visible. (Sudan Black; 1800 ×)

2.3. Niemann–Pick Disease (see also p. 554)

Large foamy vacuolated histiocytes occur in most storage disorders, and differentiation of one from another rests on subtle morphological changes and correlation of the appearances of foamy cells with other cellular changes and their histochemical staining properties. The presence of vacuoles in peripheral blood lymphocytes and the type of vacuole or their absence will sometimes need to be taken into account.

In Niemann–Pick disease type A (infantile) (Fig. 14.7), the foamy marrow storage cells stain weakly with Sudan Black, and when the Sudan Black preparations are examined in polarized light a reddish birefringence can be seen in the storage cells in most cases. The vacuoles of the storage cell are mostly small and uniform in size, and only rarely are ingested white cells or nuclear debris present. The PAS reaction is variably positive. Acid phosphatase activity is strong and mainly confined to the periphery of the vacuoles. Lymphocytic vacuolation should also be present.

2.4. Adult Niemann–Pick Disease and Sea-blue Histiocytes

In the juvenile nonneurological form of Niemann–Pick disease marrow cells similar to those in the

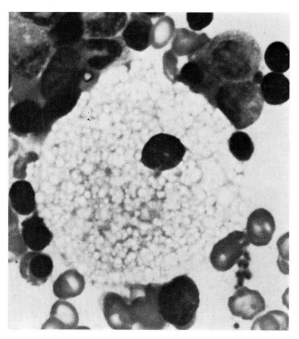

Fig. 14.7. A Niemann–Pick cell in a bone-marrow film. The fairly uniform vacuolation in the cytoplasm and the absence of other features are characteristic. (May–Grünwald–Giemsa; 1000 ×)

infantile form are found but the lymphocytic vacuolation is usually absent. Adult Niemann–Pick disease (the distinction between the adult and juvenile forms may be spurious) shows *numerous* unmistakable sea-blue histiocytes. These cells are so striking that "they should alert even the most casual of haematopathologists" (Reynolds 1973). To be of significance these cells should be numerous and easily seen in all parts of the film. The cytoplasm of the cells is packed with granules, stains deep blue with Giemsa or Wright stains, is PAS- and Sudan Black-positive, and shows strong autofluorescence. This material has none of the properties of sphingomyelin and its composition is not known. Scattered sphingomyelin-containing cells and intermediate forms are present but these need to be searched for.

Confirmation of the diagnosis of Niemann–Pick disease can be made by assay of sphingomyelinase activity in white blood cells or in cultured fibroblasts, or if these techniques are not available then a liver biopsy may be necessary. Routine histopathology in this instance is of less importance than the examination of frozen tissue by histochemistry and lipid extraction. As in all metabolic disorders, frozen tissue should be preserved for further study.

Cells similar to sea-blue histiocytes are found in lecithin–cholesterol–acyltransferase deficiency, but in much smaller numbers. Small numbers of cells of this type are occasionally present in ophthalmoplegic lipidosis.

2.5. Ophthalmoplegic Lipidosis

Some confusion may be caused by the classification of Niemann–Pick diseases and the similarity of the storage cells in the various types. In types A (infantile with neurological involvement) and B (juvenile/adult without neurological involvement), accumulation of sphingomyelin and deficiency of sphingomyelinase is well documented. In the other types (C and D) there is no such deficiency. Sphingomyelin accumulation is found in only a minority of patients, and then only in the spleen. These types (C and D) are often referred to as 'atypical Niemann–Pick disease', but since they have fairly distinctive clinical features and the pathology of the brain and viscera appear to be identical (Neville et al. 1973), the growing tendency is to put them together and apply the term 'ophthalmoplegic lipidosis', reflecting the lipid storage and the defect of vertical gaze (Lake 1977). No enzyme defect has been found and the nature of the stored substance is unknown, although Wenger et al. (1977) have found an abnormally low spingomyelinase activity in cultured fibroblasts from a group of these patients, which they prefer to label as sphingomyelin lipidosis even though sphingomyelin excess is not a constant feature. The foam cells found in the marrow (Fig. 14.8) resemble those of Niemann–Pick disease type A, but the vacuoles are of widely varying sizes and densely staining inclusions are frequently present in Giemsa preparations. The cells contain no demonstrable fat, show some PAS positivity, and have strong acid phosphatase activity. The course is long and neurological symptoms are slow to appear so it is important to be certain of the diagnosis, and to confirm the neuronal storage by rectal biopsy (see Section 4.4).

2.6. Gangliosidosis

The large foamy histiocytes found in G_{M1}-gangliosidosis type 1 have no characteristic staining reactions. Diagnosis rests on the presence of coarsely vacuolated lymphocytes and the absence of β-galactosidase activity, which must be shown by a histochemical method (Lake 1974) or by quantitative biochemical assay. No histiocytes can be found in the marrow in cases of G_{M2}-gangliosidosis (Tay–Sachs disease).

2.7. Wolman's Disease

Histiocytes that contain much neutral fat (cholesterol, cholesteryl esters, triglycerides) and stain strongly with Sudan Black or Oil Red O are present in Wolman's disease (infantile and juvenile forms), and these stain a distinctive purple colour with Nile Blue. Vacuolated lymphocytes containing neutral fat and the absence of acid esterase activity are necessary for the diagnosis.

2.8. Mucopolysaccharidosis

Although storage cells are found in the bone marrow from patients with mucopolysaccharidosis (Hansen 1972), few studies have been made in relation to the recently described enzyme defects, and it is thus difficult to relate appearances to a particular form of mucopolysaccharidosis. Bone-marrow biopsy should never be necessary except for haematological reasons. There are simpler and more reliable methods available for the diagnosis of mucopolysaccharidosis (see Tables 14.3 and 14.4 and Section 3.5).

2.9. Acquired Storage Cells

Acquired storage cells occur occasionally and can be

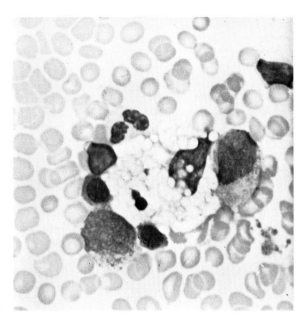

Fig. 14.8. Ophthalmoplegic lipidosis. Foamy cell in a bone-marrow film. Variable vacuole size and darkly stained inclusions differentiate these cells from other foamy storage cells. (May–Grünwald–Giemsa; 1000 ×)

related to an overload of the reticuloendothelial system in conditions such as myeloid leukaemia and thalassaemia. In histiocytosis X large foamy marrow cells may be encountered, particularly in advanced cases, but these cells, although striking in Giemsa preparations, have no demonstrable storage substance. Their acid phosphatase reaction is very strong and sharply localized, in contrast with the strong but diffuse reaction of genuine storage cells. These, however, are subtle microscopic distinctions, and the clinical history will be especially important in these cases. Conditions leading to lipid overload, e.g., infusions, may also produce foamy lipid-laden macrophages in marrow, and disorders involving lipid metabolism (hyperliproproteinaemias, hyperlipidaemia, and Tangier disease) may show similar changes.

2.10. Cystinosis

It is not always appreciated that cystine crystals, although relatively insoluble, have sufficient solubility to disappear almost completely from routinely stained films. For the diagnosis of cystinosis a slightly different approach is needed. Films should be made with great care, since the act of making the film can easily rupture the histiocytes in which the crystals are situated, in which case the crystals of cystine are much more likely to be lost. The films are air-dried, fixed in absolute alcohol, and stained with 1 % basic fuchsin in 70 % alcohol for 10 min, followed by rinsing in alcohol, clearing, and mounting. The small amount of water in the stain is insufficient to dissolve any crystine present but allows a reasonable degree of nuclear staining. The slides are then examined between partly crossed polarizers for cystine crystals, which are birefringent in their longitudinal plane. This means that the characteristic brick-shaped crystal is easily seen under these conditions, while the hexagonal end of the crystal is not so readily visible (Fig. 14.9). Most marrow samples contain a large preponderance of the brick-shaped crystals, but occasionally the less visible hexagonal shape may predominate.

A wet preparation is also invaluable for the diagnosis of cystinosis. This is made by placing one drop of the anticoagulant-treated marrow sample on a slide and covering with a large cover slip. The gently made thin preparation is ideal for searching for the intact histiocytes containing cystine crystals, and individual cystine crystals from histiocytes ruptured by the action of aspirating the marrow are also readily visible. Dirt, dust, and glass fragments (from diamond marking of the slides) are birefringent but have an irregular outline.

2.11. Bone-marrow Biopsy as an Exclusion Test

The absence of storage-type cells from an appropriately stained, adequate sample almost certainly

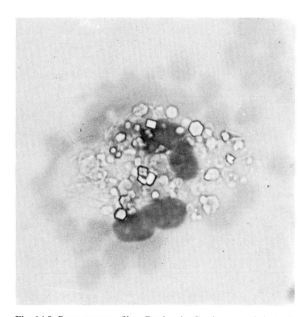

Fig. 14.9. Bone-marrow film. Cystinosis. Cystine crystals in typical hexagonal and brick shapes within a macrophage are readily visible in partially polarized light. Some fine needle-shaped crystals are also visible. The film has been lightly stained with alcoholic basic fuchsin to show nuclei. (1100 ×)

means that a storage disease can be excluded, often a useful exclusion test in a child with unexplained hepatosplenomegaly.

It is a general principle that if storage cells are seen in a bone-marrow sample and their precise identity is not known then all that should be reported is that storage cells are present. In many cases a label has been attached to a finding, and has subsequently (sometimes many years later) been proved wrong. The course of the disease may be different from that diagnosed and in some instances prenatal diagnosis has been attempted on the basis of wrong information. In all cases of storage disease enzyme assay is an essential part of the diagnosis. The histopathologist's task is to point the enzymologists in the right direction and to eliminate those cases in which no storage disease is present.

3. Urine Examination

3.1. General

The study of urinary sediment by light microscopy is of help only in metachromatic leucodystrophy and, in a limited way, in Fabry's disease. Although there have been reports on the electron microscopy of urinary sediment in Batten's disease (Armstrong et al. 1977), this must be regarded as one of the more exotic of research projects. Simpler and more reliable methods are available for routine diagnosis.

Chemical study of urinary deposit or supernatant by thin-layer chromatography can be extremely helpful in the diagnosis of the mucopolysaccharidoses, Fabry's disease, and the rarer mannosidosis, fucosidosis, and sialidoses.

3.2. Metachromatic Leucodystrophy

The presence in the urinary sediment of intracellular deposits of a substance staining golden yellow-brown after staining with the toluidine blue method as described by Bodian and Lake (1963) is pathognomonic for metachromatic leucodystrophy, although in a different clinical setting patients with mucosulphatidosis also show these deposits. The demonstration of intracellular deposits is vital to the diagnosis, but a high index of suspicion should be maintained if extracellular material is seen in the form of tubular casts. The deposits show a greenish birefringence when examined in polarized light. The cresyl–fast violet method (Lake 1965) is less useful, having the disadvantages of fading and of a poorer colour contrast between deposits and normally stained cells than with the toluidine blue method.

The appearance of the metachromatically stained deposits is identical in both metachromatic leuco-dystrophy and mucosulphatidosis. These two conditions can be differentiated in the laboratory by examination of routinely stained blood films, where Alder granulation (see Section 1.9) is present in mucosulphatidosis but absent in metachromatic leucodystrophy.

The substance inducing metachromasia in the exfoliated renal epithelial cells is a mixture of sulphatides (cerebroside sulphates) similar to the sulphatide found in the brain in metachromatic leucodystrophy. The presence of sulphatide can be confirmed by thin-layer chromatography of a lipid extract of the urinary sediment.

3.3. Fabry's Disease

Large tubular casts and mulberry-like cells staining intensely with PAS are found in the urinary sediment from patients with Fabry's disease. The cells do not exhibit metachromasia but do show a silvery birefringence. It is not always easy to see these cells and deposits, since normal urine often contains cells that stain with PAS, albeit to a lesser extent. A better procedure is to extract the deposit with chloroform/methanol (2:1 v/v) and after washing and drying the extract to perform thin-layer chromatography (TLC) (Lake and Goodwin 1976) to show the large excesses of both ceramide di- and trihexosides (Fabry's disease is X-linked); the normal individual rarely shows both di- and trihexoside, although either substance can be present separately.

3.4. Oligosaccharidoses

Water-soluble oligosaccharides can be detected by TLC in the supernatant of centrifuged urine from patients with sialidosis, mannosidosis, fucosidosis, and aspartylglucosaminuria (Humbel and Collart 1975). The patterns obtained are not always clear, but with refinements of the method better use of this route for diagnosis should be possible. The reported excess of glucocerebroside in the urine from patients with Gaucher's disease and of galactocerebroside in that of patients with Krabbe's disease is so small as not to be a reliable diagnostic test, at least in the studies performed in the author's laboratory (A. Fehily, unpublished observations).

3.5. Mucopolysaccharidoses

The excess urinary glycosaminoglycan (GAG) excretion in the mucopolysaccharidoses cannot be detected by light microscopy and is best demonstrated by one of the several precipitation methods available (Pennock 1976). The Alcian Blue precipitation method described by Whiteman (1973) is sensitive and allows quantification, and is in routine use at the Hospital for Sick Children. Further characterization of the GAG is made by two-way chromatography and electrophoresis, followed by staining by Alcian Blue. The pattern of GAG excretion is of particular importance in those cases of mucopolysaccharidosis where enzyme characterization is not readily available.

The simple spot test, applying urine to a filter paper, drying and staining with toluidine blue, is not reliable and can give negative results in confirmed cases. This method, apart from its insensitivity, cannot identify individual GAGs and cannot be used quantitatively.

4. Neuronal Storage Disease: Diagnosis by Rectal Biopsy

4.1. General Considerations on Rectal Biopsy

Rectal biopsy gives a positive indication of neuronal storage in all the neuronal storage diseases, and with the use of appropriate staining methods and electron microscopy the precise diagnosis should be possible in all cases. However, whether rectal biopsy is justifiable depends on the biochemical facilities available and the expertise of the surgeon. As originally used, rectal biopsy is a simple procedure in practised hands, but it has become outdated, for two reasons: Firstly, unless the surgeon has had experience in performing full-thickness biopsies and is familiar with the hazards involved, an unsatisfactory biopsy may be obtained and there may be surgical complications. Unsatisfactory biopsies and surgical complications can be avoided by performing an appendectomy and using the appendix as a source of neurones. This has one advantage and two disadvantages. The advantage is that much more tissue is obtained on which electron microscopy, light microscopy, and biochemical studies can be made. The two disadvantages are that patients are less tolerant of appendectomy than of rectal biopsy, and, perhaps more important, the fact that the changes in the biopsy may not exactly parallel those in rectal biopsies. The main changes of neuronal storage and smooth muscle involvement are the same but the subtle changes that help to differentiate one condition from another may not be present.

Secondly, since the inception of rectal biopsy for neurological diagnosis biochemical advances have been enormous, and in the majority of cases the diagnosis can be made by way of enzyme assay in white blood cells, serum, or cultured fibroblasts. There are a few conditions (Batten's disease, ophthalmoplegic lipidosis and the recently expanding group of sialidoses), however, in which neuronal involvement must be demonstrated before the diagnosis, with its grave prognosis, can be made.

Suction rectal biopsy of the type taken for the diagnosis of Hirschsprung's disease is usually adequate, and since it can be taken without anaesthetic is now the preferred biopsy. It has the advantage that several biopsies may be taken and repeated if necessary.

4.2. Staining Methods

The diagnostic appearances in rectal biopsies will be given for the whole range of neuronal storage diseases to provide an overall picture. Routinely prepared sections of formalin-fixed, paraffin wax-embedded tissue are of no help in differential diagnosis, because the lipids are dissolved during processing and their characteristic staining reactions are lost. Cryostat sections of fresh-frozen tissue are therefore essential and these should be stained by the following methods:

1) Haematoxylin and eosin
2) PAS (after 10-min fixation in 4% formaldehyde)
3) PAS celloidin (The slide is dipped in 0.25% celloidin in ethanol and dried; retains water-soluble compounds)
4) Luxol fast blue, neutral red
5) Sudan Black (no fixation required)
6) Feyrter's thionin method
7) Toluidine blue for brown metachromasia
8) An acid phosphatase reaction
9) An unstained, unfixed, mounted section for examination for autofluorescence (excitation 365 nm).

All these methods should be used, and if suction rectal biopsies are taken serial sections should be examined.

4.3. Gangliosidoses, Sialidoses and Farber's Disease

In the gangliosidoses the neurones are markedly enlarged and foamy, and stain strongly with both PAS methods. A rose-purple metachromasia is produced immediately with Feyrter's method, indicating the presence of the sialic acid grouping in the ganglioside. Weak staining is found with Sudan Black and luxol fast blue. There is almost no autofluorescence. Tay–Sachs disease (of all types) can be differentiated from G_{MI}-gangliosidosis by the presence of PAS-positive histiocytes in the lamina propria and vacuolation of endothelial cells in G_{MI}-gangliosidosis and by the presence of β-galactosidase activity in Tay–Sachs disease. The histochemical method for detecting hexosaminidase activity cannot demonstrate the deficiency of the A component of this enzyme in Tay–Sachs disease (Lake and Ellis 1976), but can be used to show the total deficiency of hexosaminidase activity in Sandhoff's disease.

The sialidoses (Cherry red spot–myoclonus syndrome) (Rapin et al. 1978) have very similar staining reactions, and differentiation from the gangliosidoses may not be possible by rectal biopsy. Examination of the bone marrow and/or urine or specific enzyme assay will provide the diagnosis.

In Farber's disease (Toppet et al. 1978), neuronal changes similar to those in the gangliosidoses may cause some confusion. Although ceramidase deficiency causes accumulation of ceramides there is also an increase of a ganglioside-like substance giving rise to PAS positivity and metachromasia with Feyrter's thionin. However, the diagnostic point in this condition is the silvery birefringence in polarized light, seen in the neurones after staining with Sudan Black. This is in contrast with the red birefringence given by the sphingomyelin deposition in Niemann–Pick disease.

4.4. Ophthalmoplegic Lipidosis

Patients with ophthalmoplegic lipidosis (Neville et al. 1973; Lake 1977) usually present with hepatosplenomegaly alone and do not show neurological symptoms for several years. The diagnosis, initially made by examination of bone-marrow films, needs confirmation by demonstration of neuronal involvement. Storage of the (as yet unidentified) substance in the neurones is present at an early age, and demonstration of this deposition is essential before the diagnosis, with its attendant grave prognosis, can be made.

The substance(s) accumulating in the neurones is (are) water-soluble and best demonstrated by the protected PAS reaction (PAS cell) (Fig. 14.10). The intensity of the PAS reaction is diminished by prior aqueous fixation and in some instances may be negative under these conditions. Metachromasia with Feyrter's thionin is present, indicating sialic acid residues, and apart from an intense acid phosphatase reaction the neurones display no other staining reactions. The presence of histiocytes in the

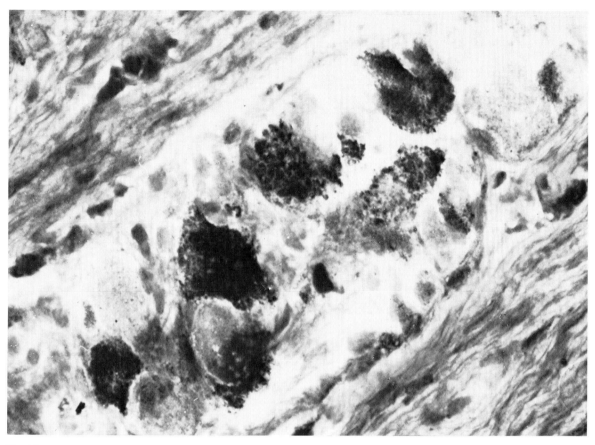

Fig. 14.10. Ophthalmoplegic lipidosis. Neurones in a cryostat section of appendix stained by the protected PAS method (PAS cell) show storage of a substance that is removed by aqueous fixatives. (800 ×)

lamina propria is a nonspecific and not uncommon finding, but in this condition they are also present in the submucosa, just beneath the muscularis mucosae.

4.5. Batten's Disease

Involvement of the smooth-muscle cells is not apparent in the conditions mentioned in the previous sections, but is found consistently together with neuronal storage in the Batten group of disorders. The neuronal staining reactions are different from group to group (Lake 1976) but are consistent within the group, and are described in Table 14.5. In addition to these reactions and the presence of smooth-muscle involvement (best indicated by autofluorescence of the deposited substance), juvenile Batten's disease always has acid phosphatase-positive histiocytes scattered among the smooth muscle cells. Proof of neuronal involvement is necessary in juvenile Batten's disease (Fig. 14.11), because the clinical situation is often that of a patient with progressive visual failure only. There may be

vacuolated lymphocytes but examination of a rectal biopsy is the only way of predicting the onset of neurological deterioration, which may occur several years later.

As with all neuronal storage disorders, the neuronal deposition is present long before neurological symptoms occur. The rectal biopsy approach can be used in a positive way to diagnose affected patients, and in a negative way to exclude the possibility of younger siblings being affected.

Table 14.5. Neuronal staining reactions in Batten's disease (rectal biopsies)

Subgroup	PAS	Sudan Black	Luxol Fast Blue	Autofluorescence
Infantile	+ +	+ +	−	+ +
Late infantile	±	+	±, +	+
Juvenile	+ +	+ +	+ +	+ +

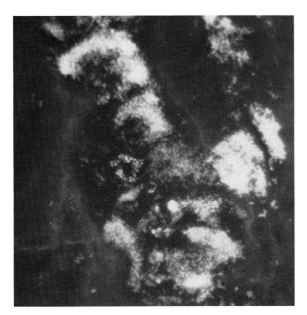

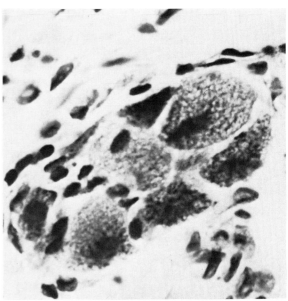

Fig. 14.11. Juvenile Batten's disease. Neurones in a cryostat section of a rectal biopsy, showing autofluorescence in an unstained unfixed section. Excitation with UG5 or BG3 filter. (800 ×)

Fig. 14.13. Rectal biopsy; Niemann–Pick disease type A. The neurones in Meissner's plexus have a distended foamy cytoplasm, an appearance also seen in the gangliosidoses. (950 ×)

4.6. Niemann–Pick Disease

Some patients with Niemann–Pick disease of the infantile type (type A) are late in showing neurological involvement, and despite proof of the disease (enzyme assay in leucocytes, liver biopsy, bone marrow) there may be some doubt as to the neuronopathic nature of the disease. Suction rectal biopsy will provide the necessary evidence, as in ophthalmoplegic lipidosis and juvenile Batten's disease.

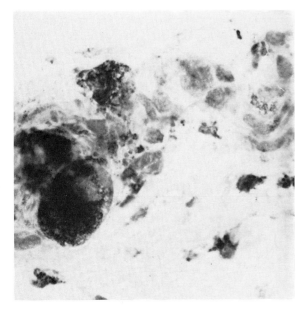

Fig. 14.12. Niemann–Pick disease type A. Cryostat section of a suction rectal biopsy stained to show acid phosphatase activity. Three neurones showing strong activity can be seen with their nerve supply. Macrophages in the loose connective tissue also show strong activity. (700 ×)

The neurones of Meissner's plexus are large and have a foamy, ground-glass cytoplasm. They are very similar in appearance to the classic neuronal storage pictures of Tay–Sachs disease (Figs. 14.12 and 14.13). The cytoplasm stains with Sudan Black (with reddish birefringence in polarized light) and has a honeycomb-like appearance in the acid phosphatase reaction. It is not always easy to be sure that the cells are neurones, but often they occur in small clusters of two or three with the tell-tale nerves leading to them.

The lamina propria is filled with histiocytes, which stain positively with Sudan Black and show reddish birefringence in polarized light, are variably PAS-positive, and exhibit strong acid phosphatase activity (Fig. 14.14). Endothelial cells are involved and this is best shown in the acid phosphatase preparation. Smooth-muscle cells contain sudanophilic deposits but this is not always marked. Numerous histiocytes are present throughout the submucosa.

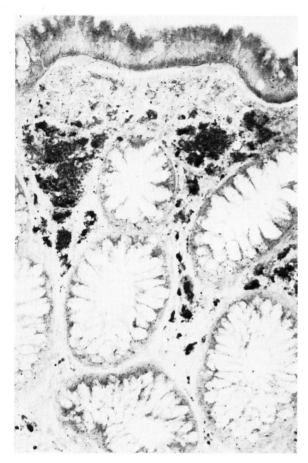

Fig. 14.14. Niemann–Pick disease type A. Cryostat section of suction rectal biopsy stained with Sudan black, showing numerous sudanophilic macrophages in the lamina propria. (280 ×)

4.7. Electron Microscopy

Ultrastructural studies of the neuronal deposits reveal membranous cytoplasmic bodies in the gangliosidoses and sialidoses (Fig. 14.15), Zebra-like bodies in Farber's disease, and pleomorphic lipid bodies in ophthalmoplegic lipidosis (not only in neurones but also in axonal swellings: Fig. 14.16). Granular osmiophilic deposits (finely granular deposits within a membrane-bound body some 1 μm in diameter) are present in infantile Batten's disease (Fig. 14.17), curvilinear bodies in the late infantile form (Fig. 14.18), and fingerprint bodies in the juvenile form (Lake 1976; Fig. 14.19).

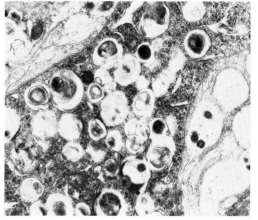

Fig. 14.16. Electron micrograph. Pleomorphic lipid bodies in a neurone from a rectal biopsy from a patient with ophthalmoplegic lipidosis. (18 000 ×)

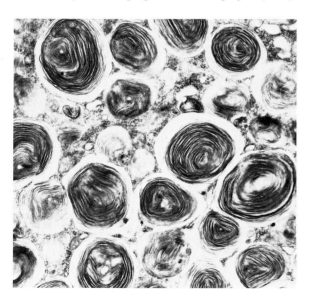

Fig. 14.15. Electron micrograph. Membranous cytoplasmic bodies (MCBs) in a neurone from the appendix of a patient with generalized gangliosidosis. The same appearance is also found in Tay–Sachs disease. (18 000 ×)

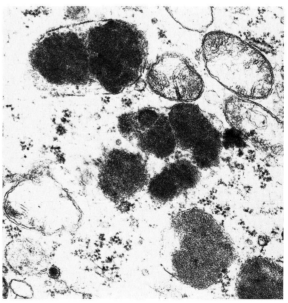

Fig. 14.17. Electron micrograph. Infantile Batten's disease. Granular osmiophilic deposits (GROD) in a neurone. (45 000 ×)

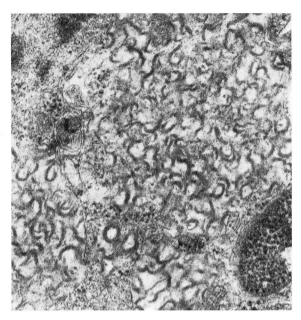

Fig. 14.18. Electron micrograph. Late infantile Batten's disease. Curvilinear bodies in a smooth muscle cell. Similar deposits are also found in neurons and lymphocytes. (68 000 ×)

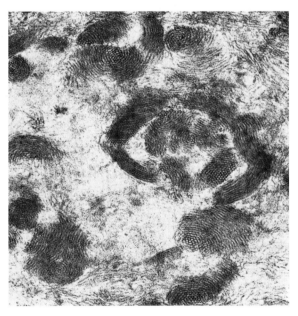

Fig. 14.19. Electron micrograph. Juvenile Batten's disease. Fingerprint bodies are present in the neuronal cytoplasm. (110 000 ×)

5. Glycogen Storage Disease (GSD)

5.1. General

Glycogen storage disease in its various forms is an important cause of failure to thrive associated with hepatomegaly. Biochemical screening (fasting blood sugar levels, glucagon stimulation in the fasting state, lactate and uric acid levels) will often give some indication of the type of GSD, and confirmation can sometimes be obtained by assay of the appropriate enzyme in red blood cells or leucocytes. A relatively large proportion of patients do not respond appropriately to glucagon, and many will need a biopsy to confirm the diagnosis. Table 14.6 shows the major types of GSD encountered. Type 5 (McArdle's disease: myophosphorylase deficiency) has been excluded from the table because it is extremely rare in children, and GSD that cannot be adequately typed is labelled type 6. From this last category there has emerged a group of patients with phophorylase kinase deficiency; to avoid confusion and proliferation of numbers this group has been designated 'type 6B'. Figure 14.20 shows the pathways of glycogen metabolism.

In many patients a liver biopsy will be necessary. This should only be performed after discussion between pathologist, surgeon, and clinician. An open liver biopsy provides most material but two cores with the Trucut needle will give adequate tissue for biochemistry and histochemistry with a small amount for routine histology. Open biopsies are divided similarly, with the piece for histology having a large surface area but little depth. The biopsies should be collected from the operating theatre and either taken directly to the laboratory or dealt with on the spot, since delay in freezing can affect the enzyme activities. It is also good practice to take a small piece of muscle (rectus abdominis or internal oblique) from the edge of the incision for freezing, so that it can be studied to determine whether there is muscle involvement. Where facilities permit, a small piece of skin can also be put into culture medium to establish a fibroblast line on which enzyme and metabolic studies can be made.

Routine histology gives only minimal information in GSD. In particular, the glycogen content cannot be related to the colour of specific stains, because the glycogens in these storage diseases have differing solubilities and much may be lost in the fixation and processing (Fig. 14.21). Cryostat sections are essential to show glycogen and enzymes, and can also give perfectly adequate histological results if the freezing and sectioning are carefully controlled.

Table 14.6. Glycogen storage diseases

Type	Enzyme defect	Signs and symptoms	Liver pathology
1A	Glucose-6-phosphatase	Hepatomegaly, extreme hypoglycaemia, acidosis, raised uric acid	Very fatty, absent G-6-Pase, normal glycogen content
1B	Unknown	Identical with 1A	As above, but normal G-6-Pase
2A	Acid α-1:4-glucosidase	No hypoglycaemia, hepatosplenomegaly, cardiomegaly, hypotonia	Increased hepatocyte glycogen, increased Kupffer cell glycogen, strong acid phosphatase activity
2B	Acid α-1:4-glucosidase	Affects skeletal muscle only	
3	Debranching enzyme	Mild hypoglycaemia, marked hepatomegaly, raised LFT	Very high glycogen content. No fat, portal fibrosis
4	Branching enzyme	Hepatomegaly, rarely hypoglycaemic jaundice	Cirrhosis, bile stasis, indigestible glycogen
6B	Phosphorylase kinase	Mild hepatomegaly, no hypoglycaemia	Very high glycogen content, mild to moderate fat, no fibrosis

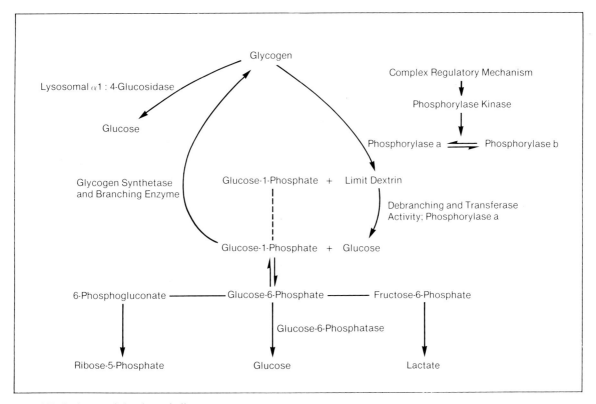

Fig. 14.20. Pathways of glycyl metabolism.

5.2. Type 1

In type 1 GSD the liver shows marked panlobular fatty change without excessive glycogen deposition. No glucose-6-phosphatase activity can be detected with the standard Gomori lead capture method, but a control liver section (rat, mouse, or human) is essential to show that the method is working. The activity must be entirely absent—not just lowered—since the other types may show subnormal activity of this enzyme with the activity confined to the periphery of the hepatocyte. The absence of glucose-6-phosphatase activity can also be demonstrated in jejunal mucosa, but very low levels are also seen in the jejunal mucosa in coeliac disease and in fructose intolerance. For this reason it is important that a

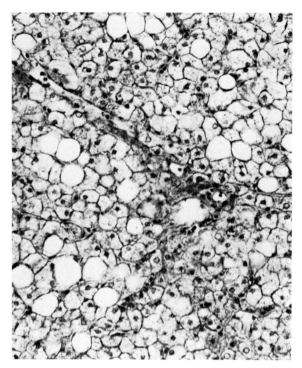

Fig. 14.21. Glycogen storage disease type I. Routine section of liver, showing fatty change. Margination of nuclei and occasional nuclear vacuolation (glycogen). (H and E; 200 ×)

known positive (i.e., normal) and a known negative (i.e., glucose-6-phosphate deficiency) should be stained at the same time if a diagnosis by jejunal biopsy is being attempted. Glucose-6-phosphatase activity is present mainly in the perinuclear and supranuclear regions of the epithelial cells, and should not be confused with the intense alkaline phosphatase activity of the brush border. Some small deposits of glycogen can be seen in the basal part of the cells, in contrast with the massive glycogen accumulation throughout the renal proximal tubular epithelium, where absence of glucose-6-phosphatase can also be demonstrated.

There is a second form of type 1 GSD, in which the activity of glucose-6-phosphatase in vitro (biochemical assay and histochemical demonstration of activity) is normal. In all other features, this disorder (termed type 1B) is identical with the more common type 1A, and the patients react as though they have no glucose-6-phosphatase activity (Igarashi et al. 1979). The enzyme has two components—one hydrolytic and one translocating the substrate through the intact endoplasmic reticulum prior to hydrolysis. Thus in vivo the hydrolytic component cannot work because the substrate is not delivered, but homogenizing or freezing and sectioning destroys the compartmentalization of the hydrolytic portion and allows hydrolysis to proceed.

5.3. Type 2

Biopsy of liver or muscle should not be necessary in Pompe's disease (type 2 GSD), because examination of the blood (light and electron microscopy and enzyme assay) makes diagnosis possible.

5.4. Type 3

In type 3 GSD the liver shows marked glycogen accumulation without fat deposition. The liver cells are enlarged and the nucleus is often off-centre, the general appearance resembling that of a plant cell. There is often portal fibrosis. Glucose-6-phosphatase activity is lowered and confined to the periphery of the hepatocytes. Histochemical methods for the demonstration of phosphorylase activity in liver give falsely low results and cannot be relied on to differentiate debranching enzyme deficiency from phosphorylase or phosphorylase kinase deficiencies.

5.5. Type 6B

Phosphorylase kinase deficiency (type 6B GSD storage disease) is becoming a relatively commonly recognized condition, and is often found incidentally. The liver shows marked glycogen storage with swollen hepatocytes and mild to moderate fat deposition. No fibrosis is found. These two latter points serve to differentiate this type of glycogen storage disease from debranching enzyme deficiency.

5.6. Type 4

The rarer type 4 GSD shows hepatic cirrhosis with bile stasis and can confidently be diagnosed by the total resistance of the glycogen present to digestion by diastase or saliva. The glycogen (long-chain-length amylopectin) shows a lasting brown-lilac colour with Gram's iodine, whereas all other glycogens give only a yellow or fleeting yellow-brown colour.

5.7. Other Types

Other forms of GSD will be encountered which do not fit into any particular category. Some 20% of patients with GSD seen at The Hospital for Sick Children, Great Ormond Street, are at present unclassifiable despite extensive biochemical investigations (Spencer-Peet et al. 1971). Frozen tissue has been kept from each biopsy so that at some future time the tissue can be assayed when newer enzyme defects are recognized.

5.8. Disorders of Fructose Metabolism

Two disorders of fructose metabolism can be confused with GSD. Fructose-1-6-diphosphatase deficiency can present in a manner resembling glucose-6-phosphatase deficiency, and in a fatty liver with glucose-6-phosphatase activity this possibility must be considered. Children with fructose intolerance (fructose-1-phosphate aldolase deficiency) who have not presented in early life with neonatal hepatitis present later with mild hepatomegaly and failure to thrive. On close questioning the information that the child has always avoided eating foods containing fructose often emerges. The similarity to the milder forms of glucose-6-phosphatase deficiency is striking, except that the glucagon stimulation test is positive, although this has also been reported in some cases of type 1 GSD (Spencer-

Peet et al. 1971). The histochemical method for the demonstration of fructose-1-phosphate aldolase activity is not very sensitive, and not all cases show the elevation of glucose-6-phosphatase reported earlier. The glycogen content may appear raised in stained sections. There is marked fatty change (Fig. 14.22) with a predominantly mid-zonal distribution, lesser amounts being found in the peripheral regions. Centrilobular areas contain only a small amount of fat.

6. Other Tissues and Techniques

6.1. Brain

In neuronal storage diseases brain biopsy has been superseded by examination of intestinal neurones (appendix or rectum), and in most instances this

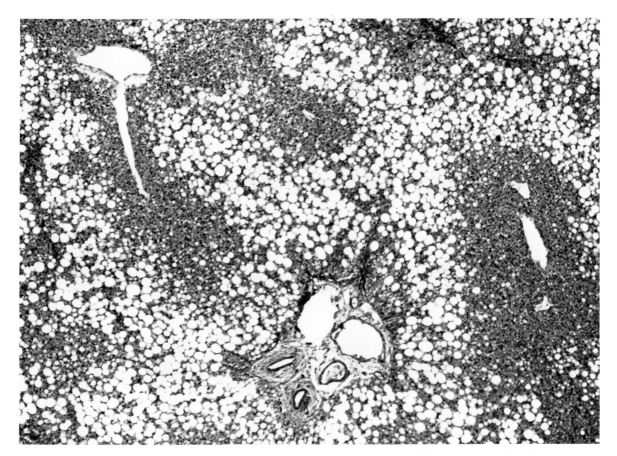

Fig. 14.22. Liver biopsy from a 5-year-old patient with fructose intolerance. Routine section. Marked mid-zonal fatty change is evident. (H and E; 70 ×)

technique has in turn been superseded by enzyme assay of white blood cells or cultured fibroblasts. In a few conditions, which can be considered to be metabolic diseases, brain biopsy is the only means of diagnosis, although some alternative sites for biopsy have been suggested. Alexander's leucodystrophy and spongiform leucodystrophy with abnormal astrocytic mitochondria (Adachi et al. 1973) are two such examples.

Neuroaxonal dystrophy is a difficult, if not impossible, diagnosis to make in a brain biopsy from a child by light microscopy alone. The axonal spheroids, although fairly common in the brain stem at post-mortem, are conspicuous by their absence in the frontal cortex on biopsy. Electron microscopy will reveal the characteristic ultrastructural features in the white matter, which are not visible on light microscopy. Recent evidence has suggested that a biopsy of peripheral nerve may provide the diagnosis and that even the smallest nerves in conjunctiva show the changes (Arsénio-Nunes and Goutières 1978). It will take several years to prove the reliability of this technique.

6.2. Adrenal

X-linked adreno-leucodystrophy can be diagnosed by examination of an adrenal biopsy (Powers and Schaumburg 1974) in which some cells of the zona reticularis and fasciculata appear striated. Electron microscope studies show that the cells contain curved needle-like crystals, which seem to be diagnostic of this disorder. Differential solubility studies (Johnson et al. 1976) and chromatography indicate that the crystalline inclusions may be cholesteryl esters with long-chain fatty acids (Moser et al. 1980). The inclusions are also reported to be present in peripheral nerves, but since similar inclusions can be seen in some otherwise normal biopsies, in demyelinations, and in Krabbe's leucodystrophy, caution should be exercised in the use of this diagnostic procedure.

6.3. Hair

In Menkes' disease there is a deficiency of copper transport. This effects all enzymes which have copper as an essential component of the enzyme. In skin biopsies from patients with Menkes' disease a lower staining intensity than normal can be shown for DOPA-oxidase and presumably also for cytochrome oxidase in other organs. A simpler test is to examine hair. The macroscopic appearance of the short, frizzy, brittle, white hair is almost diagnostic, and microscopy with a dissecting microscope is sufficient to confirm the clinical diagnosis in a classic case. The hair shows pili torti (Figs. 14.23 and 14.24) and occasional thickenings with breakage (tri-

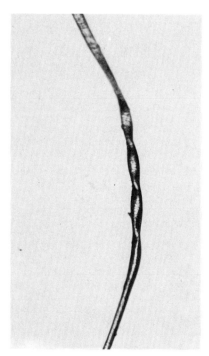

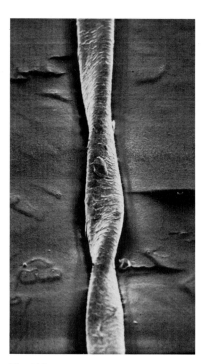

Fig. 14.23. Mankes' kinky disease. A single hair showing pili torti over a short length. This feature is not present over the whole length and is not found in every hair. (75×)

Fig. 14.24. Menkes' kinky hair disease. Scanning electron micrograph of a single hair, clearly showing pili torti. (200×)

Fig. 14.23   Fig. 14.24

chorrhexis nodosum), although the latter are not always present. Not all hairs show pili torti, so a careful search is necessary. In the older cases the hair may appear relatively normal and samples from different areas of the scalp may be necessary. Samples from obligate carriers may show an occasional pili torti but this is rare.

6.4. Skin

Metabolic disorders affecting the skin include the mucopolysaccharidoses, but the changes in this group of conditions are not specific. Other disorders (e.g., stiff-skin syndrome) are insufficiently characterized and are best not considered as metabolic diseases.

X-linked ichthyosis involves a deficiency of arylsulphatase C activity in placenta and skin. This deficiency can be demonstrated by a histochemical technique (Koppe et al. 1978) and can be confirmed by assay of steroid sulphatase activity in placenta or in cultured fibroblasts.

6.5. Other Techniques

If the approach to the metabolic disorders outlined in the previous pages has been followed (see also Table 14.7), then any biopsy taken can be used for diagnosis by the most appropriate means. In different cases this will be by biochemical assay of an enzyme, by thin layer chromatography of a lipid extract or by electron microscopy. Light microscopy, even with histochemical techniques, has distinct limitations. For example, among the growing number of disorders affecting mitochondria (Morgan-Hughes et al. 1977; Willems et al. 1977; Robinson et al. 1977; Di Mauro et al. 1980), the characteristic ragged-red fibres seen in myopathies with abnormally structured mitochondria may be absent even though there may be abundant evidence of abnormality by electron microscopy.

Electron microscopy of conventionally prepared tissue can help in showing which organelles are affected, and whether any deposited substance is membrane-bound. Most of the lysosomal storage disorders can be categorized on the basis of the appearance of the deposited substance. However, it is clear that what remains within the lysosome after the shrinkage and extraction of the stored substance caused by fixation, dehydration, and embedding is something quite different from the original content (Figs. 14.25 and 14.26). However, the artefact induced is usually constant, and consequently its appearance is a useful marker of the disease.

An abnormality of mitochondrial cytochrome content and absence of peroxisomes has been described in a patient who had a metabolic disorder similar to Zellweger's syndrome (Versmold et al.

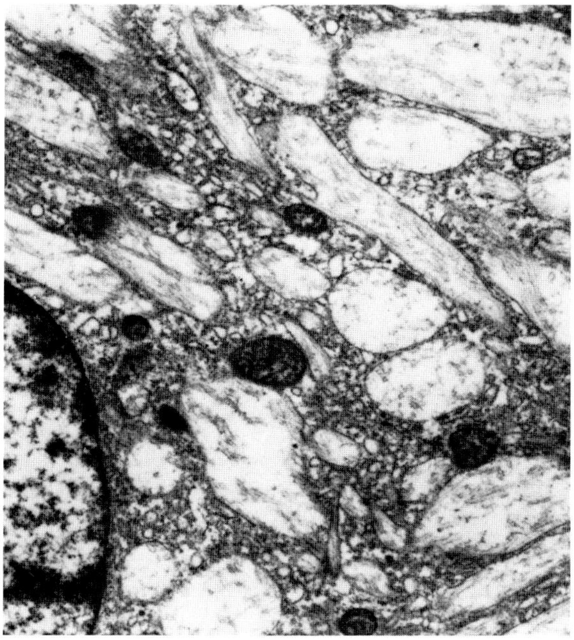

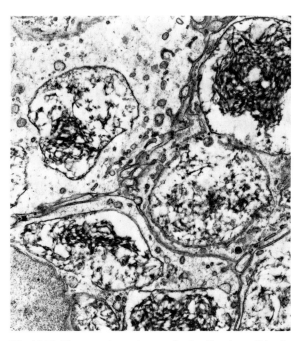

Fig. 14.25. Electron photomicrograph of portions of Niemann–Pick cells in a liver biopsy. The storage bodies are membrane-bound and contain lipid-like lamellae. Similar deposits are also present in hepatocytes. (15 000 ×)

Fig. 14.26. Electron photomicrograph of a Gaucher cell in the spleen. The elongated membrane-bound storage bodies contain tubular inclusions of cerebroside. (15 000 ×)

Table 14.7. Diagnostic routes for metabolic disorders

Disease	Tests applicable to diagnosis[a]					
Pompe's	1	10	15			
Niemann–Pick type A	1	4	10	15	(9)	(13)
Gaucher	4	10	15	(9)		
Wolman	1	4	15	(9)	(10)	
Mucopoly-saccharidosis	2	4	7	15	(10)	
Mannosidosis/-fucosidosis	1	8	15	(10)	(11)	
G_{M1}-Ganglio-sidoses						
Type I	1	4	15	(10)		
Type II	4	15	15	(13)		
G_{M2}-Ganglio-sidoses	15	(13)				
Ophthalmoplegic lipidosis	4	13	14	(9)		
Fabry	6	15				
Metachromatic leucodystrophy	5	15	Check 3			
Cystinosis	4	16				
Batten's						
Infantile	11	12	13	14		
Late infantile	11	12	13	14		
Juvenile	1	13	14			
Glycogen storage						
Type 1	17	9	15			
Type 3	17	9	15	16		
Type 6	17	9	15	16		

[a]1, Vacuolated lymphocytes; 2, Metachromatic inclusions in lymphocytes; 3, Neutrophil granulation; 4, Bone-marrow storage cells; 5, Metachromatic deposits in urine; 6, Lipid TLC of urinary deposits; 7, Urinary mucopolysaccharides; 8, TLC urinary oligosaccharides; 9, Liver biopsy—histochemistry, biochemistry; 10, Fibroblast culture; 11, Lymphocyte electron microscopy; 12, Skin biopsy—electron microscopy; 13, Suction rectal biopsy—histochemistry; 14, Suction rectal biopsy–electron microscopy; 15, Specific enzyme assay; 16, Biochemical assay of WBC or RBC; 17, Fasting blood sugar, glucagon stimulation. Numbers in parenthesis indicate tests that can also be used if specific enzyme assay is not available.

1977), and a similar absence of peroxisomes in Zellweger's syndrome has also been reported. These metabolic disorders will require electron histochemistry and biochemical investigations on fresh tissue to be certain of obtaining the right diagnosis.

An editorial in *Archives of Pathology and Laboratory Medicine* (Kornberg 1977) stresses the need for a wider horizon for anatomical pathology. This is particularly true for the study and diagnosis of metabolic disorders:

The importance of anatomic pathology remains unequivocal. However, the future of pathology does not lie in this traditional discipline, but rather in a blending of it with the newer sciences of genetics, biochemistry, and cell biology. There is a serious danger that the dominance of anatomic pathology will deprive these mutant disciplines of the nutrition they need to survive in a strange and sometimes hostile environment.

References

Adachi M, Schneck L, Cara J, Volk BW (1973) Spongy degeneration of the central nervous system (van Bogaert and Bertrand type; Canavan's disease). Hum Pathol 4: 331

Alder A (1939) Über konstitutionell bedingte Granulations veränderungen der Leukocyten. Dtsch Arch Klin Med 183: 372

Armstrong D, Wehling C, Wormer DV (1977) Diagnosis of Batten disease from urinary sediment. A brief report. Pathology 9: 39

Arsénio-Nunes ML, Goutières F (1978) Diagnosis of infantile neuroaxonal dystrophy by conjunctival biopsy. J Neurol Neurosurg Psychiatry 41: 511

Aula P, Autio S, Raivio KO, Rapola J, Thoden C-J, Koskila S-L, Yamashina I (1979) Salla disease. A new lysosomal storage disorder. Arch Neurol 36: 88

Bodian M, Lake BD (1963) The rectal approach to neuropathology. Br J Surg 50: 702

Di Mauro S, Mendell JR, Sahenk Z, Bachman D, Scarpa A, Schofield RM, Reiner C (1980) Fatal infantile mitochondrial myopathy and renal dysfunction due to cytochrome C oxidase deficiency. Neurology 30: 795

Gasser C (1950) Discussion on Alder A, Konstitutionell bedingte Granulations–Veränderungen der Leukocyten und Knochen–Veränderungen. Schweiz Med Wochenschr 80: 1095

Hagberg B, Haltia M, Sourander P, Svennerholm L, Vanier M-T, Ljunggren C-G (1978) Neurovisceral storage disease simulating Niemann–Pick disease. A new form of oligosaccharidosis. Neuropaediatrie 9: 59

Haltia H, Palo J, Autio S (1975) Aspartylglycosaminuria: a generalized storage disease. Acta Neuropathol (Berl) 31: 243

Hansen HG (1972) Hematologic studies in mucopolysaccharidoses and mucolipidoses. Birth Defects 8: 115

Haust MD, Landing BH (1961) Histochemical studies in Hurler's disease. A new method for localization of acid mucopolysaccharide, and an analysis of lead acetate 'fixation'. J Histochem Cytochem 9: 79

Humbel R, Collart M (1975) Oligosaccharides in urine of patients with glycoprotein storage diseases. I. Rapid detection by thin layer chromatography. Clin Chim Acta 60: 143

Igarashi Y, Otomo H, Narisawa K, Tada K (1979) A new variant of glycogen storage disease type 1: probably due to a defect in the glucose-6-phosphate transport system. J Inher Metab Dis 2: 45

Jenner FA, Pollitt RJ (1967) Large quantities of 2-acetamide-1-(beta-L-aspartamido)-1,2-dideoxyglucose in the urine of mentally retarded siblings. Biochem J 103: 48P

Johnson AB, Schaumberg HH, Powers JM (1976) Histochemical characteristics of the striated inclusions of adrenoleukodystrophy. J Histochem Cytochem 24: 725

Jordans GHW (1953) The familial occurrence of fat containing vacuoles in the leukocytes diagnosed in two brothers suffering from dystrophia musculorum progressiva (ERB). Acta Med Scand 145: 419

Koppe JG, Marinkovic-Ilsen A, Rijken Y, de Groot WP, Jobsis

AC (1978) X-linked ichthyosis. A sulphatase deficiency. Arch Dis Child 53: 803

Kornberg A (1977) Editorial. Arch Pathol Lab Med 101: 399

Lake BD (1965) A reliable rapid screening test for sulphatide lipidosis. Arch Dis Child 40: 284

Lake BD (1971) Histochemical detection of the enzyme deficiency in blood films in Wolman's disease. J Clin Pathol 24: 617

Lake BD (1974) An improved method for the detection of β-galactosidase activity, and its application to G_{M1}-gangliosidosis and mucopolysaccharidosis. Histochem J 6: 211

Lake BD (1976) The differential diagnosis of the various forms of Batten disease by rectal biopsy. Birth Defects 12: 455

Lake BD (1977) Histochemical and ultrastructural studies in the diagnosis of inborn errors of metabolism. Records of the Adelaide Childrens Hospital 1: 337

Lake BD, Ellis RB (1976) What do you think you are quantifying? An appraisal of histochemical methods in the measurement of the activities of lysosomal enzymes. Histochem J 8: 357

Lake BD, Goodwin HJ (1976) Lipids. In: Smith I, Seakins JWT (eds) Chromatographic and electrophoretic techniques, vol I. Heinemann, London, p 345

Morgan-Hughes JA, Darveniza P, Kahn SN, Landon DN, Sherratt RM, Land JM, Clark JB (1977) A mitochondrial myopathy characterized by a deficiency in reducible cytochrome b. Brain 100: 617

Moser HW, Moser AB, Kawamura N, Murphy J, Suzuki K, Schaumberg H, Kishimoto Y (1980) Adrenoleukodystrophy: elevated C26 fatty acids in cultured skin fibroblasts. Ann Neurol 7: 542

Muir H, Mittwoch V, Bitter T (1963) The diagnostic value of isolated urinary mucopolysaccharides and of lymphocytic inclusions in gargoylism. Arch Dis Child 38: 358

Neville BGR, Lake BD, Stephens R, Sanders MD (1973) A neurovisceral storage disease with vertical supra-nuclear ophthalmoplegia and its relationship to Niemann–Pick disease. A report of nine patients. Brain 96: 97

Pennock CA (1976) A review and selection of simple laboratory methods used for the study of glycosaminoglycan excretion and the diagnosis of the mucopolysaccharidoses. J Clin Pathol 29: 111

Pfeiffer RA, Kresse H, Baumer N, Sattinger E (1977) β-Glucouronidase deficiency in a girl with unusual features. Eur J Pediatr 126: 155

Powers JM, Schaumberg HH (1974) Adrenoleukodystrophy (sex-linked Schilder's disease). Am J Pathol 76: 481

Rampini S, Isler W, Baerlocker K, Bischoff A, Ulrich J, Plüss HJ (1970) Die Kombination von metachromatischer Leukodystrophie und Mucopolysaccharidose als selbständiges Krankheitsbild (Mukosulfatidose). Helv Paediatr Acta 25: 436

Rapin I, Goldfischer S, Katzman R, Engel J, O'Brien JS (1978) The cherry-red spot–myoclonus syndrome. Ann Neurol 3: 234

Reilly WA (1941) The granules in the leukocytes in gargoylism. Am J Dis Child 62: 489

Reynolds RD (1973) Sea-blue histiocytes (Letter). JAMA 226: 467

Robinson BH, Taylor J, Sherwood WG (1977) Deficiency of dihydrolipoyl dehydrogenase (a component of the pyruvate and α-ketoglutarate dehydrogenase complex). A cause of congenital chronic lactic acidosis in infancy. Pediatr Res 11: 1198

Spencer-Peet J, Norman ME, Lake BD, McNamara J, Patrick AD (1971) Hepatic glycogen storage disease. Q J Med 40: 95

Stanbury JB, Wyngaarden JB, Frederickson DS (1978) The metabolic basis of inherited disease, 4th edn. McGraw-Hill, New York

Toppet M, Vamos Hurwitz E, Jonniau G, Cremer N, Tondeur M, Pelc S (1978) Farber's disease as a ceramidosis; clinical radiological and biochemical aspects. Acta Paediatr Scand 67: 113

Versmold HT, Bremer HJ, Herzog V, Siegel G, von Bassewitz DB, Irle V, von Voss H, Lombeck I, Brauser B (1977) A metabolic disorder similar to Zellweger syndrome with hepatic acatalasia and absence of peroxisomes, altered content and redox state of cytochromes, and infantile cirrhosis with haemosiderosis. Eur J Pediatr 124: 261

Wenger DA, Barth G, Gittens JH (1977) Nine cases of sphingomyelin lipidosis, a new variant in Spanish–American children. Am J Dis Child 131: 995

Whiteman P (1973) The quantitative determination of glycosaminoglycans in urine with Alcian blue 8GX. Biochem J 131: 351

Willems JL, Monnens LAH, Trijbels JMF, Veerkamp JH, Meyer AEFH, van Dam K, van Haelst V (1977) Leigh's encephalomyelopathy in a patient with cytochrome C oxidase deficiency in muscle tissue. Pediatrics 60: 850

Chapter 15

Embryonic Tumours of Children

Colin L. Berry and Jean W. Keeling

Although the number of deaths resulting from tumours in infancy and childhood is small in absolute terms, neoplasms are a major cause of death in children between the ages of 1 and 15 years. Table 15.1. shows a decline in the numbers of deaths from malignant disease in this age group (1 per 1.47 million in 1962 to 1 per 1.57 million in 1975), but in general there has been little change in the last 16 years. There is a documented decline in the numbers of patients with leukaemia in Great Britain (Adelstein and White 1976), which has also been noted in the United States and Australia: as this is the largest single group of childhood malignancies it will have influenced figures considerably. However, there have been major therapeutic advances in the treatment of other tumours in children and this may also be reflected in more recent data. It is worth mentioning that deaths in the whole 0–15 age group occur largely in the first year of life—indeed mainly in the first few months; for example, of the total of 13 373 deaths in this age group in 1975 there were 11 187 in the 0–4 group (242 tumours), 1140 between 5 and 9 years (265 tumours), and 1046 in the 10–14 group (213 tumours). One further point is noteworthy: it seems likely in view of the relative constancy of the figures for deaths in the 10–14 year group that delayed deaths as a result of therapy fail to account for the fall in the first age group (0–4 years). Both declining incidence and increased 'cure' rates are probably important.

The purpose of this chapter is to give an account of the embryonic tumours of childhood, namely neuroblastoma, hepatoblastoma, nephroblastoma, medulloblastoma, teratoma, rhabdomyosarcoma, and retinoblastoma. They are not a homogeneous group, but have features in common that permit us to consider certain general aspects of oncogenesis in childhood.

1. Aetiology

In childhood malignancies the period of potential exposure to environmental carcinogens is generally short. Congenital tumours are well documented (rather more than 300 reported cases of non-leukaemic lesions) and the bulk of embryonic neoplasms occur in the first 4 years of life. Epidemiologists consider that the role of genetic factors in the induction of tumours free of confounding variables may be more readily studied in this age group, where familial tumours are not exceedingly rare and where interesting tumour/malformation syndromes occur.

Comparison with studies in adults, where factors such as age, sex, and race may be readily controlled but where climate, dietary and cultural factors, occupational changes, and variation of the intensity and duration of exposure to potential carcinogens are all independent variables, will illustrate the difficulties imposed on studies by prolonged extra-uterine existence. It is evident that the massive variation in the frequency of different tumours in different adult populations (e.g., 300× for carcinoma of the oesophagus), often thought to be attributable to environmental factors, is not seen in childhood malignancy. This effect is so marked that Innes (1972a) has suggested that the relatively constant incidence of nephroblastoma in different populations of children would allow the tumour to be used as an index of the degree of under-reporting of other tumours.

There are two main general theories of the role of genetic influence in carcinogenesis in childhood.

In 1969 Ellsworth suggested that a germ-cell *mutation* might be the first step in the development of bilateral retinoblastoma. In subsequent studies on

Table 15.1. Deaths from malignant disease in children aged 1–15 years, 1962–1975

Year	Total in 0–14 year age group (million)	Total deaths in 0–14 year group (thousands)	Deaths from malignant disease		
			0–4 years	5–9 years	10–14 years
1962	10 559.0	25 448	400	235	213
1971	11 676.5	18 517	314	308	215
1972	11 704.9	17 292	349	293	202
1973	11 602.9	15 753	296	263	230
1974	11 492.7	12 381	255	248	205
1975	11 349.9	13 373	242	265	213

retinoblastoma and neuroblastoma, and neuro-blastoma and phaeochromocytoma, Knudson (1971) and Knudson and Strong (1972) suggested that these tumours arose in a manner consistent with a two-mutation model. If we assume that the initial event in oncogenesis is mutation (itself an uncertain assumption), then according to this hypothesis two successive mutations are necessary in a somatic cell to produce a neoplasm. Hereditary cases would arise in individuals in whom one mutation has occurred in a germ cell and thus in all its progeny. One subsequent mutation in affected cells would then result in neoplasia.

In the case of retinoblastoma there are supportive data for this hypothesis in the work of Kitchin and Ellsworth (1974). These workers have shown that the retinoblastoma 'gene' has pleiotrophic effects, with an increase in second primary tumours, notably osteogenic sarcoma, in survivors of bilateral tumours. This effect is not found in unilateral cases and provides evidence for enhanced tumour susceptibility in this group. It seems likely that part of the long arm of chromosome 13 is involved in this change (Taylor 1970). New retinoblastomas did not develop after 33 months of age in Kitchin's and Ellsworth's study, and it is probable that retinal neuroblasts have completed division by this time. Finally, children with 'sporadic' bilateral retinoblastoma are more likely to have a family history of consanguinity (Hemmes 1931) and to have affected children themselves.

An alternative view of genetic factors in the aetiology of childhood tumours has been taken by Innes (1970, 1972b). He has suggested that the embryonic tumours are genetically determined characteristics in Hardy–Weinberg equilibrium. This equilibrium, an important concept in population genetics, required that if genes are widely distributed in a randomly bred population, selection pressures (e.g., death) will have little effect on their frequency (see also Berry and Keeling 1975). Innes studied the relative frequencies of leukaemia and other childhood malignancies in children of British descent in Canada, England and Wales, and New Zealand, and found that despite differences in the incidence of some adult tumours, childhood malignancies occurred at a remarkably constant rate. When comparisons were made for two periods in the same continent the specific tumour proportions were found not to change. Data in some of the groups studied were scanty, as Innes has pointed out, but the stability of the relative rates argues against an active environmental component in these tumours.

The two hypotheses are not mutually exclusive. As further data are accumulated on the progeny of survivors of childhood malignancy their relative merits may become clearer.

The pathologist has an important role to play in providing the data with which these hypotheses may be tested. It seems likely that those instances in which malformations occur in association with neoplasms are a special group; for example, despite a well-documented association we have seen only two cases of aniridia in a series of 103 nephroblastomas, and Ledlie et al. (1970) reported only one in 335 cases. In a survey of 383 embryonic tumours seen at The Hospital for Sick Children, Great Ormond Street, Berry et al. (1970) found a significant association between malformation and tumours only in the saccrococcygeal group of teratomas, where the presence of an expanding mass in intrauterine life probably resulted in the cloacal anomalies found. The general lack of association of embryonic tumours and malformation and the occurrence of a separate group of cases where such associations occur (Wilm's tumour and aniridia/hemihypertrophy, gliomas and phacomatosis, medulloblastoma and the basal cell naevus syndrome, adrenal cortical neoplasms and hemihypertrophy, etc.) suggests that careful documentation of pathological findings will permit a more accurate delineation of syndromes and may give clues to the causation by identifying associations or possible genetic linkages (see also Berry 1981).

2. Retinoblastoma

Retinoblastoma is a tumour whose frequency appears to be increasing in countries where reliable data are available (Holland and Finland), which is thought by Warburg (1974) to be attributable to an increase in bilateral lesions. The increase cannot be explained by an increase in incidence in the progeny of those surviving a lesion in their own childhood. It is the commonest primary intraocular neoplasm of childhood, representing 3% of registered cases of malignant disease occurring in children under the age of 15 years in Great Britain (Lennox et al. 1975). The tumour may be unilateral or bilateral, the bilateral cases presenting, on average, much earlier than infants with unilateral tumours: at 8 months as against 25.7 months of age in the experience of Lennox et al. (1975). The familial incidence of retinoblastoma has long been recognized (Sorsby 1962), and not surprisingly familial cases are diagnosed much earlier than sporadic ones.

The tumour is thought to be maintained by a mutation rate of around $4–6 \times 10^6$ (Briard-Guillemot et al. 1974; Czeizel and Gardanyi (1974). Around 10% of all cases are familial, but a family history is found more frequently with bilateral than with unilateral tumours (17.7% bilateral, 6.5% unilateral; Briard-Guillemot et al. 1974). The disease appears to be specifically associated with abnormalities of chromosome 13 and trisomy 21 (O'Grady et al. 1974; Orye et al. 1974).

There are no differences in sex incidence in retinoblastoma, nor does sex seem to influence survival. The age at diagnosis influences survival rate, and a mortality of 6.9% was observed in children presenting at under 1 year of age, compared with 17.9% of children presenting after that time (Lennox et al. 1975). One factor that greatly influences survival is treatment in a specialized hospital, and it seems desirable that all children with retino-blastomas should be treated in such units (Bedford 1975). The finding of Lennox et al. (1975) that the survival rate was better in children with bilateral retinoblastoma was thought to be related to the younger age at diagnosis and to a higher incidence of treatment in specialized units. However, these may not be the only factors operating; there may be biological differences between unilateral and bi-lateral retinal tumours.

2.1. Presentation and Histopathology

The tumour protrudes into the posterior chamber of the eye as solitary or multifocal papillary lesions with an irregular surface and pinkish white in colour (Figs. 15.1 and 15.2) A high proportion of the tumours are sited peripherally. The appearance on direct ophthalmoscopic examination is usually diagnostic, and biopsy is contraindicated. The histological appearance of the tumour is one composed of small dark cells with little cytoplasm, often arranged in a ribbon-like configuration. True rosette formation occurs in about half these tumours (Fig. 15.3). Necrosis and calcification are frequent findings. Extension of the tumour into the optic nerve may occur and should be sought histologically in enucleated specimens.

Invasion of the optic nerve and choroid by tumour is associated with poor prognosis, the volume of choroidal invasion probably being the most important factor (Redler and Ellsworth 1973). Histological differentiation in the tumour has been described as a useful prognostic feature (Brown 1966), but is probably not as important as choroidal infiltration. It has been suggested that survival without metastasis for 2 years after treatment of the tumour could be regarded as a cure, but there have been a number of reports of metastases occurring up to 8 years after presentation (Bedford 1975). Osteosarcoma of the orbit following radiotherapy for retinoblastoma has been reported (Lennox et al. 1975).

3. Neuroblastoma

Neuroblastomas can arise from any neuroblast (Prasad 1975). These neoplastic neuroblasts are of neural crest origin and of varying degrees of cellular maturation, but most contain osmiophilic dense-core granules 500–900 nm in diameter in their cytoplasm. Our view of the natural history of these tumours has undergone changes in recent years.

In 1963 Beckwith and Perrin coined the term in situ neuroblastoma to describe microscopic aggregates of neuroblasts in the adrenal medulla of newborns and infants up to 3 months of age. They suggested that these lesions were related to the tumour neuroblastoma, and because of their frequent occurrence (1:200 autopsies) suggested that the natural history of neuroblastoma was for involution to occur. They were supported in their assumption by the observation in such nodules of mitotic figures, peripheral invasion, and absence of a capsule. We ourselves have seen a number of similar cases in which similar findings have occurred.

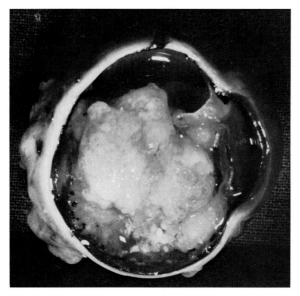

Fig. 15.1. Eye from 7-month-old male with bilateral retinoblastoma. The globe is filled by tumour. (3.5 ×)

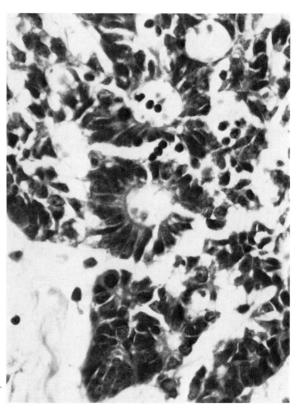

Fig. 15.3. Dark-staining tumour cells forming rosettes with well- ▷ marked internal limiting membrane. (H and E; 140 ×)

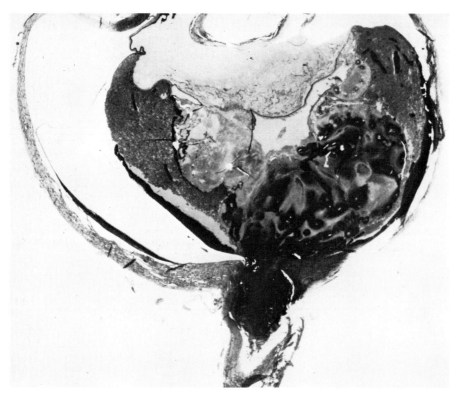

Fig. 15.2. Section shows a necrotic tumour involving the optic nerve. (H and E; 7.5 ×)

Turkel and Itabashi (1974) have since studied many human fetuses (10–30 weeks' gestation) and found neuroblastic nodules in every gland studied. These were greater than 60×60 μm in all instances and as much as 200×400 μm in one case. They pointed out that the migration pathways of neuroblasts from the paravertebral sympathetic ganglion could be traced via periadrenal sympathetic collections through the gland. This migration takes place mainly during weeks 6–7 of gestation, but it continues to a lesser extent throughout fetal life. Continuity of nodules with these pathways could be demonstrated. It seems likely that many in situ neuroblastomas are really normal developmental remnants rather than true neuroblastomas.

A well-documented and singular aspect of neuroblastoma is its tendency to regress spontaneously, by maturation to ganglioneuroma, by haemorrhagic necrosis with a calcified and fibrous remnant, or by cytolysis (see Bolande 1971). Although a number of potential immunological mechanisms have been proposed to explain these regressions, they are unsatisfactory in many ways and the significance of some studies has been questioned. Other factors concerned with the control of differentiation have also been considered in detail. Extensive studies of the effects of nerve growth factor (NGF) on neuroblastoma have been made (see review by Mobley et al. 1977). Nerve growth factor is a protein necessary for the growth and maintenance of sympathetic and some sensory neurones. From a number of experiments it seems likely that NGF acts as an agent maintaining neuronal viability. It also apparently accelerates differentiation in neurones (Levi-Montalcini et al. 1968), producing increased prominence of the Golgi apparatus, more prominent endoplasmic reticulum, and an increased number of specialized organelles (neurofilaments and neurotubules). Cultures of neuroblastoma show an ability to undergo the type of morphological development that occurs normally during growth and differentiation (Reynolds and Perez Polo 1975). A role for NGF in the process of maturation in neuroblastoma is far from certain, and the manner in which control of differentiation is regained remains an enigma.

3.1. Presentation and Histopathology

Neuroblastoma is one of the commonest embryonal tumours. Early presentation is associated with much better prognosis: there is a roughly 50% survival amongst those children presenting in the first year of life (Kinnier Wilson and Draper 1974). Survival in children with neuroblastoma is related to clinical staging at presentation (Evans et al. 1971), although this seems to be less important amongst

infants, as it is in this group that spontaneous tumour regression most often occurs (Koop 1972). The presence of histological differentiation within the tumour is a favourable prognostic feature, the presence of cellular differentiation probably being more important than the volume of differentiated tissue within a tumour (Makinen 1972).

The tumour site has prognostic implications. A neuroblastoma can arise from the adrenal medulla (Fig. 15.4) or from some part of the abdominal, thoracic, pelvic, or cervical chains of sympathetic ganglia, pelvic tumours having the best prognosis, followed in declining order by those in the thorax (Fig. 15.5), the abdomen and neck, and the adrenals. Girls seem to do better than boys, and a greater incidence of histological maturation within the tumour has been reported in girls (Kinnier Wilson and Draper 1974).

Neuroblastomas extend locally and involve adjacent structures, subsequently metastasizing to lymph nodes. Distant spread is common, especially to bone, liver, and skin (Fig. 15.6). However, the involvement of one distant site (liver, subcutaneous tissue, or bone marrow) in the absence of radiological evidence of bone involvement does not necessarily carry a poor prognosis (Koop 1972).

The tumours secrete catecholamines and their breakdown products may be detected in the urine. The number of cases in which catecholamine metabolites are detected depends on the methods used. Schweisguth (1968) found vanillylmandelic acid (VMA) or homo-vanillylmandelic acid (HVA) in 75% of 152 patients, whilst Bell (1968) found a combination of the measurement of VMA and total catecholamines used together gave a positive result in 100% of cases. Estimation of catecholamines is useful both in diagnosis and during follow-up as it allows early detection of metastases. Symptoms during pregnancy in mothers whose infants have been shown to have neuroblastomas either at birth or in the first few months of life, and which are related to catecholamine secretion by the infant's tumour, have been described. These symptoms include sweating attacks, pallor, palpitations, tingling extremities, headache, and paroxysmal hypertension. In all cases the symptoms disappear after delivery (Voute et al. 1970). Congenital neuroblastoma has been described in association with hydrops fetalis and tumour emboli in the placental vessels have been described, but invasion of the placenta has not been seen. The mothers were asymptomatic (Anders et al. 1973).

Macroscopically the tumour is usually soft, with areas of necrosis and haemorrhage. There is often extensive focal calcification, resulting in a gritty texture on cutting. Solid greyish white areas may

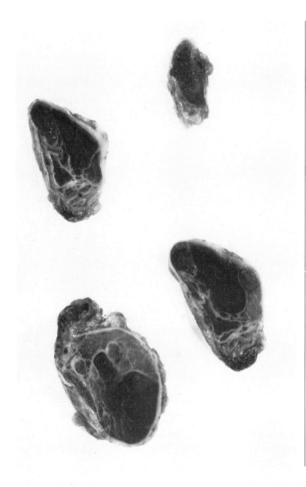

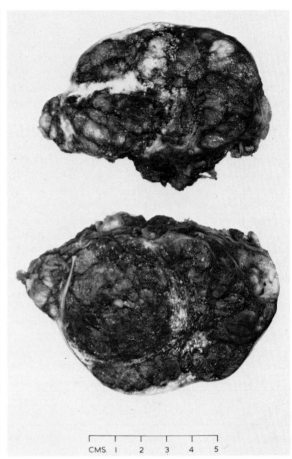

Fig. 15.5. Intrathoracic neuroblastoma from a 21-month-old male. The nodular appearance, with haemorrhages and flecks of calcification, is typical.

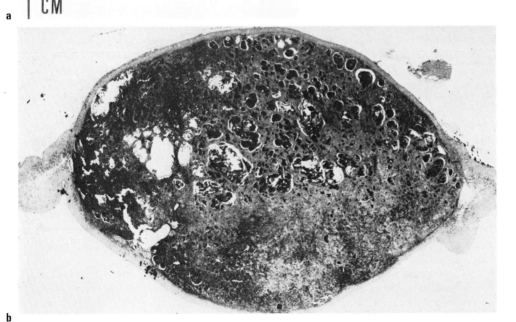

Fig. 15.4. a Slices of a small neuroblastoma in the adrenal, from a 6-month-old female with skin nodules and liver metastases at presentation. (75 ×) b Tumour, also from a 6-month-old female, discovered incidentally after death from congenital heart disease.

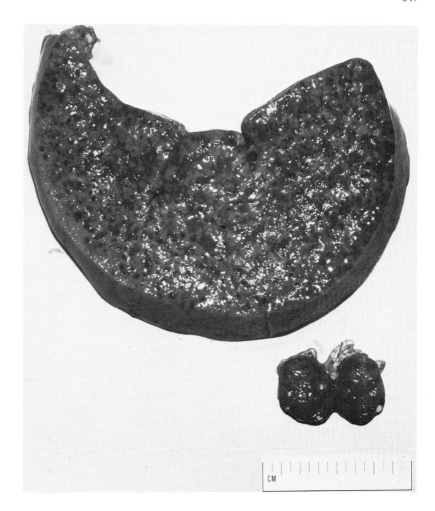

Fig. 15.6. Neuroblastoma. Female aged 6 months, with abdominal distension produced by massive hepatomegaly due to diffuse infiltration by neuroblastoma. The small adrenal primary tumour is seen in the *lower part* of the figure.

occur, which histologically contain considerable amounts of eosinophilic stroma resembling glia. Remnants of invaded or distorted local tissues may be seen.

Histologically, tumour cells are separated by fine vascular septa. Undifferentiated tumours are composed of cells like those of the primitive neural crest, and maturation results in the production of eosinophilic neurofibrillary processes and fibrillary stroma (Figs. 15.7 and 15.8). Rosette formation, consisting of an often ill-defined ring of cells around a central neurofibrillary core, is seen in some tumours. The lesion may shade imperceptibly into ganglioneuroblastoma by the formation of clumps of larger cells with abundant eosinophilic cytoplasm and well-defined nucleoli, set in a dense fibrillary tangle (Fig. 15.9). Bizarre neurones are often present. Mature ganglioneuroblastomas often appear as solid tumours with a whorled cut surface and flecks of calcification (Fig. 15.10).

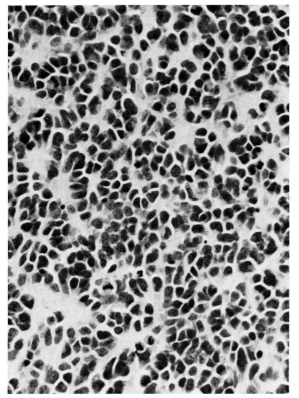

Fig. 15.7. Neuroblastoma. The tumour is composed of large darkly staining cells. The cells themselves show little differentiation but are separated by eosinophilic fibrillary material producing a loose rosettiform arrangement. (H and E; 400 ×)

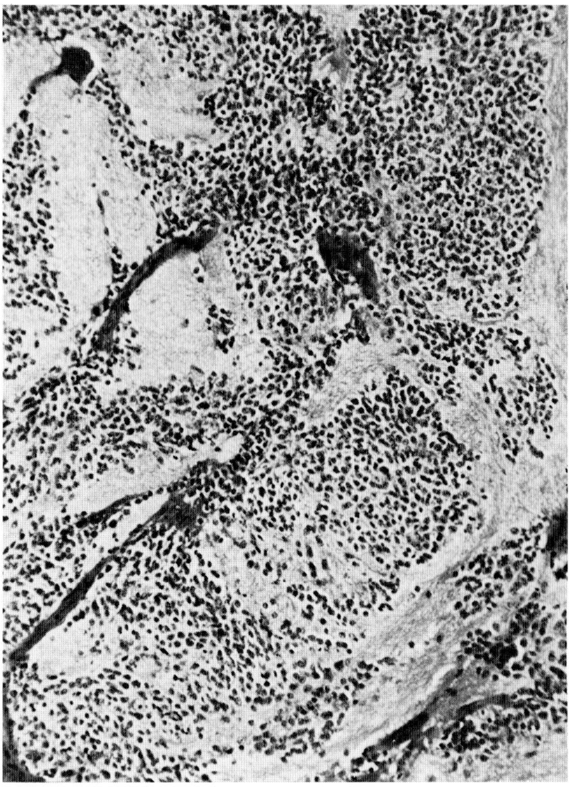

Fig. 15.8. Neuroblastoma. Early differentiation results in the production of large amounts of fibrillary material, seen here separating islands of tumour cells. (H and E; 150 ×)

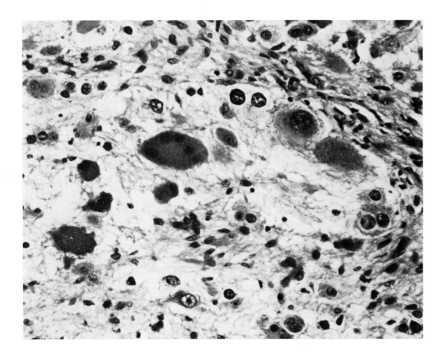

Fig. 15.9. Neuroblastoma. Differentiation within the tumour has produced large neuroblasts with abundant cytoplasm and multiple cytoplasmic processes. Some cells are multinucleate. Differentiation has also produced a mature intervening stroma.

4. Medulloblastoma

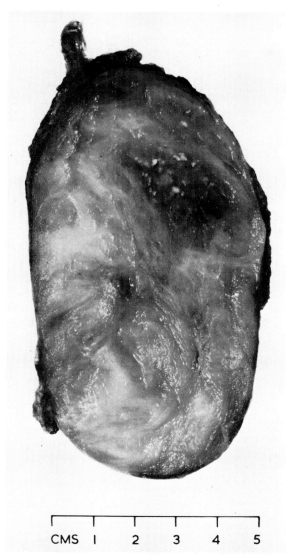

The important central nervous system tumour medulloblastoma arises in the posterior fossa. The parent cell is generally considered to be from the granular layer, a sub-pial layer of small cells present throughout the cortex at birth but disappearing by around 18 months of age. These cells may be bi-potent, able to migrate inwards to become neurones in the definitive granular cell layer but also to differentiate into neuroglia (Fujita 1967). In normal development, collections of cells morphologically similar to those of medulloblastoma were seen in 23 of 104 fetuses or neonates in which the posterior medullary velum was examined histologically, suggesting that collections of cells might become isolated at various sites on their normal migratory routes, with subsequent tumour formation.

Kadin et al. (1970) reported a case that supported the origin of these tumours from the cells of the fetal external granular layer. The spread of the tumour was studied in enough detail to show the transitional passage of the layer into true tumour formation. The case presented in the neonatal period, probably having arisen in intrauterine life, and showed irregular zones of proliferation with invasion of the molecular layer, which suggested malignant change. Electron microscopic findings (junctional complexes and cell processes containing microtubules) supported a neuroepithelial origin for the neoplasm.

Medulloblastoma has been reported to occur in siblings. Excluding cases without histological verification in both affected individuals it has been reported in two pairs of identical twins, a half-brother and -sister, two pairs of brothers, and two sisters (see Table 15.2). A striking feature of these reports is the similar age of onset of the tumour in the various sibships; in most instances there is a very close approximation. There is a well-established association of the tumour with the naevoid basal cell carcinoma syndrome (six verified cases having been reported—see Neblett et al. 1971). It is interesting to note that in these cases the prognosis of the tumour

Fig. 15.10. Cut surface of ganglioneuroblastoma, resected at the age of 3 years 6 months (male child).

Table 15.2. Occurrence of medulloblastoma in sibships

Authors	Nature of sibship	Ages at onset
Zülch (1956)	Identical twins ♀	3 months, 3 months
Griepentrog and Pauly (1957)	Identical twins ♀	8 weeks, 11 weeks
Kjellin et al. (1960)	Half-brother and -sister	10 years, 11 years
Bickerstaff et al. (1967)	Two brothers	2 years, 2 years
Belamire and Chaur (1969)	Two sisters	At birth, 15 days
Yamashita et al. (1975)	Two brothers	1.5 years, 2.5 years

appears to be good, five of the cases being alive and well 2, 5, 7, 8, and 9 years after surgery, an improvement on survival rates of around 60% in most large series.

Congenital medulloblastoma has been reported 15 times, with hydrocephalus resulting in dystocia the commonest presenting feature. Analysis of the reports suggests a definite intrauterine origin in only seven of these cases where neurological symptoms and signs were present at birth, an assumption of intrauterine growth having been made in infants presenting in the first 3 months of life (Poon et al. 1975). A predominance of females has been demonstrated in early-onset medulloblastoma, and association with the naevoid basal-cell carcinoma syndrome is also associated with early onset.

A 12-year-old girl with medulloblastoma and multiple other cerebral tumours has also been reported (Bhangui et al. 1977). This was a curious combination of tumours: medulloblastoma, optic nerve glioma, pilocytic astrocytoma, and ganglioglioma. Since the naevoid basal-cell carcinoma syndrome has been called the 'fifth phacomatosis' the presence of optic nerve glioma is interesting—the authors felt that this last lesion and the pilocytic astrocytoma might be two parts of the same tumour—they were in continuity in one area. With medulloblastoma and glial and neuronal tumour present in the same case there appears to be some support for the suggestion that bipolar differentiation of medulloblastoma may occur.

4.1. Presentation and Histopathology

This neoplasm, found in the posterior fossa of children, is over twice as common in males. Most examples in younger children are found in the midline, in the cerebellar vermis (Fig. 15.11); in the second decade they are seen in the hemisphere as well as the vermis. Although predominantly cerebellar, some examples appear to arise in the medullary velum, and extension into the fourth ventricle with consequent hydrocephalus is common. On macroscopic examination they are described as purplish grey at operation but grey after excision, with a granular cut surface. Metastasis via the cerebrospinal fluid is frequent, and in this case secondary deposits may be found in the walls of the ventricular system, in the depths of sulci, and scattered over the cord and cauda equina. Sometimes these meningeal deposits form thin grey sheets.

Microscopic examination may show a fairly uniform picture of round or oval closely packed basophilic cells resembling the granular layer of the cerebellar cortex on cursory examination. However, closer examination indicates that the cells are

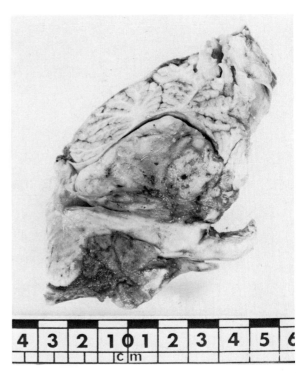

Fig. 15.11. Medulloblastoma of cerebellum extending around medulla. Courtesy of Prof. J. Smith.

somewhat larger than this type and mitoses are frequent. Sometimes the cells are grouped in trabeculae or whorls. Vascularity is variable, as is the presence of the characteristic pseudorosettes first described by Wright (1910) (Fig. 15.12). In these the carrot-like delicate processes are directed to a central focus where they merge with one another, but there is no central lumen. It is exceedingly difficult to demonstrate neurofibrils in such foci; this is occasionally possible with very rare, somewhat similar tumours that arise in the cerebrum and are more correctly classified as neuroblastomas.

In reports of large series, the occurrence of areas strongly suggestive of differentiation to oligodendroglia in a minority of tumours is a consistent feature and these areas are an integral part of the tumour (Fig. 15.13); differentiation to astrocytes and neurones is rare.

One particular feature of the local invasive properties of these tumours has aroused controversy. This is the capacity of certain examples, occurring in the lateral lobes, and usually after the first decade, to excite a marked connective-tissue reaction in the leptomeninges. Rubenstein and Northfield (1964) referred to these as desmoplastic medulloblastomas and could find no support for the thesis that some represented an independent entity, a circumscribed arachnoidal sarcoma, with a better

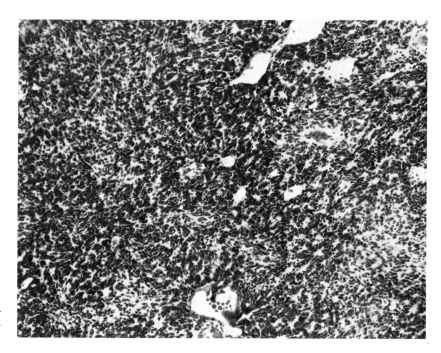

Fig. 15.12. Pseudorosette of medulloblastoma. Courtesy of Prof. J. Smith. (H and E; 400 ×)

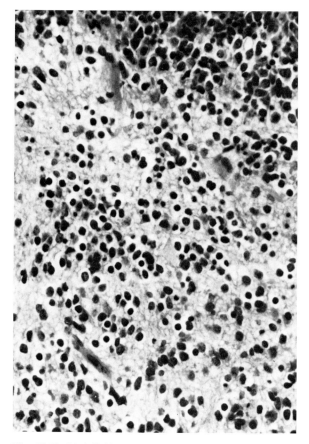

Fig. 15.13. Medulloblastoma differentiating to oligodendroglioma. (H and E; 400 ×)

prognosis. Nevertheless, occasionally older children and adolescents with tumours of this kind in the lateral lobes do survive for some years, although taken as a whole this is the most malignant group of primary brain tumours.

5. Nephroblastoma

Nephroblastoma is a common tumour of infancy, comprising around 18% of all malignant lesions in this age group. Forty percent of cases present at under 2 years of age and 85% before their fifth birthday; cases seldom occur after 12 years of age, although there are reports of this tumour in adults (Klapproth 1959). The disease is rare in adolescence: in a report by Merton et al. (1976) two adolescents with Wilm's tumours are described, although one of these was apparently atypical. In many large series, onset under the age of 2 years has been shown to be associated with a good prognosis, probably because of effects on the staging of the tumour at presentation (see Lemerle et al. [1976] for bibliography). The degree of epithelial differentiation is important prognostically (see below).

Congenital tumours are rare, most of the larger tumours described in the literature probably being mesenchymal hamartomas (Hilton and Keeling

1973). However, since Wilm's tumours, like other embryonic tumours, may occasionally originate in intrauterine life, and as the bulk of cases occur between 2 and 4 years of age, it is interesting to note the results of a study comparable to that of Beckwith and Perrin on neuroblastoma, conducted by Bové et al. (1969). Assuming that the tumour arises from metanephric blastoma during embryonic and fetal life or in early infancy, they studied material from an autopsy series. Nodular renal blastoma, defined as 'the presence in the kidney of discrete nodules of primitive undifferentiated cells which were cytologically indistinguishable from nephroblastoma, which differed unequivocally, in both size and pattern, from the tubular metanephric structures which characterize normal development of nephrons from the metanephric blastoma and which were unaccompanied by either intra-renal or extra-renal metastasis', was found to be associated with trisomy 18 and also to occur apart from this syndrome. Five of eight patients with trisomy 18 had nodular renal blastoma (NRB), but multiple congenital abnormalities were associated with NRB in all instances.

The lesions are usually sited under the cortex, and may be very extensive, causing nephromegaly. They vary in size from 50 μm to 2 mm, and are discrete although not encapsulated. Ill-defined tubular structures may be present but stomal or glomerular elements like those seen in Wilm's tumour are not found. Mitoses are extremely uncommon. As Bové et al. stress, the relationship of this lesion to nephroblastoma is uncertain. In view of more recent reports on the embryology of the adrenal and the way in which our view of so-called neuroblastoma-in-situ has changed, this note of caution is well justified. They suggest that some nodules may 'mature' into dysplastic nephrons.

Wilm's tumour can often be bilateral, when a family history is sometimes obtained. However, it is seldom practicable to decide whether an apparently multicentric origin is a genuine phenomenon or represents metastatic spread, and some bilateral Wilm's tumours may represent nephroblastomatosis, as Bové and his co-workers stressed that in five bilateral Wilm's tumours, subcapsular 'focal developmental abnormalities' were particularly common. However, in only one instance did these lesions resemble NRB.

Associations of Wilm's tumour with aniridia, hemihypertrophy, hypospadias, cryptorchidism, microcephaly, pigmented and vascular naevi, and abnormalities of the pinna have all been reported (see Miller et al. 1964), but different anomalies have been reported with NRB, mainly those of the trisomy 18 syndrome. Further, NRB is commoner in females (presumably this is related to the predominance of females in trisomy 18), whilst there is a slight male preponderance in Wilm's tumour, which is marked in those cases associated with aniridia.

Recently Stambolis (1977) has reported a case of Wilm's tumour in the right kidney, with bilateral nodular renal blastema and direct transformation of one such nodule into a benign epithelial 'nephroblastoma' consisting of tubular and glomeruloid structures, with papillary areas. Mitoses were not seen. This suggests that there are three discrete entities, NRB, benign and malignant nephroblastoma. The interrelationship of the tumours is not presently explicable in mechanistic terms.

A subsequent study of Bennington and Beckwith (1975) found 12 cases of 'persistent' metanephric blastema in 2452 consecutive paediatric autopsies (9 among 1035 cases less than 3 of months of age. This rate is much higher than the frequency of Wilm's tumours, suggesting that most instances of persistent blastema do not give rise to tumours.

De Chadarevian et al. (1977) have emphasized that massive bilateral nephroblastomatosis can be confused with Wilm's tumour. Describing four cases, all of which presented at under 2 years of age, they reported a negative family history in three cases, while one child had relatives with urinary tract disease. Following chemotherapy, hypertension, which was present in three of the four cases, disappeared and the kidneys became smaller. Bové and McAdam (1976) have studied the kidneys of 69 patients with Wilm's tumours and found evidence of abnormalities of differentiation in many of them—adenomas, hamartomas, nodular blastema, cysts, dysplastic tubules, scar, etc. This list is one that pathologists might consider to include lesions found in kidneys in many conditions and the study does not provide evidence for a general failure of control mechanisms in metanephric differentiation.

The report of Hughson et al. (1976) of two Wilm's tumour survivors who subsequently presented with benign tumours in the contralateral kidneys is also of interest. These tumours were unlike many mesenchymal renal lesions in having a large striated muscle component. The authors suggested maturation of a metastatic lesion as a possible explanation but also pointed out that the lesions may have been benign from the outset.

5.1. Presentation and Histopathology

The commonest presenting feature of nephroblastoma is an abdominal mass giving rise to distention. Vague abdominal pain is common. Abdominal trauma may result in rupture of the tumour or haemorrhage into it, the resulting pain drawing attention to the presence of a renal mass. Haematuria is a much less common symptom of renal tumour in children than in adults, being present in less than a third of cases. Symptoms due to renin secretion by the tumour include hypertension, polydipsia and polyuria, and these may be the presenting features (Sheth et al. 1978). Removal of the tumour is often followed by the regression of symptoms, but these may recur with the appearance of metastases (Bradley and Drake 1949).

The renal tumour is usually larger than the kidney in which it arises by the time it is excised. Tumour growth causes compression of surrounding renal tissue to form a fibrous pseudocapsule, dividing it from residual functioning kidney (Fig. 15.14). The surface of the involved kidney is frequently nodular. On the cut surface, fibrous septa divide the tumour into nodules, some being cystic as the result of necrosis or, rarely, because of the cystic or papillary configuration of the tumour. Focal haemorrhage is frequently present.

Nephroblastoma presents the greatest variety of histological appearance in embryonic tumours because of the wide variety of lines along which histological differentiation may occur. The most primitive or least differentiated picture is that of islands of undifferentiated, darkly stained blastema cells with oval or slightly elongated nuclei and little

cytoplasm, lying in a stroma of primitive mesenchyme, pale-staining elongated cells with a tendency towards a banded or whorled configuration. The most common type of differentiation is tubular. A wide variety of types of tubules are seen, recapitulating various stages of renal differentiation (Figs. 15.15–15.18). The tubules are lined with tumour epithelium of various types (the lining is frequently more than one cell thick) and are distinguishable from renal tubules enclosed by the advancing edge of the tumour. Glomerular differentiation is less common and seldom progresses further than a small knot of cells arising from the edge of a space lined with flattened epithelial cells (Fig. 15.19).

Some tumours have a predominantly papillary configuration, while a few consist almost entirely of cystically dilated tubules, which may be large enough to be distinguished by the naked eye. Smooth or striated muscle is occasionally seen as differentiated tissue in nephroblastoma (Figs. 15.20 and 15.21).

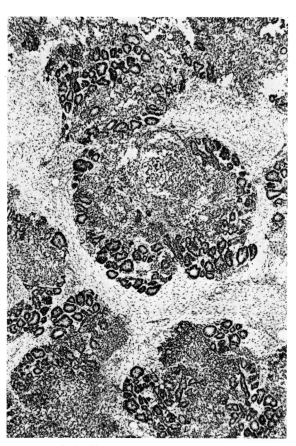

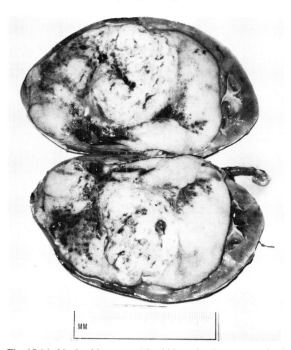

Fig. 15.14. Nephroblastoma. The kidney is almost completely replaced by an ovoid tumour mass, around which the remaining renal parenchyma is stretched. The edge of the tumour is well defined and areas of haemorrhagic necrosis are apparent on the cut surface.

Fig. 15.15. Nephroblastoma. Islands of undifferentiated darkly staining blastema cells have peripheral tubular differentiation and are separated by strands of pale-staining tumour mesenchyme. (H and E; 50×)

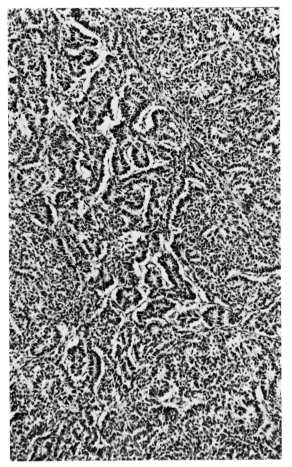

Fig. 15.16. Nephroblastoma. Ribbon-like arrangement of blastema cells in double cords but without intervening lumen. These are the earliest stage of tubular differentiation. (H and E; 120 ×)

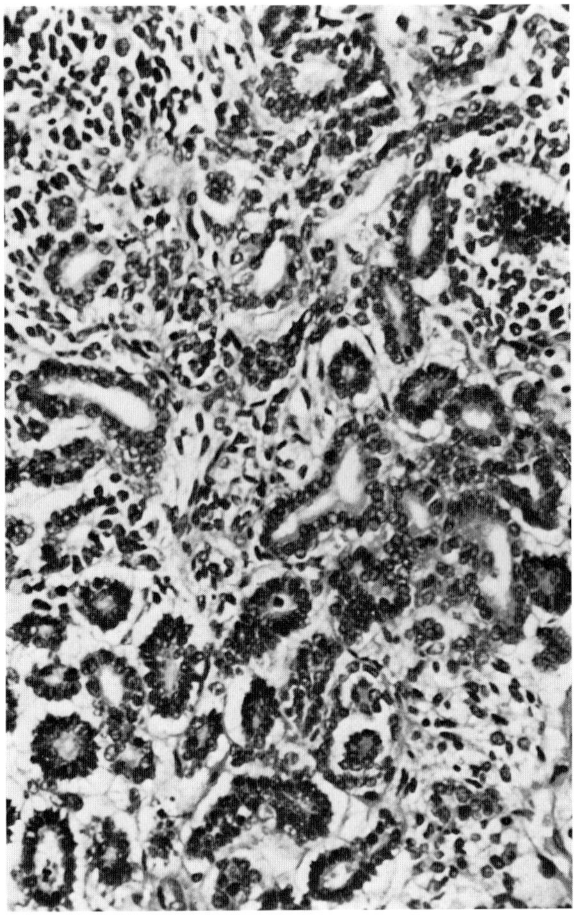

Fig. 15.18. Nephroblastoma. Tubular differentiation, undifferentiated blastema is present between tubules. The tubules have well-defined lumina. (H and E; 300 ×)

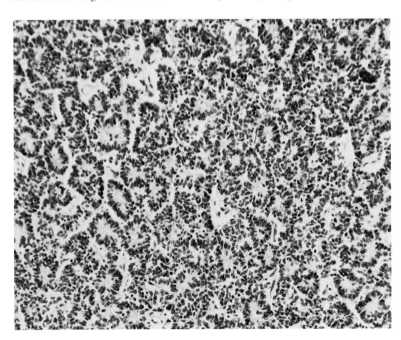

Fig. 15.17. Nephroblastoma. Incomplete tubular differentiation may produce 'rosettes'. The nuclei are more tapered than those of neuroblastoma. (H and E; 140 ×)

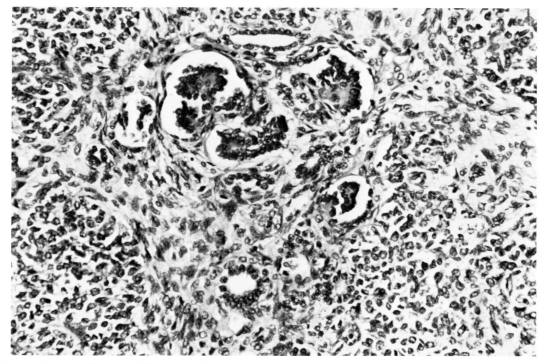

Fig. 15.19. Nephroblastoma. Glomerular differentiation does not precede further than a clump of epithelial cells protruding into a space lined with a flattened cell layer. (H and E; 300 ×)

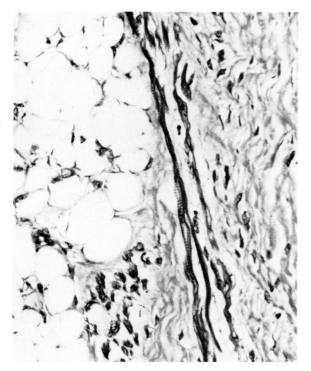

Fig. 15.20. Nephroblastoma. Differentiation with a nephroblastoma may produce mesenchymal tissues. Fatty tissue and strap-like muscle cells with well-marked cross-striations and mature collagen are intimately mixed in this tumour. (H and E; 400 ×)

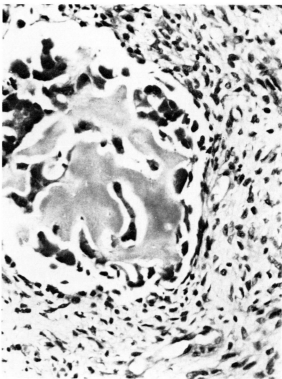

Fig. 15.21. Nephroblastoma. Same tumour as in Fig. 15.20. A circumscribed nodule of osteoid differentiation. (H and E; 400 ×)

There have been many papers on the histological classification of nephroblastoma, itemizing a large number of subgroups depending on the type and extent of histological differentiation within the tumour, some even designating a small group of tumours as 'unclassifiable'. Such classifications serve no purpose unless they are easy to apply, encompass all tumours encountered, and have some prognostic value. There have, however, been three recent studies of large numbers of cases of nephroblastoma, in which the relationship between the histological appearance of the tumour and prognosis has been examined. The experience of Lawler et al. (1977) in the first MRC nephroblastoma trial was that long survival was associated with tubular differentiation within the tumour based on a classification of the volume of differentiated tissue (from 0 to $+++$), irrespective of histological type. They also found that the presence of other types of differentiation (glomeruli, cysts or papillary structures) was associated with better survival but the association was not statistically significant. They drew attention to the 100% survival amongst patients with tumours showing extensive papillary configuration in both their own and other series, but the rarity of this type of appearance precluded statistical analysis. They found no relationship between histological differentiation and age at presentation, but infants under 1 year old at presentation were excluded from their study. Lemerle et al. (1976), in a retrospective study of 248 cases of nephroblastoma, found that the presence of differentiated structures was associated with better prognosis, but in their series it was the variety of types of differentiation rather than the volume of differentiated tissue that proved favourable. They found that haemorrhage into the tumour was an unfavourable sign, whilst necrosis was not a significant factor.

Beckwith and Palmer (1978) examined the tumour material from the American National Wilm's Tumour Study and devised a classification based on the predominant histological appearance. They divided the tumours into epithelial, blastemal, or stromal predominant and mixed types, subdividing each group by the presence or absence of anaplasia, i.e., cellular hyperchromatism, pleomorphism, and abnormal mitoses, and also recognized a sarcomatous group. They found the presence of anaplasia in any histological type and a sarcomatous pattern to be a poor prognostic sign, but found no difference in behaviour between predominantly blastemal and epithelial or mixed types. However, children presenting before 2 years of age did better than older children, and the authors note that all the differentiated tubular tumours were seen in the younger age group. Within their sarcomatous group they distinguished a 'clear-cell' sarcoma with a

predilection for metastasizing to bone. This appears to be identical with the 'bone metastasizing renal tumour of childhood' described by Lawler and Marsden (1979).

5.2. Metastasis

Tumour is found in both kidneys at presentation in between 4% and 13% of cases (Cochran and Froggatt 1967; Young and Williams 1969). It is possible, however, that the higher estimates may be weighted by referrals to specialized units. Direct extension of the tumour occurs, through the capsule to involve neighbouring viscera, into the hepatic vein and the inferior vena cava, and into the renal pelvis and down the ureter.

Lymphatic spread is commonly to hilar or para-aortic lymph nodes, although the porta hepatis and mediastinum may be involved. Haematogenous spread occurs most commonly to the lung. Solitary pulmonary metastases are not unusual, and have often been treated successfully by surgical excision. Hepatic metastases occur but are infrequent, whilst skeletal metastasis is a rare event and nephroblastoma with skeletal metastases may represent a special form of the tumour (Lawler and Marsden 1979).

A comparison of the histological differentiation seen in metastatic nephroblastoma compared with the differentiation in the primary tumour (Bannayan et al. 1971) showed more pronounced nonepithelial differentiation in metastases than in the primary tumour, where differentiation was mainly tubular. The authors considered that these changes were accelerated by radiotherapy.

5.3. Extrarenal Tumours

Extrarenal Wilm's tumours are occasionally described. These seem to be of two types, one type arising in a line from the renal bed to the scrotum supposedly arising in residual embryonic renal tissue (Bhajekar et al. 1964; Akhtar et al. 1977; Aterman et al. 1979; Orlowski et al. 1980). Clusters of mature glomeruli and tubules have been present beneath the capsule of these tumours. The second type are nephroblastomas arising within teratomas. These have been described in the mediastinum (Moyson et al. 1961) and the sacrococcygeal region (Ward and Dehner 1974) as well as in retroperitoneal tumours (Carney 1975). Whether one should regard renal differentiation in a teratoma as nephroblastoma rather than a distinctive form of maturation seems to be open to doubt; only one of the tumours described gave rise to metastases (Orlowski et al. 1980).

5.4. Fetal Rhabdomyomatous Nephroblastoma

Fetal rhabdomyomatous nephroblastoma, which occurs in infants and has a more favourable prognosis than Wilm's tumour, is described by Wigger (1976). The lesions are largely composed of bundles of immature striated muscle in a fibrous stroma, together with undifferentiated elements, fat, cartilage, smooth muscle, and bone. The author considers the tumour to be a variation of Wilm's tumour. Metastases were uncommon but death from local tumour extension occurred in a proportion of cases.

6. Rhabdomyosarcoma

The bulk of rhabdomyosarcomas (malignant tumours of striated muscle) occur in childhood, although no age is exempt. Of head and neck tumours, 80% occur in children aged 12 years or less (Dito and Batsakis 1962), most commonly in the orbital region or in the nose, mouth, or pharynx. The majority of genitourinary tumours present before the age of 4 years. There is an apparent male predominance (Legier 1961; Williams and Schistad 1964).

Li and Fraumeni (1969) reported an epidemiological study on the families of many of the 418 children dying of rhabdomyosarcoma in the United States between 1960 and 1964. In five families a second child was found to have had a soft-tissue sarcoma, three siblings and two cousins being affected. The parents and grandparents of these children had a higher incidence than normal of carcinoma of various sites and of leukaemia, and the authors suggested the existence of a familial cancer syndrome. They postulated an interaction between genetic influences and the environment and speculated on the possibility of viruses acting in this way, although no time or space clustering was found. Experimental studies have provided a good deal of information about pathogenesis and histogenesis of the tumours. Two systems of classification of rhabdomyosarcoma dependent on this work are used, that of Horn and Enterline (1958), where the lesion is divided into embryonal and botryoid, alveolar, and pleomorphic types and the system of Ashton and Morgan (1965), which has three categories, embryonal sarcoma, nonstriated embryonal rhabdomyosarcoma, and striated embryonal rhabdomyosarcoma.

Morales et al. (1972) have carried out an extensive ultrastructural study of human rhabdomyosarcoma, and have reviewed previous studies of this type.

Their findings, which should be consulted by those attempting to confirm this diagnosis, by electron microscopy, emphasize the importance of accurate identification of the fibres found in any tumour before assumptions are made about its origin. Their data suggest that the Ashton and Morgan system of classification, devised to deal with an experimentally induced tumour, will be of value in man (see Clarke and O'Connell 1973).

6.1. Pathology

In the urogenital sinus areas the tumour generally presents as a polypoid mass projecting into the vagina or bladder. The component lobules are greyish-white, opalescent and of varying size. The whole tumour is often of indeterminate origin, i.e., it has no distinct 'base' (Figs. 15.22 and 15.23). Histologically the polyps are usually covered by a layer of cuboidal or stratified squamous epithelium and may show areas of superficial ulceration. The polyps have an essentially myxomatous appearance, which may mislead the unwary, and the lesions, when solitary or infected, may be mistaken for inflammatory masses (Fig. 15.24). Examination of the cells in the zone immediately under the epithelium (Fig. 15.25) and of those scattered in the stroma will reveal a number with nuclear atypicality and eosinophilic cytoplasm, which may be arranged in strap-like forms showing cross-striation typical of muscle cells (Fig. 15.26). These are not essential for the diagnosis of rhabdomyosarcoma, as other cytological characteristics will permit the diagnosis to be made. Rhabdomyosarcomas may contain long spindle-shaped cells, with ovoid central nuclei, cells with cross-striation, or large bizarre 'tadpole' cells with their nuclei at the expanded end.

Whether present in the head and neck or pelvis, the tumour spreads rapidly by local extension and involves the local lymph nodes. Blood-borne metastases are relatively uncommon in the normally short history of the disease Nasopharyngeal tumours tend to involve bone early by local extension (Canalis et al. 1978).

Large series are few. Weichert et al. (1976) reported 35 children with rhabdomyosarcoma, 19 of the tumours occurring in the head and neck, 10 in the urogenital tract, and 6 elsewhere. They found that children with pure spindle cell tumours or completely undifferentiated tumours tended to do better than those with rhabdomyoblastic differentiation or an alveolar appearance.

Paratesticular rhabdomyosarcoma can be cured by radical surgery and radiotherapy or simple chemotherapy if they are noninfiltrating. Children with infiltrating tumours may survive if an aggressive surgical approach, i.e., retroperitoneal lymphadenectomy plus radiotherapy plus cyclic combined chemotherapy is undertaken (Malek and Kelalis 1977).

Embryonal rhabdomyosarcoma of the botryoid type may also occur in the biliary tract. In a recent review, Taira et al. (1976) reviewed 20 verified cases and added a further case of their own. Most of these tumours occur in young children (average age at onset 3.9 years) and the prognosis is poor.

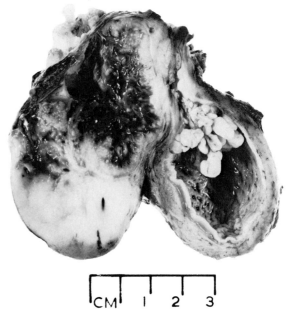

Fig. 15.23. From a 6-year-old. The tumour is infiltrating and ulcerated, with extensive secondary infection. The bladder wall is thickened.

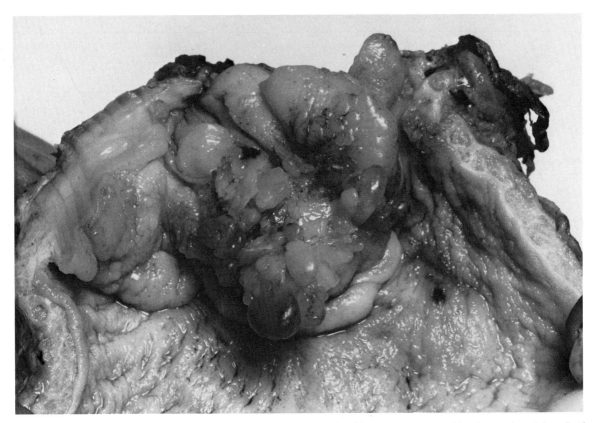

Fig. 15.22. From a 2-year-old boy presenting with strangury. Many polypoid masses are seen arising from a broad base in the trabeculated bladder.

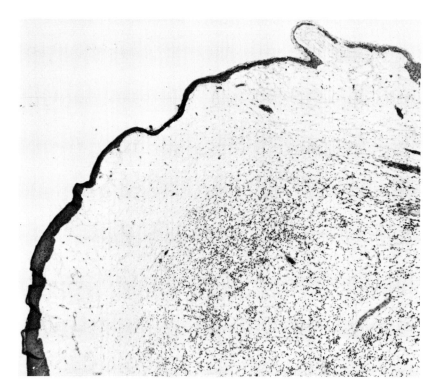

Fig. 15.24. Rhabdomyosarcoma. The botryoid polyps of rhabdomyosarcoma may be disarmingly hypocellular and the superficial part of the tumour very oedematous. Nuclei are well separated by a myxoid stroma. (H and E; 40×)

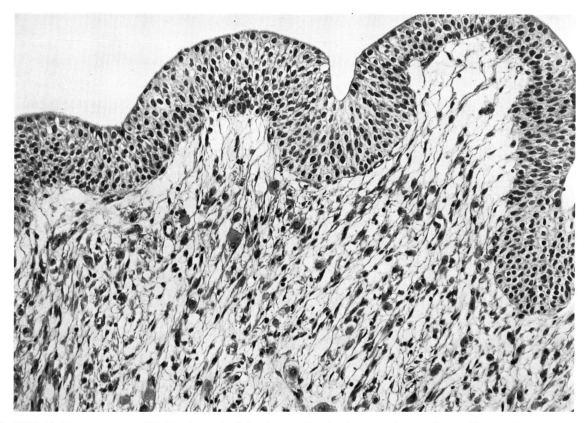

Fig. 15.25. Rhabdomyosarcoma of bladder. Marked cellular pleomorphism in a loose zone beneath the transitional epithelium. Some cells have a densely eosinophilic cytoplasm. (H and E; 250×)

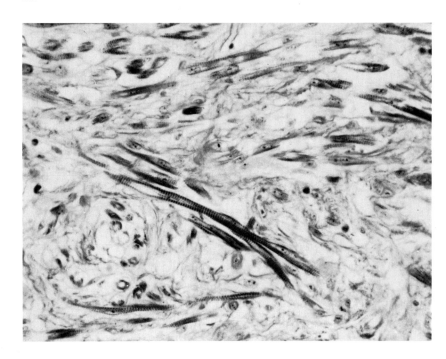

Fig. 15.26. Rhabdomyosarcoma. Cross-striations are seen in strap cells in this well-differentiated urogenital sinus tumour. (PTAH; $400 \times$)

7. Hepatoblastoma

Hepatoblastoma is much less common than neuroblastoma or nephroblastoma, accounting for less than 5% of tumours in most series from children's hospitals. It is a tumour of infancy, most cases presenting before 3 years of age. It has undoubtedly been present at birth in some instances. The usual presentations are increasing girth or the palpation of an upper abdominal mass by the mother or other attendant. Abdominal X-ray may confirm liver enlargement, and tumour calcification may be present. A liver scan, inferior vena cavagram, or hepatic arteriography may be useful in localizing the tumour and may make it possible to distinguish between a single tumour mass and multiple deposits (Clatworthy et al. 1974). Serum α-fetoprotein levels may be elevated in infants with hepatoblastoma, and may be a useful indication of recurrence in follow-up studies (Alpert et al. 1968). Chorionic gonadotrophin is produced less frequently by hepatoblastoma (Murphy et al. 1980). Hepatic lobectomy or wedge resection is the treatment of choice; addition of chemotherapy or radiotherapy may be useful but these techniques have not been fully evaluated (Clatworthy et al. 1974). The tumour is more frequently seen in the right lobe than the left (Keeling 1971; Clatworthy et al. 1974), but in about one-third of cases both lobes are involved.

Macroscopically, there is usually a firm, encapsulated, multinodular, brownish-tan tumour. Haemorrhages and cystic degeneration of necrotic areas are frequent findings (Fig. 15.27).

There is a spectrum of histological appearance; some tumours consist entirely of sheets of small cells with ovoid nuclei and narrow rim of cytoplasm resembling fetal hepatocytes (Fig. 15.28). In others, larger, better-differentiated cells with lower nuclear/cytoplasmic ratio have a trabecular or cord-like arrangement resembling liver cell plates in the developing liver. In others there appear to be two populations of cells, hepatoblasts and mesenchymal cells (Fig. 15.29) or cells resembling hepatocytes and sheets of smaller cells resembling bile duct epithelium, within which a tubular configuration may be seen. It is the duct-like cells that undergo squamous metaplasia with the production of keratin. Metaplasia to osteoid may also be seen (Fig. 15.30), and this may calcify in large enough aggregates to be visible on abdominal X-ray.

The tumour spreads locally to involve other parts of the liver, to lymph nodes in the porta hepatis, and occasionally to the duodenum and pancreas. Metastatic spread is usually to the lungs but involvement of the diaphragm and mediastinum and generalized intra-abdominal metastasis is quite common. Cerebral involvement and spread to other lymph node groups may occur (Keeling 1971).

Most recent reviews of liver tumours in children distinguish the hepatoblastoma of the infant liver from hepatocellular carcinoma occurring in older children (Ishak and Gluntz 1967; Misugi et al. 1967; Keeling 1971). Ultrastructural differences between

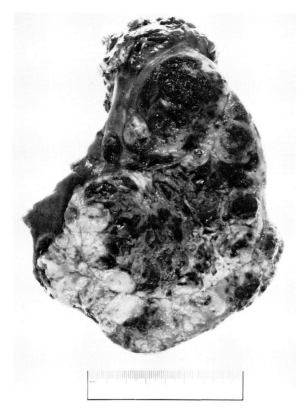

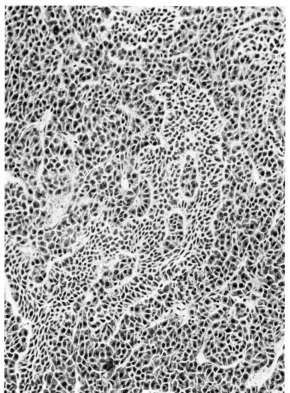

Fig. 15.27. Hepatoblastoma. Male of 6 months, presenting with abdominal distension. Hepatic lobectomy specimen, a massive lobulated tumour with extensive haemorrhage. Keeling 1971; courtesy of the Editor of the *Journal of Pathology*.

Fig. 15.28. Hepatoblastoma. Tumour cells resemble developing hepatocytes and are arranged in a cord-like configuration. Keeling 1971; courtesy of the Editor of the *Journal of Pathology*. (H and E; 100 ×)

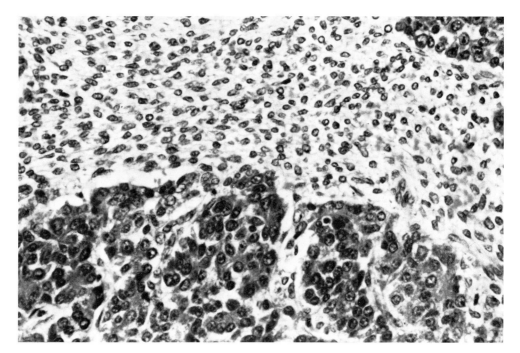

Fig. 15.29. Hepatoblastoma. A mixed cellular pattern. In the upper part of the field pale-staining elongated cells of tumour mesenchyme intervene between nodules of larger cells resembling fetal hepatocytes. (H and E; 365 ×)

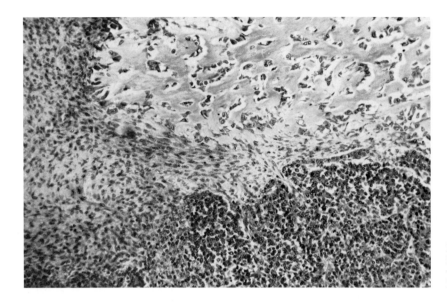

Fig. 15.30. Hepatoblastoma. An island of osteoid metaplasia is seen within tumour mesenchyme. (H and E; 145×)

the two groups are described (Misugi et al. 1967; Ito and Johnson 1969). There do not appear to be behavioural differences between the various histological types of hepatoblastoma, and Misugi et al. (1967) and Keeling (1971) consider them variations of the same embryonal tumour. Willis' (1962) division into hepatocellular, mixed, and rhabdomyoblastic tumours is probably unjustified, since thorough examination of the tumour reveals mesenchymal elements in almost every case. All hepatoblastomas could be considered to be in Willis' mixed group, and rhabdomyosarcomatous tumours, occurring as they do in older children and taking their origin from the biliary tree, should be considered a distinct tumour entity (see also p. 292).

8. Teratomas

There has always been a considerable amount of speculative literature on the origins of teratomas, which are interesting tumours derived from multiple germ layers. In recent decades there has been considerable interest in sexing teratomas, much of the work having been carried out on the basis of the presence of Barr bodies (the presence of a Barr body being considered to indicate an XX constitution). Such work has now been largely discredited. The demonstration by Atkin (1973) that all male teratomas contain a Y chromosome, whether sex chromatin-positive or -negative, and the general realization that most male tumours are hyperdiploid (they may have two Y chromosomes) suggest that parthenogenetic explanations of the origin of such tumours in males are unsatisfactory. Most female gonadal teratomas are diploid, however (Linder et al. 1975), an important distinction between male and female that has not yet been established for extragonadal tumours. Linder and his co-workers have also demonstrated, by isoenzyme and cytological studies, that the benign ovarian teratoma does arise by parthenogenesis, their study having ruled out the possibility of the tumour having arisen from a somatic cell or from an öogonium before the first meiotic division. An hypothesis for the origin of teratomas has been proposed by Erickson and Gondos (1976). These authors comment on the differences in natural history of gonadal teratomas with age—in infancy and childhood teratomas of the testis are almost always benign and those of the ovary are malignant, while the reverse is true in adults. In each gonad the peak incidence of malignancy occurs some 5–15 years after the maximal cellular proliferation phase (with peaks of meiotic and mitotic division). The authors suggest male teratomas may arise by fusion of nonmeiotically related haploid germ cells, rather than by suppression of the second meiotic division which would result in XX or YY karytypes. Benign adult female teratomas arise from cells blocked in meiosis, which are parthenogenetically activated. The rare prepubertal female malignant tumours could develop from the fusion of haploid germ cells after premature meiosis.

The frequencies of individual sites of origin of these tumours in reported series is dependent upon the age range of the population from which they were drawn. Table 15.3 gives the sites of origin of 104 teratomas seen at The Hospital for Sick Children, Great Ormond Street from 1934 to 1971 (Claireaux and Keeling 1973). At this hospital the upper age limit for new patients is 12 years and the majority of

Table 15.3. Sites of origin of 107 teratomas seen at The Hospital for Sick Children, Great Ormond Street, between 1934 and 1971

	M	*F*	*Total*
Sacrococcygeal region	22	49	71
Ovary	–	10	10
Testis	7	–	7
Basi cranium	4	2	6
Mediastinum	4	6	10
Abdomen	2	1	3
	39	68	107

tumours arise in the sacrococcygeal region. Series where the age range extends to 15 or 16 years have a larger proportion of ovarian tumours, many of which seem to present just after puberty. The majority of testicular tumours also present later, 74% of patients with these tumours undergoing orchidectomy between 20 and 49 years of age (Pugh 1976) and only about 3% of testicular teratomas presenting before 10 years of age.

8.1. Sacrococcygeal

Sacrococcygeal teratomas are tumours of the neonate and infant (Fig. 15.31) and are usually present at birth, when the tumour may be large enough to obstruct delivery (Heys et al. 1967). Presentation after 1 year of age is associated with poor prognosis (60% recurrence, compared with 10% in infants who present before that time). Immediate surgery is the treatment of choice in these infants, and observation and interval surgery are associated with an increased risk of occurrence (Berry et al. 1969). Catastrophic haemorrhage may take place into the loose connective-tissue stroma of a large tumour (Berry et al. 1969; Izant and Filston 1975). It is important to excise the mass completely, and the coccyx should be taken en bloc with the tumour; failure to do this increases the likelihood of recurrence (Berry et al. 1969; Carney et al. 1972).

The tumours are usually partially cystic masses (Fig. 15.32). Histologically, the majority are composed of differentiated tissues (Fig. 15.33). Organoid differentiation is common (Fig. 15.34). Embryonic tissue is present in the tumours in between 13% and 27% of cases in large series and is frequently neural in type, often resembling a retinal anlage (Fig. 15.35), although mesenchymal and other developing structures are frequently seen (Fig. 15.36).

Sacrococcygeal teratomas that are histologically malignant on first resection or biopsy comprise

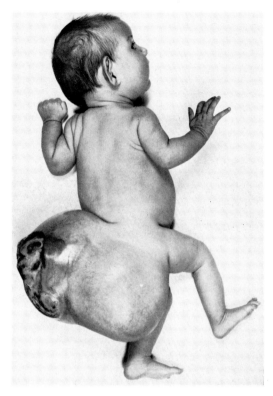

Fig. 15.31. Sacrococcygeal teratoma that was present at birth. A large ulcerated mass protrudes from the buttocks.

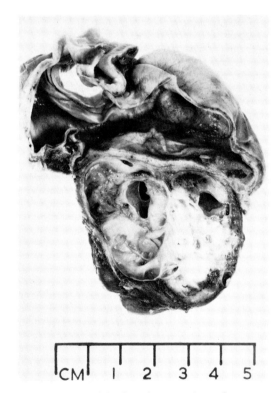

Fig. 15.32. Cystic mass arising from the sacrum in a male neonate. *Lower segment*, caesarian section for cord prolapse.

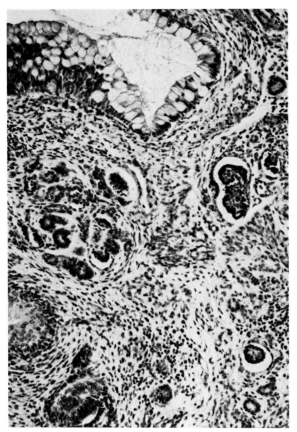

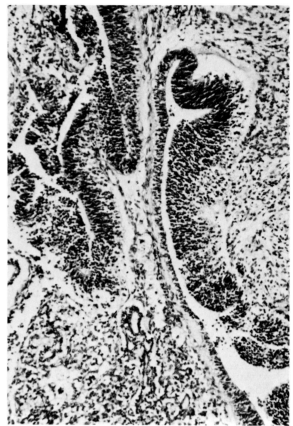

Fig. 15.33. Sacrococcygeal teratoma. A cyst lined with fully differentiated mucus secreting columnar epithelium; mature renal tubules and glomeruli are present in a stroma of immature mesenchyme. Berry, Keeling and Hilton 1971; courtesy of the Editor of the *Journal of Pathology*. (H and E; 150 ×)

Fig. 15.35. Sacrococcygeal teratoma in an infant born at 31 weeks' gestation. Embryonic neural tissue formed a major component of this tumour, here seen as retinal anlage. (H and E; 150 ×)

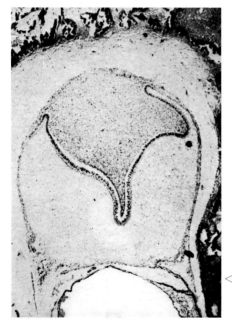

between 11 % and 27 % of the cases in reported series. The most common histological type is a large-cell carcinoma; some are anaplastic but a papillary configuration is common and the malignant element may resemble endodermal sinus (Teilum) tumour (Figs. 15.37 and 15.38).

The high incidence of malignant change in some reports is probably a reflection of secondary referral to specialist hospitals of cases treated originally elsewhere (Chretien et al. 1970). In a series composed entirely of primary referrals the incidence of malignancy is lower.

◁ **Fig. 15.34.** Sacrococcygeal teratoma. Organoid development; a developing tooth bud is present within its bony matrix. Berry, Keeling and Hilton 1969; courtesy of the Editor of the *Journal of Pathology*. (H and E; 10 ×)

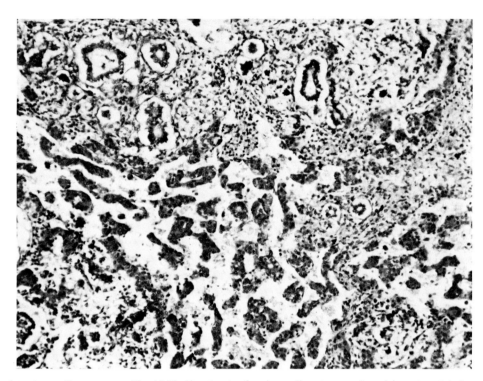

Fig. 15.36. Sacrococcygeal teratoma. Same case as Fig. 15.35. Hepatocytes forming rudimentary cords and immature tubular structures. (H and E; 150 ×)

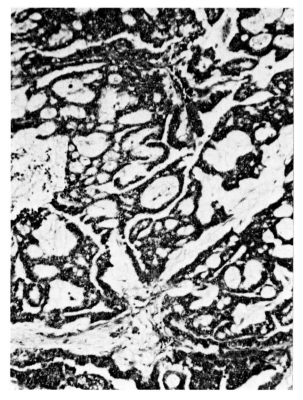

Fig. 15.37. Malignant sacrococcygeal teratoma. Adenocarcinoma with a tubular/papillary configuration. (H and E; 150 ×)

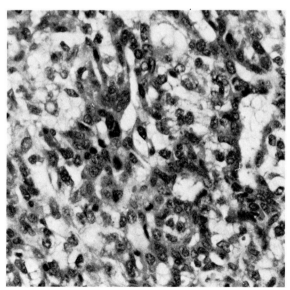

Fig. 15.38. Malignant sacrococcygeal teratoma. Solid adenocarcinoma. Some cells are mucus-secreting. (H and E; 400 ×)

8.2. Ovarian

Although a few ovarian teratomas are seen in infancy, many more are seen in older children and young adults. Histologically they are usually composed of differentiated tissues (Berry et al. 1969), but malignant ovarian teratomas are reported in children. Amongst the cases reported by Breen and Neubecker (1963), nine of seventeen malignant ovarian teratomas occurred in girls before menarche, the youngest being 14 months of age. Chorion carcinoma was seen in several tumours from young patients; differentiation to papillary carcinoma, sarcoma, and dysgerminoma was also seen. More than half these authors' young patients were dead within 1 year of presentation.

8.3. Testicular

Testicular teratomas do occur in infants and children, but as with ovarian tumours, much less commonly than in young adults. In children the tumours are usually differentiated (Testicular Tumour Panel Grade TD [teratomas differentiated]), but do not recur following surgical excision (Berry et al. 1969; Pugh 1976).

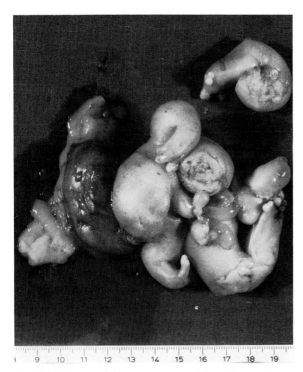

Fig. 15.39. Intracranial teratoma removed from the lateral ventricle of a 6-week-old child with hydrocephalus. One 'limb' has been removed in the surgical resection.

8.4. Mediastinal

Mediastinal teratomas are seen in both the infant and the older child. In some cases a thyroid origin is obvious and in some a thymic origin is postulated, but in many cases the exact origin of the tumour is unclear. In infants the tumours are usually composed of differentiated tissues or a mixture of differentiated and embryonic elements although the thyroid tumour reported by Heys et al. (1967), which obstructed delivery had metastasized to the liver in utero.

In older children mediastinal teratomas may be malignant, with widespread metastases and rapid downhill course. Unusual histological appearances may be present, reminiscent of embryonal sarcoma with mesenchymal and tubular elements.

Occasionally a teratoma arises within the pericardial sac. Such teratomas are tumours of infancy and usually arise from the great vessels at the base of the heart (Claireaux 1951), although the tumour may arise from the myocardium. A similar tumour has been seen in a 33-week stillbirth whose mother's previous pregnancy had resulted in twins, one dying in the neonatal period from heart failure complicating a cerebral arteriovenous malformation. Teratomas arising from the base of the skull may present as oral or intracranial masses (Fig. 15.39). Problems arise because of difficulty of excision rather than malignant change.

8.5. At Other Sites

Abdominal teratomas arising from the stomach, retroperitoneal tissues (Berry et al. 1969), or liver (Yarborough and Evashwick 1956) are uncommon; they are usually well differentiated, although a malignant hepatic teratoma has been reported (Misugi and Reiner 1965).

9. Second Malignant Neoplasms in Children Surviving Embryonic Neoplasms

There are many reports of second malignant tumours in children, with Wilm's tumour and retinoblastoma being the commonest initial lesions and osteosarcomas and chondrosarcomas the commonest second neoplasms. Many of the bone tumours in the report of Meadows et al. (1977) developed in areas previously irradiated, as did skin tumours (basal cell carcinomas) in the irradiated fields for medulloblastoma in individuals with the naevoid basal cell carcinoma syndrome. However, 33 of 102 second neoplasms were not associated with prior radiation. Twelve of these could be explained on the basis of a known inherent susceptibility but in the remaining 21 no predisposing cause was found. Associations between gliomas and leukaemia or lymphoma, and between the last two tumours and carcinomas of the colon, occurred with higher frequencies than would be expected by chance.

References

Adelstein AM, White C (1976) Population trends no. 3, p 9

Akhtar M, Kott E, Brooks B (1977) Extrarenal Wilm's tumor. Report of a case and review of literature. Cancer 40: 3087

Alpert ME, Uriel J, de Nechaud B (1968) Alpha-1-fetoglobulin in the diagnosis of human hepatoma. N Engl J Med 278: 984

Anders D, Kindermann G, Pfeifer U (1973) Metastasising fetal neuroblastoma with involvement of the placenta simulating fetal erythroblastosis. Report of 2 cases. J Pediatr 82: 50

Ashton N, Morgan G (1965) Embryonal sarcoma and embryonal rhabdomyosarcoma of the orbit. J Clin Pathol 18: 699

Aterman K, Grantmyre E, Gillis DA (1979) Extrarenal Wilm's tumour. J Invest Cell Pathol 2: 309

Atkin NB (1973) Y bodies and similar fluorescent chromocenters in human tumours including teratomata. Br J Cancer 27: 183

Bannayan GA, Huvos AG, D'Angio GJ (1971) Effect of irradiation on the maturation of Wilm's tumor. Cancer 27: 812

Beckwith JB, Palmer NF (1978) Histopathology and prognosis of Wilm's tumor. Results from the First National Wilm's Tumour Study. Cancer 41: 1937

Beckwith JB, Perrin EV (1963) In-situ neuroblastomas: A contribution to the natural history of neural crest tumours. Arch Pathol 43: 1089

Bedford MA (1975) Treatment of retinoblastoma. Adv Ophthalmol 31: 2

Belamire J, Chau AS (1969) Medulloblastoma in newborn sisters: Report of two cases. J Neurosurg 30: 76

Bell M (1968) Neuroblastoma. Newer clinical diagnostic tests. JAMA 205: 155

Bennington JL, Beckwith JB (1975) Tumours of the kidney, renal pelvis and ureter. In: Atlas of tumour pathology, 2nd, ser, Fasc 12. Armed Forces Institute of Pathology, Washington p 33

Berry, CL, Keeling JW, Hilton C (1969) Teratoma in infancy and childhood: A review of 91 cases. J Pathol 98: 241

Berry CL, Keeling JW, Hilton C (1970) Coincidence of congenital malformation and embryonic tumours of childhood. Arch Dis Child 45: 229

Berry CL (1981) The formation and behaviour of tumours in childhood. In: Davis JA, Dobbing J (eds) Scientific foundation of paediatrics. Heinemann Medical Books, London

Berry CL, Keeling JW (1975) Genetic aspects of childhood cancer. In: Symington T, Carter RL (eds) Scientific foundations of oncology. Heinemann Medical Books, London

Bhajekar AB, Joseph M, Bjat HS (1964) Unattached nephroblastoma. Br J Urol 36: 189

Bhangui GR, Roy S, Tandon PN (1977) Multiple primary tumours of the brain including a medulloblastoma in the cerebellum. Cancer 39: 293

Bickerstaff ER, Connolly RC, Woolf AL (1967) Cerebellar

medulloblastoma occurring in brothers. Acta Neuropathol (Berl) 8: 104

Bolande RP (1971) Benignity of neonatal tumours and concept of cancer repression in early life. Am J Dis Child 122: 12

Bové KE, McAdams AJ (1976) The nephroblastomatosis complex and its relationship to Wilm's tumour. A clinicopathological treatise. Perspect Pediatr Pathol 3: 185

Bové KE, Koffler H, McAdams AJ (1969) Nodular renal blastoma, definition and possible significance. Cancer 24: 323

Bradley JE, Drake ME (1949) The effect of preoperative roentgen-ray therapy on arterial hypertension in embryoma (kidney). J Pediatr 35: 710

Breen JL, Neubecker RD (1963) Malignant teratoma of the ovary. An analysis of 17 cases. Obstet Gynecol 21: 699

Briard-Guillemot ML, Nonaiti-Pellie C, Feingold J, Frezal J (1974) Étude génétique du rétinoblastome. Humangenetik 24: 271

Brown DH (1966) The clinico-pathology of retinoblastoma. Am J Ophthalmol 61: 508

Canalis RF, Jenkins HA, Hemenway WG, Lincoln C (1978) Nasopharyngeal rhabdomyosarcoma. Arch Otolaryngol 104: 122

Carney JA (1975) Wilm's tumor and renal cell carcinoma in retroperitoneal teratoma. Cancer 35: 1179

Chretien PB, Milam JD, Foote FW, Miller TW (1970) Embryonal adenocarcinomas (a type of malignant teratoma) of the sacrococcygeal region. Clinical and pathologic aspects of 21 cases. Cancer 26: 522

Claireaux AE (1951) An intraperitoneal teratoma in a newborn infant. J Pathol Bacteriol 63: 743

Claireaux AE, Keeling JW (1973) Teratomas in children (abstract). Arch Dis Child 48: 159

Clarke MA, O'Connell KJ (1973) An ultrastructural study of embryonal rhabdomyosarcoma (Sarcoma botryoides) of the bladder. J Urol 109: 897

Clatworthy HW, Schiller M, Grosfeld JL (1974) Primary liver tumours in infancy and childhood. Arch Surg 109: 143

Cochran W, Froggatt P (1967) Bilateral nephroblastoma in two sisters. J Urol 97: 216

Czeizel A, Gárdonyi J (1974) Retinoblastoma in Hungary 1960–1968. Humangenetik 22: 153

De Chadarevian JP, Fletcher BD, Chatten J, Rabinovitch HH (1977) Massive infantile nephroblastomatosis. A clinical, radiological, and pathological analysis of four cases. Cancer 39: 2294

Dito WR, Batsakis JG (1962) Rhabdomyosarcoma of the head and neck. Arch Surg 84: 582

Ellsworth RM (1969) The practical management of retinoblastoma. Trans Am Ophthalmol Soc 67: 462

Erickson RP, Gondos B (1976) Alternative explanations of the differing behaviour of ovarian and testicalar teratomas. Lancet 1: 407

Evans AE, D'Angio GJ, Randolph J (1971) A proposed staging for children with neuroblastoma. Cancer 27: 324

Fujita S (1967) Quantitative analysis of cell proliferation and differentiation in the cortex of the post-natal mouse cerebellum. J Cell Biol 22: 277

Griepentrog F. Pauly H (1957) Intra- und extrakranielle, frühmanifeste Medulloblastome bei erbgleichen Zwillingen. Zentralbl Neurochir 17: 129

Hemmes GD (1931) Untersuchungen nach dem Vorkommen von Glioma retinae bei Verwandten von mit dieser Krankheit Behafteten. Klin Monatsbl Augenheilkd 86: 331

Heys RF, Murray CP, Kohler HG (1967) Obstructed labour due to foetal tumours: Cervical and coccygeal teratoma. Two case reports. Gynaecologia 164: 43

Hilton C, Keeling JW (1973) Neonatal renal tumours. Br J Urol 46: 157

Horn RC Jr, Enterline HR (1958) Rhabdomyosarcoma: A

clinicopathological study and classification of 39 cases. Cancer 11: 181

Hughson MD, Hennigar GR, Othersen HB (1976) Cyto-differentiated renal tumours occurring with Wilm's tumours of the opposite kidneys. Am J Clin Pathol 66: 376

Innes MD (1970) Possible genetic basis of childhood neoplasia. Med J Aust 2: 187

Innes MD (1972a) Nephroblastoma, possible index tumour of childhood. Med J Aust 1: 18

Innes MD (1972b) Hereditary theory of childhood oncogenesis. Oncology 26: 474

Ishak KG, Gluntz PR (1967) Hepatoblastoma and hepatocellular carcinoma in infancy and childhood. Cancer 20: 396

Ito J, Johnson WW (1969) Hepatoblastoma and hepatoma in infancy and childhood. Light and electron microscopic studies. Arch Pathol 87: 259

Izant RJ, Filston HC (975) Sacrococcygeal teratomas. Analysis of forty-three cases. Am J Surg 130: 617

Kadin ME, Rubenstein LJ, Nelson JS (1970) Neonatal cerebellar medulloblastoma originating from the fetal external granular layer. J Neuropathol Exp Neurol 29: 583

Keeling JW (1971) Liver tumours in infancy and childhood. J Pathol 103: 69

Kinnier Wilson LM, Draper GJ (1974) Neuroblastoma, its natural history and prognosis: A study of 487 cases. Br Med J iii: 301

Kitchin FD, Ellsworth RM (1974) Pleiotrophic effects of the gene for retinoblastoma. J Med Genet 11: 244

Kjellin K. Müller K, Aström KE (1960) The occurrence of brain tumours in several members of a family. J Neuropathol Exp Neurol 19: 528

Klapproth H (1959) Wilm's tumour—A report of 45 cases and an analysis of 1351 cases reported in the world literature. J Urol 81: 633

Knudson AG Jr (1971) Mutation and cancer statistical study of retinoblastoma. Proc Natl Acad Sci USA 68: 820

Knudson AG Jr, Strong LC (1972) Mutation and cancer: Neuroblastoma and phaeochromocytoma. Am J Hum Genet 24: 514

Koop CE (1972) The neuroblastoma. In: Rickham PP, Hecker WC, Prevot J (eds) Progress in paediatric surgery. Urban & Schwarzenberg, Munich Berlin Vienna

Lawler W, Marsden HB (1979) Bone metastases in children presenting with renal tumours. J Clin Pathol 32: 608

Lawler W, Marsden HB, Palmer MK (1977) Histopathological study of the First Medical Research Nephroblastoma Trial. Cancer 40: 1519

Ledlie EM, Mynors LS, Draper GJ, Gorback PD (1970) Natural history and treatment of Wilm's tumour: An analysis of 335 cases occurring in England and Wales 1962–1966. Br Med J iv: 195

Legier JF (1961) Botryoid sarcoma and rhabdomyosarcoma of the bladder: review of the literature and report of three cases. J Urol 86: 583

Lemerle J, Tournade MF, Gerard Marchant R, Flamant R, Sarrazin D, Flamant F, Lemerle M, Junt S, Zucker J-M, Schwisguth O (1976) Wilm's tumour: Natural history and prognostic factors. A retrospective study of 248 cases treated at the Institut Gustave-Roussy 1952–1967. Cancer 37: 2557

Lennox EL, Draper GJ, Sanders BM (1975) Retinoblastoma: A study of natural history and prognosis of 268 cases. Br Med J iii: 731

Levi-Montalcini R, Caramia F, Luse SA (1968) In vitro effects of the nerve growth factor on the fine structure of the sensory nerve cells. Brain Res 8: 347

Li EP, Fraumeni JF Jr (1969) Rhabdomyosarcoma in children: Epidemiology study and identification of a familial cancer syndrome. J Natl Cancer Inst 43: 1365

Linder D, Hecht F, McCaw BK, Campbell JR (1975) Origin of

extragonadal teratomas and endodermal sinus tumours. Nature 254: 597

Makinen J (1972) Microscopic patterns as a guide to prognosis of neuroblastoma in childhood. Cancer 29: 1637

Malek RS, Kelalis PP (1977) Paratesticular rhabdomyosarcoma in childhood. J Urol 118: 450

Meadows AT, D'Angio GJ, Mike V, Banfi A, Harris C, Jenkin RDT, Schwartz A (1977) Patterns of second malignant neoplasms in children. Cancer 40: 1903

Merton DF, Yang SS, Bernstein J (1976) Wilm's tumour in adolescence. Cancer 37: 1532

Miller RW, Fraumeni JF Jr, Manning MD (1964) Association of Wilm's tumour with aniridia, hemihypertrophy and other congenital malformations. N Engl J Med 270: 922

Misugi K, Reiner CB (1965) A malignant true teratoma of liver in childhood. Arch Pathol 80: 409

Misugi K, Okajima H, Misugi N, Newton WA Jr (1967) Classification of primary malignant tumors of liver in infancy and childhood. Cancer 20: 1760

Mobley WC, Server AC, Ishü DN, Riopelle RJ, Shooter EM (1977) Nerve growth factor. N Engl J Med 297: 1096, 1149, 1211

Morales AR, Fine G, Horn RC Jr (1972) Rhabdomyosarcoma: An ultrastructural appraisal. Pathol Annu 7: 81

Moyson F, Maurus-Desmarex R, Gompel C (1961) Tumeur de Wilms mediastinale? Acta Chir Belg [Suppl] 2: 118

Murphy ASK, Vawter GS, Lee ABH, Jockin H, Filler RM (1980) Hormonal bioassay of gonadotrophin-producing hepatoblastoma. Arch Pathol Lab Med 104: 513

Neblett CR, Waltz TA, Anderson DE (1971) Neurological involvement in the naevoid basal cell carcinoma syndrome. J Neurosurg 35: 577

O'Grady RB, Rothstein TB, Romano PE (1974) D-group deletion syndromes and retinoblastoma. Am J Ophthalmol 77: 40

Orlowski JP, Levin HS, Dyment PG (1980) Intrascotal Wilm's tumor developing into a heterotopic renal anlage of probable mesonephric origin. J Pediatr Surg 15: 679

Orye E, Delbebe MJ, Vandenbeale B (1974) Retinoblastoma and long arm deletion of chromosome 13: Attempts to define the deleted segment. Clin Genet 5: 457

Poon CCS, Lim SM, Hwang WS (1975) Congenital medulloblastoma. Singapore Med J 16: 230

Prasad KN (1975) Differentiation of neuroblastoma cells in culture. Biol Rev 50: 129

Pugh R (1976) Pathology of the testis. Blackwell Scientific, Oxford London Edinburgh Melbourne, p 153, 205

Redler LD, Ellsworth RM (1973) Prognostic importance of choroidal invasion of retinoblastoma. Arch Ophthalmol 90: 294

Reynolds CP, Perez-Polo JR (1975) Human neuroblastoma: glial induced morphological differentiation. Neurosci Lett 1: 91

Rubenstein LJ, Northfield DWC (1964) The medulloblastoma and the so-called arachnoid cerebellar sarcoma. Brain 87: 379

Schweisguth O (1968) Excretion of catecholamine metabolites in urine of neuroblastoma patients. J Pediatr Surg 3: 118

Sheth KJ, Tang TT, Blaedel ME, Good TA (1978) Polydipsia, polyria, and hypertension associated with renin-secreting Wilm's tumor. J Pediatr 92: 921

Sorsby A (1962) Bilateral retinoblastoma. Br Med J ii: 580

Stambolis C (1977) Benign epithelial nephroblastoma, a contribution to its histiogenesis. Virchows Arch [Pathol Anat] 376: 267

Taira Y, Nakayama I, Moriuchi A, Takajara O, Ito T, Tsuchiya R, Hirano T, Matsushita T (1976) Sarcoma botryoides arising from the biliary tract of children—a case report with review of the literature. Acta Pathol Jpn 26: 709

Taylor AI (1970) Dq−, Dr and retinoblastoma. Humangenetik 10: 209

Turkel Susan B, Itabashi HH (1974) The natural history of

neuroblastic cells in the fetal adrenal gland. Am J Pathol 76: 225

Voute PA, Wadman SK, Van Putten WJ (1970) Congenital neuroblastoma. Symptoms in the mother during pregnancy. Clin Pediatr 9: 206

Warburg M (1974) Retinoblastoma. In: Goldberg MF (ed) Genetic and metabolic eye disease. Little Brown, Boston

Ward S, Dehner LP (1974) Sacrococcygeal teratoma with nephroblastoma—A variant of extragonadal teratoma in childhood. Cancer 33: 1355

Weichert KA, Bové KC, Aron BS, Lampkin B (1976) Rhabdomyosarcoma in children. A clinicopathologic study of 35 patients. Am J Clin Pathol 66: 692

Wigger HJ (1976) Fetal rhabdomyomatous nephroblastoma—A variant of Wilm's tumour. Hum Pathol 7: 613

Williams DI, Schistad G (1964) Lower urinary tract tumours in children. Br J Urol 36: 51

Willis RA (1962) The pathology of the tumours of children. Oliver & Boyd, Edinburgh London, p 57

Wright JH (1910) Neurocytoma or neuroblastoma, a kind of tumour not generally recognized. J Exp Med 12: 556

Yamashita J, Handa H, Toyama M (1975) Medulloblastoma in two brothers. Surg Neurol 4: 225

Yarborough SM, Evashwick G (1956) Case of teratoma of the liver with 14 years post-operative survival. Cancer 9: 848

Young DG, Williams DI (1969) Malignant renal tumours in infancy and childhood. Br J Hosp Med 8: 741

Zülch KJ (1956) Biologie und Pathologie der Hirngeschwülste. Springer, Berlin Göttingen Heidelberg (Handbuch der Neurochirurgie, vol III)

Chapter 16

Sudden Infant Death Syndrome and Nonaccidental Injury

Jean W. Keeling

A. Sudden Infant Death Syndrome

In Great Britain, about half the deaths occurring in infants between the ages of 1 week and 2 years take place outside hospital, and for this reason might be termed unexpected. The majority are reported to have had no symptoms or only trivial common symptoms such as the majority of infants exhibit at some time with no serious sequelae. In a small proportion of these infants necropsy examination will reveal the cause of death, such as an un-diagnosed congenital malformation, often of the cardiovascular system, or a serious acute infective illness, such as meningitis, where a fatal outcome is to be expected in a proportion of cases. In a further group of infants, perhaps a third of the total number, evidence of disease will be present but this will not be of sufficient severity or of a type to account for death. In the remainder no disease process is recognized, although the organs of some infants may have nonspecific histological abnormalities. In a small group there are no abnormal findings.

These deaths have been variously referred to as 'cot' or 'crib' deaths, 'sudden unexpected death' (SUD) or 'sudden infant death syndrome' (SIDS). The last term is preferred, since it encompasses those infants who are found collapsed, are resuscitated, and are subsequently unexpectedly found dead in the ensuing few weeks. A useful definition for the pathologist is 'the death of an infant or young child, which is unexpected by history and in whom a thorough necropsy examination fails to reveal a cause of death' (Beckwith 1970).

1. Epidemiology

An accurate determination of the number of infants who die suddenly and unexpectedly is not possible, partly because of the differences of opinion amongst pathologists as to what constitutes an acceptable cause of death and partly because of the reluctance to admit to being unable to find a cause of death. Sudden infant death syndrome has been accepted as a registrable cause of death in this country since 1971, which has made estimation of the number of cases easier, but some still lurk behind a variety of pseudonyms, such as viral pneumonia, bronchiolitis, laryngitis, gastroenteritis, inhalation of vomitus, and asphyxia. The last two terms are particularly unfortunate, as they imply a deficit of care on the part of the parents, compounding feelings of guilt they already have, whilst a diagnosis of asphyxia may precipitate an inquest. Estimates are further hindered by the registration of a concomitant, relatively minor congenital abnormality as the cause of death. The current estimate of the incidence of SIDS in Britain is 2–3 per 1000 live births or about 2000 deaths annually; it is the commonest mode of death in infancy outside the perinatal (1st week) period.

The majority of these deaths occur between the ages of 2 and 4 months; death from this cause is rare under the age of 1 month and uncommon over 6 months of age. Sudden infant death syndrome is more common in twins, both identical and non-identical (Carpenter 1965). Many series show an excess of males and an excess of deaths in the winter months, although this may be confined to deaths occurring after the age of 12 weeks (Fedrick 1974).

Most deaths occur during household sleeping hours, and some authors report an excess of deaths at weekends or bank holidays (Downham 1977). An association has been recorded with epidemics of viral illness, particularly influenza A_2 and B, in the community (Froggatt et al. 1971). Several series of cases show a higher rate of SIDS in urban areas than in rural ones (Cameron and Asher 1965; Valdes-Dapena 1963), but Houstek et al. (1959) and Maresch (1961) found an excess of deaths in rural areas amongst their cases.

An excess of SIDS amongst the lower socioeconomic groups has been found by several authors (Cameron and Asher 1965; Carpenter 1965). The infants are likely to have been born to young mothers of high parity, and an excess of deaths in poor immigrant families is recorded (Cameron and Asher 1965). Adverse social factors, including poor housing, were considered by several authors to be operational in families of SIDS infants (Selwyn and Bain 1963; Richards and Mackintosh 1972). Parental inadequacy was also thought to be present in about one-third of cases. The excess of SIDS deaths amongst negroes in papers from the United States was not given against the background of the racial mixture of the population (Carroll 1954), and may be a manifestation of socioeconomic factors rather than a racial predisposition. In several series, the illegitimacy rate is high, but this association has not been universally found.

The occurrence of adverse factors related to pregnancy and labour has been carefully scrutinized, particularly since the development of the concept of the recognition of a 'high-risk' group of infants shortly after birth, who are more likely to die unexpectedly during the ensuing months (Carpenter and Emery 1977). Intervention, in terms of the provision of better health care and more intensive infant supervision, might be able to prevent some of these deaths in this type of case.

Threatened abortion, antepartum haemorrhage, urinary tract infection, other infective illness in the first trimester, and surgical and other trauma have been reported in excess during pregnancies resulting in later SIDS victims. Steele and Langworth (1966) report an excess of mothers who smoked, with a large proportion of heavy smokers, during pregnancy, when compared with control mothers. Whether the effect of maternal smoking is expressed solely in low birth weight is not clear. Premature delivery, anaesthetic during labour, and short second stage of labour have been found to be associated with SIDS. An association with absence of breast feeding or the intention of breast feeding has been reported by some authors (Carpenter 1972; Carpenter et al. 1977), but others have found no difference in breast feeding practice or intention (Froggartt et al. 1971; Fedrick 1974).

Several authors have found higher morbidity during the early neonatal period amongst SIDS cases than amongst controls. Prematurity was the cause of differences in some neonatal factors, such as grunting and the need for incubator care and oxygen therapy. The reported association of cyanotic attacks and jaundice may not be related entirely to prematurity. Factors present in the neonatal period that have been associated with SIDS include feeding difficulties, respiratory abnormalities (breath holding, irregular breathing), and diarrhoea. Failure to attend follow-up clinic with the baby and hospital admission have been associated with SIDS, the latter particularly when the admission was necessitated by respiratory tract infection.

2. Necropsy Technique

The objectives of the necropsy examination in infants dying without a history of illness are two-fold. Firstly an acute disease or congenital malformation severe enough to explain death must be excluded; and secondly it is necessary to record the presence of any minor disease or malformation or other, perhaps nonspecific, deviations from the norm. Their significance may not be understood at the time, but may, when carefully collected and assessed, contribute to the better understanding of the pathogenesis or mode of death in this inadequately understood area of infant mortality.

Necropsy examination of infants who have died unexpectedly should be thorough. In addition to careful external examination with weight, crown–rump, crown–heel, and head circumference measurements and dissection of internal organs including brain and spinal cord, other investigations may prove to be of value. Total body X-ray before dissection may reveal and provide a useful accurate record of skeletal abnormalities and of recent or old fractures, in addition to yielding information about bone age and evidence of periods of growth arrest.

A sample of vitreous humour, which is easily obtained by means of a small syringe and a No. 21G needle inserted into the globe at the outer canthus with the needle directed towards the pituitary (the collapsed globe is easily reflated with water), is useful for urea and electrolyte estimation and may confirm a naked eye impression of dehydration.

An ample sterile specimen of CSF uncontaminated with blood is conveniently obtained by cisternal puncture before dissection is started. A piece of lung and/or bronchial swab and heart blood inoculated straight into a blood culture medium may be taken for bacteriological examination, in addition to gut contents and a sample of tissue or fluid from any lesion that seems to be of infective origin.

Samples for culture for viruses should include, as a minimum, swabs of the nose, brain, lung, heart, and small intestine, together with blood for virus antibody levels. In addition, specimens should be taken from the trachea or main bronchus for fluorescence examination for respiratory syncytial virus (RSV), and from the parotid, kidney, and uterine cervix for examination for evidence of cytomegalovirus (CMV) infection. Histological examination should routinely include the upper respiratory tract, a vertical laryngeal block to include the central point of the vocal cord and cross section of trachea, standard blocks of all lobes of the lungs, heart, thymus, liver, spleen, lymph nodes, gut, kidney, bladder, and the endocrine glands, and standard brain blocks. Additionally, frozen sections for fat from liver, adrenal, and corpus callosum should be prepared.

3. Necropsy Findings

The most consistent necropsy findings in SIDS cases are those in the thorax. The thymus is normal, or perhaps slightly reduced, in size and there are petechial haemorrhages in its thoracic, but rarely its cervical, part. The lungs are bulky and fill the chest. They are firm and do not deform with finger pressure. Petechial haemorrhages beneath the visceral pleura, and indeed throughout the lungs, are a frequent finding. When the lungs are sliced they are seen to maintain their shape, and blood-tinged fluid exudes from the surface on pressure. There may be 1–2 ml serous fluid in the pericardial sac, and petechiae are often present along the courses of coronary arteries. They are occasionally widespread.

On histological examination, the thymus is likely to show a minor cortical lymphocyte depletion with reduction in cortical width and the appearance of histiocytes within the cortex (the so-called starry sky appearance) of the thymus. In some cases large numbers of histiocytes are present in the cortex, usually associated with a marked reduction in cortical width.

The commonest finding on histological examination of the lungs is oedema. It is usually present in all lobes, but its distribution is patchy. The alveolar walls are diffusely thickened with a slight increase in round cells within the walls. 'Explosive desquamation' of bronchial and bronchiolar epithelium has been described in cot death cases (Bodian and Heslop 1956) and has been interpreted as the result of infection, but most pathologists now feel that this is a post-mortem artefact. Peribronchial and peribronchiolar round cell infiltration may be

present, although inflammatory exudate within the airways is scanty. Lymphoid aggregates, sometimes with well-formed germinal centres, may be present and have been interpreted as evidence of past respiratory infection (Emery and Dinsdale 1974).

In the upper airways, round cell or mixed inflammatory cell infiltration is frequently present in the nasal septum, epiglottis, and larynx and trachea, decreasing in severity in the lower parts of the airways. This may be accompanied by epithelial changes; ulceration and regeneration may both be present.

Histological abnormalities of the vocal cords are a frequent finding in SIDS, and range from ulceration of the epithelium with underlying necrosis and acute inflammatory cell infiltration, or fibrinoid necrosis beneath an intact epithelium (Fig. 16.A.1), to basement membrane thickening with minor round cell infiltration of the epithelium and deeper structures (Fig. 16.A.2).

In the heart, minor subendocardial fibroelastic thickening is sometimes present, usually in the left ventricle, though its significance is not clear.

In the liver, small collections of cells are often seen within sinusoids. These cells have been interpreted as evidence of erythropoiesis and designated a sign of hypoxia by Naeye (1976), but other authors feel that these are just circulating white cells trapped within the sinusoids.

4. Pathogenesis

Theories concerning the aetiology of cot death are legion, but it seems certain that there is no one single cause for death in these infants, although the mode of dying may be the same in many cases. In the past, when it was the usual practice to take the infant into its parents' bed, many of these deaths were ascribed to overlying (1 Kings 3.19). Although this practice has been largely discontinued, the deaths have not diminished in number.

'Status thymolymphaticus' was the fashionable diagnosis in these infants for many years, until pathologists realized that the 'enlarged' thymus that was supposed to cause death by respiratory vascular obstruction was also seen in infants dying suddenly as the result of accidents. It was thus the 'norm', and the small, flabby organ with which they were familiar was the result of cortical lymphocyte depletion secondary to the many disease processes. The presence of asphyxial haemorrhages in the thoracic viscera has given rise to a number of hypotheses for SIDS that are dependent on upper airways obstruction. The suggestion that these infants have a

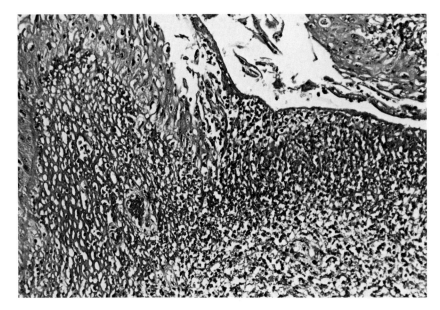

Fig. 16.A.1. 16-week-old female infant, 'perfectly well', unexpectedly found dead. Extensive inflammatory cell infiltration of vocal cords and larynx with epithelial destruction and fibrin deposition. (Martius Scarlet Blue; 240 ×)

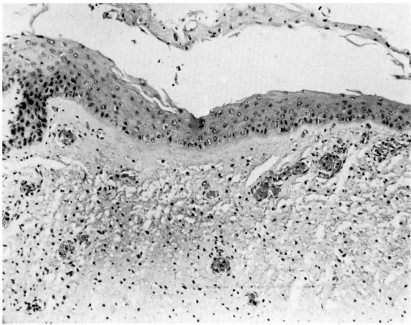

Fig. 16.A.2. 12-week-old male infant, 'cold, runny nose', found dead in his cot. Vocal cords: intact epithelium basement membrane thickenings with eosinophilic amorphous material beneath the basement membrane, scanty round cell infiltration of underlying structures. (H and E; 180 ×)

narrower larynx than normal, making them more vulnerable to obstruction by secretions during upper respiratory infections, has been disproved by careful dissection (Beckwith 1970). Similarly, unsuspected choanal atresia has been discounted as a cause of sudden death by systematic observation of the posterior nares. Accidental smothering by pillows and bed clothes has been disproved experimentally (Woolley 1945), as has the concept that a healthy infant might suffocate because it is lying prone; even a neonate is capable of adjusting his head, when lying in that position, so as to maintain an adequate airway. The possibility of nonaccidental suffocation cannot be discounted by the pathological findings if a soft object such as a pillow is used, but it is unlikely that this accounts for many of these deaths.

Several theories of the aetiology of cot death, such as epidural haemorrhage, adrenal insufficiency, congenital leukaemia, and absence of hypoplasia of the glands, can be refuted by careful necropsy examination; furthermore, it is evident from embryological considerations (p. 540) that significant parathyroid abnormality is unlikely to occur in the presence of a thymus of reasonable proportions.

The hypothesis that these deaths are due to hypersensitivity to cows' milk protein has attracted a lot of attention, and was formerly held to be supported by the low incidence of breast feeding observed in some epidemiological studies. More recent studies, which have compared social and other factors with those in control babies, have not demonstrated any difference in feeding practice between the SIDS infants and the control group. In addition, there has been a large increase in the number of mothers breast feeding over the past 5 or 6 years, which has not been accompanied by a comparable drop in unexplained infant deaths. There has been no real support for cows' milk protein hypersensitivity as a cause of cot death from immunological studies, and those infants in whom cows' milk protein hypersensitivity has been demonstrated have had a recognizable clinical illness with weight loss, diarrhoea, and general misery.

Unspecified immunological abnormality has been put forward as a possible cause of sudden infant death, but, like cows' milk protein intolerance, it has not so far been supported by laboratory investigations, although the amount of work done in this area has not been very great. It is possible that an immunological defect may be a contributory factor in some cases of cot death, and with increasing availability and comprehensiveness of screening for immunological defects further investigation in this field may be worthwhile.

The suggestion that sudden unexpected infant deaths are due to an overwhelming virus infection, which progresses so rapidly as to leave little time for tissue reaction, has had much support over the years. Reports of the success of virus isolation have been very variable and most investigations have lacked data about the prevalence of infection in the community or the isolation rate from necropsy material where death was explained. However, the success rate of virus isolation in deaths of this type has been higher in more recent studies. The appearance of the lungs at necropsy in viral pneumonia is indistinguishable from that of the lungs in SIDS, although in a number of cases of unexpected infant death examined by the present author several of those where a respiratory virus has been isolated have had histological changes, such as peribronchial and peribronchiolar inflammatory cell infiltration, inflammatory cells in the oedema fluid in alveoli, and, occasionally, epithelial changes in small airways. Positive virus isolations in these cases must, however, be critically evaluated. A positive isolation does not demonstrate a cause of death, any more than does the discovery of a minor congenital malformation.. As an alternative to overwhelming infection, it has been suggested that viruses might act as antigens and provoke an anaphylactic reaction in infants previously exposed to the virus as a result of intrauterine infection (Gunther 1966). In a recent

prospective study, however, Sever (cited in Naeye 1977) was unable to demonstrate differences in cord blood immunoglobulins between SIDS victims and controls.

Remodelling of the cardiac conducting system, an orderly process of degeneration and resorption, begins soon after birth and is completed by the end of the second year (p. 134). James (1968) postulated that this process may result in an unstable cardiac conducting system and that minor disturbances could give rise to arrhythmias and AV block, which might be fatal. There would be little to explain death on routine necropsy examination, apart from pulmonary oedema and hepatic congestion, which may result from heart failure. He postulated that cardiac arrhythmias may account for some cases of SIDS. This suggestion has prompted ECG studies on the relatives of SIDS victims and screening programmes of infants in the neonatal period. In one uncontrolled study, Maron et al. (1976) found prolongation of the Q–T interval in one parent of 26% of 42 SIDS victims and in 39% of their siblings. Kukolich et al. (1977), in a controlled study of 108 subjects from the immediate family of 26 infants dying unexpectedly, found no difference in the length of the Q–T interval between family members and controls. Southall et al. (1977) obtained ECG recordings on 2030 selected infants in the neonatal period, and found arrhythmias or other conduction abnormalities in 35 (1.8%). Abnormalities persisted for from 1 week to more than 28 weeks, although only one infant required treatment. The same group (Keeton et al. 1977) described six 'near miss' SIDS cases who had abnormalities of the conducting system, and suggests that these cases provide circumstantial evidence for a causal relationship between abnormalities of the conduction system and cot death. They postulate that a multicentre neonatal ECG screening programme with careful observation and perhaps treatment in some cases might result in a deficit of cot deaths in the monitored period. Another approach might be the careful examination of the cardiac conducting system of infants dying unexpectedly, although the number of infants with detectable conducting system anomalies on ECG testing who might be expected to exhibit histological abnormalities in the conduction system is not known. Recently Maron and Fisher (1977) have reported an abnormal arrangement of myocardial fibres in some cases of SIDS.

Most unexpected deaths occur during sleep, and Steinschneider's suggestion that an exaggeration of the episodes of apnoea that normally occur during sleep in both infants and adults might play a part in sudden infant death has resulted in a number of investigations into the regulation of respiration in infants and neonates and the mechanisms of production of apnoea at this age. Steinschneider (1972) observed the sleep state and recorded the occurrence and duration of apnoeic episodes in five infants, three of whom had recurrent episodes of apnoea and cyanosis while the other two were siblings of these infants. All had frequent periods of apnoea, which were most frequent during rapid eye movement (REM) sleep; these episodes decreased with age. Upper respiratory tract infections were associated with an increased frequency of apnoeic episodes lasting longer than 15 s, and some of these episodes were only terminated by vigorous resuscitation. Two of these infants died subsequently and their deaths were unexplained. Shannon et al. (1977) investigated ventilation and response to CO_2 in 'aborted' SIDS infants and controls, and found that hypoventilation occurred during quiet sleep and that the response to CO_2 was impaired. Three of these infants later died during sleep at home. Milner et al. (1977) have investigated the response of neonates and infants to total airway obstruction. They observed periodic respiration and were able to inhibit respiratory efforts on 15 occasions in ten premature infants with a mean gestation of 28.9 weeks whose ages ranged from 0 to 16 weeks (mean 5 weeks), but were unable to inhibit respiration in 60 investigations of 38 full-term babies. They suggest that this mechanism of respiratory inhibition may be important in the production of SIDS, not only amongst premature infants but also in those who have upper respiratory tract infections, a stimulus known to precipitate periodic respiration. Kelly et al. (1980) demonstrated an increase in periodic breathing in siblings of SIDS victims when compared with controls, both the number and the duration of episodes being increased. They suggested that these episodes might be the result of defective respiratory control which, in turn, reflects cerebral damage from mild perinatal hypoxia.

Prolonged apnoea has been produced experimentally in newborn lambs by the introduction of 'foreign' fluid into the larynx (Johnson et al. 1972). It was found that respiration was abolished if water, an acid solution, or cows' milk was introduced into the entrance of the larynx in tracheostomized lambs, but that ewes' milk or amniotic fluid had no effect on respiratory movements. The foreign fluids inhibited respiration as long as they were present, and their removal was followed by the resumption of respiration. Johnson and his colleagues found that this reflux inhibition of respiration was abolished if the superior layngeal nerves were sectioned prior to the instillation of fluid into the larynx, and postulated that it was initiated by chemoreceptors in the larynx. They found that this reflex inhibition of respiration was age-dependent and did not occur in older animals. It is tempting to speculate that the

regurgitation of acid gastric contents in the human infant might be able to produce a similar effect.

A significant increase in mucous glands in the larynx in SIDS cases when compared with infants dying from recognized causes has been demonstrated by Fink and Beckwith (1980), who measured the percentage soft-tissue area occupied by glandular elements.

Naeye (1973) has found smooth-muscle hypertrophy and hyperplasia in the media of small pulmonary arteries of SIDS victims compared with nonhypoxic controls, although the extent of the changes was significantly less than in children living at an altitude of 3010 m. He suggests that the most likely mechanism is repeated apnoeic episodes or chronic alveolar hypoventilation. Kendell and Ferris (1977), however, were unable to demonstrate any difference between the media of small pulmonary arteries and arterioles compared with nonhypoxic and acutely hypoxic controls, although medial muscular hypertrophy was demonstrated in a group of infants with chronic hypoxia from various causes.

The status of the other potential markers of chronic hypoxaemia seems to be somewhat contentious. An increase in the proportion of brown fat in periadrenal adipose tissue has been described in chronic hypoxaemic states in adults (Teplitz and Lim 1974), although Heaton (1972) found great variability from site to site in the same individual. Naeye (1974) describes a higher percentage of brown fat (cells with a clear reticular infrastructure) in the periadrenal fat of SIDS cases and infants with cyanotic congenital heart disease than in nonhypoxic controls in the age groups 2–5 months and 5–12 months, although he feels it is a poor discriminant between the ages of 1–3 months, the time when one expects to see most of the unexpected deaths. Conversely, Emery and Dinsdale (1978), in a study of the periadrenal fat in infants and children, found a higher proportion of cells with large fat vacuoles in the periadrenal adipose tissue of infants dying unexpectedly than the mean for age based on the findings of an unselected necropsy series in a children's hospital.

The role of the carotid body as a chemoreceptor that maintains the oxygen tension of systemic arterial blood is well documented. An increase in the weight and volume of the carotid bodies of man and a variety of animals living at high altitudes and of laboratory animals living in conditions simulating such a habitat have been described (Arias-Stella 1969; Laidler and Kay 1975). If infants who die unexpectedly have been chronically hypoxic, one would expect an increase in both variables. Using a point-counting technique in the examination of step sections of the carotid bifurcation, Dinsdale et al.

(1977) estimated volumes of carotid bodies in SIDS and controls and found wide variation in volume in both groups. They could not demonstrate a significantly increased volume of the carotid bodies in most of the cases of unexpected death compared with the control group, except in the few unexplained deaths occurring after 1 year of age. A further study on carotid body volume (Naeye 1976) revealed, somewhat surprisingly, that the carotid bodies of SIDS victims were smaller than those of controls.

A variety of cerebral lesions have been described in infants dying unexpectedly. Gadston and Emery (1976) describe the perivascular accumulation of fat-laden macrophages in the corpus callosum, which they associate with demyelination of the brain in response to hypoxia, in stillbirths, neonates, and infants with various conditions associated with chronic hypoxaemia, and related it to findings of fat-laden macrophages in CSF. They found similar accumulations in half of 42 children whose death was unexplained.

Naeye (1976) found an abnormal proliferation of astroglial fibres in the brain stems of 14 of 28 infants dying unexpectedly who were compared with non-hypoxic controls.

More recently, Takashima et al. (1978) described an increase in subcortical or periventricular leukomalacia in SIDS and in infants with congenital heart disease. They found that the site of the lesion was age-dependent, and suggested that the lesions were hypoxic in origin. Such damage may conceivably be the result of acute hypoxic episodes rather than as chronic hypoxia. Similar periventricular lesions are clearly related to documented discrete hypoxic episodes in neonates.

From the vast number of theories on the aetiology of SIDS, of which only a selection of the more plausible ones have been reviewed (for more detailed reviews see Valdes-Dapena 1967, 1977, 1980), and from the range of pathological pathways suggested, it is clear that we are far from solving the problem. However, as evidence from epidemiological studies accumulates and pathological changes are documented in many organs it seems very unlikely that there is any one cause of cot death. It is probable, furthermore, that in any individual case many different factors are involved, including: minor illness, the internal and external environment, developmental processes, and past insults. In future we may be able to recognize more of the factors involved and so understand their complex and potentially fatal interrelationships.

References

A. Sudden Infant Death Syndrome

Arias-Stella J (1969) Human carotid body at high altitudes. Am J Pathol 55: 82a

Beckwith JB (1970) Introduction: Discussion of terminology. In: Bergman AB, Beckwith JB, Ray CG (eds) Sudden infant death syndrome. University of Washington Press, Washington DC, p 18

Bodian M, Heslop B (1960) Sudden infant death syndrome. In: Siim J-C (ed) Proceedings of the Eighth International Congress of Paediatrics, Basel, 1956. Williams & Wilkins, Copenhagen, p 91

Cameron AH, Asher P (1965) Cot deaths in Birmingham 1958–61. Med Sci Law 5: 187

Carpenter RG (1965) Sudden death in twins. Rep Public Health Med Subj 113: 51

Carpenter RG (1972) Epidemiology. In: Camps FE, Carpenter RG (eds) Sudden and unexpected deaths in infancy. Wright, Bristol, p 7

Carpenter RG, Emery JL (1977) Final results of a study of infants at risk of sudden death. Nature 268: 724

Carpenter RG, Gardner A, McWeeny PM, Emery JL (1977) Multistage scoring system for identifying infants at risk of unexpected death. Arch Dis Child 52: 606

Carroll GJ (1974) Sudden deaths in infants. J Pediatr 45: 401

Dinsdale F, Emery JL, Gadsdon DR (1977) The carotid body—a quantitative assessment in children. Histopathology 1: 179

Downham MAPS (1977) Newcastle survey of deaths in early childhood 1974/76, with special reference to sudden unexpected deaths. Arch Dis Child 52: 828

Emery JL, Dinsdale F (1974) Increased incidence of lymphoreticular aggregates in lungs of children found unexpectedly dead. Arch Dis Child 49: 107

Emery JL, Dinsdale F (1978) Structure of peri-adrenal brown fat in childhood in both expected and cot deaths. Arch Dis Child 53: 154

Fedrick J (1974) Sudden unexpected death in infants in the Oxford Record Linkage Area. Br J Prev Soc Med 28: 164

Fink BR, Beckwith JB (1980) Laryngeal mucous gland excess in victims of sudden infant death. Am J Dis Child 134: 144

Froggatt P, Lynas MA, MacKenzie G (1971) Epidemiology of sudden unexpected death in infants ('cot death') in Northern Ireland. Br J Prev Soc Med 25: 119

Gadsdon DR, Emery JL (1976) Fatty change in perinatal and unexpected death. Arch Dis Child 51: 42

Gunther M (1966) Cot deaths; anaphylactic reaction after intra-uterine infection as another potential cause. Lancet 1: 912

Heaton JM (1972) The distribution of brown adipose tissue in the human. J Anat 112: 35

Houstek J, Benesova D, Holy J (1959) Sudden death among children of the Prague district 1956–58. Cask Pediatr 14: 590

James TN (1968) Sudden death in babies: new observation in the heart. Am J Cardiol 22: 479

Johnson P, Robinson JS, Salisbury D (1972) The onset and control of breathing after birth in foetal and neonatal physiology. Cambridge University Press, Cambridge

Keeton BR, Southall E, Rutter N, Anderson RG, Shinebourne EA, Southall DP (1977) Cardiac conduction disorders in six infants with 'near miss' sudden infant deaths. Br Med J ii: 600

Kelly Dorothy H, Walker AM, Cahen Lucienne, Shannon DC (1980) Periodic breathing in siblings of sudden infant death syndrome victims. Pediatrics 66: 515

Kendeel SR, Ferris JAJ (1977) Apparent hypoxic changes in

pulmonary arterioles and small arteries in infancy. J Clin Pathol 30: 481

Kukolich MK, Telsey A, Olt J, Motulsky AG (1977) Sudden infant death syndrome: normal QT interval on ECGs of relatives. Pediatrics 60: 51

Laidler P, Kay JM (1975) A quantitative morphological study of the carotid bodies of rats living at a simulated altitude of 4300 metres. J Pathol 117: 183

Maresch W (1961) Sudden death in childhood. Praxis 50: 804

Maron BJ, Fisher RS (1977) Sudden infant death syndrome (SIDS): cardiac pathological observations in infants with SIDS. Am Heart J 93: 762

Maron BJ, Clark CE, Goldstein RE, Epstein SE (1976) Potential role of QT interval prolongation in sudden infant death syndrome. Circulation 54: 423

Milner AD, Saunders RA, Hopkin IE (1977) Apnoea induced by airflow obstruction. Arch Dis Child 52: 379

Naeye RL (1973) Pulmonary artery abnormalities in the sudden-infant-death syndrome. N Engl J Med 289: 1167

Naeye RL (1974) SIDS—evidence of antecedent chronic hypoxia and hypoxemia in SIDS 1974. In: Robinson RR (ed) Proceedings of the Frances E Camps International Symposium on Sudden and Unexpected Deaths in Infancy. Canadian Foundation for the Study of Infant Deaths, Toronto, p 1

Naeye RL (1976) Brain-stem and adrenal abnormalities in the sudden-infant-death syndrome. Am J Clin Pathol 66: 526

Naeye RL (1977) Placental abnormalities in victims of the sudden infant death syndrome. Biol Neonate 32: 189

Richards IDG, MacIntosh HT (1972) Confidential enquiry into 226 consecutive infant deaths. Arch Dis Child 47: 697

Selwyn S, Bain AD (1963) Deaths in childhood due to infection. Br J Prev Soc Med 19: 123

Shannon DC, Kelly DH, O'Connell K (1977) Abnormal regulations of ventilation in infants at risk for sudden-infant-death syndrome. N Engl J Med 297: 747

Southall DP, Orrell MJ, Talbot JF, Brinton RJ, Vulliamy DG, Johnson AM, Keeton BR, Anderson RH, Shinebourne EA (1977) Study of cardiac arrhythmias and other forms of conduction abnormality in newborn infants. Br Med J ii: 597

Steele R, Langworth JT (1966) The relationship of antenatal and postnatal factors to sudden unexpected death in infancy. Can Med Ass J 94: 1165

Steinschneider A (1972) Prolonged apnoea and the sudden infant death syndrome: clinical and laboratory observations. Pediatrics 50: 646

Takashima S. Armstrong D. Becker LE, Huber J (1978) Cerebral white matter lesions in sudden infant death syndrome. Pediatrics 62: 155

Teplitz C, Lim YC (1974) The diagnostic significance of diffuse brown adipose tissue (B.A.T.). Transformation of adult periadrenal fat: a morphologic indicator of severe chronic hypoxemia. Lab Invest 30: 390

Valdes-Dapena M (1963) Sudden and unexpected death in infants. The scope of our ignorance. Pediatr Clin North Am 10: 693

Valdes-Dapena MA (1967) Sudden and unexpected death in infancy: A review of the world literature 1954–1966. Pediatrics 39: 123

Valdes-Dapena MA (1977) Sudden unexplained infant death, 1970 through 1975: An evolution in understanding. Pathol Annu 12: 117

Valdes-Dapena MA (1980) Sudden infant death syndrome: A review of the medical literature 1974–1979. Pediatrics 66: 597

Woolley PV (1945) Mechanical suffocation during infancy. Relation to total problem of sudden death. J Pediatr 26: 572

B. Nonaccidental Injury

Ritual sacrifice, exposure of unwanted infants, and murder of infants and children for expedience, either political or familial, have been documented during most periods of history and in most cultures, from the myth of Romulus and Remus via the Massacre of the Innocents to the murder of the Princes in the Tower. The killing of children is, in fact, but one end of the spectrum of child abuse, which ranges from severe punishment for a minor misdemeanour through the inappropriate industrial employment of untold thousands of children for long hours in abysmal conditions to passive neglect and starvation, and includes deliberate mutilation for financial gain or personal gratification.

The Battered Child Syndrome is the term coined by Kempe et al. (1962) to draw the attention of those concerned with the health and welfare of children to the clinical findings in young children who have been subjected to one or more episodes of serious physical abuse, usually at the hand of parents or those acting in a parental capacity. They pointed out the youth of affected individuals, usually below 3 years, and also remarked that multiple episodes of abuse are common. Discrepancies between history and physical findings and the failure to develop new injuries during hospital admission were important features of the syndrome. A wide variety of injuries, from bruising to multiple fractures and visceral injuries, was described, and the authors emphasized 'failure to thrive' and evidence of continued neglect in lack of cleanliness and extensive nappy rash as valuable physical signs. Kempe (1971) stressed the importance of skeletal survey in the demonstration of multiple injuries of different ages, particularly of long bones, and the frequent finding of subdural haematomas. He noted the reluctance of parents to seek medical attention for the child following injury. This is so common that delay in seeking medical aid should, in itself, give rise to suspicion of non-accidental injury. There is usually denial of any episode likely to cause injury when the child is brought for attention, but this account may later be changed and a story proffered that may try to attribute all the injuries to a single episode of 'accidental trauma'. Table 16.B.1 gives a summary of the findings of different authors in children subjected to nonaccidental injury.

The classic radiological appearances of multiple long bone fractures of different ages and the

Table 17.B.1. Cases of child abuse reviewed by various authors

	Smith and Hanson	Lauer et al.	Cameron et al.
Number of cases	134	130	29
Died	21	6	29
Permanent damage	20	NK[a]	NK[a]
Battered previously	72	57	26
Battered sibling	31	NA[a]	7
Bruises	110	92	Most
Burns/scalds	23	16	?
Skull fractures	37	29	20
Subdural haemorrhage	30	11	20
Abdominal injury	26	3	7
Long bone fractures	71	19	11
Rib fractures	20	19	14

[a]NK, not known; NA, not assessed.

association with subdural haematomas were described by Caffey (1946). His six cases had 23 long bone fractures between them. He described bone thickening following subperiosteal haemorrhage in the region of the fracture and drew attention to the delay between the injury and radiological evidence of fracture. He noted the absence of any features suggestive of metabolic or other generalized bone disease, and raised the possibility of a traumatic aetiology, although all parents of his cases denied any sort of traumatic incident. Silverman (1953) described three infants in whom radiological examination following examination for limb swelling or deformity, multiple fractures of different ages, and epiphyseal dislocations and in whose cases presentation of the evidence of past trauma resulted in the admission of 'accidental' trauma to the infant on one or several occasions.

Griffiths and Moynihan (1963) were the first to record the battered baby syndrome in this country, with a report of four cases, one of which resulted in the criminal prosecution of the father; however, the classic findings of multiple soft-tissue and skeletal lesions occurring on a number of occasions in the same infant, in siblings, and in cousins were meticulously described by West (1888), who noted recovery without the development of new lesions during stay in hospital. The possibility of a traumatic aetiology was not then considered, and the lesions were thought to be metabolic in origin.

The incidence of nonaccidental injury is difficult to assess. It is likely that many cases are not brought to medical attention, even when quite serious injury has been inflicted. This is supported by the referral of some infants to hospital by local health authority services or NSPCC (National Society for the Prevention of Cruelty to Children) officers. Most cases are missed, however, because the possibility of nonaccidental injury is not considered. There is a strong aversion amongst doctors against accepting the conclusion forced upon them by clinical and radiological evidence, namely, that the injuries were deliberately inflicted.

If Hall's experience (1975) in Preston, based on casualty department attendance of 9.6 new cases per annum with 17.2% fatality, were extrapolated to the country as a whole, this would amount to 4400 cases with 757 deaths from nonaccidental injury each year. He makes a slightly different estimate, based on Lancashire Constabulary figures of 4500 cases with 450 deaths per annum. Webb et al. (1973) estimate 4500 cases per annum in the United Kingdom, with a fatality rate of 10%–17%, permanent brain damage resulting in 30% of these cases. Arthur et al. (1976) saw only 49 cases with four deaths over a 4-year period in Derby, whereas 40 cases per annum would be expected from countrywide estimates, which suggests that the risk has been overestimated.

Smith and Hanson (1974) investigated 134 battered children admitted to Birmingham Children's Hospital. Twenty-one of these children (17%) died as a result of their injuries; in 20 cases permanent physical damage occurred; and 62 had serious injuries from which they recovered. The study of 130 battered children under 10 years of age admitted to a single hospital by Lauer et al. (1974) showed a steady increase each year over a 7-year period. Forty percent of the children had been abused previously, and six children died. The number of cases of permanent damage is not stated, but 29 had skull fractures and 11 had subdural haematomas.

Some authors suggest that males are more frequently battered than females (Gil 1969), but others have found the sex incidence to be equal (Lauer et al. 1974; Smith and Hanson 1974).

In most studies of child abuse the youth of those injured is an important finding: 110 of 134 children in Smith's and Hanson's series were under 2 years of age, and in most reports deaths are confined to children younger than this. Gil's cases have a much wider age distribution, with only 25% under 2 years and 25% over 10 years of age.

1. Necropsy Examination

The diagnosis of child abuse requires a high index of suspicion on the part of the pathologist as, despite the wide publicity given to child abuse in both the medical and the lay press, in some cases clinicians may accept the parent's account of accidental injury at face value and omit essential investigations. Parents may attempt to pass off nonaccidental injury as a 'cot death' (Macauley and Mason 1977).

If there is the slightest suspicion of child abuse, a radiological skeletal survey is essential before the necropsy examination is begun. An informed radiologist's opinion on the adequacy of the views obtained and their interpretation should be obtained and may help in deciding which bones to remove for histological examination (Figs. 16.B.1 and 16.B.2). A thorough external examination must be made, with measurement of weight and length and assessment of nutritional status. It is necessary to look for bruises, abrasions, and burns, and to pay particular attention to their distribution, also noting the general standard of cleanliness and extent of any nappy rash. Photographs of skin lesions and sketches of their distribution are useful adjuncts to the written report and are helpful in Court. The mouth and tongue should be carefully examined for laceration or abrasions, and the conjuctivae inspected for petechial haemorrhages. The eyes should be removed for examination after fixation and histological examination, particularly if abnormalities have been seen on ophthalmoscopic examination during life.

Examination of the viscera, looking for evidence of trauma and disease, retention of blood for culture and toxicological examination and of urine and liver for toxicology follows the usual pattern of the forensic paediatric autopsy. The amount and appearance of gastric contents should be carefully noted. Evidence of rib fractures should be sought after evisceration of the thorax, as anterior fractures are difficult to visualize radiologically, as is damage to the costochondral junction (Fig. 16.B.3). The brain should be fixed before examination for more accurate localization of lesions.

Histological examination of bruises and other skin lesions should be made, for evidence of vital reaction and assessment of the age of the lesion. Similarly, fractures should be removed en block together with specimens of bone from sites away from the injury to exclude bone disease and leukaemia. All organs should be examined histologically to exclude natural disease.

2. Pathological Findings

The body is usually that of an infant, and deaths over 2 years of age are uncommon. There may be evidence of poor hygiene in the form of dirty ears and flexures,

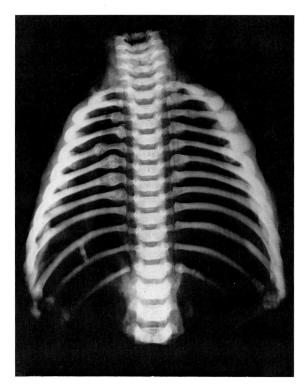

Fig. 16.B.1. Rib case with multiple fractures of the ribs on both sides. Fractures of R6–8 have the most prominent callus formation and the fracture line is obliterated, suggesting that these are of longer duration than the fractures on the left.

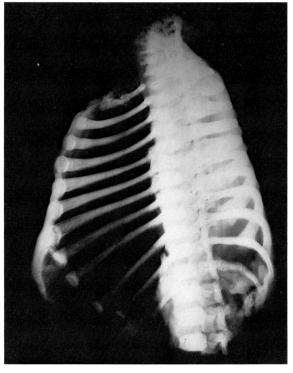

Fig. 16.B.2. Same cases as in Fig. 16.B.1: this view shows recent fracture of R1.

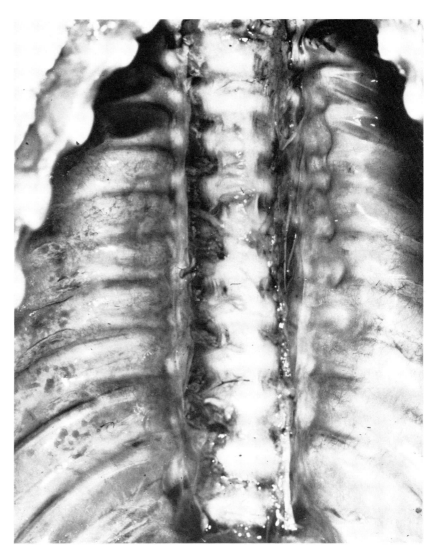

Fig. 16.B.3. Eviscerated thorax of a 9-month-old baby boy who had been punched whilst lying in his cot. Callus formation is seen on the paravertebral portions of mini-ribs on the left; there were also fractures near the anterior ends of the same ribs and dislocations of the cos-tochondral junctions on the right.

dirty, uncut nails, and extensive nappy rash. This is not invariable and some infants appear to have been well cared for. The body may be thin, which is often ascribed to neglect, but in view of the frequency of rib fractures (present in almost half the cases seen by Cameron et al. 1966) (Fig. 16.B.3), an infant so injured can be expected to suck poorly because of pain. Short stature is likely only in those infants who are chronically physically and/or emotionally deprived.

Bruises are the commonest skin lesion. The bruises of nonaccidental injury are characteristically flat without any overlying skin abrasion, but it is their distribution that betrays their origin. Bruises made by gripping tightly so as to shake the infant show a single large discolouration corresponding to the thumb, which can be matched with a line of smaller bruises caused by finger tips a few inches away. Characteristic sites are the face, where a right-handed person will inflict a large bruise over the right

eye, over the zygomatic arch, or on the mandible, with smaller bruises on the opposite side. The finger bruises matching a thumb mark over the mandible may merge into one indistinct bruise on the neck (Cooper 1975). Sets of bruises can be matched by colour and sets of bruises of different ages may be present (Fig. 16.B.4).

Black eyes are not an uncommon form of injury. These are caused by a fist or hard object being thrust into the orbit. The history is usually of an accident, but this is much more likely to cause supra-orbital bruising unless there is concomitant fracture of the roof of the orbit. Bilateral orbital bruises can never be caused by a single accident (Cooper 1975). Bruising of the ear may be present, often accompanied by petechial haemorrhages in the surrounding skin.

Petechial haemorrhages may be present in the conjunctivae. Ocular manifestions range from transient retinal haemorrhages accompanying subdural

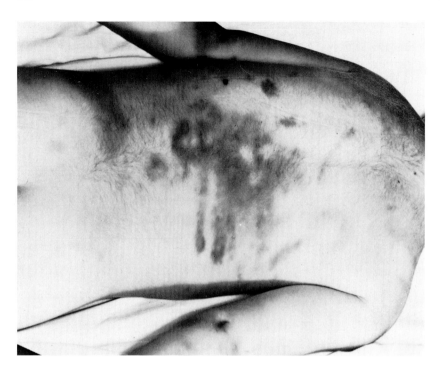

Fig. 16.B.4. Bruising of the back. The situation and linear characteristics of the bruising make accidental injury highly unlikely.

haematoma to subhyaloid, vitreous, and gross retinal haemorrhages (Fig. 16.B.5) and retinal detachment leading to extensive scarring and optic atrophy producing blindness (Mushin 1971).

When the trunk has been gripped tightly in shaking there will usually be a large bruise on either side of the mid-line, usually one higher than the other, sometimes with a second bruise on one side if the hand has moved down the body. There will be matching fingertip bruises on the opposite side of the trunk. A hand imprint may be visible on the buttock from slapping. Striking the body with a hard object may leave an impression with a pattern that can be matched to the object; sharp edges or pro-truberances will cause superimposed abrasions. Fingertip bruises may be seen on the limbs, particu-larly around the elbow and knee, if the infant has been grasped and thrown into its cot or against a hard object (Cameron 1972).

Human bites may be seen on abused children in two crescentic rows of small bruises that become confluent. They can be distinguished from self-inflicted bites by the inaccessibility of site and disparity of size (Sims et al. 1973). They can be matched to the dentition by forensic dental experts.

Burns and scalds are commonly inflicted injuries. Serious thermal injury was present in almost one-fifth of cases seen by Smith and Hanson (1974) and 12.5% of those seen by Lauer et al. (1974). Minor burns were present in other cases. Burns of the buttock and perineum caused by placing the child on a hot surface are described by Smith and Hanson

(1974) and Keen et al. (1975), who pointed out that burned and scalded children tended to be older than the rest of their battered children; and they advise caution in accepting an accidental explanation of such injury in older children. The proffered expla-nation of pulling a pan of hot liquid off a high surface should be rejected if the submental region and axilla are spared from injury. 'Dip' scalds of hands and feet are described and are unlikely to be accidental in the absence of splash scalds further up the limbs (Keen et al. 1975).

Circular burns from cigarettes are sometimes seen, and lesions of different ages may be found; this type of injury suggests premeditated insult (Simpson 1973).

Bruising of the scalp is often difficult to de-monstrate at necropsy, when the telltale tenderness on palpation of the scalp, which makes such lesions apparent clinically, is lacking. Deep bruising is more easily seen after reflection of the scalp.

Bruising and abrasions of the gums may be the result of thrusting a bottle or fist into the mouth of a crying infant. A torn frenulum may be regarded as pathognomonic of nonaccidental injury (Cameron et al. 1966). Bites on the edge of the tongue are sometimes produced accidentally.

Visceral injuries result from direct blows to the abdomen. Surface bruising may be absent in cases of serious, even fatal, visceral injury. Rupture of the liver is frequently fatal. Perforation of the small bowel, particularly the duodenum, and tearing of the mesentery are also seen (Fig. 16.B.6). Liver damage

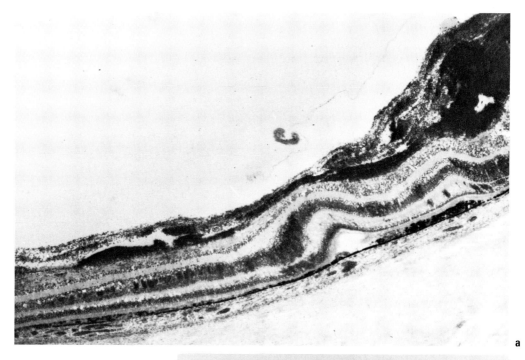

a

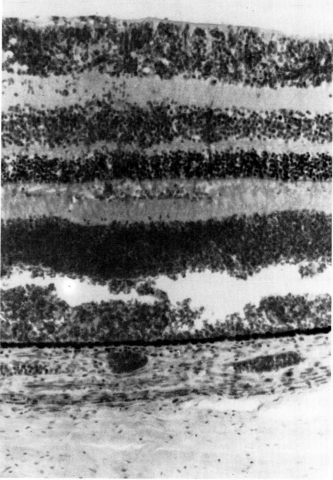

Fig. 16.B.5. a and **b** Vitreous (**a**; 30 ×) subhyaloid
(**b**; 120 ×) bleeding after repeated blows to the eye
in an 18-month-old boy. (H and E)

b

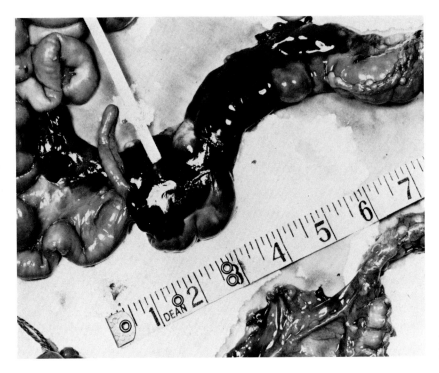

Fig. **16.B.6.** Mesenteric haemorrhage following deliberate injury.

was seen in 19% and injury of the duodenum, pancreas, or mesentery in 15% of fatal cases recorded by Camps (1969). A high incidence of liver injury in fatal cases is reported by several authors (Cameron et al. 1966; Smith and Hanson 1974). Rupture of the heart may occur in cases in which the chest is jumped on (C.L. Berry, personal communication).

Intracerebral injury may be the result of direct trauma to the head, when it may be accompanied by a fracture of the skull. Violent shaking may also damage the brain, when the likely concomitant injuries are bruises of the thorax, and perhaps fractured ribs. Subdural haematomas are the commonest intracranial injury, and comprised almost two-thirds of 37 cases of intracerebral bleeding in Smith's and Hanson's cases. Bilateral bleeding is common.

Such haemorrhage is usually acute: Macauley and Mason (1977) found chronic subdural haematoma only rarely, which is perhaps surprising in view of the large number of children who have been injured previously (more than half the children described by Smith and Hanson had evidence of previous injury). It seems likely that a proportion of these children do survive subdural haemorrhage and are seriously brain-damaged (Fig. 16.B.7). Subarachnoid and cerebral haemorrhage are seen but are less common.

Fractures are the commonest injury after bruises. Characteristically, multiple fractures of different ages are present. The skull is the commonest site for fracture; fractures were present in 28% of Smith's and Hanson's cases and 22.3% of the patients described by Lauer et al. Long-bone fractures are next in frequency, all long bones being affected with almost equal frequency. Recent fractures can be seen radiologically. Callus formation around the fracture can be seen radiologically from about the 8th day, and can be of considerable help in dating fractures. The periostium is not so firmly attached to the bone in infants as in adults, and shearing injury may be followed by subperiosteal bleeding, with subperiosteal new bone formation producing a 'double contour' to long bones (Silverman 1953). Traumatic fragmentation of the metaphysis of long bones with subsequent joint deformity has been described (Caffey 1957). Bones of the wrists, hands, and feet are rarely damaged.

Serious congenital defect is more frequent amongst abused children (7.5% of Smith's and Hanson's cases compared with 1.5% in the general population).

Poisoning as a form of nonaccidental injury should not be overlooked. The drug may be anything to which the parent has access: fenformin, diuretics, and common salt have been reported in this connection, in addition to the commonly used sedatives and tranquillizers (Rogers et al. 1976). Rogers and co-workers called attention to bizarre symptoms and signs and biochemical values and the frequency of neurological symptoms at presentation. There were two deaths amongst their six cases, and three had a dead sibling. The episodic

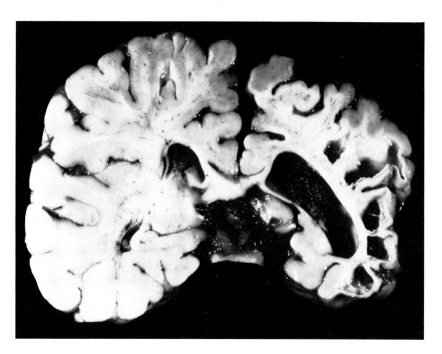

Fig. 16.B.7. Severe long-standing cerebral damage in a repeatedly injured child. From a female aged 15 months.

nature of the illness, with recurrence on returning home or following access by the mother to the child in hospital, and suspicious injury or illness in siblings are points to seek out; suspicions are confirmed by isolation of the poison.

Alcohol intoxication in the paediatric age group is usually accidental and self-administered. Forced alcohol administration as a form of child abuse is described by Grubbauer and Schwarz (1980).

Nixon and Pearn (1977) describe nonaccidental immersion in the bath as a form of child abuse. One of their cases had been injured previously and another died later with skull fractures. They distinguish nonaccidental immersion from accidental drowning in the bath in that abused children are older, of all social classes, likely to be handicapped, the eldest in the family, in the bath alone and at an odd time of day, and with a high proportion of personality defects amongst the parents. Accidental drowning, however, is usually a cause of death in the youngest of a large family of low social class (several being bathed together in the evening), together with a high incidence of family crises.

3. Dietary Abuse

It has been suggested that severe malnutrition in infancy caused by inadequate feeding because of parental adherence to certain dietary regimes, e.g., strict vegetarian (Vegan) and macrobiotic diets, is a form of child abuse. These diets are inadequate in

energy, protein, and fat-soluble vitamins for rapidly growing infants. Malnutrition, presenting as rickets, marasmus or kwashiorkor, may occur over a period of a few weeks (Roberts et al. 1979). Parents are reluctant to accept advice on infant feeding, and a care or supervision order may be necessary to ensure adequate nutrition. No deaths from this form of child abuse have so far been reported.

References

B. Nonaccidental Injury

Arthur LJ, Moncrieff MW, Milburn W, Bayliss PS, Heath J (1976) Non-accidental injury in children: what we do in Derby. Br Med J i: 1363

Caffey J (1946) Multiple fractures in the long bones of infants suffering from chronic subdural haematoma. Am J Roentgenol 56: 163

Caffey J (1957) Some traumatic lesions in growing bones other than fractures and dislocations: clinical and radiological features. Br J Radiol 30: 225

Cameron JM (1972) The battered baby syndrome. Practitioner 209: 302

Cameron JM, Johnson HRM, Camps FE (1966) The battered child syndrome. Med Sci Law 6: 2

Camps FE (1969) Injuries sustained by children from violence. In: Recent advances in forensic pathology. Churchill Livingstone, Edinburgh London, chap. 6

Cooper C (1975) The doctor's dilemma—a paediatricians view. In: Franklin AW (ed) Concerning child abuse. Churchill Livingstone, Edinburgh London, p 21

Gil DG (1969) Physical abuse of children. Findings and implications of a nationwide survey. Paediatrics 44: 857

Griffiths D, Moynihan FJ (1963) Multiple epiphyseal injuries in babies ('Battered baby' syndrome). Br Med J ii: 1558

Grubbauer HM, Schwarz R (1980) Peritoneal dialysis in alcohol intoxication in a child. Arch Toxicol (Berl) 43: 317

Hall MH (1975) A view from the emergency and accident department. In: Franklin AW (ed) Concerning child abuse. Churchill Livingstone, Edinburgh London, p 7

Keen JH, Lendrum J, Wolmon B (1975) Inflicted burns and scalds in children. Br Med J iv: 268

Kempe CH (1971) Paediatric implications of the battered baby syndrome. Arch Dis Child 46: 28

Kempe CH, Silverman FN, Steele BF, Droegemueller W, Silver HK (1962) The battered child syndrome. JAMA 181: 17

Lauer B, Brock ET, Grossman M (1974) Battered child syndrome: review of 130 patients with controls. Paediatrics 54: 67

Macauley RAA, Mason JK (1977) Violence in the home. In: Mason JK (ed) The pathology of violent injury. Arnold, London, p 218

Mushin AS (1971) Ocular damage in the battered baby syndrome. Br Med J iii: 402

Nixon J, Pearn J (1977) Non-accidental immersion in bath-water: another aspect of child abuse. Br Med J i: 271

Roberts IF, West RJ, Ogilvie D, Dillon MJ (1979) Malnutrition in infants receiving cult diets: a form of child abuse. Br Med J i: 296

Rogers D, Tripp J, Bentovim A, Robinson A, Berry D, Goulding R (1976) Nonaccidental poisoning: an extended syndrome of child abuse. Br Med J i: 793

Silverman FN (1953) The roentgen manifestations of unrecognised skeletal trauma in infants. Am J Roentgenol 69: 413

Simpson K (1973) Child abuse—the battered baby. In: Mant AK (ed) Modern trends in forensic medicine, vol 3. Butterworths, London Boston, Mass, chap. 2

Sims BG, Grant JH, Cameron JM (1973) Bite marks in the 'battered baby syndrome'. Med Sci Law 13: 207

Smith, SM, Hanson R (1974) 134 battered children: a medical and psychological study. Br Med J ii: 666

Webb J, Cooper C, Jackson H, Kelvin I, Roycroft B, Wilson D (1973) Nonaccidental injury in children. Br Med J iv: 657

West S (1888) Acute periosteal swellings in several young infants of the same family, probably rickety in nature. Br Med J i: 856

Subject Index

Current Topics in Pathology

Volume 69
Drug-Induced Pathology

Editor: E. Grundmann
With contributions by numerous experts
1981. 94 figures. VIII, 384 pages
ISBN 3-540-10415-1

Contents: Epidemiological Observation on Drug-Induced Illness. – The Pathophysiological Basis of Drug Toxicity. – Drug-Induced Liver Reactions: A Morphological Approach. – Drug-Associated Nephropathy. Part I: Glomerular Lesions. – Drug-Associated Nephropathy. Part II: Tubulo-Interstitial Lesions. A: Acute Interstitial Nephritis, Nephrotoxic Lesions, Analgesic Nephropathy. – Drug-Associated Nephropathy. Part II: Tubulo-Interstitial Lesions. B: Hypokalemic Alterations. – Drug-Induced Damage to the Embryo or Fetus. (Molecular and Multilateral Approach to Prenabal Toxicology). – Drug-Induced Cancer. – Subject Index.

Volume 68
Inflammatory Reaction

Editor: H. Z. Movat
With contributions by numerous experts
1979. 95 figures, 14 tables. VII, 296 pages
ISBN 3-540-09394-X

Contents: Ultrastructure in Acute Inflammation. – Hyperemia, Stasis, and Increase in Vascular Permeability: New Methods for Their Quantition. – The Adhesion, Migration and Chemotaxis of Leukocytes in Inflammation. – Kinetics of the Inflammatory Response in Regional Lymph. – The Kinin System and Its Relation to Other Systems. – The Complement System and Inflammation. – Phagocyclic Cells During an Acute Inflammatory Reaction. – Phlogistic Substances in Neutrophil Leukocyte Lysosomes: Their Possible Role in Vivo and Their in Vitro Properties. – Cellular Hypersensitivity and Inflammation. – The Role of Prostaglandins in Inflammation. – Subject Index.

Volume 67
Carcinogenesis

Editor: E. Grundmann
With contributions by P. Höhn, E. Kunze, K. Nomura, C. Witting, W. Schlake
1979. 112 figures, 21 tables. VI, 259 pages
ISBN 3-540-09344-3

Contents: Histogenesis of Carcinoma in the Glandular Stomach of the Rat After B 1-Resection. –
Morphology and Morphogenesis of Experimental Induced Small Intestional Tumors. – Development of Urinary Bladder Cancer in the Rat. – B-Lymphocytes in Carcinogenesis. – Subject Index.

Volume 66
Perinatal Pathology

Editors: E. Grundmann, W. H. Kirsten
With contributions by numerous experts
1979. 88 figures, 34 tables. VI, 218 pages
ISBN 3-540-09207-2

Contents: The Placenta and Low Birth Weight. – Placental Insufficiency. – Interactions Between Maternal and Fetal/Neonatal Lymphocytes. – Transfer of Humoral Secretory and Cellular Immunity from Mother to Offspring. – Single Umbilical Artery with Congenital Malformations. – C-Type Virus Expression in the Placenta. – Transplacental Effects of Diethylstilbestrol.

Volume 65*

With contributions by numerous experts.
1977. 119 figures, 24 tables. VII, 203 pages
ISBN 3-540-08330-8

Contents: Correlations Between Morphologic and Clinical Features in Idiopathic Perimembranous Glomerulonephritis (A Study on 403 Renal Biopsies of 367 Patiens). – Human Parathyroid Gland: A Freeze-Fracture and Thin Section Study. – Malignant Nephrosclerosis in Patients with Hemolytic Uremic Syndrome (Primary Malignant Nephrosclerosis). – Liver Carcinogenesis in Rats After Aflatoxin B_1 Administration. (A Light and Electron Microscopic Study). – Blastomycosis.

Volume 64*

With contributions by numerous experts.
1977. 107 figures. VI, 228 pages
ISBN 3-540-08107-0

Contents: Pulmonary Hypertension Related to Aminorex Intake (Histologic, Ultrastructural, and Morphometric Studies of 37 cases in Switzerland). – DNA Injuries, Their Repair and Carcinogenesis. – Soft Tissue Tumors in the Rat (Pathogenesis and Histopathology). – Visceral Candidosis (Anatomic Study of 34 cases).

*untitled

Springer-Verlag
Berlin
Heidelberg
New York

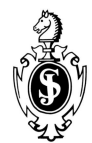